Primary Care of Women

Primary Care of Women

Editors

Karen J. Carlson, M.D.
Assistant Physician, General Internal Medicine Unit,
 Department of Medicine,
 Massachusetts General Hospital;
Director, Women's Health Associates;
Instructor, Harvard Medical School
Boston, Massachusetts

Stephanie A. Eisenstat, M.D.
Associate Physician in Medicine, Division of
 General Medicine and Primary Care,
 Department of Medicine,
 Brigham and Women's Hospital;
Associate Director, Brigham Internal Medicine Associates;
Instructor, Harvard Medical School
Boston, Massachusetts

Associate Editors

Fredric D. Frigoletto, Jr., M.D.
Chief, Vincent Memorial Obstetrics Division,
 Massachusetts General Hospital;
Charles Montraville Green and Robert Montraville Green
 Professor of Obstetrics and Gynecology,
 Harvard Medical School
Boston, Massachusetts

Isaac Schiff, M.D.
Chief, Vincent Memorial Obstetrics and Gynecology
 Service, Massachusetts General Hospital;
Joe Vincent Meigs Professor of Gynecology,
 Harvard Medical School
Boston, Massachusetts

with 85 illustrations and 10 color plates

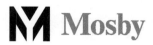 Mosby

St. Louis Baltimore Boston Carlsbad Chicago Naples New York Philadelphia Portland
London Madrid Mexico City Singapore Sydney Tokyo Toronto Wiesbaden

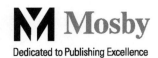

Mosby

Dedicated to Publishing Excellence

A Times Mirror Company

Editor: Stephanie Manning
Developmental Editor: Carolyn Malik
Project Manager: Dana Peick
Senior Production Editor: Catherine Albright
Designer: Amy Buxton
Manufacturing Manager: Theresa Fuchs

Printed in the United States of America
Composition by Reed Technology and Information Services, Inc.
Printing by The Maple-Vail Book Manufacturing Group.

Mosby–Year Book, Inc.
11830 Westline Industrial Drive
St. Louis, Missouri 63146

Library of Congress Cataloging-in-Publication Data
Primary care of women/editors, Karen J. Carlson, Stephanie A.
 Eisenstat; associate editors, Isaac Schiff, Fredric D. Frigoletto,
Jr.
     p.   cm.
   Includes bibliographical references and index.
   ISBN 0-8016-7677-0 (alk. paper)
   1. Women's health services. 2. Women—Health and hygiene.
3. Primary care (Medicine) I. Carlson, Karen J. II. Eisenstat,
Stephanie A.
   [DNLM: 1. Women's Health. 2. Primary Health Care. WA 309 P952
1995]
RA564.85.P754 1995
616'.0082—dc20
DNLM/DLC
for Library of Congress
                                                        95-3983
                                                        CIP

96 97 98 / 9 8 7 6 5 4 3 2

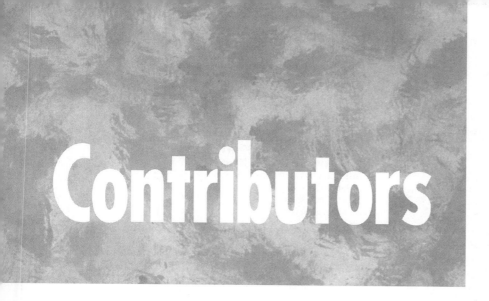
Contributors

Ronald J. Anderson, M.D.
Director of Clinical Training Programs, Department of
  Rheumatology, Brigham and Women's Hospital;
Associate Professor of Medicine, Harvard Medical School
Boston, Massachusetts
Osteoarthritis

Johnny T. Awwad, M.D.
Clinical Fellow, Reproductive Endocrinology and Infertility,
  Massachusetts General Hospital;
Harvard Medical School
Boston, Massachusetts
Dysfunctional Uterine Bleeding

Lynn A. Baden, M.D.
Instructor in Dermatology, Department of Medicine,
  Division of Dermatology, Harvard Medical School
Boston, Massachusetts
Common Dermatologic Problems

Susan E. Bennett, M.D.
Lown Cardiovascular Center, Division of General Medicine,
  Brigham and Women's Hospital;
Instructor in Medicine, Harvard Medical School
Boston, Massachusetts
Benign Breast Disease and Breast Implants
Breast Cancer Screening

Craig L. Best, M.D., M.P.H.
Division of Reproductive Immunology,
  Fearing Research Laboratory;
Department of Obstetrics, Gynecology, and Reproductive Biology,
  Brigham and Women's Hospital
Boston, Massachusetts
Early Pregnancy Disorders: Hyperemesis and Vaginal Bleeding
Early Pregnancy Disorders: Miscarriage and Recurrent
  Spontaneous Abortion

JudyAnn Bigby, M.D.
Division of General Medicine, Brigham and Women's Hospital;
Assistant Professor of Medicine, Department of Internal Medicine,
Harvard Medical School
Boston, Massachusetts
Alcohol and Drug Abuse

Susan M. Briggs, M.D.
General and Vascular Surgeon, Massachusetts General Hospital;
Assistant Professor of Surgery, Department of Surgery,
  Harvard Medical School
Boston, Massachusetts
Vascular Disorders

Linda Brubaker, M.D.
Assistant Professor and Director, Urogynecology Section,
  Department of Obstetrics and Gynecology,
  Rush Medical College
Chicago, Illinois
Chronic Bladder Disorders and Chronic Dysuria
Incontinence and Uterine Prolapse

Karen J. Carlson, M.D.
Assistant Physician, Massachusetts General Hospital;
Director, Women's Health Associates;
Instructor, Harvard Medical School
Boston, Massachusetts
Contraception
Pelvic Masses
Premenstrual Syndrome
Hysterectomy
Use of Medications in Pregnancy and Lactation
Endometrial, Ovarian, and Vulvar Cancer

David L. Carr-Locke, M.D., F.R.C.P., F.A.C.G.
Director of Endoscopy, Department of Gastroenterology,
  Brigham and Women's Hospital;
Associate Professor of Medicine, Division of Gastroenterology,
  Harvard Medical School
Boston, Massachusetts
Gallstones

Susan Cummings, M.S., R.D.
Registered Dietitian, Clinical Specialist, Department of Dietetics
  Instructor, Massachusetts General Hospital
Institute of Health Professions
Boston, Massachusetts
Obesity

Michele G. Cyr, M.D.
Division of General Internal Medicine,
  Rhode Island Hospital;
Associate Professor of Medicine, Department of Medicine,
  Brown University School of Medicine
Providence, Rhode Island
Alcohol and Drug Abuse

David M. Dawson, M.D.
West Roxbury VA Hospital;
Department of Neurology,
  Brigham and Women's Hospital;
Professor of Neurology, Harvard Medical School
Boston, Massachusetts
Stroke

Joanne M. Donovan, M.D., Ph.D.
Brockton/West Roxbury VA Medical Center;
Assistant Professor of Medicine,
   Harvard Medical School
Boston, Massachusetts
Gallstones

Barbara A. Dworetzky, M.D.
Department of Neurology and Neurophysiology,
   Brigham and Women's Hospital
Boston, Massachusetts
Stroke

Stephanie A. Eisenstat, M.D.
Associate Physician in Medicine, Brigham and Women's Hospital;
Associate Director, Brigham Internal Medicine Associates;
Instructor, Harvard Medical School
Boston, Massachusetts
Common Dermatologic Problems
Human Immunodeficiency Virus
Preconception Counseling and Nutrition
Infectious Exposure and Immunization During Pregnancy
Urinary Tract Infections in Pregnancy
Use of Medications in Pregnancy and Lactation
Domestic Violence
Sexual Assault

Bruce B. Feinberg, M.D.
Department of Obstetrics and Gynecology,
   Brigham and Women's Hospital;
Assistant Professor, Maternal-Fetal Medicine,
   Harvard Medical School
Boston, Massachusetts
Preeclampsia

Donna Felsenstein, M.D.
Director, Sexually Transmitted Disease Unit,
   Associate Physician, Department of Medicine,
   Massachusetts General Hospital;
Assistant Professor of Medicine, Harvard Medical School
Boston, Massachusetts
Sexually Transmitted Disease

Robin A. Fischer, M.D.
Assistant Professor of Obstetrics, Gynecology, and Reproductive
   Endocrinology, Department of Obstetrics and Gynecology,
   Division of Reproductive Endocrinology, University of
   Massachusetts Medical Center
Worcester, Massachusetts
Infertility

Patricia A. Fraser, M.D.
Director, Pediatric Diagnosis and Management
   of Systemic Lupus Erythematosus,
   Department of Rheumatology and Immunology,
   Brigham and Women's Hospital;
Assistant Professor of Medicine,
   Harvard Medical School
Boston, Massachusetts
Systemic Lupus Erythematosus

Andrew J. Friedman, M.D.
Department of Reproductive Endocrinology,
   Brigham and Women's Hospital;
Associate Professor of Obstetrics, Gynecology, and Reproductive
   Biology, Harvard Medical School
Boston, Massachusetts
Uterine Fibroids

Fredric D. Frigoletto Jr., M.D.
Chief, Vincent Memorial Obstetrics Division,
   Massachusetts General Hospital;
Charles Montraville Green and Robert Montraville Green, Professor
   of Obstetrics and Gynecology,
   Harvard Medical School
Boston, Massachusetts

Soheyla D. Gharib, M.D.
Division of Primary Care, Brigham and Women's Hospital;
Assistant Professor of Medicine, Harvard Medical School
Boston, Massachusetts
Abnormal Vaginal Bleeding

Elizabeth Ginsberg, M.D.
Department of Obstetrics and Gynecology,
   Brigham and Women's Hospital;
Instructor in Obstetrics, Gynecology, and Reproductive Biology,
   Harvard Medical School
Boston, Massachusetts
Renal Insufficiency

Samuel Z. Goldhaber, M.D.
Staff Physician, Cardiovascular Division, Department of
   Cardiovascular Medicine, Brigham and Women's Hospital;
Associate Professor of Medicine, Harvard Medical School
Boston, Massachusetts
Thromboembolic Disease in Pregnancy

Howard M. Goodman, M.D., FACS
Assistant Adjunct Clinical Professor, Duke University
   School of Medicine
West Palm Beach, Florida
Gynecologic Cancers

Michael F. Greene, M.D.
Director, Maternal-Fetal Medicine,
   Massachusetts General Hospital;
Associate Professor, Obstetrics, Gynecology, and Reproductive
   Biology, Harvard Medical School
Boston, Massachusetts
Hypertension in Pregnancy
Diabetes in Pregnancy

Janet E. Hall, M.D.
Assistant in Medicine, Reproductive Endocrine Unit,
   Massachusetts General Hospital;
Assistant Professor, Harvard Medical School
Boston, Massachusetts
Amenorrhea

Louise Wilkins-Haug, M.D.
Director, Antenatal Diagnostic Center, Department of Obstetrics and
   Gynecology, Brigham and Women's Hospital;
Assistant Professor, Harvard Medical School
Boston, Massachusetts
Amniocentesis and Prenatal Genetics

Linda J. Heffner, M.D., Ph.D.
Chief, Maternal-Fetal Medicine,
   Brigham and Women's Hospital;
Associate Professor of Obstetrics, Gynecology, and Reproductive
   Biology, Harvard Medical School
Boston, Massachusetts
Pregnancy in the Older Woman

Jennifer Helmick, M.S.
Senior Technical Communication Specialist,
   Eastern Research Group, Inc.;
Board Chairperson Massachusetts Coalition for Occupational
   Safety and Health
Lexington, Massachusetts
Occupational Hazards

Joseph A. Hill, M.D.
Clinical Director, Division of Reproductive Immunology,
   Fearing Research Laboratory;
Department of Obstetrics, Gynecology, and Reproductive Biology,
   Brigham and Women's Hospital;
Director, Harvard Recurrent Miscarriage Center;
Associate Professor, Harvard Medical School
Boston, Massachusetts
Early Pregnancy Disorders: Hyperemesis and Vaginal Bleeding
*Early Pregnancy Disorders: Miscarriage and Recurrent
   Spontaneous Abortion*

Keith B. Isaacson, M.D.
Chief, Vincent Memorial Division of Reproductive Endocrinology
  and Infertility, Massachusetts General Hospital;
Assistant Professor of Obstetrics, Gynecology,
  and Reproductive Biology, Harvard Medical School
Boston, Massachusetts
Endometriosis

Linda S. Jaffe, M.D.
Department of Medicine, Brigham and Women's Hospital;
Instructor in Medicine, Endocrine-Hypertension Division,
  Harvard Medical School
Boston, Massachusetts
Diabetes

Phyllis Jen, M.D.
Medical Director, Brigham Internal Medicine Associates, Brigham
  and Women's Hospital;
Assistant Professor, Department of Internal Medicine,
  Harvard Medical School
Boston, Massachusetts
Asthma in Pregnancy
Seizures in Pregnancy

Paula A. Johnson, M.D., M.P.H.
Associate Physician, Cardiovascular Division,
  Section for Clinical Epidemiology, Division of
  General Internal Medicine, Brigham and Women's Hospital;
Instructor in Medicine, Harvard Medical School
Boston, Massachusetts
Hyperlipidemia

Jeffrey N. Katz, M.D.
Assistant Professor of Medicine, Department of Rheumatology and
  Immunology, Robert B. Brigham Arthritis Center,
  Brigham and Women's Hospital
Boston, Massachusetts
Regional Musculoskeletal Disorders

Martha Ellen Katz, M.D.
Department of Medicine, Brigham and Women's Hospital;
Children's Hospital;
Clinical Instructor of Medicine,
  Harvard Institute of Reproductive and Child Health,
  Harvard Medical School
Boston, Massachusetts
Abortion

Laurence Katznelson, M.D.
Clinical Assistant in Medicine, Neuroendocrine Unit,
  Department of Medicine, Massachusetts General Hospital;
Instructor in Medicine, Harvard Medical School
Boston, Massachusetts
Hyperprolactinemia and Galactorrhea

Powel H. Kazanjian, M.D.
Assistant Professor, Department of Infectious Disease,
  University of Michigan
Ann Arbor, Michigan
Human Immunodeficiency Virus

Anne Klibanski, M.D.
Chief, Neuroendocrine Unit, Department of Medicine, Massachusetts
  General Hospital;
Associate Professor of Medicine, Harvard Medical School
Boston, Massachusetts
Hyperprolactinemia and Galactorrhea

Anthony L. Komaroff, M.D.
Director, Division of General Medicine and Primary Care, Brigham
  and Women's Hospital;
Professor of Medicine, Harvard Medical School
Boston, Massachusetts
Acute Dysuria and Urinary Tract Infections
Fatigue and Chronic Fatigue Syndrome

Irene Kuter, M.D., D.Phil.
Assistant Physician, Medical Services,
  Hematology-Oncology Unit, Massachusetts General Hospital;
Assistant Professor of Medicine,
  Harvard Medical School
Boston, Massachusetts
Breast Cancer

Carol Landau, Ph.D.
Division of General Internal Medicine, Rhode Island Hospital;
Clinical Professor, Department of Psychiatry and Human Behavior,
  Brown University School of Medicine
Providence, Rhode Island
Depression
Somatoform Disorders

Carolyn S. Langer, M.D., J.D., M.P.H.
Instructor in Occupational Medicine,
  Harvard School of Public Health
Boston, Massachusetts
Occupational Hazards

Ruth A. Lawrence, M.D.
Professor of Pediatrics, Obstetrics and Gynecology,
  Department of Pediatrics, Division of Neonatology,
  University of Rochester School of Medicine
Rochester, New York
Breastfeeding and Mastitis

Matthew H. Liang, M.D.
Director, Robert B. Brigham Multipurpose Arthritis and
  Musculoskeletal Diseases Center,
  Brigham and Women's Hospital;
Professor of Medicine, Harvard Medical School
Boston, Massachusetts
Arthralgias, Fibromyalgia, and Raynaud's Syndrome

Kathryn A. Martin, M.D.
Reproductive Endocrinology Unit,
  Massachusetts General Hospital;
Instructor in Medicine, Harvard Medical School
Boston, Massachusetts
Menopause and Estrogen Replacement Therapy

Harold Michlewitz, M.D.
Gynecology, Massachusetts General Hospital
Boston, Massachusetts
Benign Vulvar Disorders

Felise B. Milan, M.D.
Assistant Physician, Division of General Internal Medicine,
  Rhode Island Hospital;
Clinical Assistant Professsor of Community Health,
  Brown University School of Medicine
Providence, Rhode Island
Depression
Somatoform Disorders

A. Jacqueline Mitus, M.D.
Associate Physician, Hematology-Oncology Division,
  Department of Medicine, Brigham and Women's Hospital;
Instructor in Medicine, Harvard Medical School
Boston, Massachusetts
Blood Disorders

Anne W. Moulton, M.D.
Division of General Internal Medicine,
  Rhode Island Hospital;
Associate Professor, Brown University School of Medicine
Providence, Rhode Island
Chest Pain Syndromes
Coronary Artery Disease
Other Cardiovascular Diseases

David H. Nichols, M.D.
Chief of Pelvic Surgery,
  Vincent Memorial Gynecology Service,
  Massachusetts General Hospital;
Visiting Professor of Obstetrics, Gynecology,
  and Reproductive Biology, Harvard Medical School
Boston, Massachusetts
Chronic Bladder Disorders and Chronic Dysuria
Incontinence and Uterine Prolapse

Lori B. Olans, M.D., MPH
Assistant Professor of Medicine, Department of Medicine,
  Division of Gastroenterology and Internal Medicine,
  Tufts University School of Medicine
Boston, Massachusetts
Liver Disease in Pregnancy

L. Christine Oliver, M.D., M.S.
Associate Physician, Massachusetts General Hospital;
Assistant Professor of Medicine, Harvard Medical School
Boston, Massachusetts
Occupational Hazards

Rapin Osathanondh, M.D.
Department of Obstetrics, Gynecology, and Reproductive Biology,
  Brigham and Women's Hospital;
Associate Professor, Harvard Medical School
Boston, Massachusetts
Contraception
Abortion

Lela Polivogianis, M.D., MPH
Internist, Department of General Internal Medicine,
  Massachusetts General Hospital;
Instructor in Medicine, Harvard Medical School
Boston, Massachusetts
Smoking Cessation

Veronica A. Ravnikar, M.D.
Director, Reproductive Endocrinology;
Professor, Obstetrics and Gynecology,
  University of Massachusetts Medical Center
Boston, Massachusetts
Infertility

Nancy A. Rigotti, M.D.
Director, Tobacco Research and Treatment Center,
  General Internal Medicine Unit,
  Massachusetts General Hospital;
Assistant Professor of Medicine,
  Assistant Professor of Ambulatory Care and Prevention,
  Harvard Medical School
Boston, Massachusetts
Eating Disorders
Smoking Cessation

Douglas S. Ross, M.D.
Codirector, Thyroid Associates,
  Thyroid Unit, Massachusetts General Hospital;
Assistant Professor of Medicine,
  Harvard Medical School
Boston, Massachusetts
Thyroid Disease
Thyroid Disease in Pregnancy

Raja A. Sayegh, M.D.
Assistant in Gynecology, Vincent Memorial Obstetrics and
  Gynecology Service, Massachusetts General Hospital;
Instructor in Obstetrics, Gynecology, and Reproductive Biology,
  Harvard Medical School
Boston, Massachusetts
Dysfunctional Uterine Bleeding

Isaac Schiff, M.D.
Chief, Vincent Memorial Obstetrics and Gynecology Service,
  Massachusetts General Hospital;
Joe Vincent Meigs Professor of Gynecology,
  Harvard Medical School
Boston, Massachusetts
Pelvic Masses

Ellen W. Seely, M.D.
Director of Clinical Research, Endocrine Hypertension Division,
  Brigham and Women's Hospital;
Assistant Professor of Medicine, Harvard Medical School
Boston, Massachusetts
Diabetes

Linda Shafer, M.D.
Associate Psychiatrist, Department of Psychiatry,
  General Psychiatry Practice, Massachusetts General Hospital;
Instructor in Psychiatry, Harvard Medical School
Boston, Massachusetts
Sexual Dysfunction

Ellen E. Sheets, M.D.
Director, Pap Smear Evaluation Center,
  Brigham and Women's Hospital;
Assistant Professor, Department of Obstetrics, Gynecology,
  and Reproductive Medicine, Harvard Medical School
Boston, Massachusetts
Cervical Cancer and Human Papillomavirus

Robert H. Shmerling, M.D
Associate Physician, Beth Israel Hospital;
Assistant Professor of Medicine,
  Harvard Medical School
Boston, Massachusetts
Arthralgias, Fibromyalgia, and Raynaud's Syndrome

Lawrence N. Shulman, M.D.
Clinical Director, Hematology-Oncology Division,
Department of Medicine, Brigham and Women's Hospital;
Assistant Professor of Medicine,
  Harvard Medical School
Boston, Massachusetts
Nongynecologic Cancer in Pregnancy

Deborah A. Sichel, M.D.
Clinical Associate, Perinatal Psychiatry, Clinical Research Program,
  Department of Psychiatry,
  Massachusetts General Hospital;
Instructor in Psychiatry, Department of Psychiatry,
  Harvard Medical School
Boston, Massachusetts
Postpartum Psychiatric Disorders

David M. Slovik, M.D.
Chief of Medicine, Spaulding Rehabilitation Hospital;
Endocrine Unit, Massachusetts General Hospital;
Assistant Professor of Medicine, Harvard Medical School
Boston, Massachusetts
Osteoporosis

Barbara L. Smith, M.D., Ph.D.
Director, Comprehensive Breast Health Center,
  Massachusetts General Hospital;
Assistant Professor, Harvard Medical School
Boston, Massachusetts
Benign Breast Disease and Breast Implants

Valena J. Soto-Wright, M.D.
Division of Gynecologic Oncology,
  Brigham and Women's Hospital
Boston, Massachusetts
Gynecologic Cancers

Richard I. Sperling, A.M., M.D.
Associate Rheumatologist and Immunologist,
    Department of Rheumatology and Immunology,
    Brigham and Women's Hospital;
Assistant Professor of Medicine, Harvard Medical School
Boston, Massachusetts
Rheumatoid Arthritis

Egilius L.H. Spierings, M.D., Ph.D., P.C.
Division of Neurology, Brigham and Women's Hospital;
Director, Headache Section, Department of Neurology,
    Harvard Medical School
Boston, Massachusetts
Headache Syndromes

Catherine A. Staropoli, M.D.
Fellow in General Internal Medicine/Women's Medicine,
    Division of General Internal Medicine, Rhode Island Hospital;
Brown University
Providence, Rhode Island
Chest Pain Syndromes

Michael R. Stelluto
Director, Core Clinical Clerkship in Ob/Gyn,
    Brigham and Women's Hospital/Harvard Medical School;
Instructor in Obstetrics, Gynecology and Reproductive Biology,
    Harvard Medical School
Boston, Massachusetts
Contraception

Ann E. Taylor, M.D.
Reproductive Endocrinology Unit, Massachusetts
    General Hospital;
Instructor in Medicine, Harvard Medical School
Boston, Massachusetts
Hirsutism and Androgen Excess

Mari-Paule Thiet, M.D.
Department of Obstetrics, Gynecology, and Reproductive Biology,
    Brigham and Women's Hospital;
Instructor, Maternal-Fetal Medicine, Harvard Medical School
Boston, Massachusetts
Preeclampsia

Kathleen F. Thurmond, M.D.
Assistant in Gynecology, Massachusetts General Hospital;
Vincent Memorial Gynecology Service;
Instructor in Obstetrics, Gynecology, and Reproductive Biology,
    Harvard Medical School
Boston, Massachusetts
Pelvic Pain

Kathleen Hubbs Ulman, Ph.D.
Clinical Assistant in Psychiatry,
    Department of Psychiatry, Women's Health Associates,
    Massachusetts General Hospital;
Instructor in Psychology,
    Harvard Medical School
Boston, Massachusetts
Premenstrual Syndrome
Stress Management

May M. Wakamatsu, M.D.
Assistant in Gynecology,
    Massachusetts General Hospital;
Instructor in Obstetrics, Gynecology, and Reproductive Biology,
    Harvard Medical School
Boston, Massachusetts
Vaginitis

Iris Wertheim, M.D.
Division of Gynecologic Oncology,
    Brigham and Women's Hospital
Boston, Massachusetts
Gynecologic Cancers

Jacqueline L. Wolf, M.D.
Associate Physician, Division of Gastroenterology,
    Brigham and Women's Hospital;
Assistant Professor of Medicine,
    Harvard Medical School
Boston, Massachusetts
Bowel Function
Liver Disease in Pregnancy

Barbara J. Woo, M.D.
Department of Medicine, Women's Health Associates, Massachusetts
    General Hospital;
Instructor, Harvard Medical School
Boston, Massachusetts
Screening and Immunization Guidelines

To our families:
Russell, Benjamin, Samuel, and Joshua Eisenstat
and
Richard, Nicholas, and Christopher Mollica

Foreword

In the past 30 years there has been a remarkable growth of interest in the medical problems of women, as both the number of female physicians and the number of female patients who seek female physicians have increased. Thirty years ago in the United States, only 5% to 10% of medical school graduates were women, and most male and female patients (except black women) stated a strong preference for male physicians. Today, nearly one half of medical school graduates are women, and many women in the United States express a strong preference for female physicians. In addition, there is increased research support to study medical problems that predominate in or are exclusive to women, and a belated inclusion of women in studies of major diseases, such as coronary artery disease.

The past 30 years has also seen a resurgence of interest in primary care medicine. The explosion of knowledge generated by the growing investment in medical research and technology after the end of World War II led to a submersion of primary care medicine in the United States as specialties and subspecialties formed and grew. Whereas there were four primary care physicians for every specialist in the United States before World War II, there are now two specialists for every one primary care physician.

This proliferation of specialties created centrifugal forces in medicine and led to fragmentation of medical care as many patients sought and received care directly from specialized providers. For women, the fragmentation of care was compounded by very real needs for specialized care related to pregnancy and birth, menopause, cancers of the breast and reproductive organs, and other conditions that affect only women. As a result, primary care of women is provided in varied ways. Some women receive primary care from a general internist or family physician and one or more subspecialists. Other women (primarily healthy, premenopausal women) seek medical care primarily from a gynecologist and, during pregnancies, from an obstetrician. However, the growing body of knowledge about the medical problems of women is not comprehensively taught by training programs in internal medicine, family medicine, or obstetrics and gynecology.

This book successfully links and synthesizes knowledge from all of these disciplines. The section on medical disease will be of special interest to obstetricians and gynecologists, and the section on gynecology and obstetrics will be of special interest to internists and family physicians. The sections on behavioral medicine and prevention will likely be useful to doctors from all disciplines because these fields tend to get shortchanged in medical school and residency training.

The book also responds to another problem in women's health care. In this country and elsewhere, widespread variation in the treatment of conditions that are specific to women have been documented. Rates of hysterectomy vary fivefold or more from one geographic area to another. Similar variation has been documented for rates of cesarean section and for rates of mastectomy rather than breast conserving surgery for women with early-stage breast cancer. Some nonsurgical treatment decisions are equally variable: whether a woman receives hormone replacement therapy may well depend more on the training of the physician she sees than on her risk factors or personal preferences. Variations in medical practice and the questions this raises about the consistency and quality of medical decision making are not peculiar to women's health care. There is a general need for both better information about which interventions are most effective for different patients and better communication about the values and preferences of those who live with the results of medical care. However, gender differences between doctor and patient can impede effective communication about values and preferences, which is one factor behind many women's preference for female physicians. The authors of this book address this problem by being continually aware of the female patient's perspective.

The book is thorough and detailed in its treatment of all problems, yet it is organized well so that the reader can quickly find an answer to a particular question. The contributing authors, mostly from the faculties of two major teaching hospitals — Brigham and Women's Hospital and Massachusetts General Hospital, both major teaching hospitals of Harvard Medical School — have produced chapters of uniformly high quality. This book will provide an invaluable resource for any clinician who is committed to providing primary health care to women.

Anthony L. Komaroff, M.D.
Director, Division of General Medicine and Primary Care,
  Brigham and Women's Hospital;
Professor of Medicine, Harvard Medical School
Boston, Massachusetts

Albert G. Mulley, Jr., M.D., M.P.P
Chief, General Medicine Unit, Massachusetts General Hospital;
Associate Professor of Medicine, Harvard Medical School
Boston, Massachusetts

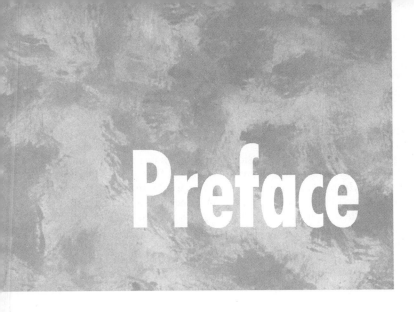

Preface

Primary Care of Women was conceived in the midst of unprecedented reform of the health care system in the United States and of the position of women within that system. A central feature of this reform has been recognition of the critical value of primary care. Particularly for women, the emphasis on subspecialization that dominated Western medicine since the 1950s has sometimes resulted in fragmentation of care. The complexities of a woman's biologic, emotional, and social functioning cannot easily be reduced to the organ-system approach of traditional medical education and practice.

A second feature of this transformation of medical practice is a recognition of the gaps in scientific knowledge that underlie clinical practice; for women, these gaps are often particularly wide. In recent years government and scientific institutions have acknowledged the exclusion of women from past medical research and the resulting uncertainty facing practicing physicians who care for women. Many efforts are now underway to establish a more scientific basis for clinical practice by studying disorders that manifest differently in or are exclusive to women.

Finally, medical practice is being changed by greater emphasis on the central role of the patient in the medical care process. An important stimulus for this change was the lay women's health movement, which has critically questioned the social and scientific practices of medicine for over 2 decades. The concurrent infusion of female physicians into the medical profession has also had a major impact on this trend.

The purpose of this book is to provide a concise, practical reference for clinicians engaged in the primary care of women. Its subject matter includes:

1) Problems commonly encountered in primary care practice that manifest differently, or respond differently to treatment, in women compared with men. Examples include coronary artery disease, human immunodeficiency virus (HIV) infection, and alcohol abuse.

2) Medical problems that occur more commonly in women (for example, osteoporosis, thyroid disease, and gallstones).
3) Problems that occur exclusively (or nearly so) in women, such as gynecologic and obstetric problems and certain endocrinopathies.

In addition to problems or diseases treated largely by the primary care clinician, the content includes problems about which the primary care provider must be knowledgeable even though care is managed by a subspecialist; for example, breast cancer. The book contains a section on psychology and behavior, which provides a framework for addressing many of the problems that prompt women to seek medical care, including depression, obesity, and domestic violence. Finally, screening and prevention, essential aspects of primary care practice, are reviewed.

An important feature is the inclusion of material on the interaction of pregnancy with medical illness. This material considers a range of issues relevant to the care of women in their childbearing years, including the effects of specific medical problems on fertility and on maternal and fetal health, the effects of pregnancy on existing diseases, the evaluation and management of problems in early pregnancy, and modification of treatment during pregnancy.

The emphasis of the book is on clinical decision making. The focus is problem-oriented and information is organized to facilitate efficient use in a busy office setting, with extensive cross-references, tables, and summaries of management recommendations. References in the text are limited to enhance readability; general and specific references are included for readers wishing to obtain more information. Although the emphasis is on practical clinical decision making, the authors have provided relevant scientific data when available. In some instances research pertaining to the female patient is sparse. The goal is to clarify what is known, what is not known, and when that is likely to matter.

Certain principles of primary care and general practice are reflected here. One such principle is attention to the costs of medical care. The cost-effectiveness of diagnostic and therapeutic interventions is implicitly and explicitly considered, and guidelines for efficient use of subspecialty resources are included. A second guiding principle is the recognition that educating patients is a vital part of primary care practice. The role of a patient's preferences in the clinical decision-making process, what the patient can expect from specific tests or treatments, and the probabilities of various outcomes of treatment are addressed.

This book is directed to all clinicians who provide primary care to adult female patients, including internists, family practitioners, obstetrician-gynecologists, nurse practitioners, subspecialists, and physicians-in-training. We recognize that the content of care varies in different settings; in some areas, obstetrician-gynecologists and subspecialists are important sources of primary care. In outlining recommendations regarding indications for referral, the convention in this book assumes that referral will be needed for many procedures, although some are performed routinely by some primary care clinicians.

We hope that the interdisciplinary and interinstitutional collaboration represented in this book will make it useful for a wide spectrum of clinicians and will promote more integrated, comprehensive, and effective care for women. For us, creating this book has been an opportunity to deepen our longstanding collaborations with our subspecialty colleagues, associate editors Dr. Fredric Frigoletto and Dr. Isaac Schiff. We are indebted to them for their essential role in shaping the sections on Obstetrics and Gynecology. We are also grateful to Dr. Anthony Komaroff, Dr. Albert Mulley, Jr., and Dr. Eugene Braunwald for their advice, support, and guidance.

We have worked side-by-side with most of the contributing authors in the care of patients at Brigham and Women's Hospital and Massachusetts General Hospital. To these valued colleagues, we owe our sincerest thanks for sharing their clinical expertise with the professional community through this book.

Our colleagues at Mosby-Year Book have been exemplary in their professionalism and support. We are grateful that Stephanie Manning, the executive editor, shared our vision for the book and provided the means to make it a reality. Carolyn Malik, our developmental editor, deserves special thanks for her unfailing support, good humor, and commitment to the book. Catherine Albright's excellent editorial efforts helped us to achieve the high standard of quality we sought.

The scientific basis for the clinical practice of primary care for women represents an evolving body of knowledge. Current research related to women's health promises to provide new answers to clinical questions and to suggest new approaches to care. We welcome comments and questions from readers to ensure that future editions of this book further address the needs of clinicians engaged in the primary care of women.

Karen J. Carlson, M.D. Stephanie A. Eisenstat, M.D.
Boston, Massachusetts

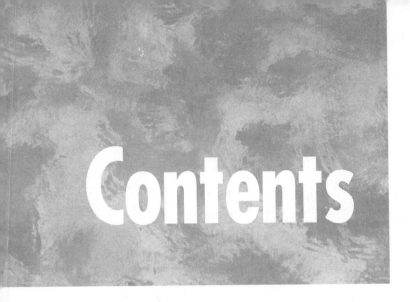

Contents

PART THREE Psychology and Behavioral Medicine

PART FOUR Preventive Medicine

APPENDIXES

Featured Plates

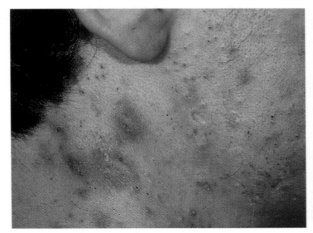

Plate 1

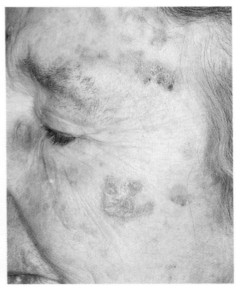

Plate 2

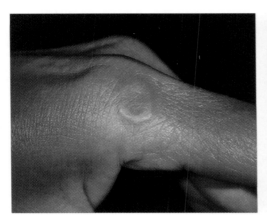

Plate 3

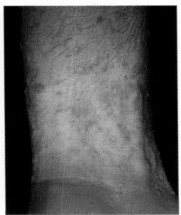

Plate 4

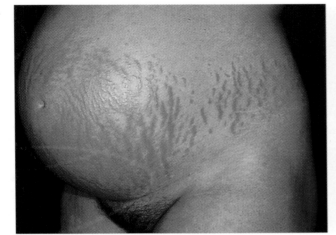

Plate 5

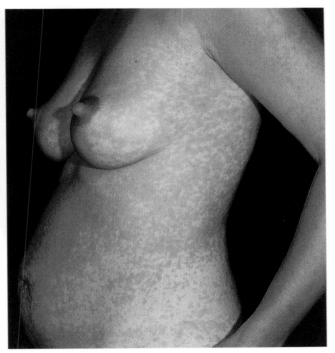

Plate 6

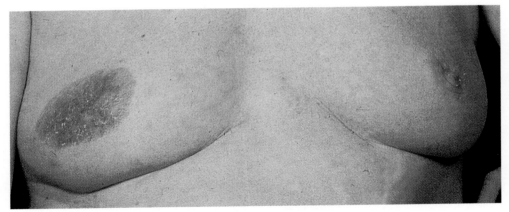

Plate 7

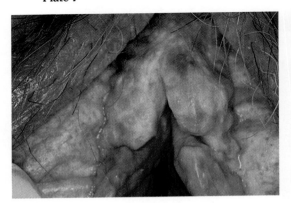

Plate 8

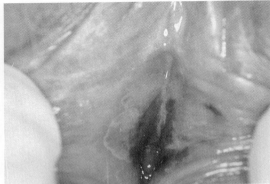

Plate 9

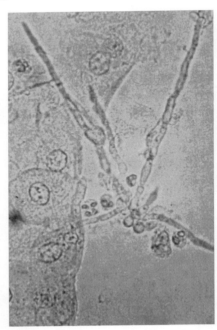

Plate 10

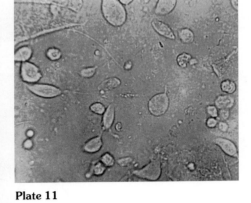

Plate 11

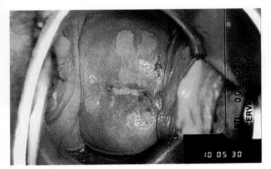

Plate 12

Featured Plates

Plate 1 Localized cystic acne. Cystic lesions appear in this patient, who has chronic comedo and pustular acne. (From Habif TP: *Clinical dermatology*, ed 2, 1990, St Louis, Mosby.)

Plate 2 Actinic keratosis. Early lesions are present on the forehead. A more advanced lesion with yellow adherent scale is seen on the cheek. (From Habif TP: *Clinical dermatology*, ed 2, 1990, St Louis, Mosby.)

Plate 3 Granuloma annulare. A ring of flesh-colored papules. (From Habif TP: *Clinical dermatology*, ed 2, 1990, St Louis, Mosby.)

Plate 4 Localized lichen planus. Early lesions are present on the flexor surface of the wrists, a common site for localized lichen planus. (From Habif TP: *Clinical dermatology*, ed 2, 1990, St Louis, Mosby.)

Plate 5 Pruritic urticarial papules and plaques of pregnancy. The abdomen is often the initial site of involvement. Initial lesions may be confined to striae. (From Habif TP: *Clinical dermatology*, ed 2, 1990, St Louis, Mosby.)

Plate 6 Pruritic urticarial papules and plaques of pregnancy. Fully evolved eruption. (From Habif TP: *Clinical dermatology*, ed 2, 1990, St Louis, Mosby.)

Plate 7 Paget's disease of the breast. (From Skarin AT, editor: *Atlas of diagnostic oncology*, 1992, New York, Gower Medical Publishing.)

Plate 8 Lichen sclerosus.

Plate 9 Lichen planus.

Plate 10 Candidal organisms in a saline wet-mount preparation under high-power magnification. Hyphae and conidia are clearly demonstrated. (From Kaufman RH, Faro S: *Benign diseases of the vulva and vagina*, ed 4, 1994, St Louis, Mosby.)

Plate 11 Trichomoniasis. Trichomonads in a wet mount prepared with physiologic saline. Usually, more immature epithelial cells are seen in the secretions of active trichomoniasis (high power). (From Kaufman RH, Faro S: *Benign diseases of the vulva and vagina*, ed 4, 1994, St Louis, Mosby.)

Plate 12 Cervical intraepithelial neoplasia (CIN) Stage I. Acetowhite appearance of part of the anterior lip of the cervix associated with CIN Stage I. This relates to mild dyskaryosis in the cervical smear. (From Symonds M, Macpherson M: *Color atlas of obstetrics and gynecology*, 1994, London, Mosby-Wolfe.)

Part One

Medical Disease in Women

1 Chest Pain Syndromes

Anne W. Moulton and Catherine A. Staropoli

EPIDEMIOLOGY

Chest pain is a common medical problem, particularly in women. Approximately 200,000 new cases of chest pain, not associated with significant coronary artery disease, are identified each year in the United States. In one study of outpatient practices two thirds of all chest pain diagnoses fell into one of three categories: angina, nonarticular chest wall pain, and pain related to the gastrointestinal tract. Of all patients entering a primary care physician's office with chest pain, 62% were diagnosed on the first visit and only 7% were referred elsewhere for consultation.

Twenty percent of patients referred for cardiac catheterization for the evaluation of chest pain have normal coronary arteries and more than half of these patients are women. Most patients with normal coronary arteries at catheterization have a benign course, with a very low incidence of myocardial infarction (1%) or cardiac death (0.6%). Although the mortality rate is low, the morbidity rate can be high, since many patients may suffer from inadequate diagnosis, persistent symptoms, and decreased function because of fear of heart disease. About 75% of these patients continue to see a physician and one half regard themselves as disabled. On average, patients with persistent chest pain of unknown cause receive 1.2 prescription medications each month, visit a primary care provider 2.2 times each year, and are hospitalized at least once each year.

Patients who consult a primary care physician have symptoms of chest pain that may be acute in onset but often are more chronic in nature. Initially acute life-threatening causes of chest pain such as unstable angina, myocardial infarction, pulmonary embolism, pneumothorax, dissecting aneurysm, and perforating ulcer or esophageal tear must be considered and may require hospitalization for evaluation. Outpatient testing and management should be tailored to the most likely causes, with attention to the following differential diagnosis (see Fig. 1-1; box, following page).

CARDIAC CAUSES

In patients who experience pleuritic chest pain the diagnosis of **pericarditis** must be considered. A viral cause is the most common in an outpatient setting. There is no evidence that women are more likely to have this entity, although it is more commonly seen in younger patients. No clinical features differentiate acute viral pericarditis and idiopathic pericarditis, and it is likely that the majority of cases of community-acquired idiopathic pericarditis are due to unrecognized viral infections. The seasonal peak of pericarditis is in the spring and fall. The most common viral causes are coxsackievirus group B and echovirus type 8. Other viruses that can cause pericarditis include mumps, influenza, mononucleosis, varicella, rubella, and hepatitis B. Acute pericarditis can be seen in human immunodeficiency virus (HIV)– positive individuals and may be idiopathic or related to specific viral pathogens, such as cytomegalovirus.

In about 50% of cases of pericarditis there is a prodrome of upper respiratory tract infection. Viral or idiopathic pericarditis should be suspected when young or otherwise healthy adults have a characteristic prodromal illness. Diagnosis is made by antibody titers and by the finding of a characteristic pericardial friction rub. Electrocardiographic changes are not specific but may include depressed PR segments and diffusely elevated ST segments. Echocardiographic documentation of a pericardial effusion is helpful. The illness, although short and dramatic, is usually self-limited, lasting 1 to 3 weeks.

Chest pain, usually in association with dyspnea, may represent the relatively rare syndrome of **hypertrophic cardiomyopathy.** Diagnosis is suggested by a systolic murmur that is increased with the Valsalva maneuver or an electrocardiogram (ECG) that reveals left ventricular hypertrophy or suggests an old myocardial infarction (MI), with no clinical history to suggest prior infarction. Echocardiography is essential for making the diagnosis and assessing the severity of the condition.

The association of **mitral valve prolapse** (MVP) with chest pain is controversial. MVP occurs in 3% to 4% or more of the population, making it one of the most common cardiovascular conditions. It is eight times more common in women than men (see Chapter 4). Despite the female predominance of MVP, chest pain associated with MVP is actually reported more frequently in men than in women. The pain has been attributed to stretching of the papillary muscle. However, in one study chest pain was found with similar frequency in patients with MVP and in control patients without MVP. Historically the chest pain with MVP has been described as an atypical angina-like pain in that it is prolonged, is not related to exertion, and can be associated with intermittent episodes of stabbing chest pain at the apex. Diagnosis is suggested by a characteristic murmur or click as well as echocardiography (see Chapter 4).

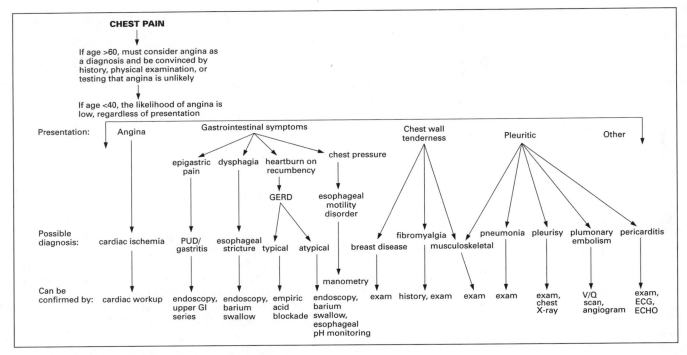

Fig. 1-1 Evaluation of chest pain in the female patient.

Dissecting **aortic aneurysm** is of acute onset, with a tearing pain noted in the anterior or posterior chest that radiates to the arms, legs, and abdomen. This process, which typically occurs in persons in their 60s and 70s, is more common in males, with a male to female ratio of 2:1. In most cases the pain is so severe that patients are taken immediately to an emergency setting, but in cases where there is a slow leak of blood through the intima the presentation may be more subtle. Women who experience symptoms from an enlarging aneurysm are more likely to be older and to seek medical attention at the time of rupture of their aneurysm. Bilateral pulses and blood pressure measurements may be unequal and there may be widening of the mediastinum indicated on chest radiograph. The definitive diagnosis is made with angiography.

Studies in the last 10 years have suggested that many patients with angina and normal coronary arteries have myocardial ischemia caused by abnormal coronary

CAUSES OF NONISCHEMIC CHEST PAIN IN WOMEN

Cardiac

Mitral valve prolapse
Pericarditis
Hypertrophic cardiomyopathy
Aortic aneurysm
Microvascular angina
Abnormal cardiac sensitivity

Pulmonary

Pneumonia
Pleurisy
Pulmonary embolism
Pneumothorax

Gastrointestinal

Esophageal disorders
    Nutcracker esophagus
    Nonspecific esophageal motility disorders
    Diffuse esophageal spasm
    Hypertensive lower esophageal sphincter
    Achalasia

Esophageal reflux
Peptic ulcer disease
Irritable bowel syndrome
Gallbladder disease

Musculoskeletal

Costochondritis/xiphoiditis
Cervical and thoracic osteoarthritis
Muscular strain
Fibromyalgia

Psychologic

Panic disorder
Anxiety/depression
Somatization
Hyperventilation
Substance abuse

Other

Chest pain associated with menopausal transition
Herpes zoster
Breast disorders

vasodilator reserve, so-called **microvascular angina**. Patients with this syndrome, the majority of whom are women, have angina-like chest pain, ischemic ST-segment depressions on electrocardiography during exercise testing, angiographically normal coronary arteries without coronary artery spasm, normal ventricular function, and an excellent prognosis (see Chapter 2).

There is also a subset of patients with chest pain and angiographically normal coronary arteries who demonstrate **abnormal cardiac sensitivity** to a variety of stimuli. It is not clear whether this syndrome is a function of abnormal activation of pain receptors within the heart or abnormal processing of visceral afferent neural impulses in the peripheral or central nervous system.

PULMONARY CAUSES

Pneumonia should be considered in any patient who has chest pain accompanied by a fever and a persistent cough that is nonproductive or productive of purulent sputum. The chest pain is described as a dull or pleuritic pain made worse by coughing or inspiration. Patients with chronic bronchitis or acute exacerbation of asthma may also complain of chest pain with cough presumed secondary to inflammation of the chest wall.

In one study of patients with chest pain in the ambulatory setting, **pleurisy** was diagnosed in women twice as much as in men. Pleurisy is described as a sharp unilateral chest pain that may be referred to the shoulders, neck, or abdomen. It is often associated with splinting of the chest wall and shallow respiration. A pleural friction rub may occasionally be auscultated over the affected area. Pleurisy is caused by inflammation of the pleura, most often related to viral infection but sometimes attributable to a collagen vascular disease.

One of the most frequently underdiagnosed conditions, **pulmonary embolism** (PE), must always be considered as a cause of chest pain. The classic presentation is pleuritic chest pain accompanied by shortness of breath, tachypnea, tachycardia, and lower extremity swelling and erythema. When the presentation is atypical a diagnosis of PE should be considered in women who have any risk factors, including oral contraceptive use, current or recent pregnancy, history of thromboembolic phenomena, cancer, systemic lupus erythematosus, antiphospholipid syndrome (see Chapter 26), recent pelvic or orthopedic surgery, hypercoagulability, or prolonged immobility. Hormone replacement therapy does not increase the risk of thromboembolism. Diagnosis is made by lung scan or pulmonary angiography. Finally **pneumothorax** is a rare cause of acute chest pain that is more common in men and easily diagnosed by physical examination and chest radiograph.

GASTROINTESTINAL CAUSES

Multiple gastrointestinal disorders have been associated with chest pain. Esophageal disorders are the most common. In studies of emergency admissions for chest pain 20% of patients with suspected myocardial infarction were given a diagnosis of esophageal disease but only 10% were believed to have an esophageal disorder that caused the chest pain. Gender has not been found to discriminate between cardiac and esophageal disease. Esophageal disorders are found in approximately one third of patients with chest pain and normal coronary arteries.

It is often difficult to distinguish esophageal chest pain from myocardial ischemia on the basis of history and physical examination findings alone. Half of patients with both known gastroesophageal reflux disease (GERD) and coronary artery disease (CAD) are unable to determine whether their chest pain is caused by a cardiac or a gastrointestinal source. Esophageal disease may manifest as classic angina, postprandial pain, pain of several hours' duration, as well as pain relieved by antacids. Chest pain on recumbency, pain not aggravated by effort, symptoms of dysphagia, and regurgitation also suggest esophageal problems. Finally, it is important to note that esophageal disease and CAD often occur in the same patient.

Two major esophageal abnormalities have been associated with chest pain–motility disorders and GERD. The **esophageal motility disorders** are diagnosed by manometry, a procedure involving the placement of pressure transducers through the nose or mouth into the esophagus. Nutcracker esophagus is the most commonly diagnosed esophageal disorder associated with noncardiac chest pain. It is diagnosed by manometric findings of elevated mean peristaltic amplitude, increased duration of muscle contraction, and normal peristaltic sequence. It is present in almost 50% of patients with abnormal motility on evaluation of chest pain. In one series a mixture of nonspecific esophageal motility disorders was present in approximately 33% of patients with abnormal manometry findings and chest pain. Diffuse esophageal spasm was found in 10%, hypertensive lower esophageal sphincter in less than 5%, and achalasia in 2%.

Abnormal motility can be detected by manometry but it is difficult to show that dysmotility itself is the cause of the chest pain. Frequently the manometric abnormalities are not temporally related to the chest pain. Provocative testing can be done with pentagastrin, hot and cold liquids, vasopressin, ergotamine, edrophonium, bethanechol, and intraesophageal balloon distention in an attempt to reproduce chest pain.

There is no gold standard test to evaluate chest pain caused by esophageal dysmotility. It is hypothesized that the esophageal abnormalities found on manometry may be a marker for other processes that may cause chest pain. The abnormal function of the coronary circulation and the esophageal muscle may be a part of a generalized abnormality in the smooth muscle, accounting for the findings of normal cardiac catheterization in patients with exertional chest pain and nutcracker esophagus.

Gastroesophageal reflux disease (GERD) is a common cause of chest pain in ambulatory practice, accounting for 30% to 60% of angiographically negative chest pain in women. The patient usually complains of angina-like pain or experiences "heartburn" as a gnawing sensation in the epigastrium. The pain can radiate to the arms or jaw. Symptoms commonly occur after meals or when recumbent. Dysphagia suggests the development of a peptic stricture. This symptom should prompt evaluation by a barium swallow. Conditions that decrease lower esophageal sphincter pressure (e.g., pregnancy, use of calcium channel blockers and other smooth muscle relaxants), as well as those which increase intraabdominal pressure (obesity) can predispose women to GERD. Since there are no identifying features of GERD on examination, the history is an important tool in diagnosis. If the history is classic for GERD the clinical consensus is to treat empirically without further evaluation and evaluate only if there is no response to therapy.

Endoscopy, barium esophagrams, and esophageal pH monitoring have all been used to help make the diagnosis of GERD. Findings of esophagitis on endoscopy or upper gastrointestinal series do not confirm that reflux is the cause of pain. **Esophagitis** may also be caused by viral, fungal, and bacterial infections, as well as pill ingestion. In immunosuppressed women the diagnosis of fungal or viral esophagitis should always be considered.

A normal endoscopy result does not rule out GERD. Two additional tests may be helpful in making the diagnosis. Esophageal acid perfusion, also known as Bernstein's test, involves infusing HCl through a nasogastric tube into the esophagus. The test result is considered positive if infusion of HCl replicates the patient's chest pain. The test has a specificity of 90% but a sensitivity of only 36%. Those patients with negative test results can undergo 24-hour esophageal pH monitoring. The specificity of this test is 85% and the sensitivity is 95%. A trial of medical therapy such as omeprazole can also be a diagnostic tool for diagnosing acid-related chest pain.

Symptoms of **irritable bowel syndrome** are reported by 10% to 20% of adults. This syndrome has a marked female predominance. Women with noncardiac chest pain are more likely then age-matched control subjects to experience the constellation of symptoms compatible with irritable bowel syndrome. Most of the symptoms are presumed to be caused by altered colonic motility. A large percentage of patients with irritable bowel syndrome report esophageal symptoms as well and on further evaluation are found to have esophageal motility abnormalities. Both irritable bowel and esophageal dysmotility may represent a spectrum of disease, the "irritable gut." Stress is known to exacerbate symptoms. Patients who seek medical attention for their symptoms have been shown to have a higher frequency of psychologic disturbances than those who do not seek medical care. Irritable bowel syndrome is discussed in Chapter 13.

Although epigastric pain is the more common presenting sign of **peptic ulcer disease** (PUD), duodenal or gastric ulcers and gastritis can manifest as chest pain. Duodenal ulcers cause pain $1\frac{1}{2}$ to 3 hours after eating. Pain is usually relieved by intake of food or antacids. Gastric ulcers may be worsened by eating. Nonsteroidal antiinflammatory drugs, which are used commonly by older women for arthritis, can predispose to PUD. Smoking is the most common risk factor for ulcers in younger women. Alcohol may cause an erosive gastritis that may be accompanied by chest pain. Diagnosis can be confirmed by endoscopy or barium examination of the upper gastrointestinal tract.

Gallbladder disease is rarely a cause of chest pain and symptoms are usually related to meals. The diagnosis of gallbladder disease is described in Chapter 14.

MUSCULOSKELETAL CAUSES

Disorders of the thoracic skeleton are among the most common causes of chest pain in the ambulatory setting. Most chest pain of musculoskeletal cause can be diagnosed by the history and physical examination alone.

Costochondritis is more common in women than men (3:1), especially African-American women. This condition may manifest as localized tenderness over the costochondral junctions, most commonly the second, third, and fourth junctions. The pain is often described as gnawing, dull, and enduring for hours or days, but it can also be characterized as sharp and fleeting. **Tietze's syndrome** has similar features but with objective signs such as swelling, warmth, and redness over one or more costochondral junctions. Pain arises on pressure over the costochondral junctions or pectoralis muscle. **Xiphoiditis** may be manifested by a deep retrosternal ache that may radiate to the epigastrium or precordium. Chest pain will be reproduced on palpation of the xiphoid process.

Cervical and **thoracic osteoarthritis** can cause nerve root compression from narrowed foramina, leading to pain referred to the dermatomes innervated by the affected nerves. The C4-T7 nerve roots innervate the chest. The quality of the pain may be similar to angina, with radiation to the jaws, arms, and neck, and the pain may be precipitated by exertion—so-called cervicoprecordial angina. Usually the pain is precipitated by motion of the upper torso and arms, or by prolonged sitting or lying. Cervical spine radiographs may reveal osteoarthritis.

Muscular strain can be precipitated by unaccustomed exercise. The pain can be felt in the costochondral junctions or in the chest wall muscles. It is reproduced on movement of the torso, arms, or ribs (as in breathing). Palpation of trigger points may also elicit pain and muscle spasm.

Fibromyalgia is a chronic syndrome of reproducible trigger point tenderness, widespread pain, fatigue, and sleep disturbance. One of the classic trigger points is the second costochondral junction. Other trigger points include the occiput, lower cervical spine, trapezius, supraspinatus, lateral epicondyle, gluteus, knee, and greater trochanter. The prevalence of fibromyalgia in the primary care setting is estimated to be 7%, with 80% of cases occurring in women, at a mean age of 50.

PSYCHOLOGIC CAUSES

Chest pain and palpitations constitute one of the top five symptom complexes unexplained by physical illness. When no obvious explanation for continuing chest pain is discovered a psychogenic diagnosis should be considered. Cardiac symptoms, including palpitations and atypical chest pain, can be a prominent component of **panic disorder.** Although this entity is found in only 1% to 3% of the population, it occurs more commonly in women. The prevalence of panic disorder in primary care practice is considerably higher precisely because of these associated somatic features. Women with this disorder are most likely to consult a primary care physician first with these complaints. Initial attacks usually occur in patients in their 20s and 30s and about 50% of episodes develop during times of stress. There is evidence that panic disorder is a biologic disorder with a strong genetic component, and there is considerable overlap of panic disorder with other causes of chest pain, including CAD, MVP, and hyperventilation syndrome, making the diagnosis and treatment more difficult. The diagnosis of chest pain secondary to panic disorder is suggested by a history of atypical chest pain (i.e., long duration, unrelated to exertion, of varying quality) in a young woman who is obviously healthy or in an older woman when an extensive evaluation has been undertaken with no results. This diagnosis is confirmed when the patient describes chest pain as accompanied by recurrent, discrete attacks of intense fear or discomfort associated with somatic or psychic symptoms of anxiety.

Chest pain and palpitations can occur as symptoms in patients with underlying **anxiety** and **depression.** Clues to diagnosis are the young age and general health of the patient or, in older women, a negative evaluation for medical causes. Detailed questioning regarding current stressors and a history of depression, anxiety, or physical or sexual abuse is essential.

Patients with **somatoform disorders** may have the symptom of chest pain in association with one or many ostensibly unrelated symptoms (i.e., no unifying diagnosis) in the presence of some degree of psychologic conflict. Somatization disorder in particular is much more common in women, whereas somatoform pain disorder is more common in men. Hypochondriasis occurs equally in both sexes (see Chapter 74).

The symptom of chest pain in conjunction with breathlessness may be caused by **hyperventilation syndrome,** which occurs more commonly in females than males. The diagnosis is suggested by an elevated respiratory rate and a shortened breath-holding time. A hyperventilation challenge test may be useful. Three minutes of forced overbreathing is followed by a 3-minute recovery period with a careful assessment of symptoms.

Any evaluation of intermittent chest pain, especially accompanied by palpitations, in women must include detailed questioning about **substance abuse,** particularly cocaine, alcohol, and benzodiazepines (see Chapter 66).

OTHER CAUSES

Symptoms of chest pain and palpitations are reported frequently by women going through **menopause.** The pain is somewhat atypical but is often brought on by exercise or episodes of stress and can occur in conjunction with hot flashes. This syndrome is thought to reflect a component of vasomotor instability that occurs as estrogen levels drop, and it may be related to microvascular angina.

Herpes zoster is characterized by unilateral pain along thoracic dermatomes for a period of days followed by rash in the same distribution. Dormant varicella viruses are reactivated in the dorsal root ganglion. The pain and rash usually disappear in weeks but the pain may persist in 10% of patients, especially in the elderly or immunocompromised, as postherpetic neuralgia.

Breast disorders can cause chest pain and are discussed in Chapter 30.

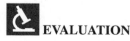 **EVALUATION**

History

A detailed history is the first step in the appropriate evaluation of chest pain. Understanding the timing, precise loca-

tion, and quality of the patient's pain and associated symptoms is essential. For example chest pain that persists for hours, is retrosternal and does not radiate, increases with lying down, is relieved by food or antacids, or is associated with heartburn, dysphagia, or reflux suggests esophageal disease. Although chest pain induced by exercise is most commonly associated with CAD, it may also accompany GERD. Pain that occurs with any movement of the chest wall suggests pulmonary or musculoskeletal causes. Pain that occurs with deep inspiration, the recumbent position (especially the left lateral decubitus), coughing, or even swallowing may represent pericarditis, especially if relief is obtained by sitting up, bending forward, or holding one's breath.

The clinician needs to obtain detailed information on medical history, cardiac risk factors, menopausal status, dietary habits, and use of alcohol, nonsteroidal antiinflammatory agents, aspirin, caffeine, or other medications. The information should include gentle questioning about a history of sexual or physical abuse, depression, anxiety, and any other current life stressors.

A knowledge of a woman's prior probability of significant cardiac disease at any age is useful. For example, women less than age 39 who exhibit typical angina have only a 26% pretest likelihood of CAD as compared with a 70% pretest likelihood of CAD in men of the same age with typical angina. Alternatively, a presentation of atypical angina in a woman above the age of 60 represents a 54% pretest likelihood of disease, not markedly different from the 67% pretest likelihood in men of the same age with atypical angina. In older patients the physician must consider angina as a diagnosis unless history, physical examination, or testing suggests this diagnosis is unlikely. More extensive discussion of the diagnosis of coronary artery disease in women can be found in Chapter 2.

Physical examination

The physical examination should begin with vital signs including bilateral pulses and blood pressure if there is a concern about a dissecting aneurysm. Examination should include careful palpation of the chest wall and costochondral junctions, looking for musculoskeletal causes with palpation and specific maneuvers. Auscultation of the lung fields may reveal findings of consolidation. Patients with pleurisy usually have a normal examination result. A careful cardiac examination may reveal murmurs, clicks, or rubs. A pericardial knock or a two- or three-component friction rub may be heard with pericarditis. Several systolic murmurs are associated with chest pain in such diseases as aortic stenosis, mitral valve prolapse with mitral regurgitation, and idiopathic hypertrophic subaortic stenosis. Pain on abdominal palpation may suggest gastrointestinal tract abnormality such as gallbladder disease or PUD. The physician should note the patient's affect to assess depression or anxiety.

SUMMARY

The differential diagnosis of chest pain poses a unique challenge to the primary care provider. Although some cases may be straightforward others may involve overlapping causes and management may be more difficult. The way in which a woman expresses her complaints has been shown to influence decisions about further evaluation. A "business-like" rather than a "histrionic" style is more likely to lead to a cardiac evaluation. The medical literature also suggests that women with chest pain are less likely than men with a comparable likelihood of CAD to receive appropriate evaluation.

Once life-threatening causes of chest pain have been ruled out, careful follow-up observation over time may yield more insight into the cause of the chest pain and direct the evaluation and treatment. Reassurance about the absence of life-threatening abnormality is often not enough. Careful attention to the diagnosis of less serious causes is necessary so that appropriate treatment can be instituted.

BIBLIOGRAPHY

Bass C; Unexplained chest pain and breathlessness, *Med Clin North Am* 75(5):1157, 1991.

Browning TH: Diagnosis of chest pain of esophageal origin, *Dig Dis Sci* 35(3):289, 1990.

Carney RM et al: Major depression, panic disorder, and mitral valve prolapse in patients who complain of chest pain, *Am J Med* 89:757, 1990.

Chambers J, Bass C: Chest pain with normal coronary anatomy: a review of natural history and possible etiologic factors, *Prog Cardiovasc Dis* 33(3):161, 1990.

Davies HA: Anginal pain of esophageal origin: clinical presentation, prevalence, and prognosis, *Am J Med* 92(S5A):S, 1992.

Diamond GA, Forrester JS: Analysis of probability as an aide in the clinical diagnosis of coronary-artery disease, *N Engl J Med* 300:1350, 1979.

An exploratory report of chest pain in primary care: a report from ASPN, *J Am Board Fam Pract* 3:143, 1990.

Kane FJ, Wittels E, Harper RG: Chest pain and anxiety disorder, *Tex Med* 86(7):104, 1990.

Katon W et al: Chest pain: relationship of psychiatric illness to coronary arteriographic results, *Am J Med* 84:1, 1988.

Lynn RB, Friedman LS: Irritable bowel syndrome, *N Engl J Med* 329(26):1940, 1993.

Reilly BM: Chest pain. In *Practical strategies in outpatient medicine, ed* 2, Philadelphia, 1984, WB Saunders.

Richter JE: Investigation and management of non-cardiac chest pain, *Bailliere Clin Gastroenterol* 5(2):281, 1991.

Richter JE, Bradley LA, Castel MDO: Esophageal chest pain: current controversies and pathogenesis, diagnosis, and therapy, *Ann Intern Med* 110:66, 1989.

Wolfe F: Fibromyalgia, *Rheum Dis Clin North Am* 16(3):681, 1990.

Yingling KW et al: Estimated prevalences of panic disorder and depression among consecutive patients seen in an emergency department with acute chest pain, *J Gen Intern Med* 8:231, 1993.

2 Coronary Artery Disease

Anne W. Moulton

■ EPIDEMIOLOGY

Cardiovascular disease is a substantial cause of mortality for women in the United States. It accounts for about 250,000 deaths each year, with 100,000 of these deaths being premature. It becomes a leading cause of death in all U.S. women after 40 years of age; one in three women will die of heart disease. In women coronary artery disease (CAD) develops approximately 10 to 15 years later in life than in men, but by the age of 70 the male/female ratio for the incidence of coronary disease starts to approach 1.

Data on the racial differences in the development of CAD are limited. Rates are the highest in black males, followed by white males, black females, and white females. However, African-American patients with CAD, especially women, have higher morbidity and mortality rates. Data also suggest that African-Americans with comparable severity of CAD are less likely to undergo coronary artery bypass procedures than whites. Rates of CAD in Hispanic populations and Asian populations in the United States are somewhat lower for both males and females.

RISK FACTORS

Risk factors for CAD in men have some predictive value in women. However, even after controlling for blood pressure, relative weight, serum cholesterol level, cigarette smoking, and glucose intolerance, men still have over 3.5 times the risk of development of CAD of women. In other words, differences in major cardiovascular risk factor levels do not account entirely for the lower incidence of CAD in women.

Role of conventional risk factors

Coronary atherosclerosis is a disease of older women, and thus **age** is truly the greatest predictor of the development of CAD in women.

Diabetes mellitus is a particularly important risk factor for CAD in women. Women with diabetes actually have a greater risk of CAD than men with diabetes, and thus diabetes eliminates any female advantage in the development of heart disease. Even after adjustment for other risk factors, the relative risk of development of CAD in women with diabetes is twice that of nondiabetic women. Studies also suggest that abnormal glucose tolerance *alone* is a risk factor for CAD in women because of a relationship between poorer glucose control (as assessed by higher level of hemoglobin A_{1c} [Hb A_{1c}]) and the risk of cardiovascular disease. Of note, this effect is seen well below diabetic levels of glycemia.

Hypertension is one of the most powerful predictors of cardiovascular and cerebrovascular disease. It is also one of the most prevalent of the major risk factors, with a prevalence ranging from 20% to 40% of the population, the higher proportion being in black women. The risk of development of CAD parallels the severity of hypertension.

Hypertension is an independent risk factor for the development of CAD, and if it is present with elevated cholesterol level or smoking, the risk of CAD increases substantially.

A portion of the sex difference in CAD susceptibility is probably related to differences in **plasma lipids** (see Chapter 3). In North America women ages 20 to 50 years tend to have lower plasma low-density lipoprotein (LDL) levels and very low-density lipoprotein (VLDL) levels and higher plasma high-density lipoprotein (HDL) levels than men of a similar age. In women there is a significant inverse correlation between HDL levels and CAD. This female advantage diminishes gradually after menopause, with increasing levels of LDL cholesterol and decreasing levels of HDL. Some studies have suggested that triglycerides may also be independently associated with the development of coronary artery disease in women, although not in men. Preliminary studies suggest that lipoprotein (a) is strongly associated with the development of atherosclerosis and coronary artery disease, especially in women. Lipoprotein (a) (Lp[a]) levels may decrease with estrogen and progesterone replacement in postmenopausal women. However, recent prospective data associating elevated levels of LP(a) and CAD in men are controversial.

Smoking is an important risk factor for the development of CAD, especially in young females. The risk for coronary death and myocardial infarction (MI) for smokers of 25 or more cigarettes per day compared to women who have never smoked is increased fivefold, even after controlling for other cardiac risk factors. When women quit smoking, their cardiovascular risk starts to drop and eventually approaches the risk for women who have never smoked, but users who continue to smoke even small amounts (one to four cigarettes per day) have an elevated risk of CAD. The relative risk of CAD for current smokers tends to be somewhat higher among older women than among younger women. The effect of cigarette smoking is substantially greater among women who have other risk factors. The decline in smoking over the last 25 years has been greater among males than females. Smoking cessation improves survival rate for both healthy women and women who have had an MI.

Obesity is a significant independent risk predictor for the development of CAD in females only. This relationship is independent of other risk factors. A masculine distribution of adipose tissue (i.e., increased waist/hip circumference) appears to increase risk of CAD in women as well as men.

A **family history of myocardial infarction** increases a woman's risk of CAD. Compared with women who have no family history of MI, women with a history of a parent who had an MI before the age of 60 have an increased risk of nonfatal and fatal MI and angina.

A **sedentary life-style** has long been thought to contribute to the risk of CAD in both males and females. There is evidence that physical activity levels decrease with age, and it has been reported that activity levels in women are lower than those in men at all age ranges. It is possible that women actually expend energy performing activities (such as work in the home) that are not typically addressed by traditional leisure physical activity questionnaires, which were developed primarily for males.

Because data on women are limited it is difficult to determine the exact impact of **psychosocial factors** on the devel-

opment of heart disease in women. There appear to be some differences from those described for men, including the fact that low socioeconomic status is associated with the development of heart disease in women. In fact, women in blue-collar occupations have over three times the rate of CAD as have women in white-collar positions. Stress is another contributing risk factor for heart disease. The multiple roles that women perform influence stress levels and indirectly influence other risk factors, such as smoking, hypertension, and obesity. CAD rates are almost twice as great among women holding clerical jobs as among women who work in the home. The predictors of CAD among clerical workers are suppressed hostility, work for a nonsupportive boss, and decreased job mobility.

Reproduction-associated risk factors

There is no association between **reproductive experiences** (i.e., parity, age at first birth) and risk of CAD. However, an association between early surgical menopause and risk for CAD is well established. Women who are postmenopausal as a result of bilateral oophorectomy have a greater risk of development of heart disease than age-matched women who have not had bilateral oophorectomy. Hysterectomy with the retention of at least one ovary is associated with little or no increase in risk of CAD, and most studies suggest no association of natural menopause with increased risk of CAD.

Studies from the 1970s and 1980s identified an increased risk of fatal and nonfatal MI for **current users of oral contraceptive pills**. This risk increases with duration of use and in the presence of other risk factors. The majority of these studies considered pills with much higher doses of estrogen and progesterone than those used in clinical practice today. More recent data indicate that the incidence of cardiovascular disease is not increased by oral contraceptive pill use in women under 30 or nonsmoking women over 30 without other cardiac risk factors. There have been multiple studies to evaluate the effect of **estrogen replacement therapy** (ERT) on risk of CAD; the majority, which are retrospective cohort or case control studies, have found a reduction in risk of CAD with ERT. The mechanism for cardiovascular protection is likely multifactorial, including alterations of serum lipid levels and direct effects on coronary arteries.

PATHOPHYSIOLOGY

The pathophysiology of CAD in women is presumed to be similar to that in men. The progression of atherosclerosis is traditionally 10 to 15 years later than it is for males; this lag is attributed to the beneficial effect of estrogen on lipid profiles. Additional positive effects of estrogen on coagulation, as well as the observation of the presence of estrogen receptors in the endothelium, suggest that other mechanisms may be at work as well. There is some clinical evidence to suggest that coronary vasospasm may be equally or more prevalent in women than in men, which accounts for the larger number of women with so-called variant angina (chest pain at rest) and with microvascular angina. The emergence of vasospasm in women as they age may be related to the declining levels of estrogen, which is known to have some vasodilatory properties. Preliminary data suggest that acute estradiol-17β administration to postmenopausal patients with CAD lowers systolic blood pressure, increases exercise time, and decreases chest pain from myocardial ischemia. This is postulated to occur through a direct vasodilatory effect, a peripheral vasodilator effect, or a combination of these mechanisms.

CLINICAL ASPECTS
Differences between males and females

There are certain anatomic, functional, and electrocardiographic characteristics that have some bearing on gender-related differences in clinical manifestations of CAD (see Table 2-1). The heart of a normal woman is smaller and lighter than that of a normal man. Although the coronary arteries are smaller in women, this is attributable to differences in heart weight. Women have a lower left ventricular end-diastolic pressure and volume, yet a higher resting ejection fraction. The ejection fraction response to exercise in healthy women is variable with less of an increase than in men. The resting electrocardiogram (ECG) reveals a PR interval and a QRS duration that are shorter in women; the R, S, and T wave amplitude in precordial leads is greater in men.

In middle age there is a higher prevalence of primary ST-T abnormalities in women than in men. The reasons for these differences are unknown, although they have been attributed to a number of factors, including change in posture, hyperventilation, hyperkinetic heart syndrome, abnormalities of left ventricular function related to mitral valve prolapse, high estrogen levels (estrogen acts as a vasodilator), and anxiety. Women with abnormal ST-T waves may have some degree of myocardial ischemia without significant CAD (so-called microvascular angina). Variant angina, produced by coronary artery spasm in the absence of fixed obstruction, is described more frequently in women. These nonspecific ST-T wave changes in women also make the interpretation of the exercise stress test result more difficult.

The literature on the correlation between clinical presentation and prevalence of CAD in women is limited. The CASS study was the first to characterize patients according to reported chest pain and then examine the prevalence of disease within these clinical subsets. The prevalences of obstructive coronary disease in women with definite angina,

probable angina, and nonspecific chest pain were significantly different (58%, 35%, and 5%, respectively) from those noted in similar subsets for males (88%, 67%, and 22%).

Clinical syndromes

Angina. In women **angina** develops twice as often as MI; in contrast, males are more likely to have acute MI as their first manifestation of CAD. It was believed initially that angina had a more favorable prognosis in women, but this probably reflects the lower prevalence of disease in women, especially in younger age groups. In women rates of angina continue upward with advancing age so that angina shifts from a predominantly male disease to a predominantly female disease after age 75 years. There appear to be some clinical differences between angina in males and females as well. Women are more likely to have anginal patterns associated with mental stress, sleep, and rest, as opposed to men, whose angina is more likely to be associated with exertion.

Women appear to experience more coronary vasospasm. There are two vasospastic entities of particular concern in women with chest pain: **variant angina** (Prinzmetal's angina) and microvascular angina (discussed later). Variant angina was first described in 1959 as an unusual syndrome of cardiac pain that occurs almost exclusively at rest and is associated with electrocardiographic ST segment elevations. It is now known to be caused by coronary artery spasm, usually of an epicardial or large septal coronary artery, resulting in myocardial ischemia in the absence of any preceding increases in myocardial oxygen demand. The reduction in arterial diameter, which can be reversed with nitroglycerin, can occur in either normal or diseased arteries and is usually focal. Patients with variant angina tend to be younger than those with chronic stable angina, and this syndrome occurs equally often in males and females. In some patients there appears to be a distinct relationship between emotional distress and episodes of coronary vasospasm, and in a few patients with variant angina this appears to be a manifestation of a generalized vasospastic disorder associated with migraine headaches, Raynaud's phenomenon, and, occasionally, aspirin-induced asthma. A large percentage of

Table 2-1 Gender differences in clinical manifestations of coronary artery disease

Manifestation	Findings in women vs. men
Electrocardiography	Higher prevalence of primary ST-T abnormalities in women
Angina	More common as first presentation of CAD Stress- and rest-related angina more common than typical exercise-induced angina Vasospasm probably more common in women
Myocardial infarction	Less likely as first presentation of CAD Silent infarction more likely Higher mortality and morbidity rates Non–Q-wave infarction more common Early reinfarction and cardiac rupture more common Higher risk for postinfarct congestive heart failure
Sudden cardiac death	Overall incidence less No increase in risk of sudden death associated with frequent or complex ventricular ectopy after acute MI

CAD, coronary artery disease; MI, myocardial infarction.

patients with variant angina are heavy smokers; this relationship supports the previous observation that cigarette smoking may influence vasomotor tone.

The diagnosis of variant angina is made in patients who demonstrate ST-segment elevations with pain. In some patients episodes of ST depressions follow episodes of ST-segment elevations and are also associated with T-wave changes. Cardiac catheterization may be helpful, and a number of provocative tests for coronary spasm have been developed. To date the ergonovine test is the most useful and sensitive, although it must be carried out in a setting where appropriate resuscitative measures are available. Other challenges include hyperventilation and administration of acetylcholine or methacholine. Nuclear scans can also be diagnostic. The drugs of choice for the treatment of variant angina are calcium channel blockers or nitrates. The natural history of variant angina is periods of frequent spasm alternating with asymptomatic periods. Long-term survival rate at 5 years is excellent (90%).

Acute myocardial infarction. Women are less likely than men to have MI as their first manifestation of CAD. They are also more likely to experience silent MI. There is limited information about gender differences in presentation with acute MI. Although equal proportions of women and men with MI have chest pain, women with acute CAD may be more likely to have gastrointestinal pain and nausea as well as more dyspnea and fatigue. Mortality and morbidity rates for acute MI are greater for women, especially African-American women. There is some disagreement about whether this excess mortality rate is a function of the older age of female patients with MI, increased comorbidity, smaller body size with smaller blood vessels, or lack of appropriate referral and treatment of women and minorities.

Women are more likely to have non–Q-wave myocardial infarction and higher postinfarction left ventricular ejection fractions after MI, but early reinfarction and cardiac rupture are also more common. The overall risk for development of postinfarct congestive heart failure is greater in women than in men, probably because of higher rates of coexisting systemic hypertension and diabetes in women with acute MI.

Sudden cardiac death. The overall incidence of sudden cardiac death among women is less than in men. However, it still accounts for 34% of CAD deaths in women. Moreover, 64% of all sudden cardiac deaths among women occur without previous CAD. The presence of frequent or complex ventricular premature beats on a Holter monitor is an independent risk factor for sudden cardiac death after acute MI in men, but not in women.

Differential diagnosis of chest pain

Differential diagnosis of chest pain is discussed in greater detail in Chapter 1. Chest pain that has a gastrointestinal cause and chest wall pain are the syndromes most commonly confused with acute cardiac ischemia in women. An additional consideration is **microvascular angina,** a diagnosis that does not constitute true angina and can only be made in a small group of patients who have had extensive cardiac testing. Patients with this entity, referred to in the past as syndrome x, have angina-like chest pain, ischemic ST-segment depressions on electrocardiography during exercise testing, angiographically normal coronary arteries without coronary artery spasm, and normal ventricular function. The

majority of patients with this constellation of findings are women, and in one large series from the National Institutes of Health, the average age was 47 years; 32% were hypertensive, 6% were diabetic, 57% had "atypical angina," 17% had "typical angina," 80% were frequently symptomatic, 11% had ischemic apparent ECG response to exercise stress, and 37% had abnormal rest ECGs. The majority of patients have attenuated coronary flow with decreased vasodilator reserve in response to metabolic and pharmacologic vasodilator stimuli; this is thought to be a consequence of dysfunction of intramyocardial periarteriolar small coronary arteries. Only a small percentage of patients have convincing evidence of myocardial ischemia based on myocardial lactate studies during stress or cardiac pacing. The infarction-free survival rate is over 90% at 10 years, but a substantial number of patients with this syndrome continue to have symptoms of chest pain.

The diagnosis of microvascular angina is usually made by some combination of exercise testing and metabolic challenge (e.g., ergonovine, dipyridamole) as well as nuclear scanning. Most patients with microvascular angina respond symptomatically to calcium channel blockers. There is preliminary evidence that this syndrome may be more likely to occur in perimenopausal or postmenopausal women, suggesting a connection with falling estrogen levels. In one small series of patients with microvascular angina who were given estrogen symptoms of chest pain disappeared with the cessation of hot flashes. Regardless of the approach taken the patient should be reassured that the absence of CAD indicates a benign prognosis with respect to mortality.

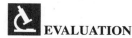 **EVALUATION**

Electrocardiographic stress testing

Over the last decade numerous studies have shown limitations in the sensitivity and specificity of electrocardiographic stress testing (EST) for the diagnosis of CAD in women as compared with men. The exercise stress test has been the most thoroughly evaluated of the noninvasive tests, but it was developed and validated, until recently, on primarily male populations. More women show exercise-induced electrocardiographic evidence of ischemia but are less likely to have significant CAD (see Table 2-2).

A summary of previous studies of EST suggests that the sensitivity is quite poor, ranging from 50% to 80% at best, and the false-positive rate (equal to 1 minus the specificity) is very high, ranging from 22% to 37% (Table 2-3). Reasons for increased false-positive results in women include a lower prevalence of CAD in women (Bayesian factors), estrogen effect (action as a vasodilator), increased pulmonary resistance, increased catecholamine release leading to increased vasospasm (microvascular angina or variant angina), decreased intramyocardial potassium levels, higher prevalence of mitral valve prolapse, and ECG changes associated with hyperventilation and anxiety. Reasons for a false-negative test result in women include the facts that women are more likely to have mild to moderate disease or single-vessel disease and are also less likely to be able to complete the full protocol (insufficient workload).

Several authors have suggested that clinicians should consider other exercise variables in addition to the presence

Table 2-2 Probability of coronary artery disease in women according to history and stress test results

History	Prevalence	Positive results		Negative results	
		EST	TST	EST	TST
Nonanginal chest pain	.05	.06	.35	.05	.02
Atypical angina	.35	.54	.85	.20	.14
Typical exertional angina	.58	.72	.93	.33	.29

Modified from Sox HC: *Post Grad Med* 743:333, 1983.
EST, exercise electrocardiographic stress testing; TST, thallium exercise electrocardiographic stress testing.

or absence of ST-segment shift in their assessment of EST results. Such factors might include duration of exercise, ability to reach target heart rate, and time required for ST-segment normalization during recovery.

Thallium stress testing

When the resting ECG is abnormal and the history suggests probable or atypical angina, thallium or other perfusion imaging improves the specificity of exercise testing in women (Table 2-2). One of the principal advantages of the exercise thallium stress test is that its validity is not affected by conditions that alter the resting ECG. As with the exercise stress test, however, a major source of false-negative results is an inadequate cardiac workload for women who are unable to exercise. The sensitivity of the thallium stress test is not quite as high in women as it is in men, but the specificity is much improved over that for the EST in women. A small percentage of false-positive results can result from attenuation of the radioactive emission by extracardiac tissues such as the breast (which produces a fixed defect in the high anteroseptal and anterolateral segments). Pharmacologic stressors in combination with nuclear testing may be useful in the evaluation of chest pain in women who are unable to exercise. The availability of new myocardial perfusion imaging agents labeled with technetium including sestamibi and teboroxime and new techniques such as single-photon emission computed tomographic (SPECT) scanning may make nuclear medicine procedures more helpful for the diagnosis of CAD in women.

The recently developed SPECT thallium imaging offers 32 images of the myocardium, as opposed to 3 projections with planar scanning. It provides better imaging of individual vessel stenosis and quantification of the extent of the abnormally perfused myocardium.

If part of the difficulty with exercise testing in women can be attributed to decreased exercise tolerance, it makes sense that studies that incorporate pharmacologic stressors (vasodilators, such as dipyridamole and adenosine) instead of exercise might be useful in the detection of coronary obstruction.

Other noninvasive studies

Exercise radionuclide ventriculography (ERV) is not routinely performed in most centers because of its cost and concern about poor test characteristics.

Cardiac fluoroscopy has been suggested as a technique that can detect the presence of coronary calcification associated with significant CAD in women. However, this diagnostic technique is no longer readily available at most institutions.

Stress echocardiography may be a sensitive technique to detect CAD in women. Exercise echocardiography, which can demonstrate the development of a new wall motion abnormality with myocardial ischemia, has been reported to have a good predictive accuracy in single-vessel CAD, a common finding in women. The advantages of exercise echocardiography are that it is easily repeatable, is noninvasive, avoids the use of a noniodinated contrast agent, and is relatively inexpensive. In addition it may provide information about the presence of other cardiac abnormalities that may cause chest pain, such as pericarditis, mitral valve prolapse, or idiopathic hypertrophic subaortic stenosis. The major disadvantage of this technique is that it requires a very experienced echocardiographer. There are concerns about the accuracy of its use and interpretation beyond university research centers.

Pharmacologic stressors have been used in combination with echocardiography. There are limited data on the accuracy of these pharmacologic stressors and their side effect profiles in males versus females. Adenosine echocardiography is more specific than dobutamine or dipyridamole echocardiography and is less likely to cause persistent

Table 2-3 Evaluation of coronary artery disease

Test	Operating characteristics in women
Electrocardiographic stress test	Women more likely to have changes suggestive of ischemia, but less likely to have significant CAD
	High rate of false-positive results (22%-37%)
	High rate of false-negative results (20%-50%), possibly related to insufficient workload or limited (single-vessel) disease
Thallium stress test	Higher specificity when resting ECG finding abnormal
Exercise echocardiography	Higher sensitivity for single-vessel disease (more common in women)
Cardiac catheterization	Higher total complication rates, arrhythmias, and hemorrhage

CAD, coronary artery disease; ECG, electrocardiogram.

symptoms. The overall sensitivity of dipyridamole echocardiography for the detection of CAD is comparable in males and females. Adverse effects are reported more in women, but they may be receiving larger relative doses of intravenous dipyridamole than men, who, in general, have greater lean body mass.

Cardiac catheterization

If gender bias occurs anywhere in the evaluation of CAD in women, it is most apparent in the lower rates of referral for invasive diagnostic testing of women for whom it is clearly indicated: those who have the combination of positive abnormal noninvasive test results, typical angina, and multiple cardiac risk factors. African-Americans, males and especially females, are also less likely to be offered coronary angiography. Data collected from large registries suggest that women undergoing angiography have more total complications, arrhythmias, and hemorrhage. There is no difference in the incidence of death, MI, stroke, vascular complications, or contrast reactions between males and females.

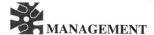 MANAGEMENT

Medical therapy

Medical treatment for women consists mainly of use of medications that have been previously shown to be effective in male populations (see Table 2-4). There is some evidence that nitrates are not as effective in women as in men with chronic stable angina in reducing the frequency or intensity of anginal symptoms. Women tend to have more symptoms of depression and fatigue with the routine use of beta blockers, and this medication is less than optimal in patients with diabetes (the majority of whom are women). Because of the potential for coexistent vasospasm, calcium channel blockers may be the preferred medical therapy for angina in women.

Thrombolytic therapy

Although thrombolytic therapy for acute myocardial infarction has been shown to have benefit in terms of survival among women, it is less than the benefit shown for men, and there are more frequent serious bleeding complications in women. Women are less likely than men to be eligible for this therapy, however, because of later presentation after the onset of symptoms of MI, as well as increased likelihood of having significant comorbid conditions (e.g., hypertension) and more advanced age. Most studies show a lower reduction in mortality rates in women than in men with thrombolysis. Reasons for the lower reduction in mortality rate in women include age, reduced myocardial salvage, resulting in less preservation of myocardial function, and more frequent cardiac events after thrombolysis. If spasm were playing a role, perhaps in younger women, thrombolysis might be less effective. The potential importance of weight, age, and gender-based dosage modification of thrombolytic agents has not been addressed by thrombolysis trials to date; this may explain some of the increased risk of bleeding. It has been suggested that a smaller percentage of eligible women than men actually receive thrombolytic therapy, and this outcome is not always a function of increased age or morbidity.

Percutaneous transluminal coronary angioplasty and other interventional devices

There is over 10 years of experience with percutaneous transluminal coronary angioplasty (PTCA) in women. Accumulated data suggest that despite the fact that men have more advanced disease indicated by angiography, women have lower clinical and angiographic success rates and higher in-hospital mortality rates. Thus female gender has been an independent predictor of reduced success with angioplasty. Initial use of a 3-mm PTCA balloon in the early 1980s was suggested as a factor in the increased morbidity and mortality rates in females. Women have had a higher incidence of intimal tears and coronary dissections. However, analysis of data using improved angioplasty techniques suggests that female gender remains a strong correlate of hospital mortality. Women may also be at a higher risk of complications because of their older age and greater degree of comorbidity. However, although acute clinical and angio-

Table 2-4 Gender differences in treatments for coronary artery disease

Treatment	Differences in women and men
Medical therapy	Limited data on effectiveness in women Nitrates somewhat less effective in chronic stable angina
Thrombolytic therapy	Less reduction in mortality rates in women Higher rates of serious bleeding complications
Percutaneous transluminal coronary angioplasty	Lower clinical and angiographic success rates Better long-term outcome, lower restenosis rates
Coronary atherectomy	Higher acute complication rates (perforation, transfusion, Q-wave MI, death) Similar restenosis rates
Coronary artery bypass grafting	Higher perioperative mortality rates Less relief of angina Less graft patency Similar 5-year to 10-year survival rates

MI, myocardial infarction.

graphic success rates appear worse in women, long-term outcome is actually better and restenosis rates are lower in women.

Data on coronary atherectomy suggest that women again have higher acute complication rates than men, but gender does not influence restenosis rates after intracoronary stenting and directional atherectomy. Procedural success of directional coronary atherectomy is significantly lower in women than it is in men. This is due to inability to engage the ostium with the guiding catheter and inability to cross the lesion with the device. Smaller vessel size in older women may be a contributing factor. Major ischemic complications are no different in men and women. Women have a significantly increased risk of angiographic and clinical complications following new device intervention, including perforation, transfusion, Q-wave MI, and death. This increased risk cannot be explained by differences in age, severity of coronary disease, reference artery diameter, lesion morphologic characteristics, or differences in stenosis reduction.

The long-term prognosis after PTCA is similar among men and women, except that more women report recurrence of angina. Among patients with severe angina men are more likely to go on to coronary artery bypass surgery. In summary, the precise reason for women's increased morbidity rate at the time of angioplasty requires further study, but favorable long-term outcome suggests that percutaneous interventions may be an excellent therapeutic option in women.

Coronary artery bypass surgery

There is some controversy about whether women with significant CAD have been less likely to be offered coronary artery bypass grafting (CABG) when indicated. Women who undergo CABG generally have more advanced disease with significant ischemia and left ventricular dysfunction. They require more emergency surgery and are referred at a later, more advanced stage of their disease process, so it is not surprising that mortality rate after bypass surgery is roughly twice that of men. Some of the gender difference in mortality rate has been attributed to differences in body size, with smaller blood vessels and thus a reduced opportunity to obtain complete revascularization. Women referred for CABG are also more likely to have diabetes, hypertension, and congestive heart failure and are less likely to have had an MI. Attempts to adjust for preoperative angina severity, number of diseased blood vessels, and body surface area have partially reduced the effect of gender on outcome.

Most of the original studies on CABG in women were made at a time when state-of-the-art care did not include use of such practices as internal mammary artery grafting, advanced cardioplegic techniques, routine antiplatelet therapy, and aggressive lipid-lowering therapy after surgery. Both internal mammary grafts and antiplatelet therapy, in particular, have been shown to be effective in women as well as in men. In the majority of studies men have found greater relief of angina after CABG than women and have shown better graft patency, but there are no apparent differences in 5- to 10-year survival rates between the sexes after successful CABG.

Psychosocial issues need to be assessed in recovery after coronary artery bypass surgery as with recovery after acute MI (see later discussion). Women are more likely to suffer from depression than men after bypass surgery and less likely to be referred to cardiac rehabilitation programs.

Diagnosis and treatment of acute myocardial infarction

Most drugs used in the treatment of acute MI appear to be equally effective in males and females. Information about sex differences in medical therapies after MI is limited because the majority of the clinical trials for patients with acute MI have excluded women, especially in the last 10 years, primarily because of restrictions of patients in the trials to age 75 or less. The literature suggests that aspirin and β-blockers have comparable effect in the prevention of reinfarction after MI, although women may be less likely to receive them. The efficacy and potential side effects of nitrates, β-blockers, and calcium channel blockers have all been studied predominantly in men. Inasmuch as coronary vasospasm may be relatively more important in females, nitrates and calcium channel blockers may be the preferred therapy in women with angina. Raynaud's phenomenon is also more common in women; thus nonselective β-blocking drugs may not provide ideal therapy in this population. In addition many women with CAD also have diabetes, which makes use of β-blockers less desirable. Women are also more likely to experience side effects with β-blockers.

Modification of risk factors in women with coronary artery disease

Current data indicate that a large proportion of MIs in women under the age of 50 (more than 60%) can be attributed to cigarette smoking. Women who stop smoking after nonfatal MI have a better long-term survival rate than those who continue to smoke. Thus smoking cessation remains the cornerstone for prevention of recurrent coronary events in women (see Chapter 73).

The incidence of hypertension in women with CAD is increased; this makes effective treatment a high priority. Control of hypertension, even mild hypertension, appears to improve survival rate in women after MI. Because of the synergistic effect of multiple coronary risk factors, hypertension control in combination with multiple risk factor modification will reduce the incidence and morbidity rate of CAD in women.

As noted previously, diabetes tends to eliminate any gender advantages women have in the development of CAD morbidity and mortality. Recently intensive therapy with insulin for type I diabetics has been shown to be effective in reducing the development of hypercholesterolemia with a trend toward decreasing cardiovascular events for women as well as men. Additional data regarding the effect of tight control in patients with type II diabetes on subsequent risk of cardiovascular disease are awaited.

Although strong prospective evidence for effective reduction in cardiovascular mortality rate by normalization of blood lipids is still lacking in women, recent studies favor this position. Clearly, increasing the HDL level in women is an important consideration. Routine exercise at moderate levels does not appear to achieve this uniformly. Nonetheless, diet and exercise remain the first line of therapy, followed by medication (see Chapter 3).

The role of alcohol in the improvement of lipid profiles in women is somewhat controversial. As compared to non-drinkers, women who consume moderate amounts of alcohol (three to nine drinks per week) have been shown to have a decreased relative risk of CAD; this finding is consistent with those of previous studies in men. An elevation of HDL level with alcohol is the best documented mechanism for the positive effect of decreasing risk of heart disease. This potential beneficial effect of drinking on lipids needs to be weighed against the risk for alcohol-related morbidity, including hypertension, alcohol dependence with end-organ damage, and possible increase in breast cancer risk, which begins to increase significantly in women with only two or more drinks per day.

The importance of obesity in the development of CAD and other risk factors for CAD in women is well known. Nonetheless, recent evidence has shown that repeated cycles of weight loss and gain may be more detrimental than maintenance of a slightly higher weight (see Chapter 71).

Women who have known CAD (or who are considered to be at high risk for the development of CAD) also constitute one of the few subpopulations of women for whom there is relatively little controversy about the use of hormone replacement therapy. Unless otherwise contraindicated, women with a uterus should be treated with estrogen and progesterone and those without a uterus with estrogen alone (see Chapter 36). There is some evidence from observational studies that use of aspirin in women ages 35 to 59 years is associated with a reduced incidence of MI.

After myocardial infarction

Women are more likely to suffer from psychologic symptoms, particularly anxiety and depression, after MI. This likelihood may be related to a variety of factors, including increased morbidity and disability after an MI. Physical symptoms, primarily cardiac, are reported more often by female patients after MI and may limit activity. Women report longer recovery time and more days lost because of cardiac symptoms than men. Women return to paid employment less often than men after an MI, although return to work is not necessarily a reflection of disease or a suitable measure of recovery in women, many of whom work in the home. Domestic responsibilities are a source of concern for recovery in women, who may return to high-demand activities in the home sooner than is advisable. Women report having more fears about resumption of sexual activities. Finally, women are referred less often to cardiac rehabilitation programs, enroll less frequently, and have poorer attendance than men. Some cardiac rehabilitation programs are now being developed with special attention to the exercise abilities and psychosocial needs of older women.

SUMMARY

Although significant CAD is rare in young women, it becomes a substantial problem for women as they age, accounting for substantial morbidity and mortality. Limited research on CAD in women has meant that much of the current diagnosis and treatment information is extrapolated from male populations. A review of the existing information about the care of women with active CAD suggests that sex-specific guidelines to evaluate cost-effective diagnosis, appropriate medical care, and the role of medical versus surgical treatment should be developed.

BIBLIOGRAPHY

Becker RC et al: Comparison of clinical outcomes for women and men after acute myocardial infarction, *Ann Intern Med* 120:638, 1994.

Bell MR, Holmes DR, Berger PB: The changing in-hospital mortality of women undergoing percutaneous transluminal coronary angioplasty, *JAMA* 269:2091, 1993.

Cannon RO: Microvascular angina: cardiovascular investigations regarding pathophysiology and management, *Med Clin North Am* 75(5):1097, 1991.

Diamond GA, Forrester JS: Analysis of probability as an aid in the clinical diagnosis of coronary artery disease, *N Engl J Med* 300:1350, 1979.

Douglas PS, editor, Brest AN, editor-in-chief: Cardiovascular Clinics, *Heart Disease in Women,* Philadelphia, 1989, FA Davis.

Eaker ED: Psychosocial factors in the epidemiology of coronary heart disease in women, *Psychiatr Clin North Am* 12(1):167, 1989.

Eaker ED et al, editors: *Coronary Heart Disease in Women,* New York 1987, Haymarket Doyma.

Eysmann SB, Douglas PS: Reperfusion and revascularization strategies for coronary artery disease in women, *JAMA* 268:1903, 1992.

Grady D et al: Hormone therapy to prevent disease and prolong life in post-menopausal women, *Ann Intern Med* 117:1016, 1992.

Graff Low K: Recovery from myocardial infarction and coronary artery bypass surgery in women: psychosocial factors, *J Women Health,* 2(2):133, 139, 1993.

Khan SS et al: Increased mortality of women in coronary artery bypass surgery: evidence for referral bias, *Ann Intern Med* 112:561, 1990.

King KB, Clark PC, Hicks GL: Patterns of referral and recovery in women and men undergoing coronary artery bypass grafting, *Am J Cardiol* 69:179, 1992.

Kuhn FE, Rackley CE: Coronary artery disease in women, *Arch Intern Med* 153:2626, 1993.

Maynard C et al: Gender differences in the treatment and outcome of acute myocardial infarction, *Arch Intern Med* 152:972, 1992.

Nwasokwa ON et al: Bypass surgery for chronic stable angina: predictors of survival benefit and strategy for patient selection, *Ann Intern Med* 114:1035, 1991.

Sarrell PM et al: Angina and normal coronary arteries in women: gynecologic findings, *Am J Obstet Gynecol* 67:467, 1992.

Shaw LJ et al: Gender differences in the noninvasive evaluation and management of patients with suspected coronary artery disease, *Ann Intern Med* 120:559, 1994.

Sox HC: Noninvasive testing in coronary artery disease, *Post Grad Med* 74:333, 1983.

Wenger NK, Speroff, Packard B: Cardiovascular health and disease in women, *N Engl J Med* 329:247, 1993.

3 Hyperlipidemia

Paula A. Johnson

Although an elevated cholesterol level is a risk factor for development of coronary heart disease, the degree of elevation that requires medical intervention, the age at which intervention is beneficial, and the population that should be screened for the abnormality continue to be studied and debated. Criteria for the evaluation and treatment of hyperlipidemia have resulted mainly from studies performed in men, such as the Lipid Research Clinics Coronary Primary Prevention Trial, the Helsinki Heart Study, and the Multiple Risk Factor Intervention Trial. It is not yet clear whether these criteria are appropriate for women, especially as women's lipid metabolism is influenced by the presence of estrogen. As the medical community begins to focus attention on women, questions regarding the evaluation and treatment of hyperlipidemia have revealed an important area requiring review of currently available data and identification of additional areas for study.

This chapter will address the following topics: the epidemiologic evidence relating cholesterol and lipoproteins to the development of coronary heart disease, screening and management of hyperlipidemia, the role of postmenopausal estrogen replacement in the hyperlipidemic patient, and the influence of oral contraceptive agents and the recently approved progesterone agents on the lipid profile. A discussion of inherited forms of hyperlipidemias is beyond the scope of this chapter.

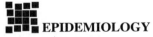

EPIDEMIOLOGY

Relationship of lipids to coronary heart disease

The Framingham Study proved the important relationship between increased total cholesterol level and increased risk of coronary heart disease (CHD). Over time it has become known that low-density lipoprotein (LDL) is the most atherogenic fraction of cholesterol. Oxidized LDL is considered significantly more atherogenic than its unoxidized precursor. This discovery has led to the investigation of antioxidants, such as vitamin E, as agents that may be useful in primary and secondary prevention of CHD. The inverse relationship between postmenopausal estrogen replacement and levels of LDL may constitute part of the basis for the finding of less CHD in women receiving post-menopausal estrogen replacement. Finally, although the positive relationship between elevated levels of LDL and the development of and mortality attributable to CHD appears to be similar in men and women, elevated LDL levels are not predictive of total cardiovascular mortality or all-cause mortality in women.

High-density lipoprotein (HDL), on the other hand, is protective against CHD. Apoprotein AI is the major component of HDL and is thought to act primarily as a transport molecule, removing cholesterol from tissue and delivering it to the liver. Data from the Framingham Study and the Lipid Research Clinics Follow-Up Study suggest that the level of HDL may be a particularly important risk factor for women and may be more predictive of the development of CHD than the level of LDL. In addition to decreasing LDL level, postmenopausal estrogen replacement may protect women against the development of CHD by producing an increase in HDL. There is a lack of specific data from clinical trials linking interventions leading to an increased level of HDL and decreased mortality and morbidity rates from CHD.

The role of triglycerides in the development of CHD has not been fully defined. Data from several prospective studies, including the Framingham Study, identify elevated triglyceride levels as a univariate predictor for the development of CHD. This association does not persist once additional risk factors, LDL, and HDL are included in multivariate models. A combined high triglyceride level and low HDL level may be a more important risk factor for the development of CHD.

A recent study examined lipid levels as predictors of cardiovascular death in white women based on a 14-year follow-up of the Lipid Research Clinics Study (Bass, 1993). In women ages 50 to 69 HDL was an independent predictor of risk of cardiovascular disease (CVD) death. LDL was a poor predictor of CVD mortality.

Lipoprotein (a) (Lp[a]), a molecule with structural similarities to LDL and plasminogen, is associated with the development of atherosclerotic vascular disease. It is thought that the majority of the population has low Lp(a) levels (less than 0.2 g/L) and only a small proportion has high (greater than 1.0 g/L) levels that are associated with atherosclerotic disease. The presence of estrogen may lower Lp(a) levels, given that postmenopausal women have been found to have significantly higher levels than premenopausal women. Women receiving postmenopausal estrogen replacement also have lower levels of Lp(a) than women not receiving hormone replacement. At present there is no standardized assay for the measurement of this protein.

SCREENING

Cholesterol levels increase with age until one reaches the age group of 54 through 74 years, during which time the total cholesterol levels tend to decline. This trend holds true for women, although there is a delay of several years before the decrease is observed. In addition, levels of total cholesterol continue to decrease for the elderly population above 75 years of age. Men tend to have higher cholesterol levels than women until middle age (45 to 55 years of age), which coincides with menopause and the decline of endogenous estrogen levels in women.

From 1960 through 1991 there was a significant decline in mean total cholesterol levels in the U.S. population. This decline is primarily attributed to reduction in LDL levels. The U.S. population's mean total cholesterol level decreased from 220 mg/dl in 1960 to 1962 to 206 mg/dl in 1988 to

1991. Data from the National Health and Nutrition Examination Survey also show that the percentage of the population with total cholesterol levels greater than 240 mg/dl decreased from 26% in 1976 through 1980 to 20% for 1988 through 1991. This decrease in total cholesterol levels was similar for men and women. Although there has been a significant decrease in the proportion of the population with elevated cholesterol levels, a large number of people still require dietary and pharmacologic intervention.

The revised guidelines of the U.S. National Cholesterol Education Program (NCEP) Expert Panel on Detection, Evaluation, and Treatment of High Blood Cholesterol in Adults recommend that *all adults 20 years of age and above undergo screening at least once every 5 years.* The screening should include measurement of total cholesterol and HDL levels and may be performed in a nonfasting state. For patients with known CHD it is recommended that a lipoprotein analysis, including measurement of LDL levels, be performed after fasting for 9 to 12 hours, with two measurements performed from 1 to 8 weeks apart. There are no specific recommendations regarding screening for hypertriglyceridemia. Triglyceride levels may increase in women who receive oral contraceptives or postmenopausal estrogen replacement, given that exogenous estrogen can lead to elevation in triglyceride levels.

These recommendations have not been without controversy in their application to specific populations, such as the elderly. Whether there is a difference in the strength of the correlation between elevation in cholesterol levels and development or rate of progression of CHD in the elderly is also controversial. Analyses of the projected cost of screening the asymptomatic elderly predict that the cost will be high and benefits unclear if this population receives lipid-lowering agents. Although these issues regarding the elderly are important, until further data prove otherwise, there are no findings to suggest that the current guidelines on screening should not be followed.

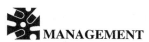

MANAGEMENT

Hypercholesterolemia

Goals of therapy. Once the initial screening for hyperlipidemia is performed, intervention should be based on the patient's level of risk for coronary artery disease. The NCEP recommends that patients be stratified into three risk groups: patients without known CHD who are at low risk because of the absence of additional risk factors (includes premenopausal women and men below the age of 35 years), patients without known CHD who are at high risk for its development as a result of the presence of additional risk factors, and the patients with known CHD or other atherosclerotic vascular disease (Fig. 3-1). Intervention in a patient without known CHD is considered primary prevention, and intervention in patients with known disease is considered secondary prevention.

There is good evidence that lowering elevated levels of serum cholesterol can lead to a decrease in morbidity and mortality rates from CHD. Several prospective studies that included women, such as the Framingham Heart Study, the Lipid Research Clinics Program Follow-Up Study, and the Rancho Bernardo Study, support that women benefit from lowering elevated levels of cholesterol with a decrease in morbidity and mortality rates from CHD. The effect of lowering cholesterol on overall mortality rate is less clear. Data from the Cardiovascular Health Study show that low levels of total cholesterol (≤160 mg/dl) have been associated with an increase in the rate of cancer diagnosed in the preceding 5 years in women. These data, combined with evidence suggesting that LDL may not be as strong a risk factor for CHD and that HDL may have a particularly strong protective effect in women compared with men, raise the question of whether treatment guidelines for hyperlipidemia should be the same for both genders. Although the NCEP guidelines may require modification for use in women, to date data are insufficient to recommend deviation from these guidelines in the treatment of hyperlipidemia in women.

For patients without known CHD risk stratification is based on total cholesterol and HDL levels. A total cholesterol of <200 mg/dl is considered a desirable blood cholesterol level. A total cholesterol level of 200 to 239 mg/dl is considered borderline-high and ≥240 mg/dl is considered a high blood cholesterol level. An HDL level of <35 mg/dl is considered a risk factor for CHD. It is suggested that patients with low levels of HDL or high blood cholesterol levels have a lipoprotein analysis performed in the fasting state to quantify the level of LDL (Fig. 3-1). Levels of LDL for patients without CHD are stratified as follows: desirable (<130 mg/dl), borderline high-risk (130 to 159 mg/dl, with or without two or more risk factors), and high-risk (≥160 mg/dl). Dietary therapy is recommended for patients in the borderline high-risk category with two or more risk factors for CHD and for those in the high-risk category (Fig. 3-2).

For patients in whom secondary prevention is undertaken, intervention is based on LDL cholesterol level. An optimal level of LDL cholesterol is ≤100 mg/dl. Dietary therapy has been suggested for patients with LDL of >100 mg/dl and <130 mg/dl, with drug therapy suggested in those with LDL of ≥130 mg/dl (Fig. 3-3). Recommendations for intervention are summarized in Table 3-1.

Other causes of lipid abnormalities, such as hypothyroidism, chronic renal failure, and nephrotic syndrome, should be considered. Lipid abnormalities resulting from these conditions are considered secondary dyslipidemias. Whereas initial treatment should be focused on the underlying abnormality, persisting lipid abnormalities should be managed according to NCEP guidelines.

Premenopausal women lose the protective effect of their premenopausal status if they have diabetes mellitus. The NCEP recommends that all patients with diabetes mellitus be screened and treated according to the guidelines developed for patients with established CHD.

Although HDL level may be a particularly important factor in the protection against CHD in women, it is not clear what steps should be followed in the case of patients with low levels of HDL and satisfactory levels of LDL. There are no good data to suggest that intervention in this population, beyond dietary and life-style changes, is beneficial. This is the case for both primary and secondary prevention.

Types of therapy

Dietary intervention. Change in diet is probably the fundamental method of lowering cholesterol level. Although

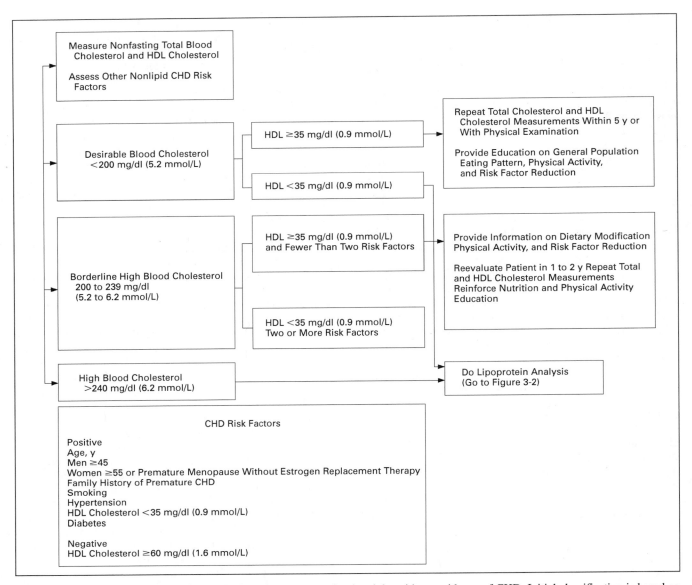

Fig. 3-1 Recommendation of the U.S. NCEP for primary prevention in adults without evidence of CHD. Initial classification is based on total cholesterol and HDL levels. CHD, coronary heart disease; HDL, high-density lipoprotein. (From *JAMA* 269:3018, 1993.)

improved over the past 20 years, the average American diet leaves room for significant refinement with regard to fat intake. For example, an average daily U.S. diet derives 37% of its caloric content from fat and 14% from saturated fat and contains 450 mg of cholesterol. Dietary cholesterol and saturated fats result in an increase in LDL level by suppressing hepatic LDL receptor activity and resulting in decreased clearance.

Diet therapy is prescribed in two steps. A Step I diet, as defined by the NCEP, includes 8% to 10% of calories from saturated fat with ≤30% of calories from fat and <300 mg of cholesterol per day. A Step II diet consists of <7% of calories from saturated fat and <200 mg of cholesterol per day. It is suggested that a 6-month trial of intensive dietary therapy, with nutritional consultation, be undertaken to achieve the desired LDL level (Table 3-1). If dietary thera-

py is not successful after this period, drug therapy should be considered. Expected rates of success in dietary intervention are not well defined.

Weight reduction, in overweight patients with abnormal lipid profiles, is an essential element of the dietary intervention. In addition to lowering LDL levels, weight reduction leads to a decrease in triglyceride level and blood pressure. Data from the Second National Health and Nutrition Examination Survey (NHANES II) show that 27% of nonpregnant women, ages 20 to 74, are overweight, compared with 24% of men.

Interestingly the distribution of the overweight population differs for men and women, with the peak prevalence in men occurring from ages 45 to 54 years (31%). The prevalence in women continues to increase through later life, peaking at ages 65 through 74 years (39%). Because of the age distrib-

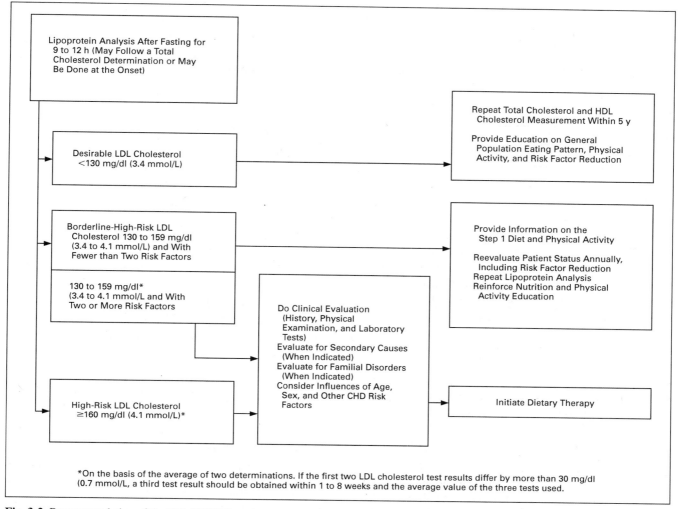

Fig. 3-2 Recommendation of the U.S. NCEP for primary prevention in adults without evidence of CHD. Subsequent classification is based on LDL cholesterol level. CHD, coronary heart disease; LDL, low-density lipoprotein. (From *JAMA* 269:3019, 1993.)

ution of overweight persons, the older female population may be more sedentary and less inclined or able to engage in regular physical exercise. It has been shown that a combination of dietary change, behavior modification, and physical exercise is the most successful strategy for achieving and maintaining weight loss. Assisting patients in achieving and maintaining weight loss is important, given that weight fluctuations (i.e., yo-yo dieting) may be an independent risk factor for mortality attributable to CHD.

A combination of weight reduction and physical exercise has been shown to lead to an improvement in the lipid profile with a decrease in LDL level, an increase in HDL level, and a decrease in triglyceride levels. Interestingly, calorie- and fat-restricted diets (NCEP Step I) and exercise may have differing effects on HDL level in women and men. Women may experience a lowering of HDL level with diet intervention alone. The addition of exercise may counter this decrease and result in an unchanged level of HDL. A combination of diet and exercise results in significant lowering of LDL levels. Once again the impact of these findings on

mortality and morbidity from coronary artery disease and on treatment recommendations warrants further investigation.

Initiating drug therapy

GOALS OF MANAGEMENT. The optimal levels of LDL, as defined by the NCEP, for patients who are treated with drug therapy are listed in Table 3-1. Given that low levels of HDL may be an important risk factor in women, it may be worthwhile to choose drug therapy aimed at both reducing LDL level and increasing HDL level.

Drug therapy as primary prevention in premenopausal women without additional risk factors for CHD should be delayed. These criteria do not apply to patients with familial hypercholesterolemia who are at high risk for the development of premature CHD.

CHOICE OF THERAPY. Cholesterol-lowering drugs can be divided into five main groups: bile acid sequestrants, nicotinic acid (niacin), 3-Hydroxy–3-methylglutaryl coenzyme A (HMG CoA) reductase inhibitors, fibric acid derivatives, and probucol. In addition, antioxidants, such as vitamin E, may prove to be beneficial in the primary and secondary pre-

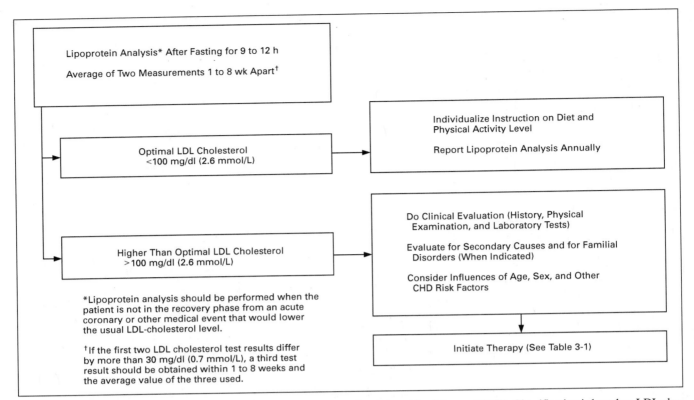

Fig. 3-3 Recommendation of the U.S. NCEP for secondary prevention in adults with evidence of CHD. Classification is based on LDL cholesterol level. CHD, coronary heart disease; LDL, low-density lipoprotein. (From *JAMA* 269:3020, 1993.)

vention of CHD. Although a detailed discussion of the mechanisms of cholesterol-lowering drugs is beyond the scope of this chapter, a brief description of the effects and side effects of the major drug classes can be found in Table 3-2.

Bile acid sequestrants and **HMG CoA reductase inhibitors** lower LDL level and slightly raise HDL level. Results of the Expanded Clinical Evaluation of Lovastatin (EXEL) Study, a multicenter, double-blind study, indicate that treatment with lovastatin led to a 24% to 40% reduction in LDL levels, a 9% to 18% decrease in triglyceride level, and a 7% to 9% increase in HDL level in 3390 women. There was no difference in effect of the drug in women receiving exogenous estrogen therapy. Whether these women were also receiving combination hormonal replacement therapy with estrogen and a progestational agent was not addressed.

Nicotinic acid (niacin) lowers LDL and triglyceride levels in addition to increasing levels of HDL. An aspirin taken a half hour before the dose and dosing with meals may decrease cutaneous flushing and increase tolerability of the drug.

The **fibric acid derivatives,** such as gemfibrizol, have their main effect on lowering triglyceride level. These agents also lead to a modest decrease in LDL and a modest increase in HDL. They are mainly used as a treatment for familial combined hyperlipidemia and hypertriglyceridemia.

MONITORING THERAPY. The NCEP guidelines recommend that the lipid profile be checked at 4 to 6 weeks and at 3 months with follow-up testing at least every 4 months.

Hypertriglyceridemia

Goals of therapy. The role that triglycerides play in atherogenesis is still unclear. Fasting triglyceride levels are stratified into four categories: normal (less than 200 mg/dl), borderline-high (200 to 400 mg/dl), high (400 to 1000 mg/dl), and very high (greater than 1000 mg/dl). Patients with very high levels of fasting triglycerides have a significant risk of pancreatitis and should be treated. Drug treatment should be aimed at lowering both triglyceride and LDL levels for patients with known elevation in LDL level and very high triglyceride level. Agents such as niacin or gemfibrizol are usually recommended. It is less clear how to treat patients with a borderline-high or high triglyceride level, a low HDL level, and a normal LDL level. It is suggested that patients undertake nonpharmacologic therapy, including weight reduction in the overweight, increased physical activity, and decreased alcohol intake.

POSTMENOPAUSAL HORMONE REPLACEMENT

Postmenopausal estrogen replacement is thought to decrease a woman's risk of morbidity and mortality from CHD. One mechanism through which estrogen replacement may provide protection is its beneficial effect on the lipid profile: a decrease in LDL level by 10% to 15% and an increase in HDL level by 10% to 15%. A first-pass effect through the liver is required for the effect on lipids. Therefore, it is necessary that oral estrogen be used to achieve these benefits. Oral estrogen may also lead to a mild increase in triglyceride level. This effect may be problemat-

Table 3-1 Recommended treatments of U.S. NCEP based on LDL cholesterol level

Patient category	Initiation level	LDL goal
Dietary therapy		
Without CHD and with fewer than two risk factors	≥160 mg/dl (4.1 mmol/L)	<160 mg/dl (4.1 mmol/L)
Without CHD and with two or more risk factors	≥130 mg/dl (3.4 mmol/L)	<130 mg/dl (3.4 mmol/L)
With CHD	>100 mg/dl (2.6 mmol/L)	≤100 mg/dl (2.6 mmol/L)
Drug treatment		
Without CHD and with fewer than two risk factors	≥190 mg/dl (4.9 mmol/L)	<160 mg/dl (4.1 mmol/L)
Without CHD and with two or more risk factors	≥160 mg/dl (4.1 mmol/L)	<130 mg/dl (3.4 mmol/L)
With CHD	≥130 mg/dl (3.4 mmol/L)	≤100 mg/dl (2.6 mmol/L)

From Expert Panel on Detection, Evaluation, and Treatment of High Blood Cholesterol in Adults: *JAMA* 269:3020, 1993.
LDL, low-density lipoprotein; CHD, coronary heart disease.

ic if the patient is hypertriglyceridemic before initiation of therapy. It may be beneficial to know a patient's triglyceride level before initiating estrogen therapy, although there are no published guidelines addressing this issue. Post-menopausal estrogen therapy may also improve the lipid profile by resulting in a decreased level of Lp(a). Therefore, in postmenopausal women with abnormal lipid profiles, hormone replacement therapy should be considered according to the recently published guidelines of the American College of Physicians.

The effect on the lipid profile and long-term outcomes in women receiving combination hormonal replacement therapy with estrogen and progesterone has not been well studied. Progesterone has an antagonistic effect on the lipid pro-file compared with estrogen, leading to an increase in LDL level and a decrease in HDL level. Cross-sectional data suggest that the addition of progesterone does not impact significantly on the beneficial effects of estrogen on the lipid profile. In fact women receiving combination therapy may have lower levels of triglycerides than those taking estrogen alone. Large-scale randomized trials to determine the risks and benefits associated with long-term hormone replacement therapy are under way with the institution of the NIH-sponsored Women's Health Initiative.

HORMONAL CONTRACEPTION

Oral contraceptive agents provide an easy and highly effective form of birth control. The widespread use of these

Table 3-2 Lipid-lowering drugs

Drug	Dose	Effects	Side effects	Indication
Bile acid sequestrants (cholestyramine and colestipol)	16-32 g/day for cholestyramine and 10 g twice daily for colestipol	Lowers LDL level, slightly increases HDL level, and reduces risk of CHD	Constipation, abdominal pain, nausea, bloating, and drug interactions	High LDL level
3-Hydroxy-3-methylglutaryl coenzyme A reductase inhibitors (lovastatin, pravastatin)	20-80 mg twice daily for lovasatin	Lowers LDL level, slightly increases HDL level	Hepatitis, myositis, and teratogenicity	High LDL level
Nicotinic acid (niacin)	0.5-2 g three times daily	Lowers LDL level, lowers TG level, raises HDL level, and reduces risk of CHD	Hepatitis, gout, hyperglycemia, ulcerogenesis, acanthosis nigricans, icthyosis, atrial arrhythmias, and insomnia	High LDL level, high TG level, and low HDL level
Fibric acid derivatives (clofibrate, gemfibrozil, and fenofibrate)	600 mg twice daily for gemfibrozil and 1 g twice daily for clofibrate	Lowers TG level, raises HDL level, and may raise or lower LDL level	Cholelithiasis, hepatitis, high LDL level, decreased libido, myositis, ventricular arrythmia, increased appetite abdominal pain, and nausea	Low HDL level, high TG level, and high LDL level
Probucol	500 mg twice daily	Lowers both LDL and HDL levels, potent antioxidant	Prolonged QT, low HDL level, diarrhea, bloating, nausea, and abdominal pain	Homozygous familial hypercholesterolemia

Modified from Blum CB and Levy RI: *JAMA* 261:3585, 1989.
LDL, low-density lipoprotein; HDL, high-density lipoprotein; CHD, coronary heart disease; TG, triglyceride.

agents has raised questions regarding their impact on patients' risk for CHD. Most oral contraceptive agents contain a combination of synthetic estrogen and progesterone. The progesterone is usually one of the several available C-19 steroids that are thought to be more androgenic than the progesterone used in hormone replacement therapy. Over the past 20 years the dose of estrogen and progesterone contained in these preparations has decreased. Different types of progestins impact patients' lipid profiles differently. For example monophasic desogestrel and low-dose norethindrone, in combination with low-dose estrogen, may have the least negative impact on HDL and LDL levels. Overall, studies of lipid profiles of women taking oral contraceptives have shown that there is little impact on the lipid profile, except in elevations in triglyceride levels. Therefore underlying hypertriglyceridemia may be exacerbated by oral contraceptive agents. If a patient has a strong family history of hyperlipidemia, it may be worthwhile to screen for hypertriglyceridemia before initiating use of an oral contraceptive agent.

There is no evidence that oral contraceptives accelerate the rate of development of atherosclerotic vascular disease. Data from the Nurse's Health Study showed no association between past oral contraceptive use and development of coronary artery disease.

Long-acting progestational agents have only recently been approved for use in the United States. These agents include subcutaneous implant of levonorgestrel (Norplant) and injectable medroxyprogesterone acetate (Depo-Provera). Their impact on patients' lipid profile has not been well described. Currently there are no guidelines for prescribing progestational agents in patients with preexisting lipid abnormalities.

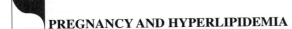

PREGNANCY AND HYPERLIPIDEMIA

Total triglyceride and cholesterol levels (including all subfractions) increase during pregnancy. Hormonal changes, such as the rise of estrogen and progesterone levels during pregnancy and the relative insulin resistance that develops in the later half of pregnancy, may be factors in the observed lipid changes. Elevated cholesterol and triglyceride levels persist during pregnancy and can remain high up to 1 year after delivery. The LDL subfraction drops at 8 weeks gestation but then continues to rise and remain elevated until 8 weeks post partum with or without breast-feeding. The HDL subfraction rises until midgestation and then levels off or declines through the remainder of the pregnancy. Therefore measurement of a women's lipid profile should be delayed until at least 6 months post partum. The effect of these lipid changes during pregnancy on development of atherosclerosis remains unclear.

BIBLIOGRAPHY

American College of Physicians: Guidelines for counseling postmenopausal women about preventive hormone therapy, *Ann Intern Med* 117:1038, 1992.

Baird DT, Glasier AF: Hormonal contraception, *N Engl J Med* 328:1543, 1993.

Barrett-Connor E, Wingard DL, Criqui MH: Postmenopausal estrogen use and heart disease risk factors in the 1980's: Rancho Bernardo, California, revisited, *JAMA* 261:1095, 1989.

Bass KM et al: Plasma lipoprotein levels as predictors of cardiovascular death in women, *Arch Intern Med* 153:2209, 1993.

Blair SN: Evidence for success of exercise in weight loss and control, *Ann Intern Med* 119 (7, pt 2):702, 1993.

Blum CB, Levy RI: Current therapy for hypercholesterolemia, *JAMA* 261:3582, 1989.

Bradford RH, Downtown M, Chremos AN: Efficacy and tolerability of Lovistatin in 3390 women with moderate hypercholesterolemia, *Ann Intern Med* 118:850, 1993.

Braunwald E: *Heart disease: a textbook of cardiovascular medicine,* ed 4, Philadelphia, 1992, WB Saunders.

Bush TL, Fried LP, Barrett-Connor E: Cholesterol, lipoproteins, and coronary heart disease in women, *Clin Chem* 34:B60, 1988.

Bush TL et al: Cardiovascular mortality and noncontraceptive use of estrogen in women: results from the Lipid Research Clinics Program Follow-up Study, *Circulation* 75:1102, 1987.

Castelli WP: Epidemiology of triglycerides: a view from Framingham, *Am J Cardiol* 70:3H, 1992.

Castelli WP: The triglyceride issue: a view from Framingham, *Am Heart J* 112:432, 1986.

Cauley JA et al: Menopausal estrogen use, high density lipoprotein cholesterol subfractions and liver function, *Atherosclerosis* 49:31, 1983.

Criqui MH et al: Plasma triglyceride level and mortality from coronary heart disease, *N Engl J Med* 328:1220, 1993.

Criqui MH et al: Postmenopausal estrogen use and mortality: results from a prospective study in a defined, homogeneous community, *Am J Epidemiol* 128:606, 1988.

Curb JD et al: Plasma lipids and lipoprotein in elderly Japanese-American men, *J Am Geriatr Soc* 34:773, 1986.

Dahlen GH et al: Association of levels of liproprotein Lp(a), plasma lipids, and other lipoprotein with coronary artery disease documented by angiography, *Circulation* 74:758, 1986.

Ettinger WH et al: Lipoprotein lipids in older people: results from the Cardiovascular Health Study, *Circulation* 86:858, 1992.

Expert Panel on Detection, Evaluation, and Treatment of High Blood Cholesterol in Adults: Summary of the second report of the National Cholesterol Education Program (NCEP) Expert Panel on Detection, Evaluation, and Treatment of High Blood Cholesterol in Adults (Adult Treatment Panel II), *JAMA* 269:3015, 1993.

Fahraeus L, Larsson-Chon U, Wallentin L: Plasma lipoproteins including high density lipoprotein subfractions during normal pregnancy, *Obstet Gynecol* 66:468, 1985.

Fahraeus L, Wallentin L: High density lipoprotein subfractions during oral and cutaneous administration of 17 beta-estradiol to menopausal women, *J Clin Endocrinol Metab* 56:797, 1983.

Foreyt JP, Goodrick GK: Evidence for success of behavior modification in weight loss and control, *Ann Intern Med* 119:698, 1993.

Fotherby K: Oral contraceptives and lipids, *Br Med J* 298:1049, 1989.

Garber AM, Littenberg B, Sox HC: Costs and health consequences of cholesterol screening for asymptomatic older Americans, *Arch Intern Med* 151:1089, 1991.

Godsland IF, Crook D, Simpson R, et al: The effects of different formulations of oral contraceptive agents on lipid and carbohydrate metabolism, *N Engl J Med* 323:1375, 1990.

Gordon T et al: High density lipoprotein as a protective factor against coronary heart disease: the Framingham Study, *Am J Med* 62:707, 1977.

Gotto AM: Practical approach to phenotyping hyperlipoproteinemia. In Kligfield PD, editor: *Cardiology reference book,* New York, 1984, Co-Medica.

Grundy SM et al: The place of HDL in cholesterol management: a perspective from the National Cholesterol Education Program, *Arch Intern Med* 149:505, 1989.

Heyden S et al: Fasting triglycerides as predictors of total and coronary heart disease mortality in Evans County, Georgia. *J Chronic Dis* 33:275, 1980.

Jacobs DR, Blackburn H: Models of effects of low blood cholesterol the public health: implications for practice and policy, *Circulation* 87:1033, 1993.

Jacobs DR, Blackburn H, Higgins M: Low cholesterol: mortality associations, *Circulation* 86:1046, 1992.

Johnson CL et al: Declining serum total cholesterol levels among US adults: the National Health and Nutrition Examination Surveys, *JAMA* 269:3002, 1993.

Kannel WB: Low high density lipoprotein cholesterol and what to do about it, *Am J Cardiol* 70:810, 1992.

Kannel WB, Castelli WP, Gordon T: Cholesterol in the prediction of atherosclerotic disease: new perspectives based on the Framingham Study, *Ann Intern Med* 90:85, 1979.

Kannel WB, Wolf PA, Garrison RJ: Framingham Study: an epidemiological investigation of cardiovascular disease, Section 36: Means at each examination and inter-examination consistency of specified characteristics: Framingham Heart Study 30-year follow-up. National Heart, Lung, and Blood Institute Publication No NIH 88-2970, 1988.

Kritchevsky D: How aging affects cholesterol metabolism, *Postgrad Med* 63:133, 1978.

LaRosa JC et al: The cholesterol facts: a summary of the evidence relating dietary fats, serum cholesterol, and coronary heart disease, *Circulation* 81z:1721, 1990.

Lipids Research Clinic Program Epidemiology Committee: Plasma lipid populations in selected North American population, *Circulation* 60:427, 1979.

Lipid Research Clinics Program: The Lipid Research Clinics' Coronary Primary Prevention Trial results. I. Reduction in incidence of coronary heart disease. II. The relationship of reduction in incidence of coronary heart disease to cholesterol lowering, *JAMA* 51:351, 1984.

Lissner L et al: Variability of body weight and health outcomes in the Framingham population, *N Engl J Med* 324:1839, 1991.

Loscalzo J: Lipoprotein(a): a unique risk factor for atherothrombotic disease, *Arteriosclerosis* 10:672, 1990.

Mannienn V, Elo MO, Frick DL: Lipid alterations and decline in the incidence of coronary heart disease in the Helsinki Heart Study, *JAMA* 260:641, 1988.

Manolio TA et al: Epidemiology of low cholesterol levels in older adults: The Cardiovascular Health Study, *Circulation* 87:728, 1993.

McLean JW et al: cDNA sequence of human apoliprotein(a) is homologous to plasminogen, *Nature* 330:132, 1987.

Meilahn EN et al: Lp(a) concentrations among pre- and post-menopausal women over time: The Healthy Women Study, *Circulation* 84:546, 1991 (abstract).

Miller NE: Associations of high density lipoprotein subclasses and apoproteins with ischemic heart disease and coronary atherosclerosis, *Am Heart J* 113:589, 1987.

Miller VT: Dyslipoproteinemia in women: special considerations *Endocrinol Metab Clin North Am* 19:381, 1990.

Mittelmark MB et al: Total blood cholesterol levels in older adult participants in community-wide screening programs, *J Am Geriatr Soc* 39:A7, 1991.

Multiple Risk Factor Intervention Trial Research Group: Multiple Risk Factor Intervention Trial: risk factor changes and mortality results, *JAMA* 248:1465, 1982.

Nabulsi AA et al: Association of hormone-replacement therapy with various cardiovascular risk factors in postmenopausal women, *N Engl J Med* 328:1069, 1993.

Rader DJ, Brewer HB Jr: Lipoprotein(a): clinical approach to a unique atherogenic lipoprotein, *JAMA* 267:1109, 1992.

Regnstrom J et al: Susceptibility to low-density lipoprotein oxidation and coronary atherosclerosis in man, *Lancet* 339:1183, 1992.

Rifkind BM: *Drug treatment of hyperlipidemia,* New York, 1991, Marcel Dekker.

Rimm EB et al: Vitamin E consumption and the risk of coronary heart disease in men, *N Engl J Med* 328:1450, 1993.

Rolengren A et al: Lipoprotein (a) and coronary heart disease: a prospective case-control study in a general population sample of middle-aged men, *Br Med J* 301:1248, 1990.

Sandkamp M, Assmann G: 1 Lipoprotein(a) in PROCAM participants and young myocardial infarction survivors. In Scanu AM, editor: *Lipoprotein(a),* New York, 1990, Academic Press.

Schaefer EJ, Levy RI: Pathogenesis and management of lipoprotein disorders, *N Engl J Med* 312:1300, 1985.

Sempos CT et al: Prevalence of high blood cholesterol among US adults: an update based on guidelines from the second report of the National Cholesterol Education Program Adult Treatment Panel, *JAMA* 269:3009, 1993.

Stampfer MJ et al: A prospective study of past use of oral contraceptive agents and risk of cardiovascular disease, *N Engl J Med* 319:1313, 1988.

Stampfer MJ et al: Postmenopausal estrogen therapy and cardiovascular disease: ten-year follow-up from the Nurses' Health Study, *N Engl J Med* 325:756, 1991.

Stampfer MJ et al: Vitamin E consumption and the risk of coronary disease in women, *N Engl J Med* 328:1444, 1993.

Steinberg D: Antioxidants and atherosclerosis: a current assessment, *Circulation* 84:1420, 1991.

Steinberg D, Witztum JL: Lipoproteins and atherogenesis: current concepts, *JAMA* 264:3047, 1990.

Steinberg D et al: Beyond cholesterol: modifications of low-density lipoprotein that increase its atherogenicity, *N Engl J Med* 320:915, 1989.

Wahl PW, et al: Distribution of lipoprotein triglyceride and lipoprotein cholesterol in an adult population by age, sex and hormone use, *Atherosclerosis* 39:111, 1981.

Williamson DF: Descriptive epidemiology of body weight and weight change in U.S. adults, *Ann Intern Med* 119 (7, pt 2):646, 1993.

Witztum JL: Current approaches to drug therapy for the hypercholesterolemic patient, *Circulation* 80:1101, 1989.

Wood PD, Stefanick ML, Williams PT: The effects on plasma lipoproteins of a prudent weight-reducing diet, with or without exercise, in overweight men and women, *N Engl J Med* 325:461, 1991.

4 Other Cardiovascular Diseases

Anne W. Moulton

This chapter considers cardiovascular diseases or syndromes that have special significance for women because of gender differences in prevalence, morbidity rate, mortality rate, or treatment (see box, below).

HYPERTENSION

Hypertension occurs commonly in women, especially as they age. It is a major cause of morbidity and mortality for elderly women, causing stroke, progressive dementia, and chronic congestive heart failure. Approximately 20% to 22% of the U.S. population has a blood pressure greater than 160/95 mm Hg. The prevalence of hypertension is higher overall in men than in women, higher in blacks than in whites, and increases progressively with age. Rates in younger white women are lower than in white men but are comparable by the ages of 60 to 74, whereas hypertension rates in black women reach those in black men by ages 45 to 54. Not only are black women more likely than white women to have hypertension, they are also more likely to have severe hypertension and earlier evidence of end-organ damage. Surveys of various other ethnic groups indicate a high rate of hypertension in Filipinos and lower rates in Chinese and Hispanic populations.

Studies of the physiologic characteristics of early hypertension in women are limited. Women have a higher resting heart rate, left ventricular ejection time, cardiac index, and pulse pressure and a lower total peripheral resistance and total blood volume than men with the same blood pressure level. Exercise appears to cause a lower rise in blood pressure in men than in women with comparable resting pressures. This suggests that women are hemodynamically

---

GENDER DIFFERENCES IN NONCORONARY HEART DISEASE

Hypertension

Women manifest end-organ damage later
Hypertension in premenopausal women less frequent and severe than in men of comparable age
Uncertainty about side-effect profiles

Aortic stenosis

Less common in women below age 70
More common in women above age 70

Mitral valve prolapse

Much more common in women
Serious complications less frequent in women

Congestive heart failure

Less common in women
Survival rate worse in women
Diastolic ventricular dysfunction more common in women

"younger" than men with an equivalent age and blood pressure level and may explain why women manifest end-organ damage from hypertension later than men do. The two types of hypertension, essential and secondary, appear to occur with the same frequency in males as in females.

EPIDEMIOLOGY

Essential hypertension

Hypertension is a heterogeneous disorder; many different factors (neurogenic, cardiac, renal, and hormonal) may play a role in its pathophysiology. Clearly a genetic predisposition and environmental factors are important in the development of hypertension. In premenopausal women hypertension appears to be less frequent and severe than in men of comparable age. However, after menopause this gender difference disappears. Hypertension is frequently associated with two other risk factors that are especially important for women: obesity and diabetes mellitus. In obese women (those who are 20% or more above their desirable weight) hypertension will develop at three times the rate of nonobese control subjects. Obesity is a particular problem for older, middle-aged women, affecting up to 60% of black and 40% of white women. White obese women are at an eightfold greater risk for development of hypertension and a tenfold greater risk for development of cardiovascular disease than nonobese white women. The strong association between obesity and blood pressure is demonstrated by the effect of weight loss on lowering blood pressure.

The relationship between diabetes and hypertension is more complex. Diabetes can result in hypertension, and hypertension can aggravate the complications of diabetes. Both conditions are associated with hyperlipidemia and obesity and can hasten the progression of atherosclerosis.

The role of race in hypertensive morbidity and mortality is significant. After the age of 40, black women have twice the incidence of hypertension of white women. Hypertensive nephrosclerosis as a cause of end-stage renal disease is four times as common in blacks as whites. It is unclear whether the hypertension is more severe or whether the vasculature is intrinsically more susceptible in blacks. Other contributing factors to the higher rates of hypertension in blacks include differences in diet (primarily sodium content), social stressors, differences in life-style (e.g., exercise), and inadequate access to medical care.

Environmental factors that are associated with hypertension in all populations include dietary intake of sodium, potassium, and calcium; use of alcohol; and socioeconomic stressors. In communities where the average salt intake is 3g/day the prevalence of hypertension is lower. Communities ingesting 8 to 12 g/day have a high prevalence of hypertension and a progressive rise in blood pressure with age. Several large cross-sectional studies have indicated a direct association of alcohol consumption with blood pressure, particularly systolic pressure. In women the relationship is J-shaped: women reporting intake of 1 to 2 drinks/day have lower pressures on average than women reporting no alcohol use and than those consuming 3 to 6 drinks/day. Psychosocial factors probably play a role in the development of high blood pressure, but the cause and effect relationship is ill defined in both males and females.

Isolated systolic hypertension is increasingly prevalent with age, especially in those ages 60 years and above. It appears to be as common in females as males. Epidemiologic studies have demonstrated an increased risk of stroke, cardiovascular disease, and death for those with isolated systolic hypertension. Treatment of isolated systolic hypertension in patients older than 60 years of age has been shown to reduce risk of stroke in both black and white women and risk of death from coronary artery disease.

Secondary Hypertension

A definitive, often correctable cause of hypertension (secondary hypertension) is present in 5% to 10% of all women with hypertension. Secondary hypertension should be considered in women whose hypertension begins in childhood or after age 50 and in those with a negative family history or who experience an acceleration of hypertension. Medical conditions causing hypertension of particular relevance to women are discussed briefly in the following sections.

Coarctation of the aorta represents 5% of congenital heart disease and generally occurs more frequently in males than in females. However, in women with Turner's syndrome who lack an X chromosome, up to 50% have associated cardiovascular abnormalities, most commonly coarctation of the aorta. The diagnosis should be readily suspected on physical examination if differences in blood pressures between arms and legs are noted in addition to absent femoral arterial pulsations (a late finding), bounding carotid pulsations, and a late systolic murmur is heard in the left second interspace and over the back. Diagnosis is confirmed by angiography. Operative resection or balloon angioplasty corrects the hypertension in 80% of cases, especially if done before the age of 20.

Renal disease is not only the most common cause of secondary hypertension in women but is one of the most common sequelae. Nephrosclerosis can develop quickly in women with malignant hypertension, especially black women. Parenchymal disease is irreversible; however identification of the condition is important because control of hypertension, especially with drugs such as angiotensin converting enzyme (ACE) inhibitors and calcium channel blockers, delays progression of renal disease. Conditions of particular importance in women include chronic pelvic nephritis resulting from vesicoureteral reflux in childhood, diabetic glomerulopathy, lupus nephritis, and analgesic nephropathy.

Renal vascular hypertension is the most common curable form of secondary hypertension in women. The obstruction of the renal artery is predominantly due to medial fibroplasia (fibromuscular hyperplasia). This lesion is more common in younger white women, whereas atherosclerotic lesions occur in older women, especially those with other risk factors for vascular disease. The diagnosis of renovascular hypertension should be suspected in any woman with significant hypertension who has no family history of hypertension, a poor response to antihypertensive therapy, or an abdominal epigastric bruit (occurs in 40% to 50% of cases). Impaired renal function is unusual because bilateral renal artery stenosis is rare. The anatomic diagnosis is made by angiography of the renal artery and assessment of the severity of stenosis by subsequent renal vein renin sampling. Balloon angioplasty has improved the management of stenotic lesions in the renal arteries, although restenoses do occur.

Takayasu's arteritis (pulseless disease) is an obliterative inflammatory arteritis of unknown cause that involves the aortic arch and great vessels in the thoracoabdominal aorta and its branches, including the renal arteries. It affects women 8.5 times more often than men and has been reported mainly in teenagers and in young women immigrants from Asia and Africa. Hypertension is present in 75% of cases and is due to both aortic coarctation and renal artery stenosis. Late manifestations include absent pulses, heart failure, and stroke. No specific therapy is available.

There are several **endocrine causes** of secondary hypertension, most of which are rare but are relevant to women. Glucocorticoid excess (Cushing's syndrome) is predominantly due to adrenocorticotropic hormone (ACTH) production by a pituitary adenoma with resulting bilateral adrenal hyperplasia (Cushing's disease). This condition affects women five to eight times as frequently as men and is usually diagnosed between the ages of 20 and 40. Diagnosis should be suspected when a woman has new hypertension with a history of some or all of the following: menstrual irregularities, emotional lability, sleep disorder, truncal obesity, peripheral muscle wasting, acne, fragile skin, purple striae, ecchymoses, delayed wound healing, abnormal hair growth, osteoporosis, peptic ulcer disease, and glucose intolerance. The diagnosis is confirmed by demonstrating excess cortisone production and lack of normal diurnal pattern and either elevated or suppressed plasma ACTH levels. Other endocrine conditions that are more common in women and are associated with hypertension include hyperparathyroidism, hypothyroidism, and hyperthyroidism.

 EVALUATION

The clinical history should focus on family history of hypertension and endocrine and renal diseases, as well as identification of other cardiac risk factors and familial diseases associated with hypertension. Physical examination should focus on careful measurement of the blood pressure in both arms, as well as a detailed examination of the optic fundi and careful palpation of the thyroid. Cardiac examination should include assessment of left ventricular hypertrophy, presence of a third or fourth heart sound, arrhythmias, left ventricular hypertrophy, and murmurs of aortic sclerosis or mitral insufficiency. The abdomen should be carefully examined for the presence of an aortic bruit. In older patients a detailed neurologic examination including a brief baseline mental status assessment is essential. Laboratory studies should include blood urea nitrogen and creatinine levels; routine urinalysis; and glucose, cholesterol, triglyceride, uric acid, and calcium levels. An electrocardiogram should be obtained and, if there is a question of left ventricular hypertrophy, an echocardiogram may be useful. Clues for the presence of secondary hypertension should be sought, with additional tests ordered only in high-risk groups or for patients in whom a particular diagnosis is more likely.

CHOICE OF THERAPY

Because of the larger number of women in the overall population particularly in the age groups in which hypertension is most common, there is a larger absolute number of women than men with hypertension. It is ironic that more studies have not assessed the relative efficacy of different therapies in women with hypertension. There remains some controversy about whether certain side effects are gender-related, although most experts in the field stress that antihypertensive drug therapy is as efficacious in women as it is in men.

Nonpharmacologic therapy

Thirty percent of American women are above ideal weight. Therefore weight reduction seems a reasonable first step in many women with mild to moderate hypertension. Reducing sodium intake may similarly be effective in women who are salt-sensitive, particularly women of African-American descent. The use of alcohol should be discouraged. Exercise has been shown to lower blood pressure effectively in both males and females. Finally, nonpharmacologic techniques such as relaxation, biofeedback, and stress management may be helpful.

Pharmacologic therapy

The most effective and best tolerated antihypertension drugs are the diuretics, β-adrenergic blockers, ACE inhibitors, and calcium channel blockers. Although diuretics and β-adrenergic blockers are the only agents that have been shown to decrease the mortality rate associated with hypertension, once-a-day doses of ACE inhibitors and calcium channel blockers have been particularly effective in controlling hypertension. Hypertensive black patients may not respond as well as whites to β-adrenergic blockers or ACE inhibitors but often respond well to diuretics or calcium channel blockers. Diabetic patients, the majority of whom are women, may be best treated with an ACE inhibitor, which does not have an adverse effect on carbohydrate metabolism and has the added benefit of preserving renal function.

VALVULAR HEART DISEASE

Below the age of 70, aortic stenosis (generally related to congenital stenosis or bicuspid valves) is more common in men. After 70 years, when the predominant cause is calcific aortic stenosis, the disorder becomes more common in women.

As women age both mitral and aortic valves tend to calcify. The calcification occurs in the annulus of the mitral valve and in the fibrosa of the aortic valve leaflets. In fact women are more likely to have calcification in either valve at a younger age than men and the mechanism for this is not understood.

In the 1990s rheumatic heart disease has been a rare cause of valvular heart disease in women in the United States. It is seen infrequently except in patients who immigrate from areas where it is common, such as Southeast Asia, South America, and Central America. For reasons that are not clear, mitral stenosis of rheumatic cause occurs predominantly in females.

Mitral valve prolapse

Mitral valve prolapse (MVP) affects 3% to 4% or more of the population, making it one of the most common cardiovascular conditions. It is eight times more common in women than in men. The prevalence of MVP is 6% in apparently healthy women but one study suggests that MVP is also widely overdiagnosed (up to 40% of patients referred to a tertiary care center with this diagnosis did not actually meet the echocardiographic criteria). For unknown reasons MVP is primarily a disorder of young women, with very low rates in elderly women. MVP exhibits a strong hereditary component, transmitted as an autosomal dominant trait.

MVP has been divided into two clinical subsets: MVP (diagnosed by echocardiographically determined systolic displacement of the mitral leaflets posteriorly and superiorly from their usual position) and "MVP syndrome," which is MVP in association with a variety of symptoms (discussed later). MVP may occur as a secondary feature of a number of conditions that either affect connective tissue (e.g., Marfan's syndrome) or cause the left ventricle to be disproportionately small in relation to the size of the mitral valve (e.g., atrial septal defect). However most cases of MVP occur independently of other recognized cardiovascular conditions and may be considered primary.

Over the last two decades investigators have reported the association of a variety of symptoms and signs with MVP, including chest pain, dyspnea, fatigue, anxiety, light-headedness, palpitations, skeletal abnormalities, altered body habitus, and electrocardiographic abnormalities. The chest pain, which is actually reported more frequently in men than women, is thought to be due to stretching of the papillary muscle. In the past some of the associated symptoms that cannot be explained by valvular abnormalities alone have been attributed to neuroendocrine and autonomic dysfunction. However recent literature suggests that this association may reflect an ascertainment bias. In one well-controlled study there was a strong association between echocardiographic and auscultatory features of MVP and thoracic skeletal abnormalities (including pectus excavatum, scoliosis, and an abnormally straight thoracic spine), low body weight, low systolic blood pressure, and palpitations. In contrast, there was no association between MVP syndrome and chest pain, dyspnea, anxiety, panic attack, or inferior lead repolarization abnormalities.

Although there is a strong female predominance in the prevalence of MVP, serious complications occur predominantly in the male population. Whereas individuals with MVP constitute 3% to 4% of the adult population they account for as much as 25% of patients who require mitral valve replacement and 13% of patients in whom endocarditis develops. Of patients with severe mitral regurgitation 50% to 90% are men, and a male predominance has also been noted in the development of endocarditis.

Congestive heart failure

Congestive heart failure (CHF) actually occurs more commonly in men than it does in women but rates increase dramatically in women as they age. After the onset of CHF, survival rates appear to be worse for women than for men, which may relate to their older age and greater prevalence of comorbidity. Important underlying causes of CHF for women include coronary artery disease, hypertension (particularly important in African-American women), valvular heart disease, and diabetes, which appears to promote heart failure to a greater extent in women than in men. After a myocardial infarction, women are more likely than men to develop CHF both in the peri-infarction period and later in their course.

There are limited data on differences in treatment for men and women with CHF. In the SOLVD trial vasodilator therapy appeared to offer similar benefit to men and women but there appeared to be a trend toward a greater reduction in mortality and CHF among men. There is some evidence that women are more likely to have diastolic ventricular dysfunction with intact systolic function and a normal ejection fraction. This could have significant implications for the choice of therapy for CHF in women as β-blockers and calcium antagonists are more beneficial in the treatment of diastolic dysfunction than conventional CHF therapy.

BIBLIOGRAPHY

Alpert MA et al: Mitral valve prolapse, panic disorder, and chest pain, *Med Clin North Am* 75(5):1119, 1991.

Amery A et al: Mortality and morbidity results from the European Working Party on High Blood Pressure in the Elderly trial, *Lancet* 1349, 1985

Anastos K et al: Hypertension in women: what is really known? *Ann Intern Med* 115:287, 1991,

Berko BA: Gender-related differences in cardiomyopathy. In Douglas PS, editor: *Heart disease in women*, Philadelphia, 1989, FA Davis Co.

Byyny RL, Speroff L: Hypertension. In *A clinical guide for the care of older women*, Baltimore, 1990, Williams & Wilkins.

Cohn LH: Valvular heart disease. In Wenger NK, Speroff L, Packard B, editors: *Cardiovascular health and disease in women*, Proceedings of an NHLBI Conference, Greenwich, Conn, 1993, Le Jacq Communications.

Devereux RB, Kramer-Fox R: Gender differences in mitral valve prolapse. In Douglas PS, editor: *Heart disease in women*, Philadelphia, 1989, FA Davis.

Frohlich ED: Coronary preventive therapy: hypertension. In Wenger NK, Speroff L, Packard B, editors: *Cardiovascular health and disease in women*, Proceedings of an NHLBI Conference, Greenwich, Conn, 1993, Le Jacq Communications.

Hall PM: Hypertension in women, *Cardiovasc Dis Women Cardiol* 77:(2):25, 1990.

Limacher MC, Yusuf S: Gender differences in presentation, morbidity and mortality in the studies of the left ventricular dysfunction (SOLVD): a preliminary report. In Wenger NK, Speroff L, Packard B, editors: *Cardiovascular health and disease in women*, Proceedings of an NHLBI Conference, Greenwich, Conn, 1993, Le Jacq Communications.

Medical Research Council Working Party: Medical Research Council trial of treatment of mild hypertension: principal results, *Br Med J* 291:97, 1985.

Medical Research Council Working Party: Medical Research Council trial on treatment of hypertension in older adults: principal results, *Br Med J* 304:405, 1992.

Raj A, Sheehan DV: Mitral valve prolapse and panic disorder, *Bull Menninger Clin* 54:199, 1990.

Schnall PL, Alderman MH, Kern R: An analysis of the HDFP trial: evidence of adverse effects of antihypertensive treatment on white women with moderate and severe hypertension, *NY State J Med* 84:299, 1984.

SHEP Cooperative Research Group: Prevention of stroke by antihypertensive drug treatment in older persons with isolated systolic hypertension: final results of the systolic hypertension in the elderly program (SHEP), *JAMA* 265:3255, 1991.

5 Stroke

Barbara A. Dworetzky and David M. Dawson

Stroke remains the third leading cause of death in the United States despite its decreasing incidence. Roughly 42% of strokes will occur in women this year. There are substantial financial costs of acute hospitalization and long-term rehabilitation of stroke survivors, with the majority of losses resulting from inability of patients to return to work and subsequent disability payments. Overall, women have fewer strokes than men at every age group with the exception of those few cases occurring in patients younger than 30. Also, there are certain conditions that predispose women to specific types of strokes that may be important in determining the pathogenesis of cerebrovascular disease. Pregnancy, use of birth control pills, and mitral valve prolapse are examples of risks for stroke that solely or predominantly affect women. Although the incidence of intracerebral hemorrhage is roughly equal in women and men, subarachnoid hemorrhage occurs more frequently in women by as much as 50%. Most of these hemorrhages in women are due to ruptured aneurysms, whereas in men they are more likely to be due to ruptured arteriovenous malformations. The topic of vascular

malformations, an important cause of subarachnoid hemorrhage, is beyond the scope of this chapter.

PATHOPHYSIOLOGY
Definition and mechanism

Current approaches to stroke diagnosis and management focus on the mechanism of stroke. There are two basic mechanisms of infarction: hemorrhagic and ischemic. Hemorrhages can be intraparenchymal or subarachnoid. Ischemic events can be defined on a time continuum. Neurologic symptoms or signs (e.g., weakness, numbness, aphasia, slurred speech, double vision) that resolve in less than 24 hours suggest that a transient ischemic attack (TIA) has occurred. Neurologic deficits that last longer than 24 hours imply that an infarction or stroke has occurred. Ischemic infarctions can be the result of systemic hypoperfusion, emboli, or thrombosis. Emboli can originate from the heart, dislodge from plaques of proximal arteries, or arise paradoxically from peripheral venous clots that cross from the right atrium to the left via a septal defect, usually a patent foramen ovale. Arterial thrombosis can occur in both large vessels (e.g., carotid, middle cerebral artery) and small vessels within the brain.

Gender differences

Recent evidence demonstrates that risks, causes, and outcomes differ between the sexes. Counseling for prevention and treatment of strokes in women requires an understanding of these gender discrepancies. Cerebral angiograms and carotid ultrasounds, for example, have demonstrated increased intracranial atherosclerosis in women and blacks, and increased extracranial (carotid and vertebral) atherosclerosis in men and whites. Autopsy studies have indicated that between the fourth and sixth decades women are more likely than men to have no atherosclerosis. This difference disappears after age 65 years, suggesting a protective effect of estrogen on the development of atherosclerosis, possibly through favorable changes in the serum lipid ratio.

Although the lifetime risk of having a stroke appears to be greater for men than for women, the lifetime risk of dying of a stroke is greater for women (16%) than for men (8%). A likely explanation for this observation is that women have longer life expectancies and have a later age of onset of stroke.

Risk factors

The most important risk factors for all strokes are hypertension, diabetes, and smoking. Additionally, prior stroke or TIA (especially a recent one) places the patient at greater risk for stroke because it implies that cerebrovascular disease has already occurred. Risk factors for stroke in general are additive, so that many victims of stroke have several determinants.

Hypertension. The Multiple Risk Factor Intervention Trial (MRFIT) showed that roughly 40% of strokes can be attributed to a systolic blood pressure of 140 or greater. Other studies have related elevated diastolic pressures to about 70% of strokes. The Framingham Study prospectively demonstrated that hypertension, whether it was labile or fixed, systolic or diastolic, was the most frequent and most powerful predictor of stroke, providing a fourfold increase in risk over normotension. Even in the young, hypertension was the most potent contributing risk, associated with approximately one quarter of strokes.

Diabetes. The Nurses's Health Study cohort (made up largely of white women 30 to 55 years old) demonstrated a significantly increased risk of both fatal and nonfatal strokes among diabetic women. Most of these strokes were ischemic in origin, although a slight increase of hemorrhages was also seen. The adverse effect conferred by diabetes appeared to be compounded by the addition of smoking, hypertension, hypercholesterolemia, or obesity. Controlling for these added risks, diabetes still posed a threefold increase in cardiovascular risk when it was present for at least 15 years.

Smoking. Smoking is a major risk factor for the development of both hemorrhagic and nonhemorrhagic strokes. More than one third of strokes can be attributed to cigarette smoking. In a prospective cohort study of women ages 30 to 55 the number of cigarettes smoked per day correlated with an increased risk of stroke, whereas the number of years of smoking did not correlate with risk. In fact smokers had the same risk for strokes as nonsmokers within 2 years of quitting, thus emphasizing the importance of the major efforts to decrease the prevalence of smoking in the United States.

Cholesterol. The role that high cholesterol level has in stroke is not as clear as its role in heart disease. The MRFIT trial revealed a modest correlation between high serum cholesterol level and nonhemorrhagic strokes. Patients younger than age 40 who have strokes have been noted to have an elevated incidence of hypercholesterolemia.

Alcohol. A prospective study of female nurses showed that moderate alcohol intake significantly lessened the risk of ischemic stroke yet increased the risk of subarachnoid hemorrhage two to three times. In nonsmokers the protective effect of alcohol was even more apparent. The mechanisms for these observations are still incompletely understood.

Uncommon risk factors

Valvular disease and atrial fibrillation. In stroke registries, about 30% of cases are embolic. Valvular disease, such as rheumatic mitral stenosis or congenital bicuspid aortic valve, may be the source of emboli in any age group. Atrial fibrillation, typically occurring in the elderly, is associated with a high risk of stroke, from 17% in those without underlying heart disease to 40% in those with valvular disease and fibrillation. In patients with idiopathic or alcoholic cardiomyopathy mural thrombi may form in the dilated left ventricle and be a source of emboli. In most instances long-term anticoagulation with warfarin (Coumadin) is the accepted mode of treatment to prevent cerebral embolism.

Mitral valve prolapse. Mitral valve prolapse (MVP) caused by myxomatous valve degeneration is a special example of cardiac valvular disease. It is common in younger individuals and is three times more common in women than in men. The risk of stroke rises fourfold in younger patients with MVP, although in older patients, as other causes of stroke rise in incidence, MVP is not a significant risk factor. Notably the subset of patients with severe MVP characterized by redundant leaflets or mitral regurgitation is at no more risk than those patients with mild disease. However, these patients are at higher risk for infectious or hemodynamic compromise. In patients without an apparent cause of stroke, patent foramen ovale leading to paradoxical embolization should be considered as the mechanism, especially if the history reveals that the onset of neurologic symptoms followed Valsalva's maneuver.

Migraine. Estimates of the frequency of migraine vary widely, but as many as 29% of women and 20% of men are subject to recurrent vascular headaches at some time in their lives. Tatemichi and Mohr summarize seven recent series of adults below the age of 50 years who had an ischemic stroke. In their total of 448 patients migraine was the presumed cause in only 4%. With such a high prevalence of migraine headaches in the population it is very hard to assess migraine as a risk factor for stroke, particularly in the middle-aged and elderly.

Two mechanisms may account for the few strokes that do occur in the migraine population: cardiogenic embolism and spasm of arteries or arterioles. Direct evidence for vasospasm in migraine, whether during the aura phase or the headache, is lacking. Cerebral blood flow is believed to be reduced during a migraine attack. Infarction, therefore, is a possible outcome. Many migraine researchers now believe that reduced blood flow is secondary, and that a biochemical event, involving serotonin and possibly other neurotransmitters, produces a zone of reduced metabolic activity preceding vascular changes.

Oral contraceptives and estrogen. In the 1960s clinical data began to suggest a relationship between use of oral contraceptives and stroke. Estimates then indicated a 4-fold to 13-fold increased risk of stroke in young women, compared with that of women not exposed to oral contraceptives. Subsequent information suggested that the risk was multifactorial and was increased by high estrogen content pills, smoking, age above 35, and hypertension. Current data do not support a relationship between use of oral contraceptives and ischemic stroke. Previous studies from prior decades all suffer from flaws in method. There is, however, evidence of a roughly fourfold increase in the risk of subarachnoid hemorrhage in women who smoke while on the pill. Nevertheless some caution in the use of oral contraceptive agents in potential stroke is still important. The package inserts for implantable subcutaneous as well as for oral agents, even those low in estrogen, advise caution in certain groups of patients:

1. Women who smoke
2. Women who have a prior history of venous or arterial thrombosis. Some of these will have a generalized hypercoagulable state (see later discussion)
3. Substance abusers, particularly users of cocaine and amphetamines

The risk of stroke in women who are postmenopausal and take estrogen is controversial: some studies show a protective effect whereas others demonstrate an increased risk. A recent study has shown no added risk for stroke with hormone replacement. Until definitive studies are done, it is advisable that women with prior TIA or stroke avoid estrogen replacement therapy.

Hypercoagulable state. Hypercoagulable states are usually inherited disorders of the hemostatic mechanism. There may also be excess coagulability in patients with cancer, disseminated intravascular coagulation, immobilization in bed, polycythemia, hyperviscosity, or pregnancy.

The **antiphospholipid syndrome** is an example of a hypercoagulable condition. Antibodies are formed against phospholipids and include lupus anticoagulant and anticardiolipin antibody. Patients may experience stroke at any age, as well as recurrent spontaneous abortion, venous thrombosis, or livedo reticularis.

Protein C, protein S, and **antithrombin III deficiencies** as well as **homocystinuria** are all rare conditions but account for some instances of hypercoagulability. Unfortunately no direct treatment is available for any of these conditions.

Dissection and vasculitis. Spontaneous arterial dissection is believed to be initiated by an intimal tear, followed by entry of blood into the media and an upward migration of blood. These events cause the vessel to be narrowed. Dissection of a carotid or vertebral artery can lead to cerebral infarction in the territory of that artery. Dissection can occur at any age and should be considered after any trauma to the neck. It is more commonly seen in women than in men. Rarely intracranial vessels are affected by primary vasculitis and cause stroke.

DETECTION OF WOMEN AT RISK FOR STROKE

Women with a history of hypertension, diabetes, atrial fibrillation, myocardial infarction, TIAs, or strokes are at an increased risk for stroke and should be monitored closely, especially when pregnant. Asymptomatic carotid bruits are markers for vascular disease and thus help identify women at risk for stroke but do not necessarily correlate with strokes that occur ipsilateral to the stenosis. An accepted practice for monitoring patients with asymptomatic bruits is to obtain yearly neck ultrasound to look for progression of the stenosis or for the onset of new neurologic symptoms referable to the stenotic vessel.

EVALUATION OF STROKE IN WOMEN

History and physical examination

Not all neurologic deficits are strokes. It is often advisable to obtain a consultation with a neurologist early in a patient's presentation to aid with the diagnosis and management. Any history of trauma, alcoholism, or use of anticoagulant medication should bring subdural hematoma into the differential diagnosis. Fever and stiff neck make infection (e.g., abscess, meningitis, encephalitis) an important consideration because therapy with antibiotics may be lifesaving. Women with multiple sclerosis may have hemiparesis or unilateral numbness. Focal seizures can mimic stroke. Migraine can produce unilateral tingling, numbness, or aphasia. Hypoglycemia and hyperglycemia can unmask old strokes. Sudden confusion is usually not due to a stroke and should initiate a search for drugs, infections, or other metabolic processes.

Approach to diagnosis

Imaging studies

CT and MRI scanning. Once it is suspected that the patient may be having a stroke, it is important to determine whether there has been bleeding. A head computed tomographic (CT) scan (Fig. 5-1), without contrast, is indicated in practically all suspected strokes to rule out hemorrhage, (see also the section, Imaging during Pregnancy). In subarachnoid hemorrhage caused by aneurysm or arteriovenous malformations the blood surrounds the brain; in primary hemorrhage within the brain blood is visible as a bright white image. CT should precede lumbar puncture. CT scan also can be useful to evaluate mass effect or shifting of brain contents from tumor or blood (raised intracranial pressure) and the need for urgent neurosurgical intervention. Bleeding into the cerebellum is particularly dangerous because the patient's condition can deteriorate quickly as a result of compression of the vital structures within the brain stem.

Magnetic resonance imaging (MRI) (Fig. 5-2) is superior to CT scan for diagnosing posterior fossa abnormality. Vascular abnormalities can be diagnosed by MRI angiography, CT scan with contrast, or cerebral angiography. MRI is not advised for critically ill patients, claustrophobic patients, or

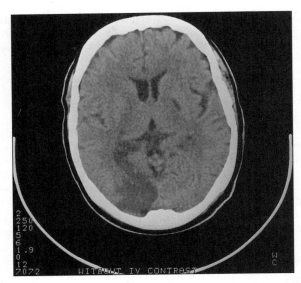

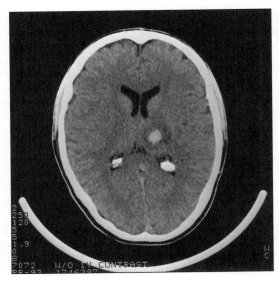

Fig. 5-1 *A,* CT scan without contrast showing a low density zone in the right occipital lobe (left side of figure), due to prior embolic infarction.

Fig. 5-1 *B,* CT scan without contrast showing a small acute hemorrhage in the left thalamus. Calcification of the choroid plexuses within the lateral ventricles is also demonstrated.

those with metallic clips or pacemakers. MRI angiography may eventually replace the more invasive cerebral angiogram when aneurysm or venous thrombosis is a concern.

If the CT scan does not show blood, the stroke is more likely ischemic in origin. It is important to remember that the CT result can be negative for the first 24 to 48 hours. If the patient experiences dizziness; is found to be pale, clam-

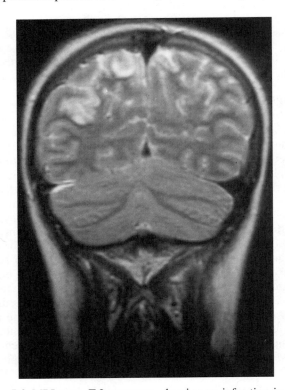

Fig. 5-2 MRI scan, T-2 sequence, showing an infarction in the right parieto-occipital region, due to eclampsia in a 15-year-old at term.

my, or near fainting; and has a history of heart disease, the differential should include arrhythmia, sepsis, and myocardial infarction. **Cerebral emboli** often appear with sudden neurologic deficits, but symptoms can improve once the embolus fragments. Echocardiogram, 24-hour Holter monitoring, and serial blood cultures can identify heart disease and an embolic cause of the stroke. **Thrombotic strokes** usually manifest as the patient awakens from sleep, revealing neurologic deficits that may subside or progress. If symptoms are referable to the carotid artery, noninvasive carotid ultrasound can evaluate the patency of this vessel and can help determine the need for endarterectomy. MRI angiography of the carotid arteries eliminates the risk of dye used during conventional angiography; however currently many surgeons will not operate without the conventional study.

New radiologic tests. There are new radiologic tests that study the in vivo flow of blood in the brain and make tissue viability estimates possible. These tests estimate cerebral territory that may be at risk for infarction even though no damage has yet been done. **Single-photon emission computed tomography** (SPECT) and **positron emission tomography** (PET) are two examples of these imaging techniques. These studies are still largely in the research phase but are beginning to be used in major medical centers. Moreover they may soon be additional tools for the diagnosis and management of stroke.

Other diagnostic testing

The abrupt onset of neurologic symptoms or signs should lead to suspicion of a stroke. These neurologic deficits can disappear, but the need for prompt evaluation is still critical because they may represent a TIA, a warning that the patient is at serious risk for stroke. Several screening blood tests should be completed on all patients with a suspected stroke or TIA. These include complete blood count, blood smear, platelets, protime, partial thromboplastin time, erythrocyte sedimentation rate (ESR), glucose, calcium, electrolytes, cholesterol, triglyceride, RPR, blood urea nitrogen, creatinine, and, if the patient is of childbearing age, a pregnancy test. Serum and urine toxic screens should also be performed on women under 45 or those with a history of illegal drug use. Later, antinuclear antibody, rheumatoid factor, anticardiolipin antibody, antithrombin III, protein C, or protein S may be useful. Lumbar puncture can help diagnose vasculitis, infection, and other more remote causes of stroke. However it is not invariably necessary in every case.

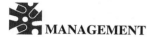

MANAGEMENT

Goals of management

The goal of treatment for bleeding in or around the brain is to prevent recurrence of hemorrhage and to prevent irreversible deterioration to coma and death from the increased pressure the blood exerts in the closed intracranial cavity. Early neurosurgical consultation for hemorrhage is extremely important to determine which patients will benefit most from surgical management.

Consideration for the treatment of ischemic stroke should focus on prevention since most neurologic deficits are not reversible. Risk factor reduction, for example, cessation of smoking and normalization of blood pressure, are important goals. Within 2 years of smoking cessation risk of stroke has declined to baseline value. Hypertension, the most potent risk for stroke, requires vigorous long-term management.

When a woman has a suspected stroke or TIA, hospitalization is often indicated to address issues related to the prevention of future strokes, to minimize the risk for increased intracranial pressure in hemorrhages and large strokes, and to maintain adequate blood pressure to ensure cerebral perfusion. Rapidly dropping the blood pressure should be prevented because this can lead to progression of the stroke by decreasing cerebral perfusion. If there is no bleeding indicated on head CT and the stroke is likely embolic and small to moderate in size, the early use of heparin should be considered while search for the embolic source is begun. Bed rest for the first 24 to 48 hours can improve blood flow to the brain in those patients whose symptoms worsen with postural changes. Once the stroke is complete (symptoms no longer fluctuate), initiation of stroke prevention measures should be considered. The following are the main agents that are available.

Choice of therapy

Use of antiplatelet agents

Aspirin. The beneficial effects of antiplatelet agents are believed to be due to prevention of aggregation by inhibiting thromboxane A_2 synthesis. Aspirin (acetylsalicylic acid [ASA]) has been used for this purpose since the mid-1970s. A metaanalysis by the Physician's Health Study Research Group has shown a slight reduction in stroke and death rate by approximately 20%. This is also noted in patients with a potential source of embolism. The ASA dose now commonly in use is one tablet a day (325 mg), although some authorities believe that a higher dose might be more effective, often with more gastrointestinal irritation. It is not current practice to prescribe ASA to patients who have not already had stroke, TIA, or other cerebrovascular events. ASA is probably effective in both sexes, although some studies, at higher doses, have shown better response in men.

Ticlopidine. Ticlopidine is an alternative therapy when a woman continues to experience stroke symptoms on ASA or cannot tolerate its side effects. Ticlopidine is a platelet antiaggregant that functions by inhibiting the adenosine diphosphate pathway. When compared to ASA 1300 mg/day, ticlopidine produces a further reduction of risk of stroke, in the overall range of 30%, and appears to be effective in both sexes. It causes severe neutropenia in 1% to 3% of patients in the first 3 months of treatment, so blood counts should be carefully monitored.

Anticoagulation. Prevention of stroke by the use of warfarin has been attempted for four decades. At the current time there is only one noncontroversial indication for the use of warfarin for stroke prevention, namely, for patients with suspected or proven cardiogenic embolism. Patients with acute stroke are usually started on heparin and then changed to warfarin. If the stroke risk persists (e.g., atrial fibrillation resistant to cardioversion), then the use of warfarin will be lifelong. Only slight prolongation of the International Normalized Ratio (INR) of 2 to 3 is required. INR, a calculated value based on a standardized reagent, is rapidly replacing the prothrombin time for monitoring coagulation time. The advantage of the INR is that it allows direct comparison of values obtained by different laboratories.

Surgical intervention. Surgical removal of plaque from the carotid bifurcation is available as a method of prevention of stroke or prevention of recurrence. Studies of the efficacy of carotid endarterectomy have been hampered by inexact knowledge of the risk of stroke with and without the operation. Recent data have been helpful. The risk of stroke recurrence after stroke or TIA is on average 10% per year and is slightly lower in women than in men. In the recent North American Symptomatic Carotid Endarterectomy Trial, a stroke rate of 26% over 2 years was reduced to 9% in carotid endarterectomy patients, provided they had stenosis of 70% or more and experienced symptoms caused by the stenotic vessel.

At present no reliable data are available on patients who have less than 70% stenosis or those who are asymptomatic (i.e., without TIA or stroke). Other surgical procedures with potential to prevent stroke include subclavian or vertebral endarterectomy and intracranial/extracranial bypass. These procedures have no proven role in stroke treatment and should be considered experimental.

Experimental therapies. There are several experimental therapies on the horizon. Some focus on reducing ischemic brain damage caused by the influx of calcium (**nimodipine**), free radical production during reperfusion of damaged brain (**21 amino steroids**), acidosis, and excitatory neurotransmitters (**glutamate receptor antagonists**). Others are concerned with the dissolution of clots (**streptokinase, recombinant tissue plasminogen activator** but increase the risk for intraparenchymal bleeding if they are not used within 90 minutes.

Rehabilitation. Rehabilitation of stroke should include a multidisciplinary approach initiated early in treatment. Physical, occupational, and speech therapies can help to maximize functional recovery, allowing many patients to return to their former environment. Rehabilitation programs help to educate patients and families about stroke and teach prevention of common stroke complications such as limb contractures, decubitus ulcers, or deep vein thromboses.

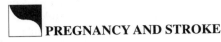

PREGNANCY AND STROKE

Epidemiology

The risk of stroke during pregnancy is believed to be quite low. However, fatal stroke, although rare in pregnancy, is a leading cause of nonobstetric maternal death. In addition, the social implications of puerperal strokes are devastating because they occur in younger women who have the major responsibility for providing care for their newborns. Still it is crucial to determine the cause of a stroke in a pregnant woman because it carries implications for treatment during the rest of the pregnancy and provides clues for counseling patients with regard to future pregnancies. It should not be assumed that pregnancy alone is a sufficient explanation for the stroke, and other causes should always be sought.

Pathophysiology

During pregnancy the mother undergoes cardiovascular changes that may increase the risk for stroke. Cardiac output rises 30% to 60% peak effects occurring in the second trimester. Blood volume can rise as much as 45% through the middle of the third trimester. Coagulability of blood elements increases as a result of a rise in fibrinogen and clotting factor levels and a decline in fibrinolysis. Platelets are more aggregable as well. All of these physiologic changes render the pregnant woman more vulnerable to both hemorrhagic and ischemic infarcts.

There is a clear increase in hemorrhagic strokes in pregnant women. Women with aneurysms or arteriovenous malformations have a fivefold to eightfold increase in the rate of rupture, primarily during the second and third trimesters, when cardiac output and blood volume are maximal. These malformations can cause subarachnoid or intraparenchymal hemorrhages, either of which can have a devastating outcome. A rare cause for stroke in pregnancy is eclampsia. Eclampsia can cause small hemorrhagic infarcts in the border zones between major arterial territories and in the occipital lobes. The mechanism is believed to be severe vasospasm that results from elevated blood pressure that overrides the upper limit of the cerebral autoregulatory system. This causes a breakdown of the blood-brain barrier with subsequent small hemorrhages and vasogenic edema.

Arterial occlusions and embolic phenomena are the most common cause of ischemic stroke in pregnancy (60% to 80%), occurring during peak "hypercoagulability" in the third trimester of pregnancy. Deep vein thromboses are common in pregnancy and can lead to embolic stroke via a patent foramen ovale. Cerebral venous thrombosis, associated with dehydration and hypercoagulation, is the most common stroke in the postpartum period. It can occur during the last week of pregnancy and up to 4 weeks postpartum. These patients usually experience severe headache, nausea, vomiting, lethargy, seizure, or diminished visual acuity caused by papilledema. Diagnosis is made by MRI or CT scan, with contrast revealing the classic "empty delta"

sign indicating a clot in the sagittal sinus. Angiography can be performed when the diagnosis is not apparent from the examinations described, but fluoroscopy time and contrast load must be kept to a minimum. Treatment employs bed rest, hydration, use of anticonvulsants, and heparinization. Mortality rate is about 25%. Fortunately those who survive usually have few sequelae. Extremely rare causes of embolic stroke are fat, air, and amniotic fluid emboli.

Stroke can also be caused by cerebral hypoperfusion from significant blood loss during delivery. Sheehan and Stanfield have described pituitary infarction by this mechanism. Peripartum cardiomyopathy, a disease more commonly seen with twin gestations, toxemia, hypertension, and births in older multiparous black women, is also an important cause of stroke from hypoperfusion. Contractions of the uterus during labor and delivery further increase cardiac output from increased venous return to the heart and from increased cardiac demand secondary to pain. Women with cardiomyopathy manifesting heart failure or arrhythmia should be treated with bed rest, digoxin, and diuretics. Subsequent pregnancy should be discouraged.

An extremely rare cause of stroke, also occurring in the postpartum period, is metastatic choriocarcinoma to the brain. This neoplasm can occlude an artery, thereby causing an infarct, or it can directly invade brain parenchyma, causing a hemorrhage. Although this neoplasm is rare, early diagnosis is crucial because it is curable with chemotherapy and whole brain radiation. Other tumors are hormonally stimulated and can appear with brain hemorrhage or infarct during pregnancy.

Evaluation of stroke in pregnancy

Imaging during pregnancy. Increased risk for stroke is not the only important issue facing physicians caring for women who are pregnant. One question that recurs is, what is the risk to the fetus of imaging when a pregnant woman exhibits acute neurologic deficits? Because radiation is known to be hazardous during the implantation and organogenesis stages in fetal development, elective imaging should be avoided during this period. However, head CT scan provides less than 1 mrad radiation to the uterus and is relatively safe during pregnancy, with proper precautions. If a pregnant woman has a suspected stroke, a head CT scan is the image of choice. Contrast agents cross the placenta and therefore should not be used if at all possible. MRI of the brain is preferred when vascular abnormality is a concern and avoids the use of contrast dye. MRI can raise body temperature by about 1° and though it is thought completely safe during pregnancy, this is not yet known.

Management

Anticoagulation during pregnancy. Another issue of concern is the use of anticoagulation for protection of stroke during pregnancy. Although no method of anticoagulation is entirely safe during pregnancy, chronic atrial fibrillation, a prosthetic valve, or an embolic source of stroke are more dangerous than the risks of anticoagulation therapy. Warfarin crosses the placenta and is known to be teratogenic, especially during the first trimester. The risk of fetal bleeding is increased. Heparin, a larger molecule, does not cross the placenta and is the preferred treatment for this reason. Subcutaneous heparin is adequate and heparin levels should be monitored.

SUMMARY

ASA appears to be of benefit in women with TIAs or strokes who have no indication for warfarin. Ticlopidine may be used for patients who remain symptomatic on ASA; however, the need for close monitoring of the complete blood count has limited its use.

Symptomatic carotid stenosis, if uncomplicated, should proceed to endarterectomy. Management of asymptomatic stenosis is an unsettled issue. Many vascular surgeons will operate on high-grade (>90%) or progressive stenoses that are clinically silent, but this practice has not been universally accepted. Data to determine the results of asymptomatic carotid endarterectomy are currently being collected.

Oral contraceptives are generally made with low estrogen content and are not considered to pose a significant risk for stroke in the absence of other stroke risk factors. There may be some increased risk for subarachnoid hemorrhage in smokers.

Postmenopausal estrogen administration does not appear to increase the risk for stroke in the absence of other risk factors for stroke.

Brain hemorrhages are neurologic emergencies because they can elevate intracranial pressure and lead to brain herniation and death. Urgent neurosurgical consultation should be obtained, even if a patient is pregnant, because intensive monitoring, evacuation of a clot, or surgical clipping of an aneurysm may often be necessary.

Head CT without contrast is the image of choice for scanning a pregnant woman who has sudden neurologic deficits.

BIBLIOGRAPHY

Ameri A, Bousser MG: Cerebral venous thrombosis, *Neurol Clin* 10:87, 1992.

Barnett HJM et al: Further evidence relating mitral valve prolapse to cerebral ischemic events, *N Engl J Med* 302:135, 1980.

Bogousslavsky J, Pierre P: Ischemic stroke in patients under age 45, *Neurol Clin* 10:113, 1992.

Bonita R: Epidemiology of stroke, *Lancet* 339:342, 1992.

Caplan LR: Diagnosis and treatment of ischemic stroke, *JAMA* 266:2413, 1991.

Caplan LR, Gorelick PB, Hier DB: Race, sex and occlusive cerebrovascular disease: a review, *Stroke* 17:648, 1986.

Colditz GA et al: Cigarette smoking and risk of stroke in middle-aged women, *N Engl J Med* 318:937, 1988.

Collaborative Group for the Study of Stroke in Young Women: Oral contraceptives and stroke in young women, *JAMA* 231:718, 1975.

Cross JN, Castro PO, Jennett WB: Cerebral strokes associated with pregnancy and the puerperium, *Br Med J* 3:214, 1968.

DiTullio M et al: Patent foramen ovale as a risk factor for cryptogenic stroke, *Ann Intern Med* 117:461, 1992.

Dunbabin DW, Sandercock PAG: Preventing stroke by the modification of risk factors, *Stroke* 21(suppl IV):iv36, 1990.

Dyken ML et al: Low-dose aspirin and stroke, *Stroke* 23:1395, 1992.

Ezekowitz MD et al: Warfarin and the prevention of stroke associated with nonrheumatic atrial fibrillation, *N Engl J Med* 327:1406, 1992.

Flora GC et al: A comparative study of cerebral atherosclerosis in males and females, *Circulation* 38:859, 1968.

The Framingham Study: Epidemiologic Assessment of the Role of Blood Pressure in Stroke, *JAMA* 214:301, 1970.

Gurwitt LJ, Long JM, Clark RE: Cerebral metastatic choriocarcinoma, *Obstet Gynecol* 45:583, 1975.

Hass WK et al: A randomized trial comparing ticlopidine hydrochloride with aspirin for the prevention of stroke in high-risk patients, *N Engl J Med* 321:501, 1989.

Howie PW: Anticoagulants in pregnancy, *Clin Obstet Gynaecol* 13(2):349, 1986.

Kannel WB, Gordon J, Dawber TR: Role of lipids in the development of brain infarction: the Framingham Study, *Stroke* 5:679, 1974.

Longstreth WT Jr, Swanson PD: Oral contraceptives and stroke, *Stroke* 15(4):747, 1984.

Manson JE et al: A prospective study of maturity-onset diabetes mellitus and risk of coronary heart disease and stroke in women, *Arch Intern Med* 151:1141, 1991.

Mantello MT et al: Imaging of neurologic complications associated with pregnancy, *Am J Roentgenol* 160(4):843, 1993.

Marks AR et al: Identification of high-risk and low-risk subgroups of patients with mitral-valve prolapse, *N Engl J Med* 320(16):1031, 1989.

Marmot MG, Poulter NR: Primary prevention of stroke, *Lancet* 339:344, 1992.

McNally LE, Corn CR, Hamilton SF: Aspirin for the prevention of vascular death in women, *Ann Pharmacother* 26(12):1530, 1992.

North American Symptomatic Carotid Endarterectomy Trial Collaborators (NASCET): Beneficial effect of carotid endarterectomy in symptomatic patients with high-grade stenosis, *N Engl J Med* 325:445, 1991.

Rothrock JF et al: Migrainous stroke, *Arch Neurol* 45:63, 1988.

Sadasivan B et al: Vascular malformations and pregnancy, *Surg Neurol* 33:305, 1990.

Schwartz RB: Neurodiagnostic imaging of the pregnant patient. Presented at New York University School of Medicine Conference on Neurologic Complications of Pregnancy, New York, Sept 18-19, 1992.

Sheehan HL, Stanfield JP: The pathogenesis of postpartum necrosis of the anterior lobe of the pituitary gland, *Acta Endocrinol* 37:479, 1961.

Stampfer MJ et al: A prospective study of moderate alcohol consumption and the risk of coronary disease and stroke in women, *N Engl J Med* 319:267, 1988.

Stampfer MJ et al: Postmenopausal estrogen therapy and cardiovascular disease: ten-year follow-up from the nurses' health study, *N Engl J Med* 325(11):756, 1991.

Steering Committee of the Physicians' Health Study Research Group: Final report of the aspirin component of the ongoing physicians' health study, *N Engl J Med* 321:129, 1989.

Sullivan JM, Ramanathan KB: Management of medical problems in pregnancy: severe cardiac disease, *N Engl J Med* 313:304, 1985.

Tatemichi TK, Mohr JP: Migraine and stroke. In Barnett HJM, editor: *Stroke,* vol 2.

Wolf PA, Kannell WB, McGee DL: Prevention of ischemic stroke: risk factors. In Barnett HJM, editor: *Stroke,* vol 2.

Wong MCW, Giulani MJ, Haley EC: Cerebrovascular disease and stroke in women, *Cardiology* 77(suppl):80, 1990.

6 Vascular Disorders

Susan M. Briggs

The true incidence and prevalence of peripheral vascular disease in women are unknown as many individuals may be asymptomatic or may present with atypical symptoms. Most studies in the literature have focused only on symptomatic women with claudication, rest pain, gangrene, or deep venous thrombosis. Nevertheless, some unique characteristics relating to the epidemiologic features, morbidity, and mortality of vascular disease in women have been described.

ARTERIAL DISEASE
Epidemiology

Traditional assessments of peripheral vascular disease in women have utilized intermittent claudication rates to determine the prevalence of vascular disease in women and male/female ratios of disease. In 1985 Criqui et al. reported intermittent claudication rates of 2.2% in men and 1.7% in women (average age 66 years). Pulse abnormalities, however, as assessed by noninvasive testing in the same group of patients, were significantly higher, reflecting occult peripheral vascular disease. Through noninvasive tests, 20.3% of men and 22.1% of women exhibited abnormalities in femoral or posterior tibial pulses. The true incidence of vascular disease in women has probably been underestimated in past studies reported in the literature.

Peripheral arterial disease, like stroke and coronary artery disease, occurs at a later age in women than in men. The important factors underlying the delayed onset of atherosclerosis in women are not well understood, but hormonal influences, particularly the effect of estrogen, are thought to be a significant factor. It is intriguing to speculate whether future studies will demonstrate a proven benefit of estrogen therapy on peripheral disease in postmenopausal women.

Risk factors for atherosclerosis in women include genetic factors, diabetes mellitus, hypertension, hyperlipidemia, and low levels of high-density lipoprotein (HDL). Several studies, including the Framingham Study, have demonstrated that the relative impact of diabetes on peripheral atherosclerotic disease may be greater for diabetic women than for diabetic men. In a series of nondiabetic patients with symptoms of vascular disease before age 60 years only 8% were women. By contrast, in diabetic women with vascular disease the male/female ratio in symptomatic patients was nearly equal for all sites of vascular disease. Peripheral vascular disease in diabetic women is more extensive than in nondiabetic women and often involves the tibial-peroneal vessels. Rest pain, ulceration, and gangrene are more common presentations of vascular disease in diabetic than nondiabetic women, and the amputation rate is significantly higher.

A consistent relationship between smoking and chronic lower extremity ischemia in women and men has been documented in numerous studies, and no significant sex differences have been well documented.

Pathophysiology

Atherosclerotic vascular disease. The characteristic pathologic finding in atherosclerosis is intimal proliferation of smooth muscle cells. Associated findings include invasion of the damaged intima by macrophages and accumulation of large amounts of connective tissue matrix and lipid. Pathologic manifestations of atherosclerotic disease present a spectrum from stenotic lesions to aneurysmal disease.

Nonatherosclerotic vascular disease. Although the majority of vascular disease in women is atherosclerotic, a significant number have nonatherosclerotic vascular disease. The main classes of nonatherosclerotic vascular disease are illustrated in the box below. Those diseases that demonstrate a female preponderance will be discussed in further detail in this section.

Immune arteritis: giant cell arteritis group. Immune arteritis, or vasculitis, is usually associated with the deposition of antigen-antibody immune complexes on the vascular endothelium, resulting in arterial wall damage. The term *arteritis* denotes a necrotizing transmural inflammation of the arterial wall. The giant cell arteritis group includes two conditions, temporal arteritis and Takayasu's arteritis, which are more common in women than men. The box on the following page contrasts the major differences between the two entities of giant cell arteritis.

Fibromuscular dysplasia. Fibromuscular dysplasia is an arterial developmental abnormality characterized by eccentric stenoses with intervening areas of dilation. Four distinct pathologic types have been identified:

1. Intimal fibroplasia
2. Medial fibroplasia
3. Medial hyperplasia
4. Perimedial fibroplasia

NONATHEROSCLEROTIC VASCULAR DISEASE

Immune arteritis
  Polyarteritis nodosa group
  Hypersensitivity arteritis group
    (includes arteritis of collagen vascular disease)
  Giant cell arteritis*
  Buerger's disease
Radiation-induced arterial damage
Arterial infections
Fibromuscular dysplasia*
Adventitial cystic disease
Popliteal entrapment syndromes
Congenital conditions affecting arteries
Hyperviscosity syndromes
Diseases affecting the arterial media
Homocysteinemia

---

*Denotes female predominance.

GIANT CELL ARTERITIS

Temporal arteritis

Elderly white female
3:1 Female/male ratio
Propensity for carotid artery and branches but may
  involve any artery
Complication: Visual disturbances (blindness)

Therapy:	Steroids
Differential:	Atherosclerosis
Diagnosis:	Elevated erythrocyte sedimentation rate, temporal artery biopsy

Takayasu's arteritis

Young Asian female
8.5:1 Female/male ratio
Propensity for aortic arch and branches, pulmonary
  artery, abdominal aorta and branches

Complications:	Cardiovascular/neurologic (hypertension/stroke)
Therapy:	Conservative
Differential:	Atherosclerosis
Diagnosis:	Fever, myalgias, anorexia, cardiovascular symptoms, angiography

Ninety percent of patients with fibromuscular dysplasia are female. The box, below left, indicates the key features of the disease.

Vasospastic diseases

Raynaud's phenomenon. Raynaud's phenomenon is characterized by episodic attacks of digital ischemia caused by cold exposure or emotional stimuli. Attacks may occur in individuals without associated diseases (primary Raynaud's disease) or with a variety of local or systemic diseases. Patients with Raynaud's phenomenon often have a triad of intermittent color changes (pallor, cyanosis, rubor) in response to cold or emotional stimuli.

Raynaud's phenomenon may be associated with occlusive vascular disease. The collagen vascular diseases, such as scleroderma, may manifest themselves by the presence of Raynaud's phenomenon. Raynaud's phenomenon is seen in approximately 20% of patients with systemic lupus erythematosus. Most individuals with diffuse scleroderma and Raynaud's phenomenon are women. The presence of digital gangrene in a young woman without evidence of atherosclerosis, particularly with normal upper extremity segmental pressures, should alert the physician to the presence of collagen vascular disease. The box, below right, lists conditions associated with Raynaud's phenomenon.

Raynaud's disease. Primary Raynaud's disease is a vasospastic phenomenon that occurs without associated local or systemic disease and primarily involves the digital

arterioles of the hands and feet. Involvement is usually bilateral and symmetric. The cause of the disease is unknown, but it is seen most frequently in women below the age of 40 years. The disease varies in severity but may progress to extremely painful ulcerations and gangrene. Treatment is conservative with amputations only in cases of severe gangrene of the digits. Vasodilators, such as nifedipine, have been used with limited success but may be tried in women with severe Raynaud's disease.

Acrocyanosis. Acrocyanosis is characterized by coolness and cyanosis of the digits and is often painless. The pathophysiologic features of the disease are unknown, but the condition is seen most commonly in women. Symptoms are more pronounced in cold weather but may be present, to a lesser degree, in warm weather. Treatment is symptomatic and vasodilators, such as nifedipine, have been effective in some women in relieving symptoms.

Livedo reticularis. Livedo reticularis is a vasospastic phenomenon, present mostly in women, characterized by bluish red discoloration of the skin of the lower extremities and hands and arms. The pathologic abnormality is thrombosis of the digital arteries with dilation of the capillaries and venules. Coldness, dull aching, and painful leg and foot ulcers of the extremity may occur, especially during the winter months. Treatment is symptomatic, and vasodilator drugs may occasionally be useful in the treatment of symptomatic women.

FIBROMUSCULAR DYSPLASIA

Incidence:	9:1 Female/male ratio
Abnormality:	Majority of cases involve renal artery (80% of cases involve right renal artery), carotid and iliac arteries also frequently involved
	Medial hyperplasia most common subtype
Cause:	Unknown
Complications:	Renovascular hypertension/transient cerebral ischemic attacks
Therapy:	Bypass grafting, percutaneous transluminal angioplasty
Differential:	Atherosclerosis
Diagnosis:	Angiography

CONDITIONS ASSOCIATED WITH RAYNAUD'S PHENOMENON

Thromboangiitis obliterans
Occupational trauma
Collagen diseases
  Scleroderma
  Dermatomyositis
  Systemic lupus erythematosus
  Polyarteritis
Frostbite, immersion foot
Sympathetic hyperactivity
Thoracic outlet syndrome
Causalgia
Cryoglobulinemia
Cold agglutinins

Differential diagnosis

Atherosclerotic vascular disease presents a wide range of symptoms from intermittent claudication, rest pain, and gangrene to embolic phenomena and aneurysmal disease. The major differential diagnoses in suspected atherosclerotic vascular disease in women are **nonatherosclerotic vascular disease,** particularly immune, arteritis and hypersensitivity arteritis, and the **vasospastic disorders.** Atherosclerosis is significantly less common in the upper extremities than in the lower extremities. Digital ischemia in the upper extremities most often results from vasospastic disorders such as Raynaud's disease, acrocyanosis, livedo reticularis, or Raynaud's phenomenon.

Venous disease of the extremities may mimic many of the symptoms of arterial occlusive disease such as pain and cyanosis. More commonly, however, arterial and venous disease may both be present in the affected extremity. Edema and stasis changes in the extremity should alert the physician to the presence of venous disease. Noninvasive arterial and venous studies will usually differentiate between the two entities.

Diagnostic testing. Numerous noninvasive tests are now available to evaluate the extent of arterial occlusive disease in women and to estimate the physiologic significance of such disease. The development of sophisticated tests such as magnetic resonance imaging (MRI) and magnetic resonance angiography (MRA) has eliminated the need for invasive angiography in many cases.

Indirect arterial pressure measurements. Noninvasive recording of extremity systolic blood pressure, using a pneumatic cuff and flow sensor (i.e., Doppler ultrasound velocity detector), is the simplest method of screening for peripheral arterial disease. Segmental blood pressure measurements allow localization of the approximate site of occlusive disease and provide a rough estimation of the extent of disease. In the lower extremity the segmental pressure measurements are performed by applying blood pressure cuffs to the thigh, to the upper calf, and above the ankle. Gradients of more than 30 mm Hg between the measurement sites suggest significant occlusive disease.

Several important limitations of the test must be kept in mind when evaluating the results. The test only measures occlusive lesions that reduce systolic blood pressure. Early occlusive arterial disease may not be detected by this method. Patients with abnormal stiffness of the arterial wall, usually from calcification, may exhibit artificially elevated extremity systolic pressures. Diabetics frequently have extensive calcification of the tibial-peroneal vessels and manifest abnormally high extremity systolic pressures. The severity of the occlusive disease is often underestimated in such cases. Finally, the size of the cuff applied to the extremity must be appropriate for the extremity as too narrow a cuff will give erroneously high pressure readings.

Measurement of the ankle pressure and the ankle pressure index are extremely valuable in evaluating the extent of occlusive disease and the likelihood that the patient's symptoms are related to arterial occlusive disease. The posterior tibial and dorsalis pedis arteries are easily measured by Doppler ultrasound. Normally peak systolic pressures increase in the lower limb as the pulse wave progresses distally. Thus ankle pressures lower than arm pressures (brachial artery measurement) suggest arterial occlusive disease. The ankle pressure divided by the arm pressure is called the ankle pressure index (AI) and should be greater than 1.0 in the absence of occlusive disease. Patients with intermittent claudication generally have an AI of 0.4 to 0.9. Patients with rest pain generally exhibit an AI of 0.3 or below. Changes in the AI with treadmill exercise testing can also be measured to delineate further the severity of the vascular disease. An AI above 1.3 or AIs that do not correlate with the severity of the patient's symptoms suggest abnormal stiffness of the arterial vessels.

Segmental plethysmography. The total blood volume of the extremity increases during systole and returns to baseline during diastole. The pulse volume recorder provides a qualitative recording of such volume changes in the extremity. Increasing severity of stenotic lesions results in loss of the dicrotic notch and flattening of the curve. As a screening modality the pulse volume recorder is used in conjunction with segmental Doppler pressure measurements.

Duplex scanning. The duplex scanning concept is a combination of real-time B-mode scanning and a pulsed Doppler device. In patients with arterial disease it is used mainly to document patency of arterial vessels, provide an estimation of the degree of stenosis, and detect arteriovenous fistulas.

Angiography. Angiography remains the gold standard for the precise delineation of the extent and anatomic location of occlusive disease of the extremity. However, the introduction of noninvasive imaging of the extremities by MRI and MRA has allowed the use of these modalities in many patients as a screening test and, with increasing frequency, as a diagnostic modality, especially in patients with renal disease, in whom injection of angiographic contrast dye presents a significant risk of renal failure.

Management of occlusive vascular disease

Early identification of women with asymptomatic vascular disease or risk factors for vascular disease is essential to decrease the incidence of significant complications of arterial disease, such as ulcerations, gangrene, and limb loss. Figures 6-1 and 6-2 illustrate guidelines for the initial management of women with symptoms of arterial disease. Pentoxifylline (Trental) has been proved effective only for the treatment of intermittent claudication, not rest pain or gangrene. No other vasodilators have been shown to be effective in the treatment of chronic lower extremity ischemia.

VENOUS DISEASE
Epidemiology

Venous disease of the extremities may be classified as acute thromboembolic disease or chronic venous insufficiency. Chronic venous insufficiency may be subdivided into primary varicose veins, superficial venous incompetence, and deep venous incompetence. Chronic venous disease occurs more frequently in women. Acute venous thromboembolic disease has been reported with equal frequency in women and men.

Pathophysiology

Venous thromboembolic disease. Virchow's triad of stasis, hypercoagulability, and injury to the vessel wall has

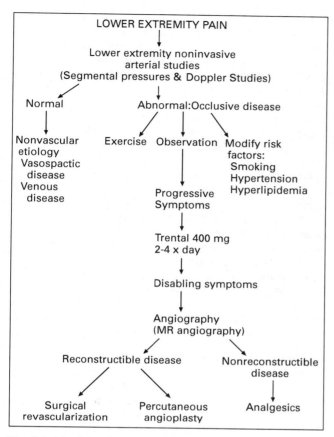

Fig. 6-1 Algorithm for management of lower extremity pain and suspected arterial occlusive disease.

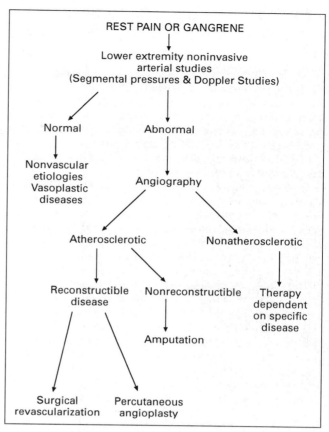

Fig. 6-2 Algorithm for management of rest pain and suspected arterial occlusive disease.

been postulated to predispose individuals to venous thromboembolic disease. Major venous thrombosis usually involves the deep venous systems of the lower extremities and pelvis. Risk factors for deep venous thrombosis (DVT) include surgical procedures, especially orthopedic operations, trauma, use of oral contraceptive pills, malignancies, and sepsis. High-dose estrogen oral contraceptives have been demonstrated to increase the risk of DVT. No such increased risk has been demonstrated with the lower-dose oral contraceptives. Estrogens increase levels of various blood procoagulant factors, which are presumed to influence the risk of DVT in women.

In a significant number of individuals with DVT, chronic venous insufficiency will eventually develop to some degree. Some studies have estimated that as many as 50% of individuals with DVT will have some evidence of chronic venous insufficiency such as edema, stasis dermatitis, induration, fibrosis, ulcerations, or pain in the affected extremity.

Serious complications of DVT include pulmonary thromboembolism, phlegmasia cerulea dolens, and venous gangrene. Of pulmonary emboli 90% originate in the lower extremities. The exact incidence of pulmonary emboli after DVT in women is unknown.

Acute massive venous thrombosis of the extremity may lead to limb-threatening arterial ischemia, followed by loss of sensory and motor function. Ischemic venous thrombosis may present with two clinical entities that are potentially

reversible if treated early, phlegmasia alba dolens and phlegmasia cerulea dolens. **Phlegmasia alba dolens** is characterized by mild pain, pitting edema, and blanching of the extremity. The hallmarks of **phlegmasia cerulea dolens,** or "painful blue leg," are severe pain, massive edema, and cyanosis, usually caused by complete occlusion of the iliofemoral venous system. Pulmonary embolus and hypovolemic shock may complicate phlegmasia cerulea dolens. Prompt treatment with elevation of the extremity, anticoagulation with heparin, fibrinolysis, and, most frequently, venous thrombectomy with fasciotomy remain the therapeutic modalities of choice. Venous gangrene is the terminal, irreversible stage of massive venous thrombosis of the extremity and may result in amputation. Venous gangrene usually develops within 7 days of the initial symptoms of extremity ischemia.

Chronic venous insufficiency. The lower extremity venous system may be divided into the superficial system (greater and lesser saphenous veins), perforating system (communicating veins), and deep system. Most chronic venous insufficiency is due to incompetency of deep system and perforating system venous valves. Primary varicose veins are due to superficial venous incompetency of the greater and lesser saphenous veins and branches. Genetic and hormonal influences have been demonstrated to influence the prevalence of varicose veins in women. Many women note a marked increase in symptoms of venous disease related to the effect of progesterone during the latter half of their menstrual cycle. Progesterone causes passive dilation of varicosities secondary to the effect of venous hypertension.

Differential diagnosis

The major differential diagnoses in the evaluation of venous disease are **occlusive arterial disease** and the **vasospastic diseases.** Lower extremity arterial noninvasive studies usually distinguish between the two entities, especially in the presence of edema and stasis changes. Nonvascular diseases such as **neuropathic diseases** and **musculoskeletal diseases** may mimic venous disease.

Once the diagnosis of venous disease is clear, the main diagnostic question is whether or not the varicosities are confined to the superficial system and are curable by compression stockings, sclerotherapy, or surgical therapy or are the end consequence of DVT with inadequate collateral circulation development. In the latter case palliative therapy, not curative therapy, remains the only course.

Diagnostic tests. Numerous noninvasive tests are available for the diagnosis of venous disease. The Doppler venous examination and duplex scan are the most frequently utilized noninvasive venous tests at present. Other tests, such as impedance plethysmography and phleborheography, are used for the diagnosis of acute venous disease but are less useful in the diagnosis of chronic venous insufficiency. Photoplethysmography may be used as an alternative to Doppler venous studies for the detection of chronic venous insufficiency.

Doppler venous examination. Doppler examination is performed with directional instruments that may measure forward or reverse flow. In the lower extremity the femoral, popliteal, and saphenous venous systems may be evaluated. Venous incompetency is demonstrated by retrograde flow during inspiration. Compression maneuvers and responses to Valsalva's maneuver may be used to detect the extent of venous obstruction and valvular incompetence further. A negative Doppler examination result is valuable as a screening test but an equivocal or positive test finding should be followed by more sophisticated screening.

Duplex ultrasound. Real-time B-mode ultrasonography has become the single most useful screening test for DVT. A negative duplex ultrasound result is highly accurate and further testing is usually not indicated. Equivocal duplex scan findings should be followed by further testing, usually a venogram. A venogram is usually not necessary in the diagnosis of DVT if the Doppler ultrasound result is positive.

Venogram. Ascending venography (more common) and descending venography (less common) may be used for the diagnosis of deep venous patency and perforator patency and competence. Descending venography is most useful to delineate the state of the venous valves.

Management of venous disease

Acute venous thrombosis is treated with anticoagulation with heparin followed by 3 to 6 months of warfarin (Coumadin) therapy. In the presence of extremity swelling compression stockings should be used. Support pantyhose rather than constricting below-the-knee support stockings are often most effective in controlling the edema. Support stockings can be ordered with zippers to facilitate their use by women who have difficulty in putting on the stockings, such as those with severe arthritic conditions. Stockings should be applied in the morning before swelling with ambulation occurs. Vena caval filters are used only when an individual has recurrent pulmonary emboli in the presence of adequate anticoagulation or when medical contraindications to anticoagulation exist.

Symptoms of chronic venous insufficiency are usually due to venous valvular incompetency of the deep and/or perforating venous system. Edema, especially at the end of the day; stasis dermatitis (eczema); pain; and ulcerations are

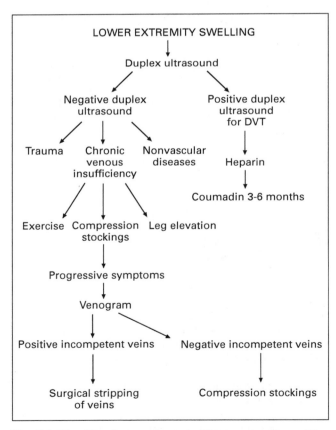

Fig. 6-3 Algorithm for management of lower extremity swelling and suspected venous disease.

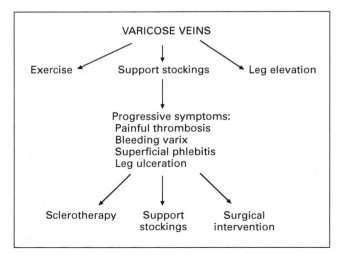

Fig. 6-4 Algorithm for management of varicose veins.

common manifestations of chronic venous insufficiency. Long-standing stasis dermatitis and edema may result in induration and fibrosis of tissues in the affected extremity. Skin changes of chronic venous disease are often most obvious in the region of the medial malleolus.

Compression stockings are the mainstay of treatment for chronic venous insufficiency. Indications for surgical therapy are recurrent superficial thrombophlebitis, bleeding varix, painful thrombosis of the superficial saphenous venous system, and ulcerations of the extremity. In the presence of DVT excision and stripping of the greater saphenous system may result in disabling edema and are usually contraindicated. Sclerotherapy and the newer laser surgery techniques are most useful for superficial varicose veins and are usually performed for cosmetic reasons. Figures 6-3 and 6-4 illustrate guidelines for the management of venous disease in women.

Management of venous thromboembolic disease in pregnancy is discussed in Chapter 58.

SUMMARY

Peripheral vascular disease, both arterial and venous, continues to be a challenging diagnostic dilemma in women. Careful history and physical examination, combined with noninvasive testing, usually elucidate the cause of the vascular insufficiency. Invasive testing is usually not indicated before consideration of surgical intervention.

BIBLIOGRAPHY

Anderson FA et al: A population-based perspective of the hospital incidence and case-fatality rates of deep vein thrombosis and pulmonary embolism, *Arch Intern Med* 151: 933, 1991.

Becker RC: Cardiovascular disease in women: introductory article, *Cardiology* 77 (Suppl):1, 1990.

Colditz GA et al: Cigarette smoking and risk of stroke in middle-aged women, *N Engl J Med* 318:937, 1988.

Criqui MH: Peripheral arterial disease and subsequent cardiovascular mortality: a strong and consistent association, *Circulation* 82:2246, 1990.

Criqui MH et al: The prevalence of peripheral arterial disease in a defined population, *Circulation* 7 1:510, 1985.

Criqui MH et al: Mortality over 10 years in patients with peripheral arterial disease, *N Engl J Med* 326:381, 1992.

Douglas PS: *Cardiovascular health and disease in women*, Philadelphia, 1993, WB Saunders.

Gerstman BB et al: Oral contraceptive oestrogen and progestin potencies and the incidence of deep venous thromboembolism, *Int J Epidemiol* 19(4):931, 1990.

Gillum RF: Peripheral arterial occlusive disease of the extremities in the United States: hospitalization and mortality, *Am Heart J* 120:1414, 1990.

Haimovici H: *Vascular surgery principles and techniques,* ed 3, Norwalk, Conn, 1993, Appleton & Lange.

Helmrich SP et al: Venous thromboembolism in relation to oral contraceptive use, *Obstet Gynecol* 69:91, 1987.

Kannel WB et al: Intermittent claudication: incidence in the Framingham study, *Circulation* 41:875, 1970.

Kerr TM et al: Analysis of 1084 consecutive lower extremities involved with acute venous thrombosis diagnosed by duplex scanning, *Surgery* 108:520, 1990.

Manson JE et al: A prospective study of aspirin use and primary prevention of cardiovascular disease in women, *JAMA* 266:521, 1991.

Moore WS: *Vascular surgery: a comprehensive review*, Philadelphia, 1991, WB Saunders.

Schroll M, Munck O: Estimation of peripheral arteriosclerotic disease by ankle blood pressure: measurements in a population study of 60-year old men and women, *J Chronic Dis* 34:261, 1981.

Scribner RG, Brown WH, Tawes RL: *Decision making in vascular surgery*, Toronto, 1987, Decker.

Wong MCW, Giuliani MJ, Haley C: Cerebrovascular disease and stroke in women, *Cardiology* 77(Suppl 2):80, 1990.

DERMATOLOGY

7 Common Dermatologic Problems

Lynn A. Baden and Stephanie A. Eisenstat

Problems related to the skin are commonly seen in the primary care office. Many of the visits that female patients make to the internist are related to a dermatologic complaint. Some of these conditions occur more frequently in women whereas others, seen exclusively in the female population. Most of the conditions seen exclusively in women are related mostly to hormonal changes associated with pregnancy or the postpartum state.

The purpose of this chapter is to review the more common dermatologic problems seen in women. For a more detailed discussion of all the possible dermatologic presentations, the reader is referred to standard textbooks.

PROMOTION OF HEALTHY SKIN

So often in the office the patient asks, "What can I do to promote normal healthy skin?" Just like any other organ, the skin needs nutrients. Balanced nutrition and exercise have been shown to promote healthy skin. On the other hand, excessive alcohol consumption, cigarette smoking, and rapid and frequent weight fluctuations can lead to deleterious and cosmetic changes, such as wrinkles and furrows, as well as predispose the person to more serious conditions such as skin cancer. Sun protection with sunscreens and avoidance of the sun between the hours of 10 AM and 2 PM are the most important factors in good skin health and the maintenance of skin to prevent these cosmetic changes and, more important, to prevent skin cancer.

PHYSIOLOGY

To better understand the skin changes that develop in women, it is helpful to understand the normal physiology of the skin and the effects that the reproductive cycle and aging have on the skin.

Effects of aging

The skin consists of two layers: the outer epidermis and the inner dermis. The stratum corneum is the outermost layer of the epidermis and is nonliving. Along with the entire epidermis, it is renewed every 3 weeks. It is this constant renewal that keeps the appearance of the skin youthful. In elderly persons this period of renewal is extended to 4 to 6 weeks, which results in thickening and yellowing of the skin, causing it to feel leathery. The inner layer or dermis is made up predominantly of blood vessels, nerves, sebaceous glands,

and fibrous tissue. The fibrous tissue is composed of 70% collagen and 30% elastin. Aging of this layer is correlated with disorganization of the collagen and elastin. These changes result in thinning of the dermis and the development of furrows, wrinkles, easy bruisability, and the appearance of telangiectasia. Not only time and gravity but sun exposure and cigarette smoking also have a deleterious effect on the dermis. Clinically, aged skin, whatever the cause, is sallow, leathery, unevenly pigmented, and furrowed.

APPROACH TO THE PATIENT WITH AGING CHANGES OF THE SKIN

There is some practical advice the clinician can give the woman who asks about interventions for the photoaging changes of the skin. In addition to sun protection, use of topical **retinoic acid (Retin-A)** has shown some benefit. The mechanism of action is that the drug accelerates cell turnover, stimulates blood vessel growth, and normalizes the collagen and elastin composition of the skin. This medication is FDA-approved for use in acne but not for photoaging. It appears to be helpful in improving fine lines but is less effective for furrows. Advice on proper application and the concomitant use of sunscreen is important because of the side effects of irritation and increased sun sensitivity. Alpha-hydroxy acids are a group of fruit-derived acids that on application are also useful in reversing some of the damaging effects of the sun and aging. The mechanism of action is likely similar to that of isotretinoic acid.

COMMON DISORDERS OF THE SKIN
Acne vulgaris and related disorders

Acne vulgaris. One of the most common disorders is acne vulgaris. It is estimated that 17 million persons, most of whom are female, have some form of acne, although the more severe cystic cases tend to occur in men. The average age of onset is 10 to 17 years; however, many women are not affected until adulthood. In many cases improvement of the acne occurs by the age of 35. Some women experience worsening of their acne during pregnancy whereas others note improvement.

A common misconception, unconfirmed in studies, is that certain foods such as greasy foods and chocolate are the cause for acne. In fact, most clinicians believe there is no relationship between dietary habits and outbreaks of acne. The cause is probably multifactorial. Defects in keratin production, obstruction of the follicular opening, increased sebum production, and overgrowth of the anaerobic bacteria *Propionibacterium acnes* contribute to the formation of acne. The production of sebum is a hormonally sensitive process, particularly androgen-sensitive. At the level of the follicle, androgen derivatives act to increase sebaceous gland size and activity whereas estrogens decrease activity. Certain drugs such as lithium or prednisone may cause acne.

Clinical presentation. The primary skin lesions of acne are comedones, papules, blackheads and whiteheads (blackheads contain oxidized keratin, not dirt). Depending on the degree of inflammation the papules of acne may progress to pustules, nodules, or cysts. Lesions are most common in areas of the body high in sebum production such as the T-zone of the face, chest, and back. (See Plate 1 of the front feature section.)

History. The first evaluation of a patient with acne should comprise a thorough history that covers age of onset, previous successful and unsuccessful treatments, and use of drugs, including oral contraceptives. The regularity of menses and any associated hirsutism should be determined so that the clinician can decide if there is a need to screen for underlying endocrine abnormalities, using tests such as free testosterone and dehydroepiandrosterone sulfate (DHEAS) levels.

Choice of therapy (Table 7-1). For mild acne, the clinician can suggest nonprescription benzoyl peroxides, salicylic acids, or alpha-hydroxy acids. If these agents are not successful, topical antibiotics may be added (clindamycin 2% or erythromycin 1%). More recalcitrant cases require oral antibiotics such as erythromycin, tetracycline, doxycycline, or minocycline. It is important to advise patients that the tetracyclines may interfere with the efficacy of the birth control pill; thus an additional means of birth control should be used. Retin-A (retinoic acid), which is the most effective topical medication for the treatment of comedonal acne, also is useful for inflammatory lesions. In addition to its irritative characteristic, it causes increased sun sensitivity. Specific instructions for use must be given.

For severe acne with a significant cystic component, oral 13-*cis*-retinoic acid (Accutane) is an option; however, many precautions apply to the use of this drug because of side effects. Accutane can produce significant and sometimes permanent clearing of lesions, even in cystic conditions. It probably works by reducing sebum production, altering keratinization, and reducing inflammation. Common side effects include dry skin, eyes, and mucous membranes; vertebral hyperostosis and abnormalities of the musculoskeletal system; and elevated liver function tests and lipid levels. It is also teratogenic, causing severe fetal craniofacial and cardiac malformations, as well as central nervous system anomalies. Because of these potentially serious side effects, strict guidelines regulate the use of Accutane, including informed consent, monthly blood evaluations, a negative result on a pretreatment pregnancy test, and use of contraception, preferably systemic. (For a more detailed discussion of Accutane, see the references at the end of this chapter.)

The combined use of daily oral spironolactone 50 to 200 mg, higher estrogen–and lower androgen–dose oral contraceptive pills (one containing the ethinyl estradiol), and low-dose daily oral prednisone 5 mg are other therapeutic options.

Treatment of acne scars includes dermabrasion, chemical peels, cosmetic surgery, and the use of injectable filler materials such as bovine collagen.

Acne rosacea. Rosacea is an inflammatory disorder of the pilosebaceous glands of the face, which results in flushing, telangiectasia, papules, and pustules, most often of the central portion of the face. It is most common in women between 30 and 50 years of age. The lesions and the symptom of the sensation of warmth are worsened with heat, caffeine, alcohol, and exercise. The skin lesions can be associated with ophthalmologic complaints such as blepharitis, conjunctivitis, episcleritis, and rosacea keratitis.

Management is relatively straightforward, but the treatment options are not always successful. Continuous use of twice-daily oral tetracycline 500 mg is the conventional treatment. Topical metronidazole gel 0.75% (Metrogel) used twice daily is quite effective but can take up to 3 months to work. Because of this long onset of action, tetracycline, 500 mg twice daily for 6 weeks, often is used concomitantly.

Hidradenitis suppurativa. This disease is a chronic disorder of the sweat glands, which leads to large purulent

Table 7-1 Therapy for acne vulgaris

Type of acne	Treatment	Minimum response time
Comedonal	Benzoyl peroxide, 2.5%, 5%, or 10% lotion or gel	2 wk
	Tretinoin (Retin-A) topical (0.025%, 0.05%, 0.1%) qd	2 wk
Papulopustular	Treatment for comedonal, *plus* antibiotics:	
	Mild cases: topical	
	Erythromycin	Until inflammation subsides
	Clindamycin	
	Tetracycline	
	Metronidazole	
	Severe cases:	
	Tetracycline or erythromycin 500 mg to 1 g/day	For at least 6 wk, then taper
	Minocycline 100-200 mg qd	
Nodulocystic	Oral isotretinoin 0.5-1 mg/kg/day	Refer to dermatologist
	(equal to 13- acis-retinoic acid)	

Modified from Graber M: *The family practice handbook,* St Louis, 1994, Mosby.

cysts, abscesses, sinus tract formation, and eventually scarring. Because it occurs in areas rich in apocrine glands, the axillae, anogenital region, and in women the inframammary skin are involved. Treatment, which is difficult for this chronic debilitating disease, includes oral antibiotics, as well as the use of intralesional and sometimes systemic steroids. Accutane is used with some success. Surgical intervention, with excision of all involved glands, sometimes is necessary and desired by the patient.

Perioral dermatitis. This entity is a fairly common facial eruption seen almost exclusively in women between 15 and 40 years of age. It is characterized by tiny erythematous, monomorphous papules and pustules that occur in the nasolabial fold. The distribution is most commonly in the chin and perioral skin, extending to but not reaching the vermilion border. Treatment includes tetracycline, 500 mg twice daily for 6 weeks. Topical antibiotics such as metronidazole gel 0.75% twice daily or clindamycin gel are less effective. Topical steroids should be avoided because they exacerbate the problem.

Eczematous disorders

Lichen simplex chronicus. Lichenification of the skin comes from the physical trauma of chronic scratching. The lesions are thickened, hyperpigmented plaques with accentuated skin markings. After 20 years of age, it is more common in women. Commonly affected areas in women include the nuchal area, the legs, and the ankles. The lesions develop over weeks to months and are associated with intense itching. The condition commonly is associated with stress. Treatment consists of moisturizers, topical steroids, and antihistamines.

Stasis dermatitis. Stasis dermatitis is a chronic, progressive skin disorder of the lower extremity associated with vascular compromise. In women it is most common after the age of 50 years. The dermatitis develops over the course of months and is itchy, painful, and associated with swelling of the ankles and nocturnal cramps. Physical examination reveals erythematous scaling plaques with exudative discharge and crusts. There is a brown-red discoloration caused by hemosiderin deposit located around the ankle. Progressive disease is associated first with superficial erosions and later with ulceration. Management includes application of moisturizers, topical steroids, and drying agents if erosions have occurred (Burow's solution). When appropriate, antibiotics for cellulitis and zinc gelatin bandages or other specialized dressings for the ulceration are instituted. Appropriate use of support hose is important adjuvant therapy.

Skin cancer

There are three relatively common types of skin cancer: basal cell carcinoma, squamous cell carcinoma, and malignant melanoma. Melanoma is potentially fatal whereas the other two do not tend to metastasize and generally are considered curable.

Basal cell carcinomas are slow-growing localized skin tumors associated with chronic sun exposure. More than 500,000 cases per year occur in the United States. The incidence is slightly higher in men than in women; however, the distribution is somewhat different because of the gender differences in areas of the body exposed to the sun. The lesions tend to be asymptomatic and appear on sun-exposed areas as translucent pearly nodules with telangiectasia. Without treatment the lesions ulcerate and destroy underlying structures, but generally the lesions are excised with resolution of the problem.

Squamous cell carcinoma is also a sun-induced skin cancer. Women have a higher incidence of these lesions in the lower extremities. The lesions develop slowly and usually are asymptomatic. The skin manifestations are indurated papules or plaques with local erosion and erythema. Lesions on the lip have the highest risk of metastasizing. Treatment is surgical removal. Squamous cell skin cancer has a precursor lesion, the **actinic keratosis.** This is a thin red scaly plaque located in sun-exposed skin. The use of sunscreens and Retin-A may be preventive. Treatment includes topical 5-fluorouracil and cryotherapy. (See Plate 2 of the front feature section.)

Melanoma is a potentially fatal type of skin cancer that usually affects persons older than 70 years of age but is seen more frequently now in younger patients. Approximately 6500 people die each year in the United States from this disease. This trend has been attributed to changes in the patterns of lifetime sun exposure, specifically intense sun exposure and resultant sun damage in persons younger than 20 years of age. Men and women are affected in equal numbers, but the distribution sites are different; in women the most common sites of occurrence are the back and legs, especially the anterotibial aspect. There are four types of melanoma: superficial spreading, (70%), nodular (16%), acral lentiginous (7%), and lentigo maligna melanoma (5%).

Risk factors for the development of melanoma include congenital nevi, a family history of melanoma, excessive sun exposure as a child, and dysplastic nevi. *Dysplastic nevi* are atypical moles characterized by varied pigmentation, irregular borders, asymmetry, and a diameter greater than 6 mm. They have an increased malignancy potential. The **dysplastic nevus syndrome** is an inherited tendency toward the development of numerous abnormal moles, increasing one's risk for the development of melanoma. Women with dysplastic nevi syndrome and all others deemed at risk for melanoma should have yearly full-skin evaluations. Worrisome features of moles include the appearance of irregular borders, changes in the color of the mole, new nodules in a mole, and itching and bleeding. Any change in a mole should be followed up with an excisional biopsy by a dermatologist. The treatment of melonoma is beyond the scope of this book.

Mammary Paget's disease is an important cutaneous sign of an underlying intraductal breast malignancy. It is important to recognize this entity because it is mimicked by a much less serious condition, eczema of the nipple. Mammary Paget's disease is commonly a missed diagnosis. It is rare in males. The clinical presentation includes red scaling plaques, often with a moist base, localized to one nipple and areola. It may be indistinguishable from chronic eczematous dermatitis of the nipple. Diagnosis is made by biopsy when there is suspicion that an "eczema" does not respond within 1 to 2 weeks of use of a topical steroid cream. Treatment, after appropriate biopsy, is surgical removal.

Inflammatory disorders

Granuloma annulare. The localized form of this disorder, whose cause is unknown, is twice as common in women as in men. It occurs mostly in young adults. The lesions, which are quite characteristic, occur as an asymptomatic ring of firm red or flesh-colored papules that develop over a course of weeks. The most common locations include the dorsa of the hands, fingers, and feet. In 75% of cases the lesions disappear within 2 years. Therapy includes intralesional or superpotent topical steroids. (See Plate 3 of the front feature section.)

Lichen planus. Lichen planus is a characteristic condition of the skin and mucous membranes that occurs perhaps more frequently in women than in men between 30 and 60 years of age. Certain drugs can induce similar-appearing eruptions. The flexor wrists, forearms, shins, and ankles are most commonly involved and have characteristic purple, pruritic, polygonal papules and plaques, often with a lacy white reticular surface. Involvement of the mucous membranes reveals lacy, white, painful lesions on the mucosa, tongue, and lips. The lesions wax and wane for years. In the mucous membranes, especially, there is a risk for the development of carcinoma. Although some cases have resolved spontaneously, that is not the norm. Treatment is difficult but initially consists of topical corticosteroids and intralesional steroids. For more persistent lesions the use of psoralens plus ultraviolet A phototherapy and oral retinoid agents for the mouth lesions is helpful. (See Plate 4 of the front feature section.)

Morphea. Morphea is a localized sclerosis of the skin seen more commonly in women. It is not associated with systemic sclerosis, although uncommonly it can be quite extensive and generalized. The lesions of morphea begin as light purple plaques that become indurated. During this purple stage the lesions are considered active. With time they become thickened, white firm plaques. Some evidence suggests an association with spirochetes (*Borrelia burgdorferi*), and therefore tetracycline or doxycycline is used for treatment. In addition to antibiotics, treatment includes topical or intralesional steroids and reassurance.

Lichen sclerosus et atrophicus. This disease is seen 10 times more frequently in women than in men. Overall, the disease, which has a predilection for the anogenital region (see Chapter 31), manifests characteristic skin lesions. These lesions are smooth, white atrophic plaques with the classic cigarette paper-like surface. The lesions reveal follicular plugs known as *delling*. Available treatments are not particularly effective but include topical steroids.

Erythema nodosum. Erythema nodosum is an inflammatory disorder of the skin characterized by tender, red, warm nodules on the extensor surfaces, specifically the shins. It is seen three times more commonly in women and most often in those between 15 and 30 years of age. The etiology is unclear, but because it is associated with a number of underlying infections, illnesses, and drugs, erythema nodosum most likely is a cutaneous hypersensitivity manifestation of an underlying systemic process. A list of disorders associated with erythema nodosum appears in the box, above right. The lesions usually appear within days of exposure and have associated symptoms of fever, malaise, and arthralgia. Generally the skin manifestations resolve spontaneously over a 6-week period. Patients often can obtain symptomatic relief with leg elevation, antiinflammatory medications, or a saturated solution of potassium iodide.

Polymorphous light eruption (PMLE). PMLE is a cutaneous disorder seen much more commonly in women. It is characterized by extremely pruritic red papules, plaques,

---

DISORDERS ASSOCIATED WITH ERYTHEMA NODOSUM

Infectious agents	*Drugs*
Tuberculosis	Sulfonamides
Coccidioidomycosis	Oral contraceptives
Histoplasmosis	Sarcoidosis
Beta-hemolytic streptococci	Ulcerative colitis
Yersinia infections	
Lymphogranuloma venereum	

---

vesicles, and urticarial lesions emerging within minutes or up to 24 hours after exposure to sunlight. Most commonly PMLE is seen at the beginning of the warmer seasons or during tropical vacations during the winter months. There may be an element of "hardening" of the skin so that after many exposures the skin no longer erupts. Ultraviolet light in the UVA, UVB, and other bands can elicit this eruption so that sunscreens are not always preventive. Treatment includes topical steroids and oral antihistamines for itch. The use of antimalarial agents and phototherapy before known sun exposure, such as before a winter vacation or in early spring, are last resorts that sometimes are used.

DISORDERS OF THE HAIR
Androgenetic alopecia

Hair loss related to circulating androgens is seen in both men and women but is often more emotionally devastating in women because it is unexpected. Unlike men, women experience androgenetic alopecia (AGA) as vertex thinning; the temporal and frontal hairlines usually are maintained. The tendency to AGA is inherited, although in multifactorial and polygenic manner. Although some persons with AGA have an underlying endocrine imbalance, the more common scenario is the presence of a genetic predisposition for the hair follicles of the scalp to process androgens in such a way that normal circulating levels become elevated at the level of the follicle only. These locally elevated levels result in scalp alopecia.

Some cases of AGA are related to elevated peripheral androgens from adrenal or ovarian sources. If elevated peripheral levels of androgens occur, there may be associated hirsutism, acne vulgaris, and menstrual abnormalities. Important tests to consider in cases of AGA include free testosterone and dehydroepiandrosterone (DHEAS) sulfate. In addition, antinuclear antibody and thyroid-stimulating hormone results may help to exclude other possible causes.

Treatment for AGA includes twice-daily use of topical minoxidil 2% solution. Antiandrogens such as spironolactone and oral contraceptives high in estrogens are also effective in certain cases. Some women opt for hairpieces whereas others undergo hair transplantation.

Telogen effluvium

Telogen effluvium is a transient loss of hair caused by the transition of growing hairs into the resting state. The causes of this transition include parturition, major stressful life events, and illness. Diffuse and sometimes quite profound hair loss is noted not when the hairs go into the resting state but when the new hairs growing underneath push the resting ones out. The hair loss is first noted about 2 to 6 months after the causal event. Although not specifically a disease of women, it is more common in women because it is most often associated with the postpartum state. Regrowth is total, and reassurance is the only treatment.

PREGNANCY AND DERMATOLOGIC DISORDERS

Pathophysiology

The skin changes that are seen during pregnancy are related to the high levels of estrogen and progesterone. The hormones stimulate melanogenesis, which leads to hyperpigmentation. There are also changes in the vascular bed and alterations in the hair growth cycles. Certain changes most commonly seen in pregnancy also can occur in the nonpregnant women and in men.

Physiologic changes

Melasma. Melasma is facial pigmentation that develops in approximately 50% to 70% of pregnant women and in 5% to 34% of women taking an oral contraceptive pill. It is characterized by macular brown hyperpigmentation accentuated by sun exposure. The changes usually fade within 1 year after delivery; however, topical hydroquinone, Retin-A, and alpha-hydroxy acids are useful in treatment.

Striae gravidarum. These are "stretch marks" that develop during the course of pregnancy. Although the color of stretch marks fade, they remain after delivery. Retin-A may be useful in treatment.

Vascular changes. Various vascular changes occur during pregnancy, including spider angioma, palmar erythema, varicosities, and cutis marmorata (an increased skin response to the cold). Resolution may occur within 1 year postpartum. The use of support hose during pregnancy may help prevent severe varicosities. Sclerotherapy may be used for leg vein treatment.

Hair. There may be increased growth of hair during pregnancy, and telogen effluvium is common in the postpartum period (see preceding disussion of hair disorders).

Specific disorders

Several cutaneous eruptions occur only during pregnancy. Classification sometimes is confusing and varies among texts. Most eruptions during pregnancy are of no danger to the developing fetus but can cause major discomfort for the mother; others are more serious. The following is one approach to classifying these disorders.

Pruritic urticarial papules and plaques. As indicated by the name, this eruption is characterized by extremely pruritic lesions that are most common in the primigravid during the third trimester. The most common presentation is that of itchy red hives and papules beginning in the striae of the lower abdomen. (See Plate 5 of the front feature section.) The eruption may remain confined to this area or become more generalized. The cause of the condition is unclear, and all symptoms and lesions resolve postpartum. There is no risk to the infant or mother. Treatments include oral diphenhydramine or topical Sarna lotion. Cool baths, if permitted by the obstetrician, are soothing.

Pruritus gravidarum. This condition results in intense itching during pregnancy. If associated with cholestasis, it is associated with increased infant mortality and prematurity. For a more detailed discussion on cholestasis of pregnancy see Chapter 14. Topical corticosteroids and oral antihistamines such as diphenhydramine, which are safe during pregnancy, are often helpful. Cholestryamine is also available for treatment.

Herpes gestationis. This is a rare blistering disease of pregnancy that may be extremely pruritic. Herpes gestationis occurs in 1:50,000 pregnancies and, despite the name, is not associated with the herpes virus. It occurs during the second or third trimester and, unlike pruritic urticarial papules and plaques may occur in subsequent pregnancies. Large red urticarial plaques and intense blisters appear on the abdomen and extremities. A 10% risk of cutaneous involvement in the fetus exists, but other fetal risks are not clear. Treatment includes administration of systemic steroids.

BIBLIOGRAPHY

Cunliffe WJ: Evolution of a strategy for the treatment of acne, *J Am Acad Dermatol* 16:591, 1987.

Ellis CN et al: Sustained improvement with prolonged topical tretinoin (retinoic acid) for photoaged skin, *J Am Acad Dermatol* 23:629, 1990.

Errickson C, Matus N: Skin disorder of pregnancy, *Am Fam Physician* 49:3, 1994.

Fitzpatrick T et al: *Color atlas and synopsis of clinical dermatology,* ed 2, New York, 1992, MeGraw-Hill.

Habif TP: *Clinical dermatology: a color guide to diagnosis and therapy,* ed 2, St Louis, 1990, Mosby.

Koh HK: Cutaneous melanoma, *N Engl J Med* 325:171, 1991.

Lasher JL, Smith JC: Anti-fungal agents in dermatology, *J Am Acad Dermatol* 17:383, 1987.

Olsen EA et al: Topical minoxidil in the treatment of androgenic alopecia in women, *Cutis* 48:243, 1991.

Parmley T, O'Brian TJ: Skin changes during pregnancy, *Clin Obstet Gynocol* 33:713, 1990.

Phillip T, Dover J: Recent advances in dermatology, *N Engl J Med* 326:167, 1992.

Rhodes AR et al: Risk factors for cutaneous melanoma: a practical method of recognizing predisposed indiciduals, *JAMA* 258:3146, 1987.

Wong RC, Ellis CN: Physiologic skin changes in pregnancy, *J Am Acad Dermatol* 10:929, 1984.

8 Diabetes

Linda S. Jaffe and Ellen W. Seely

Apart from the management of diabetes during pregnancy (see Chapter 53) many of the complications experienced by and treatment approaches in diabetic women are similar to those in men. However, in caring for diabetic women, the clinician should be aware of several issues that are unique to this population and the ways in which their disease course may differ from that of nondiabetic women and diabetic men (see Table 8-1). This chapter will focus on these issues. It is important to note, however, that available data addressing diabetes in women are limited, and it will therefore be necessary for the clinician to review new information on a regular basis as it becomes available.

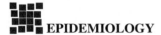

EPIDEMIOLOGY

Insulin-dependent diabetes mellitus

In childhood there is an increased incidence of insulin-dependent diabetes mellitus (IDDM) compared to that in adulthood in both women and men with a peak just prior to puberty. Between ages 12 and 14 years the incidence declines; the decrease occurs approximately 1 to 2 years earlier in girls than in boys. From this age until approximately age 30 there is a slightly lower incidence of IDDM in women (11.8/100,000/yr) compared to men (14.8/100,000/yr) with men exceeding women by approximately 25% (Fig.

8-1). The reason for this sex difference is unclear. After age 30 incidence rates appear to be similar. However, the incidence in both sexes has decreased dramatically by this time. Little information is available about the potential sex differential during the second peak of increased incidence of IDDM in the sixth and seventh decades.

Non–insulin-dependent diabetes mellitus

The incidence of non–insulin-dependent diabetes mellitus (NIDDM) according to sex is less well established than that of IDDM. Findings of studies are conflicting. Somes studies using a physician diagnosis of diabetes without specific laboratory criteria reported a higher annual incidence in women. However, other studies using more well-defined laboratory criteria show a lower incidence in women (Fig. 8-2).

EFFECT OF DIABETES ON NORMAL FEMALE PHYSIOLOGY
The menstrual cycle

Insulin sensitivity. Insulin sensitivity may vary with changes in hormonal levels during the menstrual cycle in nondiabetic women, with a fall in insulin sensitivity in the luteal phase. This normal physiologic change may be manifested more in the diabetic, who may note an increase in glucose levels, necessitating an increase in insulin requirements in the luteal phase. The diabetic population may be

Table 8-1 Medical disorders with increased frequency in diabetic women

Complication	RR*	Treatment considerations
Cardiovascular disease		Minimizing of other cardiac risk factors
Myocardial infarction	7-8	Potential benefit of estrogen replacement therapy in postmenopausal women†
Congestive heart failure	3-5	
Cardiovascular mortality	4.5	
UTI	2-3	7-day course of antibiotics
		IV antibiotics for pyelonephritis
Vaginal candidiasis	†	Improvement in glycemic control
		Topical antifungal agents
Eating disorders	†	Preventive counseling
		Metabolic stabilization to prevent/correct DKA and caloric loss via glycosuria
Necrobiosis diabeticorum	3-4	Effectiveness of topical steroids controversial

*Relative risk compared to that of nondiabetic women.
†Has not been directly determined (see text for details).
IV, intravenous; UTI, urinary tract infection; DKA, diabetic ketoacidosis.

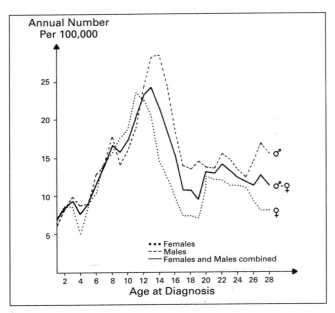

Fig. 8-1 Incidence of IDDM in females and males age 0-29 years in Denmark (From Christau B et al: *Acta Med Scand* 624:54, 1979.)

heterogeneous in this regard and some women note no changes. The potential importance of this deterioration in glucose control was demonstrated by studies in the 1970s that showed women in diabetic ketoacidosis were more likely present during or at the end of the luteal phase. Furthermore, at the time of menopause some women note a decrease in their insulin requirements.

Pathophysiology. The cause of this decrease in insulin sensitivity is not known, but a leading candidate is progesterone, which increases during this phase, and, when given

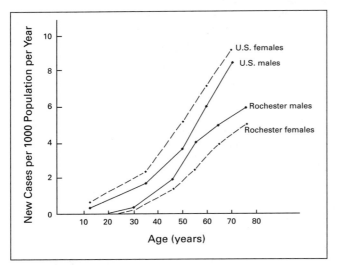

Fig. 8-2 Incidence of NIDDM in females and males in the 1975-81 National Health Interview Surveys (US females and US males) versus Rochester, Minnesota, in 1945-70 NIDDM, non–insulin-dependent diabetes mellitus. (Modified from Everhart J et al: *Diabetes in America*, National Diabetes Data Group, NIH Publication No. 85-1468, 1985, Bethesda, Md.)

exogenously, has been demonstrated to increase insulin resistance.

Issues in management. The possible influence of the menstrual cycle on diabetic control should be kept in mind in the care of all diabetic premenopausal women. In diabetics with a cyclical pattern of deterioration of glucose control a careful menstrual history should be obtained and correlated with glucose levels. Such a correlation may provide an explanation for previously unexplained erratic glycemic control and enable the patient and care provider to establish a plan for insulin regulation according to the phase of the menstrual cycle. In addition, diabetics nearing menopause should be made aware of the possible increase in insulin sensitivity after menopause and the potential need to decrease doses of insulin or oral hypoglycemic agents.

EFFECT OF DIABETES ON REPRODUCTION
Preconception and pregnancy

Pregnancy in diabetic patients with severe complications may be associated with a great increase in risk to the mother, whereas conception during poor glycemic control is associated with an increased risk of congenital malformations in the fetus. The issue of family planning for the diabetic female patient is of paramount importance because of the increased risks of unplanned pregnancies to both the mother and the fetus and therefore should be a routine part of care for these patients. Increasing the likelihood of an optimal outcome requires planning months before conception (while using some form of contraception) to achieve appropriate glucose control. For a more detailed discussion refer to Chapters 27 and 53.

Contraception

Contraception is a central issue in the care of the diabetic female patient of reproductive age. Of the contraceptive methods available today use of the oral contraceptive pills in the diabetic women has been the most controversial because of their possible effects on carbohydrate and lipid metabolism. The effects of oral contraceptive pills (OCPs) on lipid metabolism are discussed in Chapter 3.

Oral contraceptives

Pathophysiology. The alterations in carbohydrate tolerance that have been demonstrated with the use of oral contraceptives in nondiabetic women and women with a history of gestational diabetes have been attributed to the progestational agents incorporated into combination estrogen-progestin pills. The alterations are usually manifested as an increase in insulin secretion (more often than increased glucose levels) after a glucose load, consistent with an insulin-resistant state. Progestins may differ in this regard: for example, norgestrel, a gonane progestin, may have a more marked effect than norethindrone, an estrane progestin. More recent studies of subdermal progestin (levonorgestrel [Norplant]) have demonstrated similar changes in carbohydrate metabolism with an increase in insulin and glucose levels after glucose tolerance testing. The triphasic compounds afford less overall progestin exposure and have been demonstrated by some investigators to show little or no impairment in carbohydrate metabolism. Despite the hyperinsulinemia that has been attributed to the progestin in OCPs, the prior use of OCPs by nondiabetic women has not been associated with an increase in subsequent risk of the development of diabetes.

A decrease in the rate of glucose metabolism as demonstrated by euglycemic insulin clamp technique may be responsible for the impaired carbohydrate tolerance. Whether a postreceptor defect in insulin action is contributing has not been determined.

Use in the diabetic female. One study by Skouby et al. investigated the use of the combination OCPs monophasic ethinyl estradiol (EE$_2$) μg/norethindrone (500 μg) and triphasic EE$_2$ (30 to 40 μg)/levonorgestrel (50 to 125 μg) in diabetic women and demonstrated no changes in 24-hour insulin requirements, hemoglobin A$_{1c}$ levels, fasting blood glucose, or free fatty acids after 6 months of use. However, the lack of effect on insulin requirement is not a universal finding, and another study, by Rádberg et al, showed a small but statistically significant increase in insulin requirements with the use of EE$_2$ (50 μg)/lynestrenol (2.5 mg).

Vascular complications, particularly cardiac, central nervous system, and retinal, have been of concern in diabetic women on OCPs. These complications have been attributed to the high doses of estrogen previously incorporated in earlier OCP preparations. In more recent short-term prospective studies of 6 months' duration in women using combination OCPs containing 30 to 50 μg of EE$_2$, no increases in blood pressure or thrombotic complications were reported.

On the other hand a retrospective population study using similar doses of EE$_2$ has demonstrated an increase in cardiovascular complications, including stroke and venous thrombosis, in 120 diabetics who used OCPs compared to 156 diabetics who did not. Of note, the incidence was not compared to that of the nondiabetic population using OCPs. In six of the OCP users proliferative retinopathy developed and in three a rapidly progressive form developed. In contrast, another retrospective population study of 432 diabetic women found no association between past or current OCP use, or the number of years of use, and the severity of retinopathy.

Although the issue of thrombotic complications in diabetic women on OCPs needs further investigation, the concern raised by these studies has led to the examination of progestin-only preparations as an alternative means of oral contraception. Studies of several progestin-only pills in diabetics (including norethindrone 300 μg, lynestrenol 500 μg, and norethisterone 350 μg) have shown no significant effect on daily insulin requirements, despite the increase in insulin

resistance demonstrated in the experimental setting. No effect on blood pressure and retinopathy was noted with progestin-only pills in these studies. Studies of subdermal norgestrel (Norplant) in diabetic women have not yet appeared in the literature.

Intrauterine devices (IUDs). The intrauterine device may be a preferred method of contraception in diabetic women because of its lack of effects on carbohydrate and lipid metabolism. In one controlled study using the copper IUD the pregnancy rate of approximately 1% per year was the same in diabetics and control subjects. Furthermore, discontinuation rates for infection, inflammation, bleeding, and other medical conditions were similar.

Approach to contraception for the diabetic woman. A careful assessment of the risks and benefits of each type of contraception must be made on an individual basis to determine which method carries the least amount of adverse side effects and the best chance of success against conception (see Table 8-2).

Barrier methods should be strongly considered as first-line contraceptive methods for patients who seem able to comply with these methods because of the lack of effect on diabetic control. Likewise the IUD has this advantage.

The use of OCPs has generally been reserved for those patients with otherwise low cardiovascular risks profiles, including young age, normal blood pressure, normal lipid profiles, nonsmoking, and no evidence of microangiopathy. On the basis of limited studies in nondiabetics and women with a history of gestational diabetes, triphasic compounds that contain the lowest doses of progestin and preferably estranes (e.g., norethindrone) rather than gonanes (e.g., norgestrel) may have the least effect on glucose levels and insulin requirements. Despite experimental evidence supporting the development of insulin resistance none of the agents directly studied in a small number of diabetics has had any clinically significant influence on daily insulin requirements. However, there are a large number of different oral contraceptive preparations available, most of which have not been directly tested in diabetics. Furthermore, the effects of these agents on individual patients' carbohydrate tolerance may differ. Therefore, while on OCPs the diabetic patient should be counseled to monitor blood rather than urine glucose levels closely in order to assess changes in insulin requirements. Since both combination OCPs and progestin-only pills have been associated with an increase in

Table 8-2 Contraceptive methods

Method	Advantages	Disadvantages	Comments
Barrier	No effect on glycemic control	Motivation required for compliance	First-line method for patients able to comply
IUD	No effect on glycemic control	Inflammation, infection, bleeding	
Oral contraceptives	Relative ease of use vs. barrier methods	Deterioration in carbohydrate and lipid metabolism Risk of thrombotic complications	In patients with no other cardiac risk factors or microangiopathy, or when the only alternative to pregnancy
Subdermal progestin	Implanted	Deterioration in carbohydrate and lipid metabolism	Not tested in diabetics
Tubal ligation	Single procedure, permanent	Surgical procedure, permanent	For women who have completed childbearing or at very high risk for pregnancy-related complications

24-hour urinary glucose excretion, as seen in pregnancy, urinary glucose monitoring is an unreliable way of following potential changes in glucose levels and insulin requirements. Furthermore, the patient should be examined before initiation of OCPs and followed regularly for increases in blood pressure, unfavorable alterations in lipid profiles, and development or acceleration of retinopathy.

Given the effect of subdermal levonorgestrel (Norplant) on carbohydrate metabolism in nondiabetics and the delay in return to baseline carbohydrate metabolism after removal, other forms of contraception would appear to be advisable for the diabetic until more information becomes available.

Finally, for the very high-risk patient or the patient who has completed a family or does not wish to have children tubal ligation should be considered after careful counseling of the patient by her physician. It may be the best method of contraception, having the greatest efficacy rate and the least long-term risk for the diabetic patient.

DIABETES AND CARDIOVASCULAR DISEASE
Epidemiology

The incidence of cardiovascular disease (CVD) is higher in diabetics than nondiabetics. Prospective and case control epidemiologic studies demonstrate approximately a threefold increased risk of all types of CVD in diabetics versus nondiabetics. Nondiabetic women appear to be protected from manifesting CVD until they are postmenopausal. However, the diabetic female patient is at particular risk of increased morbidity and mortality rates from CVD at all ages, including ischemic heart disease, congestive heart failure (CHF), stroke, and peripheral vascular disease.

For female diabetics, as compared with female nondiabetics, the relative risk of myocardial infarction may be as high as sevenfold to eightfold, and when insulin-dependent diabetics are looked at alone, the risk is even higher. The course after acute myocardial infarction is also more complicated in diabetic women compared to both diabetic men and the nondiabetic population, despite the smallest infarct size in these patients. These women experience slightly greater in-hospital and cumulative mortality rates and a greater incidence of impaired left ventricular function, congestive heart failure, infarct extension, and fatal reinfarction.

Studies of the Framingham population demonstrate that diabetic women also have the greatest risk of congestive heart failure regardless of their underlying cardiac status. Overall, compared to nondiabetic women, these women experienced a fivefold increase in the risk of CHF, whereas the increase in the risk for diabetic men was twofold. Diabetic women with known underlying coronary artery disease (CAD) had a threefold increase in the incidence of CHF, whereas no significant increase was seen in diabetic men. When patients with a history of coronary artery disease and rheumatic heart disease were excluded, the relative risk of CHF was 5.5 for diabetic women compared to 3.8 for diabetic men. This increased risk was confined to patients using insulin therapy.

The overall cardiovascular mortality rate for diabetic women is approximately 4.5 times that for nondiabetic women, compared to the lower relative risk for diabetic men of twofold. Several studies have also demonstrated that the greatest increase in the morbidity and mortality rates attributable to CVD is confined to the subpopulation of diabetic women taking insulin. However, this area is controversial and insulin use may be primarily a marker of underlying disease severity. In summary, the relative protection that nondiabetic women experience compared to men against the morbidity and mortality attributable to CVD, particularly in the premenopausal state, is lost in the presence of diabetes, and these patients tend to have the poorest outcome (Fig. 8-3).

Pathophysiology

Diabetics have a significantly worse cardiovascular risk profile than nondiabetics. Some suggest that diabetic women may have a greater prevalence of hypertension than nondiabetics. However, even when the presence of this high-risk profile is taken into account, diabetic women still have an unexplained increased risk of cardiovascular morbidity and mortality. Several mechanisms have been proposed to explain the increase in atherogenesis in diabetes, including alterations in lipid profiles, hypercoagulability, and hyperinsulinemia.

None of these mechanisms, however, is unique to women. In fact, the association with hyperinsulinemia and CAD mortality has not been demonstrated in women although this association has not received the amount of investigation that it has in men. Both what is protective in women at baseline against the development of CVD and consequently what is lost with the development of diabetes in the female patient remain to be elucidated.

Clinical presentation

History and symptoms. A substantial number of women have silent and other atypical presentations of myocardial infarction (MI). Diabetics may also have more atypical presentations of MI, including uncontrolled diabetes, vomiting, confusion, stroke, and heart failure. Therefore in the population of female diabetics it is important to have a high clinical index of suspicion for the presence of ischemic cardiac disease when evaluating these patients' symptoms.

Issues in management

The risk of CVD attributable to diabetes is amplified in the presence of other cardiovascular risk factors. For example,

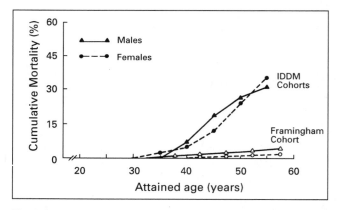

Fig. 8-3 Coronary artery disease cumulative mortality rate in females and males with IDDM compared to the nondiabetic population in the Framingham Heart Study. IDDM, insulin-dependent diabetes mellitus. (From Krowleski As et al: *Am J Cardiol* 59:750, 1987.)

the relative risk in a female diabetic smoker is over 22 times that in a nondiabetic nonsmoker. Therefore risk factors such as cigarette smoking, hypertension, and obesity must be minimized.

Postmenopausal estrogen. The issue of postmenopausal estrogen replacement and its effects on CVD has received considerable attention recently. Most prospective epidemiologic studies have shown a decreased risk of CVD among estrogen users, with a relative risk of 0.3 to 0.7 in the population-based case-control studies. Furthermore, in a cross-sectional analysis of data from the Atherosclerosis Risk in Communities Study designed to examine changes in coronary risk factors with hormone replacement therapy, nondiabetic postmenopausal women who used hormone replacement (estrogen alone or estrogen and progesterone) were found to have slightly but significantly lower fasting glucose and insulin levels than nonusers. In the Nurse's Health Study a similar benefit and no increase in adverse effects were seen in the subgroup of diabetic women who received estrogen replacement. However, no studies have been designed specifically to address the issue of the risks and benefits of estrogen replacement therapy in diabetic postmenopausal women.

Treatment of coronary artery disease. Once CAD is established, women have traditionally been considered less optimal surgical candidates for coronary artery bypass grafting (CABG), possibly because of the smaller caliber of their native vessels; they may experience less symptomatic relief and have greater operative mortality rates than men. Some but not all studies suggest that diabetics are also high-risk candidates for CABG and have higher morbidity and mortality rates than nondiabetics. This may in part be attributed to more diffuse and distally located artherosclerotic lesions found in diabetics. However, this finding has not been confirmed in all studies. Nonetheless the diabetic female patient may be at the greatest risk for this procedure. Although there appear to be more complications from percutaneous transluminal coronary angioplasty in women, it is not yet clear whether diabetic women differ from nondiabetic women or diabetic men in this regard. See Chapter 2 for further discussion of coronary artery disease.

DIABETES AND GENITOURINARY PROBLEMS
Urinary tract infections

Although there is some controversy, many studies report a twofold to threefold increased frequency of urinary tract infection (UTI) in diabetic compared to nondiabetic women. In diabetic men no difference in incidence has been noted. In addition, an increased frequency of asymptomatic UTI has been found in diabetic women but no increase in diabetic men.

Pathogenesis. The cause of this increase in frequency is not clear, and it is usually ascribed to hyperglycemia and glycosuria. It is of note that the degree of glycosuria did not appear to be a major factor in some studies. Other contributing factors include prior instrumentation and bladder dysfunction secondary to autonomic neuropathy.

Issues in management
Treatment considerations. Because of the possibility of more serious sequelae to pyelonephritis (papillary necrosis, perinephric abscess) there is a tendency to be more aggressive in the treatment of UTIs in diabetic women. Single-dose and 3-day regimens for UTIs have not been well studied in this population, and therefore a 7-day course of antibiotic therapy appears advisable. When pyelonephritis develops in a diabetic woman, parenteral rather than oral administration of antibiotics should be considered, even in patients who can tolerate oral drugs, to prevent the potential development of more serious complications. The common organisms causing UTIs in this population are similar to those in the nondiabetic.

Candida vaginitis

Although vaginal candidiasis is a common infection in all women, there is an increased incidence, in the diabetic. Despite the increased incidence, candidiasis is such a common infection in premenopausal women that it does not appear to warrant testing for diabetes if it is the only suggestive symptom. However, it is important to question women with recurrent infections as to other possible symptoms of diabetes. Given the decreased incidence of vaginal candidiasis in postmenopausal women, recurrent infections in this population would warrant evaluation for diabetes. It is of note, however, that studies have not been performed specifically to address the usefulness of this approach.

Pathogenesis. Candida growth and adherence to vaginal epithelial cells increase in the presence of glucose. The increased glucose level in the vaginal secretion of diabetics and glycosuria are the common explanations for the propensity of those women to have *candida* infections.

Issues in management
Treatment considerations. In addition to antifungal treatment improvement in glucose control should be attempted. Treatment options are shown in Tables 16-3 and 16-4.

DIABETES AND EATING DISORDERS

Eating disorders are more common in female than male adolescents and young adults and appear to be more common in patients with IDDM than the general population (see Chapter 69 for a general discussion of eating disorders). These disorders include anorexia nervosa and bulimia nervosa, as described by the DSM-III criteria, and subclinical eating disorders, in which all of the DSM-III criteria are not met. Diabetics have the unique "purge" technique of omitting or underdosing insulin available to them, which leads to glycosuria and calorie loss in the urine.

Epidemiology

Over the past decade multiple reports of eating disorders in patients with diabetes have suggested that there is an increased prevalence of eating disorders in this group. For comparison estimates of the prevalence of anorexia nervosa and bulimia in adolescent and young adult females in general range from 0.001% to 1.0% and 1.3% to 19%, respectively. In diabetics prevalence rates have been reported to range from 7% to 21%, with a predominance of females of 95%. These figures may represent ascertainment bias because when compared to nondiabetics, women with IDDM may be diagnosed more frequently with eating disorders because they are already within the medical system, and omission of insulin manifests with signs of hyperglycemia and diabetic ketoacidosis that may focus the caregiver's attention on this diagnosis.

Pathogenesis

Young women are at the greatest risk for the development of eating disorders because of greater societal pressures on women to appear thin. In addition, several factors related to diabetes may make these women even more susceptible to the development of these disorders. These include (1) chronic illness, which is associated with stress, poor self-esteem, and an altered body image; (2) dysfunctional family interactions, particularly overprotection by parents, that are not uncommon in families of diabetic patients; and (3) the treatment of IDDM, which places great emphasis on weight, dietary habits, and food.

Clinical presentation

History and symptoms. The detection of an eating disorder in a diabetic patient can be quite challenging for the clinician. Many symptoms, such as difficulty in concentrating, decreased energy level, and sleep disturbances, can also be seen in the setting of poor glycemic control alone. However, significant changes in weight, persistently poor glycemic control, and recurrent episodes of hypoglycemia or diabetic ketoacidosis should alert the physician to the possibility of an eating disorder.

Issues in management. Psychiatric consultation may be necessary to confirm the diagnosis. If an eating disorder is undiagnosed, the situation may worsen; patients with poor glycemic control may be treated with an increase in their insulin dose, leading to further weight gain, and may be pressured even more to diet. Both possibilities may predispose the patient to further disordered eating behavior or omission of insulin.

The approach is similar to that for nondiabetics, but with the physician's awareness that glucose control deserves particular attention. The long-term outcome in patients with IDDM and eating disorders is not known. Nonetheless there is an associated increased morbidity rate. Therefore management of the young diabetic female patient should emphasize prevention of eating disorders. The physician should routinely inquire about dietary habits, stress-related eating, and binging in a nonjudgmental manner. These patients should also be warned about the dangers of strict dieting and should be taught how to manage eating and drinking in social situations in the context of diabetes. Chapter 69 discusses eating disorders in greater detail.

OTHER COMPLICATIONS

In contrast to vasculopathy the other three major complications of diabetes, retinopathy, nephropathy, and neuropathy, appear to occur with similar frequency in women and men with similar duration of their diabetes. Necrobiosis diabeticorum, a skin lesion associated with diabetes whose pathogenesis is poorly understood, has a threefold to fourfold increased incidence in women.

Diabetes control and complications trial

The benefits of intensive insulin therapy (with the goal of normalizing hemoglobin A_1), including delay in the onset and progression of retinopathy and proteinuria and delay in the onset of neuropathy, were similar for women and men in the Diabetes Control and Complications Trial (DCCT), as was the risk of hypoglycemia. It is of note, however, that studies of these diabetic complications have not been specifically designed to address a sex difference.

SUMMARY

Although many complications and care issues in diabetic women are similar to those in men, important gender differences exist. These differences influence disease course and clinical care. Further research directed specifically toward female diabetics will expand our presently limited knowledge base and improve our understanding of this disease in women.

BIBLIOGRAPHY

Beard CM et al: The Rochester Coronary Heart Disease Project: effect of cigarette smoking, hypertension, diabetes, and steroidal estrogen use on coronary heart disease among 40- to 59-year-old women, 1960 through 1982, *Mayo Clin Proc* 64:1471, 1989.

Christau B et al: Incidence of insulin-dependent diabetes mellitus (0-29 years at onset) in Denmark, *Acta Med Scand* 624(Suppl):54, 1979.

Diabetes Control and Complications Trial Research Group: The effect of intensive treatment of diabetes on the development and progression of long-term complications in insulin-dependent diabetes mellitus, *N Engl J Med* 329:977, 1993.

Diamond MP, Simonson DC, DeFronzo RA: Menstrual cyclicity has a profound effect on glucose homeostasis, *Fertil Steril* 52:204, 1989.

Elkind-Hirsch KE, Sherman LD, Malinak R: Hormone replacement therapy alters insulin sensitivity in young women with premature ovarian failure, *J Clin Endocrinol Metab* 76:472, 1993.

Everhart J, Knowler WC, Bennett PH: Incidence and risk factors for non-insulin-dependent diabetes. In *Diabetes in America,* NIH Publication No. 85-1468, 1985, Bethesda, Md., National Diabetes Data Group.

Forland M, Thomas VL: The treatment of urinary tract infections in women with diabetes mellitus, *Diabetes Care* 8:499, 1985.

Garcia MJ et al: Morbidity and mortality in diabetics in the Framingham population: sixteen year follow-up study, *Diabetes* 23:105, 1974.

Godsland IF, Crook D, Wynn V: Low-dose oral contraceptives and carbohydrate metabolism, *Am J Obstet Gynecol* 163:348, 1990.

Johnson JR, Stamm WE: Urinary tract infections in women: diagnosis and treatment, *Ann Intern Med* 111:906, 1989.

Kannel WB, Hjortland M, Castelli WP: Role of diabetes in congestive heart failure: the Framingham Study, *Am J Cardiol* 34:29, 1974.

Klein BEK, Moss SE, Klein R: Oral contraceptives in women with diabetes, *Diabetes Care* 13:895, 1990.

Konje JC et al: Carbohydrate metabolism before and after Norplant removal, *Contraception* 46:61, 1992.

Krolewski AS et al: Magnitude and determinants of coronary artery disease in juvenile-onset, insulin-dependent diabetes mellitus, *Am J Cardiol* 59:750, 1987.

Lerner DJ, Kannel WB: Patterns of coronary heart disease morbidity and mortality in the sexes: a 26-year follow-up of the Framingham population, *Am Heart J* 111:383, 1986.

Maccato M, Kaufman RH: Fungal vulvovaginitis, *Curr Opin Obstet Gynecol* 3:849, 1991.

Manson JE et al: A prospective study of maturity-onset diabetes mellitus and risk of coronary heart disease and stroke in women, *Arch Intern Med* 151:1141, 1991.

Marcus MD, Wing RR: Eating disorders and diabetes. In Holmes CS, editor: *Neuropsychological and behavioral aspects of diabetes,* New York, 1990, Springer-Verlag.

Muller SA, Winkelman RK: Necrobiosis Lipoidica Diabeticorem: a clinical and pathological investigation of 171 cases, *Arch Dermatol* 93:272, 1966.

Nabulsi AA et al: Association of hormone replacement therapy with various cardiovascular risk factors in postmenopausal women, *N Engl J Med* 328:1106, 1993.

Rådberg T et al: Oral contraception in diabetic women: a cross-over study on serum and high density lipoprotein (HDL): Lipids and diabetes control during progestogen and combined estrogen/progestogen contraception, *Horm Metab Res* 14:61, 1982.

Rimm EB et al: Oral contraceptive use and the risk of Type II (Non-insulin dependent diabetes mellitus) in a large prospective study of women. *Diabetologica* 35:967, 1992.

Skouby SO, Molsted-Pedersen L, Kühl C: Contraception in diabetic women, *Acta Endocrinol* 277(Suppl):125, 1986.

Skouby SO et al: Triphasic oral contraception: metabolic effects in normal women and those with previous gestational diabetes, *Am J Obstet Gynecol* 153:395, 1985.

Skouby SO et al: Oral contraceptives in diabetic women: metabolic effects of four compounds with different estrogen/progestogen profiles, *Fertil Steril* 46:858, 1986.

Skouby SO et al: Mechanism of action of oral contraceptives on carbohydrate metabolism at the cellular level, *Am J Obstet Gynecol* 163:343, 1990.

Sobel JD: Epidemiology and pathogenesis of recurrent vulvo vaginal candidiasis, *Am J Obstet Gynecol* 152:924, 1985.

Soler NG et al: Myocardial infarction in diabetics, *Q J Med, New Series* 173:125, 1975.

Spellacy WN: Carbohydrate metabolism during treatment with estrogen, progestogen, and low-dose oral contraceptives, *Am J Obstet Gynecol* 142:732, 1982.

Spellacy WN, Ellingson AB, Tsibris JCM: The effects of two triphasic oral contraceptives on carbohydrate metabolism in women during 1 year of use, *Fertil Steril* 57:71, 1989.

Stampfer MJ et al: A prospective study of postmenopausal estrogen therapy and coronary heart disease, *N Engl J Med* 313:1044, 1985.

Stampfer MJ et al: Postmenopausal estrogen therapy and cardiovascular disease, *N Engl J Med* 325:756, 1991.

Steel JM, Duncan LJP: Serious complications of oral contraception in insulin-dependent diabetics, *Contraception* 17:291, 1978.

Steel JM, Duncan LJP: Contraception for the insulin-dependent diabetic woman: the view from one clinic, *Diabetes Care* 3:557, 1980.

Stone PH et al: The effect of diabetes mellitus on prognosis and serial left ventricular function after acute myocardial infarction: contribution of both coronary disease and diastolic left ventricular dysfunction to the adverse prognosis, *J Am Coll Cardiol* 14:49, 1989.

Vejlsgaard R: Studies on urinary infection in diabetes: bacteriuria in patients with diabetes mellitus and in control subjects, *Acta Med Scand* 179:173, 1966.

Walsh CH, Malin JM: Menstruation and control of diabetes, *Br Med J* 2:177, 1977.

Welborn TA, Wearne K: Coronary heart disease incidence and cardiovascular mortality in Busselton with reference to glucose and insulin concentrations, *Diabetes Care* 2:154, 1979.

Widom B, Diamond MP, Simonson DC: Alterations in glucose metabolism during menstrual cycle in women with IDDM, *Diabetes Care* 15:213, 1992.

Willett WC et al: Relative and absolute excess risks of coronary heart disease among women who smoke cigarettes, *N Engl J Med* 317:1303, 1987.

9 Hirsutism and Androgen Excess

Ann E. Taylor

The definitions of hirsutism and acne vary for an individual woman, depending on her personal interpretation of normal. Hirsutism, acne, and irregular menstrual cycles are the most common manifestations of excess androgen effects in women. Some hyperandrogenic women have pathologically elevated androgen levels, some have a benign functional elevation of androgen levels, and some have normal androgen levels with either increased production and clearance of androgens, increased biologic sensitivity to circulating androgens, or increased personal sensitivity to the cosmetic impact of normal androgens. Since any woman who perceives herself to have excess androgenic effects may request a hormonal evaluation for reassurance, all disorders of hyperandrogenism in women will be considered together in this chapter.

The clinician's role in the management of such women includes the identification of pathologic hyperandrogenism in women who have not complained of symptoms, the exclusion of pathologic causes of hyperandrogenism, the choice of appropriate treatment with consideration of the woman's preferences, and the prevention of other disorders that are frequently associated with hyperandrogenism. These disorders include endometrial cancer, obesity, insulin resistance, and hypercholesterolemia, which seem to occur in association with hyperandrogenism of any cause. Serious pathologic causes of hyperandrogenism are rare but usually treatable if identified. However, the majority of hyperandrogenic women have the benign condition of polycystic ovary syndrome (PCOS), which recently has been defined broadly to include any hyperandrogenic symptoms and some menstrual irregularity in premenopausal women.

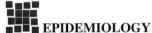

EPIDEMIOLOGY

The overall prevalence of hyperandrogenism in women is unknown, since excess androgens have previously been defined simply from the 95% confidence limits of levels in apparently normal women. Similarly, symptoms of hyperandrogenism such as hirsutism have also been defined from population studies. However, determination of the prevalence of a subjective condition such as hirsutism is difficult as a result of ethnic variation and sometimes unrealistic social norms. Ferriman and Gallwey's study of 430 women in London indicated that normal women almost never had terminal hair on the upper back or upper abdomen, and only 3% and 10% had terminal hair on the sternum and chin, respectively. Conversely, a significant number of normal women have terminal hair on the upper lip and linea alba. The majority of women with hirsutism have at least one elevated androgen level or an increased androgen production rate, if one looks hard enough. Because of more recent evidence of potential adverse consequences of hyperandrogenism, new studies are needed to determine whether there is a "safe" level of androgens for women, above which one should definitely treat the condition.

The prevalence of hyperandrogenism in specific clinical conditions has been estimated. Approximately 5% of amenorrhea and approximately 15% of female infertility in premenopausal women are estimated to be attributable to hyperandrogenism. Up to 38% of women with diffuse alopecia have evidence of hyperandrogenism, as do up to 50% of women with acne.

The distribution of hyperandrogenic symptoms varies with race. Asian and Native American women have relatively little body hair of any type, whereas women of Mediterranean extraction frequently have moderately heavy facial and body hair. Certain racial groups, particularly African-American and Hispanic women, appear to have a greater frequency of the metabolic abnormalities such as acanthosis nigricans and insulin resistance that are associated with hyperandrogenism, whereas other groups, such as Asians, appear to have a higher frequency of acne.

PATHOPHYSIOLOGY

Androgenic steroids include testosterone, the most potent androgen; dihydrotestosterone, a more potent tissue metabolite of testosterone derived especially from skin and skeletal muscle; and the weaker androgenic precursors androstenedione, dehydroepiandrosterone (DHEA), and its sulfoconjugate DHEA-S. Normal women secrete testosterone in approximately equal amounts from the adrenal glands and the ovaries; the result is a serum level that is 5% to 20% that of men. Testosterone and other androgens circulate bound to both sex hormone–binding globulin (SHBG) and other binding proteins, including albumin, so that increased amounts of SHBG result in less free and biologically available hormone. SHBG is produced in the liver, increased by estrogens, and decreased by androgens and insulin. Thus free testosterone levels are a better marker of androgenic activity than is total testosterone. Androgens are aromatized to estrogens in peripheral tissues, especially fat, so that hyperandrogenic women tend to have normal total estrogen levels.

The effects of increased androgens increase with the severity of the defect. Sebum production is increased at relatively low androgen levels, and acne, hirsutism, oligomenorrhea, male-pattern balding, deepening of the voice, increased muscle mass, and clitoromegaly sequentially become more apparent as androgen levels increase to more pathologic levels. Body hair can be classified as androgen-dependent hirsutism, including dark terminal hairs on the face, chest, abdomen, and back, and androgen-independent hypertrichosis, as on the scalp, arms, and legs. Once androgen levels are sufficient to cause differentiation of soft vellus hair to darker, thicker terminal hair, those follicles remain more sensitive to androgens thereafter. Some women with hirsutism appear to have normal androgen levels but evidence of increased peripheral conversion of testosterone to dihydrotestosterone by 5-alpha-reductase.

Androgen excess in women has several pathophysiologic consequences in addition to the cosmetic manifestations. The prolonged amenorrhea is associated with chronic endometrial stimulation by unopposed estrogens and an increased risk of endometrial hyperplasia and endometrial cancer. Most of the cases of endometrial cancer in young women occur in association with oligomenorrhea and evidence of hyperandrogenism.

Although the classic image of the woman with polycystic ovaries includes obesity, only about half of women with PCOS are obese. Still the incidence of obesity appears greater than that in the population. Hyperandrogenic women appear to have several metabolic abnormalities that are typically associated with obesity, whether or not they are obese. They are significantly more insulin resistant than normal women, independent of obesity. This relationship between androgen levels and insulin resistance is complex. Very high insulin levels appear to cause hyperandrogenemia in women with severe insulin resistance. Although elevated insulin levels are able to stimulate ovarian androgen production in vitro and to alter ovarian and adrenal androgen production *in vivo*, it is not yet clear whether the typical insulin levels in women with PCOS are the primary cause of their increased androgen production or whether the elevated androgen levels contribute to the hyperinsulinemia. The degree of insulin resistance correlates with the presence of acanthosis nigricans (Fig. 9-1), a thickening and darkening of the rugal folds of the skin most commonly seen at the nape of the neck, the axillae, and the knuckles, knees, and elbows (Fig. 9-2).

Preliminary studies have indicated that hyperandrogenic women may also have higher total cholesterol levels, and lower high-density lipoprotein (HDL) levels, than weight-matched normal women. Hyperandrogenic women also have increased waist to hip ratios compared to women with normal androgen levels. Thus multiple cardiovascular risk factors have been independently associated with female hyperandrogenism, but whether women with PCOS have an increased risk or earlier onset of cardiovascular disease is unknown. Hyperandrogenism may have some beneficial effects such as protection against osteoporosis.

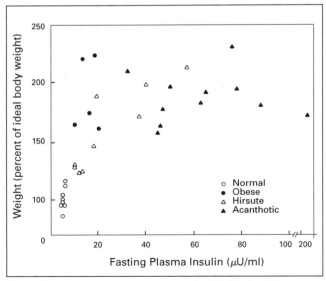

Fig. 9-1 Acanthosis nigricans is associated with the highest fasting insulin levels. (From Stuart CA et al: Insulin resistance with acanthosis nigricans: the roles of obesity and androgen excess, *Metabolism* 35:197, 1986.)

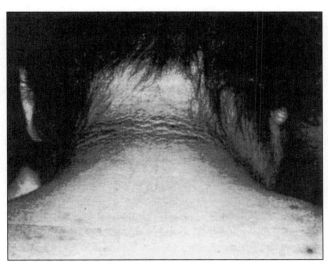

Fig. 9-2 Acanthosis nigricans. Hyperpigmented, thickened rugae of skin at the nape of the neck of a woman with severe insulin resistance. (From Yen SSC, Jaffe JB, editors: *Reproductive endocrinology*, ed 3, 1991.)

DIFFERENTIAL DIAGNOSIS

The differential diagnosis of hirsutism is outlined in the box at right. The most important differentiation for the clinician to make is between malignant and benign disease. Fortunately **androgen-secreting tumors** are rare. Steroid-secreting ovarian tumors represent approximately 5% of all ovarian tumors. Androgen-secreting adrenal tumors are similarly rare. Adrenal tumors may appear with signs and symptoms of Cushing's syndrome caused by coincident excess of cortisol production as well as of androgens. Ovarian or adrenal tumors should be suspected when the onset of hyperandrogenic symptoms is abrupt, rapid, and not associated with puberty, and when symptoms are especially severe when compared to the woman's family history.

Exogenous hormone administration should be easily determined by the clinician; it includes covert or overt androgen ingestion for muscle building or for female to male transsexual conversions. Some medications given for other purposes may have androgenic side effects. For example norgestrel is a progestin commonly used in oral contraceptives that is particularly androgenic in its actions.

Genetic defects in the androgen synthesizing enzymes of the ovary and adrenal gland that cause a clinical picture indistinguishable from that of PCOS have been identified. The most common of these is 21-hydroxylase deficiency, also known as **congenital adrenal hyperplasia** or adrenogenital syndrome. The classic form may cause salt wasting and an adrenal insufficiency crisis in a newborn female with ambiguous genitalia, whereas the nonclassic form typically presents at puberty with excess androgen production with or without menstrual irregularities. The phenotype appears to depend on both the alleles acquired and on predisposing factors, since affected members of the same family may have very different symptoms. Other forms of congenital adrenal hyperplasia involving other enzymes in the cortisol production pathway are rare but should be considered in a woman with a known family history, in a high-

DIFFERENTIAL DIAGNOSIS OF EXCESS HAIR IN WOMEN

Hirsutism (increased sexual hair)

Most common

Polycystic ovary syndrome
Idiopathic hirsutism
Medications
　Danazol for endometriosis
　Androgenic oral contraceptives (norgestrel)
Hyperprolactinemia
Hyperthecosis

Less common

Congenital adrenal hyperplasia
Ovarian tumors
　Sertoli-Leydig cell tumors
　Granulosa-theca cell tumors
　Other tumors that stimulate ovarian stroma
Adrenal tumors
　Cushing's disease
　Other tumors of the adrenal cortex
Severe insulin resistance syndromes

Hypertrichosis (increased total body hair), rare

Drugs

Dilantin
Streptomycin
Hexachlorobenzene
Penicillamine
Diazoxide
Minoxidil
Cyclosporine

Systemic illness

Hypothyroidism
Anorexia nervosa
Malnutrition
Porphyria
Dermatomyositis

---

risk ethnic group such as the Ashkenazi Jews, or in cases of unexplained hypertension.

Hyperprolactinemia has been associated with elevated DHEA-S levels and hirsutism. Typically the prolactin level elevations are mild and there is no evidence of pituitary tumor on scans. Prolactin may increase adrenal androgen production, if adrenocorticotropic hormone (ACTH) secretion is intact.

PCOS is by far the most common cause of hirsutism and other hyperandrogenic symptoms in women and is a benign condition. PCOS can be diagnosed when women have signs or symptoms of androgen excess, whether or not serum androgen levels are elevated, in association with menstrual irregularity and in the absence of any of the pathologic processes described. Both the ovaries and the adrenal glands can contribute to the excess androgen level in this heterogeneous syndrome. Obesity tends to make the hirsutism, menstrual irregularity, and insulin resistance worse, and weight loss will improve menstrual function and hirsutism scores in at least some women.

◢ EVALUATION OF HYPERANDROGENISM

History and physical examination

All women who have hyperandrogenic complaints require a detailed history and physical examination. The history should focus on the time course of the symptoms, including the age at onset and the rate of progression. A menstrual history, including menarche, regularity, conceptions, use of oral contraceptives, and symptoms of ovulation (cervical mucus, mittelschmerz, molimina), helps determine the severity of the hyperandrogenism. Also important are fluctuations and correlations of symptoms and menstrual regularity with body weight, as well as a history of all medications that might have androgenic side effects or cause hypertrichosis. Lastly, a family history of hirsutism, oligomenorrhea, infertility, and insulin resistance can be helpful in ruling out pathologic conditions or in indicating an increased likelihood of congenital adrenal hyperplasia.

Important physical examination features include height, weight, waist-to-hip ratio, and pattern of body fat distribution (abdominal, buffalo hump, supraclavicular fat). In the examination of the skin the location and quantity of terminal hair and acne should be carefully documented, so that response to therapy can be more objectively assessed. Other signs of virilization include deepening of the voice, temporal or crown balding, increased muscle mass, and clitoromegaly. A clitoral index (length × width) >35 mm² is above the normal range. In addition, a careful examination should include consideration of associated abnormalities, including elevated blood pressure, xanthomas, and acanthosis nigricans, which may be seen at the axillae, knuckles, knees, elbows, inguinal crease, and nape of the neck. Evidence of excess cortisol production, such as wide purple abdominal striae, thin skin, bruising, and proximal muscle weakness, should be documented. The breasts should be examined for galactorrhea. Finally, adrenal and ovarian masses should be ruled out by careful abdominal and pelvic examinations.

Diagnostic tests

The simplest screening laboratory tests would include free testosterone and DHEA-S levels (see box at right). If the woman has oligomenorrhea, prolactin level should be measured. Further testing, as follows, or referral to an endocrinologist is advised if there is evidence of more serious disease (see box on the following page).

Testosterone. The best validated screening test for ovarian androgen-secreting tumors is serum total and free testosterone levels. Several investigators have shown that total testosterone levels above 200 ng/dl and free testosterone levels above 2 ng/dl are relatively sensitive, but are not specific tests for identifying androgen secreting tumors. In one series all women with tumors had a total testosterone level greater than 200 ng/dl, but only 2 of 11 women with such high testosterone levels had tumors.

DHEA-S. The androgen precursor DHEA-S derives at least 95% from the adrenal gland and therefore is considered a good marker for adrenal androgen hypersecretion. The upper limit of DHEA-S for normal young women is about 500 μg/dl. Women with PCOS can have DHEA-S levels up to about 900 μg/dl without evidence of tumor. However,

DHEA-S is typically suppressed in patients with adrenal adenomas and the level is often normal in patients with adrenal carcinoma. Also adrenal androgen secretion decreases after about age 30, so age-related normal subjects must be studied to determine elevated levels in older women (Fig. 9-3).

Prolactin. All women with menstrual irregularities should have a screening prolactin level. Since the prolactin level is increased by food, stress, and breast examinations, any woman with an elevated level should have the prolactin determination repeated at a time when she is fasting and has not had an examination. Hyperprolactinemia is discussed in detail in Chapter 10.

Urine collection for 17-ketosteroids. A 24-hour urine collection for 17-ketosteroids, which will detect androgen precursors, is an important part of the evaluation for pathologic hyperandrogenism, because some tumors may not be sufficiently differentiated to synthesize the more potent androgens at the final steps of the pathway. Fewer than 1% of normal women under age 30 will have a 17-ketosteroid level greater than 17 mg/24 hr. Abdominal computed tomography (CT) may be indicated to rule out an adrenal mass. Because nonfunctioning and benign adrenal adenomas are so common, an abdominal CT should not be done unless there is a significant elevation of an adrenal androgen level. Just as with DHEA-S levels, it is critical to evaluate 17-ketosteroid levels on a nomogram that adjusts for age, because of the gradual decline in normal levels after about age 30 (Fig. 9-3).

DIAGNOSTIC TESTS

Screening laboratory tests
Free testosterone
DHEA-S
24-hour urine collection for creatinine and 17-ketosteroids (add urine-free cortisol when symptoms of Cushing's syndrome present)

Second-level tests
LH and FSH
Prolactin
Pelvic ultrasound to evaluate endometrial thickness, ovarian size, presence of abnormal ovarian masses
Oral glucose tolerance test for glucose and insulin (especially if obesity or acanthosis present)
Fasting lipids
Liver function tests if planned oral contraceptive therapy

Third-level tests (usually by an endocrinologist or gynecologist)
ACTH stimulation test for cortisol and 17-OH progesterone (to screen for congenital adrenal hyperplasia)
Dexamethasone suppression test (to screen for adrenal tumor)
Abdominal CT (to screen for adrenal tumor)
Ovarian and adrenal vein sampling
Müllerian inhibiting substance level as a marker for sex-cord tumors
Laparoscopy or laparotomy

DHEA-S, dehydroepiandrosterone sulfate; LH, luteinizing hormone; FSH, follicle-stimulating hormone; ACTH, adrenocorticotropic hormone; CT, computed tomography.

EVALUATION OF HYPERANDROGENISM

Initial screening

Free testosterone level
DHEA-S level
Prolactin level (if oligorrhea or amenorrhea present)

Indications for further evaluation or referral

History

Abrupt, rapid onset of symptoms
Symptoms of Cushing's syndrome or malaise suggestive of a tumor
Severity out of proportion to family history
Strong family history suggestive of steroidogenic enzyme dysfunction
Menstrual irregularity or infertility
Significant patient concern

Physical examination

Evidence of higher androgen levels
Terminal hair on chin, sternum, upper back, or upper abdomen
Clitoral index (height × width) >35 mm^2
Temporal balding
Deepening of voice
Evidence of associated diseases
Abdominal or pelvic mass
Acanthosis nigricans
Obesity
Galactorrhea

Diagnostic testing

Free testosterone level greater than 2 ng/dl

DHEA-S, dehydroepiandrosterone sulfate.

Pelvic ultrasound. If an ovarian tumor is suspected, new high-resolution pelvic ultrasonography, often with a transvaginal probe that gets closer to the ovaries than previous transabdominal transducers, allows identification of ovarian cysts as small as 2 to 3 mm. The sensitivity and specificity of ultrasound for the diagnosis of ovarian tumors in hyperandrogenic women are unknown, since hyperandrogenic women are typically young and intermittently grow normal physiologic cysts. Suspicious findings include large cysts and complex cysts that do not resolve spontaneously over 2 to 4 weeks. However, small hilar cell ovarian tumors can produce large amounts of androgens and still be invisible on ultrasound, and even on direct ovarian visualization at surgery. If an ovarian lesion is not seen but ovarian hyperandrogenism is suspected, selective bilateral ovarian and adrenal vein sampling has been attempted, but with significant false-positive and false-negative results.

Ultrasound can also be used to identify the classic ovarian morphology of PCOS. This morphology is identified by a ring of small peripheral follicles, typically each less than 8 mm, with an increased amount of central stroma (Fig. 9-4). Such ovaries are typically, but not always, enlarged. Of a large series of women with hirsutism, 83% had the classic appearance of polycystic ovaries on ultrasound. In addition, 23% of regularly menstruating women also had this characteristic, raising the possibilities that either the predisposition for PCOS is much more common than previously believed or that

the morphology is merely a variant of normal. The ultrasound characteristics of PCOS cannot be used to rule out other causes of hyperandrogenism, however, because the same ovarian morphology has been seen in women with hyperandrogenism of different primary causes, including exogenous androgen administration and congenital adrenal hyperplasia.

ACTH stimulation test. The best screening test for congenital adrenal hyperplasia is the 1-hour ACTH-stimulated 17-hydroxyprogesterone level. As a rule, a stimulated 17-OH progesterone level greater than 20 ng/ml is most consistent with homozygous enzyme deficiency, whereas stimulated levels less than 4 ng/ml are normal. Levels between 4 and 10 ng/ml are indeterminate: some such women are heterozygotes for 21-OH deficiency and some have a functional abnormality of androgen production that may be reversible.

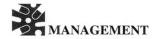 MANAGEMENT

Goals of management

The woman who has hirsutism or acne generally has one goal in mind, the clarification of her skin and normalization of her menses. The health professional has several addition-

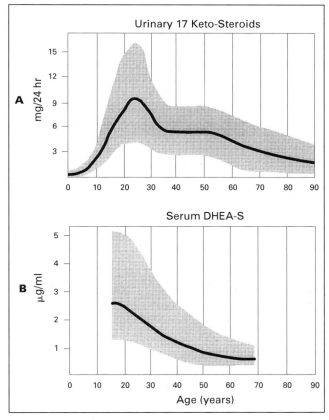

Fig. 9-3 Urinary 17-ketosteroids (mg/24 hr) (*A*) and serum DHEA-S levels (*B*) in normal women with aging. Note that there is a significant decline in both measures of adrenal androgens after age 30, long before the menopause. *A*, The shaded area represents 97% to 98% of the values in normal women. *B*, The shaded area represents the log equivalent of the mean ±2 SD and represents about 90% of the measured values. (*A*, Modified from Hamburger C: *Acta Endocrinol* 1:19, 1948; *B*, Modified from Orentreich N et al: *J Clin Endocrinol Metab* 59:551, 1984.)

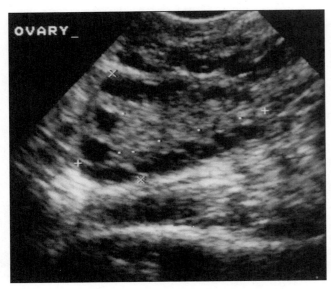

Fig. 9-4 A typical polycystic ovary on transvaginal ultrasonography. The markers represent centimeters. Note the peripheral ring of many follicles less than 1 cm in diameter. Despite the name, PCOS rarely causes growth of large cysts. (Courtesy of Ms. J. Adams.)

al management goals (see box, below) including primarily the exclusion of pathologic causes of hyperandrogenism. Women with a rapid onset of symptoms, a strong family history suggestive of a steroidogenic enzyme dysfunction, free testosterone levels greater than 2 ng/dl, or refractory response to initial treatment should be referred to an endocrinologist for further evaluation.

In the majority of women who do not have these features, the primary care provider must next consider the secondary health effects associated with hyperandrogenism such as endometrial cancer, insulin resistance, and cardiovascular risk factors. A careful history of menstrual frequency and abnormal vaginal bleeding should be obtained. Women with oligomenorrhea will need to be treated to prevent endometrial hyperplasia. All women with PCOS should also be assessed for cardiovascular risk factors, including family history, waist-to-hip ratio, blood pressure, and fasting lipid levels. It may be advisable to perform an oral glucose tolerance test for insulin levels in women who are obese or have other cardiovascular risk factors, if such information will improve a woman's motivation to lose weight or change her

diet. However, the predictive value of such testing in women with PCOS has yet to be established.

Choice of therapy

Women with hirsutism or acne and regular menses may be satisfied with cosmetic approaches such as tweezing, bleaching, and electrolysis once pathologic causes have been ruled out. Women whose primary concern is menstrual irregularity can be treated with cyclic progestins or oral contraceptives. Women with elevated adrenal androgen levels associated with elevated prolactin levels may improve with low-dose bromocriptine therapy. Most other women can be treated with one or more of the specific antiandrogen therapies available. In general these therapies can be initiated by the primary care physician, once he is convinced there is no evidence of a pathologic cause of the hyperandrogenism. All treated women should be advised that the hair follicle is viable for up to 6 months, and therefore a full 6-month trial of medication will be required before an appropriate cosmetic response can be assessed.

The optimal management of the insulin resistance associated with female hyperandrogenism has not yet been established. Since obese women with PCOS are more insulin resistant and weight loss will improve insulin resistance as well as hyperandrogenism and menstrual irregularity, they should be targeted for serious weight management. Other cardiovascular risk factors such as hypertension and hyperlipidemia should be treated directly, since potential responses to antiandrogen treatment are not yet known.

Because of their effect of regulating menses as well as reducing androgen levels, **oral contraceptives** are the drug of choice in women not currently desiring pregnancy (see box, below). Combined pills work by several additive mechanisms, including both suppression of gonadotropins leading to secondary suppression of ovarian androgen production, and increase of estrogen levels leading to increased SHBG levels and decreased free androgen levels.

In general the lowest dose pills (such as Ovcon and Modicon or Brevicon, which contain 0.4 and 0.5 mg norethindrone, respectively, with 35 μg of ethinyl estradiol) or the multiphasic pills should be tried first. In addition, pills containing the least androgenic progestins should be used. Thus the newest pills (such as Ortho-Cept, Desogen, Ortho-Tricyclen, and

---

MANAGEMENT GOALS

Identify women with hyperandrogenism
Exclude pathologic causes of hyperandrogenism
Prevent secondary disease
 Endometrial hyperplasia and endometrial cancer
Ameliorate associated diseases
 Obesity
 Insulin resistance
 Hyperlipidemia
Regulate menses
Treatment cosmetic complaints and infertility

THERAPY

Drugs

Oral contraceptives	Ethinyl estradiol 20-35 μg plus low dose of weakly androgenic progestin (0.4-1 mg norethindrone or ethynodiol diacetate, 0.15 mg desogestrel, or 0.18-0.25 mg norgestimate)
Antiandrogens	Spironolactone 50-100 mg bid
Progestins	Provera 10 mg daily × 10 days/month

Other

 Weight loss
 Cosmetic (electrolysis, bleaching, tweezing, shaving)

Ortho-Cyclen) containing desogestrel or norgestimate that have the least androgenic effect on lipids may also be the best for women with PCOS, although this assumption has not yet been formally tested. Some women with PCOS who have relatively large and active ovaries, as well as elevated luteinizing hormone (LH) levels, may need slightly higher dose pills to prevent breakthrough bleeding. For these women, higher progestin doses (such as found in Norinyl or Ortho-Novum 1/35) or the more estrogenic pro-gestin ethynodiol diacetate (found in Demulen 1/35) are more effective. Pills containing the more androgenic progestins levonorgestrel, norgestrel, and norethindrone acetate (such as Nordette, Lo-Ovral, and Lo-Estrin, respectively) should be avoided.

The use of oral contraceptives should be carefully considered in women with hyperprolactinemia, since estrogen tends to increase prolactin levels and could induce tumor growth. The suppression of androgen levels by oral contraceptives does not eliminate the possibility of an ovarian or adrenal tumor.

Women with irregular menses and fewer cosmetic symptoms may prefer **cyclic progestin therapy** to daily oral contraceptives. Medroxyprogesterone acetate (Provera) 10 mg/day for 10 to 14 days per month should induce a withdrawal bleeding in most women with PCOS because they have sufficient peripheral conversion of androgens to estrogens to induce endometrial proliferation. Some women prefer to take progestins once every 3 months, but no controlled studies have been performed to determine whether such intermittent therapy is adequate to prevent endometrial hyperplasia. Highly androgenic women may have sufficient endometrial atrophy that bleeding in response to a progestin alone will not occur and estrogen supplementation will be required.

Antiandrogens must be administered with an effective contraceptive because of their ability to cross the placenta and potentially block the normal androgen-dependent virilization of the male fetus. **Spironolactone** is the most potent antiandrogen currently available in the United States. Dosages to improve hirsutism are at least 50 to 100 mg twice a day. These dosages have been surprisingly well tolerated in normal young women, but women should have their potassium level checked within a few weeks of initiating therapy and be advised to increase their fluid intake. Spironolactone can induce menstrual irregularity in women who had previously been regular but can help normalize menses in some oligomenorrheic women, presumably by normalizing androgenic effects. The addition of an oral contraceptive to spironolactone will synergistically suppress androgens, as well as regularize menses and ensure contraception, making the combination an excellent option for many women.

Small doses of **bromocriptine** have been shown to reduce adrenal androgen levels and improve hirsutism and oligomenorrhea in some women with PCOS. It is important to start with very low doses (1.25 mg) taken with food at bedtime to prevent the nausea, drowsiness, and lightheadedness that are frequent complaints with bromocriptine. The dose can be increased by 1.25 mg increments at weekly intervals until the prolactin level is in the normal range.

Indications for referral

Referral to an endocrinologist is appropriate when a woman does not respond to the initial treatments described previously.

The initial choice of therapy for women with congenital adrenal hyperplasia is probably best determined in conjunction with an endocrinologist. Although classic therapy with glucocorticoids probably requires endocrinologic supervision, new data suggest that antiandrogens and oral contraceptives may be just as efficacious for late onset congenital adrenal hyperplasia in women who do not desire immediate pregnancy.

Women whose primary complaint is infertility also need referral to a reproductive endocrinologist. The major cause of infertility in hyperandrogenic women is anovulation, and up to 80% of anovulatory women with PCOS respond well to oral ovulation induction therapy with clomiphene citrate. Because of the risk of multiple gestations and hyperstimulation of the ovaries, the primary provider is advised to consult a specialist before considering such treatment.

The treatment for women with identified ovarian or adrenal tumors is surgical resection, which usually results in complete cure. Many small ovarian tumors can now be removed by laparoscopy, avoiding the prolonged recovery associated with laparotomy.

PROGNOSIS

Women with PCOS should be reassured that their prognosis is excellent, expecially if they are vigilant about health maintenance habits to reduce cardiovascular risk. The majority of androgen-secreting tumors have a relatively benign course. Late onset congenital adrenal hyperplasia also has a good prognosis. Many women with PCOS are very concerned that their menstrual irregularity or amenorrhea represents permanent infertility, and they are therefore reluctant to use oral contraceptives. All women should be reassured that the prospects for eventual fertility are actually quite good. One recent retrospective study of women who had had ovarian wedge resections for PCOS 20 years previously demonstrated no difference in their eventual fertility compared to that of control subjects.

BIBLIOGRAPHY

Adams J, Polson DW, Franks S: Prevalence of polycystic ovaries in women with anovulation and idiopathic hirsutism, *Br Med J* 293:355, 1986.

Dahlgren E et al: Women with polycystic ovary syndrome wedge resected in 1956 to 1965: a long-term follow-up focusing on natural history and circulating hormones, *Fertil Steril* 57:505, 1992.

Dewailly D et al: Clinical and biological phenotypes in late-onset 21-hydroxylase deficiency, *J Clin Endocrinol Metab* 63:418, 1986.

Dunaif A et al: Profound peripheral insulin resistance, independent of obesity in polycystic ovary syndrome, *Diabetes* 38:1165, 1989.

Ferriman D, Gallwey JD: Clinical assessment of body hair growth in women, *J Clin Endocrinol Metab* 21:1440, 1961.

Friedman CI et al: Serum testosterone concentrations in the evaluation of androgen-producing tumors, *Am J Obstet Gynecol* 153:44, 1985.

Futterweit W et al: The prevalence of hyperandrogenism in 109 consecutive female patients with diffuse alopecia, *J Am Acad Dermatol* 19:831, 1988.

Hamburger C: Normal urinary excretion of neutral 17-ketosteroids with special reference to age and sex variations, *Acta Endocrinol* 1:19, 1948.

Higuchi K et al: Prolactin has a direct effect on adrenal androgen secretion, *J Clin Endocrinol Metab* 59:714, 1984.

Hull MGR: Epidemiology of infertility and polycystic ovarian disease: endocrinological and demographic studies, *Gynecol Endocrinol* 1:235, 1987.

Hull MG et al: Population study of causes, treatment, and outcome of infertility, *Br Med J* 291:1693, 1985.

Laue L et al: Adrenal androgen secretion in postadolescent acne: increased adrenocortical function without hypersensitivity to adrenocorticotropin, *J Clin Endocrinol Metab* 73:380, 1991.

Maroulis GB: Evaluation of hirsutism and hyperandrogenism, *Fertil Steril* 36:273, 1981.

Meldrum DR, Abraham GE: Peripheral and ovarian venous concentrations of various steroid hormones in virilizing ovarian tumors, *Obstet Gynecol* 53:36, 1979.

Orentreich N et al: Age changes and sex differences in serum dehydroepiandrosterone sulfate concentrations throughout adulthood, *J Clin Endocrinol Metab* 59:551, 1984

Pang S et al: Worldwide experience in newborn screening for classical congenital adrenal hyperplasia due to 21-hydroxylase deficiency, *Pediatrics* 81:866, 1988.

Pasquali R et al: Clinical and hormonal characteristics of obese amenorrheic hyperandrogenic women before and after weight loss, *J Clin Endocrinol Metab* 68:173, 1989.

Polson DW et al: Polycystic ovaries—a common finding in normal women, *Lancet* 1:870, 1988.

Seppala M, Hirvonen E: Raised serum prolactin levels associated with hirsutism and amenorrhoea, *Br Med J* 18:144, 1975.

Stuart CA et al: Insulin resistance with acanthosis nigricans: the roles of obesity and androgen excess, *Metabolism* 35:197, 1986.

Tagatz GE et al: The clitoral index: a bioassay of androgenic stimulation, *Obstet Gynecol* 54:562, 1979.

Wild RA, Bartholomew MJ: The influence of body weight on lipoprotein lipids in patients with polycystic ovary syndrome, *Am J Obstet Gynecol* 159:423, 1988.

Yen SSC: Chronic anovulation caused by peripheral endocrine disorders. In Yen SSC, Jaffe JB, editors: *Reproductive endocrinology: physiology, pathophysiology and clinical management,* ed 3, Philadelphia, 1991, Saunders.

Zawadzki JK, Dunaif A: Diagnostic criteria for polycystic ovary syndrome: towards a rational approach. In Dunaif A et al, editors:*Polycystic ovary syndrome,* Boston, 1992, Blackwell Scientific.

10 Hyperprolactinemia and Galactorrhea

Laurence Katznelson and Anne Klibanski

In 1954 Forbes et al. hypothesized that the syndrome of amenorrhea and galactorrhea was caused by a lactogenic pituitary hormone. This anterior pituitary hormone was later identified to be prolactin, and we have since learned a great deal regarding both its normal physiologic function and its pathologic disorders. Prolactin has a major role in lactation and impacts on gonadal function. The pathologic hypersecretion of prolactin is the cause of secondary amenorrhea in approximately 20% of women and may be associated with galactorrhea. In this chapter we will summarize the normal physiologic control of prolactin secretion, actions of prolactin, and evaluation and management of women with hyperprolactinemic disorders.

PATHOPHYSIOLOGY
Normal control of prolactin secretion

Prolactin secretion is controlled by dual inhibitory and stimulatory factors (see Fig. 10-1). Prolactin is unique among anterior pituitary hormones because it is primarily regulated through tonic inhibition. Two decades of investigation have shown the presence of one or more **prolactin-inhibiting factors** (PIFs). **Dopamine** is the most important PIF described. Multiple studies support this hypothesis, all pointing to a direct effect of dopamine on the pituitary lactotrophs. In addition, most pharmacologic agents that cause prolactin release act by either blockade of dopamine receptors (haloperidol and phenothiazines) or dopamine depletion in the tuberoinfundibular neurons (reserpine and α-methyldopa). Other potential prolactin-inhibiting factors include gonadotropin-releasing hormone, specifically, **GnRH-associated peptide,** and γ-**aminobutyric acid**.

Stimulatory factors also regulate prolactin secretion. These substances may act directly on the pituitary or alternatively may act indirectly by dopaminergic blockade or depletion at the level of the hypothalamus. **Estrogens** are important physiologic stimulators of prolactin release. **Thy**rotropin-releasing hormone (TRH) stimulates both the synthesis and the release of prolactin *in vivo* and *in vitro* from normal, as well as tumor, lactotrophs. However, the physiologic role of TRH in prolactin secretion is unclear. Hypothyroidism results in an increase in both the thyroid-stimulating hormone and prolactin responses to TRH, and elevations in basal prolactin levels may be seen in primary hypothyroidism. **Vasoactive intestinal polypeptide** may potentiate prolactin release, although the clinical significance is unknown. GnRH may also have stimulatory properties; its administration induces the acute release of prolactin in both women with normal cycles and hypogonadal subjects. Other factors that may have stimulatory roles include **serotonin, bombesin, angiotensin II, histamine-2 antagonists,** and **opiates**.

Clinical aspects of prolactin physiology

Physiologic causes of hyperprolactinemia are summarized in the box on the following page. The following summarizes specific clinical aspects of prolactin physiology.

Diurnal and menstrual cycle variation. Prolactin is secreted in a pulsatile fashion with 4 to 9 pulses per day (60% occur during sleep). The amplitude of pulses is highly variable among individuals, with peak levels occurring during the late hours of sleep. Such rises are not associated with any specific stage of sleep. Although some studies have suggested that prolactin level varies during the menstrual cycle, the precise nature of this relationship remains unclear. Several investigators have shown that prolactin levels are significantly higher during the ovulatory and luteal phases, particularly at midcycle. This midcycle rise may be due to increased circulating periovulatory estradiol levels. Other studies have not confirmed this finding. Prolactin is probably not necessary for ovulation, since ovulatory periods may occur in females taking bromocriptine, a medication that suppresses prolactin.

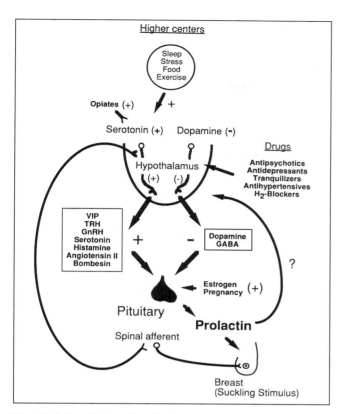

Fig. 10-1 Regulation of prolactin secretion. Prolactin release is under tonic inhibition by PIFs, predominantly dopamine. Prolactin release is stimulated by a number of factors, including VIP, TRH, and GnRH. Estrogens, pregnancy, and breast suckling stimulate prolactin release. Within the hypothalamus serotinergic and dopaminergic pathways are stimulatory and inhibitory, respectively, to prolactin release. PIFs, prolactin inhibiting factors; VIP, vasoactive intestinal peptide; TRH, thyrotropin-releasing hormone; GnRH, gonadotropin releasing hormone. (Modified from Molitch: *Endocrinol Metab Clin North Am* 21:877, 1992.)

Food. Abrupt rises in serum prolactin level occur within an hour of eating in normal and pregnant hyperprolactinemic individuals, but not in individuals with prolactinomas.

Stress. Prolactin rises during stress, including physical exertion, surgery, sexual intercourse, insulin hypoglycemia, and seizures. The significance of these changes is not known. Nipple stimulation, chest wall trauma or surgery, and herpes zoster infection of the breast may result in increases in prolactin levels.

Age. Mean levels of prolactin are slightly higher in premenopausal women than men, probably as a result of a direct

PHYSIOLOGIC CAUSES OF HYPERPROLACTINEMIA	
Pregnancy	Stress
Postpartum	Sleep
Nonnursing: days 1-7	Hypoglycemia
Nursing: with suckling	Sexual intercourse
Newborn	Nipple stimulation
Estrogens	Exercise

effect of estrogen on pituitary prolactin secretion. Some studies suggest that there is a progressive decline in prolactin levels in women with aging, particularly after the menopause. Responsiveness of prolactin to various pharmacologic agents (e.g., TRH) declines with age in women. This decline is probably due to postmenopausal estrogen deficiency.

Function of prolactin in normal states

The only established role of prolactin is to initiate and maintain lactation. Prolactin levels increase progressively with pregnancy. Estrogens play a major role in stimulation of prolactin levels. Prolactin levels rise progressively, peaking at term (100-300 ng/ml). Lactation begins when estradiol levels fall at parturition. Prolactin levels increase to 60 times higher than baseline levels in the circulation within 20 to 30 minutes of nursing. The nursing stimulus effectively promotes acute prolactin release via afferent spinal neural pathways. With continued nursing the nipple stimulation itself elicits progressively less prolactin release, and in the weeks following initiation of lactation both basal and nursing-induced prolactin pulses decrease although lactation continues. Within 4 to 6 months postpartum basal prolactin levels are normal without a nursing-induced rise.

![] EVALUATION OF HYPERPROLACTINEMIA

Clinical manifestations

The amenorrhea-galactorrhea syndrome is the classic description of the clinical manifestation of hyperprolactinemia. However, a spectrum of reproductive disorders may be seen. Prolactin level elevations are found in approximately 20% of patients with secondary amenorrhea. Women with hyperprolactinemia may have more subtle abnormalities in gonadal function, including oligomenorrhea or alterations in luteal phase function. A subset of infertile women have been described with mild or intermittent hyperprolactinemia in whom fertility was restored with bromocriptine therapy. Galactorrhea is present in only approximately 30% of female patients with hyperprolactinemia, but the presence of galactorrhea in a woman with an ovulatory disorder greatly increases the chance that hyperprolactinemia is the underlying cause of the amenorrhea.

Hypogonadism (decreased gonadal steroid levels) frequently occurs in patients with hyperprolactinemia. There are multiple potential mechanisms hypothesized for the induction of hypogonadism by prolactin, and the antigonadotrophic actions of prolactin may occur at multiple levels. Frequently the hypogonadism is associated with decreased or inappropriately normal luteinizing hormone (LH) and follicle-stimulating hormone (FSH) levels relative to the state of estrogen deficiency. Several investigations suggest that prolactin may have a suppressive effect on spontaneous LH release via decreases in endogenous GnRH levels. Prolactin appears to affect its own secretion via a short-loop negative feedback at the level of the hypothalamus. This feedback may be mediated through an increase in dopamine inhibitory tone. This increased hypothalamic dopamine tone, along with opiates and other factors, may suppress GnRH with a resultant decrease in LH pulses. The restoration of ovulatory menstrual periods in hyperprolactinemic women with pulsatile exogenous GnRH administration confirms the importance of endogenous GnRH abnormalities as the key mechanism of hypogonadism in these women.

In addition, prolactin may modulate androgen secretion at the level of both the adrenal gland and the ovary, resulting in increased secretion of dehydroepiandrosterone sulfate and testosterone. Therefore altered ratios of estrogens and androgens may further result in abnormal gonadal function, with evidence of hyperandrogenism (e.g., hirsutism). If the underlying cause of the increased prolactin level is a pituitary macroadenoma, then the adenoma could cause compression of the normal, adjacent pituitary gland with a resultant decrease in gonadotroph activity.

Hyperprolactinemia is also associated with both trabecular and cortical osteopenia. Hyperprolactinemic women may have trabecular osteopenia with spinal bone density ranging from 10% to 25% below normal. Studies have shown that the bone density in such patients may increase with normalization of prolactin levels with therapy; however, the bone density typically still remains lower than that of normal control subjects. The cause of this decrease in bone density is thought to be the hypogonadism resulting from the hyperprolactinemic state, and not the prolactin per se. Hyperprolactinemic women with normal menstrual function do not have associated bone loss. Figure 10-2 shows that hyperprolactinemic patients with hypogonadism have lower bone density than eugonadal hyperprolactinemic women.

History and physical examination

The history and physical examination should include investigation into potential causes of hyperprolactinemia in addition to its clinical manifestations.

The history should therefore screen for causes of hyperprolactinemia. (See box on the following page.) It is important to consider primary hypothyroidism and pregnancy as causes. Chronic renal disease may be associated with prolactin level elevations, likely caused by altered metabolism/clearance of prolactin and/or decreases in dopaminergic tone. A detailed history of medications may elicit a pharmacologic cause of hyperprolactinemia. Medications associated with hyperprolactinemia include reserpine, α-methyldopa, cimetidine, phenothiazines and other neuroleptics, and opiates. Estrogen therapy may lead to increases in prolactin levels, as are seen in pregnancy. However, estrogen concentrations in typical oral contraceptives (e.g., 35 μg ethinyl estradiol) are not associated with hyperprolactinemia and there is no evidence that postmenopausal replacement estrogen causes elevations in serum prolactin concentration.

In women hypogonadism related to hyperprolactinemia may cause abnormal menstrual function. The presence of oligomenorrhea or amenorrhea will have an impact on therapy. A history of infertility caused by altered luteal phase function may be present. Other hypogonadal symptoms include vaginal dryness, dyspareunia, fatigue, and diminished libido. The physical examination should include assessment of galactorrhea, which may be unilateral or bilateral.

The evaluation should also include assessment of the presence of a pituitary tumor. Hyperprolactinemia may be detected in up to 25% of patients with acromegaly and has been reported in Cushing's disease. Therefore acromegaly and Cushing's disease should be evaluated in those hyper-

prolactinemic patients with suggestive clinical manifestations. Pituitary and nonpituitary tumors may cause local mass effects, and symptoms such as headaches, diplopia, and blurry vision are common. Careful visual field examination by confrontation may reveal evidence of visual field deficits, including bitemporal hemianopsia or quadrantanopsia. These findings suggest the presence of compression of the optic chiasm by a tumor. Compression of the adjacent, normal pituitary gland may result in hypopituitarism. Symptoms attributable to hypopituitarism may include fatigue, anorexia, weight loss, dizziness, and polyuria (suggesting the presence of diabetes insipidus). Therefore in consideration of the presence of a sellar mass a careful history and physical examination should be performed to evaluate for the presence of thyroid, adrenal, and antidiuretic hormone function.

Diagnostic testing

As shown in the box on the following page, there are several causes of hyperprolactinemia. First, the prolactin level should be remeasured in a nonstimulated state, and, if pos-

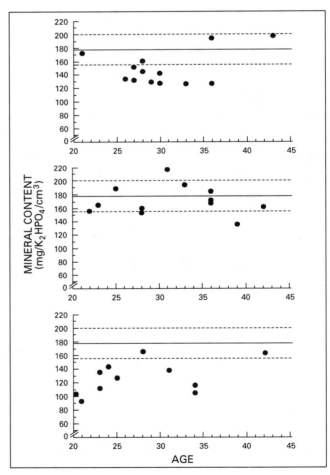

Fig. 10-2 Spinal bone density in 13 women with hyperprolactinemic amenorrhea (top panel), 12 eumenorrheic hyperprolactinemic women (middle panel), and 11 women with hypothalamic amenorrhea (bottom panel). The mean (solid horizontal line) 6 S.D. (dashed horizontal line) for 19 normal women are shown. (From Klibanski et al: *J Clin Endocrinol Metab* 67:124, 1988.)

PATHOLOGIC AND PHARMACOLOGIC CAUSES OF HYPERPROLACTINEMIA

Pituitary disease
  Prolactin-secreting tumors
  Acromegaly
  Cushing's disease
  Empty sella syndrome

Pituitary stalk section
  Clinically nonfunctioning pituitary tumors
  Trauma

Hypothalamic infiltrative or degenerative disease
  Craniopharyngiomas
  Meningiomas
  Dysgerminomas
  Gliomas
  Lymphoma
  Metastatic disease
  Tuberculosis
  Sarcoidosis
  Eosinophilic granuloma
  Irradiation

Neurogenic
  Chest wall trauma
  Chest wall lesions
  Herpes zoster
  Breast stimulation

Medications
  Phenothiazines
  Tricyclic antidepressants
  Metoclopramide
  Cimetidine
  Methyldopa
  Reserpine
  Calcium-channel blockers
  Cocaine

Other
  Renal failure
  Liver disease
  Primary hypothyroidism
  Ectopic hormone production
  Seizures

Modified from Molitch ME: *Endocrinol Metab Clin North Am* 21:877, 1992.

sible, we recommend measuring a morning prolactin level after an overnight fast in a nonstressed state. For example, prolactin may be secreted to a modest degree after a breast examination so a mild increase in prolactin levels after such an examination warrants a repeat prolactin determination.

Although a number of pathologic causes can elevate prolactin level, pituitary tumors are clinically the most important. Prolactin-secreting pituitary adenomas are the most common type of pituitary tumor and may account for up to 40% to 50% of all pituitary tumors.

Substantial elevations in prolactin level, greater than 150 ng/ml, in a nonpuerperal state are usually indicative of a pituitary tumor. There is a good correlation between radiographic estimates of tumor size and prolactin levels, and very high levels of prolactin are associated with larger tumors. Prolactinomas are classified as microadenomas (<10 mm) and macroadenomas (>10 mm). Therefore the finding of a substantial elevation in serum prolactin level in association with a pituitary lesion greater than 10 mm by radiographic analysis supports the diagnosis of a macroprolactinoma.

The majority of women with prolactinomas have microadenomas; in contrast, the majority of tumors in men are macroadenomas. This may be due to the fact that women may seek earlier evaluation than men because of menstrual disturbances.

Modest levels of prolactin elevation (e.g., 25 to 100 ng/ml) may be associated with a number of diagnoses. All causes of hyperprolactinemia should be excluded before a tumor is considered. Pregnancy should be excluded. Common causes of modest prolactin level elevations are primary hypothyroidism and chronic renal disease. Medications, including phenothiazines, metoclopramide, cimetidine, and calcium-channel blockers, may be associated with hyperprolactinemia.

One diagnostic problem is the evaluation of patients with psychiatric disease who are receiving phenothiazines and are found to have an elevated prolactin level. We recommend a magnetic resonance imaging (MRI) scan for patients whose prolactin levels are greater than 100 ng/ml and assume that levels below this value are consistent with neuroleptic administration. This strategy is based on the finding that the majority of patients receiving neuroleptics with modest prolactin level elevations have no evidence of a pituitary abnormality on scan.

Any intrasellar or suprasellar mass may lead to modest prolactin level elevations through stalk compression. Therefore any patient with modest hyperprolactinemia and no clear secondary cause, such as pregnancy or medication use, should undergo radiographic analysis. These masses include primary pituitary tumors, meningiomas, and craniopharyngiomas. In addition, hypothalamic disorder including destructive (tumors, granulomatous diseases) lesions may lead to hyperprolactinemia by interfering with normal dopaminergic tone.

When an elevated serum prolactin level is not associated with primary hypothyroidism, pregnancy, or use of pharmacologic agents, a pituitary radiographic scan should be performed to rule out the presence of either a prolactin-secreting pituitary tumor or other lesions. In addition, as described later, it is important to distinguish microprolactinomas from macroprolactinomas. An MRI scan is a more sensitive tool than a computed tomography (CT) scan for evaluating the sellar and suprasellar areas. If the scan shows normal sellar and extrasellar contents and there is no clear secondary cause of the elevated prolactin level, then the diagnosis of idiopathic hyperprolactinemia is made. These cases may represent microprolactinomas, and a small tumor may be beyond the sensitivity of the scanning technique.

MANAGEMENT

Treatment is dependent on whether the woman has hyperprolactinemia due to an underlying cause, such as drug use or hypothyroidism, or a prolactinoma. If the above evaluation suggests the presence of a microprolactinoma, there are three available treatment options: careful follow-up without treatment, medical therapy with a dopamine agonist, and, rarely, surgery. All patients with macroadenomas should be treated.

Close follow-up observation without treatment

Patients with a microadenoma and those without evidence of a pituitary tumor can sometimes be followed up without therapy if fertility is not an issue, tumor size has not increased, and normal menstrual function is not disrupted. Studies evaluating the natural history of microprolactinomas have generally shown that prolactin level elevations may remain stable and in some cases spontaneously normalize. Martin, Kim, and Malarkey (1985) studied 41 patients over 5.5 years of follow-up observation and showed that 67% of patients whose initial prolactin values were less than 57 ng/ml had normalization of the prolactin level, whereas none of the patients with initial prolactin values greater than 60 ng/ml reached normal values. These and other data suggest that the degree of prolactin level elevation is a prognostic factor for spontaneous resolution. Schlechte et al. (1989) showed that basal menstrual function is an important variable in determining progression of the prolactin level. In this study patients with normal initial menstrual function were more likely to experience normalization of prolactin values, whereas those with oligomenorrhea or amenorrhea were more likely to have no change or increases in prolactin values.

In terms of tumor size, most studies show that the majority of microprolactinomas do not increase in size. Many of these studies are not recent and must be interpreted in light of the use of less sensitive radiographic techniques such as skull films and tomograms. Studies show that tumors in patients with microprolactinomas or no radiographic evidence of tumor increase in size in 0% to 22% of patients. In a study by Webster et al. of 43 patients with presumed microadenomas with a mean follow-up period of 5.4 years, only 2 patients showed evidence of tumor progression (at 4 and 6 years of follow-up evaluation). The tumor progression was not accompanied by an increasing serum prolactin level. Follow-up evaluation of untreated patients should include both serial prolactin levels and periodic MRI scans.

Medical therapy

Medical therapy for a patient with microprolactinomas is based on the effects of hyperprolactinemia in that patient. Patients with hyperprolactinemia usually have accompanying menstrual irregularities. Bromocriptine therapy will result in a return of menstrual function in the majority of patients with amenorrhea. Luteal phase defects associated with hyperprolactinemia will also reverse with bromocriptine therapy. Ovulation rates in excess of 90% have been reported, with induced pregnancy rates in greater than 80% of patients. The presence of galactorrhea itself is not an absolute indication for bromocriptine therapy, unless the degree of galactorrhea is significantly bothersome to the patient. Hyperprolactinemia has also been associated with headaches or hirsutism, which may resolve with prolactin level normalization. If there is no evidence of hypogonadism in patients with microprolactinomas, then having no therapy is an option for some women with microadenomas who do not desire fertility.

Almost all patients with hyperprolactinemia caused by pituitary disease can be effectively treated with the dopamine agonist bromocriptine mesylate (Parlodel). Bromocriptine lowers serum prolactin levels in patients with pituitary tumors and all other causes of hyperprolactinemia. Bromocriptine is very effective in rapidly decreasing prolactin levels and both normalizing reproductive function and reversing galactorrhea. It is also useful in treating galactorrhea in patients with normoprolactinemic galactorrhea. Bromocriptine will decrease prolactin production and secretion with consequent reduction in prolactin cell size. This will result in decreased tumor size.

Therapy should be initiated slowly because side effects, including nausea, headache, dizziness, nasal congestion, and constipation, may occur. Gastrointestinal side effects may be minimized by starting with a very low dose at night (e.g., 1.25 mg ([$^1/_2$ tablet]) and increasing the dosage by 1.25 mg over 4- to 5-day intervals. This is continued until a dose that normalizes prolactin levels is reached. Taking the medication at bedtime with a snack initially will help minimize the gastrointestinal symptoms. These side effects usually improve with either continuing at the same dose or temporarily reducing the dose. If patients stop taking the medication for a few days, they may need to restart therapy at a lower dose as these side effects may return. Rarely, chronic therapy may result in side effects, including painless cold-sensitive digital vasospasm, alcohol intolerance, dyskinesia, and psychiatric reactions, such as fatigue, depression, and anxiety.

There are other dopamine agonists under investigation, including CV 205-502 and the long-acting preparations parlodel LAR and cabergoline. CV 205-502 or cabergoline may have an efficacy similar to that of bromocriptine but with fewer side effects and greater compliance.

Surgery

Although surgery is not a primary mode of management for patients with prolactinomas, in a few cases it may be useful. There are several indications for surgery, including large tumors with visual field deficits unresponsive to bromocriptine, inability to tolerate bromocriptine as a result of side effects, cystic tumors that do not to respond to medical therapy, and apoplexy of the prolactinoma. A transsphenoidal approach is almost exclusively used. When surgery is performed by experienced surgeons the morbidity rate is negligible. The main advantage of curative surgery is avoidance of long-term medication. Serri et al. (1983) reported that of 28 patients with microprolactinomas 24 were cured with transsphenoidal surgery as determined by normalization of serum prolactin levels. However, after approximately 4 years 50% of these initially cured patients experienced a recurrence of hyperprolactinemia, although there was no radiographic evidence of tumor. Another group found a recurrence rate of 39% after approximately 5 years. These data suggest that although surgery may normalize prolactin levels initially in patients with microprolactinomas, there is a relatively high recurrence risk. A serum prolactin level greater than 9 ng/ml 1 to 3 days after surgery indicates surgical failure.

Conventional radiotherapy (4500 to 5000 rad) or proton beam therapy may be indicated in patients with larger tumors in whom immediate control of symptoms and fertility is not a high priority and in those who are not able to tolerate medical therapy.

Macroprolactinomas

In contrast to patients with microprolactinomas patients with macroprolactinomas need more definitive therapy. Patients with macroadenomas may have evidence of local mass effects caused by the expanding tumor, with resultant visual field abnormalities and hypopituitarism resulting from compression of the normal pituitary gland. Therefore it is very important to be aggressive in management to prevent or reverse these complications. Bromocriptine will produce significant tumor shrinkage in up to 75% of patients. Size reduction may occur in weeks or over many months. This is frequently accompanied by improvement in visual field abnormalities and pituitary function. Molitch et al. (1985) treated 27 such patients with bromocriptine and found reduction in tumor size by at least 50% in 64% of patients. Tumor shrinkage often occurred within 6 weeks in this study. Sixty-six percent of patients had normalization of prolactin levels, but the fall in prolactin level did not necessarily correlate with reduction in tumor size.

Transsphenoidal surgery is not used as a primary therapy for patients with macroprolactinomas except in neurosurgical emergency. Surgical cure is inversely proportional to serum prolactin levels and tumor size. There are no data directly comparing bromocriptine to surgery as primary therapy for macroadenomas. Specific circumstances, such as the presence of a cystic prolactinoma (which often does not respond fully to bromocriptine therapy), may predict a poor initial response to bromocriptine therapy in all such patients. Bromocriptine is a useful adjunct therapy in patients with large tumors when complete resection has not been possible.

Pregnancy and prolactinomas

Many women with hyperprolactinemia are infertile. Bromocriptine is typically used to normalize prolactin levels and allow normal ovulation to occur. We recommend discontinuing bromocriptine when pregnancy is detected. There is concern, however, that during pregnancy the high levels of estrogens may lead to lactotroph stimulation and tumor growth. Pregnancy in a normal woman will lead to increased pituitary size through estrogen-stimulated lactotroph hyperplasia. Therefore pituitary enlargement may lead to local complications including visual field deficits, headaches, and diabetes insipidus. Molitch (1985) reviewed the series on pregnancy outcomes in hyperprolactinemic patients. Up to 5% of patients with microprolactinomas experience clinically significant tumor enlargement (headaches or visual deficits or both). Therefore patients with microprolactinomas may be followed carefully without therapy during pregnancy. Patients should receive close follow-up observation, and visual field analysis performed at monthly intervals is recommended.

In contrast, 15% to 36% of patients with macroadenomas are at risk for clinically significant tumor enlargement in any trimester. Some centers therefore recommend transsphenoidal resection of the macroadenomas before conception. However, prior surgery does not prevent tumor enlargement during pregnancy. We do not recommend a preventive sur-

gical approach and instead follow these patients closely, as noted for patients with microprolactinomas. Monitoring of serum prolactin levels throughout pregnancy is not clinically useful because prolactin levels increase markedly during pregnancy and a decision to reinstitute therapy is dependent upon clinical symptoms. The published data suggest that if a complication does occur, it is rapidly reversible with the reinstitution of bromocriptine, which is then continued through term.

The outcome of bromocriptine-induced pregnancies is comparable to that of normal pregnancies. A large international experience with bromocriptine and pregnancy suggests that bromocriptine therapy does not result in complications for the fetus. Breast-feeding after delivery appears to be safe. Patients with macroadenomas should continue to be followed closely and the decision to institute therapy is based on tumor size and clinical symptoms.

Indications for referral

The routine evaluation and management of hyperprolactinemia may be performed by the primary caregiver. There are several indications for referral to an endocrinologist; the presence of a macroprolactinoma is one. These patients often have visual field dysfunction, cranial nerve deficits, and hypopituitarism. The urgency of these situations dictates that the therapy be managed by a caregiver with much experience in bromocriptine dosing and monitoring of side effects. In addition, medical therapy may be complicated by the presence of anterior and posterior pituitary insufficiency, and management may require an endocrinologist with experience in such therapy. Hyperprolactinemia that does not respond to bromocriptine should also be an indication for referral. Management of these patients may require reinitiation of bromocriptine therapy instead of attempted therapy with other dopamine agonists. Again these other dopamine agonists should be administered by physicians with experience with such medications. Finally, patients considered for surgery should also have the indications for surgery reviewed with an endocrinologist.

SUMMARY

In summary, patients with hyperprolactinemia need to have a complete evaluation to determine the underlying cause of the elevated prolactin level. If either idiopathic hyperprolactinemia or prolactinoma is the cause, then dopamine agonist therapy is highly efficacious in lowering prolactin levels, restoring gonadal function, and reversing local tumor complications.

BIBLIOGRAPHY

Bassetti M et al: Bromocriptine treatment reduces the cell size in human macroprolactinomas: a morphometric study, *J Clin Endocrinol Metab* 58:268, 1984.

Bergh T, Nillius SJ, Wide L: Bromocriptine treatment of 42 hyperprolactinemic women with secondary amenorrhea, *Acta Endocrinol* 88:435, 1978.

Blackwell RE: Hyperprolactinemia: evaluation and management, *Endocrinol Metab Clin North Am,* 21:105, 1992.

Forbes AP et al: Syndrome characterized by galactorrhea, amenorrhea and low urinary FSH: comparison with acromegaly and normal lactation, *J Clin Endocrinol Metab* 14:265, 1954.

Franks S et al: Incidence and significance of hyperprolactinemia in women with amenorrhea, *Clin Endocrinol* 4:597, 1975.

Klibanski A, Greenspan SL: Increase in bone mass after treatment of hyperprolactinemic amenorrhea, *N Engl J Med* 315:542, 1986.

Klibanski A et al: Effects of prolactin and estrogen deficiency in amenorrheic bone loss, *J Clin Endocrinol Metab* 67:124-30, 1988.

Koppelman et al: Vertebral body bone mineral content in hyperprolactinemic women, *J Clin Endocrinol Metab* 59:1050, 1984.

March CM et al: Longitudinal evaluation of patients with untreated prolactin-secreting pituitary adenomas, *Am J Obstet Gynecol* 139:835, 1981.

Martin TL, Kim M, Malarkey WB: The natural history of idiopathic hyperprolactinemia, *J Clin Endocrinol Metab* 60:855, 1985.

Molitch ME: Pregnancy and the hyperprolactinemic women, *N Engl J Med* 312:1364, 1985.

Molitch ME: Pathologic hyperprolactinemia, *Endocrinol Metab Clin North Am* 21:877, 1992.

Molitch ME et al: Bromocriptine as primary therapy for prolactin-secreting macroadenomas: results of a prospective multicenter study, *J Clin Endocrinol Metab* 60:698, 1985.

Noel GL, Suh HK, Frantz AG: Prolactin release during nursing and breast stimulation in postpartum and nonpostpartum subjects, *J Clin Endocrinol Metab* 38:413, 1974.

Schlechte JA et al: Long term follow-up of women with surgically treated prolactin-secreting pituitary tumors, *J Clin Endocrinol Metab* 62:1296, 1986.

Schlechte J et al: The natural history of untreated hyperprolactinemia: a prospective analysis, *J Clin Endocrinol Metab* 68:412, 1989.

Serri O et al: Recurrence of hyperprolactinemia after selective transsphenoidal adenectomy in women with prolactinoma, *N Engl J Med* 309:280, 1983.

Sisam DA, Sheehan JP, Sheeler LR: The natural history of untreated microprolactinomas, *Fertil Steril* 48:67, 1987.

Webster J et al: Low recurrence rate after partial hypophysectomy for prolactinoma: the predictive value of dynamic prolactin function tests, *Clin Endocrinol* 36:35, 1992.

Weiss MH et al: Natural history of microprolactinomas: six-year follow-up, *Neurosurgery,* 12:180, 1983.

11 Osteoporosis

David M. Slovik

Osteoporosis is a major medical problem, which leads to increased morbidity and mortality, loss of function, long-term physical and emotional disability, and suffering. It is estimated that more than 25 million persons in the United States have osteoporosis; 1.3 million fractures are attributable to osteoporosis each year and the annual cost of caring for patients with osteoporosis-related fractures is $10 billion.

Osteoporosis is a systemic skeletal disease characterized by low bone mass and microarchitectural deterioration of bone tissue, with a consequent increase in bone fragility and susceptibility to fracture. Bone has a normal ratio of mineral to matrix. **Osteomalacia** refers to a group of disorders characterized by an abnormality in bone mineralization. The ratio of mineral to matrix is diminished as a result of an excess of unmineralized osteoid. **Osteopenia** is a general term referring to bone density that is lower than that seen in healthy young adults. Osteopenia can be caused by many disorders, including osteoporosis, and predisposes bone to fragility fractures. A **fragility fracture** is one that occurs without any trauma, or it can occur after a fall from a height of less than 12 inches or after abrupt deceleration from a speed slower than a run.

EPIDEMIOLOGY

The hip, vertebrae, and distal portion of the forearm are the most common sites of osteoporotic fractures, although fractures of other sites, including the pelvis, femur, tibia, and humerus, also occur with increased frequency. Of the estimated 1.3 million osteoporotic fractures annually, more than 500,000 are of the vertebrae and 250,000 are of the hip.

The incidence of hip fractures increases with advancing age. This is due to a combination of factors, including low bone mass, increased falls, and decreased protection from falls. At 50 years of age, the average white woman has a lifetime risk of 17.5% for hip fracture, and the lifetime risk for any fracture of the hip, spine, or distal forearm is almost 40%. After the age of 60 years, the age-specific incidence of proximal femur fractures increases almost exponentially. By the ninth decade of life, the cumulative incidence of fractures of the proximal femur is approximately 32% for women and 17% for men.

The lifetime risk for a 50-year-old white women to be clinically diagnosed with a vertebral fracture is 15.6%. This figure is probably low because many of these fractures are asymptomatic.

PATHOPHYSIOLOGY OF AGE-RELATED BONE LOSS

Most of the bone mass in adults is laid down during adolescence. Even though bones have stopped growing in length after puberty with closure of the growth plates, radial bone growth continues, the bone mineral content increases, and bones become stronger.

Trabecular (cancellous) bone attains its peak bone mass in the late 20s and cortical (compact) bone shortly thereafter. After a transient period of equilibrium, bone loss may begin sometimes by the late 30s or early 40s and accelerates for several years after the menopause.

Age-related bone loss occurs in both genders and affects trabecular and cortical bone, although to different degrees.

Risk factors for bone loss

Genetics. Bone density is more highly correlated in monozygotic than in dizygotic twins. Daughters of women with osteoporosis have lower spinal bone mass than normal control subjects of similar age. Osteoporosis is more common in whites and Asians compared with blacks. During early adulthood, bone mass generally is 5% to 10% higher in blacks than in whites and the subsequent fracture incidence is lower.

Aging. A steady age-related decline in bone mass occurs in all persons after skeletal maturity, although the rates vary.

Peak bone mass. The amount of bone attained at the time of skeletal maturity is very important. If the rate of bone loss with age is constant, then those women with the lowest bone density at skeletal maturity will be at greatest risk for sustaining fractures later in life.

Nutrition and life-style factors. Good nutrition is important to bone health. Adequate calcium is especially important in the years of growth and development and also is important in the postmenopausal years. Diets high in protein, phosphorus, fat, fiber, sodium, and caffeine may be harmful, either by increasing the excretion of calcium in the urine or interfering with the intestinal absorption of calcium. Alcohol abuse and cigarette smoking also are harmful to bone.

Exercise and physical activity. Immobilization can cause significant bone loss.

Hormones. Many hormones are important in bone development and maintaining a normal skeleton. These include estrogens, androgens, parathyroid hormone, vitamin D and its metabolites, calcitonin, insulin, glucocorticoids, prolactin, growth hormone, and thyroid hormone.

Deficiencies of gonadal steroids during the time of bone development will lead to thinner bones later in life; deficiencies later in life will produce severe bone loss and osteoporosis. Estrogen deficiency in premenopausal women as a result of gonadal dysgenesis, anorexia nervosa, prolonged amenorrhea, excessive exercise, or gonadotropin-releasing hormone (GnRH) therapy may reduce peak bone mass. Excesses of thyroid hormone or glucocorticoids can lead to bone loss. (See box, below.)

Bone remodeling

Bone remodeling is the cellular process that allows continuous removal of old bone and replacement with new bone. In remodeling there is cyclic erosion and repair of microscopic cavities, with long periods of quiescence between cycles. The adult skeleton is composed of two types of bone tissue: cortical (compacta, lamella) or trabecular (spongiosa, cancellous). Cortical bone constitutes approximately 80% of the total skeletal mass but only one third of the total surface. It forms the outer wall of all bones, but the bulk of cortical tissue is in the shafts of long bones of the appendicular skeleton. Trabecular bone provides the remaining 20% of total skeletal mass and about two thirds of its surface. Trabecular bone consists of plates that are distributed in relatively uniform manner. In osteoporosis there is a reduction in the number of plates, and there is conversion of plates to rods. Trabecular bone is found mainly in the bones of the axial skeleton and in the ends of the long bones.

Bone remodeling is a complex process regulated by hormones and growth factors. Any time that bone resorption is greater than bone formation, bone loss occurs. The imbalance can be in absolute or relative terms.

RISK FACTORS AFFECTING BONE LOSS

Genetics	Nutrition and life-style
Aging	Exercise and physical activity
Peak bone mass	Hormones

CLASSIFICATION

Age-related osteoporosis accounts for 80% to 90% of osteoporosis in women. There are many secondary causes of osteoporosis that may affect the amount of bone seen at the time of skeletal maturity or the amount of bone that subsequently is lost, (see box, below).

 EVALUATION

Two groups of patients usually seek medical evaluation:

*   Those with no history of osteoporosis. These women are usually young and healthy and are either premenopausal or in their early menopausal years. They

---

CLASSIFICATION OF OSTEOPOROSIS

Unknown causes
Primary osteoporosis (postmenopausal, senile)
Juvenile osteoporosis
Idiopathic osteoporosis

Endocrine causes
Hypogonadism
Glucocorticoid excess (endogenous or exogenous)
Thyrotoxicosis
Primary hyperparathyroidism
Hyperprolactinemia
Diabetes mellitus

Hematologic malignancies
Multiple myeloma
Leukemia
Lymphoma

Systemic mastocytosis
Heritable disorders of connective tissue
Osteogenesis imperfecta
Homocystinuria
Ehlers-Danlos syndrome

Immobilization
Drugs
Alcohol
Chronic heparin administration

Nutrition
Calcium deficiency
Scurvy
Malnutrition

Localized
Posttraumatiac (Sudeck's osteodystrophy)
Postfracture
Regional (migratory) osteolysis

Miscellaneous
Primary biliary cirrhosis
Rheumatoid arthritis
Chronic obstructive pulmonary disease

From Slovik DM. In Barbieri R, Schiff I, editors: *Reproductive endocrine therapeutics,* New York, 1988, Alan R Liss.

are concerned about developing osteoporosis and want to know whether they are at risk and what they can do to prevent it.
- Those with evidence of osteoporosis on the basis of clinical problems (e.g., fractures), bone density measurements, or radiographs.

Patients with hip fractures seek treatment for pain and deformity after a fall. After successful treatment and rehabilitation, many are left with limitation of function and the need for an assistive device (e.g., a walker or cane). In women with vertebral fractures, the most frequent symptoms are back pain, loss of height, and the development of a dorsal kyphosis. Back pain may be of acute onset following ordinary physical activity such as bending or lifting. The pain may be severe and usually is located over the fractured vertebrae. It often radiates in a radicular pattern laterally and is accompanied by severe paraspinal muscle spasm. The pain may be sufficient to produce shortness of breath and may be increased by minimal movements such as turning in bed, flexing the spine, or taking a deep breath. On examination, a dorsal kyphosis usually is evident, especially if prior fractures have occurred, and spasm with guarding may significantly limit spinal motion. Additional problems include nausea, anorexia, abdominal distention, and constipation.

The acute pain usually subsides after 1 to 2 weeks but is often present for as long as 4 to 6 weeks, and it may take even longer before normal activities can be resumed. Chronic back pain in these patients can be very troublesome. It is usually more diffuse and difficult to localize compared with the acute pain and is often described as a dull ache. This chronic pain usually is due to muscle strain and results from changes in the normal structure of the back with the development of a kyphosis and an increased lumbar lordosis. Acute sudden back pain may be due to additional fractures, microfractures, or muscle spasm. Progressive loss of height occurs as a result of these fractures. In severe cases the rib cage may come to rest on the iliac crest.

In evaluating patients for osteoporosis, it is important to diagnose treatable and reversible causes, determine the extent of bone loss, and establish baseline data that can be followed. The evaluation of osteoporosis can be divided into several areas.

History and physical examination

A detailed history and physical examination is necessary to identify risk factors and the secondary causes of osteoporosis. This should include looking for evidence of disorders that cause osteomalacia (see box, above right). Other causes of chronic low back pain, including degenerative arthritis and disk disease, should be sought. An extensive history of medications, diet, and exercise and activity level should be obtained. Height should be measured.

Laboratory tests

Laboratory tests should be completed to help in the differential diagnosis of osteoporosis and osteomalacia. These general laboratory tests include a complete blood cell count, sedimentation rate, chemistry profile, serum and urine protein electrophoresis, and thyroid-stimulating hormone value. A 24-hour test of urine calcium and creatinine levels is also

---

CLASSIFICATION OF RICKETS AND OSTEOMALACIA

I. Vitamin D deficiency
  A. Dietary
  B. Insufficient sunlight exposure
II. Gastrointestinal disorders
  A. Postgastrectomy
  B. Small intestinal diseases with malabsorption (e.g., celiac disease)
  C. Hepatobiliary disease (e.g., biliary atresia)
  D. Pancreatic insufficiency
III. Disorders of vitamin D metabolism
  A. Pseudovitamin D deficiency (vitamin D dependent)
  B. Anticonvulsants
IV. Hypophosphatemic rickets and osteomalacia
  A. X-linked hypophosphatemic rickets (vitamin D resistant)
  B. Sporadic or adult-onset
  C. Fanconi syndrome
  D. Tumor-induced
  E. Phosphate depletion
V. Acidosis
  A. Distal renal tubular acidosis
  B. Ureterosigmoidostomy
  C. Drug-induced (e.g., chronic acetazolamide therapy)
VI. Chronic renal failure
VII. Mineralization defects
  A. Hypophosphatasia
  B. Aluminum
  C. Medications: fluoride, bisphosphonates
VIII. Defective matrix synthesis
  A. Fibrogenesis imperfecta ossium
IX. Miscellaneous
  A. Axial osteomalacia

From Slovik DN, Ritter JS. In Aronoff GM, editor: *Evaluation and treatment of chronic pain*, Baltimore, 1992, Williams & Wilkins.

---

helpful. A serum 25-hydroxyvitamin D level should be obtained in those women suspected of having vitamin D deficiency. This group most commonly includes elderly persons living in northern climates, those with evidence of malabsorption, and those taking medications known to affect vitamin D metabolism, for example, phenytoin (Dilantin). A parathyroid hormone level should be obtained in suspected cases of primary (serum calcium is high) or secondary (serum calcium is low) hyperparathyroidism.

Blood and urine test results usually are normal in uncomplicated cases of osteoporosis. After a fracture the alkaline phosphatase level may be elevated. Very high levels of alkaline phosphatase suggest other metabolic bone diseases, including Paget's disease and osteomalacia. Liver disease also can elevate the alkaline phosphatase, but measuring the bone-specific fraction can differentiate the bone component from other sources. A small group of patients with osteoporosis has hypercalciuria.

Radiologic evaluation

Osteopenia is difficult to diagnose on spine radiographs because a decrease of at least 30% of bone mass may be necessary before osteopenia is evident. In osteoporosis, thinning and accentuation of the cortex and a relative increase in the vertical trabeculae (caused by a relatively greater loss of the horizontal trabeculae) may be evident. If a fracture is evident on x-ray film, then severe bone loss already has occurred unless the fracture was traumatic in nature. A radiograph of a tender area of the spine may show a fracture, but other vertebrae also may show deformities. The types of fractures identified are (1) anterior wedge fractures caused by loss of anterior height, (2) biconcave fractures caused by the expansive forces of the intervertebral disks, primarily in the lumbar region, and (3) compression fractures with loss of both anterior and posterior height of the vertebrae. On occasion, bone scans are required to assess for stress fractures, metastatic disease, or other abnormalities.

Bone density measurements

Noninvasive techniques. Plain spine radiographs can identify vertebral deformities but are unable to provide quantitative information. Thus various methods to measure bone density were developed. The amount of cortical and trabecular bone and the rate of bone loss vary in different parts of the body (Table 11-1.) There is a more rapid loss of trabecular bone in the vertebrae in the early menopausal years compared with cortical bone loss in other sites of the body.

Single-photon absorptiometry (SPA) is based on the transmission of photons from an external radioisotope source (I^{125}) through bone to a detector. SPA measurements are obtained primarily of the shaft of the forearm where there is predominantly cortical bone. In disorders in which cortical bone is reduced more than trabecular bone (e.g., primary hyperparathyroidism), a cortical bone density measurement is helpful.

Dual-photon absorptiometry (DPA) can measure total body calcium and the bone mineral content of regional areas of the body (e.g., lumbar spine and hip). This technique uses either two different isotopes or a single isotope such as gadolinium-153, which emits photons at two energy levels. This technique has generally been replaced by dual-energy x-ray absorptiometry (DXA).

DXA uses an x-ray source instead of a radionuclide. This technique measures areas similar to those obtained with DPA, and the measurements of the lumbar spine are highly correlated (0.98) on the basis of the two techniques. DXA however, is superior to DPA because it has clearer image resolution, better reproducibility, faster measurement time, and lower radiation, and it avoids the problems of changes

Table 11-1 Approximate proportions of cortical and trabecular bone at various sites in the skeleton

Site	Cortical (%)	Trabecular (%)
Hip		
Trochanteric region	50	50
Femoral neck	75	25
Vertebrae	40-60	40-60
Forearm		
Shaft	95	5
Distal	30-50	50-70

Modified from Cummings SR et al: *Epidemiol Rev* 7:178, 1985.

in the measurements when the radioactive source is changed. Measurements of the lumbar spine (in the anterior, posterior, and lateral projection), hip, total body, and forearm can be made using this technique. Because of its superior reproducibility, spinal DXA is preferred for the follow-up of osteopenia.

Quantitative computer tomography (QCT) has been adapted to measure the mineral content in the axial skeleton. A volumetric density is obtained. Usually L1 to L4 are scanned and the values compared with a standard solution of potassium phosphate. This technique measures trabecular bone. Because trabecular bone is lost most rapidly after the menopause, QCT is the best technique for diagnosing osteopenia, although other techniques also are appropriate. A comparison of the four techniques is shown in Table 11-2.

Clinical use. The strength of a bone is related to its mass, mineral content, and density. Bone strength is a determinant of fracture susceptibility. The bone mineral content of the spine and hip is inversely related to the risk of fracture. Bone density measurements can be used to diagnose osteopenia before a fracture has occurred and can identify patients at risk of developing future fractures. Bone density tests cannot distinguish osteoporosis from osteomalacia. Bone density measurements can be compared with those of a young, normal population (to determine if significant osteopenia has developed); to age-matched control subjects (to determine if there has been excessive loss of bone); or to a "fracture threshold," a level below which fractures are more likely to occur.

Bone density measurements should be obtained when the results will influence the physician's therapeutic recommendations or the patient's compliance with them. Specific recommendations from a task force of the National Osteoporosis Foundation for bone mass measurements are listed in the box on the following page. In estrogen-deficient women, bone mass measurements may be helpful in influencing the physician's decision to prescribe estrogens or the patient's tendency to take them. The task force suggested that if a measurement is 1 SD or more below the mean for that site compared with premenopausal women, hormone replacement should be recommended. If the measurement if more than 1 SD above the mean for such younger women, no intervention is needed. Women with values between these limits should be followed up and the measurement repeated after 2 to 5 years (depending on initial bone mass). These are only guidelines, and other factors should be considered. In addition, bone mass measurements may be helpful in women with hypogonadism as a result of excessive exercise or anorexia nervosa if the results will help the person alter her exercise program or eating habits or take hormone-replacement therapy. If a woman refuses estrogen therapy regardless of her bone density, then there is no need for this test.

Bone mass measurements need not be obtained (1) for women who are on or are about to be placed on long-term hormone replacement therapy unless changes in therapy are being considered; (2) as an isolated screening program without an organized plan for patient management; or (3) for patients with established osteoporosis unless the measurement is being used as a baseline to evaluate subsequent treatment. There are many other potential indications.

Table 11-2 Techniques for the measurement of bone mass

Technique	Site	Precision* (%)	Accuracy†	Examination time (min.)	Absorbed dose of radiation‡ (mrem)
Single-photon absorptiometry	Proximal and distal radius, calcaneus	1-3	5	15	10-20
Dual-energy photon absorptiometry	Spine, hip, total body	2-4	4-10	20-40	5
Dual-energy x-ray absorptiometry	Spine, hip, total body	0.5-2	3-5	3-7	1-3
Quantitative computed tomography	Spine	2-5	5-20	10-15	100-1000

Modified from Johnston CC Jr., Slemenda CW, Melton LJ III: Clinical use of bone densitometry, *N Eng J Med* 324:1105, 1991.
*Precision is the coefficient of variation (standard deviation divided by the mean) for repeated measurements over a short period of time in young, healthy persons.
†Accuracy is the coefficient of variation for measurements in a specimen whose mineral content has been determined by other means (e.g., measurement of ashed weight).
‡To convert millirems to millijoules per kilogram of body weight, multiply by 0.01.

Measurements of bone density at any site can be used as a predictor of fracture risk at other sites. It appears, however, that site-specific measurements are better; for example, DXA measurements of the proximal femur predict hip fracture risk better than measurements at other sites.

PREVENTION AND TREATMENT

Preventing bone loss and the subsequent development of osteoporosis is of major importance because at present, there are no effective, safe, and proved means for strengthening the skeleton and restoring skeletal integrity. Thus any agent or means of achieving the maximum amount of bone at the time of skeletal maturity and reducing postmenopausal bone loss will have long-term beneficial effects.

Calcium and nutritional factors

Calcium is essential for the development of a normal skeleton and for achieving peak bone mass. Inadequate calcium can reduce peak bone mass and hasten bone loss later in life. With advancing age, there is (1) a decrease in the dietary intake of calcium, (2) a decrease in intestinal absorption of calcium, and (3) a decreased ability to adapt to the low-calcium diets common in the postmenopausal years by increasing $1,25-(OH)_2$ vitamin D production and intestinal calcium

---

RECOMMENDED CLINICAL USES OF BONE-MASS MEASUREMENTS

1. In estrogen-deficient women—to diagnose significantly low bone mass in order to make decisions about hormone replacement therapy
2. In patients with vertebral abnormalities or roentgenographic osteopenia—to diagnose spinal osteoporosis in order to make decisions about further diagnostic evaluation and therapy
3. In patients receiving long-term glucocortoid therapy—to diagnose low bone mass in order to adjust therapy
4. In patients with primary asymptomatic hyperparathyroidism—to diagnose low bone mass in order to identify those at risk of severe skeletal disease who may be candidates for surgical intervention

From Johnston CC et al: *J Bone Miner Res* 4 (suppl 2):1, 1989.

---

absorption. The usual dietary calcium intake for postmenopausal Amercian women ranges from 400 to 500 mg/day, much below the recommended daily allowance of 800 to 1000 mg/day for adults. There is increasing evidence that calcium supplementation to approximately 1500 mg/day may slow down bone loss in some healthy postmenopausal women with osteoporosis and in elderly women. However, it has no demonstrated protective effect in the immediate postmenopausal period.

On the basis of a recent consensus development conference on osteoporosis (1993), the recommended elemental calcium intake for white women is 1000 mg/day for adults, 1500 mg/day for postmenopausal women, and 1200 mg/day for adolescents. Adequate calcium intake is important in the growing years to attain the maximum amount of bone. To achieve adequate calcium intake, consumption of foods with a high calcium content such as milk and dairy products is recommended.

If sufficient calcium cannot be obtained from food sources, then calcium supplementation is necessary. The amount of elemental calcium varies with the different calcium salts. The calcium content of several common preparations is as follows: carbonate, 40%; citrate, 21%; lactate, 13%; and gluconate, 9%. Therefore 1 g of calcium carbonate contains 400 mg of elemental calcium, but 1 g of calcium gluconate contains only 90 mg of calcium. Many calcium preparations are poorly absorbed, especially in older persons. Calcium supplements are best taken with meals inasmuch as food helps absorption. Calcium carbonate preparations are the most commonly used because of the higher calcium content in each tablet and their lower cost, thus making compliance easier. Other preparations such as calcium citrate are perhaps better absorbed, especially in patients with achlorhydria. In postmenopausal women whose estrogen level is adequate, a total calcium intake of 1000 mg/day is appropriate, whereas in those women with estrogen depletion an intake of 1500 mg/day is necessary. In healthy persons with no personal or family history of nephrolithiasis and who are not hypercalciuric, calcium supplements appear to be associated with minimal risk of nephrolithiasis. Patients with a personal or family history of calcium-containing kidney stones need to be evaluated before increasing their calcium intake.

Vitamin D

Numerous factors and disorders affect vitamin D metabolism in postmenopausal women. Any factor that reduces skin exposure to sunlight will diminish endogenous vitamin D synthesis. In elderly persons, vitamin D ingestion may be insufficient to compensate for the reduced exposure to sunlight. In addition, vitamin D deficiency may result from interference with the intestinal absorption of vitamin D.

Vitamin D deficiency is common in elderly persons, especially those who are chronically ill, housebound, and poorly nourished. Perhaps 10% to 20% of elderly osteoporotic women have mild vitamin D deficiency, and some have an osteomalacic component to their bone problems.

Many therapeutic programs for osteoporosis include vitamin D in various doses, although its use in osteoporosis is based on scant scientific data. High doses of vitamin D can increase the intestinal absorption of calcium, but when it is given along with calcium supplementation, the risk for developing hypercalcemia and hypercalciuria is increased. Lower doses of vitamin D in the range of 400 to 800 IU (10 to 20 μg) per day should generally be sufficient to prevent vitamin D deficiency.

In contrast to calcium, which is quite abundant in foods, vitamin D is not generally available in sufficient quantities in unfortified foods. Thus, in postmenopausal women, especially older women, 400 to 800 units of vitamin D in the form of multivitamins is appropriate, especially if they receive insufficient sunlight exposure.

Exercise

Physical exercise is important both in bone development and in the maintenance of the skeleton. Immobilization can produce rapid and significant bone loss. There is increasing evidence that exercise is beneficial to bone. Exercise also helps strengthen back muscles, improve agility and mobility, and helps one develop a sense of well-being. There is no consensus as to which exercise programs are best, nor how frequently and for how long one should participate in them. Weight-bearing exercises are necessary, although water exercises or swimming can be helpful if the patient has a vertebral fracture associated with pain. A referral to a physical therapist is sometimes necessary to initiate a program and ensure that it is properly instituted. This program should include gentle abdominal and back-strengthening exercises but should avoid exercises that produce flexion and sudden rotational movement of the spine. An exercise program for 30 minutes, three times a week if tolerated, would seem appropriate, but this regimen must be individualized. Walking briskly for 1 hour, three or four times weekly, also may help.

Estrogens

Estrogen-replacement therapy continues to be the gold standard in preventing postmenopausal bone loss and is the only agent to demonstrate a reduction in fractures. Numerous controlled, randomized, double-blind studies from around the world have consistently shown beneficial effects of estrogen-replacement therapy in slowing bone loss. The beneficial effect of estrogen is most dramatic when instituted as close to the onset of the menopause as possible. Most studies have shown a reduction in bone loss and mainte-nance of bone mass when estrogen therapy is instituted, but there may be a small transient increase in bone mass within the first year when previous activated bone remodeling units are filled in.

Estrogen replacement therapy may slow down bone loss when instituted many years after the menopause and in women with established osteoporosis. Thus, even when postmenopausal women begin hormone therapy later in life, the rate of bone loss can be reduced. In this setting, estrogen is not really a "replacement" as it may be when instituted close to the menopause but acts rather as a pharmacologic antiresorptive agent.

Bone loss may begin several years before the actual menopause, but estrogen-replacement therapy should not be started in the premenopausal years unless there is evidence of estrogen deficiency or bone loss with repeated bone density measurements. Estrogen-replacement therapy will maintain the structural integrity and architecture of bone. Epidemiologic studies have reported a reduction of 50% to 60% in hip, distal forearm, and vertebral fractures in women receiving estrogen-replacement therapy. The beneficial effects of estrogen on bone continue for as long as estrogen is taken, and recent evidence suggests that for a long-term beneficial effect, estrogens need to be taken for at least 7 years.

The minimum dose of estrogen to prevent bone loss appears to be 0.625 mg of conjugated equine estrogen daily or equivalent doses of other estrogen preparations. The beneficial effect of estrogen on bone is independent of its route of administration.

The risks, benefits, indications, and various treatment regimens are discussed in Chapter 36. In women who are undecided about whether to take estrogen-replacement therapy to prevent bone loss, a bone-density measurement may be helpful (see section on clinical uses of bone-density measurements).

Calcitonin

Calcitonin is a peptide hormone secreted by the parafollicular cells of the thyroid gland. Its physiologic role in calcium metabolism is unclear, but as a therapeutic agent it inhibits osteoclast function. Synthetic salmon calcitonin is approved by the Food and Drug Administration (FDA) for the treatment of postmenopausal osteoporosis. Studies have shown maintenance of bone mass with doses of salmon calcitonin between 50 and 100 U administered subcutaneously daily or every other day. The best regimen for administering calcitonin is not established nor are there sufficient data regarding fracture prevention. Salmon calcitonin may be more beneficial in patients with "high" turnover rather than "low" turnover osteoporosis, but bone markers are not sufficiently sensitive at this time to consistently distinguish the two states. Several reports suggest that calcitonin has analgesic properties and thus may offer an additional benefit to patients with pain after vertebral fractures.

Salmon calcitonin has a good safety profile. Initiating treatment with a dose of 25 U daily or every other day and then slowly increasing by 25 U every week until the desired treatment dose is achieved will minimize side effects and improve compliance. Side effects include facial flushing, nausea, and dizziness. If side effects occur, the dose can be lowered. The side effects usually are transient and diminish in intensity with time despite continuing the same dose of medication. Supplementation with 1000 mg of calcium and a multivitamin is necessary to prevent the development of secondary hyperparathyroidism with calcitonin administration.

The major drawback of calcitonin is the need for subcutaneous injections. Salmon calcitonin comes in a concentration of 200 U/ml, but insulin syringes, which are generally used for administration, are calibrated at a concentration of 100 U/ml. Therefore, orders must be clear as to how much calcitonin is required (e.g., 100 U of calcitonin is 50 U on the insulin syringe, or 0.5 ml). Calcitonin also is expensive, but beneficial responses may be seen with 50 to 100 U every other day or by some intermittent treatment regimens. Nasal spray formulations have been developed and currently are being evaluated.

Other potential therapies

There are many pharmacologic agents under active investigation for the treatment of osteoporosis. Some of these are approved by the FDA for indications other than osteoporosis. Until they are proved to be effective in the treatment of osteoporosis and approved by the FDA, they should be considered experimental.

Bisphosphonates. The bisphosphonates, a group of compounds related chemically to pyrophosphate, are potent inhibitors of osteoclastic bone resorption. They appear to bind to hydroxyapatite crystals, and when these crystals are taken up by osteoclasts, the osteoclast's ability to resorb bone is impeded.

The bisphosphonates have been used therapeutically for two disorders characterized by increased bone turnover: Paget's disease and hypercalcemia of malignancy. Recent studies of women with postmenopausal osteoporosis have shown a small increase in vertebral bone mineral content and a short-term reduction in the incidence of vertebral fractures. In these studies etidronate was administered in a dose of 400 mg/day for 2 weeks, followed by an 11- to 13-week drug-free period for 2 to 3 years. During the period when etidronate was not administered, calcium was given in a dose of 1000 to 1500 mg/day. Long-term efficacy and additional data are required before it is approved.

The bisphosphonates are very poorly absorbed and must be given on an empty stomach to maximize absorption. Currently, there are many more potent bisphosphonates under active investigation, with initial results very encouraging.

Fluoride. The skeletal effects of excessive fluoride have been known for 60 years and include sclerosis of bones, ligaments, and muscle attachments. The first clinical reports using sodium fluoride for the treatment of osteoporosis appeared in the early 1960s. Since then, numerous studies have appeared, but only a few were of sufficient size and design to warrant adequate interpretation. Dosages of 50 to 80 mg/day of sodium fluoride produce an increase in spinal bone density of 5% to 10% per year for several years in many subjects. Despite the increase in trabecular bone density, cortical bone density continues to decline, calcium balance improves very little, and total body calcium does not change—all suggesting a redistribution of calcium within the body.

A 4-year prospective trial of postmenopausal women with osteoporosis was conducted in which sodium fluoride, 75 mg/day, was shown to increase trabecular bone but to decrease cortical bone density (Riggs, 1992). The number of new vertebral fractures was similar in the sodium fluoride and placebo groups, but there was a threefold increase in the number of peripheral fractures in the sodium fluoride group. Side effects of sodium fluoride include nausea, vomiting, epigastric pain, gastritis, periarticular pain, and a painful plantar fascial syndrome. Stress fractures also occur. Further investigation with the use of lower doses of sodium fluoride or different preparations, including enteric-coated tablets, slow-release forms, and monofluorophosphates, needs to be undertaken.

Anabolic steroids. A reduction in the blood levels of weak androgens has been reported with aging and in women with osteoporosis. Anabolic steroids or synthetic derivatives of testosterone appear to inhibit bone resorption and may weakly stimulate bone formation. Significant side effects can occur. These include liver abnormalities, sodium and fluid retention, and masculinizing effects. They can adversely affect serum lipid levels by reducing the high-density lipoproteins and elevating the low-density lipoproteins.

Vitamin D analogs. In recent years the active metabolites of vitamin D have been synthesized and used in clinical trials for postmenopausal osteoporosis. A recent report suggested a beneficial effect with the use of 1,25-dihydroxy vitamin D (calcitriol). The results have not been consistent with those of other studies, and one of the major drawbacks is the potential development of hypercalciuria and hypercalcemia.

Thiazide diuretics. These agents reduce urinary calcium excretion, and in some patients a positive effect on calcium balance and a reduction in bone loss and fractures have been reported. Thiazide diuretic therapy is indicated in patients with hypercalciuria but should not be instituted at this time specifically to prevent bone loss. Caution should be used in hypertensive, osteoporotic persons who may be receiving high doses of calcium and vitamin D in addition to a thiazide diuretic, because hypercalcemia may occur in this setting.

Antiestrogens. Tamoxifen, a synthetic antiestrogen, has come to play a major role in the treatment of patients with breast cancer. Tamoxifen is not a pure antiestrogen. It has some estrogen-agonist effects on bone. Initial studies have reported a decrease in bone turnover and the maintenance of vertebral bone density in women receiving tamoxifen.

Other agents. Other agents to stimulate bone formation are being evaluated. Parathyroid hormone, when administered intermittently either alone or with other agents, is anabolic to bone. Growth hormone and growth factors are other potential agents for use in osteoporosis.

Fall prevention

The potential for falls can be minimized by the person avoiding medications that produce drowsiness or confusion and surveying the home to remove hazards.

SUMMARY

In recent years great strides have been made in our understanding of the biology of the bone cells, the pathophysiology of bone loss, and our ability to diagnose and treat osteoporosis. Because of the size of the population either having developed osteoporosis or at risk for developing it, all physicians and health care workers caring for this group should be familiar with the basic management of these patients.

However, a referral to a physician specializing in osteoporosis is appropriate (1) when a case is unusual or complicated, (2) if there are difficulties in interpreting bone density results or other laboratory tests, or (3) when difficult therapeutic or diagnostic decisions need to be made.

Recommendations are as follows:

A. For women without established osteoporosis who are seeking risk assessment:

- Clinical risk factors are not sensitive for detection of women with low bone mass who may be at increased fracture risk. Therefore bone density measurements can be used to assess for subsequent fracture risk inasmuch as low bone mass is a major determinant of fracture. However, bone density measurements should be obtained only when the results would influence treatment.
- Ensure adequate calcium: 1000 mg for women on estrogen therapy and 1500 mg for those not taking estrogen.
- Ensure adequate supply of vitamin D either from sunlight or from a multivitamin containing 400 units of vitamin D.
- Exercise.
- Estrogen therapy in appropriate women.

B. For women with established osteoporosis:

- Although 80% to 90% have age-related osteoporosis, it is important to consider other causes.
- Bone density measurements are helpful to follow so that changes in treatment can be made when necessary.
- Ensure adequate calcium, vitamin D, and exercise.
- Specific therapy with estrogen or calcitonin should be considered.
- Although other agents certainly will become available in the future, agents such as etidronate are still considered experimental for the treatment of osteoporosis.
- Avoid medications that can increase the tendency to fall, and survey the home to remove hazards.

BIBLIOGRAPHY

Bonjour J-P et al: Bisphosphonates in clinical medicine. In Heersche JNM, Kanis JA, editors: *Bone and mineral research,* ed 8, Amsterdam, 1994, Elsevier Science BV.

Chapuy MC, Arlot ME, Duboeuf F: Vitamin D_3 and calcium to prevent hip fractures in elderly women, *N Engl J Med* 327:1637, 1992.

Consensus Development Conference on Osteoporosis: *Am J Med* 95(suppl 5A), 1993.

Dawson-Hughes B et al: A controlled trial of the effect of calcium supplementation on bone density in postmenopausal women, *N Engl J Med* 323:878, 1990.

Dempster DW et al: Anabolic actions of parathyroid hormone on bone, *Endocri Rev* 14:690, 1993.

Gowen M: Cytokines and cellular interactions in the control of bone remodeling. In Heersche JNM, Kanis JA, editors: *Bone and mineral research,* ed 8, Amsterdam, 1994, Elsevier Science BV.

Grady D et al: Hormone therapy to prevent disease and prolong life in postmenopausal women, *Ann Intern Med* 117:1016, 1992.

Heaney RP: Nutritional factors in osteoporosis, *Annu Rev Nutr* 13:287, 1993.

Johnston CC Jr, Slemenda CW, Melton LJ III: Clinical use of bone densitometry, *N Eng J Med* 324:1105, 1991.

Kleerekoper M, Mendlovic DB: Sodium fluoride therapy of postmenopausal osteoporosis, *Endocri Rev* 14:312, 1993.

Lindsay R, Cosman F: Primary osteoporosis. In Coe FL, Favus MJ, editors: *Disorders of bone and mineral metabolism,* New York, 1992, Raven Press.

Love RL et al: Effects of Tamoxifen on bone mineral density in postmenopausal women with breast cancer, *N Engl J Med* 326:852, 1992.

Lukert BP, Raisz LG: Glucocortoid-induced osteoporosis: pathogenesis and management, *Ann Intern Med* 112:352, 1990.

McDermott MT, Kidd GS: The role of calcitonin in the development and treatment of osteoporosis, *Endocri Rev* 8:377, 1987.

Parfitt AM: Bone remodeling: relationship to the amount and structure of bone, and the pathogenesis and prevention of fractures. In Riggs BL, Melton LJ III, editors: *Osteoporosis: etiology, diagnosis, and management,* New York, 1988, Raven Press.

Riggs BL et al: Effect of fluoride treatment on the fracture rate in postmenopausal women with osteoporosis, *N Engl J Med* 322:802, 1990.

Rigotti NA et al: Osteoporosis in women with anorexia nervosa, *N Engl J Med* 311:1601, 1984.

Sinaki M: Exercise and physical therapy. In Riggs BL, Melton LJ III, editors: *Osteoporosis: etiology, diagnosis, and management,* New York, 1988, Raven Press.

Slovik DM: Endocrine therapy of postmenopausal osteoporosis: calcium, vitamin D, calcitonin, fluoride and parathyroid hormone. In Barbieri R, Schiff I, editors: *Reproductive endocrine therapeutics,* New York, 1988, Alan R Liss.

Watts NB et al: Intermittent cyclical etidronate treatment of postmenopausal osteoporosis, *N Engl J Med* 323:73, 1990.

12 Thyroid Disease

Douglas S. Ross

EPIDEMIOLOGY

Virtually all types of thyroid dysfunction are more common in females than in males. Hypothyroidism resulting from autoimmune thyroiditis is three to five times more common in women than in men. Population surveys indicate a prevalence of hypothyroidism of 6% to 7% in older women, whereas up to 17% of women over age 60 have been reported to have positive antithyroid antibodies. Data on the true prevalence of hyperthyroidism are more difficult to interpret, since sensitive thyroid-stimulating hormone (TSH) measurements have only recently allowed for the detection of mild hyperthyroidism. Prevalence estimates have varied from 0.4% to 2.0% of the female population. Hyperthyroidism is 5 to 10 times more common in females than in males. Postpartum thyroid dysfunction occurs in 4% to 7% of women. Sporadic goiter or clinically solitary thyroid nodules are present in 5% to 7% of women in the United States and are at least four times more common in women than men. Differentiated thyroid cancer accounts for 1.6% of cancers in women and is three to four times more common than in men.

THYROID FUNCTION TESTS

The introduction and widespread use of sensitive TSH assays over the past several years have made the correct interpretation of thyroid function considerably more reliable than in the past. TSH is the pituitary hormone that regulates thyroid hormone production through negative feedback. The relationship between TSH and free thyroxine (T_4) concentrations is log-linear. Therefore relatively small changes in free T_4 concentrations are associated with large changes in serum TSH concentrations. With rare exceptions in ambulatory patients, elevated serum TSH concentrations indicate hypothyroidism, and subnormal or undetectable TSH concentrations indicate hyperthyroidism.

Screening thyroid function

The most precise single test to screen thyroid function is a serum TSH level. Many laboratories measure TSH and automatically add a free T_4 level if the TSH level is high to assess the degree of hypothyroidism, or add free T_4 and T_3 levels if the TSH level is subnormal to assess the degree of hyperthyroidism. TSH levels alone are not a reliable indicator of thyroid function if the patient has pituitary or hypothalamic disease. Patients with a TSH-producing pituitary adenoma or partial pituitary resistance to thyroid hormone may have a normal or elevated TSH level associated with hyperthyroidism. Patients with non–thyrotropin-producing pituitary tumors or hypothalamic disease may have secondary or central hypothyroidism with subnormal, normal, or even elevated TSH values. Therefore some recommend that both TSH and free T_4 be measured as screening tests. A more cost-effective approach is to add free T_4 measurements to TSH levels only when there is a strong suggestion of thyroid dysfunction in a patient with a normal TSH level, or when there is a history suggestive of past or present pituitary or hypothalamic dysfunction. For example, TSH alone would be an inappropriate screening test in a woman complaining of fatigue who has galactorrhea or amenorrhea.

Free T_4 measurements

Measurement of serum T_4 and triiodothyronine (T_3) concentrations is complicated by protein binding to thyroxine-binding globulin (TBG), thyroxine-binding prealbumin (TBPA), and albumin. The free hormone hypothesis states that only the unbound or free hormone is readily available for uptake into tissues. Since over 99% of T_4 is bound, the free hormone level is a very small fraction of the total hormone level and is difficult to measure. Free T_4 and T_3 measurements are estimated by several different techniques. Equilibrium dialysis is too tedious for routine measurements. Commercial kits estimating "direct" free hormone levels may give misleading values for patients with nonthyroidal illness or unusual binding protein abnormalities. The free T_4 index is calculated by multiplying the total T_4 by the T_3 resin uptake, a measure of the inverse of unoccupied sites on T_4-binding proteins. Because this test has been confused with serum T_3 measurements, it has been renamed the thyroid hormone–binding ratio (THBR), or index (THBI). This ratio is the patient's T_3 resin divided by the average T_3 resin for the laboratory.

$$\text{Free } T_4 \text{ index} = \text{Total } T_4 \times \frac{\text{Patient's } T_3 \text{ resin}}{\text{Average normal } T_3 R}$$

The free T_4 index corrects abnormal total T_4 values caused by high or low serum levels of the major binding protein, TBG. TBG excess, the most common abnormality, is seen in hyperestrogenic states including pregnancy and in oral contraceptive or conjugated estrogen therapy. TBG excess is associated with a normal serum TSH level, a high total T_4 level, a low THBI, and a normal free T_4 index. In contrast hyperthyroidism is associated with a subnormal TSH level, a high total T_4 level, a high THBI, and a high free T_4 index. The box on the following page lists other causes of hyperthyroxinemia and hypothyroxinemia seen in euthyroid patients.

Thyroid function in hospitalized patients

Assessment of thyroid function is considerably more difficult in critically ill hospitalized patients. Such patients have reductions in serum T_4 and T_3 values, and estimates of free T_4 levels are frequently unreliable. Serum TSH values may be subnormal in severely ill patients and may be slightly elevated during recovery from severe illness. Therefore both TSH and thyroid hormone measurements are required, and mild abnormalities in test results warrant repeat testing after full recovery from the acute illness.

CAUSES OF ABNORMAL SERUM T₄ VALUES IN EUTHYROID PATIENTS

Euthyroid hyperthyroxinemia

TBG excess
  Hereditary, estrogens, hepatitis, acute intermittent
    porphyria
  Drugs (5-FU, perphenazine, clofibrate, heroin,
    methadone)
Familial dysalbuminemic hyperthyroxinemia
Abnormal TBPA
Autoantibodies to thyroxine
Peripheral resistance to thyroid hormone
High altitude
Amphetamines
Inhibition of T_4 to T_3 conversion
  Amiodarone, ipodate, iopanoic acid, propranolol

Euthyroid hypothyroxinemia

TBG deficiency
  Hereditary, androgens, glucocorticoids, acromegaly,
    nephrosis, drugs (danazol, colestipol-niacin,
    L-asparaginase), nonthyroidal illness
Displacement of T_4 from binding proteins
  Phenytoin, salicylates, fenclofenac, furosemide,
    phenylbutazone
Triiodothyronine (T_3) therapy

T_4, thyroxine; 5-FU, 5-fluorouracil; TBPA, thyroxine-binding prealbumin; T_3, triiodothyronine; TBG, thyroxine-binding globulin.

HYPERTHYROIDISM
Clinical presentation

Few women with moderate to severe hyperthyroidism delay seeking medical advice. However, mild and subclinical hyperthyroidism may be unnoticed for years. The most common complaints are weight loss, palpitations, tremulousness, heat intolerance, and sweating. Increased cardiac output may aggravate angina or congestive heart failure. Up to 20% of older patients may have atrial fibrillation, and such patients should have anticoagulation to prevent embolic sequelae.

Dyspnea may result from increased oxygen consumption and CO_2 production, respiratory muscle weakness, congestive heart failure, exacerbation of asthma, or tracheal narrowing caused by goiter. Increased gut motility results in hyperdefecation, malabsorption, and steatorrhea. Rarely anorexia or vomiting may occur.

A normochromic normocytic anemia develops primarily as a result of increased plasma volume. Ferritin levels are elevated. Graves' disease may be associated with leukopenia caused by antineutrophilic antibodies, idiopathic thrombocytopenic purpura, or pernicious anemia.

Hyperthyroidism increases the level of sex hormone–binding globulin, which increases the total estradiol level but decreases the unbound estradiol level. LH level is increased, but the midcycle LH surge is reduced and oligomenorrhea is common.

Thyroid hormone has a direct resorptive effect on bone, increasing the serum ionized calcium level and suppressing parathyroid hormone and 1,25-dihydroxyvitamin D levels; the result is a negative calcium balance. Alkaline phosphatase level may rise and remain elevated for months during and after treatment, presumably reflecting remineralization of osteoporotic bone.

Tremor, hyperactivity, emotional lability, insomnia, and proximal muscle weakness are commonly seen. Diagnosis of elderly patients may be difficult because conduction system disease masks the tachycardia; they may be more apathetic than hyperactive, and a goiter may not be readily appreciated.

Ophthalmopathy occurs only in Graves' disease. Most patients have mild periorbital swelling and proptosis. More severe orbitopathy results in limitation of extraocular muscles and diplopia. Corneal ulceration from exposure and loss of vision caused by compression of the optic nerve are rare severe manifestations of autoimmune ophthalmopathy.

Differential diagnosis

Conceptually there are two groups of disorders: hyperthyroidism caused by de novo synthesis of thyroid hormone associated with a *high* radioiodine uptake, and hyperthyroidism caused by release of preformed hormone from an inflamed gland associated with a *low* radioiodine uptake. Since treatment of these two groups of disorders differs, it is critical to obtain a radioiodine uptake in most hyperthyroid patients to prevent inappropriate therapy. (See Table 12-1.)

Hyperthyroidism with an elevated radioiodine uptake. Graves' disease is the most common form of hyperthyroidism in all age groups in the United States. It is due to stimulation of the TSH receptor by a specific thyroid-stimulating immunoglobulin (TSI). Some patients with autoimmune thyroiditis initially have a short-lived hyperthyroid phase presumably mediated by TSI ("Hashitoxicosis"). Toxic adenoma and toxic multinodular goiter are more common in older patients and result from autonomy of thyroid follicular cells. TSH-producing pituitary adenomas, partial pituitary resistance to thyroid hormone, and trophoblastic disease are rare causes of hyperthyroidism with an elevated radioiodine uptake.

Hyperthyroidism with a low radioiodine uptake. Hyperthyroidism produced by inflammation and destruction of thyroid parenchyma with release of stored hormone is associated with a low radioiodine uptake (usually less than 1%). Subacute granulomatous thyroiditis (de Quervain's thyroiditis) frequently follows a viral respiratory illness; the patient is acutely ill with fever and elevated sedimentation rate, and the thyroid is exquisitely tender. Subacute lymphocytic thyroiditis (silent or painless thyroiditis) is part of the spectrum of autoimmune thyroid disease, is not associated with thyroid tenderness, and may occur in the postpartum period or may recur in the same patient. Both classically appear with a hyperthyroid phase, followed by a hypothyroid phase and then recovery (Fig. 12-1). Occasionally the hyperthyroid or hypothyroid phase is mild and asymptomatic. In the absence of ophthalmopathy it is impossible to differentiate painless thyroiditis from mild Graves' disease without radioiodine uptake testing. Other rare causes of hyperthyroidism with a low radioiodine uptake are factitious ingestion of thyroid hormone (thyroglobulin will be suppressed), struma ovarii (the uptake is elevated over the pelvis), and large deposits of metastatic thyroid follicular carcinoma.

Iodine-induced hyperthyroidism. The mechanism of iodine-induced hyperthyroidism is a substrate-induced

Table 12-1 Differential diagnosis of hyperthyroidism

Disorder	Radioactive iodine uptake	Confirmatory findings
Graves' disease	Increased	Thyroid scan: diffuse bilateral homogeneous uptake
Autoimmune thyroiditis ("Hashitoxicosis")	Increased	Clinical course: hypothyroidism often follows
Toxic adenoma	Increased	Thyroid scan: focal uptake corresponding to a palpable nodule
Toxic multinodular goiter	Increased	Thyroid scan: patchy areas of increased and decreased uptake, possibly corresponding to palpable nodules

Rare causes
  TSH-producing pituitary adenoma
  Partial pituitary resistance to thyroid hormone
  Trophoblastic disease
	Increased	

Subacute granulomatous thyroiditis	Decreased	Tender thyroid, fever, elevated ESR
Subacute lymphocytic thyroiditis (painless thyroiditis)	Decreased	Nontender thyroid; may occur postpartum

Rare causes
  Factitious ingestion of thyroid hormone
  Struma ovarii
  Metastatic follicular thyroid carcinoma
	Decreased	

Iodine-induced hyperthyroidism	May be decreased if iodine load recent	History of radiocontrast dye, kelp tablets, povidone-iodine (Betadine) douche, amiodarone use

TSH, thyroid-stimulating hormone; ESR, erythrocyte sedimentation rate.

increase in hormone synthesis, usually occurring in a nodular goiter with areas of autonomous function. If the iodine load was recent, however, the radioiodine uptake may be low as a result of washout of the tracer by the nonradioactive iodine. It is unusual for the uptake to be less than 1%, however. Common causes of iodine loads include radiocontrast dye, kelp tablets, povidone-iodine (Betadine) douches, iodine-containing expectorants, and amiodarone.

Diagnostic tests

The diagnosis of hyperthyroidism is made by measuring serum TSH and thyroid hormone levels as described previously. A radioiodine uptake is necessary to distinguish hyperthyroidism caused by new hormone synthesis from hyperthyroidism caused by subacute thyroiditis. This may be inconvenient in the postpartum period since it would interrupt nursing. The serum T_3/T_4 ratio [ng/μg]) is usually greater than 20 in hyperthyroidism caused by Graves' disease or toxic goiter, and usually less than 20 in hyperthyroidism caused by subacute thyroiditis. Therefore one could defer the radioiodine uptake test in a mild case of suspected postpartum lymphocytic thyroiditis and follow the patient's course. A thyroid scan is necessary if one wishes to differentiate Graves' disease (diffuse bilateral homogeneous uptake) from a toxic nodule (focal uptake corresponding to a palpable nodule) or toxic multinodular goiter (patchy areas of increased and decreased uptake, possibly corresponding to palpable nodules).

Management of hyperthyroidism

β-Blockers are useful in all causes of hyperthyroidism unless contraindicated. Hyperthyroidism causes an increased number of β-adrenergic receptors, and β-blockers reduce tachycardia and tremulousness (see Table 12-2).

Graves' disease. The three major treatment options for Graves' disease are antithyroid drugs, radioiodine, or surgery. Antithyroid drugs are administered for one of two reasons. Most patients opting for surgery are pretreated with antithyroid drugs so that they are euthyroid preoperatively. Many patients opting for radioiodine are also pretreated with antithyroid drugs to alleviate symptoms more rapidly and prevent a transient radiation-induced exacerbation of hyperthyroidism. Alternatively one can take antithyroid drugs for 1 to 2 years or longer with the hope of obtaining a remission.

Antithyroid drugs. Propylthiouracil (PTU) and methimazole (Tapazole), the two antithyroid drugs available in the United States, inhibit iodination of tyrosyl residues on thyroglobulin, thus preventing new hormone synthesis. Therefore 2 to 8 weeks of therapy is necessary to exhaust preformed thyroid hormone stores and control hyperthyroidism. Initial doses are high (PTU 100 mg tid or Tapazole 10 mg tid or 30 mg qid) to be certain that iodination is inhibited. Doses are then reduced to maintenance levels (PTU, 50 to 100 mg

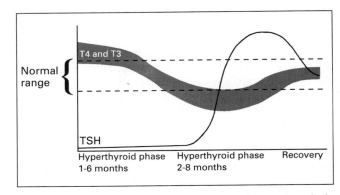

Fig. 12-1 Time course of changes in thyroid function test results in patients with subacute thyroiditis. A similar course is seen in patients with subacute granulomatous thyroiditis (de Quervain's thyroiditis), subacute lymphocytic thyroiditis (painless, silent, or postpartum thyroiditis), or radiation-induced thyroiditis.

Table 12-2 Management of hyperthyroidism

Disorder	Choice of therapy
Graves' disease	
Young women	Radioactive iodine often preferred; thionamides or surgery
Young women anticipating pregnancy	Radioiodine or surgery to ensure euthyroidism before pregnancy
Pregnant women	Propylthiouracil
Toxic multinodular goiter or toxic adenoma	Usually radioactive iodine preferred
	Surgery if nodule or goiter presents cosmetic or obstructive problem
	Thionamides only as adjunctive therapy before or after ablative procedure
Subacute granulomatous or lymphocytic	No therapy or β-blockers only
thyroiditis	Steroids possibly helpful in severe cases
Iodine-induced hyperthyroidism	Discontinuation of iodides
	β-blockers if mild; thionamides if moderate to severe

bid or methimazole, 5 to 15 mg qid), allowing some hormone to be synthesized to maintain a euthyroid state. Both drugs are poorly tolerated by 5% to 10% of patients because of nausea, vomiting, rashes, hives, joint pains, or fevers. There is a 0.25% or less risk of reversible agranulocytosis, and rarely PTU causes hepatocellular necrosis and methimazole causes cholestatic jaundice. Many physicians prefer methimazole to PTU because of its longer half-life, once-daily dosing regimen, and possible lower incidence of serious toxicity. Methimazole has been associated with a rare scalp defect, aplasia cutis, if administered during pregnancy, and PTU is therefore preferred for the pregnant hyperthyroid patient (see Chapter 59). PTU, unlike methimazole, is protein bound; it crosses the placenta less readily and is poorly concentrated in breast milk. It is therefore also preferable for a mother who wishes to nurse while on antithyroid medication.

Patients who have been taking antithyroid drugs for 1 to 2 years have a 20% to 30% remission rate in the United States. This rate is higher for women with small glands, mild hyperthyroidism, high antimicrosomal antibody titers, and glands that shrink on antithyroid drug therapy. Remission rates are higher if antithyroid drugs are taken for 10 years, and a recent study also suggested that remission rates are greater if higher doses of antithyroid drugs are administered simultaneously with levothyroxine to maintain a suppressed serum TSH level.

Radioiodine. Radioiodine is widely used in the United States. The only known complication of therapy is a 1% risk of radiation thyroiditis. This results in 2 to 3 weeks of thyroid pain, as well as exacerbation of the hyperthyroidism as a result of release of hormone stores from the radiation-induced inflammation. Patients with cardiovascular disease, elderly patients, or patients who are not tolerating the hyperthyroidism well are pretreated with antithyroid drugs to deplete hormone stores and ameliorate symptoms more rapidly. Radioiodine averages 8 to 16 weeks or longer for its full therapeutic effect. There is no increased risk of cancer after radioiodine treatment of hyperthyroidism; the dose to the ovaries is similar to that of pelvic computed tomography (CT), barium enema, or other diagnostic procedures; and a small study failed to show any increased risk in birth defects in babies of mothers who had previously received radioiodine. Radioiodine cannot be administered during pregnancy, however, since it would ablate the fetal thyroid tissue.

Surgery. Surgery has become an unpopular treatment for Graves' disease. There is a 1% risk of hypoparathyroidism or recurrent laryngeal nerve damage, it requires general anesthesia and a hospital admission, and it leaves a scar. Patients allergic to antithyroid drugs can be safely operated on by using β-blockade and 10 days of saturated solution of potassium iodide (SSKI) treatment preoperatively.

Many centers consider the goal of radioiodine or surgical therapy to be permanent hypothyroidism. When this approach is taken, recurrent hyperthyroidism is rare and thyroid hormone levels are easily controlled by levothyroxine administration. Some centers attempt to maintain a functioning remnant so that the patient is euthyroid. Many such patients may become asymptomatic but have persistent subclinical hyperthyroidism with its associated risks (see later discussion). Treatment failure, recurrent hyperthyroidism, or late development of hypothyroidism is more likely when a partially ablative approach is chosen.

Choice of therapy. Young women with hyperthyroidism should be encouraged to avoid pregnancy until the condition has resolved. If they opt for a trial of antithyroid drugs, it is optimal that they wait for a year after stopping therapy, to prevent recurrent hyperthyroidism during a pregnancy. Thus the onset of Graves' disease could delay a desired pregnancy for 3 years or longer, and women should consider more definitive therapy. It is generally advised that women wait for 6 months after receiving radioiodine before conceiving; however, this recommendation is not based on any data. Pregnancy plans can proceed shortly after a thyroidectomy.

New mothers may want to delay definitive therapy, since surgery and radioiodine treatment both result in a short absence from their baby and interrupt nursing. Patients who receive radioiodine are advised to avoid close contact with children and pregnant women for about 5 days.

Very large goiters may best be approached surgically. Very small glands and mild hyperthyroidism are more likely to be associated with a remission after a course of antithyroid drugs. Otherwise the choice of initial therapy is best discussed with the patient and many find one approach more attractive than another.

Toxic nodules and toxic multinodular goiter. Unlike Graves' disease, autonomous thyroid function rarely goes into remission (although iodine-induced hyperthyroidism may resolve). Ablative therapy is therefore offered early. When appropriate, patients are pretreated with antithyroid drugs, and when euthyroidism is achieved, one can proceed with surgery or radioiodine. For large goiters, especially if there is substernal extension, surgery may be more appropriate than radioiodine. Hypothyroidism after radioiodine administration is uncommon after ablation of a toxic nodule and is less commonly seen in patients with toxic nodular goiter.

Subacute thyroiditis. Spontaneously resolving hyperthyroidism from subacute thyroiditis does *not* respond to antithyroid drugs or radioiodine since there is no *de novo* hormone synthesis. β-Blockers are usually sufficient to ameliorate the symptoms of hyperthyroidism. In subacute granulomatous thyroiditis pain is best treated with salicylates or nonsteroidal antiinflammatory agents; however, severe pain and hyperthyroidism respond to a course of steroids. Steroids may also ameliorate the course of subacute lymphocytic thyroiditis in the rare patient who is not tolerating the hyperthyroidism. The hypothyroid phase is treated with levothyroxine.

Management of hyperthyroidism in pregnancy is discussed in Chapter 59.

HYPOTHYROIDISM
Clinical presentation

Hypothyroid symptoms frequently have an insidious onset and the diagnosis may be delayed for years. Most commonly patients complain of weight gain, fatigue, cold intolerance, and muscle cramps. These complaints are sufficiently nonspecific that many euthyroid patients are screened for possible hypothyroidism. Hypothyroidism is associated with a reduced cardiac output. Serum cholesterol and triglyceride levels are markedly elevated, thereby increasing the risk of atherosclerosis. In severe myxedema there may be pericardial and pleural effusions. Alveolar hypoventilation caused by a blunted response to both hypercapnea and hypoxia occurs. Sleep apnea may develop.

Decreased gut motility leads to constipation. Anemia may be normochronic as a result of hypoproliferation or may be related to iron malabsorption or associated pernicious anemia. Decreased free water clearance may lead to hyponatremia. Abnormal LH and FSH dynamics result in menorrhagia. In severe hypothyroidism increased prolactin and galactorrhea levels may be present.

Patients may be hypothermic and lethargic, with severe myxedema leading to coma. Peripheral neuropathies, abnormal visual-evoked responses, neurosensory deafness, carpal tunnel syndrome, and myopathies are all common. Patients characteristically have facial puffiness, hyperkeratosis and carotenemia, hair loss including the lateral third of the eyebrows, and brittle nails.

Differential diagnosis

Worldwide the most common cause of hypothyroidism is iodine deficiency. However, endemic goiter is no longer found in the United States because of the iodination of the food supply. Virtually everyone in the United States with hypothyroidism has chronic lymphocytic thyroiditis (Hashimoto's disease), or the hypothyroidism is due to prior treatment of hyperthyroidism. Most patients with Hashimoto's thyroiditis have a characteristically symmetric and rubbery goiter, frequently with a palpable pyramidal lobe.

Some patients, however, have an atrophic variant. Dietary goitrogens are not a cause of hypothyroidism in the United States but may play an important role in Third World countries. Lithium may cause goiter and hypothyroidism, frequently with positive titers of antithyroid antibodies. It is controversial as to whether all such patients have underlying autoimmune thyroid disease. Patients taking lithium should be monitored periodically with serum TSH level determinations. Iodine in large doses can also cause hypothyroidism in patients with underlying autoimmune thyroid disease. Amiodarone and other iodine-containing medications may be the cause of iodine-induced hypothyroidism. (Note that iodine can cause hyperthyroidism in nodular goiter with autonomy and can cause hypothyroidism in autoimmune thyroiditis.) (See box, below.)

Rarely patients with partial biosynthetic defects in thyroid hormone biosynthesis have goiter and mild hypothyroidism. The thyroid can be damaged through external radiation therapy. Hypothyroidism may be secondary or central, caused by pituitary or hypothalamic disease. Since subacute lymphocytic thyroiditis (silent thyroiditis) may present minimal symptoms, one should also consider the possibility that the hypothyroidism is transient, especially if it occurs in the postpartum period.

Diagnostic tests

The evaluation of hypothyroidism is straightforward. If there is no history of radioiodine therapy, surgery, external radiation, or pharmacologic intervention, an elevated TSH level and a low free T_4 level strongly suggest autoimmune (Hashimoto's) thyroiditis. Antimicrosomal or anti–thyroid peroxidase (anti-TPO) antibodies (TPO is the microsomal antigen) are inexpensive and confirm the diagnosis of autoimmune thyroiditis. If the thyroid is symmetric and nonnodular, a thyroid scan adds little information and is not necessary. Although many "nodules" in a patient with hypothyroidism represent focal thyroiditis or fibrosis, both nodular goiter and Hashimoto's thyroiditis are common and can coexist. Hypothyroid patients with nodular thyroids therefore require further evaluation.

Management

Most endocrinologists prefer to use levothyroxine (T_4) preparations to treat hypothyroidism (Table 12-3) because

---

DIFFERENTIAL DIAGNOSIS OF HYPOTHYROIDISM

More common causes
  Chronic lymphocytic thyroiditis (Hashimoto's thyroiditis)
  Prior treatment of hyperthyroidism (radioactive iodine or surgery)

Less common causes
  Lithium
  Iodine-containing medications (in setting of underlying autoimmune thyroid disease)
  Congenital thyroid hormone biosynthetic defects
  External radiation therapy
  Transient hypothyroid phase of subacute granulomatous or lymphocytic thyroiditis

their long half-life (6 to 7 days) results in very stable serum levels, even when a dose is inadvertently omitted. In contrast the half-life of T_3 is about 1 day, and frequently patients who are taking T_3 or T_3-containing preparations (thyroid extract or liotrix) have hypertriiodothyronemia shortly after ingestion of the hormone and may have subnormal concentrations before the next dose. Occasionally patients who take their medication in the morning may note palpitations or tremulousness.

Conflicting recommendations relate to the rapidity with which thyroid hormone replacement is initiated. The degree of myxedema is not solely dependent upon the measurement of free T_4 and TSH levels but rather is assessed clinically on the basis of the duration and end-organ effects of hypothyroidism. One patient with a T_4 level of 0.5 μg/ml and a TSH level of 80 mU/ml may have minimal symptoms, whereas another with similar values may be nearly comatose. Patients with more severe symptoms, elderly patients, and those with coexisting cardiopulmonary or other complicating illness are started gradually on thyroid hormone, whereas younger patients may be started on close to full replacement doses. For example, an 80-year-old hypothyroid woman with congestive heart failure and coronary artery disease might be started on 0.025 mg of levothyroxine, with 0.025-mg increments every 3 to 6 weeks. A 65-year-old woman with no known cardiac disease might be started on 0.050 mg of levothyroxine with 0.025- to 0.050-mg increments every 4 to 6 weeks. In contrast, a healthy 21-year-old woman discovered to have hypothyroidism can safely be started on 0.100 mg of levothyroxine that is then titrated to achieve a normal TSH concentration. Changes in serum TSH level after a dose adjustment may take 4 to 6 weeks before a steady state is obtained. More frequent adjustments in levothyroxine dose can be made, but TSH values obtained earlier than 4 to 6 weeks after a dose adjustment do not fully reflect the effects of the prior change in dose. Levothyroxine dose should be titrated to normalize serum TSH concentrations to prevent subclinical hyperthyroidism and adverse skeletal and cardiac effects.

Management of hypothyroidism in pregnancy is discussed in Chapter 59.

SUBCLINICAL THYROID DISEASE
Subclinical hyperthyroidism

Subclinical hyperthyroidism is a subnormal or undetectable serum TSH concentration with normal serum free T_4 and T_3 concentrations. The majority of these patients are asymptomatic. The largest group are receiving thyroid hormone preparations. Many are being inappropriately treated with overzealous replacement therapy for hypothyroidism. Oth-

ers are purposely given suppressive doses of levothyroxine to prevent growth of goitrous tissue.

Patients taking levothyroxine in doses that result in subclinical hyperthyroidism may have a reduction in bone density of 5% to 15% after 5 to 10 years. The femoral neck, femoral trochanter, and radius are affected more than spinal trabecular bone. It is therefore critical that women receiving replacement doses of thyroid hormone have the dose titrated to normal serum TSH concentrations. Measurement of serum T_4 concentration alone is inadequate, since changes in serum free T_4 concentrations are insensitive and may not detect even 40% overtreatment with levothyroxine.

Another group of patients with subclinical hyperthyroidism includes those with very mild endogenous hyperthyroidism. Some of these patients have autoimmune thyroid disease; however, the majority are older women with multinodular goiters and autonomous function. In addition to reduction in bone density older patients with subclinical hyperthyroidism have an increased risk of atrial fibrillation, and subclinical hyperthyroidism may also exacerbate angina or congestive heart failure. Thus it appears appropriate to consider treatment of patients with endogenous subclinical hyperthyroidism, especially in the presence of coexisting cardiovascular disease, osteoporosis, or a well-defined autonomous nodule.

Subclinical hypothyroidism

Patients with an elevated TSH and normal free T_4 levels have subclinical hypothyroidism. In the United States most of these patients have Hashimoto's thyroiditis. In two randomized trials women with subclinical hypothyroidism did better on symptom scoring and psychometric testing when treated with levothyroxine. A subgroup with initial abnormal systolic time intervals became normal with treatment. There was no change in cholesterol levels, although subsequent studies have reported an improvement in HDL- and low-density lipoprotein (LDL)-cholesterol levels in patients with subclinical hypothyroidism after treatment. If a patient with subclinical hypothyroidism caused by Hashimoto's thyroiditis also has a goiter, suppression of the TSH level to normal values will usually cause regression of the goiter.

SPORADIC NONTOXIC GOITER AND THYROID NODULES

Nodular thyroid disease is extremely prevalent in women. By palpation 6% of women have thyroid nodules. However, ultrasound demonstrates nodules in 21% of patients, and an autopsy series reports nodularity in 57% of patients. Unselected series suggest that the risk of cancer in a thyroid nodule is about 5%. The risk may be smaller in patients with

Table 12-3 L-thyroxine therapy

Type of therapy	Indications	Clinical guidelines
Replacement	Hypothyroidism	Average replacement dose is 0.112 mg Aim for normal TSH level; T_4 level may be modestly elevated
Suppression	Thyroid nodule	Use lowest dose necessary to suppress TSH level to subnormal values Aim for TSH level 0.05-0.5 mU/L (third-generation TSH assay)
	Thyroid cancer	Generally suppress TSH level to <0.01 mU/L

TSH, thyroid-stimulating hormone; T_4, thyroxine.

multinodular goiter, but it is not negligible. Therefore any solitary nodule or any dominant nodule within a multinodular goiter requires further evaluation. Dominant nodules are either larger, more firm, or particularly nonfunctional on thyroid scintigraphy.

Diagnostic tests

Fine needle aspiration is frequently the initial diagnostic procedure. Fine needle aspiration (FNA) is an office procedure done with local (Xylocaine) anesthesia and generally uses a 25 g needle. An adequate cytologic specimen is obtained in 90% of aspirates. "Macrofollicular lesions" (which include normal thyroid, colloid goiter, and true macrofollicular neoplasms) are benign and do not require surgery unless they are large and cause obstructive symptoms or are cosmetically unacceptable. Papillary cancer is readily diagnosed by needle aspirate and accounts for about 4% of nodules. "Microfollicular or cellular lesions" are problematic, since they may represent benign microfollicular adenomas, well-differentiated follicular carcinomas, or benign hyperfunctioning adenomas. Therefore a thyroid scan is needed to distinguish the hyperfunctioning ("hot") nodules. Nonfunctioning ("cold") microfollicular lesions are excised to exclude capsular or vascular invasion consistent with the diagnosis of follicular carcinoma.

Alternatively one can start the evaluation with a thyroid scan. Five percent or more of thyroid nodules may be hyperfunctioning, and these nodules do not require further evaluation by needle aspiration. Nodules that are indeterminate on thyroid scan can be rescanned while the patient is taking levothyroxine ("suppression scan") to determine whether they are truly autonomous. Ultrasound adds little to the initial evaluation of the thyroid nodule. It is useful, however, in following nodule size when the examination is difficult or in defining anatomic characteristics and dominance in a multinodular goiter.

Management

Until recently levothyroxine has been widely used to suppress pituitary TSH production and to reduce or inhibit growth of goitrous tissue. Suppressive therapy by definition results in subclinical hyperthyroidism and may therefore be a risk for reduced bone density (see previous discussion). Randomized trials have supported the use of suppressive therapy for nontoxic goiter. However, three recent short-term trials have failed to demonstrate a reduction in the size of solitary nodules in patients taking suppressive doses of levothyroxine. Since many apparent solitary nodules are associated with multinodularity when the thyroid is examined by ultrasound, it is possible that suppressive therapy may interrupt further goitrogenesis. Until further long-term studies clarify this issue, levothyroxine may be given in doses that result in subnormal but detectable TSH concentrations with the hope of minimizing any adverse effects of subclinical hyperthyroidism (see Table 12-3).

BIBLIOGRAPHY

Carr D et al: Fine adjustment of thyroxine replacement dosage: comparison of the thyrotropin releasing hormone test using a sensitive thyrotropin assay with measurement of free thyroid hormones and clinical assessment, *Clin Endocrinol* 28:325, 1988.

Cooper DS: Subclinical hypothyroidism. In Mazzaferri EL, Bar RS, Kreisberg RA, editors: *Advances in endocrinology and metabolism,* vol 2, St Louis, 1991, Mosby-Year Book.

Farrar JJ, Toft AD: Iodine-131 treatment of hyperthyroidism: current issues, *Clin Endocrinol* 35:207, 1991.

Ross DS: Subclinical thyrotoxicosis. In Mazzaferri EL, Bar RS, Kreisberg RA, editors: *Advances in endocrinology and metabolism,* vol 2, St Louis, 1991, Mosby-Year Book.

Ross DS: Evaluation of the thyroid nodule, *J Nucl Med* 32:2181, 1991.

Ross DS: Thyroid hormone suppressive therapy of sporadic nontoxic goiter, *Thyroid* 2:263, 1992.

Spencer et al: Applications of a new chemiluminometric thyrotropin assay to subnormal measurement, *J Clin Endocrinol Metab* 70:453, 1990.

13 Bowel Function

Jacqueline L. Wolf

Normal bowel function elicits little attention. However, alterations in bowel function may consume inordinate amounts of time and energy. Such focused attention on the bowels often results in frequent consultations with physicians. In the United States, Canada, and Northern Europe women are more likely than men to seek the advice of their physicians for changes in bowel function.

Women report many changes in bowel function throughout their life. Anecdotal reports of variations during the perimenstrual period, in pregnancy, and posthysterectomy have stimulated clinical and basic research studies on the effect of these states and concomitant changes in female sex hormone levels on normal gastrointestinal physiologic processes. Three disorders of bowel function—irritable bowel syndrome, functional bowel disorder, and intractable constipation—are more common in women than in men, lending further support to the possible effect of female hormones on bowel function.

This chapter will focus upon (1) three disorders that are more common to women than to men (irritable bowel syndrome, functional bowel disorder, and intractable slow transit constipation), (2) the effect on bowel function of three states with different levels of sex hormones (the menstrual cycle, pregnancy, and posthysterectomy), and (3) the effect of sexual and physical abuse on symptoms of abdominal and pelvic pain.

DEFINITION OF NORMAL BOWEL FUNCTION

Normal bowel function is quite difficult to define and varies greatly from person to person. In the general population normal bowel frequency varies from three times per week to two to three times per day. However, to an individual, abnormal bowel function may mean a change in the frequency of stool; a change in the consistency or ease in elimination of the stool; the occurrence of gas, cramping, or pain; or a general belief that the bowel movements should be different from what they are.

SYNDROMES THAT ARE MORE COMMON IN WOMEN
Irritable bowel syndrome

Epidemiology. Irritable bowel syndrome (IBS) occurs in about 15% to 20% of the population. However, the exact incidence is difficult to estimate because most people with symptoms do not consult a physician. In industrialized countries female patients predominate: twice as many women as men report symptoms in large studies. In less developed countries such as India males constitute the majority of patients. Cultural biases in the use of the health care system raise the question of the true incidence and gender frequency of IBS.

Definition of irritable bowel syndrome. Definitions for IBS vary from physician to physician and from study to study. In an attempt to standardize the definition a consensus conference was held in Rome in 1988. The proposed definition of IBS, which is based on symptoms, is continuous or recurrent symptoms for at least 3 months of (1) abdominal pain or discomfort relieved with defecation, or associated with a change in frequency or consistency of stool, and (2) disturbed defecation at least 25% of the time with three or more of (a) altered stool frequency, (b) altered stool form (hard or loose/watery), (c) altered stool passage (straining or urgency, feeling of incomplete evacuation), (d) passage of mucus, or (e) bloating or a feeling of abdominal distention (see box, below). If all criteria for irritable bowel syndrome are not met the symptom complex may be called functional bowel disorder (FBD). However, often the terms irritable bowel syndrome and functional bowel disorder are used interchangeably.

Pathogenesis. The cause of IBS has not been determined and is likely multifactorial. A subgroup of IBS patients clearly have increased visceral sensitivity. Balloon distention of different colonic segments causes pain in about 50%

DEFINITION OF IRRITABLE BOWEL SYNDROME

Continuous or recurrent symptoms for at least 3 months of:
1. Abdominal pain or discomfort relieved with defecation *or* associated with a change in frequency or consistency of stool *and*
2. An irregular (varying) pattern of defecation at least 25% of the time (three or more of the following)
   a. altered stool frequency
   b. altered stool form (hard or loose, watery stool)
   c. altered stool passage (straining or urgency; feeling of incomplete evacuation)
   d. passage of mucus
   e. bloating or feeling of abdominal distention

From Drossman DA, Thompson WG: *Ann Intern Med* 116:1010, 1992.

of IBS patients compared to only 10% of control subjects. However, with balloon distention in the rectum, only IBS patients who predominantly have diarrhea experience gas, distention, urgency, and the desire to evacuate. During a normal day some patients with IBS are aware of distal and proximal small bowel contractions. Occasionally when patients with IBS or FBD undergo a routine colonoscopy they are aware of the exact position of the colonoscope and actually feel the pinch of a biopsy (personal observation). Whether this sensation is more common in IBS or FBD patients than in the general population is not known. Colonic and small bowel motility abnormalities have been noted in some patients who meet all the criteria for IBS. However, colonic motility abnormalities do not correlate well with clinical findings. Small bowel motility abnormalities correlate better with symptoms. There is a strong association of altered jejunal and ileal motility with abdominal pain and of small bowel transit time with constipation or diarrhea. Stress clearly exacerbates symptoms of IBS and FBD, but how this happens is not known. It is postulated that many hormones and peptides, such as vasoactive intestinal polypeptide, substance P, cholecystokinin, and enkephalins found in both gut and brain play a role in the exacerbation of symptoms.

Clinical presentation

History and symptom presentation. Although IBS is defined by the lower abdominal complaints (see box, p. 79), there is an increased incidence (25% to 50%) of upper gastrointestinal complaints such as reflux, heartburn, dyspepsia, and respiratory and urinary complaints. Urinary tract symptoms such as frequency, nocturia, and urgency are common in patients with IBS. To determine the cause for these symptoms urodynamic studies were done in 30 patients with irritable bowel syndrome and 30 matched control subjects. Bladder distensibility was the same in both IBS and control patients. Detrusor instability, which is involuntary detrusor muscle contractions, appeared to be playing a major causative role: it occurred in 30% of IBS patients but only 3% of controls.

Abdominal pain is one of the two major criteria for IBS. Distinguishing a gastrointestinal from a gynecologic source of abdominal pain can be difficult. In one study up to 60% of women who reported pain to a gynecologist and had a negative laparoscopy result had symptoms suggestive of IBS (Prior, 1989). In a 12-month study of 71 women complaining of abdominal pain who sought medical attention at gynecology clinics in Manchester, England, those with symptoms of IBS were less likely to have had a definitive diagnosis made or have resolution of their pain during the study period. In the study 52% of the patients had IBS. Only 8% of the women with IBS compared to 44% of those without it had a definitive gynecologic diagnosis. At the end of the year 65% of women with and 32% of women without IBS still had abdominal pain. Determining how far to pursue a definitive diagnosis with costly and invasive tests in patients with IBS requires a careful history, physical examination, and clinical acumen.

History that would rule out the diagnosis of IBS and should prompt further evaluation includes onset in old age, unexplained weight loss, abdominal pain or diarrhea that awakens the patient from sleep, steatorrhea, melena, hematochezia except when documented from hemorrhoids or fissure, and fever. A careful history of drug (laxatives and other medications) ingestion should be obtained.

Physical examination. The physical examination by itself is not helpful in making the diagnosis of IBS but may help by arousing suspicion of another diagnosis. Findings incompatible with the diagnosis of IBS are rebound tenderness, involuntary abdominal boardlike rigidity, an abdominal mass, a succussion splash, high-pitched tinkling bowel sounds in rushes, fever, or guaiac-positive stool.

Diagnostic tests. There is no test for diagnosing IBS. As with the physical examination the tests are useful for ascertaining that another diagnosis is not more likely. The routine blood tests that should be done in most patients are a complete blood count which includes a white blood cell count, hemoglobin, hematocrit, and platelet count; an erythrocyte sedimentation rate; and certain chemical determinations, including glucose, electrolytes, amylase, lipase, and liver function tests. A protime and partial thromboplastin time are helpful in patients with diarrhea. Tests for malabsorption should be individualized. A urinalysis is useful for patients with urinary tract symptoms. A stool volume greater than 200 ml is not consistent with IBS. In patients with frequent stools an examination of stool for leukocytes, ova and parasites (three samples), culture and sensitivity (three samples), and Sudan stain for qualitative stool fat should be done. A flexible sigmoidoscopy should be done in all patients with hematochezia, sudden constipation, or diarrhea and in all patients over the age of 40. A barium enema or colonoscopy is indicated for some patients to exclude neoplastic or obstructive lesions or colitis. An oral lactose tolerance test or hydrogen breath test for lactase deficiency may be indicated in patients with bloating or frequent stools. Further diagnostic tests may be indicated, but a detailed discussion is beyond the scope of this chapter. For a review see Schuster (1991).

Differential diagnosis. The final diagnosis of irritable bowel syndrome is one of exclusion. Other identifiable and potentially specifically treatable causes should be excluded, including neoplasms, inflammatory bowel disease, endometriosis, sorbitol intolerance, malabsorption, pseudoobstruction, and pancreatic and hepatic disease. A full differential diagnosis is beyond the scope of this chapter. However, the diagnosis of lactose intolerance is worth special consideration.

LACTOSE INTOLERANCE. In patients with bloating the clinician should first ascertain that the patient does not have a lactose intolerance. In those with a lactase deficiency the onset of bloating with or without abdominal pain may occur several minutes to hours after lactose ingestion. For diagnosis, a 1- to 2-week trial of a completely lactose-free diet, a hydrogen breath test after lactose ingestion, or serial blood glucose levels after lactose ingestion can be done. If the patient is lactose-intolerant avoidance of lactose-containing foods and medications should help decrease or eliminate flatulence. Foods with lactose are milk, cream, cheese, butter, whey, cassein, lactalbumin, milk solids, yogurt, ice cream, ice milk, and prepared foods that contain these substances. If lactase deficiency is not complete many patients tolerate milk products pretreated with or ingested with exogenous lactase (Lactaid and Dairyease) and yogurt.

FIBER PREPARATIONS

Content	Preparation
Psyllium	Fiberall: powder, wafers
	Konsyl
	Maalox daily fiber
	Metamucil: powder, wafers, effervescent, sugar-free
	Mylanta natural fiber
Methylcellulose	Citrucel
Pectin	Certo, Sure-Jell, pectin powder, apple pectin capsules
Calcium polycarbophil	Fibercon tablets

Management

Goals of therapy. Because of the probable multifactorial causes of IBS treatment is directed toward symptomatic relief and stress management. No one therapy will help all patients. Some need no therapy as they spontaneously become asymptomatic without treatment. Most IBS patients continue to have intermittent symptoms for years. Many require therapy for their symptoms.

Choice of therapy

FIBER THERAPY. One of the mainstays of therapy is fiber. A good healthy diet should contain 25 to 30 g/day of fiber, but many people eat far less fiber. Dietary manipulation with the aim of increasing the fiber intake to 30 to 40 g of fiber should be one of the first treatments undertaken for both constipation and diarrhea. The increased stool fiber content results in increased water retention and a bulkier stool. There are two sources of fiber—**insoluble** (wheat bran, lignin, methylcellulose, hemicellulose, or calcium polycarbophil) and **soluble** (oat bran, psyllium, gums, or pectin). Many over-the-counter preparations containing these fiber sources exist and are useful for fiber supplementation. The box above lists some of the more common preparations. Patients may tolerate one type of fiber and not others. Bloating and gas are common after ingestion of some sources of fiber, but it is difficult to predict which source of fiber will produce no or minimal side effects in an individual. Personal observation suggests that methylcellulose (Citrucel) or pectin may be better tolerated, but this has not been proved.

THERAPY FOR BLOATING. Bloating may respond to elimination of foods likely to cause gas. These include beans, brussels sprouts, carrots, celery, onions, apricots, bananas, prunes, raisins, pretzels, and wheat germ (see box, below). Beano, an over-the-counter preparation of the enzyme α-galactosidase, may partially metabolize the insoluble sugars

FOODS LIKELY TO PRODUCE FLATULENCE

Beans	Apricots	Pretzels
Brussels sprouts	Bananas	Wheat germ
Carrots	Prunes	Milk and
Celery	Raisins	milk products
Onions		

Modified from Sutalf LO, Levitt MD: *Dig Dis Sci* 248:652, 1979.

Table 13-1 Preparations for controlling flatulence

α-Galactosidase	Beano	3-8 drops with food
Activated charcoal	Charcoal Plus	400 mg (2 tabs) tid
Simethicone	Gas X chewables Mylicon Phazyme	80-160 mg tid or 125 mg qid

in beans and peas, thereby decreasing the amount of sugar available for bacterial fermentation in the colon. Because the bacterial fermentation of the sugar causes gas, a decrease in available sugar should decrease flatulence. Decreased flatulence may also follow ingestion of **activated charcoal,** which may absorb gas, and **simethicone,** which changes the surface tension of liquids, allowing easier elimination of gas bubbles (Table 13-1).

PROKINETIC AGENTS (Table 13-2). In some patients with constipation and/or bloating the prokinetic agents **cisapride, metoclopramide,** and **domperidone** (not yet available in the United States) may be helpful. Metoclopramide increases upper gastrointestinal tract motility but does not affect colonic motility.

ANTICHOLINERGIC AGENTS (Table 13-3). Anticholinergic agents are the most frequently used agents for the treatment of IBS. They may be beneficial for abdominal pain and diarrhea associated with IBS. However, no well-designed placebo-controlled trials have proved them to be beneficial. Initial doses of anticholinergics should be small and administered $1/_2$ hour before meals and at bedtime. Anticholinergics exist alone or as combination medication. They are often combined with a mild tranquilizer in a single tablet or capsule.

ANTIDIARRHEAL AGENTS (Table 13-4). For chronic diarrhea or frequent stools cholestyramine (a binder of bile acids), diphenoxylate, and loperamide, may be useful. Lactose-intolerant patients should ascertain that the medication is lactose-free. The loperamide liquid preparation (Imodium) is lactose-free.

ANXIOLYTICS AND TRICYCLIC ANTIDEPRESSANTS (Table 13-5). Anxiolytic medications such as buspirone HCL (Buspar), chlordiazepoxide (Librium), lorazepam (Ativan), and diazepam (Valium) may help diminish the IBS symptoms associated with stress and anxiety, but their use poses the risk of dependency. Tricyclic antidepressants in low doses may help abdominal pain. The usual doses for this use are smaller than for treating depression: amitryptaline 10 to 50 mg at bedtime and desipramine 50 mg at bedtime.

Table 13-2 Prokinetic agents

Drug	Dosing	Precautions
Cisapride	5-20 mg tid-qid	Diarrhea
Metoclopramide	10 mg qid	Restlessness, drowsiness, fatigue, lassitude in 10%; dizziness, insomnia, headache, confusion, depression, acute dystonic reactions

Table 13-3 Anticholinergic agents

Agent	Dose	Side effects (for all medications)
Belladonna	5-10 GTT PO tid	Dry mouth, decreased sweating, blurred vision, mydriasis, cycloplegia, increased ocular tension, drowsiness, urinary hesitancy and retention, tachycardia, palpitations, loss of taste, headache, nervousness, dizziness, insomnia, nausea, vomiting, constipation, bloating, decreased lactation, allergic reactions.
Clinidium bromide (Quarzan)	2.5-5 mg PO tid to qid	
Dicyclomine hydrochloride (Bentyl)	10-20 mg PO qid	
Hyoscyamine sulfate (Levsin)	0.125-0.25 mg SL or PO q4h or time released 0.375-0.75 mg PO q12h	
Propantheline bromide (Probanthine)	7.5-15 mg PO qid	

*For tid or qid dosing give 3 doses 15-30 min before meals.
†Note: use with care in the elderly and patients with other diseases.

STRESS MANAGEMENT. Stress management and in selected cases more extensive counseling are often of benefit and should be considered in patients with IBS and FBD.

Intractable constipation

Definition and pathogenesis. Constipation causes much consternation and often results in a significant amount of time spent in trying to produce a bowel movement. Patients with severe, intractable idiopathic constipation are predominantly young women of reproductive age. These patients have one or fewer bowel movements per week and a colon of normal diameter. Their gastrointestinal motility is less than those of normal women or men.

Gastrointestinal transit can be determined by measuring the amount of time radiopaque markers take to traverse the distance from mouth to anus. After ingestion of 20 radiopaque markers, 95% of normal people eliminate all markers by 5 days. In contrast, patients with slow transit constipation retain more than four or five markers at 5 days and may retain markers at 8 days. As in IBS, women with intractable constipation have had reported associated abnormal bladder function and esophageal motility.

Clinical presentation. The evaluation of patients with intractable constipation is similar to that of patients with constipation predominant IBS. The diagnosis is one of exclusion and demonstration of abnormal gut transit time. A history of drug ingestion, age of onset of symptoms, speed of onset (i.e., sudden versus progressive), and other associated symptoms should be elicited. Gastrointestinal bleeding and weight loss are incompatible with the diagnosis. The physical examination is remarkable for palpable stool in the colon. Diagnostic tests should center around excluding the diagnosis of obstructing lesions, volvulus, pseudoobstruction, hypothy-

roidism, and chronic laxative abuse. A barium enema and sigmoidoscopy or colonoscopy with or without biopsy is usually done. A sitzmarker study should be done as follows: A patient is given a sitzmarker capsule at night. Abdominal supine and lateral radiographs are taken to enumerate and locate the markers the next day, at 5 days, and, if any marker remains, at 7 to 8 days after ingestion. To exclude other motility disorders rectal and esophageal studies may be helpful.

Management

Choice of therapy (Table 13-6). Treatment is difficult and often meets with limited success. Increased fiber should be the first line of therapy, but fiber use alone may not be successful. Adequate hydration and exercise are important. Avoidance of bowel stimulating laxatives, which when used may result in dependence, should be the aim of therapy. Treatment trials with a nonabsorbable sugar or short-term therapy with mineral oil should precede treatment with milk of magnesia, magnesium citrate, castor oil, bisacodyl USP (Dulcolax), senna, or cascara sagroda. The prokinetic agent cisapride could be useful. Why slow transit constipation occurs more commonly in young women is unknown and under investigation.

MENSTRUAL CYCLE AND GASTROINTESTINAL FUNCTION

Menstruating women undergo many physiologic changes throughout the month. Recent studies have examined the effects of the variable levels of estrogen and progesterone on

Table 13-4 Antidiarrheal agents for treatment of irritable bowel syndrome

Agent	Dose
Cholestyramine	½ to 1-g scoop or packet qd-qid
Loperamide	2 mg qd-qid
Diphenoxylate HCL	2.5 mg qid

Table 13-5 Anxiolytics and antidepressants used in the treatment of irritable bowel syndrome

Medication	Dose
Anxiolytics	
Buspirone HCL (Buspar)	5-10 mg tid
Diazepam (Valium)	2-5 mg bid-qid
Chlordiazepoxide (Librium)	5-10 mg tid or qid
Lorazepam (Ativan)	0.5-2 mg bid-tid
Phenobarbital	15 mg tid
Antidepressant	
Amitryptyline	10-50 mg qhs
Desipramine	50 mg qhs

Table 13-6 Choice of therapy for intractable constipation

Drug	Dose	Side effects/precautions
Fiber (including supplements)	30-40 g/day	
Beano or activated charcoal (for gas)	(See Table 13-1)	
Lactulose	1-2 tsp qd-qid	Bloating
Mineral oil	1-2 tbsp qd-tid	Do not use in the elderly, or patients with reflux (because of lipoid pneumonia associated with reflux). Use over long period may interfere with absorption of fat-soluble vitamins
Cisapride	10-20 mg tid	Diarrhea
Laxatives	Use sparingly	Bowel may become dependent on laxatives
Milk of magnesia	Begin with minimum dose	
Magnesium citrate		
Castor oil	PO	
Bisacodyl (sodium or calcium)	Suppositories or tablets	
Senna	PO	
Cascara sagrada	PO	
Glycerin	Suppositories	

gastrointestinal function. However, based on the results of these studies, whether gastrointestinal function is altered during different phases of the menstrual cycle is controversial.

Small intestinal transit

One parameter that has been examined is small intestinal transit. Small intestinal transit affects bowel frequency and consistency of stool. Measurement of expired breath hydrogen after ingestion of lactulose estimates the length of time a substance takes to reach the proximal colon. As lactulose is not absorbed in the small intestines, it passes unchanged into the colon. It is metabolized by colonic bacteria, releasing H_2 gas that is absorbed through the colonic wall, is exhaled by the lungs, and then can be measured. That this mainly determines small intestinal transit is based upon the assumption that there is not delayed gastric emptying. Wald et al. (1981) found significantly increased small intestinal transit time in the luteal phase compared to that in the follicular phase in 15 women who ingested lactulose mixed in water. Although the mean transit times were 25% longer, five women had no prolongation of the transit times in the luteal phase. Turnbull et al. (1989) could not confirm these results. Measurements of intestinal transit after ingestion of a test meal mixed with lactulose showed no variations with the menstrual cycle.

Colonic motility

The effect of the menstrual cycle on colonic motility has also been examined. In the colon water is absorbed from the intestinal contents, decreasing stool volume. Hence colonic motility may impact the volume and frequency of the stool. The measurement of whole gut transit using unabsorbable markers is mainly a measurement of colonic motility. Because the solid markers mixed with feces reside in the colon for a significantly longer period than in the rest of the gastrointestinal (GI) tract, investigators use the time taken to eliminate the markers after their ingestion as a gross estimate of colonic transit. Colonic transit has been reported to be both equal in men and women and slower in women. Measurements of colonic transit during the menstrual cycle of women have shown both slowing and no change in the luteal phase compared to that in the follicular phase.

Common bowel complaints

Normal menstruating women often report periods of constipation or diarrhea that seem to fluctuate with the menstrual cycle. However, these symptoms are often subjective and cannot be confirmed in prospective studies. Whitehead et al. (1990) attempted to estimate bowel complaints at menstruation in patients from a family planning clinic and women referred to a gastroenterology clinic with IBS or FBD. Thirty-four percent of Planned Parenthood subjects without IBS or FBD reported one or more bowel symptoms with menstruation. These included increased gas (14%), increased diarrhea (19%), and increased (11%) and decreased (16%) constipation. Significantly more patients with FBD and IBS than control subjects had increased gas at menstruation, and significantly more patients with IBS than control subjects had increased diarrhea or constipation at menstruation. In smaller studies, 64% (Hinds, 1989) and 96% (Rees, 1976) of women reported a change in bowel habits with menses. To determine whether the retrospective recall of menstrual symptoms was accurate, Heitkemper and Jarrett (1992) prospectively examined gastrointestinal symptoms and select mood and somatic symptoms in a small number of women with and without FBD. Confirming the observations of Whitehead et al. (1992) they found a significant increase in abdominal pain at menses compared to that in the follicular or luteal phases in both groups. Patients with FBD had increased abdominal pain, nausea, and diarrhea compared to women without FBD. No significant differences were noted in stool consistency and frequency across the menstrual cycle, although in a previous study Heitkemper, Shaver, and Mitchell (1988) found decreased consistency of the stool in women at menses. Bloating and cramping abdominal and pelvic pain were worse during menses in the FBD group. Other complaints of poor work or school performance and backache paralleled the increase in abdominal pain in the premenstrual period through the third day of menses. More women with FBD (39%) than control subjects (28%) had sought health care for perimenstrual distress. Dysmenorrheic women report more menses-related gastrointestinal symptoms than do control subjects.

HYSTERECTOMY AND BOWEL FUNCTION

If bowel function is affected by the hormonal state of a woman, changes in bowel function should follow hysterectomy. In a case-control study of Scottish women with and without hysterectomy, Taylor, Smith, and Fulton found that women who had had a hysterectomy reported less frequent bowel movements than control subjects. Also reported were more laxative use, harder stools, and constipation in women with a hysterectomy, but these findings were not statistically significant. Increased urinary frequency concomitant with decreased bowel frequency was noted in 10 of 91 women after hysterectomy. A criticism of the study is that no control was included for patients with IBS. Because IBS patients have an increased risk of hysterectomy this may have biased the findings. A prospective study of bowel function in 205 women before, 6 weeks after, and 6 months after hysterectomy examined the effect of hysterectomy on bowel function (Prior et al., 1992). Only 13 women had bilateral oophrectomy. Twenty-two percent of patients had symptoms of IBS before surgery. After surgery 10% of normal women complained of new gastrointestinal symptoms occurring more than once per week and 5% of the women experienced constipation. Of the women with preexisting IBS 6 months after hysterectomy, 33% were asymptomatic, 27% had improved symptoms, and 20% complained of increased symptoms. Although no relationship could be found between the development of de novo constipation and de novo urinary dysfunction, 29 of the 205 women had an increase in frequency, urgency, and/or incontinence. The cause of development of constipation after hysterectomy is unclear. It is thought to be due to injury of the autonomic nerves that are located on the lateral side of the rectum, cervix, and vaginal fornix. However, constipation not only occurs after a radical hysterectomy, in which the nerves may be damaged, but also after a simple hysterectomy, in which presumably the nerves are left intact. The effect of hysterectomy on sphincter and colonic motility has been examined and the results are controversial. One report noted failure of the internal anal sphincter to relax to baseline in 60% of patients after radical or simple hysterectomy for cervical cancer, whereas others found no change in the sphincter. Studies by Barnes and Smith reported the finding of increased rectal volume required to trigger the rectal-anal sphincter inhibitory response; however, a study by Roe did not. An increased paradoxic reaction of the colonic motility gradient to the prokinetic agent Prostigmin that created a functional obstruction was found in patients after hysterectomy with ovaries left *in situ*. From the data obtained from these small studies it would appear that women may experience constipation and urinary symptoms after hysterectomy, but they occur only in a minority of patients. For a further discussion of the effects of hysterectomy refer to Chapter 44.

RELATIONSHIP BETWEEN ABUSE AND PELVIC AND ABDOMINAL PAIN

Physical and sexual abuse not only affect the psychologic well-being of a patient but often result in gynecologic and gastrointestinal symptoms. Abuse is a major epidemic in the United States. Estimates of the incidence of childhood sexual abuse in the United States vary from 15% to 38%. Women outnumber men by 2:1 to 4:1. Physician awareness of the abuse is poor; as few as 2% of physicians in one study and 17% in another were cognizant of the abuse. Only 20% to 50% of abuse episodes come to the attention of authorities. Because the history is rarely volunteered and may impact medical therapy, physicians should routinely ask patients about abuse. Suspicion of possible abuse (sexual and physical) should be aroused by a patient who has chronic pelvic or abdominal pain, frequent visits to a physician for seemingly minor or unexplainable complaints, drug abuse, panic attacks, or frequent ecchymoses. Up to 80% of severely sexually abused girls report sexual abuse as women. The risk of sexual abuse appears to be higher in patients with IBS than in the general population. In a referral-based gastroenterology clinic practice, Drossman et al. (1990) found a 44% incidence of abuse. In a random sampling of healthy residents of Olmsted County, Minnesota, in which 70% of the queried group responded, 28% of 830 residents reported abuse and 23% reported sexual abuse (Talley, Zinsmeister, and Melton, 1993). Those who reported sexual abuse were twice as likely to have IBS or FBD as those without abuse. All patients with abuse were more likely to have seen a physician within the past year than nonabused patients. In another large study in which members of a health maintenance organization in California were queried sexual abuse was reported by 19% of women and 6% of men (Longstreth and Shragg, 1992). Sexual abuse was reported in 10% of the population without IBS, in 21% of IBS patients who reported constipation or diarrhea as predominant symptoms, and in 36% of IBS subjects with pain as the predominant symptom. Most studies report significantly more physician visits by both IBS patients and subjects reporting sexual abuse and increased surgical procedures among patients who have been abused. For more detailed discussion of abuse see Chapters 68 and 72.

Knowing about abuse can potentially affect decisions about surgery, endoscopy, and other invasive tests. Every patient, male or female, should be asked whether he or she has ever had unwanted sexual attention, been forced to perform sexual acts, or has had physical acts of abuse such as hitting, pushing, or kicking directed against him or her. Posttraumatic syndrome can develop after either physical or sexual abuse. Psychologic intervention may be of benefit for such patients.

PREGNANCY AND BOWEL FUNCTION

Epidemiology

It is commonly believed that constipation is a frequent complaint in pregnancy. However, many studies have failed to show that a majority of women have constipation. In a study by Levy (1971) of bowel function in 1000 healthy pregnant Israeli women, 55% had no change in bowel frequency, 34% had increased frequency, and 11% had decreased frequency. Other surveys showed an increase in constipation. In Anderson's study of 200 British women interviewed in the third trimester, 38% of women reported having had constipation sometime during their pregnancy and 18% still had it at the time of the interview. Because of constipation and other ill-defined gastrointestinal complaints 70% of the women reported dietary modification, primarily increasing fiber intake, which likely improved the symptoms of constipation.

Physiologic changes in gastrointestinal function during pregnancy

Small bowel transit time appears to be prolonged in pregnancy. In a study using mercury-filled balloons, prolongation of small intestinal transit time (58 ± 12 hours vs. 52 ± 10 hours) in 12- to 20-week pregnant women compared to that in control subjects, was noted. Use of H_2 breath tests after lactulose ingestion in 15 women revealed prolongation of transit time in the third trimester compared to the postpartum period (131 ± 14 minutes vs. 93 ± 7 minutes) (Everson, 1992). Lawson, Kern, and Everson (1985) found a statistically significant increase in the mean transit time from the first to the second trimester with an increase that was not significant in the third trimester and a subsequent fall in the postpartum period. Although the postpartum mean transit time was less than in the first trimester, the difference was not significant. Transit times increased as progesterone levels increased from <1 ng/ml to 80 ng/ml but not as levels increased further.

Evaluation of colonic motility or transit in pregnant women has not been done, but studies in rats have examined the effects of hormones and pregnancy on colonic transit. Rats that are in a high estrogen-progesterone state or that have been ovariectomized and pretreated with estrogen and progesterone show significantly slower transit times than animals in a low hormonal state or ovariectomized without hormone replacement. Pregnant rats have transit times similar to those of the ovariectomized animals pretreated with hormones.

Management

Treatment of constipation in pregnancy should be aimed at dietary modification through increased fiber intake and adequate liquid consumption. Supplementation of fiber ingested in the diet with psyllium (Metamucil, Konsyl, Effersyllium), methylcellulose (Citrucel), calcium polycarbophil (Fibercon), or pectin to 30 to 40 g/day of fiber is safe and often effective. Bloating may occur with some sources of fiber but not others. Therefore, if bloating occurs changing the source of fiber may be beneficial. Nonabsorbable sugars such as lactulose, sorbitol, and glycerin are safe if dietary manipulation fails. Use of mineral oil should be limited to short periods, only in patients without a risk of aspiration, and only in the morning or at lunch. Saline solution containing laxatives may result in sodium retention in the mother. Other laxative use should be limited because of the risk of dependence. Laxatives to avoid are castor oil, which may induce uterine contractions in the mother; cascara sagrada, which may cause diarrhea in the neonate; and the anthraquinones. The other stimulant laxatives appear to be safe. Although many women attribute some of their constipation to use of prenatal vitamins that contain iron, the vitamins should be continued if at all possible.

Hormonal fluctuations throughout the menstrual cycle and in pregnancy may affect bowel function, causing changes in frequency of bowel movements and periodic complaints of abdominal discomfort and bloating.

SUMMARY

Women with IBS or FBD may have increased symptoms at the time of their menstrual periods. Pregnant women often complain of constipation, but studies proving an increased incidence are lacking. However, part of the discrepancy between patient reporting and the findings of retrospective studies may be due to dietary manipulation by the patient. After an abrupt fall in levels of female sex hormones posthysterectomy most women have no change in their bowel function. However, a small number experience marked constipation requiring therapeutic intervention. A problem that affects many women and results in increased gastrointestinal and gynecologic complaints is sexual and physical abuse. Women who have been abused have more frequent visits to physicians and more surgical procedures. Awareness of the history of abuse may greatly impact the care of a patient. Physicians should be aware of the gastrointestinal symptoms that may fluctuate with hormonal changes and stress in women. These complaints should be taken seriously and evaluated and treated in a thoughtful way.

BIBLIOGRAPHY

Anderson AS: Constipation during pregnancy: incidence and methods used in its treatment in a group of Cambridgeshire women, *Health Visit* 12:363, 1984.

Arhan D et al: Segmental colonic transit time, *Dis Colon Rectum* 24:625, 1981.

Bachmann GA, Moeller TP, Benett J: Childhood sexual abuse and the consequences in adult women, *Obstet Gynecol* 71:4:631, 1988.

Bailey LD Jr, Stewart WR, McCallum RW: New directions in the irritable bowel syndrome. In Friedman G, editor: *Gastroenterology clinics of North America,* Philadelphia, 1991, WB Saunders.

Barnes W et al: Manometric characterization of rectal dysfunction following radical hysterectomy, *Gynecol Oncol* 42:116, 1991.

Baron TH, Ramirez B, Richter JE: Gastrointestinal motility disorders during pregnancy, *Ann Intern Med* 118:366, 1993.

Davies GJ et al: Bowel function measurements of individuals with different eating patterns, *Gut* 27:164, 1986.

Drossman DA, Thompson WG: The irritable bowel syndrome: review and a graduated multicomponent treatment approach, *Ann Intern Med* 116:1009, 1992.

Drossman DA et al: Bowel patterns among subjects not seeking healthcare: use of questionnaire to identify a population with bowel dysfunction, *Gastroenterology* 83:529, 1990.

Drossman DA et al: Sexual and physical abuse in women with functional or organic gastrointestinal disorders, *Ann Intern Med* 113:828, 1990.

Everson GT: Gastrointestinal motility in pregnancy. In Reily CA, Abell TL, editors: *Gastroenterology clinics of North America,* Philadelphia, 1992, WB Saunders.

Friedman G: Treatment of the irritable bowel syndrome. In Friedman G, editor: *Gastroenterology clinics of North America,* Philadelphia, 1992, WB Saunders.

Heitkemper MM, Jarrett M: Pattern of gastrointestinal and somatic symptoms across the menstrual cycle, *Gastroenterology* 102:505, 1992.

Heitkemper MM, Shaver JF, Mitchell ES: Gastrointestinal symptoms and bowel patterns across the menstrual cycle in dysmenorrhea, *Nurs Res* 37:108, 1988.

Hinds JP, Stoney B, Wald A: Does gender or the menstrual cycle affect colonic transit? *Am J Gastroenterol* 84:123, 1989.

Kamm MA, Farthing MJG, Lennard-Jones JE: Bowel function and transit rate during the menstrual cycle, *Gut* 30:605, 1989.

Lawson M, Kern F Jr., Everson GT: Gastrointestinal transit time in human pregnancy: prolongation in the second and third trimesters followed by postpartum normalization, *Gastroenterology* 89:996, 1985.

Leserman J et al: The relationship of abuse history with health status and health care use in a referral GI clinic, *Gastroenterology* 104:A541, 1993.

Levy N, Lemberg E, Sharf M: Bowel habit in pregnancy, *Digestion* 4:216, 1971.

Lind CD: Motility disorders in the irritable bowel syndrome. In Friedman G, editor: *Gastroenterology clinics of North America,* vol 20, Philadelphia, 1991, WB Saunders.

Longstreth GF, Shragg GP: Irritable bowel syndrome and childhood abuse in HMO health examinees, *Gastroenterology* 102:A477, 1992.

Lynn RB, Friedman LS: Current concepts: irritable bowel syndrome, *N Engl J Med* 329:1940, 1993.

Metcalf AM et al: Simplified assessment of segmental colonic transit, *Gastroenterology* 92:40, 1987.

Preston DM, Lennard-Jones JE: Severe chronic constipation of young women: idiopathic slow transit constipation, *Gut* 27:41, 1986.

Prior A, Marton DG, Whorwell PJ: Anorectal manometry in irritable bowel syndrome: differences between diarrhea and constipation predominant subjects, *Gut* 31:458, 1990.

Prior A, Whorwell PJ: Gynaecological consultation in patients with the irritable bowel syndrome, *Gut* 30:996, 1989.

Prior A et al: Relation between hysterectomy and the irritable bowel: a prospective study, *Gut* 33:814, 1992.

Rao SSC et al: Studies on the mechanism of bowel disturbance in ulcerative colitis, *Gastroenterology* 93:934, 1987.

Rees WDW, Rhodes JWT: Altered bowel habit and menstruation, *Lancet* 2:475, 1976.

Roe AM, Bartolo DCC, Mortensen NJM: Slow transit constipation: comparison between patients with or without previous hysterectomy, *Dig Dis Sci* 33:1159, 1988.

Ryan JP, Bhojwani A: Colonic transit in rats: effect of ovariectomy, sex steriod hormones, and pregnancy, *Am J Physiol* 251:G46, 1986.

Schuster MM: Diagnostic evaluation of the irritable bowel snydrome. In Friedman G, editor: *Gastroenterology clinics of North America,* 1991, vol 20, Philadelphia, 1991, WB Saunders.

Springs FE, Friedrich WN: Health risk behaviors and medical sequelae of childhood sexual abuse, *Mayo Clin Proc* 67:527, 1992.

Smith AN et al: Disordered colorectal motility in intractable constipation following hysterectomy, *Br J Surg* 77:1361, 1990.

Stanhope CR: *Gynecol Oncol* 42:114, 1991 (editorial).

Sutalf LO, Levitt MD: Follow-up of a flatulent patient, *Dig Dis Sci* 248:652, 1979.

Talley NJ, Zinsmeister AR, Melton LJ III: Sexual abuse is linked to functional bowel disorders in the community, *Gastroenterology* 104:A590, 1993.

Taylor T, Smith AN, Fulton PM: Effect of hysterectomy on bowel function, *Br Med J* 299:300, 1989.

Turnbull GK et al: Relationships between symptoms, menstrual cycle and orocaecal transit in normal and constipated women, *Gut* 30:30, 1989.

Wald A et al: Effect of pregnancy on gastrointestinal transit, *Dig Dis Sci* 27:1015, 1982.

Wald A et al: Gastrointestinal transit: the effect of the menstrual cycle, *Gastroenterology* 80:1497, 1981.

Walker EA et al: Medical and psychiatric symptoms in women with childhood sexual abuse, *Psychosom Med* 54:658, 1992.

West L, Warren J, Cutts T: Diagnosis and management of irritable bowel syndrome constipation, and diarrhea in pregnancy. In Reily CA, Abell TL, editors: *Gastroenterology clinics of North America,* Philadelphia, 1992, WB Saunders.

Whitehead WE et al: Evidence for exacerbation of irritable bowel syndrome during menses, *Gastroenterology* 98:1485, 1990.

Whorwell PJ et al: Bladder smooth muscle dysfunction in patients with irritable bowel syndrome, *Gut* 27:1014, 1986.

Wingate DL: The irritable bowel syndrome. In Friedman G, editor: *Gastroenterology clinics of North America,* vol 20, Philadelphia, 1991, WB Saunders.

Zighelboim J, Talley NJ: What are functional bowel disorders? *Gastroenterology* 104:1196, 1993.

14 Gallstones

Joanne M. Donovan and David L. Carr-Locke

Gallbladder and biliary tract diseases that result from gallstones are major causes of morbidity and mortality in the United States and other industrialized countries and are twice as common in women as in men. Cholesterol gallstone formation is a multifactorial process that requires cholesterol supersaturated bile and rapid formation of cholesterol crystals, both of which are frequently accompanied by impaired motor function of the gallbladder. As epidemiologic observations have suggested and as clinical studies have confirmed, estrogens and progesterones potentiate formation of cholesterol stones. The range of therapeutic options is broad and includes laparoscopic and open cholecystectomy, surgical bile duct exploration and choledocholithotomy, interventional peroral endoscopy, shock wave lithotripsy, percutaneous transhepatic and direct access gallbladder techniques, and direct and oral pharmacologic dissolution. Cholecystectomy represents one of the most common operations on women, with approximately 500,000 performed annually in the United States. This chapter outlines the pathophysiologic and epidemiologic characteristics and treatment of gallstones, with particular emphasis on why women are more prone to their development.

PATHOPHYSIOLOGY
Types of gallstones

There are three major classes of gallstones: cholesterol stones, black pigment stones, and brown pigment stones.

Cholesterol and black pigment stones are formed exclusively in the gallbladder, although their clinical presentation may occur after migration to the bile ducts. **Cholesterol stones,** which constitute more than 80% of gallstones in the United States, are composed predominantly of crystalline cholesterol, cemented together in a mucin gel framework together with small amounts of inorganic and organic calcium salts. **Black pigment stones** are largely composed of polymerized calcium bilirubinate (unconjugated bilirubin), together with inorganic calcium salts. Clinical risk factors for black pigment stones include conditions in which increased quantities of conjugated bilirubin are excreted into bile, such as hemolytic anemia and cirrhosis. **Brown pigment stones** are formed almost exclusively in the bile ducts, are associated with bacterial infection of the biliary tree, and are predominantly formed of bacterial degradation products such as calcium salts of lipids degraded by bacteria, including fatty acids and bilirubin. Their pathogenesis is usually secondary to infection, and the only major risk factor is mechanical bile stasis, most often caused by cholesterol gallstones in the Western world. Additional factors may play a part in Southeast Asia, such as biliary parasite infestation and bile duct strictures, since ductal stones often appear without coexisting gallbladder stones in this area of the world. The pathophysiologic character of pigment stone formation will not be discussed further since sex differences do not appear to affect their formation directly.

Mechanisms of gallstone formation

Several defects interact to initiate gallstone formation: the presence of cholesterol-supersaturated bile, rapid formation of cholesterol crystals, and gallbladder hypomotility. Because of its extreme insolubility in water, cholesterol is excreted from the body almost entirely via biliary secretion, as cholesterol or after transformation into bile salts. In the gallbladder, bile salts, together with the major biliary phospholipid lecithin, solubilize cholesterol in micellar lipid aggregates or in fragments of lipid bilayers called *vesicles*. Cholesterol gallstone patients secrete cholesterol-supersaturated bile, which can spontaneously form cholesterol crystals, the building blocks of gallstones. Much recent work has identified both pronucleating and antinucleating factors in the bile of healthy persons as well as those who have cholesterol gallstones. However, qualitative differences in the balance of pronucleating and antinucleating proteins in gallstone patients are only beginning to be identified.

Cholesterol hypersecretion. Cholesterol homeostasis is controlled by hepatocytes, which synthesize cholesterol and regulate its excretion directly as cholesterol or bile salts. Biliary cholesterol supersaturation can be produced by imbalances in the enzymes regulating cholesterol flux. The sensitivity of these processes to hormonal regulation accounts for an excess of gallstone disease in women, as well as higher high-density lipoprotein (HDL) levels, one of the factors associated with a decreased risk of cardiovascular disease in women. As Fig. 14-1 depicts, the pool of free cholesterol in the hepatocyte is derived from lipoproteins and cholesterol synthesis. Although total liver free cholesterol does not vary substantially, a subset of this pool is thought to control cholesterol secretion into bile. Hence biliary cholesterol secretion and saturation vary in proportion to the size of the free cholesterol pool. Chylomicrons containing dietary cholesterol in the form of cholesterol esters undergo endocytosis by the apolipoprotein B/E receptor as well as an independent chylomicron remnant receptor. The apolipoprotein B/E receptor also regulates the uptake of low-density lipoprotein (LDL), which contains endogenously synthesized cholesterol. After hydrolysis by neutral cholesterol ester hydrolase, cholesterol from cholesterol esters joins free cholesterol from the lipoprotein surface to supply the free cholesterol pool. The hepatocyte also synthesizes cholesterol from acetate, with the rate-limiting step controlled by hydroxymethylglutarylcoenzyme A (HMG-CoA) reductase. After esterification by the enzyme acyl:cholesterol:acyl transferase (ACAT), the hepatocyte secretes cholesterol esters in the core of newly synthesized lipoproteins—principally very low-density lipoprotein (VLDL) and HDL. Cholesteryl esters are reversibly stored in the hepatocytes and, after hydrolysis by neutral cholesterol ester hydrolase, free cholesterol is restored to the hepatocyte for synthesis or excretion. Net excretion of cholesterol occurs either by direct secretion into bile as free cholesterol, or after transformation into bile salts via the rate-limiting enzyme 7-α-hydroxylase.

Effects of estrogen and progesterone. Several of the enzymes regulating cholesterol homeostasis are affected by either endogenous and exogenous estrogens or progesterone.

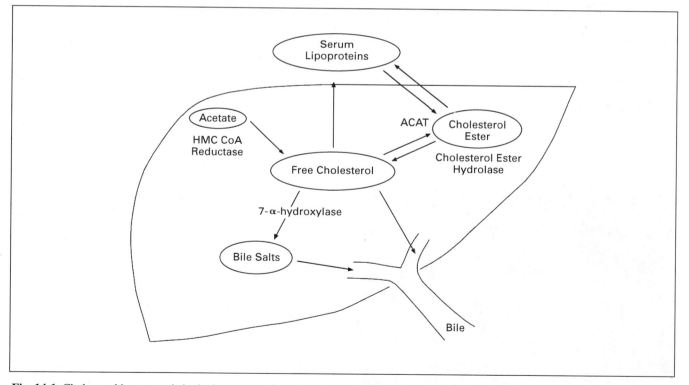

Fig. 14-1 Cholesterol homeostasis in the hepatocyte. Input into the pool of free cholesterol within the hepatocyte occurs via synthesis and from uptake of low-density lipoprotein and chylomicron remnants containing cholesterol esters. The rate limiting step in cholesterol synthesis is HMG-CoA reductase. Cholesterol esters are hydrolyzed by lysosomal cholesterol ester hydrolase. Cholesterol is used by the hepatocyte for synthesis of VLDL and HDL. Net excretion of cholesterol occurs directly into bile or after conversion via 7-α-hydroxylase to bile salts. Cholesterol can also be stored within the hepatocyte in the form of cholesterol esters synthesized by ACAT. HMG CoA, hydroxymethylglutaryl coenzyme A; VLDL, very low-density lipoprotein; HDL, high-density lipoprotein; ACAT, acyl: cholesterol: acyl transferase.

However, their net effect on biliary cholesterol secretion depends upon the dose and differs for acute and chronic exogenous administration. Estrogens, whether in oral contraceptives, at puberty, or as estrogen replacement therapy, increase biliary cholesterol saturation. Estrogen-mediated increases in hepatic cholesterol uptake via LDL and chylomicrons are largely matched by increases in biliary cholesterol secretion, but not bile salt synthesis. Progesterones inhibit the enzyme ACAT and increase the biliary free cholesterol pool and, consequently, biliary cholesterol secretion. Although HMG CoA reductase is not affected by sex hormones, its activity is increased in obesity and hypertriglyceridemia, with consequent increases in cholesterol synthesis and secretion into bile. Estrogens and progesterones do not significantly alter the rate-limiting enzyme of bile salt synthesis, 7-α-hydroxylase, the activity of which decreases with age.

Biliary sludge. An important intermediate step in the formation of gallstones is the development of biliary sludge. Sludge can be detected ultrasonographically (Fig. 14-2) and is composed of microcrystals of cholesterol and calcium bilirubinate in a thick mucin gel. Although sludge may evolve to gallstone formation, in the majority of cases it disappears spontaneously. Occurrence of biliary sludge is more common in pregnancy, and its clinical implications will be discussed later in this chapter.

Gallbladder hypomotility and emptying. Gallbladder hypomotility prevents the complete clearance of cholesterol crystals by the gallbladder and can predispose to cholesterol gallstone formation. In a vicious cycle cholesterol-supersaturated bile itself induces gallbladder hypomotility. Progesterones, but not estrogens, directly impair both the rate of gallbladder emptying and the maximum ejection fraction. Gallbladder volume is increased and ejection fraction is impaired in pregnancy but both return to normal in the postpartum period.

EPIDEMIOLOGY AND RISK FACTORS

In general, the clinical groups at risk for gallstones reflect the pathophysiologic processes of gallstone formation (see box at right). Although ultrasound studies have shown a great deal of geographic and ethnic variation in the prevalence of gallstone disease, the overall prevalence of gallstones in women is about twice that in men in all ethnic groups. Native American populations, in particular the Pima, constitutionally hypersecrete biliary cholesterol and hyposecrete bile salts. Consequently, gallstone disease is frequent in this population, reaching a prevalence of about 80% in older women. In Asian and African black populations gallstone disease is much rarer, with prevalences of less than 10%. European populations have intermediate prevalences of 10% to 25%.

After childhood, when gallstones are equally rare in both sexes, gallstone prevalence increases sharply with age, as shown in Fig. 14-3 in a large prospective ultrasound survey of over 4500 adult Danish subjects. In all postpuberty age groups the relative risk of gallstones in women exceeds that in men, but in younger age groups the relative risk is greater. Gender differences in the prevalence of gallstones are largely attributable to the consequences of pregnancy. As shown in Fig. 14-4 the risk of gallstone disease rises with each pregnancy, and the relative risk is highest for younger women. Although parity is a strong risk factor for gallstone disease in young women, the relative risk diminishes in the postmenopausal age group.

Exogenous estrogens also promote the development of gallstones in females as well as males treated with supraphysiologic estrogen doses. Shortly after the introduction of oral contraceptives case-control studies noted a twofold to threefold increase in the incidence of gallstone disease, but more recent studies have shown a lower relative risk of 1.1 (age-adjusted), with the highest relative risks in the youngest women. The effect of pregnancy is confounding, since initiation of oral contraceptives may follow recent pregnancy, and studies did not use ultrasound to detect asymptomatic gallstones. However, a dose-related response was demonstrated, with the risk for use of products with >50 μg of estrogen daily of 1.21, and a risk of 0.97 for those with <50 μg estrogen. Prospective ultrasound studies of prevalence have shown an elevated risk for users of oral contraceptives, but the effect was not significant after multivariate analysis. With current use of lower estrogen doses the relative risk for users of oral contraceptives is thought to be minimal.

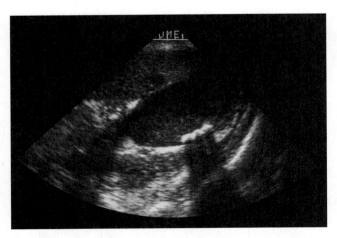

Fig. 14-2 Ultrasonographic appearance of hyperechoic gallbladder sludge without acoustic shadowing, layering above three stones with distinct acoustic shadows.

RISK FACTORS FOR GALLBLADDER DISEASE IN WOMEN

Ethnic origin: Native American
Age
Estrogen
  Pregnancy
  Parity
  Exogenous estrogen
    Oral contraceptives
    Postmenopausal estrogen
Hypertriglyceridemia
Drugs
  Fibric acid derivatives
  Nicotinic acid
Obesity and rapid weight loss
Gallbladder stasis

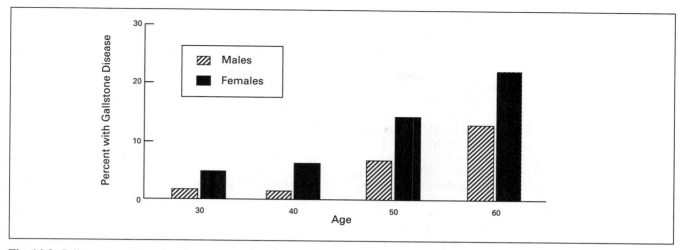

Fig. 14-3 Gallstone prevalence in a large prospective ultrasound survey of over 4500 adult Danish subjects increases sharply with age. At younger ages there is a female preponderance that narrows in older age groups. (From Jorgensen T: *Am J Epidemiol* 126:912, 1987.)

Postmenopausal estrogen replacement therapy is associated with a 2.5-fold increase in surgical gallstone disease. The risk of gallstone disease persists after stopping estrogen therapy, since gallstones seldom spontaneously dissolve or pass. In contrast to oral estrogens, which undergo first pass metabolism in the liver, transdermal estrogens do not increase biliary cholesterol saturation and probably do not increase the risk of gallstones.

Since the body's cholesterol is almost exclusively excreted through the bile, there has been much study on the interrelationship between serum lipid levels and cholesterol gallstones. Hypertriglyceridemia is associated with an increased risk of gallstones. Increased total serum cholesterol level is not associated with an increased risk, but high levels of HDL cholesterol and low levels of serum cholesterol are probably associated with a decreased risk of gallstone disease. Not surprisingly, pharmacologic agents that alter serum lipid levels have important effects on biliary cholesterol secretion and hence on cholesterol gallstone formation.

The fibric acid derivatives clofibrate and gemfibrozil both increase the amount of cholesterol secreted into bile and have been associated with statistically significant differences in the prevalence of gallstone disease and biliary tract complications. Nicotinic acid has also been associated with a modest increase in biliary tract disease. In contrast, HMG-CoA reductase inhibitors such as mevinolin or lovastatin decrease cholesterol synthesis and also markedly reduce cholesterol secretion into bile. Biliary cholesterol saturation therefore decreases markedly, and preliminary studies demonstrate that HMG-CoA reductase inhibitors accelerate pharmacologic dissolution of gallstones.

Obesity is considered an independent risk factor for cholesterol gallstones, independent of the effect on serum lipids. In the Nurses' Health Study cohort, relative weight was associated with an increased incidence of symptomatic gallstones (sixfold higher for the highest quintile) for women, but not for men. A confounding factor in the association of obesity with gallstones is that reducing diets are

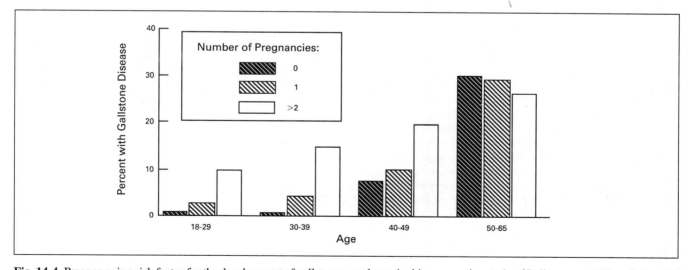

Fig. 14-4 Pregnancy is a risk factor for the development of gallstones, as shown in this prospective study of Italian women. The relative risk is highest for young women but increases in all premenopausal groups with each successive pregnancy. (From Barbara L et al: *Hepatology* 7:913, 1987.)

associated with a very high risk of development of gallstones. Patients undergoing rapid weight loss, of greater than 15 kg total, over several weeks, are at extremely high risk of development of gallstones, with gallstone developing in 20% in this short time. Increased biliary cholesterol excretion as well as failure of low levels of dietary fat to contract the gallbladder interact synergistically to accelerate formation of cholesterol gallstones. Ursodiol has been successful in preventing the formation of biliary sludge and gallstones, suggesting that prophylaxis of gallstone formation in this very high-risk group is warranted.

Gallbladder stasis potentiates gallstone development by preventing clearance of biliary sludge and microgallstones. Patients with subnormal cholecystokinin (CCK) release caused by decreased duodenal stimulation (e.g., those on total parenteral nutrition or fat-restricted diets) or with neuropathy (e.g., spinal cord injury patients and diabetics with autonomic dysfunction) have impaired gallbladder motility. Progesterone, but not estrogen, impairs gallbladder emptying and acts synergistically to accelerate gallstone development while cholesterol secretion is increased during pregnancy.

NATURAL HISTORY OF GALLSTONES

The natural history of gallstones has been studied in asymptomatic and symptomatic patients. In several studies subjects have been retrospectively identified with gallstones, and the risk of development of symptoms or biliary complications such as acute cholecystitis or cholangitis, common duct obstruction, or pancreatitis was determined. The risk of symptom development is from 20% to 40% over 20 years, with the highest risk in the first 5 years and decreasing risk the longer the stones remain asymptomatic. Importantly patients did not have complications as their initial manifestation of gallstones.

In several studies gallstones in women appear to have a higher risk of causing symptoms than in men. Although this effect has been ascribed to the greater use of ultrasonography in women, with incidental identification of gallstones, prospective studies have also observed higher rates of development of symptoms, but not complications, in women. The number or size of stones does not appear to correlate with the development of symptoms.

Patients who are already symptomatic are more likely to continue to have symptoms than those who were initially asymptomatic. Moreover, the risk of complications in previously symptomatic patients, including common bile duct obstruction, cholecystitis, cholangitis, and pancreatitis, is 15% to 20% over 5 years. Gallbladder nonvisualization on oral cholecystogram confers an additional risk of worsening symptoms or biliary complications.

Pancreatitis is a well-known complication of gallstones. In contrast to other causes of pancreatitis that are more common in males, gallstone pancreatitis has the same epidemiologic patterns as gallstones and is twice as common in women as in men. Recently it has been established that biliary sludge is present in the majority of patients with recurrent idiopathic pancreatitis. Although follow-up evaluation has been limited, cholecystectomy or treatment with ursodiol may be successful in preventing further recurrences.

A rare but significant long-term complication is gallbladder carcinoma, which accounts for about 2% of all malignancies in the United States. The majority of patients with gallbladder cancer have gallstones, usually of the cholesterol type. Common risk factors for gallstones and gallbladder cancer include older age, female sex, and American Indian ancestry. The highest risk is found in gallbladders harboring large gallstones, with the size of the largest gallstone correlating with the risk of development of gallbladder cancer. The relative risk rises for stones from 1 to 2 cm in diameter and reaches a relative risk of about 10 for gallstones greater than 3 cm in diameter. It should be noted that very large gallstones are relatively rare, constituting only 6% of all gallstones in one study in the Native American Indian and white populations. However, because of the high relative risk of gallbladder cancer in patients with large stones, about one third of all gallbladder cancers have been estimated to occur in patients with stones greater than 3 cm. In populations in whom cholesterol stones are less common a disproportionate number of patients with gallbladder cancer harbor cholesterol stones. The actual risk of cholesterol versus pigment stones is unknown. However, since cholesterol stones form at a younger age, the duration of gallstone disease may be the important variable, and gallstone size may simply be a marker for duration of gallstone disease.

CLINICAL PRESENTATION
History and symptom presentation

Gallstones cause symptoms only when migration occurs into the cystic or common bile duct. Biliary pain, caused by stones intermittently obstructing or passing through the cystic duct, bile duct, or papilla, is a constant, noncolicky, abdominal pain lasting from 30 minutes to several hours. The location is most often epigastric, rather than right upper quadrant, and may radiate to the back or scapulae. A history of postprandial or nocturnal symptoms is helpful. There is no correlation between the presence of gallstones and symptoms such as nausea, dyspepsia, diarrhea, constipation, heartburn, irregular bowel habits, or bloating. Additional symptoms are present when gallstone disease has led to complications, including acute cholecystitis, biliary obstruction, pancreatitis, and cholangitis.

Physical examination

Physical examination is most helpful during an acute attack of biliary colic or cholecystitis. Abdominal tenderness localized to the midclavicular line below the costal margin has been termed *Murphy's sign*. Ultrasonic demonstration of tenderness over the gallbladder, the radiographic equivalent of Murphy's sign, is very helpful in confirming the diagnosis. Cholecystitis or cholangitis is typically accompanied by fever, but in cholangitis localizing abdominal signs may be absent.

Diagnostic tests

The logical application of diagnostic tools for the documentation of suspected gallstone disease naturally depends upon the correct recognition of clinical presentation. It cannot be overemphasized that a carefully taken history is essential before embarking on what should be a thorough assessment of the biliary tract when indicated. Technology should complement, not substitute for, good clinical practice.

Laboratory tests. During biliary colic results of laboratory tests may be entirely normal. Transient partial or complete obstruction of the biliary tree may produce abnormalities in levels of serum transaminase, alkaline phosphatase, and bilirubin. After passage of a gallstone serum transaminase levels may be elevated to 10 to 20 times normal but rapidly decrease to normal. Alkaline phosphatase level is characteristically disproportionately elevated during partial or complete biliary obstruction. Serum bilirubin level rises during complete biliary obstruction, but the rise occurs more slowly over days.

Radiographic tests

Plain abdominal radiography (KUB). The plain film will detect between 10% and 30% of gallstones within the gallbladder and 2% or less in the bile duct. This simple procedure carries no risk; it has a very low sensitivity but high specificity, making this an initial investigation of limited benefit. Detection of calcification in gallstones, however, has implications for nonoperative therapy.

Oral cholecystography (OCG). OCG was the principal method for gallstone evaluation until the advent of ultrasound. Radiographic imaging of the gallbladder area is obtained 12 to 15 hours after ingestion of contrast medium (Fig. 14-5) and is usually followed by induction of gallbladder contraction achieved by ingestion of fat or by intravenous injection of cholecystokinin or its octapeptide, sincalide. Serious morbidity from orally administered contrast agents is rare, but minor symptoms of nausea, vomiting, and diarrhea occur in up to 50%. Renal toxicity may occur in patients receiving large doses or a simultaneous intravenous agent, and this combined examination is therefore contraindicated. A technically satisfactory OCG will allow

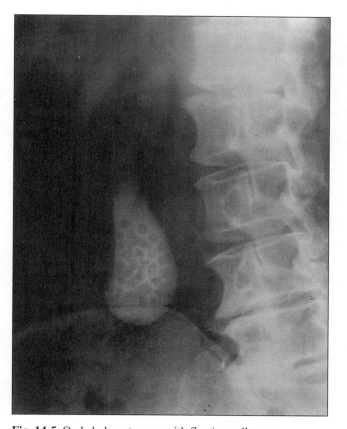

Fig. 14-5 Oral cholecystogram with floating gallstones.

diagnosis of radiolucent gallstones with a sensitivity of more than 90%. In the absence of interfering factors a nonopacified gallbladder has a positive predictive value of disease of over 90%. However, at least 10% of patients with complete nonopacification and 60% with poor opacification after single-dose OCG have normal gallbladders. Nonopacification may result from failure of contrast medium absorption, uptake or excretion by the liver, or failure of entry into the gallbladder, implying mechanical obstruction of the cystic duct. OCG is now commonly used to assess cystic duct patency for proposed medical therapy.

Ultrasound. Ultrasound now represents the first-line investigation of suspected biliary disease and uses high-frequency sound of 3.5 to 5 MHz for imaging by reflection. Gallbladder stones have a characteristic appearance of high-amplitude intraluminal reflections casting acoustic shadows with gravity-dependent movement (see Fig. 14-2). The patient must fast for at least 8 hours before the examination in order to allow maximal distention of the gallbladder. Ultrasound detects gallbladder stones with sensitivity and specificity of more than 95% but is somewhat less sensitive for biliary sludge. Nonimaging of the gallbladder may be due to its being packed with stones with very little surrounding bile, a small contracted gallbladder, lack of fasting, obesity, or an atypical gallbladder position. Ultrasound is far less sensitive (40% to 70%) for bile duct stones, because of the relative inaccessibility of the lower bile duct to sound waves that results from surrounding structures and bowel gas.

Radionuclide scanning (scintigraphy). Scanning with a technetium-labeled derivative of iminodiacetic acid (IDA) has become the most popular form of radionuclide scanning, in which 3 to 5 mCi of the radionuclide is injected intravenously. After an interval of 20 to 60 minutes the radionuclide is taken up by the liver and excreted into bile, where it readily produces a representation of the biliary tract on gamma camera imaging. Patient preparation is minimal as the test is employed only in suspected acute cholecystitis. In the absence of chronic liver disease and parenteral feeding the sensitivity exceeds 95% and the specificity approaches 100% for cystic duct obstruction if the gallbladder fails to image. The presence of mild cholestasis with bilirubin levels up to 4 mg% does not preclude use of this technique and some IDA analogs are excreted in the presence of a level greater than 15 mg%. The negative predictive value of a normal scan finding is greater than 98%.

Computed tomography (CT). The CT scan is capable of demonstrating the biliary tree and gallstones, but pure cholesterol stones may not be distinguishable from surrounding bile by CT. Diagnosis of gallbladder disease is likely to be 80% accurate, and in the presence of jaundice the distinction between a dilated and a nondilated system is possible with a sensitivity of up to 88% and a specificity of up to 97%. Sensitivity and specificity of identification of the cause of obstruction are equivalent to those of ultrasound, although CT demonstrates the lower bile duct more accurately. CT assessment of stone density has improved the results of medical dissolution with bile acids with or without shock-wave lithotripsy.

Endoscopic retrograde cholangiopancreatography (ERCP). ERCP was developed in the early 1970s as a method for direct cholangiography by instillation of contrast medium across the papilla and directly into the biliary tree. Its advantages over percutaneous transhepatic cholangiography are the additional information gained from endoscopic examination of the upper GI tract and papilla, the ability to perform biopsy, the concomitant pancreatogram, and the potential for immediate biliary therapy. Endoscopy also allows collection of bile for microscopic examination for cholesterol crystals or bilirubin granules and is the most sensitive method for diagnosing biliary sludge. Attention to detail and the need for high-quality radiographs make for improved accuracy in the diagnosis of calculous disease, and it is vital that no barium studies have been undertaken within 3 days of the ERCP as residual barium in the colon commonly overlies the pancreas and lower bile duct. In experienced hands successful cholangiography should be achieved in more than 95% of cases irrespective of bile duct diameter and is a highly accurate method for identifying stones in the bile ducts and gallbladder. Sensitivity and specificity for stone disease exceed 90%. ERCP fails in a small number of attempts because of inaccessibility of the duodenal papilla, presence of pyloric or duodenal stenosis, and some cases of duodenal diverticulum or Billroth II partial gastrectomy. Morbidity rate for diagnostic ERCP should be less than 1% with a mortality rate of less than 0.1%. Sepsis was once the most serious complication but has been minimized by the introduction of immediate endoscopic therapy. Acute pancreatitis now represents the most common complication, but no preprocedure pharmacologic manipulations have proved effective in preventing this.

APPROACH TO THE PATIENT WITH GALLSTONES

For a patient with a history of recurrent biliary pain without jaundice, ultrasound is likely to be the only modality needed. ERCP may occasionally be required when abdominal ultrasound does not show gallstones and symptoms continue. OCG and CT may be useful for assessment before nonoperative therapy (Fig. 14-6).

For the woman with suspected cholecystitis, urgent ultrasound and/or radionuclide scanning has a high success rate

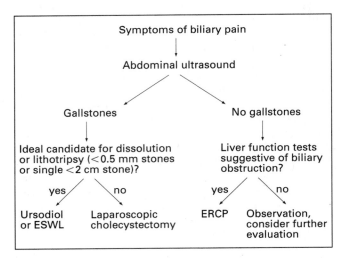

Fig. 14-6 Approach to the woman with uncomplicated gallstones. ESWL, extracorporeal shock-wave lithotripsy; ERCP, endoscopic retrograde cholangiopancreatography.

for diagnosis. Only in the presence of significantly abnormal liver function test results or overt jaundice is cholangiography necessary. The presence of a gallbladder mass may be further defined by CT.

Characterization of obstructive jaundice is now possible in all patients by logical and judicious use of initial noninvasive studies such as ultrasound and CT followed by direct cholangiography by percutaneous transhepatic cholangiography or ERCP with a view to therapy if indicated. In a patient with acute pancreatitis without obvious cause the diagnosis of gallstones is important, and urgent ultrasound combined with biochemical predictive tests allows a diagnosis in up to 80%. This allows selection of patients for emergency ERCP when appropriate and elective treatment for those who recover from the initial attack.

Today very few cases of gallstone disease are not amenable to modern imaging methods, but all modalities have some limitations, and clinical suspicion remains imperative in pursuing the correct diagnosis.

MANAGEMENT

Goals of management

Once clinical symptoms of gallstones develop, treatment algorithms, as summarized in Fig. 14-6, are the same for both sexes, with the exception of treatment during pregnancy. Treatment options range in degrees of invasiveness from oral pharmacologic dissolution with ursodiol, extracorporeal shock-wave lithotripsy with ursodiol, endoscopic interventions and percutaneous techniques, to surgery.

Choice of therapy

Noninvasive therapies

Ursodiol. Ursodiol, or ursodeoxycholic acid, is a naturally occurring bile acid, is present in minor quantities in bile, and dissolves cholesterol gallstones when given in doses of 8 mg/kg/day. Only selected patients are suitable candidates for dissolution therapy: the stones must be cholesterol, as determined by their ability to float on an OCG (see Fig. 14-5), and demonstrate no calcification on KUB or CT; the cystic duct should be patent (gallbladder opacification on OCG) for the bile salts to reach the gallstones; and ideally the stones should be less than 1 cm in diameter. Although larger stones have been successfully treated, the success rate is much lower, and these patients should be treated by lithotripsy followed by dissolution therapy. For patients who meet these criteria dissolution is successful in about two thirds but takes up to 2 years, typically proceeding at 1 mm per month. Dissolution is monitored by abdominal ultrasound, and ursodiol is continued for 3 months after a negative ultrasound result to ensure dissolution of small fragments. During ursodiol administration intestinal cholesterol absorption decreases and biliary cholesterol secretion decreases, but bile salt synthesis and serum lipoprotein levels are unchanged. Ursodiol has no significant toxicity and only occasionally causes diarrhea. Only patients with infrequent symptomatic biliary pain, without urgent complications of gallstones, should be considered for dissolution therapy.

Methyl tert-butyl ether. Methyl tert-butyl ether is an ether that remains liquid at body temperature and rapidly dissolves cholesterol. Clinical studies have shown that stones of any size and number can be dissolved if they have high enough cholesterol content and if direct access to the gallbladder can be achieved by percutaneous or transpapillary approaches (Fig. 14-7). The main disadvantages are those of many volatile organic solvents, namely, damage to gastrointestinal mucosa, anesthetic properties, and flammability. Currently this solvent and the method required to administer it remain in the research arena.

Other chemical therapies. Chemical dissolution of bile duct stones has been attempted by perfusing the common bile duct with solvents administered via an indwelling nasobiliary tube, percutaneous transhepatic catheter, cholecystostomy tube, or existing T-tube. Initial results with the semisynthetic vegetable oil, monooctanoin, and methyl tertbutyl ether have been disappointing because of incomplete stone dissolution and the potential for complications. Therefore, because of its low efficacy and high morbidity, contact chemical dissolution therapy has not assumed an important role in cases of refractory common bile duct stones and should be reserved for patients for whom other adjuvant endoscopic techniques have failed and who are poor operative candidates. Newer agents with better methods for instillation are awaited.

Extracorporeal shock-wave lithotripsy. Extracorporeal shock-wave lithotripsy fragments cholesterol gallstones by high-energy shock waves into smaller fragments (Fig. 14-8) that can either pass spontaneously through the cystic and common bile ducts or dissolve with ursodiol 45. Postlithotripsy treatment with ursodiol must be continued until 3 months after the gallbladder is clear of fragments. For the ideal candidate with a single gallstone of less than 2 cm in diameter, the success rate approaches 80%. Lithotripsy can also be used for patients with up to three stones with a total diameter of 2 cm, but with a lower success rate. The

rate of complications, including common bile duct obstruction or pancreatitis secondary to fragment passage, is less than 5%.

Risk of recurrence. After lithotripsy or dissolution therapy the risk of gallstone recurrence is high, up to 50% after 5 years. Patients should be followed with periodic ultrasound every 6 months, and therapy with ursodeoxycholic acid should be reinstated if asymptomatic gallstones recur, since dissolution is more rapid for small stones.

Endoscopic therapy. Endoscopic treatment of choledocholithiasis has gained widespread acceptance since the first independent reports of endoscopic sphincterotomy in 1974. Endoscopic sphincterotomy was initially considered justifiable only in elderly postcholecystectomy patients with recurrent or retained common bile duct stones who were at high risk of serious complications from conventional surgical common bile duct exploration. With improved efficacy, demand, and training in therapeutic biliary endoscopic techniques, however, there has been an expanding role for the endoscopic management of choledocholithiasis (Fig. 14-9). There is now general agreement among surgeons and gastroenterologists that endoscopic removal of common bile duct stones is preferable to surgery (1) in patients who have undergone previous cholecystectomy, (2) in high-risk surgical patients when the gallbladder is still present, (3) in patients with severe acute cholangitis, (4) in selected patients with acute biliary pancreatitis, and (5) in special circumstances for the average risk surgical patient with suspected choledocholithiasis before laparoscopic cholecystectomy (see Fig. 14-6). Up to 15% of patients undergoing cholecystectomy have common duct stones. Unlike those with gallbladder stones the majority of individuals with asymptomatic common duct stones will ultimately become symptomatic, in either the early or the late perioperative period, with the development of one or a combination of symptoms, including biliary pain, jaundice cholangitis, or pancreatitis. The natural history has mitigated in favor of an active treatment approach rather than expectant management for all patients with detected common bile duct stones. In the early postoperative period T-tube extraction is an option. However, endoscopic sphincterotomy can be safely and effectively performed without the need for T-tube maturation, allowing timely discharge from the hospital, and is the procedure of choice for common bile duct stones that appear in the late perioperative period.

Management in the elderly. In the elderly a deliberate decision is often made to leave the gallbladder in situ after endoscopic removal of common bile duct stones. The short- and long-term results in such patients do not differ from those in the postcholecystectomy patient and can be managed expectantly unless symptoms dictate otherwise. Careful follow-up observation for 5 to 10 years indicates that approximately 10% will experience gallbladder symptoms or complications sufficient to warrant cholecystectomy, the majority of which occur in the first year. The risk of development of biliary symptoms appears to be dependent on the continuing presence of stones in the gallbladder, and these results suggest that the low risk of subsequent gallbladder complications after endoscopic bile duct clearance mitigates against routine cholecystectomy in this group.

ERCP and laparoscopic cholecystectomy. Optimal management of patients with suspected common bile duct stones

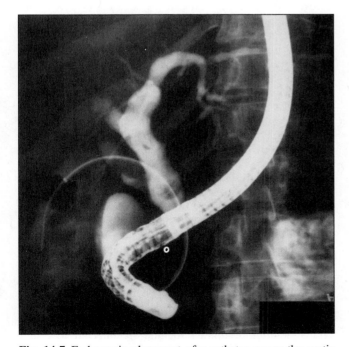

Fig. 14-7 Endoscopic placement of a catheter across the cystic duct into the gallbladder for the delivery of methyl tert-butyl ether.

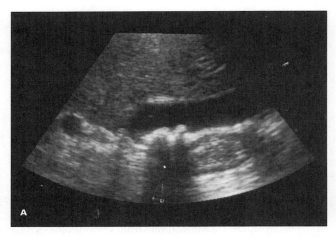
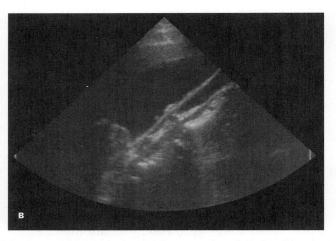

Fig. 14-8 Ultrasonographic appearances before and after extracorporeal shock-wave lithotripsy showing fragmentation. *A,* Before lithotripsy; *B,* after lithotripsy.

has yet to be determined in those undergoing laparoscopic cholecystectomy. The place of preoperative ERCP and treatment of duct stones in young, good surgical risk patients has been examined in two prospective, randomized controlled trials, with the conclusion that no advantage was conferred by initial endoscopic bile duct clearance before cholecystectomy. Patients with a high likelihood of common bile duct stones based on established clinical and biochemical indicators, including elevated liver function tests, a dilated common bile duct greater than 8 mm on a sonogram, and a history of jaundice or pancreatitis, should undergo preoperative ERCP and stone extraction. Small asymptomatic stones may be of minor clinical relevance as their natural

history is not known, and conceivably many, if not most, of these calculi would pass spontaneously without ever coming to clinical attention.

Gallstone pancreatitis. The majority of patients experience mild pancreatitis caused by transient impaction of a stone in the ampulla followed by spontaneous migration into the duodenum. These individuals do well with conservative therapy alone and are unlikely to benefit from urgent intervention. In contrast, it has been proposed that the more severe cases of pancreatitis result from persistent stone impaction or choledocholithiasis with infected bile, offering the hope that early stone extraction by surgical or endoscopic techniques would halt progression of the acute event and prevent the development of future attacks. An endoscopic approach offers the theoretic advantage of immediate relief of ampullary obstruction and ductal clearance without the risks of general anesthesia or the surgical procedure. Two randomized, controlled trials have demonstrated that those with mild pancreatitis had favorable outcomes regardless of treatment strategy, but in patients with severe pancreatitis urgent ERCP and endoscopic sphincterotomy reduced the morbidity and mortality rates compared to those of conservatively managed patients.

Cholangitis. The majority of patients with calculous cholangitis have mild disease and typically respond rapidly to conservative therapy consisting of intravenous fluids and antibiotics. For these individuals further treatment should be based on their fitness for surgery. Emergency ERCP is the treatment of choice for those individuals with severe cholangitis at presentation, as well as those not responding within 24 hours to conservative treatment. Emergency surgery should be reserved for those in whom endoscopic therapy fails, as conventional surgical treatment is associated with morbidity and mortality rates of 10% to 50%, depending upon the severity of illness and the presence of comorbid illnesses. Endoscopic decompression can be performed successfully in 85% to 95% of cases, with lower morbidity and mortality rates than percutaneous transhepatic or surgical drainage.

Percutaneous techniques. In percutaneous transhepatic cholangiography, contrast medium is injected to obtain direct cholangiography. In experienced hands it is techni-

Fig. 14-9 Endoscopic retrograde cholangiopancreatography demonstrating *A,* choledocholithiasis, and *B,* basket capture of the stone before extraction.

cally successful in nearly 100% of attempts in the presence of a dilated biliary system and over 70% when not dilated. The reported accuracy for detecting the level of biliary obstruction is over 95% and for defining the cause 90%. Morbidity is reported in up to 30% but serious complications occur in 3% to 10% as a result of sepsis, bile leakage, hemorrhage, pneumothorax, bile embolization, and adverse reactions to contrast medium and result in a mortality rate of up to 0.3%.

Surgery. The gold standard has been conventional open cholecystectomy, which carried an overall mortality rate of 0.2% in a large recent study. Although only introduced into clinical practice in 1988, laparoscopic cholecystectomy has rapidly replaced conventional open cholecystectomy as the standard. Rapid advances in surgical technique and equipment have made possible laparoscopic transcystic stone extraction and endoscopic exploration of the common duct although these techniques are not yet routine. Laparoscopic cholecystectomy has a 5% rate of conversion to open cholecystectomy that is primarily due to local complications, usually bleeding, or to technical difficulties that prevent adequate dissection. Common bile duct injuries are currently more frequent than in open cholecystectomy, 0.2% to 0.5%; most occur during the first 25 procedures by an individual surgeon. The introduction of laparoscopic cholecystectomy should not alter the indications for cholecystectomy, but overall numbers of cholecystectomies seem to be increasing.

PREGNANCY AND GALLSTONES

Epidemiology

Prospective ultrasonographic study has demonstrated that the incidence of sludge and gallstone formation increases progressively with each trimester of pregnancy (Fig. 14-10). During pregnancy biliary cholesterol saturation increases, mediated at least partly through the effects of estrogens. Gallbladder stasis also occurs secondary to the effects of high progesterone levels. The additive effects contribute to a very high incidence of cholesterol gallstone formation during pregnancy that is several times that for age-matched women. Stones tend to be multiple and small.

Natural history

The natural history of gallstones in pregnant and postpartum women differs from that in the general population. In contrast to longitudinal studies in the general population that suggest that the annual incidence of new symptoms is 2% to 3%, symptoms develop in about one third of pregnant women with gallstones. Moreover, the most common cause of pancreatitis during pregnancy is gallstone or biliary sludge. Hence biliary disease should be high on the differential diagnosis of abdominal pain during pregnancy.

In the first postpartum month approximately one half of women have either gallbladder sludge or stones (see Fig. 14-5). However, in the next year at least 75% of the patients with biliary sludge the gallbladder will revert to normal and about one third of the women with gallstones will spontaneously pass or dissolve the gallstones.

Management

During pregnancy. In general, therapy is aimed at temporizing and delaying surgical intervention until the postpartum period. Patients with symptoms thought to be due to common bile duct stones causing cholangitis, obstruction, or severe pancreatitis should be treated without delay by ERCP and sphincterotomy, using appropriate radiologic safety precautions to the fetus. In experienced hands the risk of complications is low. If unavoidable, conventional cholecystectomy does not seem to pose significant risks to the pregnancy in the first or third trimester. Surgery during the second trimester has been associated with premature labor. Laparoscopic cholecystectomy has been undertaken during pregnancy but may be limited by technical considerations as pregnancy advances and, if possible, should be deferred until the postpartum period.

Postpartum. In view of their high frequency of spontaneous clearance of gallstones women with postpartum biliary pain may be considered for ursodiol therapy if they have small (<5 mm) gallstones or biliary sludge as documented by ultrasound. Once the high-risk period of pregnancy has passed, these women are most likely at lower risk of gallstone recurrence. Case reports have shown that ursodiol is not excreted in breast milk, although no controlled data are available.

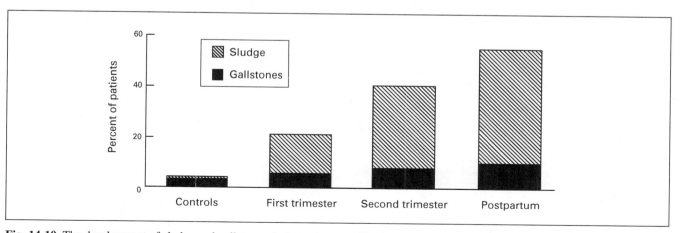

Fig. 14-10 The development of sludge and gallstones during pregnancy. The incidence of sludge increases with each trimester, and gallstones developed in almost 10% by delivery. (From Maringhini A et al: *Gastroenterology* 95:1160, 1988.)

SUMMARY

Women are at higher risk for the development of gallstones because of their exposure to estrogens after puberty, during pregnancy, with oral contraceptives, and with post-menopausal estrogen replacement therapy. Although the risk of symptomatic gallstone disease may be higher than in men, therapy is similar for both sexes. For asymptomatic individuals with gallstones no therapy is warranted, with rare exceptions. For mildly symptomatic patients the risks of expectant management are minimally higher than those of surgical or nonsurgical therapy. However, for patients with severe symptoms or complications of gallstones the risk of further morbidity is high and gallstone ablation should be recommended. For the majority of patients laparoscopic cholecystectomy is the treatment of choice for cholelithiasis, although for selected patients pharmacologic dissolution therapy with or without lithotripsy is an alternative. Emergency management of cholangitis and pancreatitis and elective management of choledocholithiasis in the era before, and now during, laparoscopic cholecystectomy are optimally endoscopic. When there are therapeutic alternatives the patient is perhaps best served by evaluation in a center where all modalities are available.

BIBLIOGRAPHY

Barbara L et al: A population study on the prevalence of gallstone disease: the Sirmione study, *Hepatology* 7:913, 1987.

Bennion LJ et al: Effects of oral contraceptives on the gallbladder bile of normal women, *N Engl J Med* 294:189, 1976.

Bennion LJ, Mott DM, Howard BV: Oral contraceptives raise the cholesterol saturation of bile by increasing biliary cholesterol secretion, *Metabolism* 29:18, 1980.

Boston Collaborative Drug Surveillance Program: Oral contraceptives and venous thromboembolic disease, surgically confirmed gallbladder disease, and breast tumours: report from the Boston Collaborative Drug Surveillance Program, *Lancet* 1:399, 1973.

Boston Collaborative Drug Surveillance Program: Surgically confirmed gallbladder disease, venous thromboembolism, and breast tumors in relation to postmenopausal estrogen therapy, *N Engl J Med* 290:15, 1974.

Braverman DZ, Johnson ML, Kern F Jr: Effects of pregnancy and contraceptive steroids on gallbladder function, *N Engl J Med* 302:362, 1980.

Cahalane MJ, Neubrand MW, Carey MC: Physical-chemical pathogenesis of pigment gallstones, *Semin Liver Dis* 8:317, 1988.

Carey MC: Pathogenesis of gallstones, *Am J Surg* 165:410, 1993.

Carey MC, LaMont JT: Cholesterol gallstone formation. 1. Physical-chemistry of bile and biliary lipid secretion, *Prog Liver Dis* 10:139, 1992.

Carr-Locke DL: Endoscopic approaches. In Blumgart LH, editor: *Surgery of the liver and biliary tract,* London, 1987, Churchill Livingstone.

Carr-Locke DL: Role of endoscopy in gallstone pancreatitis, *Am J Surg* 165:519, 1993.

Cooper AD: Metabolic basis of cholesterol gallstone disease, *Gastroenterol Clin North Am* 20:21, 1991.

Coronary Drug Project Research Group: Gallbladder disease as a side effect of drugs influencing lipid metabolism, *N Engl J Med* 296:1185, 1977.

Diehl AK: Epidemiology and natural history of gallstone disease, *Gastroenterol Clin North Am* 20:1, 1991.

Donovan JM, Carey MC: Pathogenesis of cholesterol and pigment gallstone formation, *Gastroenterol Clin North Am* 20:47, 1991.

Everson GT, McKinley C, Kern F Jr: Mechanisms of gallstone formation in women: effects of exogenous estrogen (Premarin) and dietary cholesterol on hepatic lipid metabolism, *J Clin Invest* 87:237, 1991.

Fan ST et al: Early treatment of acute biliary pancreatitis by endoscopic papillotomy, *N Engl J Med* 328:228, 1993.

Friedman GD: Natural history of asymptomatic and symptomatic gallstones, *Am J Surg* 165:399, 1993.

Grodstein F et al: A prospective study of symptomatic gallstones in women: relation with oral contraceptives and other risk factors, *Obstet Gynecol* 84:207, 1994.

Hay DW, Carey MC: Chemical species of lipids in bile, *Hepatology* 12:6S, 14S, 1990.

Henriksson P et al: Estrogen-induced gallstone formation in males: relationship to changes in serum and biliary lipids during hormonal treatment of prostatic carcinoma, *J Clin Invest* 84:811, 1989.

Jacobson IM: Endoscopic sphincterotomy in patients with intact gallbladders. In Jacobson IM, editor: *ERCP—diagnostic and therapeutic applications,* New York, 1989, Elsevier.

Janowitz P et al: Gallbladder sludge: spontaneous course and incidence of complications in patients without stones, *Hepatology* 20:291, 1994.

Jorgensen T: Gallstones in a Danish population: fertility period, pregnancies, and exogenous female sex hormones, *Gut* 29:433, 1989.

Jorgensen T: Prevalence of gallstones in a Danish population, *Am J Epidemiol* 126:912, 1987.

Lai ECS et al: Endoscopic biliary drainage for severe acute cholangitis, *N Engl J Med* 326:1582, 1992.

LaMont JT, Carey MC: Cholesterol gallstone formation. 2. Pathobiology and pathomechanics, *Prog Liver Dis* 10:165, 1992.

Lee SP, Maher K, Nicholls JF: Origin and fate of biliary sludge, *Gastroenterology* 94:170, 1988.

Lee SP, Nicholls JF, Park HZ: Biliary sludge as a cause of acute pancreatitis, *N Engl J Med* 326:589, 1992.

Lowenfels AB et al: Gallstone growth, size, and risk of gallbladder cancer: an interracial study, *Int J Epidemiol* 18:50, 1989.

Maclure KM et al: Weight, diet, and the risk of symptomatic gallstones in middle-aged women, *N Engl J Med* 321:563, 1989.

Maringhini A et al: Biliary sludge and gallstones in pregnancy: incidence, risk factors, and natural history, *Ann Intern Med* 119:116, 1993.

Maringhini A et al: Sludge, stones and pregnancy, *Gastroenterology* 95:1160, 1988 (letter).

Maringhini A et al: Sludge and stones in the gallbladder after pregnancy: prevalence and risk factors, *J Hepatol* 5:218, 1987.

May GR, Sutherland LR, Shaffer EA: Efficacy of bile acid therapy for gallstone dissolution—a meta-analysis of randomized trials, *Aliment Pharmacol Therapeut* 7:139, 1993.

McSherry CK: Cholecystectomy: the gold standard, *Am J Surg* 158:174, 1989.

Neoptolemos JP et al: Controlled trial of urgent endoscopic retrograde cholangiopancreatography and endoscopic sphincterotomy versus conservative treatment for acute pancreatitis due to gallstones, *Lancet* 2:979, 1988.

NIH Consensus conference: Gallstones and laparoscopic cholecystectomy, *JAMA* 269:1018, 1993.

O'Donnell LDJ, Heaton KW: Recurrence and re-recurrence of gallstones after medical dissolution: a longterm follow-up, *Gut* 29:655, 1988.

Petitti DB, Sidney S, Perlman JA: Increased risk of cholecystectomy in users of supplemental estrogen, *Gastroenterology* 94:91, 1988.

Ransohoff DF, Gracie WA: Treatment of gallstones, *Ann Intern Med* 119:606, 1993.

Ros E et al: Occult microlithiasis in idiopathic acute pancreatitis: prevention of relapses by cholecystectomy or ursodeoxycholic acid therapy, *Gastroenterology* 101:1701, 1991.

Ros E et al: Symptomatic versus silent gallstones—radiographic features and eligibility for nonsurgical treatment, *Dig Dis Sci* 39:1697, 1994.

Ros E et al: Utility of biliary microscopy for the prediction of the chemical composition of gallstones and the outcome of dissolution therapy with ursodeoxycholic acid, *Gastroenterology* 91:703, 1986.

Sackmann M et al: The Munich gallbladder lithotripsy study: results of the first five years with 711 patients, *Ann Intern Med* 114:290, 1991.

Schoenfield LJ: Oral and contact dissolution of gallstones, *Am J Surg* 165:427, 1993.

Scragg RKR, McMichael AJ, Seamark RF: Oral contraceptives, pregnancy, and endogenous oestrogen in gall stone disease: a case-control study, *Br Med J* 288:1795, 1984.

Slivka A et al: Endoscopy during pregnancy, *Gastrointest Endosc* 1994 (abstract).

Southern Surgeons Club: A prospective analysis of 1518 laparoscopic cholecystectomies, *N Engl J Med* 324:1073, 1991.

Steigmann GV et al: Precholecystectomy endoscopic cholangiography and stone removal is not superior to cholecystectomy, cholangiography, and common duct exploration, *Am J Surg* 163:227, 1992.

Strasberg SM, Clavien PA: Cholecystolithiasis—lithotherapy for the 1990s, *Hepatology* 16:820, 1992.

Strasberg SM, Clavien PA: Overview of therapeutic modalities for the treatment of gallstone disease, *Am J Surg* 165:420, 1993.

Valdivieso V et al: Pregnancy and cholelithiasis: pathogenesis and natural course of gallstones diagnosed in early puerperium, *Hepatology* 17:1, 1993.

15 Blood Disorders

A. Jacqueline Mitus

There is no gender difference in the approach to hematologic problems in women. However, certain disorders occur more frequently in women, and their special clinical implications form the main focus of discussion. Abnormalities unique to pregnancy are addressed at the end of this chapter.

ABNORMALITIES OF RED BLOOD CELLS
Anemia

Epidemiology. Rates of anemia vary according to age and gender. The National Health and Nutrition Examination Survey (NHANES II) provided data on the prevalence of anemia in the United States from 1976 to 1980; anemia was highest among teen-age girls between 15 and 17 years (5.9%) and young women 22 to 44 years of age (5.8%). Men in these age groups were less severely affected, 2.6% and 2.9%, respectively, mainly because iron deficiency is less common in this subset (Dallman, 1984).

Definition of anemia in women. The normal range of hemoglobin (Hb) and hematocrit (Hct) differs for women and men: Hb >12 g/dl (Hct >36%) in females and Hb >14 g/dl (Hct >40%) in males. However, these parameters demonstrate racial variation. For example, normal Hb concentrations in African-Americans are 1 g/dl lower than in white persons (Meyers, 1979). Consequently, anemia occurs when Hb levels fall below 11g/dl (Hct <33%) in women and below 13 g/dl (Hct <36%) in men.

Pathophysiology. Anemia results from decreased red cell production or increased destruction as a result of hemolysis or hemorrhage. These two fundamental pathophysiologic processes are distinguished by the reticulocyte count, a marker of red cell proliferative activity (see box, right). The hypoproliferative anemias (low reticulocyte count) can be classified into different categories, including: "building block" deficiency (iron, folate, vitamin B$_{12}$, erythropoietin deficiency), infiltrative marrow processes (fibrosis, metastatic cancer, granuloma), marrow suppression (toxin, virus), and primary hematologic conditions (aplastic anemia, myelodysplasia, leukemia).

In acute bleeding or hemolysis, compensatory erythroid hyperplasia is detected by an elevated reticulocyte count. Hemolysis stems from a defect in the red cell itself or from some alteration in the red cell environment. Intrinsic erythrocyte abnormalities generally are inherited, and comprise disorders of hemoglobin (e.g., thalassemia), cell membrane (e.g., hereditary spherocytosis), and cellular enzymes (e.g.,

glucose-6-phosphate dehydrogenase deficiency). Environmental changes leading to premature destruction of an otherwise normal erythrocyte tend to be acquired. Hypersplenism, antierythrocyte antibodies, red cell parasites, and mechanical fragmentation are some examples of these "extrinsic" red cell abnormalities.

APPROACH TO ANEMIA

Decreased production (low reticulocyte count)
"Building block" deficiency
   Iron
   Folate
   Vitamin B$_{12}$
   Erythropoietin

Infiltrative marrow processes
   Metastatic cancer
   Fibrosis
   Granuloma
   Necrosis

Bone marrow suppression
   Toxin
   Virus
   Radiation

Primary hematologic conditions
   Aplastic anemia
   Acute leukemia
   Myelodysplastic syndromes

Increased destruction (elevated reticulocytes)
Intrinsic red blood cell abnormalities
   Hemoglobinopathies (e.g., thalassemia)
   Enzymopathies (e.g., glucose-6-phosphate dehydrogenase [G6PD] deficiency)
   Membrane defects (e.g., hereditary spherocytosis)

Extrinsic red blood cell defects
   Hypersplenism
   Antibody deposition
   Mechanical fragmentation
   Intraerythrocytic infection (e.g., malaria)

Clinical presentation. The clinical manifestations of anemia vary on the basis of the rate of its development and its causative factors. Specific findings particularly relevant to women are highlighted in the sections to follow. In general, however, most patients complain of fatigue; 5% of persons at a large outpatient practice who reported fatigue were discovered to have anemia (Spaulding, 1964). Cardiopulmonary symptoms reflect the degree of anemia, the rapidity of its onset and the compensatory capacity of the cardiovascular system. A sudden drop in the hematocrit level precipitates dizziness, lightheadedness, when the person stands, and syncope whereas symptoms of chronic anemia are dyspnea on exertion or at rest and palpitations. An interesting "rushing" or pounding in the ears has led an occasional patient with anemia to an otolaryngologist.

History. The history is directed to ascertain the acuity of anemia. Prior blood counts or a history of blood donation (implying normal blood counts at that time) may prove invaluble in dating onset. Questions regarding the patient's general health, with specific emphasis on signs or symptoms of bleeding, should be explored. Dietary habits, hobbies, and occupational and social history may provide important clues concerning possible toxic suppression of the marrow, nutritional deficiency, and risk for human immunodeficiency virus (HIV), as well as other relevant findings. A hereditary anemia may become obvious with a careful family history. Even if the patient is unaware of the genetic disorder, frequent splenectomy or cholecystectomy in successive generations point to an inherited hemolytic process.

Physical examination. Pallor and icterus—indicative of hemolysis—are best detected by examination of the conjunctiva, mucous membranes, and palmar creases. Glossitis suggests an underlying vitamin deficiency (e.g., vitamin B_{12} deficiency) and should prompt careful neurologic testing of the posterolateral columns (position and vibratory sense). The spleen enlarges in an inferomedial direction and is best detected with the patient in the right lateral decubitus position.

Diagnostic tests. As previously noted, the reticulocyte (retic) count is pivotal in classifying anemias as a process of decreased production or accelerated destruction. Generally reported as a percentage of total red cells, in an anemic patient this value should be corrected to account for a decrease in the absolute erythrocyte number:

retic corrected = retic observed $\times$ (observed Hct/normal Hct)

Without this adjustment, a mild reticulocytosis may be misinterpreted as an elevation whereas in fact it may be inappropriately low for the degree of anemia present.

RED BLOOD CELL INDEXES. An assessment of red cell size, Hb concentration, and shape is useful in the evaluation of anemia. Automated cell counters now have the capacity to directly measure red cell volume (previously it was a calculated value). Histograms of these data provide the mean corpuscular volume (MCV), as well as an assessment of size variation, that is, the red cell distribution width (RDW). The normal MCV ranges from 80 to 100 fl, and diagnostic possibilities are refined on the basis of the MCV value—whether it is normal (normocytic) microcytic (MCV <80 fl), or macrocytic (MCV >100 fl) (see box, above right). The RDW is abnormal when greater than 14, implying a

---

MEAN CORPUSCULAR VOLUME AND ANEMIA

Decreased (MCV <80 fl)
  Iron deficiency
  Thalassemia
  Anemia of chronic disease (25%)
  Sideroblastic anemia
  Lead poisoning

Normal (MCV 80-100)
  Infiltrative processes
  Anemia of chronic disease (75%)
  Bleeding

Increased (MCV >100 fl)
  Folate deficiency
  Vitamin B_{12} deficiency
  Hypothyroidism
  Drugs (e.g., alcohol)
  Liver disease
  Aplastic anemia
  Myelodysplasia
  Reticulocytosis

---

wide range of erythrocyte size. Decreased hemoglobin content of the erythrocytes (hypochromia) results from a defect in hemoglobin synthesis and hence a problem with globin chain production or iron availability. Less commonly, hyperchromia implies loss of cell membrane and ensuing increased surface-to-volume ratio. The appearance of red cells gives further insight into the nature of anemia. Infiltration of the bone marrow (tear drop red cells), disturbance of the vascular endothelium (fragmentation), and congenital hemolysis (bite cells) are but a few of the many disorders that can be diagnosed by review of the peripheral smear.

SERUM CHEMISTRY TESTS. Several serum chemistry tests are helpful as general screens for hemolysis. Destruction of red cells occurs most commonly in the reticuloendothelial system (extravascular hemolysis) but also may develop within the vascular tree (intravascular hemolysis). In both instances there is elevation of indirect bilirubin and serum lactate dehydrogenase and depression of haptoglobin. In contrast, detection of free hemoglobin in the plasma (hemoglobinemia) or urine (hemoglobinuria) or the presence of iron-laden tubular epithelial cells in the urine sediment (urine hemosiderin) is specific for intravascular lysis of erythrocytes. More refined studies follow to delineate the specific cause of hemolysis.

SPECIFIC TYPES OF ANEMIA
Iron deficiency

Pathogenesis. Iron stores are meticulously conserved by the body and represent a carefully regulated balance between dietary intake and physiologic requirements. There is no normal mechanism for excretion; daily losses of approximately 1 mg result from sloughing of epithelial cells from the skin and from the gastrointestinal and genitourinary tracts. Iron is best absorbed as the heme moiety found in meats and fish. Vegetables and grain products provide small amounts of ferrous (Fe^{2+}) and ferric (Fe^{3+}) iron, the absorption of which is less efficient than heme iron and is dependent on intestinal pH and food ligands. Despite iron fortification in many commercial food products, in a normal, well-balanced diet only 10% of ingested iron is absorbed. Consequently persons with restricted dietary intake (e.g., vegetarians) may consume an inadequate amount of this element.

Although decreased oral intake, increased demand (pregnancy), abnormal absorption (achlorhydria), and urinary loss of iron (chronic hemolysis) should be considered in the differential diagnosis, by far the most common cause of iron deficiency is bleeding—physiologic or pathologic. Men and women enter adulthood with marginal iron reserves because of the demands imposed by growth spurts during childhood and adolescence. In women, obligatory iron loss is compounded by menstrual bleeding, which claims an additional 20 to 40 mg per month (40 to 80 ml blood). As a result monthly requirements for women approach 50 to 70 mg compared with only 30 mg for men. Consequently, most menstruating women, if not overtly iron deficient, will have borderline stores. In a postmenopausal woman (or in a man of any age), the presence of iron deficiency mandates a search for occult blood loss.

Clinical presentation. Absence of iron leads to decreased manufacture of hemoglobin, as well as abnormal epithelial growth. Glossitis, angular cheilosis, and koilonychia (spooned, ridged, and brittle nails) signal advanced deficiency. Dysphagia can result from the unusual development of an esophageal web, the **Plummer-Vinson syndrome**, which usually does not reverse itself with iron replacement. **Pica**, the abnormal craving of anything, remains a puzzling but at times dramatic symptom in some patients. Although ice craving (pagophagia) is most common and benign, ingestion of clay-rich soils (geophagia) or starch (amylophagia) is particularly hazardous because these materials interfere with normal iron absorption.

Diagnostic tests. Microcytic, hypochromic erythrocytes with occasional "pencil" and target forms are hallmarks of iron deficiency. Laboratory confirmation of iron deficiency (Table 15-1) includes the finding of depressed serum iron and ferritin levels. The total iron-binding capacity (TIBC), a reflection of transferrin level, is elevated in a compensatory response. Of these, the serum ferritin value is both more sensitive (90%) and specific (100%) for iron deficiency (Van Zeben et al., 1990). Because these laboratory values can be altered by concomitant systemic illness (see following discussion), a bone marrow examination for assessment of iron stores may be necessary. Less commonly relied upon, the RDW also has been shown to aid in the diagnosis of iron deficiency; in one study an elevated RDW was the most sensitive indicator (94%) of this condition.

Differential diagnosis. Two clinical situations may be mistaken for iron deficiency, thalassemia trait and anemia of chronic disease (see Table 15-1). Thalassemias comprise a group of congenital disorders caused by deficient or absent production of alpha or beta globin chains (α- or β-thalassemia, respectively). Imbalanced globin synthesis leads to hypochromic cells and precipitation of unmatched chains within the erythrocyte, causing its premature destruction. This process occurs both within the peripheral circulation and in the bone marrow (ineffective erythropoiesis). The clinical manifestations of α-thalassemia, prevalent in black and Asian persons, depend on how many of the four alpha globin genes have been deleted. One gene deletion is phenotypically silent. When two genes are affected, microcytosis is observed, which can be misinterpreted as a sign of iron deficiency. Three- and four-gene deletion leads to more pronounced clinical and laboratory findings, rendering the correct diagnosis more obvious. In β-**thalassemia trait**, common in persons of Mediterranean descent, microcytosis and mild anemia also are potentially confused with iron deficiency anemia. For the purposes of genetic counseling and because it may be harmful to prescribe iron for patients with

Table 15-1 Differential diagnosis of iron deficiency: clinical and laboratory features

History/physical examination	Iron	Total iron-binding capacity	Ferritin	Smear	Red cell distribution width	Marrow iron
Iron deficiency Bleeding Pica Angular cheilosis Koilonychia Dysphagia	↓	↑	↓	Microcytosis Hypochromia Pencil shapes	↑	Absent
Anemia of chronic disease Chronic infection or inflammation	↓	↓	↑	RBC normal (¼ microcytosis)	Normal	↑ (in reticuloendothelial system, not RBC precursors)
Thalassemia trait Family history Splenomegaly (±)	Normal/↑	Normal	↑	Microcytosis Targets Hypochromia	Normal	↑

RBC, red blood cells.

thalassemia (who have a tendency to overabsorb iron), it is important to distinguish between these processes (see Table 15-1). In addition to obtaining iron studies (iron, TIBC, and ferritin) the RDW can be helpful in this distinction; it is elevated in iron deficiency and typically normal in thalassemia trait. Although findings on Hb electrophoresis confirm the presence of β-thalassemia (elevated levels of hemoglobin A_2 and hemoglobin F), results are normal in α-thalassemia, which remains a diagnosis of exclusion.

Chronic disease also gives rise to a hematologic profile easily confused with iron deficiency. Through mechanisms incompletely defined, chronic inflammation leads to sequestration of iron within reticuloendothelial tissue, thus rendering it unavailable for incorporation into hemoglobin. Consequently the terms *anemia of ineffective iron reutilization* and *anemia of inflammation* are better reflections of the true pathophysiologic mechanism (Huarani, 1992; Schilling, 1991). Anemia is usually mild (Hct in the low 30s) and, although usually normocytic, may be microcytic in up to one quarter of cases. Even though distinctions are not always straightforward, differentiation of iron deficiency from anemia of chronic disease can be accomplished from review of laboratory data (see Table 15-1). In both situations, the serum iron level is depressed, but the TIBC typically is high in iron deficiency and low in anemia of chronic disease. Although determination of the serum ferritin level remains the best noninvasive test, it is an acute-phase reactant and thus may be mildly elevated even in the setting of low iron stores. It has been argued, however, that ferritin levels greater than 50 μg/L rarely indicate iron deficiency (Schilling, 1991). In equivocal cases an empiric trial of iron therapy may be warranted before a bone marrow examination is performed.

Management. In addition to replacing lost iron, thus improving the patient's well-being, the most important aspect in the assessment of iron deficiency is defining the source of blood loss. In premenopausal women, menstrual bleeding is the likely cause; however, further evaluation may be dictated by the clinical, social, and family history. The gastrointestinal tract is a common site of hemorrhage, and the finding of iron deficiency in postmenopausal women (or men) mandates a thorough radiographic or endoscopic evaluation.

Iron supplementation. Iron stores usually can be replenished by oral supplementation. Many iron preparations are poorly tolerated because of bloating, constipation, and/or diarrhea; however, ferrous gluconate or polysaccharide-iron complexes seem to cause fewer side effects than does ferrous sulfate. Peak reticulocytosis occurs at variable time periods after institution of therapy, and complete correction of anemia and restoration of iron reserves requires up to 8 or 9 months.

Alternatively, total body iron can be rapidly replaced by a single intravenous administration of iron: (iron dose [mg] = 150 × [13-pretreatment Hb]). Peak reticulocytosis occurs after about 10 days; although normalization of the Hct level takes 4 to 5 weeks, most patients experience symptomatic improvement within 1 to 2 weeks. Because the major drawback of this approach is the small risk of anaphylaxis and transient arthralgias, intravenous dosing should be reserved for patients whose condition is refractory to oral replacement, who are unable to absorb iron, or in whom a more rapid normalization of Hb and Hct levels are desired.

Pernicious anemia

Epidemiology. Pernicious anemia (PA) traditionally has been regarded as a disorder affecting older persons of northern European descent. As a result, it probably has been underrecognized in other populations, in particular young black women; one series documented that 21% of cases involved black females, one quarter of whom were younger than 40 years of age (Carmel and Johnson, 1978).

Pathogenesis. Because of the abundance of cobalamin (vitamin B_{12}) in red meats and dairy products, deficiency of this vitamin on a dietary basis is extremely rare, occurring only in fastidious ovolactovegetarians (vegans). Instead, depletion usually results from defective absorption. Once ingested, cobalamin binds to intrinsic factor, produced by gastric parietal cells, whereby it is protected from enzymatic degradation until it reaches its site of absorption in the terminal ileum. Any disturbance along this pathway can lead to vitamin B_{12} deficiency; surgical absence of the stomach or ileum, inflammation (e.g., sprue), or bacterial overgrowth of the ileal mucosa. Antibodies produced against intrinsic factor or parietal cells also interfere with cobalamin absorption and result in a condition named for its formerly lethal potential, pernicious anemia.

Absence of cobalamin, a critical cofactor in DNA synthesis, leads to arrest of nuclear division that is most apparent in tissues with rapid turnover. In the bone marrow these effects are striking. While cytoplasmic maturation proceeds unimpaired, nuclear division comes to a halt (nuclear-cytoplasmic dysynchrony), leading to the formation of large cells with an immature and noncondensed nucleus (megaloblasts). These abnormal cells are destroyed within the marrow cavity, resulting in ineffective erythropoiesis. Although morphologic findings are most pronounced in the erythroid lineage, all marrow elements are equally affected, leading to anemia, leukopenia, and thrombocytopenia; *megaloblastic pancytopenia* is perhaps a more accurate description of this process.

Clinical presentation (See box on following page.)

History. Because anemia develops slowly in PA, compensatory cardiac mechanisms often protect the patient from symptoms until the hematocrit has fallen to very low levels. Easy bruising and bleeding may be noted. A number of patients report glossitis, diarrhea, heartburn, and bloating, which reflect changes in gastrointestinal epithelial division. Abnormal cervical Pap results also may be found. Neurologic abnormalities develop in a percentage of persons with cobalamin deficiency, but these do not correlate with the severity of anemia. Bilateral, symmetric paresthesias of the fingers and toes, imbalance, and ataxia reflect classic involvement of the posterolateral columns (subacute combined system disease). Less commonly, slowed mentation, irritability, depression, and impaired memory mimic dementia. Other autoimmune disorders such as vitiligo and hypothyroidism are diagnosed with increased frequency in patients with PA and in their relatives.

Physical examination. Jaundice as a result of intramedullary hemolysis superimposed on the pallor of anemia explains the unusual lemon-yellow hue of persons with untreated cobalamin deficiency. The tongue typically is depapillated, smooth, and shiny, producing a classic "beefy

CLINICAL PRESENTATION OF PERNICIOUS ANEMIA

History
Fatigue
Dyspnea
Bleeding
Gastrointestinal complaints

Examination
Lemon-colored skin
Glossitis
Neurologic changes (combined system disease)

Laboratory tests
Pancytopenia
Macrocytosis
Hypersegmented neutrophils
Elevated indirect bilirubin level
Elevated lactic dehydrogenase level
Low vitamin B_{12} level
Abnormal bone marrow (megaloblasts)

red" appearance. Abnormal position and vibratory sense point to nervous system involvement.

Diagnostic tests. The peripheral blood smear findings are characteristic, revealing large, oval-shaped red cells (macroovalocytes) and hypersegmented neutrophils. Indirect hyperbilirubinemia and markedly elevated serum lactic dehydrogenase (LDH) levels attest to the profound intramedullary hemolysis underlying this condition. The availability of serum B_{12} assays has largely replaced the need for bone marrow examination.

A Schilling test can be performed to help define the cause of cobalamin deficiency and establish a diagnosis of PA. Vitamin B_{12} stores are replaced by intramuscular injection, and then oral radiolabeled B_{12} is administered. The presence of radioactivity in the urine confirms absorption and subsequent excretion of the vitamin. A patient with PA is unable to absorb vitamin B_{12} when it is given alone (the first phase of the test), which is corrected by coadministration of intrinsic factor (second phase). Rarely, bacterial overgrowth of the ileum accounts for malabsorption, and if findings of the first two parts of the Schilling test are abnormal, a course of antibiotics is prescribed as a last measure (third phase). Because the Schilling test is somewhat cumbersome (requiring several 24-hour urine collections) and despite the causative factors, parenteral B_{12} administration is the therapy of choice; thus most practitioners treat empirically without obtaining this study.

Therapy. Replacement of vitamin B_{12} is accomplished by intramuscular injection (1000 μg cobalamin), initially weekly and then monthly for life.

Anemia of starvation

The hematologic changes associated with anorexia nervosa have been recognized for decades but remain unexplained. Anemia can be profound and is characterized by prominent acanthocytosis (spiculation of red cells). Varying degrees of leukopenia and thrombocytopenia also are noted. Gelatinous degeneration of the bone marrow with focal cellular necro-

sis appears to underlie these hematologic abnormalities, all of which improve upon increase in caloric intake and weight gain. (Chapter 69 covers anorexia and bulimia in detail.)

Hemolytic anemia

Infrequently, disorders inherited as sex-linked recessive may affect women. One of the more common of these is glucose-6-phosphate dehydrogenase (G6PD) deficiency. Because of unequal inactivation of the X chromosome (lyonization), some women have a relative deficiency of this enzyme. As a result, hemoglobin is abnormally susceptible to oxidative stress such as occurs on exposure to certain medication (e.g., antimalarial agents, dapsone). When oxidized, hemoglobin denatures, forming rigid aggregates, Heinz bodies, that impede the red cell's pliability and that are removed in the macrophage-lined sinusoids of the spleen. Bitelike deformation of the erythrocyte and extravascular hemolysis ensue.

ABNORMALITIES OF THE PLATELET COUNT
Thrombocytopenia

Pathophysiology. Thrombocytopenia on the basis of underproduction results from megakaryopoiesis that is ineffective (e.g., myelodysplasia) or that has been disrupted by infiltration of the marrow by malignant or infectious processes. Isolated absence of platelet precursors (amegakaryocytosis) is extremely rare. In contrast, increased destruction of platelets accompanies a variety of clinical situations, including hypersplenism, disseminated intravascular coagulation (DIC), immune thrombocytopenic purpura (ITP), and thrombotic thrombocytopenic purpura (TTP). Because the last two conditions appear to affect women disproportionately compared with men (3:1), they are discussed in greater detail later in this section.

Clinical presentation

History. Normal hemostasis hinges on complex interactions among platelets, coagulation proteins, and the vessel wall. Platelets play a central role in this process through the formation of a hemostatic plug that subsequently is stabilized by the coagulation proteins to produce a firm fibrin clot. In patients with thrombocytopenia, bleeding occurs immediately on injury and typically involves mucocutaneous surfaces: epistaxis, oral and gastrointestinal hemorrhage, menorrhagia, petechiae, and ecchymoses. Deep-seated bleeding (e.g., hemarthrosis) is unusual and suggests a factor deficiency such as hemophilia. Platelet counts greater than 50,000/mm^3 rarely are associated with spontaneous bleeding, and patients usually have no symptoms or note only mild excessive bruising after trauma. In contrast, when severe depression occurs (platelets <20,000/mm^3), pronounced and often unprecipitated hemorrhage ensues.

All patients with thrombocytopenia should be carefully queried as to symptoms of underlying illness; collagen vascular diseases and human immunodeficiency virus (HIV), infection may first occur with ITP. A meticulous list of all medications must be obtained (prescription and nonprescription), inasmuch as both immune thrombocytopenia and, less commonly, direct suppression of megakaryopoiesis have been reported with myriad drugs. Rarely, a family history may suggest a form of congenital thrombocytopenia.

Physical examination. Physical findings depend on the degree of thrombocytopenia. With significant platelet depression, petechiae, mucosal bullae, and hematomas, as well as retinal and gastrointestinal bleeding, may be noted. Evaluation of a patient with thrombocytopenia should include careful palpation for the presence of an enlarged spleen and a search for stigmata of underlying systemic illness.

Specific causes

Immune thrombocytopenic purpura. ITP results from deposition of antibody or antigen-antibody complexes on the platelet and their subsequent consumption within the reticuloendothelial system. Women, particularly in their childbearing years, appear to have a higher incidence of idiopathic autoimmune thrombocytopenia for reasons that remain unclear. The degree of thrombocytopenia is variable as is the propensity for bleeding. Often a diagnosis is made incidentally after a complete blood count obtained for unrelated purposes.

The diagnosis of ITP remains one of exclusion, resting on the careful consideration of other causes of thrombocytopenia and the finding of normal or increased numbers of megakaryocytes in the bone marrow. The peripheral smear typically reveals decreased numbers of platelets, some of which appear larger than normal. Assays for antiplatelet antibodies may help confirm the diagnosis but are neither specific nor sensitive enough to stand alone as a diagnostic test.

MANAGEMENT. No therapy is required when thrombocytopenia is mild. If the platelet count falls below 50,000/mm^3 or if bleeding develops, treatment with corticosteroids is initiated. Although usually effective, steroids rarely are curative, and relapse often occurs after the drug is discontinued. Splenectomy is generally the next step, resulting in remission in about 70% of cases. Infusion of intravenous gammaglobulin, another therapeutic option, is highly likely to improve platelet number, but its effects are transient and a treatment course very expensive. Therefore it is best reserved for the setting of acute bleeding refractory to steroids. Management of pregnancy in a women with ITP poses additional considerations and therapeutic dilemmas (see later discussion).

Thrombotic thrombocytopenic purpura

DEFINITION. TTP is a rare condition with a classic pentad of fever, neurologic change, uremia, microangiopathic hemolysis, and thrombocytopenia. For reasons that remain poorly understood, as with ITP, woman are affected about two to three times more frequently than are men.

PATHOPHYSIOLOGY. The cause of TTP remains unknown. Widespread thrombotic occlusion of arterioles and capillaries involve predominantly the brain, kidneys, heart, pancreas, spleen, and adrenal glands. It is presumed that after some inciting event, endothelial damage results in the formation of platelet-rich microthrombi that occlude vascular flow and cause shearing fragmentation or red blood cells. TTP has been associated with a variety of systemic conditions, including infection, pregnancy, and collagen vascular illness, as well as the use of such drugs as cyclosporine.

CLINICAL PRESENTATION. Clinical symptoms can be subtle or absent at onset. Vague neurologic findings are often present at some point during the course of the disease and include headache, visual changes, neuropathies, seizures, and coma. Fever and bleeding are variable in severity.

Although the diagnosis may be apparent when all symptoms are present, the full pentad occurs in only 30% of cases; especially when complaints are mild, this disorder can be overlooked.

DIAGNOSTIC TESTS. Thrombocytopenia, abnormal renal function, and hemolytic anemia are the hallmarks of TTP. Examination of the peripheral smear is pivotal inasmuch as it will reveal fragmentation of red cells consistent with microangiopathic destruction. Intravascular hemolysis is confirmed by the finding of an elevated indirect bilirubin and LDH, depressed haptoglobin, presence of plasma, and urine-free hemoglobin.

MANAGEMENT. Immediate recognition of TTP is crucial because delay in therapy results in significant mortality. Although the pathogenesis of this condition remains largely unknown, empiric treatment with plasma infusion or plasma exchange results in remission in about 80% of instances.

Thrombocytosis

Thrombocytosis is a normal response to a number of systemic conditions, including iron deficiency, chronic inflammation, infection, and hyposplenism. However, an elevated platelet count may indicate aberrant marrow production and suggest a disorder such as essential thrombocythemia (ET).

Essential thrombocythemia

Epidemiology and definition. ET is a chronic myeloproliferative disease characterized by marked elevation in platelet number and an unpredictable pattern of hemorrhage or thrombosis. Although it affects older men and women equally, it seems to be more common in young females.

Clinical presentation. Hemorrhage and recurrent thrombosis punctuate the course of patients with ET. Bleeding tends to occur at mucocutaneous surfaces reflective of the defect in primary hemostasis. Thrombosis can develop in the venous or arterial tree and involve large and small vessels. Although deep venous thrombosis and pulmonary embolus are most common, occlusion at unusual sites (sagittal and portal vein, subclavian and coronary artery) has been described. Headache, transient ischemic attack, and other neurologic symptoms represent microthrombotic obstruction. Previously regarded as a benign condition in young persons, several studies have documented severe and life-threatening complications in this cohort. Splenomegaly is present in one third of cases; otherwise findings on physical examination are unremarkable.

Diagnostic tests. Platelets typically exceed 1 million in number and exhibit a variety of functional abnormalities. No single clinical finding is specific for ET, and thus diagnosis remains one of exclusion. First, reactive causes of thrombocytosis must be eliminated. Among laboratory data helpful in this regard are iron studies (normal in ET), sedimentation rate (often very low in ET), and fibrinogen level (normal in ET). Elimination of other myeloproliferative conditions is the next step, and more detailed hematologic testing is required.

Therapy. Management of patients with ET remains controversial. In the absence of symptoms, it is reasonable to monitor clinical developments carefully without intervention. Platelet-lowering agents such as hydroxyurea, anagrelide and interferon are reserved for the development of hemorrhage or thrombosis. Aspirin and other antiplatelet drugs should be used with caution inasmuch as they can exacerbate the underlying hemorrhagic diathesis.

ABNORMALITIES OF WHITE BLOOD CELLS
Leukopenia

Normal white blood cell (WBC) count and granulocyte number differ among races. Approximately one quarter of African-Americans have WBC fewer than 5300/mm^3 and an absolute granulocyte count less than 2700/mm^3 (Broun, Herbig, and Hamilton, 1966). Although it has been demonstrated that granulocyte reserve (as measured by neutrophil increment after hydrocortisone administration) is depressed in this group, neutropenia does not correlate with an increased risk of infection and represents a normal variant (Mason, Lessin, and Schechter, 1979).

Immune neutropenia. As with anemia and thrombocytopenia, neutropenia results from decreased production or increased destruction. Rare congenital disorders and primary bone marrow diseases (e.g., myelodysplasia, leukemia) are the major conditions leading to diminished synthesis of granulocytes. More often, neutropenia arises from increased clearance by an autoantibody and occasionally, a drug may be implicated. Idiopathic neutropenia is of particular relevance to women inasmuch as it may be the first sign of an underlying illness such as systemic lupus erythematosus. When it is accompanied by rheumatoid arthritis and splenomegaly, the triad of Felty's syndrome is met. Although many patients with neutropenia remain asymptomatic, the risk of life-threatening bacterial infection mandates close observation and the immediate institution of antibiotics in the presence of fever.

Bone marrow examination is indicated to exclude a primary hematologic condition. Tests for antineutrophil antibodies remain unreliable, and the diagnosis of immune neutropenia remains one of exclusion.

Leukocytosis

Although leukocytosis usually implies infection, it may be noted in otherwise healthy women. In women who are obese, smoke, and use oral contraceptives, the WBC count has been shown to range between 5800 and 14,200/mm^3 (Fisch and Freeman, 1975). Of these associations, smoking causes the most marked abnormalities and has a dose-dependent effect.

PREGNANCY AND BLOOD DISORDERS

Normal pregnancy results in expected alteration of the hematologic profile (see box, right). Some changes, however, are not benign and reflect pathologic developments during gestation.

Physiologic changes

Red blood cell changes. Hb concentrations fall during normal pregnancy because of a disproportionate rise in plasma volume over red cell mass. Between weeks 34 and 36, plasma volume has expanded by about 1250 ml whereas red cell mass increases more slowly and less dramatically, 250 to 400 ml at term. This physiologic or dilutional change accounts for second and third trimester Hct values in the low-30 range (Hb 10 to 11 g/dl), although 3% to 5% of apparently healthy women have even lower levels. The MCV typically rises 1 to 4 fl in pregnancy and can mask underlying iron deficiency.

Pregnancy places extreme demands on the iron reserves of women; approximately 250 mg of iron is utilized by the developing fetus and an additional 100 mg is sequestered in the placenta. Expansion of maternal red cell mass consumes another 500 mg, with variable amounts lost at delivery. Overall about 1 g of iron is required for normal gestation. Consequently, iron supplementation is mandatory during routine prenatal care and should be continued for many months thereafter.

White blood cell changes. Nearly 50% of women develop leukocytosis (WBC >10,000) or some abnormality of the white cell differential during pregnancy. Circulating myelocytes and metamyelocytes are noted in 25% of CBC's even when the absolute white count is normal. These changes seem to be most prominent the third trimester and resolve postpartum (Kuvin and Brecher, 1962).

Changes in platelets. Thrombocytopenia in the pregnant woman presents a complex series of diagnostic and management issues that have been summarized in a recent review by McCrae and others. Mild depression in platelet number can accompany normal, uncomplicated gestation. Eight percent of healthy women have platelet counts that range between 100,000 and 150,000/mm^3, and a small percentage drop below 50,000/mm^3 (Burrows and Kelton, 1988; 1990). Infants born to these women are at low risk for complications inasmuch as neonatal thrombocytopenia and bleeding are rare. The cause of this process remains unclear but probably represents accelerated activation and consumption of platelets in the uteroplacental circulation. Benign pregnancy-associated thrombocytopenia must be distinguished from other conditions in which depressed platelet number can lead to serious hemorrhage.

Pathologic processes

Folate deficiency. Folate is second only to iron as the most common cause of nutritional anemia in the gravid female (Pryor and Morrison, 1990). Derived from green leafy vegetables and legumes, folate stores are depleted within weeks to months if intake is restricted or demand is increased. In pregnancy, minimal daily requirements rise twofold or higher over nongravid needs and thus exogenous supplementation should be provided. Except for the absence of neurologic abnormalities, the clinical and hematologic

---

NORMAL HEMATOLOGIC CHANGES DURING PREGNANCY

Red blood cells
Dilutional anemia
Elevated MCV (1-4 fl)

White blood cells
Leukocytosis
Early myeloid forms

Platelets
Mild thrombocytopenia

findings in folate deficiency are identical to those of megaloblastic anemia caused by vitamin B_{12} deficiency.

Preeclampsia. Preeclampsia, defined by hypertension and proteinuria during pregnancy, is accompanied by thrombocytopenia in 15% to 50% of cases. Probably a variant of this condition, the HELLP syndrome (hemolysis, elevated liver enzymes, and low platelet count), also is characterized by microangiopathic hemolytic anemia and accelerated consumption of platelets. Because of high maternal and fetal mortality, these disorders must be promptly recognized and treated. Expeditious delivery of the fetus and aggressive transfusional support form the mainstay of therapy. These syndromes are covered in detail in Chapter 51.

Immune thrombocytopenic purpura. As previously noted, ITP is particularly common in women of childbearing years. Because maternal antiplatelet antibodies can cross the placenta, management is complicated by the additional risk posed to the fetus. The optimal mode of delivery in these cases remains controversial. It has been argued that because passage through the birth canal places the thrombocytopenic infant at risk for intracranial hemorrhage, cesarean section should be performed in this setting. However, it may be unnecessary in the woman whose fetus is unaffected. Further complicating delivery decisions, neither maternal platelet count nor antibody titer reliably predicts thrombocytopenia in the neonate. Consequently, some clinicians advocate obtaining fetal blood (via fetal scalp vein or percutaneous umbilical blood sampling, PUBS). If thrombocytopenia is absent in the neonate, normal vaginal delivery can be undertaken.

Antiphospholipid antibodies and habitual abortion. The antiphospholipid antibodies comprise a heterogeneous family of proteins associated with recurrent arterial and venous thrombosis. Although involvement of the uteroplacental vessels has been implicated in habitual abortion, the precise risk of miscarriage in this setting is not known. Clinical studies are hampered by fluctuating antibody titers and imperfect assays. It does appear, however, that those women with repeatedly positive assay results incur an increased risk of fetal loss (see Chapter 48).

BIBLIOGRAPHY

Bridges KB: Iron imbalance during pregnancy. In Frigoletto FD Jr, Bern MM, editors: *Hematologic disorders in maternal-fetal medicine,* New York, 1990, Wiley Liss.

Broun GO, Herbig FK, Hamilton JR: Leukopenia in negroes, *N Engl J Med* 275:1410, 1966.

Burrows RF, Kelton JG: Incidentally detected thrombocytopenia in healthy mothers and their infants, *N Engl J Med* 319:142, 1988.

Burrows RF, Kelton JG: Thrombocytopenia at delivery: a prospective study survey of 6715 deliveries, *Am J Obstet Gynecol* 162:731, 1990.

Carmel R, Johnson CS: Racial patterns in pernicious anemia, *N Engl J Med* 298:647, 1978.

Chanarin I, McFadyen IR, Kyle R: The physiologic macrocytosis of pregnancy, *Br J Obstet Gynaecol* 84:504, 1977.

Dallman PR, Yip R, Johnson C: Prevalence and causes of anemia in the United States, 1976-1980, *Am J Clin Nutr* 39:437, 1984.

Feinstein DI: Lupus anticoagulant, anticardiolipin antibodies, fetal loss and systemic lupus erythematosus *Blood* 80:859, 1992 (editorial).

Fisch IR, Freedman SH: Smoking, oral contraceptives and obesity: effects on white blood cell count, *JAMA* 234:500, 1975.

Ginsberg JS, et al: The relationship of antiphospholipid antibodies to thromboembolic disease in systemic lupus erythematosus: a cross sectional study, *Blood* 80:975, 1992.

Handin RI: Disorders of the platelet and vessel wall. In Wilson JD et al, editors: *Harrison's principles of internal medicine,* ed 12, New York, 1991, McGraw-Hill.

Haurani FI: Anemia of chronic disease: a misnomer, *Ann Intern Med* 116:520, 1992 (letter).

Koller O, Haram K, Sagen N: Maternal hemoglobin concentration and fetal health. In Frigoletto FD Jr, Bern MM, editors: *Hematologic disorders in maternal-fetal medicine,* New York, 1990, Wiley Liss.

Kuvin SF, Brecher G: Differential neutrophil counts in pregnancy, *N Engl J Med* 266:877, 1962.

Mason BA, Lessin L, Schechter GP: Marrow granulocyte reserves in black Americans, *Am J Med* 67:201, 1979.

McCrae KR, Samuels P, Schreiber AD: Pregnancy-associated thrombocytopenia:pathogenesis and management, *Blood* 80:2697, 1992.

Meyers LD, Habicht JP, Johnson CL: Components of the difference in hemoglobin concentrations in blood between black and white women in the United States, *Am J Epidemiol* 109:539, 1979.

Mitus AJ et al: Hemostatic complications in young patients with essential thrombocythemia, *Am J Med* 88:371, 1990.

Mitus AJ, Schafer AI: Thrombocytosis and thrombocythemia, *Hematol Oncol Clin North Am* 4:157, 1990.

Pryor JA, Morrison JC: Nutritional anemias. In Frigoletto FD Jr, Bern MM, editors: *Hematologic disorders in maternal-fetal medicine,* New York, 1990, Wiley Liss.

Ridolfi RL, Bell WR: Thrombotic thrombocytopenia purpura: report of 25 cases and review of the literature, *Medicine* 60:413, 1981.

Schilling RF: Anemia of chronic disease: a misnomer, *Ann Intern Med* 115:572, 1991 (editorial).

Spaulding WB: The clinical analysis of fatigue, *Appl Therapeutics,* p 911, Nov 1964.

Teferi A, Hoagland HC: Issues in the management of essential thrombocytosis, *Mayo Clin Proc* 69:651, 1994.

Thompson CE et al: Thrombotic microangiopathies in the 1980's: clinical features, response to treatment and the impact of the human immunodeficiency virus epidemic, *Blood* 80:1890, 1992.

van Zeben D et al: Evaluation of microcytosis using serum ferritin and red blood cell distribution width, *Eur J Haematol* 44:105, 1990.

INFECTIOUS DISEASES

16 Human Immunodeficiency Virus

Powel H. Kazanjian and Stephanie A. Eisenstat

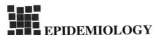

EPIDEMIOLOGY

Women represent the fastest-growing segment of persons with acquired immunodeficiency syndrome (AIDS) in the United States. In 1981, 3.2% of reported AIDS cases occurred in women, but that proportion increased to 11.5% of new cases by 1990 (Table 16-1). These trends will likely continue—seroprevalence studies show that rates of human immunodeficiency virus (HIV) infection among women applying to the Job Corps have already exceeded that of men. By the year 2000 it is projected that more women than men will have AIDS in this country, as is presently the case worldwide. Currently in the United States there are 20,000 women with AIDS and 140,000 who are HIV-infected. At present AIDS is the fifth leading cause of death in African-American women in the United States and is the leading cause of death in women of childbearing age in New Jersey and New York City (Table 16-2).

This chapter reviews the epidemiology, demographics, and natural history of HIV infection in women and offers management strategies of the asymptomatic woman. Indications for immunizations, antiretroviral agents, and medications used for prophylaxis against opportunistic infections are summarized.

DEMOGRAPHIC FEATURES

The demographic features of women with HIV infection differ from those of HIV-infected men. More women with AIDS are persons of color than are men with AIDS; 52% of women with AIDS are African-American, 21% are Hispanic, and 27% are white (Fig. 16-1). Also, the risk behavior for seropositive women differs from that of HIV-infected men overall and from that of their heterosexual male counter-parts. HIV-infected women are less likely than are HIV-infected heterosexual men to be intravenous drug users (IVDUs) (51% vs. 70%) but are more likely to be the sex partners of IVDUs (21% vs. 3%). Thus, IV drug use directly or indirectly accounts for a minimum of 70% of HIV infection in women (Fig. 16-2).

According to recent studies, most of the women who are seropositive for HIV are of reproductive age, married, monogamous, and poor.

Heterosexual transmission has increased from 3% of all AIDS cases among women in 1983 to 16% in 1990; up to 50% of women who acquire HIV by heterosexual activity did not know that they had been exposed to HIV. Factors associated with increased transmission include lack of condom use, anal intercourse, number of contacts, advanced disease state, and genital ulcerative disease (see box on the following page). The incidence of transmission of HIV from an infected man to a female partner in a fixed relationship after unprotected sex over a sustained period of time is 20%.

CLINICAL PRESENTATION

Recent reports suggest that important gender differences exist in the type and frequency of complications of HIV infection. HIV-infected women develop a different pattern

Table 16-1 Number and percentage of reported cases and male-to-female ratio for women and heterosexual men with AIDS in the United States

Year	No. (%) of all AIDS cases Women	Heterosexual men	Ratio
1981	6(3.2)	24(12.7)	4.0
1987	1701(8.1)	4127(19.7)	2.4
1990	4890(11.5)	11,632(27.3)	2.4

Modified from Ellerbrock TV: *JAMA* 265:2971, 1991.

Table 16-2 Death rates and leading causes of death among African-American women ages 15 to 44 years

Rank	Cause of death	Adjusted death rate (age-adjusted deaths/100,000 1980 U.S. population)
New Jersey, 1987		
1	AIDS	40.6
2	Cancer	30.1
3	Heart disease	23.1
4	Injuries	20.3
5	Homicide	10.2
New York, 1987		
1	AIDS	29.5
2	Cancer	23.1
3	Homicide	17.5
4	Heart disease	16.3
5	Liver disease and cirrhosis	10.5

Modified from Chu S, Buehler JW, Berkelman RL: *JAMA* 264:225, 1990.

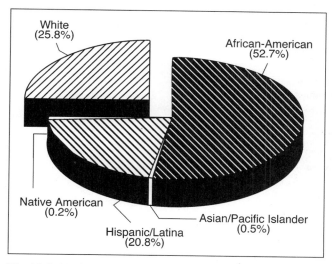

Fig. 16-1 AIDS in women by ethnicity. (From Centers for Disease Control, Jan 1992.)

of complications early in the course of their infection and meet criteria for AIDS earlier in their illness than do men. Lack of access to care and attention to the health care of the child in favor of self-care may contribute to less early detection and intervention.

Preliminary evidence suggests that the chronic consequences of HIV infection may affect women more adversely than men; female gender, nonwhite race, and IVDU as a risk behavior were associated with low quality-of-life scores on the Medical Outcomes Study Short Form Health Survey. However, reports from the Centers for Disease Control (CDC) suggest that survival time of women and heterosexual men is similar.

Most of the information regarding the natural history of HIV infection and management of the HIV-infected person is derived from studies of infected men. Symptoms of the acute infection that occur 2 to 6 weeks from the time of viral transmission are mild and do not provoke the patient to seek medical attention. Positive HIV serology (ELISA

and Western blot) will first appear 1 to 3 months later. CD4 cells will then decline on an average of 50 to 80/cu mm/yr (Fig. 16-3).

Surveillance data from the CDC of more than 16,000 diagnosed cases of AIDS in women (1981 through 1990) reveal a different spectrum of opportunistic infections commonly seen in women with AIDS: the five most common are listed in the box on the following page.

For the clinician caring for women at all stages of HIV infection, it is important to recognize that many gynecologic conditions are not only more common in women with HIV but also may take a more aggressive course and require more intensive intervention (see box on the following page). Cervical dysplasia and recurrent vaginosis caused by *Candida albicans* is associated with the early stage of HIV infection (CD4 cell count as high as 500/cu mm).

In one study cervical cytologic findings revealed that 40% of 35 HIV-positive women had squamous intraepithelial lesions compared with 9% of 32 HIV-negative women. Another study showed that colposcopic examination associated with biopsy increased the detection of cervical abnormalities. The CDC includes invasive cervical cancer but not carcinoma in situ or cervical dysplasia as an AIDS-defining illness (see box, p. 109). The definitions become important for reporting statistics and for classification. Once classified as having AIDS, the patient is eligible for disability compensation. Vaginal candidiasis is a frequent disorder in women and is especially prevalent in HIV-infected women. Women with HIV and vaginal candidal infection had a mean CD4 cell count of 504/cu mm whereas those with esophageal candidal infection had a CD4 count of 30. New and unexpected or more frequent or refractory candidal infection in the absence of antibiotics, as well as other sexually transmitted diseases and abnormal Pap smear results, should prompt physicians of these affected women to recommend HIV testing (see box, p. 109).

Severe ulcerative genital lesions as a result of herpes simplex was the AIDS-defining diagnosis in 18% of 44 women prospectively followed who developed AIDS (see box, p. 109). Genital herpes simplex viral infections are prevalent in the general population and may be particularly refractory in HIV-infected men and women. Menstrual irregularities are seen with greater frequency in HIV-infected women than in those who are not infected (41% vs. 24%). Amenorrhea and

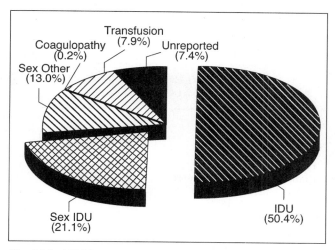

Fig. 16-2 AIDS in women by exposure category. IDU, intravenous drug user. (From Centers for Disease Control, Jan 1992.)

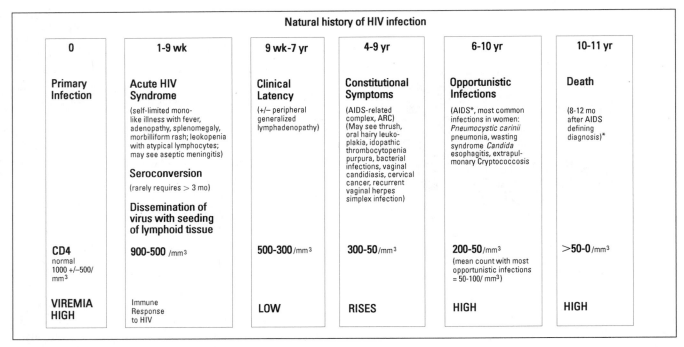

Fig. 16-3 Natural history of HIV infection.
*AIDS-defining diagnoses utilize the CDC criteria of 1992 (*MMWR* 41:RR-17, 1992).

between-period bleeding were noted particularly; however, more complete documentation of the types of menstrual irregularity is needed.

Diffuse lymphadenopathy is often present during moderate stages of immunosuppression (CD4 cell count of 300/cu mm). The enlarged glands are nontender, persist for a minimum of 3 months, and are characterized by the presence of two or more extrainguinal sites of involvement. Other diseases that occur in the middle stage of HIV infection include extrapulmonic *Mycobacterium tuberculosis* infections, recurrent herpes zoster, persistent mucocutaneous herpes simplex infections, and recurrent bacteremias caused by *Streptococcus pneumoniae* and *Salmonella sp.* The oral manifestations of HIV infection—candidiasis and hairy leukoplakia—make their first appearance at this time.

Kaposi's sarcoma, seen frequently in homosexual men, is found in fewer than 2% of HIV-infected women as an initial AIDS diagnosis. When Kaposi's sarcoma has occurred in women, it has been associated with sex with a bisexual man. The incidence of non-Hodgkin's lymphoma in HIV-infected women is unknown. There is an increased occurrence and aggressiveness of cervical cancer in infected women.

OPPORTUNISTIC INFECTIONS IN WOMEN AND MEN: (CDC AIDS SURVEILLANCE DATE 1981-1990 [161,073 CASES; 16,778 WOMEN])

Five most common infections in women with AIDS

Pneumocystis carinii pneumonia
Wasting syndrome
Esophageal candidiasis
Extrapulmonary cryptococcosis neoformans
Herpes simplex

Modified from Murrain M: *J Women's Health* 2:243, 1993.

Important gender-related differences exist in the types of diseases to which women are susceptible when HIV infection is advanced (CD4 cell count <200/cu mm). In men, *Pneumocystis carinii* pneumonia (PCP) is the dominant infection whereas in women, bacterial pneumonia caused by *Streptococcus pneumoniae* or *Haemophilus influenzae* is predominant. Other opportunistic infections occurring in the late stage of HIV infection in men or women include cerebral toxoplasmosis, esophageal candidiasis, and cryptococcal meningitis. Disseminated cytomegalovirus infection and *Mycobacterium avium* complex infection occur at the most terminal period, often when the CD4 cell count falls below 50/cu mm.

No significant differences exist in the clinical presentation of any of these opportunistic infections or, on the basis of present data, in the response to therapy between men and women with AIDS.

COMMON GYNECOLOGIC PROBLEMS IN HIV-INFECTED WOMEN

Candidal vaginitis
Genital herpes
Syphilis
Pelvic inflammatory disease
Human papillomavirus disease
  Condyloma acuminatum
  Cervical dysplasia
  Cervical carcinoma
Primary HIV ulcers
Chancroid
Menstrual irregularities
  Amenorrhea
  Intercyclic bleeding

AIDS-DEFINING GYNECOLOGIC DIAGNOSES

Invasive cervical cancer
Severe ulcerative genital lesions from herpes simplex

APPROACH TO THE WOMAN WITH ASYMPTOMATIC HIV

Overview

Recent data suggest that HIV-infected women seek medical care later than do men. Inasmuch as women frequently use emergency rooms, family planning clinics, sexually transmitted disease clinics, youth guidance centers, jail clinic facilities, and drug treatment units, these are the sites at which to target efforts at early diagnosis and use of early intervention. The management strategies of HIV infection during pregnancy should not differ from that for nonpregnant women.

History and physical examination

A thorough history and physical examination are important for all women whose test results are positive for HIV, not only to identify the stage of the disease but to aid prognosis. The history should focus on HIV exposure, signs and symptoms of systemic disease, and gynecologic complaints. The initial physical examination should include a vaginal examination and Pap smear, as well as a complete physical.

Diagnostic tests

Initial testing helps in staging of the disease because it is clear that the risk for developing opportunistic infections is closely associated with the fall in CD4 counts. The CD4 cell count should be measured every 3 to 6 months to guide therapeutic decisions regarding the use of zidovudine and PCP prophylaxis (see later discussion). A Pap smear is repeated every 6 to 12 months because of the possibility that HIV infection may accelerate the progression of cervical abnormalities. In addition, initial testing also should identify infections previously acquired by the patient that may become reactivated as a result of progressive loss of T cell function. Tests such as serologic reaction to *Toxoplasma gondii* (IgG), Venereal Disease Research Laboratory test (VDRL), and a purified protein derivative (PPD) skin test may reveal a latent infection that could show progression to cerebral toxoplasmosis, neurosyphilis, and tuberculosis,

respectively. Finally, hepatitis B virus (HBV) serologic testing for surface or core antibody (anti-HBs or anti-HBc) should be measured and hepatitis C (see box, below).

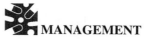

MANAGEMENT

Choice of therapy

Gynecologic complications

Vaginal candidiasis. Topical clotrimazole is sometimes effective in the treatment of vaginal infections caused by *Candida* spp. There may be some advantage to using the newer antifungal preparations with a greater spectrum against yeast species, such as Femstat or Terazol (*C. glabrata* as well as *C. albicans* (Table 16-3). Cases refractory to topical treatment occur with a greater frequency than in non–HIV-infected women, and fluconazole has been shown to be effective under these circumstances. In cases of frequent recurrences, 5-day courses of fluconazole each month for 6 months have been used; there are no controlled data to guide therapy of this disease or the value of long-term suppressive therapy with oral fluconazole. Ketoconazole also can be used if fluconazole is unavailable (Table 16-4).

Genital herpes. Infection with herpes simplex is very common. Suspected infection should be confirmed by culture. If the patient has *severe* symptoms such as urinary retention, pain, fever, or CNS complaints, the clinician should consider intravenously administered acyclovir. Otherwise, for *acute* infection, oral acyclovir, 400 mg every 4 hours for 7 to 10 days, is recommended. For *recurrent* herpes simplex infection the oral therapy is the same as for the acute episode. The evidence is unclear as to the efficacy of the addition of acyclovir ointment, but it may be used (5% ointment applied topically every 8 hours) to relieve symptoms. Prophylaxis with a maintenance dose of acyclovir, 200 mg orally twice a day (or three times a day), is then used indefinitely. It is important to monitor renal function while the patient is on acyclovir therapy. Some studies have shown an increase in resistant strains of herpes simplex. For resistant recurrent herpes simplex IV foscarnet (40 mg/kg at 8-hour intervals) can be used for 3 weeks if initial treatment with acyclovir is ineffective, but foscarnet has many side effects. Treatment options are summarized in Table 16-5.

Menstrual irregularities. Intervention for menstrual irregularities is covered in Chapter 28 and 29.

Human papillomavirus

Abnormal Pap smear findings. The current recommendations for Pap smear screening in the woman with HIV infection is every 6 months. Any evidence of abnormal results on

WHEN TO REFER FOR HIV COUNSELING AND TESTING

Persistent/recurrent/severe vaginal candidiasis
Recurrent/severe genital herpes simplex
Genital ulcer disease (syphilis, chancroid)
Recalcitrant or multisite condyloma acuminatum
Abnormal Pap smear result (moderate to severe cervical dysplasia, carcinoma in situ, or squamous cell carcinoma)
Persistent/recurrent pelvic inflammatory disease
Pregnancy

INITIAL EVALUATION OF WOMEN WITH POSITIVE HIV SEROLOGY

Complete physical examination and Pap smear
Baseline complete blood cell count and liver function tests
CD4 counts
IgG titers for *Toxoplasma gondii*
Venereal Disease Research Laboratories (VDRL) tests
Purified protein derivative (PPD) test with controls
Hepatitis B: anti-HBs or anti-HBc
Hepatitis C

Table 16-3 First-line topical vaginal antiinfective agents

Antifungal	Type	Dose	Contraindications/comments
Sulfanilamide (AVC)	Cream 15% (4 oz)/ suppository 1.05 g	1 applicator or suppository 1-2/day for 30 days	Do not use in pregnancy
Butoconazole (Femstat)	Cream 2% (28 g)	1 applicator qhs × 3 days (if necessary, 6 days)	No studies in first trimester OK in third trimester
Miconazole nitrate (Monistat 3)	200-mg suppositories Cream 2%	1 suppository qhs for 3 days qhs × 7 days	Efficacy in diabetics not clear
Clotrimazole (Mycelex)	Cream 1% (45, 90 g) Vaginal tablets (100, 500 mg)	1 applicator cream × 7 days 1 500-mg tab qhs	Give during first trimester only if necessary
Nystatin vaginal tablets (Mycostatin)	100,000 units	1 vaginal tablet qd × 2 wk	
Sulfathiazole, Sulfacetamide, and Sulfabenzamide triple sulfa (Sultrin)	78-g cream or vaginal tablets	1 applicator bid 4-6 days 1 tab qhs × 10 days	Increases risk for cleft palate; do not use in pregnancy
Terconazole (Terazol)	Vaginal cream 0.4% (45 g) 0.8% (20 g) Suppositories 80 mg	1 applicator 0.4% qhs × 7 days 1 suppository or 0.8% cream qhs × 3 days	
Tioconazole (Vagistat-1)	Ointment 6.5%	1 applicator qhs	
Clotrimazole (Femcare)	Vaginal cream 1%(45 g)/ vaginal inserts 100 g	1 insert qhs × 7 days	
Clotrimazole (Gyne-Lotrimin)	Vaginal cream 1% (45 g)/ vaginal tablets 100 mg	2 tab qd qhs × 3 days	
Miconazole nitrate (Monistat 7)	Vaginal cream 2% (45 g)/ suppositories 100 mg		
Boric acid	600-650 mg gelatin capsule of powder	Apply qd × 14 days	

a Pap smear, including atypia, koilocytosis, or inflammation, should be referred to a gynecologist for further evaluation and consideration of colposcopy. After colposcopic examination, careful screening with Pap smears should be performed every 3 months (see Chapter 77 for more details on management of abnormal Pap smear results).

Condyloma. Cervical and vaginal warts (or condyloma) are very common in these patients, and various treatment options are available for human papillomavirus. These are summarized in Table 16-6. (Chapter 17 covers the management of sexually transmitted disease in detail.)

Pelvic inflammatory disease (PID). PID may be a marker for HIV infection, and therefore women who manifest PID should be offered HIV testing. The course of the disease varies, depending on the degree of immunocompetence reflected by the CD4 count. Women with lower CD4 counts (<200 cu/mm) have a more aggressive course than those with counts less than 200 cu/mm. Among women with HIV infection who have PID, there is a higher incidence of abscess formation and surgical intervention for the PID. (For a detailed discussion on PID, see Chapter 17.)

Choice of prophylaxis

Prevention of reactivation of a latent infection may be possible with the use of specific agents (Table 16-7).

Toxoplasmosis. It has been estimated that one third of patients who have a reactive IgG serology to *T. gondii* will experience a recrudescence of their chronic latent infection.

Table 16-4 Second-line antifungal therapy: oral preparations

Antifungal agent	Type	Dose	Contraindications/comments
Ketoconazole (Nizoral)	Cream Tablets 200 mg (oral)	Simple *Candida* or recurrent: 200 mg/day or bid	GI effect, allergy, liver involvement
		Maintenance: 200 mg PO qd 5 days/mo at onset menses × 6 mo or 100 mg PO qd × 6 mo Severe ulcerative: 800 mg PO qd	Possible risk for osteoporosis Many drug interactions Avoid during pregnancy
Fluconazole (Diflucan)	Tablets 200 mg (oral)	Simple *Candida* or recurrent: PO qd × 7 days or until asymptomatic Maintenance: 100 mg PO qd × 5 days at onset of menses × 6 mo or 50 mg PO qd × 6 mo Severe ulcerative: 400 mg PO qd	Allergic reaction, GI, headache, drug interactions, liver involvement Avoid during pregnancy

Table 16-5 Treatment for common HIV-related gynecologic condition: herpes simplex infection

	Dose	Side effects
Acute	Oral acyclovir 400 mg q4h for 7-10 days	Leukopenia Anemia
Recurrent	Oral acyclovir 400 mg q4h *plus* topical acyclovir ointment 5% q3h for 7-10 days followed by prophylaxis with oral acyclovir 200 mg bid or tid	Same
Resistant	IV acyclovir 10 mg/kg q8h × 10 days If ineffective, then consider: IV foscarnet 40 mg/kg q8h for 3 wk	Hypocalcemia, renal dysfunction, leukopenia
Prevention	For recurrent herpes, or if patient has history of herpes and CD4 count <200, oral acyclovir 400 mg bid	

The reactivation of toxoplasmosis may be prevented by trimethoprim-sulfamethoxasole (TMZ-SMZ) used as prophylaxis for pneumocystis carinii pneumonia (PCP) (see later discussion).

Syphilis. Because patients with a reactive VDRL test may experience a rapid progression to neurosyphilis, it has been advocated that a lumbar puncture be performed on all persons whose test is reactive; benzathene penicillin should be administered only to those whose cerebrospinal fluid (CSF) formula is entirely normal. Treatment for tertiary neurosyphilis with either daily intramuscular procaine penicillin or intravenous penicillin for 10 days should be administered if the VDRL test result shows CSF positivity or if there is pleocytosis, elevation of protein, or presence of hypoglycorrhachia.

Mycobacterium tuberculosis. HIV-positive patients with PPD positivity (induration of 2 mm or greater) should receive isoniazid (INH) in a dose of 300 mg/day for a period of at least 12 months. With INH intolerance or INH-induced hepatitis, oral rifampin, 600 mg daily for 12 months, has been advocated. Rifampin plus pyrazinamide has been recommended for those with skin test conversion after contact with multiply resistant strains of *Mycobacterium tuberculosis.*

Prophylactic agents. Guidelines established for prophylaxis against PCP and antiretroviral therapies are derived from large national studies conducted on men and women. Although men predominate in these studies, the results led

Table 16-6 Treatment of human papillomavirus–related conditions

Condition	Therapy
Condyloma acuminatum	
Vaginal flat condyloma	Topical 5-fluorouracil cream once a week for 10 wk or qd for 5 days
Vulvar/perianal lesions <2 cm	Trichloroacetic acid (95%) topically
Cervical lesions	Topical 5-fluorouracil, then if not effective consider: Cryosurgery CO$_2$ laser treatment
Abnormal Pap smear	
Atypia, koilocytosis, inflammation or dysplasia, cervical intraepithelial neoplasia	Refer for colposcopy After treatment, follow-up Pap smear every 3-4 mo

to licensure of these agents and established recommendations for persons of both genders.

PCP prophylaxis. Three prophylactic regimens have been shown to dramatically reduce the incidence of PCP in persons with CD4 cell count below 200/cu mm. Because the most extensive published clinical experience is with trimethoprim-sulfamethoxazole (TMP-SMZ) (one double-strength tablet daily), the CDC recommends this as the first-line prophylaxis for PCP. As a single agent, TMP-SMZ also provides partial protection against reactivation of latent *Toxoplasma gondii* infections. On the basis of in vitro data, TMP-SMZ also may protect against infections caused by *Nocardia* sp., *Salmonella* sp., *Haemophilus influenzae,* and *Listeria monocytogenes.* However, the incidence of severe adverse reactions to TMP-SMZ, including gastrointestinal distress, fever, rash, and leukopenia, is estimated to be as high as 40% to 60% and results in cessation of drug administration in half of those who have the experience of an adverse reaction. More recently, one double-strength tablet 3 times weekly has been shown to reduce the incidence of adverse reactions. More than 70% of patients who experience an adverse reaction to TMP-SMZ are able to tolerate dapsone (25 mg/kg/day), an agent that has been recently shown in retrospective studies to be effective in preventing PCP. It has not been determined, however, whether dapsone is as effective as TMP-SMZ in preventing PCP. Aerosolized pentamidine, 300 mg/mo, is considered a third-line regimen because it is less effective than TMP-SMZ in reducing the incidence of PCP, increases the incidence of extrapulmonic pneumocystis, and threatens the transmission of *Mycobacterium tuberculosis* from patient to health care worker. The use of these agents is not contraindicated in pregnancy.

Antiretroviral therapy (Table 16-8). At a dosage of 500 mg/day, zidovudine (AZT, or ZDV) delays the onset of opportunistic infections in persons with CD4 cell counts less than 500/cu mm, although survival is not prolonged in this group of patients. AZT has been shown to prolong survival in patients with AIDS or in those with a CD4 cell count less than 200/cu mm. AZT results in a delay in the rate of decline of CD4 cells such that, following an initial small increase in CD4 counts, counts will decline to levels noted at the initiation of therapy after an average of 10 months of treatment. Patients should be seen in 2 weeks, then monthly thereafter to monitor for commonly occurring side effects such as anemia. Initially, many patients experience transient myalgias, headache, and fatigue, which often disappear more quickly if AZT is begun at a dose of 300 mg/day and increased to 500 mg/day over a 2-month period.

A multicenter trial in pregnant women suggests that AZT reduces the transmission rate of HIV from mother to fetus.

Table 16-7 Prophylaxis of some important opportunistic infections in women

Infection	Primary prophylaxis	Secondary prophylaxis
Vulvovaginal candidiasis	Not indicated	May consider weekly or monthly micronazole or clotrimazole suppositories Ketoconazole or fluconazole
Herpes simplex	Not known	May consider acyclovir 400 mg twice daily or 200 mg three times daily if recurrences frequent
Pneumocystic pneumonia	If CD4 <200, oral thrush or unexplained fevers >2 wk: sulfamethoxazole (Bactrim) 160 mg/800 mg 1-2 times daily or three times weekly Aerosolized pentamidine 300 mg every 4 wk Dapsone 50-100 mg qd	Same as primary prophylaxis
Tuberculosis	If PPD positive, isoniazid (INH) for at least 12 mo (consider INH in high-risk patients with anergy or PPD >2 mm induration)	Probably unnecessary after standard treatment for active disease
Mycobacterium avium complex	In patients with CD4 count <100, consider: Rifabutin Clarithromycin	Not applicable

Modified from Jewett JF, Hecht FM: *JAMA* 269(9): 1143, 1993.

To date, no specific adverse effect to mother or child has been reported. Interim analysis of this study has shown that AZT reduces the transmission rate of HIV from mother to fetus from 25% to 8%. In this trial, intravenous AZT was administered intrapartum because of the possibility that acquisition of the virus may occur as the fetus traverses the birth canal.

Macrocytosis occurs universally with AZT but does not interfere with therapy. The frequency of the major complications, leukopenia and anemia, is related to the degree of suppression of CD4 cells. The rate of dose-limiting marrow suppression ranges from 3% a year in asymptomatic patients to 40% a yr in patients with AIDS. Available therapeutic options include reinitiating AZT following a temporary discontinuation of the drug after the hemoglobin level has risen to baseline (usually above 8 g/dl) and absolute neutrophil count (ANC) increases above 750/cu mm; continuation of AZT with periodic transfusions and granulocyte stimulating factor (G-CSF) administration; or change to dideoxyinosine (ddI) therapy. Other adverse reactions less commonly encountered with AZT treatment include confusion and myopathy, which are late complications of AZT treatment.

Drug-resistant strains of HIV emerge in patients with AIDS treated with AZT for more than 6 months. Although unproved, many physicians have observed that patients classified as having a poor clinical response to AZT have developed resistance. Resistance to AZT is less pronounced when treatment is given early in the course of infection. Because resistance is conferred by a site-specific alteration in binding of AZT to reverse transcriptase, strains resistant to AZT retain susceptibility to other nucleoside analogs, including dideoxyinosine (ddI) and dideoxycytidine (ddC).

Two recent studies indicate that the initial clinical benefit of an initial course of AZT can be extended by a subsequent switch to ddI. In one study, patients who had a CD4 cell count less than 300/cu mm and signs of clinical deterioration while taking AZT for at least 6 months had an improved outcome—in terms of delay in the onset of a new AIDS-defining diagnosis, in the number of opportunistic infections, and in an increase in CD4 cell counts—when they were switched from AZT to ddI. In another study, a similar benefit was shown in patients who had a CD4 cell count less than 300/cu mm and in asymptomatic patients with a CD4 cell count less than 200/cu mm who had received at least 16 weeks of prior treatment with AZT. One study (AIDS Clinical Trial Group 116A), however, comparing AZT with ddI in patients who had never taken AZT, showed no difference in clinical outcome and demonstrated that ddI is not a superior drug when used as initial therapy. Viral resistance to ddI occurs after prolonged treatment; the degree of resistance may be lower than that with AZT.

Significant toxicity to ddI includes pancreatitis and peripheral neuropathy, which occur in approximately 10%

Table 16-8 Summary of antiretroviral therapy

Medication	Dose	Indication	Common side effects
Zidovudine (AZT)	500 mg/day	CD4 <500	Anemia, leukopenia
Dideoxyinosine (ddI)	200 mg/day	No response to AZT Complications from AZT	Pancreatitis, peripheral neuropathy, diarrhea
Dideoxycytidine (ddC)	0.75 mg PO q8h	No response to ddI or complications from both AZT and ddI	Peripheral neuropathy
Stavudine	200 mg PO bid	No response to ddI or complications from both AZT and ddI	Peripheral neuropathy

of patients. The drug should be stopped immediately if there is evidence of clinical or chemical pancreatitis (pancreatic amylase elevation greater than 1.5 × baseline value). Severe pain and numbness that characterize peripheral neuropathy are related to the cumulative dose and occur an average of 9 months after initiation of therapy. Neuropathy is reversible upon prompt discontinuation of ddI. Diarrhea is common but mild and usually does not interfere with continued therapy. Unlike AZT, cytopenias rarely occur. Neither ddI nor ddC has been used during pregnancy; the teratogenic effects of these agents are unknown.

A recent study has shown that monotherapy with ddC is as effective as ddI in delay of disease progression in persons who previously had received AZT and had a CD4 cell count of less than 300/cu mm. The major adverse reaction observed with ddC is peripheral neuropathy, which develops in 30% of patients in a dose-related fashion. Pancreatitis occurs much less frequently than with ddI (estimated incidence 1%).

Stavudine (deoxyfluorothymidine, D4T) is a non–FDA-approved nucleoside reverse transcriptase inhibitor that is available by a compassionate release protocol from the manufacturer to those patients with CD4 count less than 300 cells/cu mm who have had intolerance to or in whom approved antiretroviral therapy with AZT and ddI failed. This agent has in vitro activity against HIV that is comparable to AZT, and initial clinical studies have demonstrated improvement in surrogate markers of HIV infection at a dosage of 0.5 mg/kg/day. Adverse reactions occur in less than 10% of patients and include peripheral neuropathy and elevations of transaminase tests. Another RT inhibitor, 3-thiacytidine (3TC), is currently being investigated in limited clinical trials.

Combination therapy. Although monotherapy delays disease progression and reduces viral burden, combination therapy is under investigation because of the limitations of monotherapy—failure to achieve cure or eradicate viral replication. Theoretic benefits of combination therapy include achieving a potential synergistic effect on viral suppression, preventing the emergence of resistant strains, and reducing toxicity (synergistic combinations of antiretroviral drugs may reduce the dose of each drug required for virus inhibition).

One study showed that persons with a CD4 cell count less than 400 cells/cu mm who had received 16 weeks of prior treatment with AZT had improvements in surrogate markers of HIV infection when ddI was added. Because clinical end points were not monitored, this study provides no guide as to whether patients would benefit by having ddI added to or alternated with AZT if no toxicity to AZT has occurred. Three other small studies of AZT-ddI combinations demonstrated that surrogate markers of HIV infection, CD4 cell counts, and quantitative HIV-1 cultures improve more significantly than with monotherapy.

ddC 0.75 mg every 8 hours, when given in combination with AZT 200 mg every 8 hours, resulted in a larger initial elevation in CD4 cell counts and more sustained elevation of CD4 counts when compared with AZT alone in patients who had advanced HIV disease but were AZT naive. On the basis of this study, which did not include clinical end points, ddC may be offered in combination with AZT to patients who have advanced HIV infection—CD4 cell count less than 300/cu mm—and demonstrate clinical or immunologic deterioration.

There are two ongoing trials to investigate the clinical utility of a new nonnucleoside reverse transcriptase inhibitor, delavirdine (DLV), a piperazine derivative, in combination with a nucleoside drug to be administered before the development of resistance to that agent. In vitro, DLV demonstrates synergistic antiviral activity with AZT, ddI, and ddC. Other than transient rash (25% of patients), this agent causes minimal toxicity in human beings. In one double-blinded study, patients with CD4 counts between 200 and 500/cu mm who have previously received AZT for less than 6 months receive AZT with or without DLV. In the other study, persons with counts less than 300/cu mm who have received ddI for less than 4 months receive ddI with or without DLV.

How and when to combine available antiviral agents optimally are under active investigation. Two studies that address this issue are being completed. ACTG 155 assesses the effectiveness of AZT combined with ddC for symptom-free persons with CD4 cell counts less than 200/cu mm or for those with symptomatic disease and CD4 counts less than 300/cu mm who had been taking AZT by itself for less than 6 months. Another study of patients with CD4 cell counts between 200 and 500/cu mm (ACTG 175) includes an additional ddI plus AZT arm.

The clinician's options. The optimal use of antiretroviral agents remains unestablished since they have become available before adequate data about their efficacy are complete. The indications for monotherapy are evolving, but there are insufficient data at present to determine whether and when to combine the nucleosides. However, clinicians must make decisions now because many patients are interested in combining antiviral agents on the basis of the limited effectiveness of monotherapy and the promising early data regarding combination therapy.

One option is to administer AZT when the CD4 count falls below 500/cu mm. ddI or ddC should be substituted for AZT if there is significant toxicity to AZT or when the CD4 cell count falls below 300/cu mm. If there is rapid immunologic deterioration (decline in CD4 cell count >100/cu mm/yr) or marked progression of clinical disease with AZT therapy, combination antiviral therapy can be used by adding ddI to AZT. AZT can be used in combination with ddC under these circumstances when ddI cannot be used (e.g., if the patient has pancreatitis or severe diarrhea). If ddC cannot be tolerated by the patient in this setting and AZT either has failed or caused toxicity, the clinician can obtain D4T from the manufacturer through a compassionate-release protocol.

Convergent combination therapy. One strategy is based on the use of combination chemotherapy, with drugs targeted at the same enzyme; for example, RT uses nucleoside (AZT and ddI) and nonnucleoside (nevirapine) RT inhibitors. The desired intention is to exploit the mutational interactions of AZT, ddI, and nevirapine and force the RT into a dysfunctional state that results in poorly replicating virus. This has been demonstrated experimentally, in one laboratory, but the results have not been reproduced in others. Nevertheless, clinical trials evaluating convergent combination therapy have not been completed.

New agents. Among the novel approaches under investigation is inhibition of HIV protease, the enzyme that is responsible for the cleaving of viral precursor polypeptides into a mature and infective virus. By acting to reduce viral replication after insertion into the human genome, the protease inhibitors may act synergistically with drugs that act before integration—the RT inhibitors. These agents are active in vitro and have not demonstrated toxicity in early studies. Larger clinical trials are in design to evaluate their clinical efficacy.

Unique treatments of HIV infection that inhibit regulatory proteins, such as *tat* or *rev*, are in progress. Tat inhibitors work by blocking RNA viral protein synthesis. A potential clinical advantage is that the tat or rev inhibitors are active against AZT-resistant isolates. Clinical trials have shown that tat is ineffective, and trials to investigate rev are in design.

Preventive interventions

Immunizations. HIV-infected persons should receive annual influenza vaccine in November. Because the frequency of *Streptococcus pneumoniae* and *Haemophilus influenzae* infections are increased in HIV-infected persons, Pneumovax and recombinant *H. influenzae* type B (HIB) vaccine are recommended by the Advisory Committee on Immunization Practices (ACIP) and the Centers for Disease Control (CDC) for all persons with HIV infection. Revaccination should be administered every 3 years. Hepatitis B vaccine is recommended for persons who lack evidence of HBV markers and have any of the following risk factors: active IV drug use, sexually active women, and household or sexual contacts of HBV surface antigen carriers. Tetanus-diphtheria vaccine boosters should be given every 10 years. Mumps and rubella vaccines are recommended for susceptible adults, and measles vaccine is advocated for nonimmune adults born after 1956.

Other strategies. All patients who are sexually active are potentially at risk for contracting HIV disease. However, some patients are at higher risk than others. Although it is important to discuss safe sex practices with all patients, particular patients should be offered HIV testing as well. The box on p. 109 summarizes current recommendations concerning when to refer women for HIV testing. It is important to counsel the patient so as to ensure confidentiality in testing.

The primary care of women with HIV infection is very important. The box, above right, summarizes the basic primary care management for these women.

A vaginal sheath, or female condom, has been licensed for use as a contraceptive device that a woman controls. Its efficacy, however, remains unestablished. Although nonoxynol-9, the ingredient in spermicides, has activity against HIV, it does not reduce the transmission of HIV to women during vaginal intercourse.

 PREGNANCY AND HIV DISEASE

One study suggested that CD4 counts fall more during pregnancy in an HIV-infected woman than in the nonpregnant state. It is unknown whether the pregnancy-associated decreases in CD4 cell counts show the same increase in development of opportunistic infections as in the nonpregnant state.

Although the agents used to treat opportunistic infections in pregnancy are potentially teratogenic, the benefits of treatment to the mother outweigh the potential risk to the fetus. At present, standard use of CD4 values for initiation

---

SUMMARY OF PRIMARY CARE MANAGEMENT OF WOMEN WITH HIV INFECTION

Pelvic examination and Pap smear every 6 months
Chlamydia/gonococcal screening for women at high risk
CD4 counts every 3-4 mo
Tuberculin testing (PPD every year)
Early intervention with AZT therapy
Vaccinations:
  Pneumococcal once every 3 yrs
  Haemophilus influenzae once every 3 yrs
  Influenza once a year
  Hepatitis B if hepatitis antibody–negative and have risk
    factors (see text)
Counseling on safe sex practices and pregnancy

---

of antiviral therapy and prophylaxis for PCP is recommended. Opportunistic infections, such as those caused by *Pneumocystis carinii, Toxoplasma gondii,* and *Cryptococcus neoformans,* are life-threatening. Others, such as those caused by *cytomegalovirus* or *Mycobacterium avium* complex, may result in significant morbidity. Trimethoprim sulfamethoxazole appears safe and effective for both prophylaxis and therapy of PCP in pregnancy. Detailed information on the agents used to treat these specific infections is beyond the scope of this chapter.

SUMMARY

This chapter outlines the distinct features of HIV infection in women. It outlines the important gender differences that exist in risk factors and in the type and frequency of complications of HIV infection. It provides the physician with a strategy for staging HIV infection and for managing the asymptomatic patient. The indications for the use of antiviral agents and medications used for prophylaxis against opportunistic infections has been reviewed. Innovative methods for enrolling HIV-infected pregnant and nonpregnant women into epidemiologic and clinical trials are required to obtain more accurate information regarding the epidemiology, transmission, and perinatal infection associated with HIV.

BIBLIOGRAPHY

Adachi A et al: Women with human immunodeficiency virus infection and abnormal papanicolaou smears: a prospective study of colposcopy and clinical outcome, *Obstet Gyncol* 81:372, 1993.

Bartlett JG: *The Johns Hopkins Hospital guide to medical care of patients with HIV infection,* ed 4, Baltimore, 1994, Williams & Wilkins.

Bartlett JG: *1992–1993 recommendations for the medical care of persons with HIV infection,* Baltimore, 1992, Critical Care Co.

Biggar R et al: Immunosuppression in pregnant women infected with HIV, *Am J Obstet Gyncol* 161:1239, 1989.

Brettle RP, Leen CLS: The natural history of HIV and AIDS in women, *AIDS* 5:1283, 1991.

Carpenter CJ et al: Human immunodeficiency virus infection in North American women: experience with 200 cases and a review of the literature, *Medicine* 70:307, 1991.

Centers for Disease Control: 1993 revised classification system for HIV infection and expanded surveillance: case definition for AIDS among adolescents and adults, *MMWR* 41(PR-17), Dec 18, 1992.

Chu SY, Buehler JW, Berkelman RL: Impact of the human immunodeficiency virus epidemic on mortality in women of reproductive age, United States, *JAMA* 264:225, 1990.

Corey L, Fleming T: Treatment of HIV infection; progress in perspective, *N Engl J Med* 326:483, 1992.

Cotton D: AIDS in women. In Broder S, Merrigan T, Bolognesi D, editors: *Textbook of AIDS medicine,* Baltimore, 1994, William & Wilkins.

Dattel BJ et al: AIDS (HIV) risk assessment in an inner city women's clinic, *J Reprod Med* 37:821, 1992.

Ellerbrock TV et al: Epidemiology of women with AIDS in the United States, 1981-1990: a comparison with heterosexual men with AIDS, *JAMA* 265:2971, 1991.

Fauci A: Combination therapy for HIV infection: getting closer, *Ann Intern Med* 116:85, 1992.

Friedland GH et al: Survival differences in patients with AIDS, *AIDS* 4:144, 1991.

Gold J: HIV-1 infection: diagnosis and management, *Med Clin North Am* 76:1, 1992.

Graham NM, Zeger SL, Park LP: The effects on survival of early treatment of human immunodeficiency virus infection, *N Engl J Med* 326:1037, 1992.

Hankins CA, Handley MA: HIV disease and AIDS in women: current knowledge and a research agenda, *J AIDS* 5:957, 1992.

Jewett JF et al: High risk of human papilloma virus infection and cervical squamous intraepithelial lesions among women with symptomatic human immunodeficiency virus infection, *Am J Obstetrics and Gynecology,* 165(2):392, 1991.

Jewett JF, Hecht FM: Preventive health care for adults with HIV infection, *JAMA* 269(9):1143, 1993.

Kahn JO et al: A controlled trial comparing continued zidovudine with didanosine in human immunodeficiency virus infection, *N Engl J Med* 327:581, 1992.

Lazzarin A et al: Italian study group on HIV heterosexual transmission man-to-woman sexual transmission of the human immunodeficiency virus, *Arch Intern Med* 151:2411, 1991.

Masur H: Prevention and treatment of *Pneumocystis* pneumonia, *N Engl J Med* 327:1853, 1993.

Meng T et al: Combination therapy with zidovudine and dideoxycytidine in patients with advanced HIV infection: a phase II study, *Ann Intern Med* 116:13, 1992.

Minkoff ML, DeHovir JA: Care of women infected with the human immunodeficiency virus, *JAMA* 266:2253.

Murrain M: Differences in opportunistic infection rates in women with AIDS, *J Women's Health* 2:243, 1993.

Padian NS, Shiboski SC, Jewell NP: Female to male transmission of human immunodeficiency virus, *JAMA* 226:1664, 1991.

Rich J et al: The effect of chemoprophylaxis for *Pneumocystis carinii* pneumonia on development of reactivation toxoplasmosis. In Program and abstracts of the Eighth International Conference on AIDS, Amsterdam, 1992 (abstract no. B3244).

Rompalo A, Anderson J, Quinn T: Reproductive tract infections and their management in women infected with the human immunodeficiency virus, *Infectious diseases in clinical practice,* p 277, 1992.

Safrin S et al: Seroprevalence and epidemiologic correlates of human immunodeficiency virus infection in women with acute pelvic inflammatory disease, *Obstet Gynecol* 75:666, 1990.

Spence MR, Reboli AC: Human immunodeficiency virus infection in women, *Ann Intern Med* 115:827, 1991.

Sperling R et al: A survey of zidovudine use in pregnant women with human immunodeficiency virus infection, *New Engl J Med* 326 (13):857, 1992.

St. Louis ME et al: Human immunodeficiency virus infection in disadvantaged adolescents: findings from the US Job Corps, *JAMA* 226:2387, 1991.

US Department of Health and Human Services: *HIV/AIDS/Surveillance: US AIDS cases reported through December 1992,* year-end ed, Washington, DC, 1993, US Government Printing Office.

Wachtel T et al: Quality of life in persons with human immunodeficiency virus infection: measurement by the medical outcomes study instrument, *Ann Intern Med* 116:129, 1992.

Wofsy C: Therapeutic issues in women with HIV disease. In Sande MA, Volberding PA, editors: *The medical management of AIDS,* Philadelphia, 1992, Sanders.

Yarchoan R, Pluda J, Perno C: Antiretroviral therapy of human immunodeficiency virus infection: current strategies and challenges for the future, *Blood* 15:859, 1991.

Yarchoan R et al: Therapy of AIDS or symptomatic HIV infection with simultaneous or alternating regimen of AZT and ddI. In Program and abstracts of the Eighth International Conference on AIDS, Amsterdam, 1992, (abstract no. A15).

17 Sexually Transmitted Disease

Donna Felsenstein

Each day 33,000 persons in the United States (12 million annually) contract one or more sexually transmitted infections. Of these infections 86% occur in persons between 15 and 25 years old, an age-group just entering the reproductive years. Women are at greater disadvantage than men; because the infections can be asymptomatic, most women who are infected do not realize that they need medical help. In addition, physical examination may reveal no signs of infection. Unless screening techniques are used to identify infection, these women are at significant risk for the development of complications, including infertility, adverse pregnancy outcomes, chronic abdominal pain, and cervical cancer. The primary care clinician needs to know who to screen, which tests to use, and how to interpret the test results. In addition, practitioners must know how to educate their patients regarding the modes of transmission of infection and methods to decrease the risk of acquiring a sexually transmitted disease (STD).

RISK FACTORS

Although a woman may contract a sexually transmitted infection at any age, the incidence of STD is greatest in those younger than 25 years of age. Any woman in this age-group who has had at least one sexual encounter should undergo the appropriate screening tests for STD. Regardless of age, other risk factors include a history of multiple partners, a previous STD, a sex partner with other partners in the preceding 3 months, use of illicit drugs, and use of nonbarrier contraceptives.

To identify those women at risk, the practitioner must use a frank, nonjudgmental approach in obtaining a sexual history. Unfortunately, clinicians often are uncomfortable asking patients about numbers of sexual partners, sexual preferences, and sexual practices, and thus prevent their patients from feeling free to respond truthfully. In addition, many professionals use terminology that their patients may neither understand nor interpret correctly. Questions should be phrased simply to avoid misinterpretation. Giving patients latitude in answering the questions facilitates obtaining more truthful responses. Being specific as to a patient's actual sexual practices helps the practitioner determine from which areas of the body to obtain a specimen to rule out potential infection (see box, below).

APPROACH TO THE WOMAN

All women whose sexual history determines them to be at risk for an STD should receive appropriate screening. The physical examination should include evaluation of the oral cavity, skin, lymph nodes, and external genitalia, as well as a pelvic and bimanual examination. A wet preparation of the vaginal secretions should be obtained to search for hyphae, *Trichomonas* organisms, clue cells, and polymorphonuclear leukocytes (PMNs). Specimens should be obtained from the cervix for identification of gonorrhea and chlamydia. A Gram's stain of the cervical secretions allows identification of mucopurulent cervicitis by the presence of at least 10 to 20 PMNs per oil-immersion field ($\times$1000) in an area of cervical mucus and a minimal number of epithelial cells. A positive Gram's stain or the finding of mucopus on a cotton swab of the cervical os has been shown to correlate with infection caused by *Chlamydia trachomatis*. Alternatively, it may indicate the presence of infection with organisms such as *Neisseria gonorrhoeae*, or herpes simplex. Specimens from the oral cavity and rectum should be obtained when indicated by the sexual history or dictated by signs or symptoms. All women at risk for STD should be screened for syphilis (see later discussion). Human immunodeficiency virus (HIV) testing should be considered.

PATHOGENS

The list of sexually transmitted pathogens is long. Infections are caused by a variety of organisms:

- Bacteria—*Neisseria gonorrhoeae, Haemophilus ducreyi* (chancroid), *Calymmatobacterium granulomatis* (granuloma inguinale, donavanosis), *Gardnerella vaginalis, Chlamydia trachomatis*
- Mycoplasma—*Mycoplasma hominis, Ureaplasma urealyticum*
- Fungi—*Candida albicans*
- Spirochetes—*Treponema pallidum*
- Viruses—herpes simplex virus, human papillomavirus (warts), hepatitis A, B, and C, cytomegalovirus, human immunodeficiency virus (HIV)
- Protozoa—*Trichomonas vaginalis, Entamoeba histolytica, Giardia lamblia*
- Ectoparasites—*Phthirus pubis* (crab louse), *Sarcoptes scabiei* (scabies)

Several of the major pathogens are discussed here; human papillomavirus is discussed in Chapter 78.

Neisseria gonorrhoeae

Gonorrhea is caused by the bacteria *Neisseria gonorrhoeae*, a gram-negative diplococcus. The actual incidence of gonorrhea is believed to be 1 to 2 million cases annually, significantly more than the roughly 500,000 cases reported each year. Transmission of infection with *N. gonorrhoeae* occurs readily. There is a 20% risk of a man acquiring urethral infection after one exposure to an infected woman. The likelihood of transmission from a man to a woman is probably higher.

Clinical presentation. The incubation period for gonorrhea is difficult to define in women, but symptoms may occur within 10 days. Unlike men, most infected women have no symptoms. Although the endocervical canal is the primary site of infection in women, colonization of the urethra also occurs in up to 70% to 90% of women. In women who have undergone a hysterectomy, the urethra is the primary site of infection. Gonococcal **urethritis** is one of the causes of the sterile pyuria syndrome. Symptoms may include dysuria and urinary frequency. Discharge may be expressed from the infected urethra.

Women with symptomatic **cervical infection** may report vaginal discharge, dysuria, abnormal uterine bleeding, or labial pain or swelling (Bartholin's gland abscess). The cervix may be normal in appearance, or there may be evidence of mucopurulent cervicitis, including edema, erythema, friability, or a discharge from the cervical os. **Endometritis** results from ascension of infection from the cervical canal.

Fitz-Hugh–Curtis syndrome, or perihepatitis, is an inflammatory process involving the surface of the liver. Patients have right upper quadrant abdominal pain that can be pleuritic. Fever, nausea, and symptoms of lower tract infection may be present. The liver is tender on examination. Evidence of salpingitis sometimes is present. The white blood cell (WBC) count and erythrocyte sedimentation rate (ESR) may be elevated. Liver function tests reveal elevated levels in 50% of patients. Normal findings on a right upper quadrant ultrasound can help distinguish this syndrome from acute cholecystitis. A culture specimen of the cervix may be positive for *N. gonorrhoeae*. A definitive diagnosis is established by laparoscopic findings of patchy purulent or fibrinous deposits on the surface of the liver.

N. gonorrhoeae causes 20% to 40% of cases of **salpingitis (pelvic inflammatory disease** [PID]). Other causes of PID

TAKING A SEXUAL HISTORY

1. Do you have sex with men or women, or both?
2. How many sexual partners do you have at present, for example, 1, 2, 5, 10?
3. How many partners have you had in the past 6 months? year? lifetime? 1, 5, 10, 50?
4. How old were you when you first had sex?
5. When did you have sex last?
6. Do you put your mouth on someone's penis? rectum? vagina?
7. Does someone put his penis in your vagina? mouth? rectum?
8. Do you use birth control? What kind? Do you use birth control all the time?
9. Do you use condoms? Do you use them all the time with each partner?
10. Have you ever had a sexually transmitted infection such as gonorrhea, herpes, chlamydia, warts, syphilis, or pelvic inflammatory disease?

include *Chlamydia trachomatis* and anaerobic bacteria. The role of other organisms such as *Trichomonas vaginalis, Gardnerella vaginalis, Ureaplasma urealyticum,* and *Mycoplasma hominis* has yet to be clarified. Regardless of the cause, the signs and symptoms generally are similar (see discussion under *C. trachomatis*). Complications of salpingitis include infertility, an increased propensity for ectopic pregnancies, and chronic abdominal pain as a result of scarring and adhesions. One episode of PID can predispose a patient to recurrent episodes of PID caused by vaginal flora, presumably because of an alteration of host defense mechanisms within the salpinx.

Pharyngeal infection is more readily transmitted by fellatio than by cunnilingus. Of heterosexual women with gonorrhea 10% to 20% have infection of the pharynx. The sexual history and results of subsequent screening cultures are important in making this diagnosis because more than 90% of cases are asymptomatic. Patients with symptoms often report a mildly to moderately sore throat. Cervical lymph nodes may be painful. The pharynx may be normal in appearance or mildly inflamed, or an exudative pharyngitis may be present. The anterior cervical nodes may be enlarged and tender on examination. Indeed, it is difficult to distinguish gonococcal pharyngitis from that caused by group A streptococcus. The diagnosis of gonococcal pharyngitis must be specifically sought by obtaining a sexual history from patients with a sore throat. The diagnosis of pharyngeal gonococcal infection can be made by placing a specimen from the posterior pharynx on agar containing modified Thayer-Martin (MTM) medium. Culture media used to diagnose group A streptococcal infection do not permit the growth of the gonococcus. Several of the newer rapid tests for *N. gonorrhoeae* may be used as well.

If untreated, **pharyngeal infection** will resolve spontaneously within 12 weeks. Treatment, however, is necessary to eliminate the pharynx as a reservoir of infection. More important, treatment can prevent dissemination of the organism, a complication of pharyngeal infection.

Infection of the rectum occurs in 30% to 50% of women with gonorrhea. The most common cause is contamination of the rectum by infected vaginal secretions, and in a smaller percentage of women, by rectal intercourse. Although most infected women are asymptomatic, symptoms of proctitis can occur. These include constipation, tenesmus, anorectal pain, and anorectal bleeding or discharge. The discharge may be purulent or mucoid. On examination, there may be mild erythema around the anus. Findings on anoscopic or proctoscopic examination may be insignificant or may reveal involvement of the lower end of the rectum. The mucosa may show inflammatory changes, may be friable, and may bleed easily. A mucopurulent exudate may be present. Gonococcal proctitis should be differentiated from infection caused by *Chlamydia trachomatis,* herpes simplex, *Treponema pallidum,* and *Entamoeba histolytica.*

A positive Gram's stain rectal smear can be found in 60% to 80% of infected patients. Although this smear is difficult to read, its specificity is extremely high. Diagnosis also can be made by obtaining a specimen for culture or by using one of the newer techniques described later.

Gonococcal ophthalmia neonatorum, a severe, bilateral purulent conjunctivitis, occurs in the neonate 1 to 7 days after the infant's passage through an infected birth canal.

This infection is prevented by the instillation of 1% silver nitrate in each conjunctival sac at birth. Adult **ocular infection** often is due to autoinoculation. Both infections require treatment with systemic antibiotics.

Disseminated gonococcal infection (DGI) occurs in 1% to 3% of infected patients. The incubation period is variable, ranging from 7 to 30 days after mucosal infection. In women, DGI often occurs around the time of menses or during pregnancy. Women may be at greater risk for dissemination than are men. Other risk factors include pharyngeal infection and complement deficiency. Patients have symptoms of systemic illness, including fever, anorexia, and malaise. Skin lesions are the most common manifestation of DGI. They occur predominantly on the extremities and range from 5 to 30 in number. The upper extremities are involved more often than the lower extremities. The lesions occur most often near the joints of the hands and feet. Their initial appearance is nonspecific, beginning as an erythematous macule or papule, which evolves into a pustule that ultimately may develop a hemorrhagic or necrotic center.

Infection with *N. gonorrhoeae* is the most common cause of acute septic arthritis in young adults and most often involves the knees, elbows, ankles, and wrists. Migratory polyarthralgias are more common in DGI than is septic arthritis. Tenosynovitis may occur at one or several sites. Other manifestations of DGI include hepatitis, myopericarditis, and, rarely, endocarditis, meningitis, osteomyelitis, and pneumonia.

Blood cultures are positive in only 25% of patients with DGI. Cultures of skin lesions may be positive in a small percentage of patients. The diagnosis is made by culturing all potentially infected sites, including the cervix, urethra, rectum, and pharynx.

Diagnostic tests. Gram's stain remains the most rapid and inexpensive method of diagnosing gonococcal infection; it is highly sensitive in specimens obtained from men with symptomatic urethritis. Although the sensitivity of Gram's stain is only 40% to 60% for cervical and anal specimens, the specificity of this test is 95%.

Culture remains the gold standard of diagnosis. The bacteria *N. gonorrhoeae* are small gram-negative diplococci with flattened abutting sides that on a Gram's stained smear have the appearance of a pair of kidney beans. The organism is extremely sensitive to drying and temperature. Specimens must be placed on the appropriate medium within minutes; the organism will die on the tip of a cotton swab. Cultures will not survive unless they are rapidly placed at 35° to 37°C in 3% to 5% carbon dioxide. When a carbon dioxide environment is not readily available, the planted specimen can be put in a candle jar and placed in an incubator. Selective culture media such as Thayer-Martin or modified Thayer-Martin (MTM) agar are used to culture *N. gonorrhoeae* to prevent its overgrowth by other saprophytic organisms present in the specimen. Some strains will fail to grow on these media, and thus specimens from relatively sterile sites (such as cerebrospinal fluid, blood, joints) should be plated on chocolate media that do not contain antibiotics. Special transport media are necessary when a laboratory is not immediately available. Because the organism is extremely sensitive to drying, temperature, and the level of carbon dioxide, cultures can be falsely negative if the specimen is not processed rapidly and correctly.

The newer diagnostic techniques, including the use of direct immunofluorescence and indirect enzyme immunoassays, are neither more sensitive nor more specific than culture. Sensitivity and specificity of the DNA probe range from 88% to 99%. False-positive results may be obtained with these rapid tests, particularly in the assessment of cure. In addition, culture remains an important means of identifying antibiotic-resistant strains of *N. gonorrhoeae*. The use of newer technologies is preferable to culture only when logistic problems prevent culturing a specimen.

Choice of therapy. For decades, penicillin was the drug of choice for the treatment of gonococcal infections. Strains of penicillin-resistant *N. gonorrhoeae* appeared in the United States in the 1970s, where overall, more than 8% of the strains of *N. gonorrhoeae* are resistant to penicillin; the prevalence increases to 25% to 35% of strains in certain urban areas. Thus, recommended regimens no longer include the use of penicillin. Because 35% to 50% of women infected with *N. gonorrhoeae* also are coinfected with *Chlamydia trachomatis,* any regimen for treating gonorrhea should include empiric treatment for *C. trachomatis.* The regimens noted in the box at right are effective for eradicating infection, with cure rates of 92% to 98%.

Preliminary studies have shown that ceftriaxone may be effective in treating incubating syphilis. Thus this regimen would be preferable to the use of the fluoroquinolones, which are not effective in the treatment of incubating syphilis. The fluoroquinolones should not be used during pregnancy, in lactating women, or in patients younger than 18 years of age.

All patients with gonorrhea are at risk for syphilis and should receive appropriate screening. All partners of patients with gonorrhea within the preceding 30 days should be evaluated and treated.

Chlamydia trachomatis

Infection with *Chlamydia trachomatis* is the most commonly occurring STD in the United States, with 4 million cases each year. It is the cause of one quarter to one half of the cases of PID. It is the most common cause of neonatal conjunctivitis and interstitial pneumonia in infants younger than 6 months of age born to an infected mother. The prevalence of chlamydial infection ranges from 3% to 5% of asymptomatic women seen in general medical clinics to 15% to 20% of those seen in STD clinics.

Chlamydia organisms are a special type of bacteria. There are many serotypes of *C. trachomatis.* Serotypes A, B, and C cause trachoma, the most common cause of blindness in the world. Serotypes D through K are sexually transmitted and are responsible for the clinical syndromes described in this section. Serotypes L1 to L3 also are sexually transmitted and are the etiologic agents of lymphogranuloma venereum.

Transmission of chlamydial infection is not uncommon; 60% to 75% of women whose male partners have chlamydial urethritis are infected with *C. trachomatis.* Most women with chlamydial cervicitis are asymptomatic. Thus routine screening of women at risk, as well as notification of female partners of infected men, is of utmost importance in helping to identify most of the women infected with this organism.

Clinical presentation. A large proportion of women with genital chlamydial infection have normal findings on cervical examination. If results of the examination are abnormal, there may be evidence of **mucopurulent cervicitis.** The cervix may be erythematous and edematous with increased friability. The mucopurulent discharge may be evident on visual inspection of the cervical os, or yellowish mucopus may be present on a cotton swab of the os. A Gram's stain of a cervical smear that reveals more than 10 to 20 PMNs per oil-immersion field in the presence of cervical mucus that is free of contamination with vaginal secretions has been shown to correlate with the presence of *C. trachomatis.* Recent data, however, suggest a greater correlation when more than 30 PMNs per oil field are seen.

TREATMENT OF GONORRHEA

Uncomplicated endocervical, urethral, or rectal infection

Ceftriaxone 125 mg IM once or
Cefixime 400 mg PO once

plus

Empiric treatment for *C. trachomatis* with
　　Doxycycline 100 mg PO bid × 7 days or
　　Tetracycline 500 mg PO qid × 7 days or
　　Erythromycin base or stearate 500 mg PO qid × 7 days or
　　Azithromycin 1 gm PO once

The patient allergic to cephalosporins

Spectinomycin* 2 g IM or
Ciprofloxacin† 500 mg PO once or
Norfloxacin† 800 mg PO once or
Ofloxacin† 400 mg PO once

plus

Empiric treatment for *C. trachomatis*

In pregnancy

Ceftriaxone 125 mg IM

plus

Empiric treatment for chlamydia with
　　Erythromycin base 500 mg PO qid × 7 days

Disseminated infection

Initial treatment

Recommended

Ceftriaxone 1 g IV daily

Alternatives

Cefotaxime 1 g IV q8h or
Ceftizoxime 1 g IV q8h or
Spectinomycin 2 g IM q12h

After 24-48 hr of improvement, therapy may be switched to one of the following regimens to complete 7 days of treatment:

Continuing treatment

Recommended

Cefixime 400 mg PO bid

Alternatives

Cefuroxime axetil 500 mg PO bid or
Ciprofloxacin 500 mg PO bid

All regimens should include treatment for *C. trachomatis*

---

* Not adequate in the treatment of pharyngeal infection.
† Cannot be used during pregnancy or in patients younger than 18 years of age.

C. trachomatis is one of the etiologic agents of the **acute urethral syndrome** and is a cause of sterile pyuria in the sexually active woman. The symptoms of dysuria and frequency can be misdiagnosed as a bacterial urinary tract infection. Urethritis may occur without cervicitis. A urethral discharge, meatal erythema, or swelling can be present. A Gram's stained smear of the urethral discharge may reveal more than 10 PMNs per oil field. Infection of Bartholin's ducts may result in abscess formation and a **Bartholin's gland abscess** similar to that seen with gonococcal infection.

Fitz-Hugh–Curtis syndrome was initially thought to be caused only by *N. gonorrhoeae*. Evidence now suggests that *C. trachomatis* may be a more common pathogen. (See preceding discussion of *N. gonorrhoeae* for clinical signs and symptoms.)

Of the cases of **PID** that occur annually in the United States 25% to 50% are due to *C. trachomatis*. Women complain of unilateral or bilateral abdominal pain, which may be mild or severe. Other symptoms include a vaginal discharge, dyspareunia, and menorrhagia. Fever sometimes occurs. Abdominal tenderness may be mild, or peritoneal signs may suggest an acute abdominal process. Pelvic examination may reveal a mucopurulent discharge from the cervical os. Cervical motion tenderness, uterine tenderness, or unilateral or bilateral adnexal tenderness can be detected on palpation. Adnexal swelling, if present, indicates a possible tuboovarian abscess, a condition that must be distinguished from an ectopic pregnancy. Laboratory tests may not be helpful in the diagnosis of PID. An elevated ESR and a leukocytosis can be seen; however, a normal ESR or WBC does not rule out the diagnosis. Specimens for cultures or for other diagnostic tests for chlamydia and gonorrhea must be obtained from the cervical os.

A woman with one episode of PID has a 10% to 20% risk of infertility and a sevenfold increased risk of an ectopic pregnancy should she become pregnant. In addition, some women subsequently experience chronic lower abdominal pain because of scarring and adhesions. Recent studies have demonstrated the presence of *C. trachomatis* DNA in the fallopian tubes of infertile women who have never had a clinical episode of PID. Thus asymptomatic PID caused by *C. trachomatis* may indeed occur.

Chlamydial infection during pregnancy raises special concerns; 8% to 12% of pregnant women are infected with chlamydia. The prevalence approaches 20% to 30% in unwed teen-agers in inner-city regions. An infant passing through an infected birth canal has a 35% to 50% chance of developing chlamydial inclusion conjunctivitis and a 25% risk of developing chlamydial neonatal pneumonia. Because of an increased incidence of chlamydial cervicitis and a decreased incidence of gonorrhea, in many hospitals erythromycin is now instilled into the conjunctival sac of newborn infants instead of 1% silver nitrate. This prevents the development of chlamydial conjunctivitis; however, nasopharyngeal colonization still occurs and infants remain at risk for the development of chlamydial pneumonia.

Inclusion conjunctivitis can develop in the sexually active adult as a result of spread from the genital region. It manifests by an acute, copious mucopurulent discharge and inflamed edematous conjunctivae. Symptoms may be mild, however, and can mimic other causes of bacterial conjunctivitis.

Lymphogranuloma venereum (LGV), which is due to chlamydial serotypes L1 to L3, is endemic in developing countries in Asia, Africa, and South America. Several hundred cases are reported annually in the United States, although the exact incidence is unknown and is likely to be higher. It is seen more commonly in men than women in a ratio of 5:1 inasmuch as women tend to have asymptomatic infection. LGV is a systemic illness that begins 3 days to 3 weeks after exposure. A primary lesion appears on the labia or vagina as a papule, a shallow ulcer, or an erosion. This lesion may go unnoticed. Two to six weeks after exposure the second stage begins with the development of painful, swollen lymph nodes that drain the involved site. One third of lymph nodes become fluctuant (buboes) and go on to suppurate with the development of draining fistulas. Constitutional symptoms may occur. Left untreated, progressive ulceration, fistulae formation, and abnormal lymphatic drainage of the genitals can occur. If the rectum is involved, rectal strictures can develop. In addition to genital ulcerative disease, serotypes L1 to L3 also can cause urethritis, cervicitis, and proctitis.

Treatment of LGV consists of the use of doxycycline, tetracycline, or erythromycin at doses similar to that for other chlamydial infections (see discussion later in this section); however, antibiotics should be taken for 3 to 4 weeks.

Diagnostic tests. Evaluation of potentially infected sites can be accomplished through a variety of diagnostic tests. Regardless of the technology used, it is of paramount importance that the specimen be obtained in the appropriate manner. The organism is an intracellular host parasite, and thus host cells must be obtained. Swabs must be adequately rotated or the site gently rubbed or scraped to obtain an adequate specimen. Obtaining superficial "pus" will give a false-negative result.

Tissue culture always has been the gold standard for diagnosing chlamydial infection. Samples for isolation, which are collected with use of swabs that are not toxic to the tissue monolayer, are placed in transport media. Specimens inoculated onto cell monolayers are evaluated in 48 to 72 hours for evidence of the development of chlamydial inclusions. This technique is expensive to perform and requires the expertise of trained laboratory personnel.

More rapid tests based on newer technologic methods have become available in recent years. Direct monoclonal antibody staining (fluorescent antibody [FA]) is a rapid test that takes 30 to 60 minutes to perform. Samples are placed directly onto a slide, stained with a fluorescein-labeled monoclonal antibody, and evaluated for the presence of fluorescing elementary bodies. The sensitivity rate of this assay depends greatly on the skill of the technician reading the slide. In addition, host cells can be seen on the slide, thus confirming the adequacy of the obtained specimen and eliminating one cause of false-negative results.

The enzyme immunoassay (EIA) is an automated test; thus the need for a highly trained laboratory technician is obviated. Numerous specimens can be processed at one time. The quality of the specimen is especially important because it cannot be assessed as it can with the FA test. Poorly acquired specimens will give false-negative results. In those EIA tests that use polyclonal antichlamydial antibodies, antigen cross-reactivity between lipopolysaccharides of *Acinetobacter, Escherichia coli,* and *Klebsiella* species can occur, causing a false-positive result.

A nonisotopic DNA probe is commercially available. It utilizes a single-stranded DNA that is complementary to the ribosomal ribonucleic acid (rRNA) of *C. trachomatis.* This assay seems to have a high false-positive rate and thus is not recommended for screening purposes, particularly in low- or moderately low-risk groups. The use of polymerase chain reaction (PCR) technology is now being applied to chlamydial detection and is commercially available. The sensitivity is 95% to 98%, with a specificity of 96% to 100% (Table 17-1).

Use of the ligase chain reaction in the detection of chlamydial infection is presently under investigation. Compared with PCR, the ligase chain reaction may have increased sensitivity and specificity. Further studies are in progress.

The diagnosis of LGV is best made by use of serologic evaluation. A complement fixation (CF) titer of at least 1:64 or a microimmunofluorescence (micro-IF) titer of at least 1:512 is consistent with a diagnosis of LGV. The organism can be isolated from a suppurative lymph node or primary lesion, although this is not commonly recommended.

Although serologic evaluation is useful in the diagnosis of LGV, it is not particularly helpful in the diagnosis of the sexually transmitted syndromes caused by *C. trachomatis* serotypes D through K. Only 50% of patients will have CF titers greater than 1:16. The micro-IF test, however, is more sensitive than the CF test because it can measure IgM or IgG to specific serotypes when this information is needed. Few laboratories, however, perform this test.

Practitioners occasionally receive results of Pap smears that show inclusions caused by *C. trachomatis.* The finding of chlamydial inclusions is highly specific; unfortunately, sensitivity is limited. Chlamydial inclusions also can be seen on Giemsa stain of scrapings of the conjunctivae and are helpful in diagnosing active inclusion conjunctivitis.

Choice of therapy. *C. trachomatis* has a long life cycle, and thus therapeutic levels of antibiotics are required at the intracellular site for an extended period. The tetracyclines and erythromycin have been highly successful in the treatment of chlamydial infections. Because these drugs commonly have side effects, including gastrointestinal disturbance, alternative regimens have been sought.

The fluoroquinolones have been shown to have good activity against *C. trachomatis* in vitro. Their high oral bioavailability, long half-life, and high concentration in tissues make them good treatment candidates. Despite these characteristics, few fluoroquinolones have been demonstrated to be clinically effective in the treatment of chlamydial infection. Only one quinolone presently available, ofloxacin, has been shown to be effective against *C. trachomatis,* although various clinical studies have shown a failure rate up to 19%. The fluoroquinolones are contraindicated during pregnancy and in those younger than 18 years of age.

Azithromycin is an azalide with a low minimal inhibitory concentration (MIC) against *C. trachomatis* (<0.06 to 0.25 mg/L) and an ability to achieve high intracellular levels. Thus this antibiotic is highly effective in erradicating the organism. Azithromycin's long half-life of 60 hours allows infrequent dosing. Its one-time dosing schedule makes treatment convenient for patients and significantly decreases the problem of patient noncompliance. At present, however, the cost of azithromycin is higher than that of the tetracyclines or erythromycin, making it less affordable for many patients.

The drug of choice for the treatment of chlamydial infection during pregnancy is erythromycin. The estolate preparation should be avoided in pregnancy. The fluoroquinolones are contraindicated during pregnancy as are the tetracyclines. Although azithromycin is classified as a category B drug, little data are available on its use in pregnancy and at present, it is not recommended in pregnancy (see box, below).

Although some women with PID require hospitalization, many do not. Patients should be hospitalized if the diagnosis is uncertain, if surgical emergencies such as appendicitis or ectopic pregnancy cannot be ruled out, if a tuboovarian abscess is suspected, or if the patient is severely ill, an adolescent, pregnant, HIV-positive, unable to tolerate or comply with an outpatient regimen, or unable or unlikely to return for clinical follow-up within 72 hours. Treatment of PID should consist of an antibiotic regimen adequate to treat gonorrheal as well as chlamydial infection (see box on following page).

All partners of patients with chlamydial infection or PID should be evaluated and treated.

Genital ulcers

Practitioners in primary care practice frequently must treat a woman with genital ulcers. A clinical diagnosis often is based on appearance. When multiple lesions are present, a diagnosis of herpes simplex infection frequently is made; a painless singular lesion is diagnosed as syphilis. Generalizations such as these often can be misleading and result in misdiagnosis and mistreatment. Practitioners must be aware

Table 17-1 Diagnostic tests used for *Chlamydia trachomatis*

	Sensitivity (%)	Specificity (%)
Tissue culture	85	100
Fluorescent antibody test*	75-90	90-99
Enzyme immunoassay	80-90	95
DNA probe	70-92	97-98
Polymerase chain reaction	95-98	99-100

*Sensitivity may vary and depends on the skill of the laboratory technician.

TREATMENT OF UNCOMPLICATED GENITAL INFECTION CAUSED BY *C. TRACHOMATIS*

Doxycycline* 100 mg PO bid for 7 days or
Tetracycline* 500 mg PO qid for 7 days or
Erythromycin base or stearate 500 mg PO qid for 7 days
Alternative agents:
Azithromycin* 1 g PO once or
Ofloxacin[†] 300 mg PO bid for 7 days or

---

*Should be avoided in pregnancy.
[†]Should be avoided in pregnancy and in those younger than 18 years of age.

of the various causes of genital ulcers, incubation periods, and the clinical presentations, both typical and atypical. A thorough understanding of the diagnostic tests available is necessary.

A full discussion of all causes of genital ulcers is beyond the scope of this text (see box at right). Syphilis and herpes simplex are discussed in detail in the next section.

Genital ulcers are a significant risk factor for the transmission of the human immunodeficiency virus (HIV). Practitioners must take the time to discuss this concern with their patients and to consider HIV testing.

Syphilis

One in every 10,000 infants born in the United States has congenital syphilis. The increase in the number of cases of congenital syphilis over the past decade is indicative of an increase in the incidence of primary and secondary syphilis in women of childbearing years and in heterosexual men. Between 40,000 to 50,000 cases of syphilis are now seen annually in the United States, the highest incidence since 1949.

Transmission of the spirochete, *Treponema pallidum,* the causative agent of syphilis, generally occurs through sexual contact, with an acquisition rate of 30% after one exposure to an infected person. Transmission can occur transplacentally, after contact with mucous membranes (including kissing), by transfusion of infected blood, and possibly by direct inoculation. Patients are most infectious during the initial stages; however, potentially they can transmit the organism by sexual contact for an extended period, up to 4 years after acquisition of the disease.

The incubation period is variable, ranging between 3 and 90 days after an exposure. The primary manifestation is the appearance of the chancre, which begins as a macule or

---

TREATMENT OF PELVIC INFLAMMATORY DISEASE

Ambulatory regimen

Cefoxitin 2 g IM plus probenecid, 1 g PO concurrently or
Ceftriaxone 250 mg IM (alternative: ceftizoxime or cefotaxime 500 mg IM
plus
Doxycycline 100 mg PO bid × 14 days
(erythromycin may be substituted for doxycycline)

Inpatient treatment

Cefoxitin 2 g IV q6h or cefotetan IV 2 g q12h
plus
Doxycyline 100 mg IV or PO bid
Continue this combination treatment for at least 4 days and 48 hr after clinical improvement, followed by doxycycline 100 mg PO bid to complete 14 days.

Alternate regimen

Clindamycin 900 mg IV q8h *plus* gentamicin 1.5 mg/kg IV q8h for at least 4 days and 48 hr after clinical improvement.
Continue clindamycin 450 mg PO qid to complete 14 days.
(This regimen has good activity against anaerobes but may be less effective against gonorrheal and chlamydial infection.)

APPROACH TO THE PATIENT WITH GENITAL ULCERS

Causes

Infectious

Treponema pallidum
Herpes simplex virus
Chlamydia trachomatis L1-L3 (lymphogranuloma venereum)
Haemophilus ducreyi (chancroid)
Cytomegalovirus (CMV)
Epstein-Barr virus (EBV)
Human immunodeficiency virus (HIV)
Calymmatobacterium granulomatis (granuloma inguinale)

Noninfectious

Trauma
Fixed drug reactions
Behçet's syndrome
Neoplasm

Evaluation

Syphilis serology*
Tzanck test or direct immunofluorescence for herpes simplex virus (HSV)
Viral culture for HSV
Serology for lymphogranuloma venereum (*H. ducreyi*)
Gram's stain for *H. ducreyi*†

---

*Rapid plasma reagin (RPR), Venereal Disease Research Laboratory (VDRL), or automated reagin test (ART) should be performed initially and, if negative, repeated in 1 and 3 months.
†A scraping of the edge of the ulcer is placed on a slide; after staining, the smear is evaluated for "tracking" of small gram-negative rods.

---

papule, progressively erodes, and forms an ulcer. Although the chancre usually is painless and indurated, it can be painful (particularly when secondarily infected), soft, and nonindurated. Although usually thought of as a single lesion, multiple chancres can be present and can be mistaken for herpes simplex infection. Chancres most commonly occur in the genital region but can be found on other parts of the body as well. When they appear on the cervix or rectum, they often go unnoticed and thus undiagnosed. Painless regional lymphadenopathy sometimes is present. Without treatment, the chancre resolves spontaneously within 5 weeks.

The secondary phase of the infection is due to the hematogenous spread of the organism. The signs of secondary syphilis appear 2 to 8 weeks after the appearance of the chancre and may occur while the chancre is still present. Patients have nonspecific flulike symptoms of malaise, fever, arthralgias, headache, and pharyngitis.

The most characteristic finding on physical examination is the rash of secondary syphilis, which often appears as an erythematous macular or maculopapular rash on various parts of the body, including the palms and the soles. The appearance of the rash can vary from papular, papulosquamous (scaling), to pustular. Classically, the rash is described as nonpruritic, although cases of pruritic rash have been mistaken for dermatologic conditions such as eczema. The rash must be distinguished from a drug allergy (which also can involve the palms and soles), pityriasis rosea, viral exanthems, and other skin conditions. Other findings can include generalized lymphadenopathy, hepatosplenomegaly, and alopecia. Mucous patches may be present in the oral cavity. Condyloma latum in the genital region needs to be distinguished from genital warts (condyloma accuminatum).

Several complications of disseminated infection can occur, including syphilitic meningitis, which manifests as an aseptic meningitis. Ocular involvement can result in the development of uveitis, and the patient complains of a painful, red eye.

Without treatment, the uncomplicated manifestations of secondary syphilis resolve within 2 to 10 weeks and the infection becomes latent. The finding of seropositive syphilis in the absence of clinical manifestations is consistent with the diagnosis of latent syphilis. Within the first 4 years after infection, clinical relapses may occur, with the appearance of lesions at the site of the initial chancre (chancre redux) or other cutaneous manifestations.

Since the use of penicillin for the treatment of syphilis began, the rate of tertiary syphilis, including cardiovascular involvement (coronary disease, aortic aneurysms, aortic insufficiency), gummatous lesions, and neurosyphilis, has been significantly reduced. Recently, however, an increase in the number of cases of neurosyphilis has occurred, particularly in patients with HIV infection. The manifestations of neurosyphilis vary. Syphilitic meningitis, which often occurs early after infection, can mimic the symptoms of bacterial meningitis. Meningovascular syphilis most often occurs within the first few years after infection and can result in a cerebrovascular accident, or stroke. The later manifestations of neurosyphilis, such as general paresis (mental status changes) and tabes dorsalis (loss of position and vibration sensation), occur after many years. In addition, asymptomatic involvement of the nervous system can persist for many years.

Diagnostic tests. *T. pallidum* is a tightly coiled helical cell that is too small to be visualized by the use of light microscopy. Thus darkfield microscopy, an easy and excellent method of diagnosing primary syphilis, is needed. The newer models of office microscopes can be made into a darkfield microscope with the addition of an attachment to the condenser. Serous material from the abraded ulcer is placed in a normal saline wet mount and evaluated under the darkfield microscope for the presence of the typical, motile, coiled organisms. Results of a darkfield test will be negative if the patient has applied local antiseptics to the chancre or has recently taken systemic antibiotics. When possible, initial negative results should trigger repeat tests on 2 or 3 consecutive days.

Serologic findings can be used to diagnose primary syphilis, although nontreponemal test results may be negative in up to 40% of patients at the time they seek evaluation for a syphilitic chancre. Thus initial seronegativity should prompt consideration of repeat syphilis testing in 3 to 4 weeks in a patient with a genital ulcer.

The nontreponemal tests—the Venereal Disease Research Laboratory (VDRL), rapid plasma reagin (RPR), and the automated reagin test (ART)—are nonspecific tests used to screen patients for syphilis. They are nonspecific tests because they detect a group of antibodies directed against the cardiolipin antigen found on both *T. pallidum* and host

cells, which increases in many inflammatory conditions such as systemic lupus erythematosus and tuberculosis. Thus confirmation of the diagnosis of syphilis must be made by a positive treponemal test result—for example, the fluorescent treponemal antibody absorption test (FTA-ABS), the microhemagglutination–*Treponema pallidum* assay (MHA-TP), the *Treponema pallidum* immobilization test (TPI), and the hemagglutination treponemal test for syphilis (HATTS), which assay for the presence of antibody to the organism *T. pallidum.*

At all stages of infection the treponemal tests are more sensitive than the nontreponemal tests. In most patients, the treponemal test results remain positive despite therapy, although 15% to 25% of patients treated during the primary stage may revert to seronegativity after 2 to 3 years. A patient's response to therapy can be determined by following nontreponemal tests, the titer of which should decline after treatment.

The diagnosis of neurosyphilis can be difficult. It is made on the basis of clinical manifestations and a lumbar puncture that reveals one or more of the following findings in the cerebrospinal fluid (CSF): an elevated white cell count (>4 WBC/mm^3), an elevated protein level, or positive VDRL finding. However, a negative CSF VDRL result has been shown in up to 50% of patients with neurosyphilis, and thus does not rule out the diagnosis of neurosyphilis. New techniques to aid in the diagnosis of neurosyphilis, such as PCR, are being investigated.

Women with any sexually transmitted infection should be screened for syphilis. Pregnant women are in a special category. *All* pregnant women, regardless of their sexual history, should be screened for syphilis early in the first trimester. Women at high risk for acquiring syphilis and those who reside in communities where the prevalence of syphilis is high should be retested during the second and third trimesters and at the time of delivery.

Choice of therapy. The treatment of syphilis requires the presence of adequate antibiotic levels for an extended period of time. Thus a penicillin with a long half-life, such as benzathine penicillin, must be used (see the following box).

Pregnant women should be treated with the appropriate dose of penicillin for their stage of syphilis. Erythromycin no longer is recommended to treat syphilis in the penicillin-allergic pregnant female because it fails to eradicate fetal infection. Instead, pregnant women with syphilis who have a history of penicillin allergy should undergo skin testing to the major and minor penicillin determinants. If skin testing results are positive, desensitization to penicillin should be considered in consultation with an expert and undertaken in an appropriate intensive care setting.

All patients with primary or secondary syphilis should receive follow-up with serologic testing every 3 months for at least 2 years after treatment to ensure that the titer of the nontreponemal test falls appropriately. Patients with primary syphilis should show a fourfold decline in the nontreponemal titer within 3 months, and 97% of treated patients should have a negative nontreponemal test result within 2 years. The greater the duration of untreated infection, the greater the time needed to achieve seronegativity. Patients with latent syphilis should be tested every 6 months. The possibility of treatment failure should be considered in patients with latent

TREATMENT OF SYPHILIS

Early syphilis (primary, secondary, or duration less than 1 year)

Benzathine penicillin G 2.4 million units IM × once (CDC recommendation)

Benzathine penicillin G 2.4 million units IM weekly × 2 wk (Mass. State Department of Health)*

Alternative regimens—nonpregnant penicillin-allergic patient

Doxycycline 100 mg PO bid × 2 wk

Tetracycline 500 mg PO qid × 2 wk

Erythromycin 500 mg PO qid × 2 wk

Latent syphilis (duration greater than 1 year or unknown)

Benzathine penicillin G 2.4 million units IM weekly × 3 wk†

Alternative regimen—nonpregnant penicillin-allergic patient

Doxycycline 100 mg PO bid × 30 days†

Tetracycline 500 mg PO qid × 30 days†

---

*Many experts recommend the longer treatment regimen.

†Neurosyphilis should be ruled out by physical examination. A lumbar puncture should be considered in all patients.

Patients treated with alternative antibiotics such as tetracy-cline or doxy-cycline should undergo a lumbar puncture before treatment.

---

syphilis if there is an increase in the nontreponemal titer or if a fourfold decline does not occur within 12 to 24 months in those patients with a titer of 1:32 or more. Failed treatment of syphilis at any stage requires that the patient be retreated. A lumbar puncture to rule out asymptomatic neurosyphilis must be performed before retreatment.

Pregnant women require closer follow-up, with monthly serologic testing for syphilis repeated throughout the pregnancy. Retreatment should be considered in a pregnant woman if a fourfold decrease in the nontreponemal titer does not occur within a 3-month period.

All partners of infected patients should be appropriately evaluated and treated when indicated. Partners of patients with primary and secondary syphilis who have been exposed within the preceding 90 days should be screened for syphilis but should be treated empirically for possible infection at the time that they are seen. Partners exposed more than 90 days earlier should be screened for syphilis as should partners of patients with latent syphilis. Partners of patients with syphilis of unknown duration with titers of 1:32 or more should be screened and treated presumptively for possible infection.

Genital ulcer disease is a risk factor for HIV infection. Because there is an increased incidence of HIV infection in patients with syphilis, and vice versa, all patients with syphilis should be counseled on HIV infection, and HIV testing should be considered. HIV infection generally does not affect syphilis serology, although nontreponemal titers have been shown to be falsely negative in some patients with HIV. Thus biopsy specimens of skin rashes and lesions that suggest syphilis should be obtained in HIV-positive patients with initial negative syphilis serology. Standard regimens for syphilis have been noted to fail in patients with HIV, and the optimal treatment for syphilis in these patients is unclear. A lumbar puncture should be performed in the HIV-positive patient with syphilis of more than 1 year's duration or when the duration of infection is unknown. At present, some authorities believe that examination of the CSF should be considered to rule out asymptomatic neurosyphilis before treating HIV-positive patients with early syphilis. After treatment, serologic status should be followed monthly. Retreatment should be considered if the nontreponemal titer does not decrease by two dilutions within 3 months for primary and secondary syphilis or if a rise in titer occurs.

Herpes simplex infection

Herpes simplex virus (HSV) is a member of the herpesvirus group, which includes HSV 1, HSV 2, cytomegalovirus, Epstein-Barr virus, varicella-zoster virus, and Herpesvirus 6. These viruses have the ability to establish a latent state within host cells and to cause recurrent disease. Genital herpes simplex virus infection is due predominantly to HSV 2, although 5% to 30% of cases can be caused by HSV 1. Serologic studies have shown that 30% to 60% of young adults have antibody to HSV 2. Transmission of HSV 1 and 2 occurs through close contact with someone who is shedding the virus in secretions, from skin lesions, or from mucous membranes. The incubation period ranges from 2 to 7 days.

Clinical presentation. Most patients with primary infection have nonspecific systemic symptoms, including fever, chills, malaise, headache, and myalgias and appear to have "the flu." Pain or itching may accompany or precede the appearance of the herpetic lesions, which can involve the labia, vagina, cervix, perineum, buttocks, urethra, and bladder. More than 70% of women with genital lesions have cervical involvement as well. Lesions begin as papules or vesicles on an erythematous base that go on to ulcerate and heal spontaneously. Often, vesicles will not be present at the time a woman is examined because vesicles located on the labia become macerated and open to form an ulcer. Lesions may manifest as small linear fissures and can be mistaken for trauma or irritation. Tender inguinal lymphadenopathy often is present. Patients may report vaginal discharge and can be misdiagnosed as having vaginitis. With involvement of the urethra and bladder, patients may experience symptoms of urethritis or cystitis.

Symptoms may last for 2 days or for more than 3 weeks. Symptoms associated with primary infection may be milder in women who have previous antibody to HSV 1. Viral shedding from genital lesions may persist for 12 days. Lesions can take up to 3 weeks to heal. Complications of genital HSV infection include sacral radiculopathy that results in urinary or fecal retention. Aseptic meningitis may occur. HSV proctitis can occur in women who have rectal intercourse.

Symptoms do not develop in all women who acquire genital HSV infection. Serologic studies have shown that 60% of women infected with HSV 2 may not have symptomatic outbreaks and may be unaware of their infection. These patients can remain asymptomatic or manifest their first episode of clinical genital herpes infection later in life.

Recurrent outbreaks occur most frequently during the first year after infection. Some patients never experience a clinical recurrence, whereas others have frequent recurrences, some as often as once or twice each month. Many women have recurrences around the time of menses. The degree of severity of the recurrence varies from patient to patient; 50% of women experience prodromal symptoms, including tingling, itching, or pain at the site of the eruption as early as 30 minutes to 2 days before an outbreak. Recurrences generally are milder and shorter in duration than the primary infection. A clinical "recurrence" may occur without a previous primary outbreak.

Asymptomatic cervical viral shedding can occur in the absence of vulvar lesions. The true rate of asymptomatic shedding has yet to be determined. In one study asymptomatic shedding of HSV occurred in 11% to 23% of women screened intermittently during the first year after clinical presentation. The true rate is likely to be higher.

Lesions of genital HSV infection in the immunocompromised patient (those on a regimen of chemotherapy or infected with HIV) may appear as progressively enlarging ulcers, several centimeters in size. They can be present for weeks to months. Reactivation of infection occurs more frequently in these patients. Prolonged treatment with antiviral agents is needed for complete healing to occur.

Issues regarding neonatal HSV infection often arise during the counseling of women with herpes. Neonatal infection with HSV can occur when an infant passes through an infected birth canal, resulting in significant neonatal morbidity and mortality. Fortunately, this uncommon event is estimated to occur in 1 in 3000 to 20,000 live births. The greatest risk to the neonate occurs in those women who contract a primary infection around the time of delivery; 10% of pregnant women are at risk of contracting primary HSV 2 infection from their HSV 2–seropositive partners. Infection of the neonate can occur during a recurrent outbreak, but this is a less frequent event. Particular care needs to be taken at and around the time of delivery for those women with a previous history of HSV infection, a history of exposure to a male partner with HSV, or evidence of active lesions that on examination suggest HSV infection.

Diagnostic tests. Viral culture is the gold standard test used to confirm the clinical diagnosis of herpes simplex infection. The fluid from a vesicle or a rubbing of the base of an ulcer can be obtained with a Dacron swab, placed in transport media, and forwarded to the tissue culture laboratory. Cultures may show positivity in 1 to 2 days but may take several days if the inoculum is low. The sensitivity of culture is over 90% if vesicles are present but falls to 30% when lesions are crusted.

The Tzanck test, which can be performed while the patient is in the office, provides rapid results. A scraping taken from the base of an unroofed vesicle or from the base of an ulcer is placed on a slide and then stained with Wright or Giemsa stain. The presence of multinucleated giant cells is diagnostic of a herpetic infection, but this finding does not differentiate between infection with HSV or varicella-zoster. The sensitivity of the Tzanck test ranges from 40% to 80% depending on the skill of the person reading the slide. An alternative to the Tzanck test is the use of direct immunofluorescence staining of the prepared slides.

Serologic testing may be helpful in diagnosing primary infection when there is evidence of conversion from seronegativity to seropositivity. Cross-reactivity between antibody to HSV 1 and HSV 2 occurs with many currently used tests. For patients who have had previous HSV 1 infection, a diagnosis of primary HSV 2 infection is difficult to make with present serologic techniques. If determination of specific antibody for HSV 1 and HSV 2 is needed, this can be requested from laboratories capable of assaying these antibodies with the use of Western blot technology.

Choice of therapy. At present there is no cure for genital HSV infection. The antiviral agent acyclovir has been shown to be helpful in the treatment of primary HSV infection. Topical acyclovir can decrease the duration of local symptoms but does not reduce the systemic symptoms often associated with primary infection. It should not be placed intravaginally and thus does not affect cervical lesions and cervical viral shedding. Oral acyclovir, however, decreases systemic and local symptoms, viral shedding, and time to healing and thus is of greater benefit in the treatment of primary infection. A dose of 200 mg orally five times daily for 10 days is recommended in women who are not immunocompromised. A higher dose of 400 mg five times daily until healing is complete is needed in HIV-positive patients. Intravenous acyclovir (5 mg/kg every 8 hours) is necessary when patients require treatment for complications of HSV infection such as urinary retention.

Oral acyclovir, when initiated at the onset of a clinical recurrence, decreases time of viral shedding and duration of lesions. It may help in decreasing duration of local symptoms, although this has been less well established. Treatment of recurrent outbreaks should be started during the prodrome, or with the onset of lesions. Dosing regimens include oral acyclovir 200 mg five times daily for 5 days, 400 mg three times daily for 5 days, or 800 mg twice daily for 5 days.

When taken daily, oral acyclovir has been shown to be effective in decreasing clinical recurrences by up to 75%. Most patients with recurrent infection do not require ongoing treatment with acyclovir; some benefit from intermittent therapy begun at the onset of an outbreak. Suppressive daily therapy should be reserved for those patients with frequent or severe recurrences or for those patients whose emotional well-being may require a break from recurrences. Regimens include oral acyclovir 200 mg three times daily or 400 mg twice daily. Suppressive therapy has been approved for up to 5 years. Information is being gathered on the safety of longer treatment regimens. Suppressive therapy should be discontinued on an annual basis to determine if the pattern and number of recurrences have decreased with time, as is often the case. Patients should be informed that a severe outbreak is likely to occur immediately after discontinuation of suppressive therapy. Patients should be aware that despite the use of suppressive therapy with acyclovir, both symptomatic outbreaks, as well as asymptomatic viral shedding, can still occur.

Newer antiviral therapies are being evaluated in the treatment of genital HSV infection. Famcyclovir recently has been approved in the treatment of herpes zoster infection. Its use in genital HSV infection is under investigation. The active metabolitic of famcyclovir has been shown to have a longer half-life than does acyclovir, and thus less frequent doses are effective.

Despite adequate therapy, some women have an extremely difficult time accepting the diagnosis of genital HSV infection. Patients often feel stigmatized. They may have concerns regarding new relationships and are fearful of being rejected. They may become depressed. In addition to making a diagnosis and prescribing medication, each medical provider is obligated to offer all patients appropriate education and counseling regarding HSV infection, as well as appropriate supportive help to those patients in need.

SAFER SEX PRACTICES

Despite all the public awareness of STD and HIV infection, some patients continue to place themselves at increased risk of infection. What can a practitioner do to help patients decrease the likelihood of acquiring an STD? Women must be educated to avoid sex with a casual contact. Numbers of sexual partners must be limited. Patients should know their partners well before entering into a sexual relationship. Frank and explicit discussions should be encouraged between partners regarding previous sexual contacts, history of previous STD, and use of recreational drugs. Couples considering a sexual relationship can be counseled together regarding modes of transmission of STD and incubation periods. Testing for STD in both partners can be performed at the same time.

The practitioner must stress the need for condoms to be used during each and every sexual encounter. Although condoms may decrease transmission rates, women must understand the correct use of condoms and their limitations. Not all condoms are alike, and different brands have been shown to be more effective in preventing transmission of HIV than others. (A rating list can be obtained from the CDC). Petroleum-based lubricants can react with latex, causing breakage of the condom. In addition to condoms, spermicide that contains nonoxynol-9 should be used to decrease transmission of some infections. The female condom may be helpful to those women whose male partners refuse to comply with condom use.

Aside from abstinence, there are no totally safe sex practices. Medical providers, however, must play an active role in educating their patients about safer sex practices and in decreasing their risk for STD.

BIBLIOGRAPHY

Augenbraun MH, McCormack WM: Current treatment options for *Neisseria gonorrhoeae* and *Chlamydia trachomatis* anogenital infections, *Curr Opinion Infect Dis* 6:5, 1993.
Brunham RC et al: Mucopurulent cervicitis—the ignored counterpart in women of urethritis in men, *N Engl J Med* 311:1, 1984.
Bryson YJ et al: Risk of acquisition of genital herpes simplex virus type 2 in sex partners of persons with genital herpes: a prospective couple study, *J Infect Dis* 167:942, 1993.
Bryson YJ et al: Treatment of first episodes of genital herpes simplex virus infection with oral acyclovir: a randomized double-blind controlled trial in normal subjects, *N Engl J Med* 308:916, 1983.
Campbell LA et al: Detection of *Chlamydia trachomatis* deoxyribonucleic acid in women with tubal infertility, *Fertil Steril* 59:45, 1993.
Centers for Disease Control: 1993 sexually transmitted diseases treatment guidelines, *MMWR* 42 (RR-14)1, 1993.
Centers for Disease Control: Recommendations for the prevention and management of *Chlamydia trachomatis* infections, *MMWR*, 42 (RR-12):1, 1993.
Douglas JM et al: A double-blind study of oral acyclovir for suppression of recurrences of genital herpes simplex virus infection, *N Engl J Med* 310:1551, 1984.
Frenkel LM et al: Clinical reactivation of *herpes simplex* virus type 2 infection in seropositive pregnant women with no history of genital herpes, *Ann Intern Med* 118:414, 1993.
Holmes KK et al, editors: *Sexually transmitted diseases*, ed 2, New York, 1990, McGraw-Hill.
Hook EW III, Marra CM: Acquired syphilis in adults, *N Engl J Med* 326:1060, 1992.
International Society for STD Research: Proceedings of the tenth international meeting, *Sex Transm Dis* 21:S1, 1994.
Ison CA: Laboratory methods in genitourinary medicine: methods of diagnosing gonorrhea, *Genitourin Med* 66:453, 1990.
Iwen PC, Blar TMH, Woods GI: Comparison of the Gen-Probe PACE 2 system in cervical specimens, *Am J Clin Pathol* 95:578, 1991.
Kihlström E, Danielsson D: Advances in biology, management and prevention of infections caused by *Chlamydia trachomatis* and *Neisseria gonorrhoeae*, *Curr Opinion Infect Dis* 7:25, 1994.
Kostman JR, Stull TL: Molecular techniques in the diagnosis of sexually transmitted diseases, *Curr Opinion Infect Dis* 5:5, 1992.
Koutsky LA et al: Underdiagnosis of genital herpes by current clinical and viral-isolation procedures, *N Engl J Med* 326:1533, 1992.
Martin DH et al: A controlled trial of single dose of azithromycin for the treatment of chlamydial urethritis and cervicitis, *N Engl J Med* 327:921, 1992.
Mertz GJ et al: Risk factors for the sexual transmission of genital herpes, *Ann Intern Med* 116:197, 1992.
Norgard MV: Clinical and diagnostic issues of acquired and congenital syphilis encompassed in the current syphilis epidemic, *Curr Opinion Infect Dis* 6:9, 1993.
Romanowski B et al: Serologic response to treatment of infectious syphilis, *Ann Intern Med* 114:1005, 1991.
Straus SE et al: Suppression of frequently recurring genital herpes: a placebo-controlled double-blind trial of oral acyclovir, *N Engl J Med* 310:1545, 1984.
Toomey KE, Barnes RC: Treatment of *Chlamydia trachomatis* genital infection, *Rev Infect Dis* 12(S6):S645, 1990.

Section VII

NEPHROLOGY

18 Acute Dysuria and Urinary Tract Infections

Anthony L. Komaroff

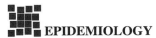 **EPIDEMIOLOGY**

One quarter of all adult women experience an episode of acute dysuria each year. It is one of the most common clinical problems seen by clinicians in the developed Western nations. Our knowledge about the causes, diagnosis, and treatment of dysuria has been expanded greatly in the past 20 years.

The classic teaching about women with dysuria without symptoms or signs of acute pyelonephritis has included the following:

1. Such patients have bacterial cystitis.
2. The responsible microorganisms are almost always the gram-negative coliform bacteria.
3. The single most important test is a urine culture.
4. Greater than 100,000 bacteria/ml (a positive culture) constitute proof of a urinary infection.
5. Patients with positive cultures should receive 7 to 14 days of treatment with any of several relatively benign antimicrobial agents.

Recent evidence seriously challenges these assumptions.

This chapter summarizes this evidence and proposes a scheme for categorizing the condition of women with acute dysuria. The discussion pertains only to the problem of dysuria in an office practice as it is most commonly seen and is not applicable to dysuria in adolescents or nosocomial urinary tract infections. (For a more detailed discussion on urinary tract infection during pregnancy see Chapter 60.) Chronic dysuria is discussed in Chapter 19.

CAUSES OF ACUTE CYSTITIS

The clinical syndrome called acute cystitis is now recognized to consist of at least six different conditions, each of which is managed differently. These conditions are summarized in Table 18-1. Each category has important differences from the rest with respect to diagnostic testing, treatment, and prognosis.

Specific conditions included in acute cystitis

Subclinical pyelonephritis. Acute pyelonephritis is clinically distinct from cystitis. However, another common and related entity is not: **subclinical pyelonephritis.** Several studies indicate that among women with the presenting complaint of dysuria without symptoms or signs suggesting acute pyelonephritis, up to 30% in most office settings (and up to 80% of women in emergency rooms serving indigent populations) nevertheless have *upper* tract infection, or at least tissue invasion of the urinary tract.

Such patients have subclinical pyelonephritis. Subclinical pyelonephritis may produce minimal symptoms, may smolder for long periods of time, and may be difficult to eradicate. Indeed, the unrecognized presence of subclinical pyelonephritis may explain, in retrospect, why some studies of treatment for cystitis have shown 10% to 15% initial failure rates and high rates of recurrent infection.

At present there is no practical way of accurately diagnosing subclinical pyelonephritis at the time of the initial visit. Clinical features can increase the likelihood of this condition, as discussed later, but easily available diagnostic tests are of little help. For practical purposes, subclinical pyelonephritis is diagnosed after the fact, by the detection of treatment failure on follow-up urine cultures. Although patients with subclinical pyelonephritis usually have a prompt symptomatic response, relapse may occur in 10% to 50% after the traditional 7-day to 14-day course of treatment, even when the organism is sensitive to the antimicrobial used. The optimal antimicrobial regimen for subclinical pyelonephritis has not been established.

Lower urinary tract bacterial infection. Many women with acute dysuria have lower tract bacterial infection. That is, they have no clinical or laboratory evidence of acute or subclinical pyelonephritis but have some degree of bacteriuria. The only specific physical examination abnormality seen with any frequency is suprapubic tenderness. Usually patients with lower tract bacterial infection have a positive culture. However, in recent years it has become apparent that in 30% to 50% of women who clinically have cystitis the urine culture is negative by the traditional criteria: either bacterial pathogens are found in concentrations less than 100,000/ml or the urine culture is sterile. Some observers postulated that low-count bacteriuria was caused by infection involving only the urethra and the periurethral glands, and not the bladder (the **acute urethral syndrome**). It now is clear that the bladder and urethra usually are infected simultaneously but that there simply is a lower concentration of organisms.

Thus the traditional definition of significant bacteriuria—greater than 10^5 organisms per milliliter of urine—has been

Table 18-1 Categorization of women with acute dysuria

Category	Location			Colony count[†]	Pyuria[‡]	Effectiveness of antimicrobial treatment
	Upper tract*	Bladder	Urethra			
Acute pyelonephritis	+	+	±	>100,000[§]	+	+
Subclinical pyelonephritis	+	+	±	>100,000[§]	+	+
Lower urinary tract bacterial infection	—	+	+	>100	+	+
Chlamydial urethritis	—	—	+	0-100	+	+
Gonococcal urethritis	—	—	+	0-100	+	+
Other urethritis	—	—	+	0-100	+	+
No recognized pathogen	—	?	+	0-100	—	—
Vaginitis	—	—	—	0-100	—	+

Modified from Komaroff AL: *N Engl J Med* 310:368, 1984.
* Or tissue-invasive infection.
§ True in almost all patients.
† Colony count in colonies per milliliter.
‡ Pyuria typically is seen with gonorrheal and trichomonal urethritis but is not typically seen with monilial urethritis.

shown to be of little value in *symptomatic* cases. In fact, it is preferable to use 10^2 to 10^3 organisms per milliliter ml of urine as the threshold for defining significant bacteriuria. The work of Stamm and his colleagues has shown that dysuric women with such low colony counts really are infected. They found that 46% of acutely dysuric women with negative clean-voided specimen cultures nevertheless were truly infected; that is, urine obtained by suprapubic aspirate or catheter specimen, and hence free of contamination, contained bacteria—but in concentrations less than 100,000/ml. Not only *Escherichia coli* but also *Staphylococcus saprophyticus* and *Proteus* spp., can produce low-count bacteriuria and real infection. (The threshold of greater than 10^5 organisms per milliliter of urine is still useful in identifying women with asymptomatic bacteriuria, the purpose for which the threshold was originally intended.) Moreover, randomized, controlled trials have shown that patients with low-count bacteriuria benefit from antibacterial therapy.

E. coli accounts for 70% to 90% of community-acquired urinary tract infections (UTIs) in women. In most recent studies, *S. saprophyticus*—a coagulase-negative, novobiocin-resistant organism that sometimes is identified imprecisely by microbiology laboratories as *S. albus* or *S. epidermidis*—is the second most frequent cause of lower tract infection. Thus *S. saprophyticus* should never be dismissed as a contaminant when it grows in pure culture from a urine specimen. (*S. aureus* is only an occasional urinary pathogen, and hematogenous spread to the urinary tract from some other septic focus should always be considered with *S. aureus* UTIs.) The other gram-negative coliform bacteria, group B streptococci and the enterococci, are the other urinary pathogens that are seen with some frequency in community-acquired UTIs. Diphtheroids, alpha-hemolytic streptococci, and lactobacilli—organisms that often are grown from a clean-voided urine specimen—are rarely if

ever true urinary pathogens. Although uncomplicated UTIs in women usually involve one organism, polymicrobial UTIs may occur more often than had been thought.

Chlamydial urethritis. *Chlamydia trachomatis* urethritis accounts for 5% to 20% of cases of dysuria, and its presence may be especially likely when urine cultures are sterile. Risk factors that increase the likelihood of chlamydial infection include (1) a sexual partner with recent urethritis, (2) a new or recent sexual partner, (3) the stuttering onset of symptoms over a period of days rather than abruptly, and (4) the absence of hematuria.

Gonococcal urethritis. Gonococcal urethritis may account for up to 10% of cases of dysuria among inner-city women. Pyuria is usually present. Even in the absence of symptoms suggesting pelvic inflammatory disease, there may be purulent discharge from the urethral or cervical os. Risk factors that increase the likelihood of gonococcal urethritis are (1) a history of gonorrhea, (2) a recent sexual partner with urethral discharge, and (3) being an indigent inner-city women.

Other urethral infections. *Trichomonas vaginalis, Candida albicans,* and *herpes simplex* virus all can occasionally cause urethritis. Other associated symptoms and signs (e.g., cervicitis or vaginitis, vesicular eruptions) can suggest the diagnosis. Trichomonal urethritis typically produces pyuria, whereas candidal urethritis usually does not. Laboratory testing and standard treatment regimens for these organisms are discussed in Chapters 17 and 42.

No recognized pathogen. Despite extensive studies, no recognized pathogen can be found in some women with dysuria. Often these patients also do not have pyuria and do not respond to antimicrobial treatment. This raises the possibility that they suffer from a urethritis caused by noninfectious factors. Postmenopausal, estrogen-deficient women may develop dysuria secondary to desiccation of the urethral and vaginal mucosa. Therefore the patient with acute dysuria, but without pyuria, ordinarily should not be given immediate treatment with antimicrobial agents.

Vaginitis. Vaginitis is an important and often neglected cause of dysuria and "negative" cultures. A patient with vaginitis may not mention vaginal symptoms as a presenting complaint, stating only that she has dysuria perhaps because some patients are embarrassed to speak of symptoms affecting the genital organs. Vaginitis may be the most common cause of dysuria in some settings. Dysuria caused by vaginitis typically is perceived as an external sharp somatic type of pain, caused by the impact of the stream of urine as it hits the irritated labia. Dysuria associated with urethritis, on the other hand, typically is perceived as an internal, burning visceral type of pain. Also, urinary frequency and urgency are very unusual in patients with vaginitis.

Recurrent dysuria

The preceding discussion involves the management of a single episode of dysuria. Every clinician knows, however, that some women are prone to recurring episodes of dysuria from repeated UTIs. The repeated episodes of UTI often seem to "cluster" during several-month periods of apparently increased susceptibility.

Recurrent UTIs traditionally have been categorized as either reinfections with a new organism or relapses with the same organism. Reinfections generally indicate lower tract infection and account for most recurrences. Relapses are formally defined as occurring within 14 days of completing treatment, although many clinicians regard recurrent infection with the same organism occurring up to 2 months later as being relapses. Relapses are important to distinguish from reinfections because they generally signify uneradicated upper tract infection.

There is one practical problem that frequently arises in distinguishing a reinfection from a relapse. Although a recurrent infection with most bacterial species (e.g., a recurrent infection with enterococcus) indicates a relapse, a recurrent infection with *E. coli* may be either a reinfection with a new strain or a relapse from the old, uneradicated strain of *E. coli*. Relapse with the same strain can be assumed if both the former and the current isolate have an identical antibiogram. Another way of recognizing a relapse with *E. coli* involves the biotype, the pattern of sugar fermentations that is used by most bacteriology laboratories to characterize bacterial species. The biotype usually is written as a seven-digit number on the urine culture report. If at least five of the seven digits are identical, the patient is very likely to have a relapse with the same strain of *E. coli*.

In the past 15 years, research has begun to identify the pathogenetic mechanisms that explain recurrent infection, at least for coliform infection. Most of the insights have involved *host cell* factors. Vaginal and periurethral colonization has long been identified as the first step in UTI. From the periurethral "beachhead," organisms can begin their ascending spread up the urethra and into the rest of the urinary tract.

Several factors seem to facilitate periurethral colonization. The uroepithelial cells of girls and women prone to recurrent infection have glycolipid receptors that increase the adherence for *E. coli*; these receptors, which are present in greater

numbers even when these persons are uninfected, are genetically determined. Women who carry a gene that promotes the display of ABO and Lewis blood group antigens on the surface of epithelial cells are protected against recurrent UTIs, perhaps because these blood group antigens prevent bacteria from binding to the cell-associated receptors.

There also appear to be bacterial virulence factors that influence the course of UTI. A special kind of pili (*Gal-Gal pili* or *P fimbriae*) is almost always found in patients with acute pyelonephritis and urosepsis and in about 50% of patients with cystitis, but is seen in only about 20% of fecal isolates. Another virulence factor is the ability of *E. coli* to produce hemolysin, which appears to enhance injury of uroepithelial cells after the bacteria attach to them.

Certain behavioral factors also influence recurrence. Sexual intercourse transiently increases the concentration of bladder bacteria by as much as tenfold. Intercourse encourages the retrograde movement of periurethral organisms up the urethra and into the bladder. Women who deliberately defer urination when they first experience the need to urinate, because responsibilities in the workplace or at home make that necessary, may be at greater risk for recurrent infection. Use of a contraceptive diaphragm more than doubles the risk of developing UTIs. The spermicidal jelly (as well as spermicidal foam and condoms, but not oral contraceptives) dramatically increases vaginal and periurethral colonization. Oral contraceptive users have an increased frequency of asymptomatic bacteriuria, but it is not clear if this association is independent of sexual activity.

Sometimes, recurrent dysuria may be caused by chlamydial, gonorrheal, trichomonal, monilial, or herpetic urethritis. The natural history and proper management of these conditions are poorly understood. Interstitial cystitis, a disorder of uncertain cause, diagnosed by cystoscopic examination, occasionally causes recurrent cystitis (see Chapter 19).

 EVALUATION OF ACUTE DYSURIA

How does the clinician approach a woman with acute dysuria (an initial or a recurrent attack) on the basis of the preceding information? Clinical data and easily available laboratory data allow the clinician to categorize the individual patient's condition with reasonable, although imperfect, accuracy.

History and physical examination

The clinical history guides the extent of the physical examination and laboratory testing (Table 18-2). The severity and duration of dysuria—urgency and frequency—should first be assessed.

The patient should always be asked about symptoms of vaginal discharge and irritation. Such symptoms strongly suggest vaginal infection; therefore a pelvic examination should be performed.

Risk factors suggestive of subclinical pyelonephritis should be sought: a known underlying urinary tract abnormality, diabetes mellitus or other conditions or therapies producing an immunocompromised state, a history of urinary tract infections in childhood, documented relapsing UTI in the past, symptoms for 7 to 10 days before seeking care (this also suggests chlamydial urethritis), three or more

Table 18-2 Key factors in the history and physical examination

History	Physical examination
History of vaginal discharge or pelvic pain or infertility	Pelvic examination
History of prior UTIs	
History of diabetes	
Immunocompromised host	
Signs and symptoms of pyelonephritis	Examine for costovertebral-angle tenderness

UTIs in the past year, or acute pyelonephritis in the past year. Subclinical pyelonephritis also may be more likely in indigent, inner-city residents.

The symptoms and signs of acute pyelonephritis—fever, rigors, flank pain, and costovertebral-angle tenderness, nausea and vomiting—reliably indicate the presence of acute pyelonephritis.

If by history one suspects chlamydial infection (see Chapter 17 for a more detailed discussion on diagnosis of chlamydial infection), a pelvic examination is warranted. Chlamydial urethritis often is seen in combination with chlamydial cervicitis, an entity characterized by mucopurulent cervical discharge and edematous areas on the ectocervix. Although chlamydial cervicitis is generally responsive to the same therapeutic regimen as chlamydial urethritis, it is theoretically possible that patients with cervicitis are more likely to have indolent chlamydial pelvic infection; these patients might benefit from a careful history relating to infertility and might be counseled explicitly about returning for medical care in the case of symptoms that might suggest pelvic inflammatory disease.

Diagnostic tests

Urinalysis and urine culture. Patients with likely acute or subclinical pyelonephritis should have urinalysis (including Gram's stain) and urine culture performed (see box, below). If the patient's temperature is greater than 101° F or the patient appears toxic, blood cultures should be obtained. A Gram's stain of uncentrifuged urine is considered indicative of greater than 100,000 bacteria per milliliter of urine if any organisms are seen. Gram's stain of sediment may be preferable because even in acute pyelonephritis there can be fewer than 100,000 organisms per milliliter of urine.

DIAGNOSTIC TESTS

Urinalysis
Urine culture
If indicated (patient toxic, temperature >101° F), obtain blood cultures
Gram's stain of uncentrifuged urine: if positive for organisms, indicates urine bacterial colony >100,000/ml
Chlamydial screening if clinically indicated
Urethral culture for gonorrhea if clinically indicated

If there is no evidence to suggest any of the aforementioned conditions, the "diagnosis by exclusion" is still lower tract bacterial infection— which accounts for 60% to 70% of patients with dysuria. In such patients a urinalysis provides immediately useful information because patients who have pyuria will likely require only single-dose/short-course therapy. A urine culture is of less value in patients with presumptive lower tract bacterial infection, except in those patients with one or two previous symptomatic urinary infections during the past year. In such patients the possibility of relapse (and hence of upper tract infection) needs to be pursued by comparing the results of past urine cultures with a current culture.

Chlamydial screening. In patients with the risk factors for chlamydial urethritis (described earlier) chlamydial screening during pelvic examination should be performed.

Screening for gonorrhea. In patients with risk factors for gonococcal urethritis (described earlier) a urethral culture for gonorrhea should be obtained. When purulent discharge from the urethral (or cervical) os is present, it should always undergo a Gram's stain: a positive Gram's stain result is a reliable indicator of gonorrhea and should lead to immediate treatment. When urethral or cervical discharge is not present, which can occur in gonococcal urethritis, the urethra should be swabbed. The swab needs to be inserted several millimeters into the urethra. The tip of a regular cotton swab is too large; therefore a calcium-alginate-tip swab should be used. The swab should be plated promptly on an appropriate medium (Thayer-Martin agar, or New York City agar) that has been prewarmed to room temperature.

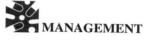 **MANAGEMENT**

Choice of therapy

Uncomplicated lower urinary tract bacterial infection
Single-dose therapy. In women with uncomplicated lower urinary tract bacterial infection a single dose of oral therapy is nearly as effective as the traditional 7- to 14-day course in patients with lower tract infection (Table 18-3).

The benefits of single-dose/short-course therapy are as follows:

1. A lower rate of medication side effects, particularly vaginal candidiasis, rash, and diarrhea
2. A reduced problem with noncompliance
3. A lower rate of emergence of resistant bacteria
4. Lower cost, as summarized elsewhere.

The single-dose regimen that appears to be most effective is trimethoprim-sulfamethoxazole (TMP-SMX), 160 mg-800 mg (one double-strength tablet) or 320 mg-1600 mg (two double-strength tablets) by mouth. In patients allergic to sulfonamides, trimethoprim alone (200 mg) or amoxicillin (2 or 3 g) is effective.

Short-course therapy. The best 3-day regimens are TMP-SMX 160 mg-800 mg twice daily or (if allergic to TMP-SMX) amoxicillin 500 mg four times daily.

Three-day short-course regimens appear slightly more effective than single-dose regimens in eradicating bacteriuria and are still associated with low rates of adverse drug reactions.

Table 18-3 Treatment for uncomplicated urinary tract infection

Medication	Dosage
Single-dose treatment	
Trimethoprim-sulfamethoxazole (TMP-SMX)	160 mg-800 mg (one double-strength tablet) or 320 mg-1600 mg (two double-strength tablets)
TMP	200 mg
Amoxicillin	2-3 g
Short-course treatment	
TMP-SMX	160 mg-800 mg bid for 3 days or
Amoxicillin	500 mg 4 times a day for 3 days

Acute pyelonephritis. The treatment of acute pyelonephritis is still a controversial area (Table 18-4). When the patient has a community-acquired case of acute pyelonephritis, is younger than 55 years of age, is not diabetic, has no known underlying urinary tract abnormality, has no past history of acute pyelonephritis, is not pregnant, and is not very sick (temperature less than 101° F, normotensive, no rigors), outpatient management with oral antimicrobial agents is preferable. If gram-negative bacilli are present, treatment with TMP-SMX for 14 days is effective and clearly preferable to ampicillin. An alternative is to give one parenteral injection of gentamicin in the office or emergency room followed by these oral antimicrobials. If the Gram's stain result suggests enterococcal infection, ampicillin or amoxicillin is the treatment of choice.

When the patient with community-acquired acute pyelonephritis is older than 55 years of age, has a known or suspected urinary tract abnormality, is experiencing a recurrence of acute pyelonephritis, is diabetic or is immunocompromised in some way, or is very sick, she should be hospi-

talized and started on intravenous therapy. If the patient is having a recurrent UTI, particularly if a prior episode has occurred within the past 6 months, the results of the urine culture and sensitivities from the prior episode (along with the Gram's stain of the current urine) should guide therapy. When the patient is having her first case of gram-negative bacillary acute pyelonephritis, intravenous TMP-SMX may be the preferred first-line treatment, having been found superior to the combination of intravenous gentamicin and ampicillin in one trial. Given current community-resistance patterns, neither intravenous ampicillin nor amoxicillin are any longer acceptable first-line therapy for acute pyelonephritis caused by gram-negative bacilli. Amoxicillin is the treatment of choice for suspected enterococcal infection. If the Gram's stain finding does not clearly indicate gram-negative bacilli or enterococci, or if it suggests a polymicrobial infection, treatment with a quinolone is indicated. Of the quinolones, ciprofloxacin may be the preferred agent; it provides broad-spectrum coverage against both gram-negative and most gram-positive organisms, is particularly good in the rare case of community-acquired *Pseudomonas* UTI, has excellent tissue penetration even in patients with renal failure, and has relatively little toxicity. If the patient refuses hospitalization, treatment with oral ciprofloxacin is probably the best option except if the patient is pregnant or considering pregnancy. If one is unable to obtain a clear menstrual history to ensure that the patient is not pregnant or if the patient is not practicing appropriate contraception, an alternative treatment is advised.

Treatment of pyelonephritis during pregnancy is covered in Chapter 60.

Subclinical pyelonephritis. For suspected subclinical pyelonephritis, immediate treatment for 10 to 14 days should be initiated before the culture result returns (see box on the next page). Pooled data from several trials indicates that 10 days of therapy with TMP-SMX may be the most effective, having only a 1% failure rate (in contrast, single-dose TMP-SMX had a 16% failure rate). There are no good randomized studies comparing alternative antimicrobial regimens in

Table 18-4 Treatment options for acute pyelonephritis

Type	Management
Uncomplicated	*Gram-negative bacteria* TMP-SMX 160 mg-800 mg bid for 14-day course Gentamicin IM in office (or emergency room) followed by TMP-SMX for 14 days *Enterococcus* Ampicillin 500 mg q8h Amoxicillin 500 mg q8h

Complicated
  Toxic (temperature >101° F, Hypotensive or rigors)
  Diabetic patient
  Immunocompromised state
  Older than age 55 years
  Known underlying urinary tract abnormality
	Gram-negative bacteria
	TMP-SMX 160 mg-800 mg IV q12h or
	Gentamicin 1 mg/kg of body weight IV q8h and ampicillin 500 mg IV q8h
	Enterococcus
	Amoxicillin 500 mg IV q8h
	Unclear pathogen or polymicrobial
	Ciprofloxacin 500 mg PO q12h or 200-400 mg IV q12h

Pregnancy	See Chapter 20

Modified from Stamm W, Hooton T: *N Engl J Med* 329:1328, 1993.

patients with subclinical pyelonephritis. When the urinalysis indicates gram-positive cocci in chains, indicating the likelihood of enterococcal infection, ampicillin or amoxicillin would be the treatment of choice. When gram-negative bacilli are seen, the treatment of choice is more controversial. This subject is discussed later in the section on use of new antimicrobial agents.

Every effort should be made to obtain a follow-up culture 2 to 4 days following the end of therapy, because patients with subclinical pyelonephritis may be particularly prone to relapse. In patients with recurrent infection caused by the same organism (relapsing infection), treatment for 6 weeks may be indicated, although this is another poorly studied area. In patients who experience relapse after a 6-week course of therapy, diagnostic studies to look for a cause of the persistent infection (e.g., intravenous pyelogram and retrograde studies) are indicated.

Chlamydial urethritis. Patients with chlamydial urethritis, as well as those with low-count bacteriuria, usually will achieve clinical and microbiologic cure by treatment with doxycycline, 100 mg twice a day for 10 days (see box, below). Less-expensive regimens of tetracycline hydrochloride, 500 mg four times daily for 7 days, or erythromycin, 500 mg four times daily for 7 days, probably would be equally effective. Because chlamydial infections tend generally to be hard to eradicate, it is unlikely that single-dose therapy would be effective. Also, patients with chlamydial urethritis should be counseled to return promptly if dysuria recurs. Partners of these patients need to be treated, and the

clinician should counsel the woman to abstain from sexual intercourse until the partner has been treated.

Gonococcal urethritis. For gonococcal urethritis diagnosed by a positive finding on Gram's stain or culture should be treated with ceftriaxone, 250 mg IM once plus oral doxycycline, 100 mg twice daily for 7 days. Again, partners need to be treated, and the woman needs to abstain from sexual intercourse until completion of the partner's therapy.

RECURRENT URINARY TRACT INFECTION
Diagnostic tests

A single episode of relapsing infection, as previously defined, or three or more infections in the past year with the same organism (persistent infection), can reasonably be pursued with intravenous pyelography (IVP) and cystoscopic examination.

IVP and cystoscopy are less clearly indicated when patients have three or more infections in the past year with different organisms (reinfections). Three studies of the yield of IVP and cystoscopic examination in women with recurrent UTI have been conducted in recent years, but unfortunately none clearly distinguishes relapse from reinfection in the patients studied. On the basis of other studies it is likely that most of the patients studied were experiencing reinfections. The three studies found that IVP revealed a surgically correctable lesion in fewer than 1% of patients, although cystoscopic examination revealed a correctable lesion (e.g., urethral diverticulum) in up to 4% of patients. Because these studies suggest a somewhat higher yield from cystoscopic examination, without the radiation exposure and dye risk of IVP, cystoscopy is recommended before IVP, although this may not be a choice because urologists often insist on an IVP before performing cystoscopy. When the patient has experienced three or more reinfections in a year, a referral to a urologist should be considered, although the yield of urologic evaluation still will be low.

Although IVP has been the standard imaging technique for years, one recent study indicates that contemporary ultrasound is at least as accurate. In another study, 158 consecutive patients (men and women) with UTI were simultaneously evaluated by use of both IVP and ultrasonography combined with a plain abdominal radiograph. Ultrasonography detected an early bladder tumor that had been missed on IVP and clarified the nature of several renal cysts seen on IVP; IVP detected one case of mild papillary necrosis that had been missed by ultrasonographic examination.

Management
Choice of therapy

Antibiotic prophylaxis. Antimicrobial prophylaxis can be recommended in a woman who has had three or more bacterial infections in a year. Antimicrobial prophylaxis greatly reduces the frequency of recurrent infection during the period of prophylaxis and for a few months thereafter. TMP-SMX, one half of a regular-strength tablet (40 mg-200 mg) each day, appears to be the most effective regimen (Table 18-5). In women whose recurrences are clearly related to sexual activity, the one-time use of an antimicrobial at the time of intercourse also is demonstrably effective, and may be a more attractive option for many women than taking a

Table 18-5 Prophylactic therapy for recurrent urinary tract infections

Medication	Dosage
TMP-SMX	One half regular-strength tablet (40 mg-200 mg) PO qd
	If associated with sexual activity, take at time of intercourse
TMP-SMX	One half regular strength tablet (40 mg-200 mg) or one regular strength tablet 80-400 mg PO
Cephalexin	250 mg PO qd

daily antimicrobial dose. Oral TMP-SMX 40-200 mg (half of a single-strength dose) to 80-400 or oral cephalexin 250 mg is effective. A third approach, for women with recurrent infections who are not on a daily prophylaxis regimen, is to keep an antimicrobial in the medicine cabinet: most women with recurrent UTI can reliably identify symptoms indicating that a recurrent UTI is beginning and can quickly eradicate the infection by the immediate use of antimicrobial agents.

New antimicrobial agents. In most patients with community-acquired UTIs, including acute pyelonephritis, there is no need to consider using as initial therapy a variety of antimicrobial agents introduced in recent years. Several newer agents with excellent coverage of gram-negative bacilli—third- and fourth-generation cephalosporins and aztreonam—provide relatively poor coverage of gram-positive pathogens and are not more effective than TMP-SMX. Other newer agents with good gram-negative and gram-positive coverage—amoxicillin-clavulanate, the extended-spectrum penicillins, and the quinolones—also are not superior as first-line agents to TMP-SMX. Community isolates in the 1980s were sensitive to TMP-SMX in about 95% of cases, to first-generation cephalosporins in about 85% to 90% of cases, and to ampicillin in about 65% of cases. All of the newer antimicrobial agents are much more expensive than TMP-SMX. More important, unnecessary use of these newer agents will encourage the development of resistance to these drugs among organisms in the community. In my judgment, the quinolones have a place in the treatment of acute pyelonephritis, as already discussed, but not in the other kinds of bacterial UTIs. This could change if resistance to TMP-SMX becomes more common in the 1990s. There is currently no convincing evidence that the new macrolides, such as azithromycin and clarithromycin, are superior to tetracyclines, doxycycline, or erythromycin in treating suspected chlamydial infection.

BIBLIOGRAPHY

Brunham RC et al: Mucopurulent cervicitis—the ignored counterpart in women of urethritis in men, *N Engl J Med* 311:1, 1984.

Fihn SD et al: Association between diaphragm use and urinary tract infection, *JAMA* 254:240, 1985.

Fowler JE, Pulaski ET: Excretory urography, cystography, and cystoscopy in the evaluation of women with urinary-tract infection: a prospective study, *N Engl J Med* 304:462, 1981.

Guze LB, Beeson PB: Observations on the reliability and safety of bladder catheterization for bacteriologic study of the urine, *N Engl J Med* 255:474, 1956.

Johnson JR, Stamm WE: Urinary tract infections in women: diagnosis and treatment, *Ann Intern Med* 111:906, 1989.

Komaroff AL: Acute dysuria in women, *N Engl J Med* 310:368, 1984.

Komaroff AL et al: Management strategies for urinary and vaginal infections, *Arch Intern Med* 138:1069, 1978.

Latham RH, Running K, Stamm WE: Urinary tract infections in young adult women caused by *Staphylococcus saprophyticus, JAMA* 250:3063, 1983.

Norrby SR: Short-term treatment of uncomplicated lower urinary tract infections in women, *Rev Infect Dis* 12:458, 1990.

O'Hanley P et al: Gal-Gal binding and hemolysin phenotypes and genotypes associated with uropathogenic *Escherichia coli, N Engl J Med* 313:414, 1985.

Rubin RH et al: Single-dose amoxicillin therapy for urinary tract infection: multicenter trial using antibody-coated bacteria localization technique, *JAMA* 244:561, 1980.

Schaeffer AJ, Jones JM, Dunn JK: Association of in vitro *Escherichia coli* adherence to vaginal and buccal epithelial cells with susceptibility of women to recurrent urinary-tract infections, *N Engl J Med* 304:1062, 1981.

Sheinfeld J et al: Association of the Lewis blood-group phenotype with recurrent urinary tract infections in women, *N Engl J Med* 320:773, 1989.

Souney P, Polk BF: Single-dose antimicrobial therapy for urinary tract infections in women, *Rev Infect Dis* 4:29, 1982.

Spencer J, Lindsell D, Mastorakou I: Ultrasonography compared with intravenous urography in investigation of urinary tract infection in adults, *Br Med J* 301:221, 1990.

Stamm WE, Hooton TM: Management of urinary tract infections in adults, *N Engl J Med* 329:1328, 1993.

Stamm WE et al: Causes of the acute urethral syndrome in women, *N Engl J Med* 303:409, 1980.

Stapleton A et al: Postcoital antimicrobial prophylaxis for recurrent urinary tract infection, *JAMA* 264:703, 1990.

Tolkoff-Rubin NE, Rubin RH: Ciprofloxacin in management of urinary tract infection, *Urology* 31:359, 1988.

Wong ES et al: Management of recurrent urinary tract infections with patient-administered single-dose therapy, *Ann Intern Med* 102:302, 1985.

19 Chronic Bladder Disorders and Chronic Dysuria

David H. Nichols and Linda Brubaker

The pathophysiologic mechanisms of lower urinary tract disorders are varied, encompassing many neurologic, anatomic, hormonal, and infectious causes. Similarly, symptom complexes may vary somewhat for each disorder, although they may overlap among different disorders. Imagining a continuum between purely sensory symptoms (i.e., dysuria, dyspareunia, urgency) and purely motor symptoms (incontinence) may simplify the initial approach. Most symptom complexes fall somewhere between the two but show a predominance of one symptom type. Loosely, then, urinary tract disorders may be categorized as primarily sensory or primarily motor.

This chapter considers the primarily sensory disorders: those associated with chronic irritative symptoms of dysuria, frequency, urgency, and, occasionally, pelvic pain and dyspareunia. Lower urinary tract bacterial infections and urethritis, which sometimes cause chronic irritative symptoms, are discussed in greater detail in Chapter 18. Evaluation of dysuria in pregnancy is discussed in Chapter 60. Chapter 34 addresses the predominantly motor disorders (incontinence) and prolapse.

CAUSES OF CHRONIC IRRITATIVE SYMPTOMS
Interstitial cystitis

Interstitial cystitis is a poorly understood disorder characterized by chronic irritative voiding symptoms, sterile urine, and bladder mucosal abnormalities on cystoscopic examination. Until recent years, research on the epidemiology, etiology, and treatment of this sometimes disabling condition has been sparse. Among urologists, interest and expertise in the management of interstitial cystitis have been limited to a small number of specialty centers.

What is known of the epidemiology of interstitial cystitis is based on case series from specialty clinics. The prevalence of the condition is unknown. The disorder is diagnosed most frequently in white women. Women with interstitial cystitis have a higher frequency of immunopathologic abnormalities (sensitivities or allergies to medications, allergic rhinitis, asthma, food allergies, and rheumatoid arthritis) and irritable bowel syndrome than do control subjects. Hysterectomy is also more common among women with the disorder.

The symptoms most commonly reported by women with interstitial cystitis include urgency, frequency, pelvic pain or pressure, bladder spasms, dyspareunia, burning, nocturnal awakening by pain, and a sensation of incomplete voiding. Symptoms typically wax and wane; they may worsen during the premenstrual phase of the cycle.

Studies of the etiology of interstitial cystitis suggest that it is a syndrome of bladder inflammation initiated by a variety of stimuli, possibly including bacterial infection, autoimmune processes, or contact irritants. Pathologic findings include mild edema and hyperemia of the mucosa, with characteristic petechiae (extravasations of blood from small capillary defects) or, less commonly, ulcerations. Mast cell proliferation within the mucosa is often seen.

Diagnosis of interstitial cystitis is based on the history and results of urodynamic studies and cystoscopic examination. Urodynamic evaluation, performed to exclude involuntary bladder contractions and other abnormalities, usually shows decreased bladder capacity and hypersensitivity. Cystoscopic examination should be accompanied by hydrodistention of the bladder, which is sometimes therapeutic. Bladder biopsy is performed to exclude malignancy.

Bacterial cystitis

Occasionally, persistent bacterial infection of the bladder may manifest as chronic dysuria. Diagnosis generally is straightforward, based on the presence of pyuria and growth of bacterial culture (see Chapter 18).

Urethritis

Urethritis, an inflammatory condition of the urethra, may be present with or without infectious agents. Pyuria usually is present on urinalysis, but standard bacterial urine cultures are negative. Infectious agents include trichomonads, gonococci, and yeast. With urethritis alone, in the absence of cystitis, culture may show low levels of the causative bacteria, yet the infection may be significant.

Chronic urethritis that is not associated with an infectious agent and that is refractory to empiric antibiotic therapy should be evaluated further. Environmental allergens, similar to those causing vulvitis, and dietary exacerbants, including cranberry juice, should be considered as potentially offending agents.

Urethral syndrome

Although the symptoms of urethral syndrome are the same as those that characterize other sensory disorders of the urinary tract (dysuria, frequency, urgency, and pelvic pain), urethral syndrome occurs on a chronic basis and without any obvious cause. Urethral syndrome is a diagnosis of exclusion, to be made following a search for infectious agents and environmental allergens. It is possible that urethral burning is a form of chronic pain mediated by small, unmyelinated sympathetic nerves.

The physical examination in women with urethral syndrome reveals a tender urethra, and urodynamic evaluation (a urethral pressure profile) may show spasm of the urethral voluntary sphincter.

Urethral diverticulum

Although an unusual finding, a clinician should suspect a urethral diverticulum in any patient with a history of recurrent lower urinary tract infections, even those without a classic triad of dribbling, dysuria, and dyspareunia. As many as 70% of patients with a urethral diverticulum report a combination of dysuria, frequency, and urgency, whereas a smaller number complain of dribbling, dyspareunia, or hematuria.

Postmenopausal atrophy

Because the tissues of the distal third of the urethra are estrogen-sensitive, lack of estrogen in postmenopausal women may cause chronic irritative symptoms. Atrophic changes also may predispose the woman to recurrent bacterial urinary tract infections.

Trauma

Inadequate lubrication during sexual activity may result in trauma to the lower urinary tract.

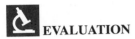 **EVALUATION**

History

The physician can learn a great deal about any patient's urinary problems by taking a thorough history. The clinician must appreciate the patient's perception of the problem and must determine how much the symptoms bother her, how long they have been occurring, whether they are recurrent or progressive, how they relate to her general overall health, what has relieved them in the past, and what tends to aggravate the condition.

The 24-hour voiding diary (urolog) is helpful in reviewing fluid intake and output. A sample diary is shown in Fig. 19-1. The urolog can be helpful in determining exacerbating medications, activities, or fluid intake. The woman's use of common bladder irritants (including alcohol, caffeine, and carbonated drinks) should be ascertained. The clinician should assess the relationship of symptoms to any sexual activity and to the type of contraceptive method used. Menopausal status should be noted.

The clinician also should investigate the effects that any previous pregnancies and deliveries have had on both urinary function and bowel function and should ask about any prior surgery.

Physical examination

A pelvic examination is an important part of the evaluation of chronic urinary symptoms. If the urethra is infected, physical examination may demonstrate the exudation of pus through the meatus on urethral stripping with the index and middle finger in the vagina, and inspection or palpation may reveal an anterior vaginal mass or sacculation, indicative of a urethral diverticulum. The clinician should evaluate the endocrine state of the vaginal mucosa, noting any atrophy or loss of rugal folds. Any tenderness beneath the base of the bladder should be noted and the adequacy of pelvic supports assessed.

DAILY VOIDING DIARY (UROLOG) Starting at midnight								

A Name_____ Date_____

Time	Intake		Amount voided	Leaking?			Urge to void?	
	Amount	Type		Small	Medium	Large	Weak	Strong

B COMMON BLADDER IRRITANTS

Alcoholic beverages
Carbonated beverages
Chocolate
Coffee (including decaffeinated coffee) and tea
Fruits and fruit juice (especially citrus and cranberry)
  Exceptions: apricots, papaya, pears, watermelon
Nutrasweet
Tomatoes
Vitamin B complex

Fig. 19-1 *A*, Daily voiding diary. A typical bladder voiding diary (urolog) indicates the amount and circumstances regarding intake and leakage episodes. *B*, Bladder irritants frequently reported by patients.

Diagnostic tests

The initial evaluation includes a urinalysis (to detect hematuria and pyuria and to assess specific gravity) and urine culture (to rule out chronic bacterial infection). Subsequent testing is guided by the results of these tests. Detection of microhematuria requires that a malignant condition be excluded by means of urine cytology, cystopic examination, and intravenous pyelography or renal ultrasound. Detection of pyuria should prompt a search for infectious causes of urethritis, including chlamydial infection (detectable by immunofluorescence techniques from urethral swabs) and gonorrheal infection (detectable by cultures of the urethra or cervix).

Referral for cystoscopic examination and urodynamic testing is necessary in some cases. If interstitial cystitis is suspected by history, cystoscopic examination is appropriate to rule out other disorders and to look for the bladder mucosal abnormalities associated with this disease. Urethroscopic examination sometimes is indicated for the evaluation of chronic urethral inflammation, urethral diverticula, a hypoestrogenic state within the urethra, and urethral tone. Urodynamic testing may be useful in selected cases if incontinence is associated with irritative symptoms (see Chapter 34).

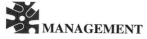

MANAGEMENT

Interstitial cystitis

Initial management of suspected interstitial cystitis in the primary care setting emphasizes patient education and self-care. A diary of food and fluid intake and voiding habits is useful to identify dietary precipitants for symptom flares. (Figure 19-1 lists common bladder irritants.) In women with minimal pain symptoms, bladder retraining may be undertaken to increase the interval between voiding episodes (described in Chapter 34).

To establish the diagnosis of interstitial cystitis, referral for cystoscopic examination with hydrodistention of the bladder is necessary. This procedure has therapeutic value in some patients but also has the potential to exacerbate symptoms.

There are few controlled studies of medical therapy for interstitial cystitis. Antihistamines, anticholinergics (such as propantheline bromide [Pro-Banthine] and oxybutinin), and tricyclic antidepressants have been tried with limited success. Sodium pentosanpolysulfate (Elmiron) is an oral analog of heparin in investigational use that has demonstrated effectiveness in relieving symptoms of interstitial cystitis.

Specialty referral for intravesical therapy is needed for more severe cases of interstitial cystitis. Intravesical dimethyl sulfoxide (DMSO) is the only drug therapy approved by the Food and Drug Administration (FDA). Other intravesical therapies under study include silver nitrate and sodium oxychlorosene (Clorpactin). Intravesical administration of heparin, which has antiinflammatory and surface-protective actions on the bladder mucosa, sometimes is used for maintenance therapy.

Major surgical interventions have little if any place in the management of interstitial cystitis. Augmentation cystoplasty, ileal reservoirs, and nerve resection are experimental procedures that should be reserved for patients whose quality of life warrants such drastic measures. Interstitial cystitis may occur coincidentally in a patient with a demonstrable cystocele or another form of genital prolapse. Correction of the hernial defect is unlikely to have any effect on the symptoms produced by the interstitial cystitis.

Psychosocial support and self-care regimens have been useful in the care of women with interstitial cystitis, including self-administered bladder instillations, nutritional supplements, bladder retraining, and relaxation training.

Urethral diverticula

There is no need to treat asymptomatic diverticula, although the physician should tell the patient about the condition so that she may seek periodic reevaluation of it. Symptoms may include dysuria, dribbling, and dyspareunia. The treatment of symptomatic diverticula is transvaginal surgical excision, which is not without risk of urethral stenosis, fistula, or urinary incontinence.

Other conditions

For discussion of management of cystitis and urethritis, see Chapter 18; and of postmenopausal atrophy, see Chapter 36.

BIBLIOGRAPHY

Bavendam TG: A common sense approach to lower urinary tract hypersensitivity in women, *Contemp Urol* 4:25, 1992.

Hanno PM: Diagnosis of interstitial cystitis, *Urol Clin North Am* 21:63, 1994.

Koziol JA: Epidemiology of interstitial cystitis, *Urol Clin North Am* 21:7, 1994.

Murakami S et al: Strategies for asymptomatic microscopic hematuria: a prospective study of 1034 patients, *J Urol* 144:99, 1990.

Ratliff TL, Klutke CG, McDougall EM: The etiology of interstitial cystitis, *Urol Clin North Am* 21:21, 1994.

Sant GR, LaRock DR: Standard intravesical therapies for interstitial cystitis, *Urol Clin North Am* 21:73, 1994.

Testa GM: The urethral syndrome—why what we do works, or doesn't, *Med J Aust* 157:549, 1992.

Whitmore KE: Self-care regimens for patients with interstitial cystitis, *Urol Clin North Am* 21:121, 1994.

20 Renal Insufficiency

Elizabeth Ginsberg

Renal insufficiency can have a tremendous impact on the endocrinologic, reproductive, and sexual function of women. This chapter focuses on the various effects in women of acute renal insufficiency, chronic renal insufficiency, dialysis, and renal transplantation, as well as pregnancy in the women with renal dysfunction.

APPROACH TO THE PATIENT WITH AN ABNORMAL CREATININE LEVEL

Determining an abnormal creatinine level

There are no prospective studies that follow women with mild elevations in the serum creatinine level to determine the incidence of clinically significant renal failure. Neither are there established recommendations for routine screening of renal function in the nonpregnant woman.

Many factors can affect the measurement of blood urea nitrogen (BUN) and creatinine. The BUN is affected by protein intake, corticosteroids, and renal perfusion. Serum creatinine reflects muscle catabolism, dietary protein intake, and urinary excretion. Because of this, the normal creatinine level is greater in men because of their greater muscle mass. In addition, the serum creatinine level is increased (and therefore urine creatinine decreased) by medications such as cimetidine and trimethoprim. This may be due partially to the competition for renal tubular secretion. Cephalosporins and acetoacetate can artifically raise measurement of serum creatinine because these are agents measured by colorimetric assays (Table 20-1).

When assessing these values, one must keep in mind that women have smaller muscle mass than men, and therefore in the normal state, they have lower serum creatinine levels. Thus for each level of creatinine, there is potentially more compromise of the glomerular filtration rate (GFR) for women than for men, necessitating further evaluation for underlying etiologic factors. This is also important when one is considering the use of potentially nephrotoxic medications such as aminoglycosides. A serum creatinine value

of 1.5 may be normal in a man but reflects renal insufficiency in a woman and would be an indicator for adjusting the dose of a nephrotoxic agent. Table 20-2 gives the laboratory reference ranges for renal function tests in women compared with men.

Evaluation of an abnormal creatinine level

Once an elevation in creatinine has been established on serial testing (even if mild), an estimation of the GFR should be obtained by ordering a 24-hour urine collection for creatinine clearance. Because little data are available on the natural history of abnormal creatinine levels in women, there are no standard recommendations for follow-up. Generally, follow-up monitoring of BUN, creatinine, and electrolytes is performed every 3 to 4 months until stable, then annually. Evaluation for potential causes must be pursued when renal insufficiency is diagnosed, because the probability of renal insufficiency progressing to renal failure depends on the etiology identified. Causes and procedures for evaluation appear in the box on the following page. Evaluation of an abnormal creatinine value in the pregnant woman is addressed later in this chapter.

ACUTE RENAL FAILURE
Epidemiology and etiology

A recent population-based study reported the incidence of acute renal failure (ARF) to be 172 per 1 million adults. ARF is defined as serum creatinine greater than 6.56 mg/dl. Prostatic disease has accounted for the largest proportion of the cases. After excluding these cases, men still have been found to be 2.8 times more likely to have renal failure than are women. The incidence increases with age, regardless of gender. The overall survival of patients with renal failure has been found to be 54% at 3 months and 34% at 2 years, which in part is attributed to the number of elderly persons in the geographic area studied. The etiologic factors in ARF are somewhat different in women than in men. Table 20-3 highlights the causes of ARF more commonly seen in women.

Table 20-1 Factors affecting creatinine measurement

Effect on creatinine level	
Increase	**Decrease**
Cimetidine	Muscle wasting
Trimethoprim	
Increased muscle mass	
Cephalosporins*	
Acetoacetate*	

Modified from Wyngaarden J, Smith L: *Cecil's textbook of Medicine* ed 19, Philadelphia, 1988, WB Saunders.
*Falsely increases measurement because of assay.

Table 20-2 Laboratory reference range for renal function tests in men and women

Test	Reference range	
	Female	**Male**
Creatinine:		
serum or plasma	0.5-1.1 mg/dl	0.6-1.2 mg/dl
Creatinine clearance:	88-128 ml/min/	97-137 ml/min/
serum or plasma plus urine	1.73 m^2	1.73 m^2
Uric acid: serum	2.6-6.0 mg/dl	3.5-7.2 mg/dl

ABNORMAL CREATININE VALUES IN WOMEN

Causative factors

Vascular depletion
Nephrotoxic drugs
Obstruction
Sepsis and infection
Contrast dyes
Hypertension
Metabolic

Evaluation techniques

Serial serum BUN and creatinine levels every 3-4 mo
24-hour urine collection for creatinine clearance (with
  simultaneous serum creatinine measurement)
Serum electrolyte levels if creatinine value is rising

Definition

The definition of ARF is a fall in GFR that occurs over a period of hours or days.

Clinical presentation

History and physical examination. In addition to obtaining a complete history and performing a physical examination, there are some particular areas to address, which are summarized in the box, below.

Diagnostic tests. The general diagnosis of renal insufficiency is made by evaluation of serum BUN, creatinine, and electrolyte values. Evaluation of the 24-hour urine collection will allow calculation of the BUN and creatinine clearance and an analysis of urinary protein losses. Plotting the serial creatinine levels and creatinine clearance values over time on a graph in the office may be helpful in determining the rate of renal function loss. Examination of the urinary sediment may be helpful as well and, although not pathognomonic for specific disease processes, may indicate possible etiologic factors. The key findings for the urinary sediment, although not consistently seen in all situations, appear in Table 20-4 (For a more detailed discussion, see Isselbacher reference.)

**EVALUATION OF WOMAN WITH
ACUTE RENAL FAILURE**

Key factors in history

Medical history
Pregnancies past and present
Medications

Key factors in physical examination

Volume status
Evidence of volume overload

Diagnostic tests

BUN, creatinine
Electrolytes and uric acid
Urinalysis
Renal ultrasound (for suspected obstruction)

Table 20-3 Causes of acute renal failure in women

	General causes	Additional causes more prevalent in women
Prerenal	Hypovolemia	Severe hyperemesis
	Hemorrhage	Placenta previa
		Placental abruption
	Sequestration of fluid into extra-cellular compartment	Ovarian hyperstimulation syndrome
	Other	Fatty liver of pregnancy
	Cardiovascular	
	Decreased cardiac output	Peripartum cardiomyopathy
	Hepatorenal syndrome	Severe preclampsia
Renal	Vascular diseases (thrombotic microangiopathy)	
	Vasculitis	Lupus nephritis
		Scleroderma
	Toxin-induced (tubular injury)	Antibiotics
		Aminoglycocides
		Pregnancy related:
		Septic abortion
		Hemorrhage
		Placenta previa
		Placental abruption
		Uterine rupture
		Eclampsia/preeclampsia
	Cortical necrosis	Placental abruption
		Placenta previa
Postrenal		Pyelonephritis
	Extrarenal obstruction	Incarcerated uterus
	Extraureteral obstruction	Cervical carcinoma
		Ovarian carcinoma
		Endometriosis
		Complication with pelvic surgery (hysterectomy)

Specific types

In general, history, physical, and serum/urine renal indices can be helpful in differentiating among the various types of ARF. The urinary findings in ARF help to differentiate between specific types: prerenal versus renal (Table 20-5).

Prerenal. The most common cause of ARF in women is the same as in men, acute tubular necrosis (ATN) secondary to shock. Hemorrhagic and septic complications of pregnancy and gynecologic surgery can lead to ARF but are not common. When hemorrhage occurs in women of childbearing age who have no other underlying disease, and leads to renal failure, the prognosis for recovery of renal function is good for ATN but poorer for cortical necrosis. The pathologic diagnosis of ATN occurs in the setting of hemorrhage because of extreme volume loss, hypotension, and the resulting hypoperfusion of the kidneys. Hemodialysis is indicated if the BUN value is greater than 120 to 140 mg/dl and the serum creatinine level is greater than 8 to 10 mg/dl or if uremic symptoms—specifically hyperkalemia, acide-

Table 20-4 Urinary sediment and causes of renal disease

Findings	Differential diagnosis
Hematuria Red cell casts Proteinuria	Glomerular disease Vasculitis
Renal tubular cells Tubular granular/epithelial casts	Acute renal failure: acute necrosis
Pyuria White cell casts No/mild proteinuria	Tubular Interstitial disease Obstruction Pyelonephritis
Hematuria Pyuria No casts	Glomerular disease Obstruction, infarction Interstitial
Hematuria alone	Vasculitis Glomerular disease
Pyuria alone	Pyelonephritis

Modified from Isselbacher: *Harrison's principles of interal medicine*, ed 13, New York, 1994, McGraw Hill.

mia, pericardial effusion, to or volume overload—are present. Renal function in this setting generally begins to improve in 4 to 20 days.

Renal. Nonpregnancy-related causes are beyond the scope of this chapter, but pregnancy causes are covered later in the text (See Isselbacher reference for a thorough discussion of renal causes of ARF.)

Postrenal. In postrenal ARF, azotemia can occur only if the outflow of both kidneys is obstructed. In women bilateral ureteral obstruction is rare but is seen with malignant tumors of the pelvis, such as advanced cervical cancer (see Table 20-3). Ultrasonography is an excellent method to diagnose the level and potential cause of obstruction and to evaluate dilation of the ureters and renal collecting systems. Computed tomography (CT) scanning can provide similar information but is poor at delineating pathologic conditions of the uterus and ovaries and is more costly. Treatment initially is directed at bypassing the obstruction, initially with retrograde stents placed by use of cystoscopy under fluoroscopic examination. If this is unsuccessful, then drainage of the urine proximal to the block must be performed percutaneously.

Management

The underlying cause of the renal failure and electrolyte abnormalities should be treated as promptly as possible by

Table 20-5 Urinary findings in acute renal failure

Index	Prerenal	Renal (acute tubular injury)
Urine osmolality mOsm/kg H_2O	>500	<350
Urine sodium mEq/L	<20	>40
Urine/plasma creatinine	>40	<20
Fractional sodium excretion	<1	>1

From Wyngaarden J, Smith L, editors: *Cecil's textbook of medicine*, Philadelphia, 1988, WB Saunders.

SIGNS AND SYMPTOMS OF UREMIA

Hyperkalemia
Metabolic acidosis
Hyperuricemia
Evidence for volume overload
Congestive heart failure
Pericarditis
Anorexia, nausea, diarrhea, vomiting
Gastrointestinal bleeding
Weakness
Fatigue

means of the protocols noted in standard medical textbooks. As stated before, the most common causes of death in women are infection and hemorrhage, both gastrointestinal and pregnancy-related. Regardless of the diagnosis, hemodialysis is started if the BUN value is 100 to 120 mg/dl and the creatinine level is greater than 8 to 10 mg/dl. Severe uremic symptoms are an indication for dialysis as well (see box, above).

Prognosis and outcome

The mortality associated with ARF has remained relatively constant since the 1950s because of an increase in the age of patients affected and in the number of patients with underlying illness. The prognosis for recovery of renal function also depends on the severity of the insult that caused the ARF. The best prognosis has been seen in obstetric cases in which there are no other medical co-morbidities. Mortality from ATN has been reported to be 50% lower for women than for men because the causes of ATN in women are associated with lower mortality rates.

Often the only advice that the clinician can offer the patient is to monitor the renal function tests closely and observe for stability over time. Consultation with a nephrologist is often helpful.

CHRONIC RENAL FAILURE
Epidemiology

Chronic renal failure occurs with equal frequency in women and men. The box, below, lists the most common causes of chronic renal failure, and Table 20-6 lists those most prevalent in women. Diseases that occur more commonly in women, such as sarcoidosis, lupus nephritis, amyloidosis, and other immunologic vasculitidies, also account for a higher proportion of renal disease in women. Urinary tract

MOST FREQUENT TREATABLE CAUSES OF END-STAGE RENAL FAILURE

Diabetes	Malignant disease
Hypertension	Metabolic diseases
Glomerulonephritis	Congenital/hereditary
Cystic kidney diseases	Sickle cell
Interstitial nephritis	AIDS nephropathy
Obstructive nephropathy	Other
Collagen vascular diseases	

Modified from the US Renal Data System: *Incidence and causes of treated ESRD*, Bethesda, Md, 1993, National Institutes of health.

Table 20-6 Female-to-male ratio of incidence of treated causes of end-stage renal disease 1987-1990

Disease	Ratio	
	Female	Male
Collagen vascular disease	2.9	1
Interstitial nephritis	1.2	1
Diabetes	1.1	1
Cystic kidney diseases	1	1.1
Sickle cell	1	1.3
Hypertension	1	1.4
Malignant disease	1	1.7
Other	1	1.7
Metabolic diseases	1	1.6
Glomerulonephritis	1	1.6
Obstructive nephropathy	1	2.5
Congenital	1	2.6
AIDS nephropathy	1	5.9
All causes	1	1.2

Modified from US Renal Data System: *Methods of ESRD Treatment,* Bethesda, Md, 1993, National Institutes of Digestive and Kidney Disease.

Table 20-7 Rate of progression to uremia

Disease	Months to uremia	Percent of patients with terminal uremia at end of first year
Chronic pyelonephritis	13.6 (0.7-52.4)	56 (Total N = 52)
Glomerulonephritis	10.1 (0.7-36.8)	70 (Total N = 40)
Diabetic nephropathy	6.0 (0.5-14.2)	88 (Total N = 24)
Polycystic kidney disease	18.1 (5.6-40.8)	36 (Total N = 11)
Nephrosclerosis	5.7 (2.0-9.0)	100 (Total N = 8)
Amyloidosis	5.3 (0.2-19.6)	88 (Total N = 8)

From Ahlmen J: *Acta Med Scan* (suppl) 582:1, 1975.

infections occur more commonly in women but in the absence of other factors, such as pregnancy, renal calculi, obstruction, or diabetes, rarely cause renal failure.

Approximately 50% of the patients with end-stage renal disease (ESRD) are women. The yearly incidence of ESRD is slightly higher in men according to data from the 1993 United States Renal Data System (USRDS). The exception is Native-American women who are slightly more likely to develop ESRD than are men. Diabetes is the most common cause of ESRD in the United States and also has a slight female preponderance. Women also have a higher incidence of interstitial nephritis, lupus nephritis from lupus erythematosus, scleroderma, and hemolytic uremic syndrome/TTP thrombotic thrombocytopenic purpura. After adjustment for the diagnosis, age, and race of the patient, women maintained on peritoneal or hemodialysis therapy have been found to have a slightly higher survival than do men (approximately 3% higher), but this difference in the most recent USRDS report seems to be less pronounced.

Progression to end-stage renal failure and dialysis

In one prospective study by Ahlmen, the rate of disease progression to ESRF from a persistent abnormal creatinine value of 5.0 mg/dl was dependent on the underlying disease (Table 20-7). A review of gender differences revealed that women became uremic in 5.9 months compared with 11.6 months for men, but the difference was not statistically significant. A recent study showed that when women are on hemodialysis for ESRD, they survive longer, possibly because they receive proportionally more dialysis than do men who have higher muscle mass and therefore more nitrogenous waste to clean.

Clinical issues in end-stage renal failure

Although ESRD causes many hormonal aberrations in women, only a few clinical studies focus on the endocrinologic function of women with renal insufficiency or renal failure.

Menstrual function and reproduction. Amenorrhea, irregular menses, and regular menses have all been reported in women with ESRD. As many as 90% of premenopausal women undergoing chronic hemodialysis may have menstrual irregularities. Clinically patients can have either an increase or a decrease in menstrual frequency, and the data are not clear as to what the natural course of menstrual dysfunction is for these women. The *new* onset of menstrual irregularity and amenorrhea in a woman with renal disease often indicates worsening renal function and uremia. In fact, the onset of uremic symptoms (see box, p. 138) correlates with the onset of menstrual irregularity and is seen when the creatinine clearance falls between 10 and 15 ml/min. Amenorrhea occurs with a creatinine clearance of less than 4 ml/min. Amenorrhea appears to be a common presentation except in women receiving continuous ambulatory peritoneal dialysis (CAPD); research data suggest that despite the elevation of serum prolactin levels in CAPD, amenorrhea may be less frequent. It is unclear from the data whether the age of true menopause is different for women with ESRD. Because of the difficulty in diagnosing menopause in amenorrheic women, one needs to document an elevated serum follicle-stimulating hormone (FSH) to ascertain menopausal status.

Pathophysiology. The menstrual irregularities seen in patients with severe renal insufficiency reflect **chronic anovulation** (for more detail on the pathophysiology of anovulation see Chapter 29). There appear to be abnormalities at various levels in the hypothalamic-ovarian feedback loop. In small studies of luteinizing hormone (LH) and FSH pulsatility in premenopausal patients, on dialysis therapy, anovulatory patterns with no midcycle peaks have been observed. Because LH and FSH are glycoproteins that are not cleared by dialysis, renal failure rather than the dialysis itself is the most likely cause of the abnormal ovulatory cycling. In addition, hypothalamic stimulation of LH and FSH release appears to be abnormal, possibly because of the excessive endorphin activity that occurs in chronic renal insufficiency. Endorphins are known to inhibit release of gonadotropin-releasing hormone (GnRH), thereby diminishing release of LH and FSH. Prolactin elevation has been shown to cause hypoestrogenism by inhibition of hypothalamic pulsatile GnRH release and is associated with lower estradiol levels than those found in women with normal prolactin levels.

Interestingly, in response to the lack of ovarian estradiol secretion that occurs with menopause, gonadotropins have been found to be appropriately elevated in postmenopausal patients who are receiving dialysis or who have undergone oophorectomy. This indicates that the negative feedback effects of estradiol on the hypothalamus are intact. Other observed hormonal changes include low serum estradiol and testosterone levels in premenopausal dialysis patients and predictably low progesterone in women with oligomenorrhea, which again reflects anovulation. In contrast, some studies have found that menstruating or irregularly menstruating women on dialysis therapy have normal estradiol levels.

Prolactin. Serum prolactin levels rise as the severity of renal failure progresses. Most women, but not men, have elevated prolactin levels by the time ESRD occurs and dialysis is instituted. The high prolactin levels inhibit release of GnRH from the hypothalamus and therefore also inhibit pulsatile pituitary FSH and LH release, thus inhibiting ovulation. The cause of the hyperprolactinemia is multifactorial. In small studies, prolactin levels normalize in patients on erythropoietin therapy, but regular menstrual bleeding occurs in only half the women observed. Because serum prolactin is positively correlated with the degree of renal insufficiency, decreased renal clearance is a factor. In addition, increased production of prolactin secondary to a primary pituitary abnormality and to abnormal hypothalamic function with a decrease in the prolactin inhibitory factor has been demonstrated. This inhibitory factor is thought to be dopamine; therefore the combination of decreased clearance, increased secretion, and decreased responsiveness to inhibition leads to increased prolactin levels in the most women on dialysis therapy.

Clinical issues (see box, below). Anovulation may manifest as amenorrhea, oligomenorrhea (menses occurring less than every 35 days), or polymenorrhea (uterine bleeding occurring more frequently than every 21 days). For the dialysis population who do have menses, heparin given during dialysis increases the amount and duration, but not the frequency, of menstrual flow.

Although the absence of menses (and therefore ovulation) in a group of patients who are chronically anemic to begin with may appear beneficial, the consequences of chronic anovulation are significant. For one thing the chronic anovulation can lead to the development of endometrial hyperplasia and carcinoma. Whether menses are absent or irregular this group is at increased risk of endometrial cancer. Clinically, it is important that a gynecologist determine whether an endometrial biopsy and interventional therapy are necessary (see later discussion in management section). It is unknown whether hypoestrogenemia, which occurs in some dialysis patients, is a significant cause of osteoporosis in a population already affected by metabolic bone disease.

Regarding the elevation of prolactin, the practitioner faces a clinical dilemma: whether patients with renal insufficiency need to have further evaluation of the elevated prolactin. If renal failure has not occurred, an elevated prolactin level suggests the possibility of a pituitary adenoma. Although

there are no published studies addressing the prevalence of pituitary microadenoma or macroadenoma in patients with chronic renal failure, prolactin levels of greater than 100 ng/ml are uncommon. Prolactin levels greater than 100 ng/ml or levels that are associated with galactorrhea or visual disturbance are abnormal and merit further evaluation with pituitary imaging to exclude prolactinoma.

Infertility. It is unusual for women receiving either peritoneal dialysis or hemodialysis to conceive because anovulation is common. In addition, hyperprolactinemia, which is associated with anovulation and abnormal endometrial maturation, are all contributory to infertility. The uremic environment also may be toxic to developing embryos and may inhibit implantation. Pregnancy occurs infrequently, in as few as 0.9% of female hemodialysis patients of childbearing age. One study by Souqiyyeh et al. found a pregnancy rate of 7% (27 pregnancies in 380 women) in a young female hemodialysis population. These women were not hypertensive and had had prior pregnancies; thus it may be that young patients without vascular disease have a better chance for conception.

Sexual function. Severe chronic renal insufficiency requiring dialysis is associated with decreased sexual desire, frequency of intercourse, and sexual satisfaction in women as well as in men. Hyperprolactinemic dialysis patients have a significantly lower frequency of sexual intercourse and orgasm than those with normal prolactin levels.

It is unclear what the cause of changes in sexual function are. Some have suggested that in the amenorrheic hemodialysis population the lower estradiol levels may be involved. Low estrogen levels cause vaginal atrophy and dryness, which can lead to dyspareunia. Decreased sexual desire and function also may be due to prolactin itself. Bromocriptine has been tried in some small studies with male dialysis patients and seems to improve sexual function. There are no studies using this therapy in women dialysis patients.

Relevant studies have found a significant psychologic component to the decreased libido experienced by women on dialysis and an association with depression.

Bone metabolism. Chronic renal failure impairs the metabolism of vitamin D to the biologically active 1,25-hydroxyvitamin D_3, resulting in hypocalcemia. This, compounded by hyperphosphatemia and poor nutrition, causes secondary hyperparathyroidism. Renal osteodystrophy, a combination of osteitis fibrosa, osteosclerosis, osteomalacia, and osteoporosis, results. Although dialysis itself lowers the serum phosphate level, aluminum in the dialysate may exacerbate osteomalacia. The overall bone density for postmenopausal women receiving dialysis is lower than that of men. It is unclear whether this is due to the hypoestrogenemia of menopause or because women receiving dialysis achieve lower-peak bone density than do men. There are no data as to whether amenorrheal premenopausal women have lower bone densities than do eumenorrheal women. Neither are there data on the efficacy of estrogen-replacement therapy in retarding bone loss as a result of osteoporosis in menopausal women with ESRD.

Thyroid function in women receiving hemodialysis. The diagnosis of hypothyroidism in the dialysis patient can be difficult. The symptoms associated with hypothyroidism are similar to many of the symptoms of uremia. In addition,

---

SUMMARY OF CLINICAL ISSUES FOR WOMEN WITH CHRONIC RENAL FAILURE

Anovulation	Bone loss
Infertility	Anemia
Sexual function	

results of the thyroid function tests can be abnormal, even though the patient is clinically euthyroid, because of problems with measurement. Some studies have suggested that the total triiodothyronine (T_3) and total and free thyroxine (T_4) are lower in the dialysis population compared with control subjects. One study found that 43% of the dialysis patients had T_3 levels in the hypothyroid range but not necessarily associated with clinical symptoms (Lim et al., 1977). Reverse T_3 can be normal, elevated, or low, and the T_3 uptake has been found to be normal or elevated. The abnormalities may be related to the loss of albumin and transferrin protein, thus affecting the measurement. Thyroid-stimulating hormone (TSH) has been found to be higher in patients on dialysis compared with age-matched control subjects (5.2 +/− 0.4 μU/ml for study group vs. 3.0 +/− 0.2 μU/ml) but is still generally within the upper normal laboratory range. Various studies have shown a higher prevalence of clinically enlarged thyroid or goiter in this group.

The difficulty one encounters is diagnosing hypothyroidism. When symptoms are severe and suggest hypothyroidism, the TSH value should be measured; if it is above 15 μU/ml the patient should be treated for hypothyroidism.

Anemia. Because of the lack of renal erythropoietin production in patients with ESRD, anemia results despite iron therapy. Erythropoietin (EPO) replacement has taken the place of repeated transfusion therapy for the anemia associated with ESRD. An added benefit is the decreased risk of exposure to hepatitis and HIV infection and the decrease in the development of antigens/antibodies from repeated blood transfusions. Despite its widespread use, there are limited data on the effect of EPO on the menstrual and ovulatory patterns of dialysis patients. One small study suggested a regularization of the menses, but there were no data on ovulation and conclusions could not be drawn from so small a study.

Management

Prevention. Women with severe chronic renal failure often do not receive routine health maintenance examinations such as pelvic examinations, Pap smears, and mammograms (see box, below). There may be a tendency for physicians to focus on the renal disease or to assume that the patient's life span is limited and therefore diagnosing an occult malignant condition will not significantly affect her longevity. Data indicate that dialysis patients may be at an increased risk of developing solid tumors and that patients who have undergone renal transplantation are at increased risk for leukemia and lymphoma. Therefore it is important that routine health maintenance be addressed, as well as these patients' daily medical needs.

MANAGEMENT ISSUES OF WOMEN WITH CHRONIC RENAL FAILURE: PREVENTION

Routine physical examinations
Pap smears and pelvic examinations
Mammograms

Menstrual dysfunction (menometrorrhagia)

Goals of management. The goal of treatment is to regulate the menstrual cycle as close to normal as possible to decrease the significant effects of chronic anovulation. After excluding pathologic changes of the endometrium by biopsy, it is important to control the abnormal bleeding that can be very aggravating and frustrating to the patient.

Choice of therapy. After a screening endometrial biopsy has been completed, a number of treatment options are available to control irregular bleeding in this population. One option is to use exogenous progesterone therapy such as medroxyprogesterone acetate (dose: 10 mg orally for 10 days) given at least four times per year. This schedule will effectively interrupt the proliferation-hyperplasia-carcinoma cycle.

Alternatively, the physician could use combination oral contraceptives. Given present knowledge, it is unclear whether these medications increase the incidence of arteriovenous shunt clotting, but it is unlikely that low-dose pills (<30 μg of estrogen) would have a significant effect.

A newer treatment, endometrial ablation, or the destruction of the tissue lining the uterus by means of either electrocautery or laser energy, is available and is appropriate for patients with significant medical problems. Treatment requires only local anesthesia and takes less than 1 hour to complete. A single treatment is effective in significantly diminishing or permanently eliminating uterine bleeding in 80% of the cases. Repeat treatment is necessary in the remainder of patients.

Despite the aforementioned interventions, some patients continue with profuse menstrual bleeding and thus will require hysterectomy.

Erythropoietin. EPO is routinely prescribed for patients with severe anemia secondary to ESRD. EPO is given intravenously at the time of dialysis. Studies indicate that although EPO may be associated with hypertension, patients have improved well-being after institution of therapy. EPO therapy reverses the anemia and corrects the prolonged bleeding time in hemodialysis patients. In about half of the premenopausal women treated, there is a regularization of menstruation as well.

EPO therapy appears to result in more regular menstruation and presumably ovulation in women receiving dialysis and may improve fertility. It also has been reported to improve the general well-being of dialysis patients and to improve libido and sexual performance in men despite a lack of change in hyperprolactinemia or in testosterone, LH, or FSH levels. These parameters have not been completely assessed for women receiving EPO therapy.

Calcium supplementation. Chronic renal failure (CRF) causes secondary hyperparathyroidism as a result of decreased 1,25-dihydroxyvitamin D_3 synthesis by the diseased kidney, which results in decreased intestinal calcium absorption. This is compensated for by an increase in parathyroid hormone secretion. As GFR decreases, serum phosphate rises, increasing calcium deposition in bone, decreasing serum calcium levels, and exacerbating parathyroid hormone production. It is important to provide calcium supplementation to the patient with CRF. Sometimes to ensure serum calcium levels of 10.5 to 11 mg/dl and to suppress parathyroid hormone, parathyroidectomy is necessary to halt the progression of the bone disease. The potential roles for exercise and estrogen replacement in this population have not been established.

RENAL TRANSPLANTATION

Epidemiologic studies indicate that women, especially those in minority groups, are less likely to undergo renal transplantation than are men, with a ratio of 1:1.3. When women undergo transplantation, they do as well as men, with excellent long-term graft survival and prognosis. In 60% to 89% of these patients, menstrual function regularizes as the uremic state improves. Sexual interest and libido often return to pre-CRF levels as well. Hypertrichosis (excess body hair growth) is also common and may be a problem cosmetically.

 PREGNANCY AND RENAL DYSFUNCTION

Normal renal physiology in pregnancy

Parameters for renal function. Various physiologic changes occur during normal gestation of which the clinician needs to be aware (see box, below). In normal pregnancy blood volume increases by 45% by term, with the greatest increase occurring during the second trimester. The glomerular filtration rate (GFR) increases by approximately 50% by the beginning of the second trimester and remains elevated until delivery. Renal plasma flow does not increase quite as much and actually decreases during the third trimester. Creatinine clearance is also elevated, peaking in the early third trimester at approximately 150 ml/min, down to 130 ml/min at term. Total body water is increased with a resultant decrease in plasma osmolality that is seen from the fifth week of gestation until delivery. Urea clearance is increased, leading to relative hypouricemia, which is more pronounced in the first two trimesters. The renal glucose excretion increases up to a factor of 10, resulting in glycosuria in pregnant women (for more details about abnormal glycosuria in pregnancy and the diagnosis of diabetes see Chapter 53). The supine position, which is associated with decreased urinary flow and sodium excretion, has not been shown to consistently decrease glomerular filtration and renal plasma flow.

Anatomic changes with pregnancy. Anatomic changes include (1) the dilation of the renal calyces, pelves, gestation, and ureters and (2) a decrease in peristalsis as a result of uterine and iliac artery pressure on the ureters (especial-

---

NORMAL RENAL PHYSIOLOGY IN PREGNANCY

Sodium and water retention
Lowering of blood pressure
Reduction in peripheral vascular resistance
Normal GFR increased 30%-50%
Decrease in creatinine to 0.5 mg/dl
Decrease in BUN to 9 mg/dl
Decrease in plasma osmolality to 270 mOsm/kg H_2O-1
Decrease in plasma uric acid to 3-4 mg/dl
Decrease in plasma bicarbonate to 20 mEq/l
Dilation of the ureters

---

ly the right) and the muscle-relaxing properties of progesterone (produced by the placenta), respectively. Urinary stasis occurs, which increases the risks of bacteriuria (often asymptomatic) and pyelonephritis. In fact, pyelonephritis is a common cause of ARF in the pregnant woman and is the reason why pyelonephritis is a more common cause of ARF in women than in men (see Table 20-3).

Abnormal renal physiology during pregnancy

Proteinuria. Normal urinary protein is less than 300 mg/24 hours in pregnancy. Higher urinary losses indicate inherent renal disease. If proteinuria is present with hypertension after week 20 of gestation the diagnosis of preeclampsia must strongly be considered, (see Chapter 51 for a detailed discussion of preeclampsia and eclampsia).

Urine output. It is difficult to know what amount of urine output defines an oliguric state, but any calculation less than 700 ml/24 hours should be suspect.

Specific renal disorders in pregnancy

Acute renal failure

Epidemiology and etiology. The incidence of ARF in pregnancy has been estimated at less than 0.01% and accounts for 2.8% of all cases of ARF. The incidence peaks in the late third trimester, between 35 and 40 weeks, and is due mainly to preeclampsia and bleeding complications. However, before the legalization of abortion, the distribution of ARF was bimodal, with an early peak in the second trimester around 16 weeks as a result of septic abortion. At that time it was also a major cause of maternal mortality. Now because of sterile procedures, ARF from septic abortion is rare.

Specific causes of acute renal failure. The box, below, presents a list of causes of ARF in pregnancy.

HEMORRHAGE. The bleeding complications that cause ARF include hemorrhage from the uterus as a result of placental abruption, placenta previa, or uterine rupture. The greatest occurrence of these life-threatening conditions is during the third trimester, from 24 to 40 weeks of gestation.

Postpartum hemorrhage because of uterine atony, retained placental fragments (preventing uterine contraction around the raw placental bed), lacerations of the cervix or vagina, uterine inversion, and rupture have all been reported to cause ARF as a result of volume loss.

INCARCERATED UTERUS. Urinary obstruction that results from an incarcerated uterus occluding the bladder outlet is an uncommon event, but when it does happen, it can produce ARF. The affected women has a retroverted uterus and manifests acute urinary retention in the late first—or early second—trimester of pregnancy. Uterine incarceration in the third trimester has been reported. The urinary obstruction occurs as the enlarging retroverted uterus becomes

---

ACUTE RENAL FAILURE IN PREGNANCY

Placental abruption	Pyelonephritis
Placental previa	Preecalmpsia eclampsia
Septic abortion	Ovarian hyperstimulation syndrome
Incarcerated uterus	Hyperemesis

wedged between the sacrum and the pubic symphysis, with subsequent obstruction of the bladder outlet. On physical examination, the cervix is lodged beneath the pubis and often cannot be seen on speculum examination. The bladder is distended and tender. In the second trimester on abdominal examination the uterus may feel smaller than expected for dates. In some cases the uterus can be dislodged by exerting pressure vaginally on the posterior aspect of the uterus, usually under general anesthesia because of the tenseness of the abdominal wall and extreme pain experienced by the woman. Occasionally the clinician needs to perform laparoscopy or laparotomy. Once the uterus is seated in the abdomen and dislodged from the pelvic bones, it will not incarcerate again. A postobstructive diuresis then occurs, which is similar to that seen in women with uteri enlarged with fibroids that have been removed.

If incarceration is not corrected, the BUN and creatinine levels will rise.

PYELONEPHRITIS. Pyelonephritis is the most common infectious complicaton of pregnancy and also a cause of renal failure in women. Complete ureteral obstruction by the uterus, causing oliguria, anuria, and partial obstruction, has been reported in pregnant women with pyelonephritis. (For a more detailed discussion on urinary tract infection and pyelonephritis see Chapter 60.)

PREECLAMPSIA. Any woman with preeclampsia should be closely monitored for renal failure. A more detailed discussion on this condition appears in Chapter 51.

OTHER CAUSES. Hyperemesis has resulted in ARF if there is severe volume depletion. In addition, ARF in association with fatty liver of pregnancy and prolonged retention of a dead fetus in the uterus has been described.

OVARIAN HYPERSTIMULATION SYNDROME. Ovarian hyperstimulation syndrome may occur after ovulation induction with human menopausal gonadotropins or purified follicle-stimulating hormone and, rarely, after administration of clomiphene citrate when human chorionic gonadotropin is given to induce ovulation. The syndrome, which is characterized by capillary leaks, has clinical manifestations of cystic ovarian enlargement, ascites, weight gain, and pleural effusions. Because of the intravascular volume loss, prerenal azotemia, with elevated BUN and creatinine levels, may result. The condition is self-limited, and therapy is supportive, with intravenous hydration and bed rest.

Prognosis and outcome. Kennedy et al. reviewed 251 patients with ARF, of whom 43 were pregnant. The obstetric group was oliguric for 1 to 28 days, with a mean of 11 days, and the average rate of rise of blood urea was 41 mg/100 ml. In similar studies by Hawkins et al. and Sibai et al. the researchers found that if the women survived, renal function ultimately returned to normal regardless of etiologic factors. In approximately 12% of 81 women followed up by Stratta et al., permanent renal insufficiency occurred—most of the cases because of preeclampsia and eclampsia.

Placental abruption and prolonged intrauterine fetal death may increase the likelihood that cortical necrosis will develop. If cortical necrosis occurs, maternal mortality may be as high as 100%. Survival is even poorer with increasing maternal age. It has been suggested that factors predisposing women to cortical necrosis, such as hypertenion and

advancing maternal age, explain the poorer prognosis associated with cortical necrosis as compared with acute tubular necrosis. Fetal mortality in ARF caused by hemorrhage and eclampsia is 71% and 76%, respectively.

Survival after ARF in an obstetric population treated in one dialysis center was 78.8% at 1 year and 72.5% at 5 years, including women with cortical necrosis. If the women with cortical necrosis were excluded, survival increased to 85.8% at 1 year and 85% at 5 years.

Chronic renal failure in pregnancy

Management. Miscarriage, premature labor and delivery, intrauterine growth retardation, placental abruption (premature placental separation), and intrauterine fetal death can occur in women with CRF. Hydramnios (excessive amniotic fluid accumulation) is seen in women receiving hemodialysis. The morbidity and poorer pregnancy prognosis for pregnant women receiving dialysis are not associated with the use of heparin during the dialysis. Preeclampsia is common but difficult to diagnosis in women with renal insufficiency and hypertension.

The prognosis for the pregnancy is better in the woman with chronic renal insufficiency who conceives and is subsequently placed on dialysis therapy than it is for the woman who conceives while already on maintenance hemodialysis. In the woman with CRF who is contemplating pregnancy, dialysis generally is started when the serum BUN level is greater than 80 mg/dl; the goal is to keep it less than 50 mg/dl. The assumption is that decreased azotemia improves the fetal environment, decreases the incidence of hydramnios, and improves pregnancy outcome. Late in pregnancy fetal urea production increases and may necessitate increased dialysis frequency or duration to maintain the same maternal serum urea nitrogen values. Peritoneal dialysis and hemodialysis appear to be equally useful.

THERAPEUTIC ABORTION. A woman's decision to carry or to terminate her pregnancy may hinge on the long-term impact it will have on her health and her survival. The physician who recommends therapeutic abortion because of poor pregnancy prognosis, poor maternal health, or a fear that pregnancy may lead to further deterioration of maternal renal function must bear in mind that termination of the pregnancy does not necessarily halt the progression of the underlying renal disease. It is unknown whether therapeutic abortion prevents sensitization to transplantation antigens. If end-stage renal disease occurs and renal transplantation is pursued, this could complicate finding a compatible kidney.

DIALYSIS. In the rare instance that a woman on maintenance dialysis therapy conceives, the prognosis for her pregnancy is bleak. Only 19 of 820 successful pregnancies were reported in this group in the 1990 European dialysis registry. Most conceptions occur in women who have some residual renal function before dialysis. The literature indicates that therapeutic abortions are performed in up to 45% of pregnancies in women on dialysis therapy. Miscarriage occurs in 11% to 54% of the pregnancies, and up to 61% of the infants are delivered prematurely. Hydramnios is common and increases the risk of premature labor because of excess uterine distention. Cesarean section is performed for worsening fetal or maternal condition in up to 46% of reported cases. Reasons for early delivery include premature labor, placental abruption, ruptured membranes, fetal distress, growth retardation, and worsening maternal hypertension. Preeclampsia often develops before 37 weeks of gestation, leading to premature iatrogenic delivery. In one registry report, from 42% to 90% of newborn infants had evidence of growth retardation, with an average fetal weight of 1900 g at 33.2 weeks. Counseling patients appropriately about pregnancy prognosis is hindered by the fact that some series report only live births. Available—although limited—data reveal live birth rates to be 19% to 63%, with the highest rate in a series in which 8 of 14 women were receiving peritoneal dialysis. This does not imply that peritoneal dialysis is the safer method of dialysis for pregnant women. It is not clear which method of dialysis is superior in pregnancy inasmuch as fetal and maternal complications occur with both. Hemodialysis may be associated with more severe anemia, as well as hypotensive episodes, which may result in decreased placental perfusion. Perritoneal dialysis may be complicated by peritonitis leading to premature labor and delivery and by obstruction of the peritoneal catheter. Erythropoietin successfully treats the anemia of ESRD in pregnant hemodialysis patients; however, the same pregnancy complications occur as in the non-EPO-treated pregnancies. EPO has been documented to exacerbate chronic hypertension.

Prognosis and outcome

Mild renal insufficiency. Pregnancy outcome in women with mild renal insufficiency as defined as a serum creatinine value less than 1.5 mg/dl is generally good, in the range of 90%. In a study by Katz and colleagues, 89 pregnant women in a total study group of 121 with biopsy-confirmed diagnoses had mild renal insufficiency. They were found to have a fetal survival rate of 94%, stillbirth rate of 4.1%, and neonatal death rate of 4.9%. Neonatal mortality was four times that seen in the general population. The preterm birth rate (less than 36 weeks) was 20%, compared with 13% nationally and 5.7% for the local population; 24% of the infants were small for gestational age, a rate 500% greater than that in normal infants. It is unclear whether fetal and neonatal deaths are increased in women with mild renal insufficiency who have glomerulonephritis, because the data included women with more severe renal dysfunction and the study was conducted at a time when less advanced neonatal care was available.

Moderate renal insufficiency. Pregnancy and fetal outcome are less favorable in patients with moderate renal insufficiency (serum creatinine greater than 1.4 mg/dl) than in women with mild disease (see box, above right). Therapeutic abortion rates were higher, ranging from 13% to 24%. Premature delivery occurs in 54% to 63% of cases, with a significant number of the deliveries performed because of signs of maternal or fetal compromise such as worsening renal function, hypertension, placental abruption, and fetal distress (Bear, 1976; Cunningham, 1988). Cesarean section rates range from 47% to 61%, and up to 40% of the infants demonstrate evidence of growth retardation, with an even higher percentage in women with hypertension. Intrauterine death has been reported in 3% to 10% and neonatal deaths in 3% to 13% of the pregnancies in this population. Overall fetal survival is 60% to 92%, with the higher rates being reported in more recent series. The advent of modern maternal and neonatal care has contributed to the improvement in survival rate.

PREGNANCY AND FETAL OUTCOME IN WOMEN WITH MODERATE RENAL INSUFFICIENCY

Higher cesarean section rates
Increased rate of premature delivery
High rate of growth retardation
Increased risk fetal death
Decreased fetal survival

In general, the presence of hypertension is an indicator of poorer fetal prognosis. In a study by MacKay (1963), there were no fetal survivors among 13 patients with serum creatinine levels less than 28 mg/dl.

Severe renal insufficiency or renal failure. Pregnancy outcomes in women with severe renal insufficiency, especially those who conceive while on dialysis therapy, are poor. The knowledge that the chance of carrying a fetus to viability is low and that the pregnancy may be emotionally devastating and medically complicated does not deter all women. For some women the desire to bear a child outweighs the risks. In these cases, the support and expertise of the medical staff, as well as the general health of the mother and the cause of the renal disease, all play a significant role in obtaining the best maternal and fetal outcome.

The effect of pregnancy on future renal function

Interpretation of the literature regarding the effect of pregnancy on long-term renal function is hindered by the grouping of patients into groups with "mild" and "moderate" degrees of renal insufficiency that include overlapping levels of serum creatinine. In addition, patient numbers are small and no statistical analyses were obtained in any series. Taking into account the limitations of published series, it seems likely that patients with serum creatinine levels of less than 1.5 mg/dl are not at significant risk of harming themselves by conceiving. The data are less clear for higher levels, with postpregnancy deterioration reported in 23% to 50% of these cases. Until the effect of pregnancy on future renal function is better defined, appropriate counseling of women considering childbearing will not be possible.

RENAL TRANSPLANTATION

Pregnancy is not uncommon in women who have undergone renal transplantation, as they generally are ovulatory. The prognosis for pregnancy is excellent in transplant patients inasmuch as immunosuppressive agents tend to be well-tolerated by the fetus.

SUMMARY

The course of renal insufficiency is similar in men and women. Some differences in disease frequencies exist between men and women. However, renal insufficiency in women often is complicated by derangements of hormonal, menstrual, and therefore reproductive function. Like men, women with severe renal insufficiency whose disease progresses to a need for dialysis suffer from depression and sexual dysfunction. Unfortunately, treatment of sexual dysfunction in women on dialysis therapy has not been studied. Pregnancy outcome generally is good in women with serum creatinine levels below 1.4 to 1.5 mg/dl, and pregnancy does not appear to alter the course of their renal disease. However, pregnancy might be detrimental in women with higher serum creatinine levels. Pregnancy outcome in women who conceive while on dialysis therapy is poor. Renal transplantation reverses the reproductive dysfunction seen in women on dialysis and is associated with good pregnancy outcome. Until prospective studies focusing on women better elucidate the endocrinologic abnormalities and natural progression of renal diseases in women, optimal management and counseling will not be possible.

BIBLIOGRAPHY

Abu-Romeh SH et al: Recombinant human erythropoietin (rHuEPO) and fertility in women on dialysis, *Nephrol Dial Transplant* 5:834, 1990 (letter).

Ahlmen J: Incidence of chronic renal insufficiency: a study of the incidence and pattern of renal insufficiency in adults during 1966-1971 in Gothenburg, *Acta Med Scan (Suppl)* 582:1, 1975.

Anderson RJ, Schrier RW: Acute renal failure. In Wilson JD et al, editors: *Harrison's principles of internal medicine*, 12 ed, New York, McGraw Hill, 1991.

Barry AP et al: Renal failure unit: obstetrical and gynaecological admissions, *J Obstet Gynaecol Br Commonwealth* 76:899, 1964.

Bear RA: Pregnancy in patients with renal disease, *Obstet Gynecol* 48:13, 1976.

Bierman M, Nolan GH: Menstrual function and renal transplantation, *Obstet Gynecol* 49:186, 1977.

Bleumle LW, Webster GD, Elkington JR: *Acute tubular necrosis, AMA Arch Intern Med* 104:180, 1959.

Bobik A et al: Evidence for a predominantly central hypotensive effect of alpha-methyldopa in humans, *Hypertension* 8:16, 1986.

Bommer J et al: Improved sexual function in male hemodialysis patients on bromocriptine, *Lancet* 8:496, 1979.

Bommer J et al: Improved sexual function during recombinant human erythropoietin therapy, *Nephrol Dial Transplant* 5:204, 1990.

Boyle JA et al: Serum uric acid levels in normal pregnancy with observations on the renal excretion of urate in pregnancy, *J Clin Pathol* 19:501, 1966.

Brandes JC, Fritsche C: Obstructive acute renal failure by a gravid uterus: a case report and review, *Am J Kidney Dis* 18:398, 1991.

Brenner BM, Rector FC Jr, editors: ed 4, *The kidney*, 2 vols, Philadelphia, 1991, WB Saunders.

Buvat J: Influence de l'hyperprolactinemie primaire sur le comportement sexuel humain, *Nouv Presse Med* 11:3561, 1982.

Chopra IJ et al: Reciprocal changes in serum concentrations of 3,3´,5´-triiodothyronine (reverse T_3) and 3,3´,5-triiodothyronine (T_3) in systemic illnesses, *J Clin Endocrinol Metab* 41:1043, 1975.

Chugh KS et al: Acute renal failure of obstetric origin, *Obstet Gynecol* 48:642, 1976.

Coe FL, Brenner BM: Approach to the patient with diseases of the kidneys and urinary tract. In Isselbacher KL, editor: *Harrison's principles of internal medicine*, 13, New York, 1994, McGraw-Hill.

Cohen D et al: Dialysis during pregnancy in advanced chronic renal failure patients: outcome and progression, *Clin Nephrol* 29:144, 1988.

Cowden EA et al: Hyperprolactinemia in renal disease, *Clin Endocrinol* 9:241, 1978.

Cunningham FG: Acute pyelonephritis complicating pregnancy. In Pritchard JA, MacDonald PC, Gant NF, editors: *Williams obstetrics,* (suppl 18), East Norwalk, Conn, 1988, Appleton & Lange.

Cunningham FG et al: Chronic renal disease and pregnancy outcome, *Am J Obstet Gynecol* 163:453, 1990.

Dandona P, Newton D, Platts MM: Long-term haemodialysis and thyroid function, *Br J Med* 1:134, 1977.

Davison JM, Dunlop W: Changes in renal hemodynamics and tubular function induced by normal human pregnancy, *Semin Nephrol* 4:198, 1984.

Davison JM, Hytten FE: Glomerlular filtration during and after pregnancy, *J Obstet Gynaecol Br Commonwealth* 81:588, 1974.

Dunlop W: Serial changes in renal hemodynamics during normal human pregnancy, *Br J Obstet Gynaecol*, 8:1, 1981.

Dunlop W et al: Clinical relevance of coagulation and renal changes in preeclampsia, *Lancet* 2:346, 1978.

Eika B, Skajaa K: Acute renal failure due to bilateral ureteral obstruction by the pregnancy uterus, *Urol Int* 43:315, 1986

Eschbach JW et al: Treatment of the anemia of progressive renal failure with recombinant erythropoietin, *N Engl J Med* 321:158, 1989.

Evans AJ, Anthony J, Masson GM: Incarceration of the retroverted gravid uterus at term, *Br J Obstet Gynaecol* 93:883, 1986 (case report).

Feest TG, Round A, Hamad S: Incidence of severe acute renal failure in adults: results of a community-based study, *Br Med J* 306:481, 1993.

Finkelstein FO, Finkelstein SH: Evaluation of sexual dysfunction of the patient with renal failure, *Dial Transplant* 10:921, 1981.

Finkelstein FO, Finkelstein SH, Steele TE: Assessment of marital relationships of hemodialysis patients, *Am J Med Sci* 271:21, 1976.

Finkelstein FO, Steele TE: Sexual dysfunction and chronic renal failure, *Dial Transplant* 7:877, 1978.

Finn WF: Recovery from acute renal failure. Lazarus JM, Brenner BM, editors: *Acute renal failure* 3 ed, New York, 1993, Churchill Livingstone.

Frank E, Anderson C, Rubinstein D: Frequency of sexual dysfunction in "normal" couples, *N Engl J Med* 299:111, 1978.

Gadallah MF et al: Pregnancy in patients on chronic ambulatory peritoneal dialysis, *Am J Kid Dis* 20:407, 1992.

Geerlings W et al: Combined report on regular dialysis and transplantation, *Europe Nephrol Dial Transplant*, 6, suppl, 4:5, 1991.

Ginsberg ES, Owen WF: Reproductive endocrinology and pregnancy in women on hemodialysis, *Semin Dial* 6:105, 1993.

Ginsberg JS et al: Heparin therapy during pregnancy, *Arch Intern Med* 149:2233, 1989.

Gladziwa U et al: Pregnancy in a dialysis patient under recombinant human erythropoietin, *Clin Nephrol* 37:215, 1992.

Gomez F et al: Endocrine abnormalities in patients undergoing long-term hemodialysis, *Am J Med* 68:522, 1980.

Goodwin NJ et al: Effects of uremia and chronic hemodialysis on the reproductive cycle, *Am J Obstet Gynecol* 100:528, 1968.

Grunfeld J-P, Ganeval D, Bournerias F: Acute renal failure in pregnancy, *Kidney Int* 18:179, 1980.

Hagen C et al: Comparison of circulating glycoprotein hormones and their subunits in patients with oat cell carcinoma of the lung and uraemic patients on chronic dialysis, *Acta Endocrinol* 83:26, 1976.

Handelsman DJ et al: Ovarian function after renal transplantation: comparison of cyclosporin A with azathioprine and prednisone combination regimens, *Br J Obstet Gynaecol* 91:802, 1984.

Hankins GD, Cedars MI: Uterine incarceration associated with uterine leiomyomata: clinical and sonographic presentation, *J Clin Ultrasound* 17:385, 1989.

Harkins JL, Wilson DR, Muggah HF: Acute renal failure in obstetrics, *Am J Obstet Gynecol* 118:331, 1974.

Hershman JM et al: Thyroid function in patients undergoing maintenance hemodialysis: unexplained low serum thyroxine concentrations, *Metabolism* 27:755, 1978.

Herwig KR et al: Chronic renal diseases and pregnancy, *Am J Obstet Gynecol* 92:1117, 1965.

Hess LW et al: Incarceration of the retroverted gravid uterus: report of four patients managed with uterine reduction, *South Med J* 82:310, 1989.

Hou S: Pregnancy in women requiring dialysis for renal failure, *Am J Kid Dis* 9:368, 1987.

Hou S, Grossman SD: Pregnancy in chronic hemodialysis patients, *Semin Dial* 3:224, 1990.

Hou SH, Grossman SD, Madias NE: Pregnancy in women with renal disease and moderate renal insufficiency, *Am J Med* 78:185, 1985.

Hou SH, Grossman S, Molitch ME: Hyperprolactinemia in patients with renal insufficiency and chronic renal failure requiring hemodialysis or chronic ambulatory peritoneal dialysis, *Am J Kid Dis* 6:245, 1985.

Howmans DC et al: Acute renal failure caused by a gravid uterus, *JAMA* 246:1230, 1980.

Imbasciatti E et al: Pregnancy in women with chronic renal failure, *Am J Nephrol* 6:193, 1986.

Isselbacher KJ, editor: *Harrison's principles of internal medicine*, ed 13, New York, 1994, McGraw-Hill.

Jackson RC: Acute renal failure and the artificial kidney in obstetrics and gynaecology, *Proc R Soc Med* 56:107, 1962.

Jones SR: Acute renal failure in adults with uncomplicated acute pyelonephritis: case reports and review, *Clinical Infectious Dis* 14:243, 1992.

Kaptein EM et al: The thyroid in end-stage renal disease, *Medicine* 67:187, 1988.

Katz AI, Lindheimer MD: Effect of pregnancy on the natural course of kidney disease, *Semin Nephrol* 4:252, 1984.

Katz AI et al: Pregnancy in women with kidney disease, *Kidney Int* 18:192, 1980.

Kennedy AC et al: Factors affecting the prognosis in acute renal failure, *Q J Med* 42:73, 1973.

Brenner BM, Rector FC Jr, editors: *The kidney,* 2 vols, Philadelphia, 1991, WB Saunders.

Kincaid-Smith P, Fairley KF, Bullen M: Kidney disease and pregnancy, *Med J Aust* 2:1155, 1967.

Kincaid-Smith P, Whitworth JA, Fairley KF: Mesangial IgA nephropathy in pregnancy, *Clin Exp Hypertens* 2:821, 1980.

Kioko EM et al: Successful pregnancy in a diabetic patient treated with continuous ambulatory peritoneal dialysis, *Diabetes Care* 6:298, 1983.

Kitzmiller JL et al: Diabetic nephropathy and perinatal outcome, *Am J Obstet Gynecol* 141:741, 1981.

Kohara N: Clinical study concerning factors of decreased bone mineral content in hemodialysis patients, *Nippon Jinzo Gakkai Shi* 33:587, 1991.

Kokot F, Wiecek A, Grzeszczak W: Role of endogenous opioids in the pathogenesis of endocrine abnormalities in chronic renal failure, *Semin Dial* 1:213, 1988.

Kunin CM: Natural history of "lower" urinary tract infections, *Infection* (supp) 2:s44–9, 1990.

Lapata RE, McElin TW, Adelson BH: Ureteral obstruction due to compression by the gravid uterus, *Am J Obstet Gynecol* 106:941, 1970.

Lazarus JM, Brenner BM, editors: ed 3, *Acute renal failure,* New York, 1993, Churchill Livingstone.

Leader L et al: Haemodialysis in pregnancy , *S Afr Med J* 53:871, 1978.

Levy NB: Sexual adjustment to maintenance hemodialysis and renal transplantation: national survey by questionnaire preliminary report, *Trans Am Soc Artif Organs* 19:138, 1973.

Lim VS, Kathpalia SC, Frohman LA: Hyperprolactinemia and impaired pituitary response to suppression and stimulation in chronic renal failure: reversal after transplantation, *J Clin Endocrinol Metab* 48:101, 1979.

Lim VS et al: Gonadal function in women with chronic renal failure: a study of the hypothalamo-pituitary-ovarian axis, *Proc Dial Transplant Forum* 7:39, 1977.

Lim VS et al: Thyroid disfunction in chronic renal failure, *J Clin Invest* 60:522, 1977.

Lim VS et al: Ovarian function in chronic renal failure: evidence suggesting hypothalamic anovulation, *Ann Intern Med* 93:21, 1980.

Lim VS et al: Blunted peripheral tissue responsiveness to thyroid hormone in uremic patients, *kidney Int* 31:808, 1987.

Lind T, Hytten FE: The excretion of glucose during normal pregnancy, *J Obstet Gynaecol Br Commonw* 79:961, 1972.

Lindheimer, MD et al: Acute renal failure in pregnancy. In Lazarus JM, Brenner BM, editors: *Acute renal failure,* ed 3, New York, 1993, Churchill Livingstone.

Lindsay RM et al: The endocrine status of the regular dialysis patient. In Kerr DNS, editor: *Proceedings of the European Dialysis and Transplant Association,* Amsterdam, 1968, Excerpta Medica Foundation.

Lowrie EG, Lew NL: Death risk in hemodialysis patients: the predictive value of commonly measured variables and an evaluation of death rate differences between facilities, *Am J Kidney Dis* 15:458, 1990.

MacKay EV: Pregnancy and renal disease, *Aust NZ J Obstet Gynaecol* 3:21, 1963.

Maher JF: Modifications of endocrine-metabolic abnormalities of uremia by continuous ambulatory peritoneal dialysis, *Am J Nephrol* 10:19, 1990.

Mastrogiacomo I et al: Hyperprolactinemia and sexual disturbances among uremic womenon hemodialysis, *Nephron* 37:195, 1984.

McGregor E et al: Successful use of recombinant human erythropoietin in pregnancy, *Nephrol Dial Transplant* 6:292, 1991.

Meislin HW: Incarceration of the gravid uterus, *Ann Emerg Med* 16:1177, 1987.

Meyers SJ, Lee RV, Munschauer RW: Dilatation and nontraumatic rupture of the urinary tract during pregnancy: a review, *Obstet Gynecol* 66:809, 1985.

Mitch WE, Bender WL, Walker WG: Management of progressive and end-stage renal disease. In Harvey AM et al, editors: *The principles and practice of medicine,* 22 ed, East Norwalk, Conn, 1988, Appleton & Lange.

Mitra S et al: Periodic hemodialysis in pregnancy, *Am J Med Sci* 259:333, 1970.

Morley JE et al: Menstrual disturbances in chronic renal failure, *Horm Metab Res* 11:68, 1979.

Morrin PAF et al: Acute renal failure in association with fatty liver of pregnancy, *Am J Med* 42:844, 1967.

Munk B, Rasmussen KL: Acute urinary retention caused by incarcerated fibromyoma in the eight week of pregnancy, *Ugeskr Laeger* 150:1937, 1988.

Murray MD et al: Ibuprofen-associated renal impairment in a large general internal medicine practice, *Am J Med Sci* 299:222, 1990.

Nageotte MP, Grundy HO: Pregnancy outcome in women requiring chronic hemodialysis, *Obstet Gynecol* 72:456, 1988.

Nelson MS: Acute urinary retention secondary to an incarcerated gravid uterus, *Am J Emerg Med* 4:231, 1986.

Ober WE et al: Renal lesions and acute renal failure in pregnancy, *Am J Med* 21:781, 1956.

Olgaard K, Hagen C, McNeilly: Pituitary hormones in women with chronic renal failure: the effect of chronic intermittent haemo- an peritoneal dialysis, *Acta Endocrinol* 80:237, 1975.

Orme BM et al: The effect of hemodialysis on fetal survival and renal function in pregnancy, *Trans Am Soc Artif Organs* 14:402, 1968.

O'Shaughnessy R, Weprin SA, Zuspan FP: Obstructive renal failure by an overdistended pregnant uterus, *Obstet Gynecol* 55:247, 1980.

Owen WF Jr et al: The urea reduction ratio and serum albumin concentration as predictors of mortality in patients undergoing hemodialysis, *N Engl J Med* 329:1001, 1993.

Parsons FM: The results of haemodialysis in acute renal failure of pregnancy, *Proc R Soc Med* 56:111, 1962.

Pepperell RJ, Adam WR, Dawborn JK: Haemodialysis in the management of chronic renal failure during pregnancy, *Aust NZ Obstet Gynaecol* 10:180, 1970.

Pride SM, James CStJ, Ho Yuen B: The ovarian hyperstimulation syndrome, *Semin Reprod Endocrinol* 8:247, 1990.

Pritchard JA: Changes in the blood volume during pregnancy and delivery, *Anesthesiology* 26:393, 1965.

Pritchard JA, MacDonald PC, Gant NF, editors: Maternal adaptation to pregnancy. In *Williams Obstetrics,* East Norwalk, Conn, 1989, Appleton & Lange.

Ramirez G et al: Thyroid dysfunction in uremia: evidence for thyroid and hypophyseal abnormalities, *Ann Intern Med* 84:672, 1976.

Redrow M et al: Dialysis in the management of pregnant patients with renal insufficiency, *Medicine* 67:199, 1988.

Registration Committee of the European Dialysis and Transplant Association: Successful pregnancies in women treated by dialysis and kidney transplantation, *Br J Obstet Gynaecol* 87:839, 1980.

Renschler HE, Bach HG, Baeyer H: The urinary excretion of glucose in normal pregnancy, *German Med Monthly* 12:24, 1961.

Rice GG: Hypermenorrhea in the young dialysis patient, *Am J Obstet Gynecol* 116:539, 1973.

Rosenthal T, Insler V, Iaine A: Haemodialysis in acute renal failure following hyperemesis gravidarum, *Aust NZ Obstet Gynaecol* 14:57, 1975.

Roxe DM, Parker J: Report of a survey of reproductive function in female hemodialysis patients. Proceedings of the National meeting of the American Nephrology Nursing Association, New Orleans, 1985.

Schaefer RM et al: Improved sexual function in hemodialysis patients on recombinant erythropoietin: a possible role for prolactin, *Clin Nephrol* 31:1, 1989.

Schiffer MA, Dunn I: Jaundice with hepatorenal failure associated with pregnancy or gynocologic procedures, *Obstet Gynecol* 39:241, 1972.

Shimamoto K et al: Permeability of antidiuretic hormone and other hormones through the dialysis membrane in patients undergoing chronic hemodialysis, *J Clin Endocrinol Metab* 45:818, 1977.

Sibai BM, Villar MA, Mabie BC: Acute renal failure in hypertensive disorders of pregnancy: pregnancy outcome and remote prognosis in thirty-one consecutive cases, *Am J Obstet Gynecol* 162:777, 1990.

Sievertsen GD et al: Metabolic clearance and secretion rates of human prolactin in normal subjects and in patients with chronic renal failure, *J Clin Endocrinol Metab* 50:846, 1980.

Slater DN, Hague WM: Renal morphologic changes in idiopathic acute fatty liver of pregnancy, *Histopathology* 8:567, 1984.

Smalbraak I et al: Incarceration of the retroverted gravid uterus: a report of 4 cases, *Eur J Obstet Gynecol Reprod Biol* 39:151, 1991.

Smith K et al: Renal failure of obstetric origin, *Br Med Bull* 24:49, 1968.

Souqiyyeh MZ et al: Pregnancy in chronic hemodialysis in patients in the kingdom of Saudi Arabia, *Am J Kid Dis* 19:235, 1992.

Soyannwo MAO, Armstrong MJ, McGeown MG: Survival of the foetus in a patient in acute renal failure, *Lancet* 2:1009, 1966.

Stratta P et al: Pregnancy-related acute renal failure, *Clin Nephrol* 32:14, 1989.

Strickler RC et al: Serum gonadotropin patterns in patients with chronic renal failure on hemodialysis, *Gynecol Invest* 5:185, 1974.

Strober W, Waldmann TA: The role of the kidney in the metabolism of plasma proteins, *Nephron* 13:35, 1974.

Surian M et al: Glomerular disease and pregnancy: a study of 123 pregnancies in patients with primary and secondary glomerular diseases, *Nephron* 36:101, 1984.

Swamy AP, Woolf PD, Cestero RVM: Hypothalamic-pituitary-ovarian axis in uremic women, *J Lab Clin Med* 93:1066, 1979.

Swartz EM, Komins JI: Postobstructive diuresis after reduction of an incarcerated uterus, *J Reprod Med* 19:262, 1977.

Transactions of the Annual Meeting of the Society of the Alumni of the Sloane Hospital for Women: Symposium on the "social problem" of abortion, *Bull Sloane Hosp Women* 11:65, 1965.

Turney JH, Ellis CM, Parsons FM: Obstetric acute renal failure 1956–1987, *Br J Obstet Gynaecol* 96:679, 1989.

Turney JH et al: The evolution of acute renal failure, 1956–1988, *QJ Med* 74:83, 1990.

Unzelman RF, Alderfer GR, Chojnacki RE: Pregnancy and chronic hemodialysis, *Trans Am Soc Artif Organs* 19:144, 1973.

US Renal Data System: Incidence and causes of treated ESRD, *USRDS 1993 Annual data report,* National Institute of Diabetes and Digestive and Kidney Diseases, Bethesda, Md, March 1993, National Institutes of Health.

US Renal Data System: Methods of ESRD treatment, *USRDS 1993 annual report,* National Institute of Diabetes and Digestive and Kidney Diseases, Bethesda, Md, March 1993, National Institutes of Health.

US Renal Data System: Patient survival, *USRDS 1993 annual data report,* National Institute of Diabetes and Digestive and Kidney Diseases, Bethesda, Md, March 1993, National Institutes of Health.

van Eijkeren MA et al: Measured menstrual blood loss in women with a bleeding disorder or using oral anticoagulant therapy, *Am J Obstet Gynecol* 162:1261, 1990.

Van Winter JT et al: Uterine incarceration during the third trimester: a rare complication of pregnancy, *Mayo Clin Proc* 66:208, 1991.

Walker WG, Mitch WE: Pathophysiology of uremia and clinical evaluation of renal function. In Harvey AM et al, editors: *The principles and practice of medicine,* 22 ed, East Norwalk, Conn, 1988, Appleton & Lange.

Whalley PJ, Cunningham FG, Martin FG: Transient renal dysfunction associated with acute pyelonephritis of pregnancy, *Obstet Gynecol* 46:174, 1975.

Winearls CG et al: Effect of human erythropoietin derived from recombinant DNA on the anaemia of patients maintained by chronic haemodialysis, *Lancet* 2:1175, 1986.

Woodrow G, Turney JH: Cause of death in acute renal failure, *Nephrol Dial Transplant* 7:230, 1992.

Wyngaarden J, Smith L, editors: *Cecil's textbook of medicine,* ed. 19, Philadelphia, 1988, WB Saunders.

Yasin SY, Bey Doun SN: Hemodialysis in pregnancy, *Obstet Gynecol Surv* 43:655, 1988.

Zingraff J et al: Pituitary and ovarian dysfunctions in women on haemodialysis, *Nephron* 30:148, 1982.

21 Headache Syndromes

Egilius L. H. Spierings

Seventy-five percent of women of reproductive age experience headaches, and most of them experience headaches more than once each month. In 15% the headaches are severe enough to affect daily activities, and in 5% the headaches are associated with vomiting. However, up to the age of 30, only 25% of the women with headaches have sought medical advice.

In their presentation headaches in women do not differ significantly from those in men. However, in women headaches occur more frequently, are more intense, last longer, and are more disabling. The estrogens, both endogenous and exogenous, play an important role because they are among the most potent chemicals that cause headaches. Headaches occur especially when estrogen levels change, and women with headache are more prone to headaches during menstruation and ovulation. It is also during these times of the menstrual cycle that headaches are generally more intense and last longer. Headaches that occur with menstruation or ovulation are also often more difficult to treat, both abortively and preventively.

Women with menstrual headaches are more likely to experience the onset of headache at menarche and are more likely to improve during pregnancy but not with menopause. These women are also more likely to experience aggravation of their headaches with the use of an oral contraceptive.

DEFINITION OF HEADACHE SYNDROMES

The majority of headaches in the general population are accounted for by three headache syndromes. These headache syndromes are muscle-contraction headache, migraine, and muscle-contraction vascular headache (Table 21-1). Muscle-contraction headache is equally common in men and women. Migraine, on the other hand, is two to three times more common in women. A rare headache condition is cluster headache, which mostly affects men. It consists of severe, unilateral headache that lasts from $\frac{1}{2}$ hour to 2 hours. It occurs daily, once or twice each day, for 2 to 8 weeks with remissions of 6 to 12 months.

Muscle-contraction headache

Muscle-contraction headache is the most common headache syndrome. It consists of mild or moderate headaches, diffuse in location, and pressing in quality. The headaches usually lack significant associated symptoms, such as nausea, vomiting, photophobia, and phonophobia, because of their relatively low intensity. Muscle-contraction headache is divided

into episodic and chronic, depending on frequency of occurrence. In episodic muscle-contraction headache the headaches occur up to two or three times each week. They begin during the day, usually in the late afternoon and last for several hours. In **chronic muscle-contraction headache,** the headaches occur daily or almost daily. They are usually present on awakening in the morning or occur shortly after getting up. The headaches gradually build in intensity as the day progresses and last for most or all of the day.

Migraine headache

In migraine the headaches are moderate or severe in intensity; are localized, usually to the temple and/or behind the eye; and are throbbing in nature. They are generally associated with other symptoms, such as nausea, vomiting, photophobia, and phonophobia. The headaches occur in attacks that last from 4 to 6 hours to 2 or 3 days. The attacks occur with variable frequency, ranging from once each year to weekly. In women the migraine attacks often occur once or twice each month, in relation to menstruation or ovulation. The headaches begin during the day and build to their maximum intensity within several hours. However, the migraine

Table 21-1 Differentiating symptoms of the three most common headache syndromes

Headache type	Symptoms
Muscle-contraction	Mild/moderate headaches
	Diffuse in location
	Pressing in quality
	Not associated with nausea or vomiting
Migraine	Moderate/severe headaches
	Localized in the temple and/or behind the eye
	Throbbing in quality
	Associated with nausea and sometimes with vomiting
Muscle-contraction vascular	Daily or almost daily headaches
	Frequently moderate/severe in intensity
	Regularly awaken the patient out of sleep early morning
	Associated with nausea and sometimes with vomiting

can also be present on awakening in the morning or wake the patient at night.

Migraine is divided into two forms: **migraine, with or without aura.** The type the patient has depends on the occurrence of transient focal neurologic symptoms before the headache. These symptoms usually last between 10 and 30 minutes and occur within 1 hour before the onset of the headache. The symptoms are always sensory in nature and are either visual or somatosensory. The visual symptoms are usually unilateral, affecting both eyes and one visual field. Their typical presentation is the scintillating scotoma, which is schematically shown in Fig. 21-1. It generally begins near the center of vision as a small spot surrounded by bright, often flickering and sometimes colorful, zigzag lines. After slight enlargement, the circle of zigzag lines breaks open on the inside to take the form of a horseshoe. The horseshoe then gradually expands into the periphery of a visual field and ultimately fades away.

The somatosensory symptoms typically present themselves in the form of digitolingual paresthesias (Fig. 21-1). These paresthesias consist of a feeling of numbness or pins-and-needles that starts in the fingers of one hand. They gradually extend upward into the arm, ultimately involving the face, especially the nose and mouth area, on the same side. The paresthesias are always unilateral in location and have to be differentiated from the bilateral numbness of hyperventilation syndrome. Migraine with aura (classic migraine) constitutes 5% to 10% of migraine; the remainder is migraine without aura (common migraine).

Muscle-contraction vascular headache

Muscle-contraction vascular headache is a headache syndrome in which migraine headaches are superimposed upon chronic muscle-contraction headache. The headaches occur daily or almost daily and with a certain regularity, often once or twice weekly, which build in intensity to cause migraine headaches with the features mentioned. The condition may,

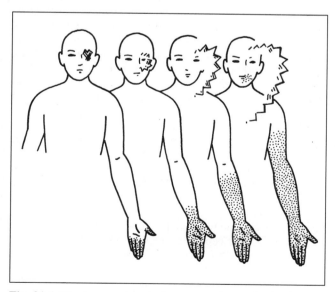

Fig. 21-1 The two most typical aura symptoms of migraine, the scintillating scotoma and digitolingual paresthesias, in their successive stages of development (*left to right*).

however, be presented as intermittent severe headaches, and the erroneous diagnosis of migraine may then be made. The suggestion of this syndrome should be made when a migraine condition is presented with a relatively high frequency (i.e., more than two attacks per month).

Muscle-contraction vascular headache is, like chronic muscle-contraction headache, often associated with the frequent use of analgesics. It has been shown that frequent use of analgesics for headache is associated with perpetuation of the headaches and ineffectiveness of preventive treatment. It needs to be addressed before preventive treatment is initiated and often results, by itself, in a significant improvement of the headaches.

PATHOPHYSIOLOGY
Headache mechanisms

The two most common mechanisms in headache are muscle contraction and extracranial arterial vasodilation. Muscle contraction causes pain through the accumulation of waste products in the muscles as a result of the prolonged contraction. The pain caused by prolonged muscle contraction is mild or moderate in intensity and diffuse in location. It is often described as an ache more than a pain and tends to be pressing in nature. The dilation of the extracranial arteries causes pain by a stretching of the nerve fibers that coil around them. In response to being stretched the nerve fibers become activated and send impulses to the central nervous system. At the same time the nerve fibers release chemicals into the peripheral tissues, such as substance P, neurokinin A, and calcitonin–gene-related peptide. These chemicals have inflammatory properties and cause a so-called neurogenic inflammation. The neurogenic inflammation is associated with further dilation of the arteries and a lowering of the pain threshold. The extracranial arterial vasodilation causes a localized pain, usually in the temple or behind the eye but sometimes in the back of the head. The pain is moderate or severe in intensity and described as sharp, steady, or throbbing.

The two headache mechanisms interact in two ways. Muscle contraction can lead to extracranial arterial vasodilation when the mechanical interference with muscle circulation extends beyond a critical point. Extracranial arterial vasodilation can cause muscle contraction through a voluntary and involuntary contraction of the muscles as a result of the intense pain. A vicious cycle can thus be created, that over time leads to a progression of the headaches. The involvement of a muscular mechanism in headache, including migraine, can often be ascertained by asking about the state of contraction of the neck muscles.

With regard to the two headache mechanisms in the three headache syndromes described, the muscular mechanism is predominantly involved in muscle-contraction headache, the vascular mechanism in migraine, and both mechanisms are involved in muscle-contraction vascular headache. However, the matching of the headache mechanisms and the headache syndromes is far from perfect, and, for example, the muscular mechanism is more important in migraine than is generally realized. Consequently, many patients who are diagnosed as having migraine in actual fact suffer from muscle-contraction vascular headache although their headaches are severe and intermittent as in migraine.

Headache continuum

As a result of the interaction of the headache mechanisms, the three headache syndromes (i.e., muscle-contraction headache, migraine, and muscle-contraction vascular headache) fall on a continuum that is schematically shown in Fig. 21-2. The episodic form of muscle-contraction headache stands on one side of the continuum and migraine on the other. In between are chronic muscle-contraction headache and muscle-contraction vascular headache. Patients can experience headaches anywhere on the continuum and can in the course of time move along it as indicated by the arrows.

Episodic muscle-contraction headache can over time develop into chronic muscle-contraction headache as a result of a gradual increase in frequency of the headaches. The increase in frequency is in turn associated with a progressive earlier onset of the headaches, ultimately leading to a daily and continuous headache. The most common cause of progression of episodic into chronic muscle-contraction headache is treatment of the headaches with analgesics. Analgesics, whether obtained with or without prescription, only address the symptom of headache and neglect the underlying mechanisms. This neglect of the underlying mechanisms results in the gradual deterioration of the headaches as described. The chronic muscle-contraction headache that develops out of episodic muscle-contraction headache is referred to as secondary. In case of primary chronic muscle-contraction headache there is often a precipitating physical event causing the headaches, such as a whiplash injury of the neck or a flulike illness.

With further progression of the condition, chronic muscle-contraction headache may develop into muscle-contraction vascular headache. The change in headaches underlying this progression is a gradual increase in their intensity resulting in severe headaches. The severe headaches in muscle-contraction vascular headache are similar to those in migraine. They have the same features, such as unilateral location and throbbing quality, and the same associated symptoms, that is, nausea, vomiting, photophobia, and phonophobia. The suggestion of this condition, as opposed to migraine, should be raised when the frequency of the severe headaches is high and/or the onset of the severe headaches occurs late in life. Migraine generally has its onset early in life (i.e., within the first three decades), with an average age of onset of 18 in women.

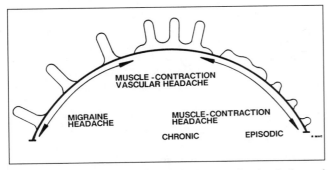

Fig. 21-2 The continuum of muscle-contraction headache and migraine.

Muscle-contraction vascular headache may, however, also develop out of migraine as a result of a gradual increase in frequency. An increase in frequency of migraine headaches is generally associated with a progressive interposition of the headaches with muscle-contraction headaches. This ultimately leads to a daily and continuous headache with regular buildup in intensity to cause severe headaches. Again treatment of the headaches with analgesics and vasoconstrictors, including caffeine, is often the cause of the progression.

Finally with regard to the headache continuum, under appropriate treatment patients may move back along it. Muscle-contraction vascular headache, under treatment, may improve to either migraine or muscle-contraction headache, depending on the nature of the original condition. In the same way chronic muscle-contraction headache, either primary or secondary, may improve to episodic muscle-contraction headache when treatment is effective.

 EVALUATION OF HEADACHE SYNDROMES

History

A good history is the key to the diagnosis of the previously described headache syndromes. Patients have a tendency to talk only about the severe headaches although the information regarding their mild headaches is at least equally important. The following are important questions to ask the patient: When did the headaches start? How often did they occur initially and how long did they last? Were the headaches severe in intensity or could they be easily treated with simple analgesics? Were they initially associated with nausea or vomiting? How often do the headaches, including the mild ones, occur presently? If the present frequency of the headaches is different from the initial frequency, how did they change over time? Did the headaches gradually become more frequent and more intense? Was there a sudden change, and, if so, was it related to any particular event? Do the headaches come about during the day or are they present on awakening in the morning? How often do they awake the patient out of sleep at night? How long do the headaches take to build up to their maximum intensity? How often are they severe and how long do the severe headaches last? Do the severe headaches relate to the menstrual cycle? How often are they associated with nausea or vomiting? Where are the headaches located? Do they have a preferential location? What is the nature of the headaches? Are the neck and shoulder muscles tight or sore? Are they tight or sore all the time or only with the headaches? What makes the headaches worse and what makes them better? Does physical activity or exertion make them worse? What about coughing, sneezing, straining, and bending over? Does lying down make the headaches better? Does applying a cold pack or a heating pad help? What can bring on a headache? In particular does fatigue, lack of sleep, oversleeping, skipping a meal, or physical exertion bring on headache? When headache is brought on by stress, does it occur during or after the stressful event? Can a headache be brought on by dietary products, such as chocolate or aged cheese?

As important as the headache questions are the questions related to the intake of medications, whether obtained with prescription or not. It is very important to know exactly how often a certain medication is taken: how many tablets or capsules each day and how many days each week or month. Of the nonprescription medications the headache and sinus medications especially are important. How much caffeine does the patient use, in both medications and dietary products? Does the patient use an oral contraceptive? If so, have the headaches been worse since use of the contraceptive was initiated? Are the headaches worse during the week that the oral contraceptive is not taken and the vaginal bleeding occurs? If the patient is menopausal, is she on estrogen replacement therapy? Are the estrogens taken cyclically, and, if so, are the headaches worse on the days that the estrogen replacement is not taken?

Special consideration should always be given to headaches of recent onset, that is, headaches that started within weeks or months before consultation, especially when they have progressed in frequency or intensity. When a patient complains of an acute severe headache, the onset of the headache is important. When did the headache start and how long did it take to build up to its maximum intensity? Did the headache build up to its maximum intensity in a matter of seconds, minutes, or hours? Also of special concern are the headaches that are always located on the same side of the head: always on the left or always on the right. This fixed lateralization to one side of the head must be explored. The explanation can sometimes be found in skeletal asymmetry or ipsilateral tightness of the neck muscles. At other times an ipsilateral chronic sinusitis is the cause, but the fixed lateralization can also be due to an intracranial lesion on the side of the headaches. When transient focal neurologic symptoms occur in association with the headaches, it is important that these symptoms alternate sides. If the headaches are fixed to only one side, especially the contralateral side, an intracranial lesion is likely.

Physical examination and diagnostic testing

Patients who have headache should always be given a screening neurologic examination at the least. Any abnormality found on the examination should be a reason for further diagnostic testing, in particular neurodiagnostic imaging. When computed tomography is performed, it should always be conducted with intravenous contrast enhancement unless the headache is acute and subarachnoid hemorrhage is suspected. Magnetic resonance imaging is an alternative to computed tomography with contrast; it is not necessary to conduct both.

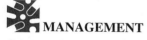 **MANAGEMENT**

Goals of therapy

The treatment of headache can be divided into abortive and preventive. **Abortive treatment** aims at the individual headaches to decrease their intensity and duration, if possible within 1 or 2 hours. **Preventive treatment** aims at decreasing the frequency of occurrence of the headaches. Abortive treatment is generally indicated when the headaches are moderate or severe in intensity. Whether preventive treatment is also indicated depends on the frequency, intensity, and duration of the headaches as well as on the

effectiveness of the abortive treatment. In general preventive treatment should be considered when severe headaches occur more often than twice each month.

Abortive and preventive treatments of headache will be discussed as they relate to the three most common headache syndromes: muscle-contraction headache, migraine, and muscle-contraction vascular headache. Only treatments that have been shown, in double-blind, placebo-controlled studies, to have an efficacy of at least 50% (Tables 21-2 and 21-3) will be discussed.

Choice of therapy

Abortive headache therapy

Oral abortive treatment. Medications that can be used for the abortive treatment of headache can be divided into oral and nonoral. Common oral medications that are prescribed for the abortive treatment of headache are, in order of increasing potency, Midrin, Tylenol with Codeine #3, Fiorinal/Fioricet and Percodan/Percocet.

MIDRIN. Midrin is a combination preparation that contains 65 mg isometheptene mucate, 100 mg dichloralphenazone, and 350 mg acetaminophen. Isometheptene is a mild sympathomimetic vasoconstrictor and dichloralphenazone is a mild sedative. It is an effective medication for the treatment of mild to moderate headaches and is generally tolerated well without adverse effects. Midrin is contraindicated in patients who use a monoamine-oxidase inhibitor. The recommendations to the patient are to take two capsules at the onset of the headache, followed by one capsule as needed every half-hour to a maximum of six in a 24-hour period.

NONSTEROIDAL ANTIINFLAMMATORY AGENTS. Instead of Midrin, a nonsteroidal antiinflammatory analgesic can be prescribed, such as naproxen sodium (Anaprox), which is absorbed relatively rapidly. Commonly the dose prescribed is 550 mg, followed, if necessary, by 275 mg every one-half hour to a maximum of 1100 mg.

MEDICATIONS WITH ADDICTIVE POTENTIAL. Tylenol with Codeine #3, Fiorinal/Fioricet, and Percodan/Percocet are potentially addicting medications. **Tylenol with Codeine #3** contains 300 mg acetaminophen and 30 mg codeine phosphate. It is mildly addicting as it produces some euphoria, and readily causes nausea and constipation as adverse effects. Patients are generally recommended to take one or two tablets as needed every 4 to 6 hours. Tylenol #3 can be used when oral treatment is required and Midrin or equivalent analgesics are not sufficiently effective in aborting the headaches.

Fiorinal contains 50 mg butalbital, 40 mg caffeine, and 325 mg aspirin. Fioricet has the same composition as Fiorinal except that it contains acetaminophen instead of aspirin. Fiorinal and Fioricet are moderately addicting medications as they cause euphoria and generally do not produce adverse effects. Generally these medications are avoided because of the addictive potential. One should rely on the nonoral abortive medications (discussed later) when Midrin or Tylenol #3 is not sufficiently effective.

Percodan contains 4.5 mg oxycodone hydrochloride, 0.38 mg oxycodone terephthalate, and 325 mg aspirin. **Percocet** contains 5 mg oxycodone hydrochloride and 325 mg acetaminophen. Percodan and Percocet are addictive medi-

Table 21-2 Summary of abortive headache treatments

Treatment	Dose and schedule	Contraindications	Adverse effects
Oral abortive treatment			
Isometheptene mucate (Midrin)	2 capsules at the onset of headache followed by 1 every $1/2$ hr to a maximum of 6/day	Use of MAO inhibitor, glaucoma	Drowsiness, restlessness, dizziness, rash
Naproxen sodium (Anaprox)	550 mg followed by 275 mg every $1/2$ hr to a maximum of 1100 mg/day	Peptic ulcer disease, bleeding disorders, aspirin allergy	Dyspepsia, indigestion
Acetaminophen with codeine (Tylenol #3)	1-2 tablets every 4-6 hrs	Liver disease in high doses	Nausea, constipation, lightheadness, dizziness
Sumatriptan succinate (Imitrex)	100 mg every hour to a maximum of 300 mg/day	Hypertension, coronary artery disease, use of MAO inhibitor	Tingling, tightness, lightheadedness, nausea
Nonoral abortive treatment			
Indomethacin (Indocin)	50 mg suppository: 1 every $1/2$ hr to a maximum of 4/day	Peptic ulcer disease, bleeding disorders	Dyspepsia, indigestion
Ergotamine tartrate (Cafergot)	2 mg suppository: $1/3$ every $1/2$-1 hr to a maximum of 2/day	Pregnancy, peripheral artery disease, coronary artery disease, hypertension	Nausea, vomiting, leg cramps
Sumatriptan succinate (Imitrex)	6-mg injection: 1 every hour to a maximum of 2/day	Hypertension, coronary artery disease, use of MAO inhibitor	Tingling, tightness, lightheadedness, nausea
Dihydroergotamine mesylate (DHE 45)	0.5 mg IM or 1 mg SC injection: 1 every $1/2$-1 hr to a maximum of 2/day	Hypertension, coronary artery disease, peripheral artery disease, pregnancy	Nausea, vomiting, leg cramps

MAO, monoamine oxidase.

cations and, therefore, should never be used for the treatment of headache.

SUMATRIPTAN SUCCINATE. An oral medication for the abortive treatment of headache that is not yet available in the United States is sumatriptan succinate (Imitrex). This medication is a serotonin analog that potently constricts the extracranial arteries and also reduces neurogenic inflammation. The oral tablet available in Europe and Canada contains 100 mg of the medication. It can be taken at intervals of 1 hour to a maximum of three tablets each day. Sumatriptan is contraindicated in patients with hypertension or coronary artery disease. Its most common adverse effects are a warm, hot, tingling, or tight sensation, generally in the upper half of the body, and lightheadedness. It is available in an injection form and has been used successfully to abort a headache. The patient can be taught how to administer the subcutaneous injection. This is discussed later in the chapter.

When abortive therapy is ineffective. The most common reason that abortive treatment of headache is ineffective is the dysfunction of the gastrointestinal tract that is associated with moderate and severe headaches. This dysfunction consists of atony and dilation of the stomach with closure of the pyloric sphincter (Fig. 21-3). It has been shown to impair significantly the absorption of medications that are taken by mouth. Prior administration of 10 mg metoclopramide hydrochloride (Reglan) has been shown to improve this impaired absorption. Prior administration of metoclopramide is possible when the headache comes about during the day and gradually builds up in intensity. The metoclo-

pramide can then be given first and followed, after 15 minutes, by Midrin or Tylenol with Codeine #3. Metoclopramide generally does not cause adverse effects, in particular drowsiness, and prevents the nausea caused by the headache or the Tylenol #3. However, this approach is not feasible when the headache is present on awakening in the morning or wakes the patient out of sleep at night. In those cases it is better to use a nonoral medication for the abortive treatment rather than to increase the potency of the oral medication.

Nonoral abortive therapy. The nonoral medications for the abortive treatment of headache can be divided into rectal and parenteral.

RECTAL PREPARATIONS. Rectal medications include indomethacin and Cafergot. The **indomethacin** (Indocin) suppository contains 50 mg indomethacin. Indomethacin is a potent nonsteroidal antiinflammatory analgesic and a mild cranial vasoconstrictor. It is contraindicated in patients with peptic ulcer disease or bleeding disorders. General recommendation to the patient is one suppository as needed every half-hour to a maximum of four. The **Cafergot** suppository contains 2 mg ergotamine tartrate and 100 mg caffeine. Ergotamine is a potent vasoconstrictor and also reduces neurogenic inflammation. It is contraindicated in patients with hypertension or coronary artery disease. It also should not be given during pregnancy as it is uterotonic. The patient is generally recommended to take one third of a suppository as needed every half-hour to 1 hour to a maximum of two. Common adverse effects of the Cafergot suppository are

Table 21-3 Summary of preventive headache treatments

Treatment	Dose and schedule	Contraindications	Adverse effects
Serotonin antagonists			
Methysergide maleate (Sansert)	2 mg 2-4 times/day	Hypertension, vascular disease, valvular heart disease, chronic pulmonary disease, fibrotic conditions	Nausea, indigestion, fibrosis
Pizotifen hydrogen maleate (Sandomigran)	0.5-3 mg at bed time	Glaucoma, prostate hypertrophy	Sedation, weight gain
Beta-adrenoceptor blockers			
Atenolol (Tenormin)	25-200 mg once/day	Sinus bradycardia, atrioventricular block, congestive heart failure, diabetes mellitus	Fatigue
Metoprolol tartrate (Lopressor)	50-100 mg 2 times/day	Sinus bradycardia, atrioventricular block, congestive heart failure, diabetes mellitus	Fatigue
Nadolol (Corgard)	40-160 mg once/day	Sinus bradycardia, antrioventricular block, congestive heart failure, diabetes mellitus, obstructive pulmonary disease	Fatigue
Propranolol hydrochloride (Inderal)	80-160 mg LA once/day	Sinus bradycardia, atrioventricular block, congestive heart failure, diabetes mellitus, obstructive pulmonary disease	Fatigue, depression, insomnia,
Timolol maleate (Blocadren)	10 mg 2 times/day	Sinus bradycardia, atrioventricular block, congestive heart failure, diabetes mellitus, obstructive pulmonary disease	Fatigue
Tricyclic antidepressants			
Amitriptyline hydrochloride (Elavil)	25-75 mg at bed time	Epilepsy, cardiac arrhythmia, glaucoma	Sedation, dry mouth, constipation, weight gain
Doxepin hydrochloride (Sinequan)	25-75 mg at bed time	Epilepsy, cardiac arrhythmia, prostate hypertrophy, glaucoma	Sedation, dry mouth, constipation, weight gain
Calcium-entry blockers			
Verapamil hydrochloride (Isoptin)	120-240 mg SR 2 times/day	Atrioventricular block, sick sinus syndrome	Constipation, pedal edema,
Flunarizine chloride (Sibelium)	10 mg at bed time	Depression	Sedation, weight gain
Miscellaneous medications			
Acetylsalicylic acid (Aspirin)	325 mg/day	Peptic ulcer disease, bleeding disorders	Dyspepsia
Sodium valproate (Depakote)	1000-1500 mg/day	Liver disease	Nausea, indigestion

LA, long-acting; SR, slow release.

nausea, vomiting, and leg cramps. Ergotamine is also available for administration in an oral tablet (Cafergot) but this is generally ineffective because of poor absorption. The sublingual ergotamine tablet (Ergostat), although effective, is generally poorly tolerated.

PARENTERAL MEDICATIONS: DIHYDROERGOTAMINE MESYLATE AND SUMATRIPTAN SUCCINATE. The parenteral medications that can be used for the abortive treatment of headache are dihydroergotamine mesylate and sumatriptan succinate. Dihydroergotamine mesylate (D.H.E. 45) can be administered by intravenous, intramuscular, or subcutaneous injection. Intravenous administration of the medication is not recommended because, like ergotamine, it is a potent arterial vasoconstrictor. In the office or emergency room the general approach is to recommend intramuscular administration of the medication in a dose of 0.5 mg that can be repeated after

a half-hour to 1 hour. As nausea is also a common adverse effect of dihydroergotamine prior administration of an antiemetic (e.g., 10 mg metoclopramide hydrochloride [Reglan] intramuscularly) is advisable. For administration by the patient at home the general recommendation is to use subcutaneous administration of a 1 mg dose.

Sumatriptan succinate (Imitrex) is administered by subcutaneous injection in a dose of 6 mg. It works relatively rapidly when given parenterally and, when administered in this way, generally provides relief within half-hour to 1 hour. The medication can be repeated after 1 hour, but it has been shown that this generally does not increase its efficacy. Its half-life is short (i.e., 2 hours) and as a result the headache may return after 8 to 12 hours. At that point the injection can be repeated and equally good relief generally is obtained. Its most common adverse effects are a warm,

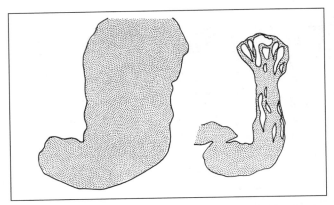

Fig. 21-3 The stomach during (*left*) and after (*right*) migraine showing dilation and atony with closure of the pyloric sphincter during the attack.

hot, tingling, or tight sensation, usually in the upper half of the body, and lightheadedness. Dihydroergotamine and sumatriptan are, like ergotamine, contraindicated in patients with hypertension or coronary artery disease. Dihydroergotamine also should not be used during pregnancy as it is uterotonic.

Preventive therapy. The four prototypical medications used for the preventive treatment of headache are methysergide maleate, propranolol hydrochloride, amitriptyline hydrochloride, and verapamil hydrochloride. Of these medications methysergide is probably the most effective but least tolerated and verapamil the least effective but best tolerated. Propranolol and amitriptyline have intermediate efficacy and are therefore most commonly used. Propranolol is particularly effective in migraine and muscle-contraction vascular headache. Amitriptyline is particularly effective in muscle-contraction headache and muscle-contraction vascular headache. It always should be tried first to treat the headache condition preventively with a single medication. However, in muscle-contraction vascular headache the combination of propranolol and amitriptyline often is most effective. Combinations of preventive medications that should be avoided are propranolol with either methysergide (vasoconstriction) or verapamil (bradycardia).

Methysergide maleate. Methysergide maleate (Sansert) is available in 2-mg tablets. Treatment is usually initiated with a dose of one tablet twice daily, after which it is increased to one tablet four times daily. The medication causes nausea and indigestion as adverse effects; therefore it is advisable to take it with meals and also at bedtime with some food. With long-term use the medication can cause retroperitoneal, pleuropulmonary, or endocardial fibrosis. Methysergide should therefore not be taken for longer than 4 to 6 months, after which it must be discontinued for 2 to 4 weeks. The medication is contraindicated in patients with hypertension, vascular disease, valvular heart disease, chronic pulmonary disease, or fibrotic conditions. Another serotonin antagonist that has been shown to be effective in headache prevention is **pizotifen hydrogen maleate** (Sandomigran; not available in the United States).

β-Blockers. **Propranolol hydrochloride** (Inderal) is usually prescribed in dosages ranging from 80 to 160

mg/day. When the long-acting (LA) capsule is prescribed, the medication can be given once daily. Generally treatment is initiated with 80 mg LA/day, after which the dose is gradually increased until satisfactory headache prevention results or the pulse rate has decreased to between 50 and 60. Common adverse effects of propranolol are fatigue, depression, and insomnia in women. Other β-receptor blockers that have been shown to be effective in headache prevention are **atenolol** (Tenormin), **metoprolol tartrate** (Lopressor), **nadolol** (Corgard), and **timolol maleate** (Blocadren). The feature shared by the β-blockers effective in headache prevention is a lack of intrinsic sympathomimetic or partial agonist activity. Atenolol and metoprolol are cardioselective and therefore can be used, although with care, in patients with obstructive pulmonary disease, such as asthma. The β-blockers in general are contraindicated in patients with sinus bradycardia, atrioventricular block, congestive heart failure, or diabetes mellitus.

Antidepressants. **Amitriptyline hydrochloride** (Elavil) is usually prescribed in dosages ranging from 25 to 75 mg per day. It is long-acting and therefore can be given once daily, preferably at bedtime, as it causes sedation. Treatment is generally initiated with 25 mg at bedtime with a gradual increase in the dose until satisfactory headache prevention is obtained or a dry mouth has developed. Amitriptyline is the only medication that has been shown to be effective in the preventive treatment of both chronic muscle-contraction headache and migraine. It can therefore be considered a broad-spectrum preventive antiheadache medication. A medication related to amitriptyline that has proved effective in the preventive treatment of muscle-contraction vascular headache is **doxepin hydrochloride** (Sinequan). Amitriptyline and doxepin are both tricyclic antidepressants and are therefore contraindicated in patients with epilepsy, cardiac arrhythmia, prostate hypertrophy, or glaucoma. In addition to sedation and dry mouth, common adverse effects are constipation and weight gain.

Calcium channel blockers. **Verapamil hydrochloride** (Isoptin) is usually prescribed in dosages from 240 to 480 mg/day. When the slow release (SR) tablet is prescribed, the medication can be given once or twice daily. Treatment usually begins with 120 mg SR twice daily, gradually increasing the dose to 240 mg SR twice daily. Common adverse effects of verapamil are constipation and impotence. The medication is contraindicated in patients with atrioventricular block or sick sinus syndrome. Another calcium-entry blocker that has been shown to be effective in headache prevention is **flunarizine chloride** (Sibelium; not available in the United States).

Other preventive therapies. **Aspirin** (acetylsalicylic acid) has also been shown to be effective in headache prevention. However, its efficacy is low and amounts to approximately 20%. A recent addition to the headache preventive medications is the antiepileptic **sodium valproate** (Depakote). Its exact place in headache management, however, is yet to be established.

When preventive therapy is ineffective. The most common reason that preventive headache treatment is ineffective is too-frequent use of abortive medications. Abortive treatment of headache with analgesic and/or vasoconstrictor medications should not be used commonly more than 1 or 2 days each week. An exception to this are the ergot medications, ergotamine and dihydroergotamine, which should not be used more frequently than once or twice each month. If used more frequently abortive treatment will over time aggravate the headache condition and render preventive treatment ineffective. Therefore patients with frequent headaches and frequent use of abortive treatment should first be withdrawn from their analgesic and/or vasoconstrictor medications before preventive treatment is initiated. Withdrawal from analgesic and/or vasoconstrictor medications is generally best accomplished abruptly. Corticosteroids can be used to mitigate the withdrawal headache. Often prednisone is prescribed, 60 mg the first day, 40 mg the second, and 20 mg the third, in four divided dosages taken with meals and also at bedtime with some food.

Controlling trigger factors. Headaches often have a hereditary basis. The familial occurrence of headache is not limited to migraine, as is often assumed. However individual headaches are often brought about by endogenous or exogenous factors (see box, below). The menstrual cycle is an important endogenous trigger factor of headaches, as mentioned. Other important endogenous trigger factors are fatigue, lack of sleep, oversleeping, and lack of food. Exogenous trigger factors are stress, weather changes, dietary products, and alcoholic beverages. The trigger factors often need each other to bring on headache and, therefore, one strategy for decreasing headache frequency is to prevent them from compounding.

In the dietary products and alcoholic beverages the relevant chemicals are caffeine, ethanol, sympathomimetic amines, and additives. **Caffeine** as a dietary ingredient is significant in coffee (50 to 100 mg/8 ounces), tea (25 to 50 mg/8 ounces), and cola drinks (15 to 25 mg/12 ounces). The headache caused by caffeine is probably a withdrawal headache caused by decreasing of the vasoconstrictor effect of the chemical. Caffeine withdrawal often occurs on weekends partially because of oversleeping, which delays the first cup of coffee. It is therefore advisable to limit the total daily caffeine intake to 100 or 200 mg. **Ethanol** probably causes headache, directly or indirectly, through its vasodilator effect. However, it also causes the so-called hangover headache in those otherwise not subject to headaches. The hangover headache occurs several hours after the ethanol consumption, usually the next morning, and is not caused by the ethanol itself. Chemicals in alcoholic beverages other than ethanol have also been implicated, the so-called congeners.

The **sympathomimetic amines** that are present in dietary products are tyramine and phenylethylamine. These chemicals are present in aged cheese, red wine, and dark chocolate. They act on the sympathetic nerve fibers to release the neurotransmitters norepinephrine and epinephrine. Once released, the transmitter substances act on their target tissues to produce the sympathetic effects. One of these sympathetic effects is a constriction of the blood vessels that may lead to an increase in blood pressure. The headache follows as the vasoconstriction wears off and rebound vasodilation of extracranial arteries occurs. The **food additives** are sodium nitrite, monosodium glutamate, and aspartame. Sodium nitrite is often added to meat to preserve its red color. It is present in cured-meat products, such as frankfurters, bacon, salami, and ham. Monosodium glutamate is a food additive used extensively in the preparation of some Chinese dishes. Aspartame is an artificial sweetener that is present in diet food products. The mechanism by which the food additives cause headache is not known.

PREGNANCY, LACTATION, AND HEADACHE

In general the use of medications during pregnancy and lactation should be discouraged because of potential effects on the embryo, fetus, or infant. With regard to abortive treatment **promethazine hydrochloride** (Phenergan) can be used safely. When prescribed as a rectal suppository of 50 mg it is often at least somewhat effective. It is generally recommended that patients take one suppository as needed every 2 to 4 hours. The medication is also helpful in relieving nausea and vomiting and, in addition, causes drowsiness. The drowsiness makes it easier for patients to sleep, thereby facilitating the recovery from the headache. With regard to preventive treatment medications should be avoided if at all possible. In the presence of tightness of the neck and shoulder muscles physical therapy or relaxation exercises can be prescribed. Fortunately headaches often improve by themselves once the pregnancy has progressed into the second trimester. In the third trimester a tricyclic antidepressant (e.g., amitriptyline or doxepin), may be used in low dosages also to secure restful sleep. The β-blockers should be avoided because of decreased placental blood flow and growth retardation of the fetus.

ESTROGENS AND HEADACHE

Oral contraceptives are currently the second most common method of contraception. Most women use oral contraceptives that contain less than 50 μg ethinyl estradiol. Headache is one of the most common adverse effects of use of oral contraceptives and is related to the dose of the estrogen. With oral contraceptives that contain less than 50 μg ethinyl estradiol headaches occur in 5% to 10%. However, oral contraceptives can also aggravate preexisting headaches in 40% to 50% of users, whereas actual improvement occurs in 10% to 20%. Conversely, discontinuing oral contraceptives has been shown to reduce headache frequency by at least 60% in 70% of patients. It is therefore important to inquire about the

---

COMMON TRIGGER FACTORS FOR HEADACHES

Menstrual cycle
Diet
  Caffeine
  Tyramine and phenylethylamine in aged cheese, red wine,
    and dark chocolate
Food additives
  Sodium nitrate
  Monosodium glutamate
  Aspartame
Alcohol

occurrence of headaches in women who are considering or are taking oral contraceptives. In women with significant headaches, especially when they are related to the menstrual cycle, aggravation of the headaches should be considered against the potential benefits of using an oral contraceptive.

Estrogens are also used in menopause to treat hot flashes and vaginal dryness and to prevent osteoporosis and coronary artery disease. The estrogens used here are either conjugated estrogens obtained from the urine of pregnant mares (Premarin) or synthetic estradiol (Estrace, Estraderm). They are often given cyclically (i.e., for 3 weeks and then discontinued for 1 week), to decrease the increased risk of endometrial cancer associated with their use. However headaches with the use of estrogens occur specifically or are particularly intense during the week off the estrogens. Therefore it is preferable that women with preexisting headaches or headaches that develop on estrogens be given the hormones noncyclically. The increased risk of endometrial cancer can then be decreased by combining the estrogens with a small dose of progestin, such as 2.5 mg medroxyprogesterone acetate (Provera). Also under these circumstances the lowest dose of estrogens possible should be used. For titration of the dose of the hormones the menopausal symptoms of hot flashes and vaginal dryness can be used. It has been shown that decreasing the dose of the estrogens by at least one-half and giving the hormones noncyclically can reduce headache frequency by at least 60% in 60% of patients. In women with significant headaches aggravation of the headaches should again be considered against the potential benefits of estrogen replacement therapy (see Chapter 36).

BIBLIOGRAPHY

Arthur GP, Hornabrook RW: The treatment of migraine with BC 105 (pizotifen): a double blind trial, *NZ Med J* 73:5, 1971.

Breslau N, Davis GC, Andreski P: Migraine, psychiatric disorders, and suicide attempts: an epidemiologic study of young adults, *Psychiatr Res* 37:11, 1991.

Buring JE, Peto R, Hennekens CH: Low-dose aspirin for migraine prophylaxis, *JAMA* 264:1711, 1990.

Buzzi MG, Moskowitz MA: The antimigraine drug, sumatriptan (GR43175), selectively blocks neurogenic plasma extravasation from blood vessels in dura mater, *Br J Pharmacol* 99:202, 1990.

Cady RK et al: Treatment of acute migraine with subcutaneous sumatriptan, *JAMA* 265:2831, 1991.

Celentano DD, Linet MS, Stewart WF: Gender differences in the experience of headache, *Soc Sci Med* 30:1289, 1990.

Chapman LF et al: A humoral agent implicated in vascular headache of the migraine type, *Arch Neurol* 3:223, 1960.

Couch JR, Hassanein RS: Amitriptyline in migraine prophylaxis, *Arch Neurol* 36:695, 1979.

Dalton K: Migraine and oral contraceptives, *Headache* 15:247, 1976.

Diamond S: Treatment of migraine with isometheptene, acetaminophen, and dichloralphenazone combination: a double-blind, crossover trial, *Headache* 15:282, 1976.

Diamond S, Baltes BJ: Chronic tension headache treated with amitriptyline—a double-blind study, *Headache* 11:110, 1971.

Epstein MT, Hockaday JM, Hockaday TDR: Migraine and reproductive hormones throughout the menstrual cycle, *Lancet* 1:543, 1975.

Friedman AP, DiSerio FJ: Multicenter investigation of Fioricet and acetaminophen with codeine, *Clin Ther* 10:69, 1987.

Gomersall JD, Stuart A: Amitriptyline in migraine prophylaxis: changes in pattern of attacks during a controlled clinical trial, *J Neurol Neurosurg Psychiatry* 36:684, 1973.

Graham JR: Rectal use of ergotamine tartrate and caffeine alkaloid for the relief of migraine, *N Engl J Med* 250:936, 1954.

Graham JR: Methyseride for prevention of migraine: experience in five hundred patients over three years, *N Engl J Med* 270:67, 1964.

Graham JR: Cardiac and pulmonary fibrosis during methysergide therapy for headache, *Am J Med Sci* 254:23, 1967.

Graham JR, Wolff HG: Mechanism of migraine headache and action of ergotamine tartrate, *Arch Neurol Psychiatry* 39:737, 1938.

Hartman MM: Parenteral use of dihydroergotamine in migraine, *Ann Allergy* 3:440, 1945.

Hering R, Kuritzky A: Sodium valproate in the prophylactic treatment of migraine: a double-blind study versus placebo, *Cephalalgia* 12:81, 1992.

Jansen I et al: Sumatriptan is a potent vasoconstrictor of human dural arteries via a 5-HT$_1$-like receptor, *Cephalalgia* 12:202, 1992.

Jensen R, Brinck T, Olesen J: Sodium valproate has a prophylactic effect in migraine without aura: a triple-blind, placebo-controlled cross-over study, *Neurology* 44:647, 1994.

Kaufman J, Levine I: Acute gastric dilation of stomach during attack of migraine, *Radiology* 27:301, 1936.

Klapper JA, Stanton J: Clinical experience with patient administered subcutaneous dihydroergotamine mesylate in refractory headaches, *Headache* 32:21, 1992.

Kudrow L: The relationship of headache frequency to hormone use in migraine, *Headache* 15:36, 1975.

Kudrow L: Paradoxical effects of frequent analgesic use, *Adv Neurol* 33:335, 1982.

Lance JW, Curran DA: Treatment of chronic tension headache, *Lancet* 1:1236, 1964.

Lebbink J, Spierings ELH, Messinger HB: A questionnaire survey of muscular symptoms in chronic headache: an age- and sex-controlled study, *Clin J Pain* 7:95, 1991.

Louis P: A double-blind placebo-controlled prophylactic study of flunarizine (Sibelium) in migraine, *Headache* 21:235, 1981.

Markley HG, Cheroms JCD, Piepho RW: Verapamil in prophylactic therapy of migraine, *Neurology* 34:973, 1984.

Markush RE et al: Epidemiologic study of migraine symptoms in young women, *Neurology* 25:430, 1975.

Mathew NT: Prophylaxis of migraine and mixed headache: a randomized controlled study, *Headache* 21:105, 1981.

Messinger HB et al: Headache and family history, *Cephalalgia* 11:13, 1991.

Morland TJ, Storli OV, Mogstad TE: Doxepin in the prophylactic treatment of mixed "vascular" and tension headache, *Headache* 19:382, 1979.

Nelemans F: Een technisch gelukt onderzoek met indomethacine bij patienten lijdende aan migraine: een dubbelblind onderzoek versus placebo, *Huisarts Wetenschap* 14:337, 1971.

Oral Sumatriptan Dose-Defining Study Group: Sumatriptan: an oral dose-defining study, *Eur Neurology* 31:300, 1991.

Pedersen E, Moller CE: Methysergide in migraine prophylaxis, *Clin Pharmacol Ther* 7:520, 1966.

Preston SN: A report of a collaborative dose-response clinical study using decreasing doses of combination oral contraceptives, *Contraception* 6:17, 1972.

Ross-Lee L et al: Aspirin treatment of migraine attacks: plasma drug level data, *Cephalalgia* 2:9, 1982.

Saadah HA: Abortive headache therapy with intramuscular dihydroergotamine, *Headache* 32:18, 1992.

Shekelle RB, Ostfeld AM: Methysergide in the migraine syndrome, *Clin Pharmacol Ther* 5:201, 1964.

Sicuteri F, Michelacci S, Anselmi B: Termination of migraine headache by a new anti-inflammatory vasoconstrictor agent, *Clin Pharmacol Thera* 6:336, 1965.

Soelberg Sorensen P, Hansen K, Olesen J: A placebo-controlled, cross-over trial of flunarizine in common migraine, *Cephalalgia* 6:7, 1086.

Solomon GD, Steel JG, Spaccavento LJ: Verapamil prophylaxis of migraine: a double-blind, placebo-controlled study, *JAMA* 250:2500, 1983.

Southwell N, Williams JD, Mackenzie I: Methysergide in the prophylaxis of migraine, *Lancet* 1:523, 1964.

Spierings ELH: Migraine and "the pill," *J Drug Res* 5(Nov suppl):67, 1980.

Spierings ELH: Headache caused by medications and chemicals, *Headache Q* 3:403, 1992.

Spierings ELH, Saxena PR: Antimigraine drugs and cranial arteriovenous shunting in the cat, *Neurology* 30:696, 1980.

The Subcutaneous Sumatriptan International Study Group: Treatment of migraine attacks with sumatriptan, *N Engl J Med* 325:316, 1991.

Tokola RA, Neuvonen PJ: Effect of migraine attacks on paracetamol absorption, *Br J Clin Pharmacol* 18:867, 1984.

Turner P: Beta-blocking drugs in migraine, *Postgrad Med J* 60(suppl 2):51, 1984.

Volans GN: Absorption of effervescent aspirin during migraine, *Br Med J* 4:265, 1974.

Volans GN: The effect of metoclopramide on the absorption of effervescent aspirin in migraine, *Br J Clin Pharmacol* 2:57, 1975.

Weerasuriya K, Patel L, Turner P: Beta-adrenoceptor blockade and migraine, *Cephalalgia* 2:33, 1982.

Yuill GM, Swinburn WR, Liversedge LA: A double-blind, cross-over trial of isometheptene mucate compound and ergotamine in migraine, *Br J Clin Pract* 26:76, 1972.

22 Arthralgias, Fibromyalgia, and Raynaud's Syndrome

Robert H. Shmerling and Matthew H. Liang

▦ EPIDEMIOLOGY

There has been little study of the epidemiology, pathogenesis, natural history, or unique features of musculoskeletal complaints in women. Approximately one of every seven visits to the primary care physician is for musculoskeletal symptoms. In women, most visits are probably for aches and pains or low back pain, the so-called nonarticular rheumatic syndromes. Diffuse connective tissue disease as a cause of arthritis is infrequent in the general population but more common in women than in men (Table 22-1). For example, in the United States 1% of the population is afflicted with rheumatoid arthritis (RA), which is two to three times more common in women than in men. The differences are even greater for systemic lupus erythematosus (SLE). In contrast, spondyloarthropathies and gout are less common in women.

Why these conditions that are considered to be immune-mediated occur more frequently in women is unknown, but it is suspected that sex hormones (estrogen, progesterone, testosterone) may be important.

⚗ EVALUATION

The goals of evaluating patients with musculoskeletal complaints irrespective of gender are to rule out treatable illness, to identify which patients need more extensive diagnostic tests and follow-up, and to prevent disability. Laboratory tests are rarely diagnostic in rheumatic disease but serve as adjuncts to a detailed history and physical examination. Similarly, x-ray studies are rarely diagnostic at initial presentation. Laboratory tests may be deferred at the initial visit except when a systemic rheumatic condition is suspected. Radiographs early in disease are most likely to be helpful only in select situations (see box, below).

⤨ APPROACH TO THE PATIENT WITH RHEUMATOLOGIC COMPLAINTS

History

The history should determine the location of pain (by having the patient point) and whether the pain is likely to be articular, inflammatory, or part of a systemic illness. How and when the pain started, what makes the pain worse or better, its temporal pattern, and the presence of constitutional symptoms (such as fever or weight loss) are important details.

Pain originating from joint structures should be improved by resting the joint and made worse by stretching the joint or by weight bearing. **Stiffness after prolonged immobility ("gelling")** suggests inflammatory joint disease or synovitis. This symptom probably results from altered viscosity of inflammatory joint fluid but is also experienced by older patients, as well as by patients with hypothyroidism, fibromyalgia, Parkinson's disease, and disorders with only a minor inflammatory component such as osteoarthritis. Clinically significant gelling lasts at least 15 to 30 minutes. In inflammatory disease the length of gelling may be propor-

Table 22-1 Diffuse connective tissue diseases

Disease	Estimated prevalence (%)	Female: male
Rheumatoid arthritis	1	2-3:1
Systemic lupus erythematosus	0.054	3-8:1
Systemic sclerosis	0.014	12:1
Polymyositis/dermatomyositis	0.006	2:1
Ankylosing spondylitis	0.13	1:3
Gout	1.6	1:7

INDICATIONS FOR RADIOGRAPHIC EVALUATION OF MUSCULOSKELETAL COMPLAINTS

No antecedent history, with abnormal joint examination
Significant trauma (especially near joint in prepubertal patient)
Age younger than 15 years
Progressive symptoms and failing conservative management
Symptoms not relieved by rest of involved area
Symptoms in patient with weight loss, prior malignant disease, fever, immune dysfunction
Recurrent acute monoarthritis

---

tional to the severity of the inflammatory process and may shorten as the patient's condition improves. The physician, in ascertaining morning stiffness, should ask about the usual time of awakening and the time when the patient is as limber as she will be during the day. The time elapsed is probably the most reliable way of eliciting this symptom.

Night pain may be a clue to a diagnosis and is also a major factor in impairing sleep, an important component of quality of life. Pain that awakens the patient may be infectious, neurogenic, vascular, or crystal-induced (e.g., gout or pseudogout) or may result from movement of a joint with severe structural damage during sleep. Tendinitis and bursitis also may awaken a patient. Synovitis without structural damage rarely causes night pain.

Neurogenic pain is often described in vague terms ("I can't describe it") or as numbness, an extremity falling asleep, shooting or burning pain, or pins and needles. Pain from vascular insufficiency is brought on by use and is relieved with rest within a few seconds. In neuroclaudication or spinal stenosis, use-related pain usually is bilateral, does not radiate below the knee, and improves slowly with sitting or bending forward.

A complaint of **locking of a joint** suggests a mechanical derangement of the fingers, knees, and occasionally the hip or shoulder. It may occur without warning when caused by ligamentous disruption or muscle weakness, or with pain when caused by a meniscal tear or loose bodies within the joint. Locking is the inability to move a joint smoothly through its complete range of motion because of an internal derangement (loose body, torn cartilage, or meniscus) or an extraarticular soft tissue block such as a tendon nodule, the cause of trigger finger.

Review of systems. A brief review of systems should be undertaken to determine whether the musculoskeletal symptoms might be related to a systemic illness or a systemic rheumatic illness. This can be done simply by asking the following questions: "If you didn't have this [complaint], would you be feeling well?" "Do you have any other medical problems?" "Do you have any other joints involved?"

Functional assessment. Inability to function is the final common pathway of all rheumatic illness; dysfunction and pain are the issues that most concern patients. The clinician should always assess how the symptoms affect the person in child-rearing responsibilities, work, home activities, and sexual function. The presence of functional impairment may point the physician toward different or more aggressive treatment. In the patient with polyarthritis, for example, a joint that is symptomatically out of proportion to the others may indicate advanced structural damage or possibly even infection. Screening for functional problems can be accomplished quickly with five questions, and a more detailed inventory can be used to complete the assessment (see box, above right). For patients with cognitive difficulties or multiple disabilities, direct observation of essential activities usually is needed to identify specific deficits.

When self-reported function is compared with observed ability to perform certain tasks, women report more disability than do men for the same level of musculoskeletal impairment. This also appears to be true for pain reporting. Studies of decompression laminectomy for lumbar spinal

---

FUNCTIONAL ASSESSMENT

Screening
- Which activity is most difficult for you?
- Are you worse, better, or the same as before?
- What can't you do now that you could do before?
- What can't you do but need to or want to do?
- How do you sleep? Can you sleep through the night?

Specific Activities of Daily Living
- Ask about difficulties with the following:
  Child-rearing responsibilities
  Ambulation
  Dressing
  Eating
  Personal hygiene
  Transfer
  Sexual activity

---

stenosis and total joint arthroplasty show that although the outcomes of the surgery for pain relief and functional improvement are the same, women tend to have more severe symptoms with their surgery.

Physical examination

The history, physical examination, and duration of symptoms are the three most important and useful "tests" in the diagnosis and management of rheumatic disorders. The goal of the examination is to locate the anatomic site, to identify whether the symptoms come from inside the joint or an extraarticular source, and to determine whether the problem is inflammatory or noninflammatory. The cardinal signs of true joint inflammation (**synovitis**) are effusion (fluid), warmth, palpable swelling over the joint line, diminished range of motion in all directions of the joint, and pain over all palpable areas of the joint capsule.

Point tenderness over anatomic sites of bursa is **bursitis** or a tear in a muscle or tendon. **Tendinitis,** on the other hand, is suggested by linear swelling, warmth, tenderness over the course of tendon, and occasionally an audible rub. Stretch of the tendon should reproduce the pain, although active motion is typically more painful than passive motion in tendinitis. In the examination the patient is asked to imitate the examiner taking the major joints through an active range of motion. If the active range of motion is limited, the examiner should note whether it is limited by pain, weakness, or mechanical block. The joint should then be taken through a passive range of motion. If the passive range is normal and active range is limited, disease of soft tissue—muscle or nerve—should be suspected, for example, tendinitis, myopathy, torn ligament or muscle, or peripheral neuropathy. If the active and passive ranges of motion are equally limited, a soft tissue block such as in a frozen shoulder or synovitis should be considered.

Women tend to have more spine and joint morbidity than do men until about the fourth or fifth decade. It is also a clinical impression that rheumatoid synovitis in women leads to more deformity and dysfunction than in men, perhaps because of the relatively smaller-sized joints and thinner bone structure in women.

Diagnostic tests

Laboratory tests

Acute-phase reactants. Acute-phase reactants are a heterogenous group of proteins synthesized in the liver whose levels appear to reflect inflammation or tissue necrosis. The most commonly used of these is the erythrocyte sedimentation rate (ESR). The ESR can be high or low in the absence of a pathologic condition, it increases with age and anemia, and it is higher in women than in men. A rough rule of thumb is that an ESR's age-adjusted upper limit of normal for men is the age divided by 2; for women, it is the age plus 10 divided by 2.

The ESR is important in the diagnosis and monitoring of giant cell arteritis (GCA) and polymyalgia rheumatica (PMR) inasmuch as it is part of the criteria for the clinical diagnosis of these disorders. However, up to 10% of patients with GCA/PMR may have a normal ESR. The ESR generally is elevated in systemic vasculitis but is often normal in certain vasculitides such as primary central nervous system (CNS) angiitis or Henoch-Schönlein purpura.

Autoantibodies. Autoantibodies—immunoglobulins directed against autologous intracellular, cell surface, and extracellular antigens—are seen in a number of rheumatic illnesses. The intracellular antigens include nuclear components (antinuclear antibody [ANA]) and cytoplasmic components (e.g., antineutrophilic cytoplasmic antibodies [ANCA]).

Antibodies to cell-surface antigens react with a variety of antigens, including human leukocyte antigen (HLA) molecules. Other antibodies may react with plasma components such as coagulation factors (e.g., lupus anticoagulant). Low titers of autoantibodies are present in a small proportion of the normal population; therefore a diagnosis of rheumatic disease should not be based solely on the presence of an autoantibody.

ANTINUCLEAR ANTIBODIES (ANA). Testing for ANA is helpful in the evaluation of suspected systemic lupus erythematosus (SLE) inasmuch as the test is highly sensitive (95% to 99%) in this disease. Certain ANA types—for example, Sm and dsDNA—are highly specific for SLE. The ANA's predictive value is highest when the titer and pattern of the ANA are considered in the context of the clinical presentation. The pattern of the ANA (diffuse, peripheral, speckled,

or nucleolar) correlates with the antigen against which the antibody is targeted (Table 22-2). For example, anti-dsDNA antibody generally produces a peripheral staining in ANA, whereas anti-Ro antibody produces a speckled ANA. Although some of these precipitins add to the specificity of the test, they possess variable and limited sensitivity. When SLE is highly suspected and the ANA is negative, an anti-Ro antibody and a hemolytic complement (CH$_{50}$) assay should be obtained because some SLE patients with a negative ANA will have a positive anti-Ro antibody and others may be complement-deficient.

Although anti-Sm and anti-dsDNA antibodies are highly specific (but not highly sensitive) for SLE, the ANA's most important limitation is its lack of specificity. Rheumatic disorders such as systemic sclerosis, Sjögren's disease, and rheumatoid arthritis also are associated with ANA positivity, although the sensitivity of the test in these diseases is much lower than in SLE. Patients without rheumatic disease, including healthy elders, patients with infectious illness (e.g., mononucleosis, AIDS), or those taking certain medications (procainamide, hydralazine, phenytoin), also may be seropositive for ANA. Although false-positive ANA results tend to be in low titer, a proportion will be of medium to high titer. The ANA titers of patients with SLE also may be low. Thus the ANA test should be ordered only when the pretest probability is appreciable. (For a more detailed discussion on ANA and SLE see Chapter 26.)

ANTICYTOPLASMIC AUTOANTIBODIES. The detection of serum IgG antibodies against cytoplasmic granules of neutrophils and monocyte lysosomes (ANCA) is extremely valuable in the diagnosis of suspected Wegener's granulomatosis (sensitivity is up to 95% in the context of active diffuse disease) and crescentic glomerulonephritis. These antibodies may also have a pathogenic role. The most frequently used method for detecting ANCA is indirect immunofluoresence microscopy in which two fluorescence patterns are observed: cytoplasmic (C-ANCA) and perinuclear (P-ANCA). ANCA also may be detected by enzyme-linked immunosorbent assay, which detects the antigens PR-3 and MPO that frequently are responsible for the immunofluorescent patterns, C-ANCA or P-ANCA, respectively. Patients who demonstrate C-ANCA with PR-3 specificity are likely to have

Table 22-2 Antinuclear antibodies in rheumatic disease

Disease	ANA(%)	Pattern*	Titer	anti-dsDNA(%)	anti-Sm(%)	anti-RNP(%)	anti-Ro(%)	anti-La(%)
SLE	95-99	P,D,S,N	50% >1:640	20-30	30	30-50	30	15
Sjogren's	75	D,S	Low	5	0	15	50	25
RA	15-35	D	10% >1:640	<5	0	10	10	5
Scleroderma	50-90	S,N,D	Often high	0	0	30	5	1
DILE	100	D,S	May be high	0	<5	<5	<5	0
MCTD	95-99	S,D	May be high	0	0	95	<5	5
Normal	<5	D	Rarely >1:80	0	0	<5	<5	Rare

From Schumacher HR, ed: *Primer on the rheumatic diseases*, Atlanta, Arthritis Foundation, 1993.
* P, peripheral; D, diffuse; S, speckled; N, nucleolar. Presented in order of decreasing frequency.
SLE, systemic lupus erythematosus; RA, rheumatoid arthritis; DILE, drug-induced lupus erythematosus; MCTD, mixed connective tissue disease.

active Wegener's granulomatosis whereas P-ANCA directed against MPO suggests pauciimmune glomerulonephritis or other systemic vasculitis. Non-MPO P-ANCAs have been observed in a variety of disorders, including inflammatory bowel disease and other inflammatory disorders.

Rheumatoid factor (RF). Rheumatoid factors are antibodies directed against serum gammaglobulins. These autoantibodies appear to be synthesized in response to immunoglobulin that has been conformationally altered after reaction with an antigen. The most commonly found rheumatoid factor is an IgM antibody to IgG.

The RF is one of the most frequently ordered tests in the evaluation of patients with suspected rheumatic disease, but its clinical utility is limited. The estimated sensitivity of the test among patients with RA is 75% to 90%, but such estimates are derived from highly selected populations in whom the prevalence of RA is relatively high. Other rheumatic diseases may be accompanied by the presence of RF, but the sensitivity in most of these conditions is even lower. The assay technique and titer of the RF may alter the sensitivity, but use of a more sensitive assay or setting a lower titer as a cutoff for a positive test result will produce lower specificity.

Results of the RF test exhibit low specificity and low positive predictive value in a primary care practice. A variety of nonrheumatic diseases are associated with the presence of RF. Rheumatic diseases such as Sjögren's, SLE, and cryoglobulinemia may have clinical features in common with RA and may manifest RF. The test's usefulness is largely determined by the prevalence of RA and the prevalence of diseases associated with a false-positive test in the population seen by the clinician. For patients older than 75 years of age, the reported incidence of false-positive RF reactions is 2% to 25%.

Given the modest sensitivity and specificity of the RF test, it should be ordered only for patients with a moderate likelihood of RA.

Complement. Serum complement represents a series of more than 20 biologically active proteins and inhibitors produced in the liver and comprises 2% to 3% of the total plasma protein concentration. The best screening test for a complement abnormality is the CH_{50}, which is a functional assay of the entire classic pathway. A low level would suggest either consumption of complement or a deficiency of one or more components. Complement activation and consumption generally are triggered by exposure of the host to a foreign protein, especially when bound to host antibody (immune-complex disease).

Conditions with immune-complex formation are those in which measurement of complement may be useful, including SLE (especially with nephritis), cryoglobulinemia, chronic infections that cause glomerulonephritis (GN) or vasculitis (e.g., endocarditis or hepatitis B), generalized vasculitis (e.g., rheumatoid vasculitis or active polyarteritis nodosa [PAN]), and serum sickness. In SLE nephritis, serial measurement of complement may prove useful in monitoring patients inasmuch as complement levels may decrease just before or concomitant with disease flare and return to normal over weeks to months when disease activity diminishes. The correlation of lupus nonrenal disease activity with complement is variable, however, and thus complement should be considered in the context of the clinical picture.

HLA-B27. The association between the HLA-B27 allele and the spondyloarthropathies makes this genetic marker a potentially useful test in evaluating patients with possible spondyloarthropathy. The diagnostic sensitivity of this test is approximately 95% in ankylosing spondylitis, 80% in Reiter's disease, 70% in patients with the spondylitis of psoriatic arthritis, and 50% in symptomatic spondylitis associated with inflammatory bowel disease. Moreover, patients without rheumatic symptoms but with HLA-B27 positivity have an increased relative risk (although low absolute risk) for the development of these spondylitides compared with those who are seronegative to HLA-B27. The background prevalence of this genetic marker (approximately 6% to 10% in white populations) and the fact that only a small number of persons who are seropositive to HLA-B27 will ever develop a spondyloarthropathy limit the utility of the test. In general, because spondyloarthropathies are uncommon in women, HLA-B27 testing should not be ordered unless there is at least a moderate pretest probability.

Assessment of organ damage or involvement

Overview. In patients with systemic rheumatic disorders, extraarticular involvement is often the rule even in the absence of signs or symptoms. In addition, agents used in their treatment may have systemic toxicity. Such involvement can be deduced by appropriate laboratory testing, such as renal or liver function tests, blood counts, muscle enzyme values, or urinalysis. For selected patients, more elaborate testing may be indicated, such as a 24-hour urine collection for protein and creatinine clearance, imaging studies (e.g., head magnetic resonance imaging [MRI]), or lumbar puncture, depending on the suspicion of specific organ systems involved and diagnosis under consideration.

Joint fluid analysis. Synovial fluid analysis can differentiate infection, crystal-induced disease, or hemarthrosis and characterizes the process as inflammatory or noninflammatory (Table 22-3).

The routine joint fluid analysis should include a white blood cell count and differential, Gram's stain, and culture and crystal examination by polarizing microscopy. The mucin clot, complement, and sugar and protein determinations on joint fluid have little or no usefulness. If gonococ-

Table 22-3 Rapid joint fluid examination

Method	Noninflammatory	Inflammatory
Gross appearance	Clear Can read print through joint fluid	Cloudy Print difficult to read through joint fluid
String test	Strings 1-2 inches	Drips like water from syringe
Wet preparation unspun joint fluid	Less than 2 WBC/hpf ($\leq$2000/cmm)	Greater than 2 WBC/hpf (>2000/cmm)

WBC/hpf, white blood cell count per high-power field.

cal or tuberculosis infection is suspected, appropriate culture media should be utilized.

Normal or noninflammatory joint fluid has the consistency and color of egg white and is clear; inflammatory fluid tends to be cloudy. The string sign is elicited after the syringe has been withdrawn by pressing slowly on the plunger with the syringe held parallel to the floor until a drop appears at the end of the needle and falls. Normally the fluid should string for about 2 to 3 inches. The more inflammatory the fluid, the more waterlike the consistency and the fluid will fall in drops. Inspecting the fluid for cells and crystals can be accomplished quickly by placing a drop of fluid on a slide with a cover glass and examining it at low and higher power (wet preparation). White blood cell counts greater than 2 per high-power field suggests inflammation, and this can be confirmed by the formal cell count, in which fluids with more than 2000 cells or more than 75% polymorphonuclear leukocytes are considered inflammatory.

A search for crystals requires careful scrutiny of the slide. Crystals may be seen without a polarizing microscope. The light source should be reduced by closing the diaphragm of the light source and lowering the condenser. In most fluids that contain urate crystals, pine needle-shaped crystals in and outside of white blood cells will be seen; under polarizing microscopy, they will be yellow when parallel to the axis of the polarizer. Pseudogout crystals are scanty, less brightly birefringent, and pleomorphic in appearance; blunt-ended rhomboids are most typically seen. They are blue when parallel to a polarizing lens.

Radiographs. In contrast to arthrocentesis, radiographs for a new joint complaint are rarely helpful, and, accordingly, the indications are limited (see box, p. 158). Plain radiographs show changes in bone best and in soft tissue less well. The soft tissue findings usually confirm the physical examination. The changes in bone include erosions, joint space narrowing, osteophytes, fractures, and primary or metastatic bone tumors. Because it takes 4 to 6 months of inflammation for chronic synovitis to cause erosions that are radiographically evident, a film taken before this is rarely helpful. One exception is the patient who has had recurrent attacks of acute arthritis in a joint. A radiograph may demonstrate an erosion typical of gout. X-ray films of septic joints show abnormal findings 10 days to 2 weeks into the course: the process should have been detected by arthrocentesis well before radiographic changes are evident.

CLINICAL PATTERNS OF ARTHRITIS
Monarthritis

A woman reporting pain or stiffness of a single joint may have an extraarticular problem, systemic rheumatic disease such as monarticular rheumatoid arthritis, a crystal-induced disease, or an infection. The differential diagnosis in approximate order of frequency in a primary care setting is noted in the following box.

The patient's age is key in interpretation of the history. Monarticular complaints in prepubertal patients require careful evaluation for traumatic conditions and congenital defects such as a slipped capital epiphysis and hip dysplasia. A sexually active woman may have gonococcal or reactive arthritis. Crystal-induced arthritis is rare in premenopausal

DIFFERENTIAL DIAGNOSIS OF MONARTHRITIS
Infection
Crystalline synovitis (rare in premenopausal women) (particularly first metatarsophalangeal joint)
Systemic rheumatic illness (knee in rheumatoid arthritis)
Hemarthrosis

women. In postmenopausal women, gout may be related to use of diuretics.

The degree of pain and the circumstances with which it occurs are helpful clues to diagnosis. Severe pain, especially during rest, narrows the differential diagnosis but is infection until proved otherwise. Mild to moderate pain is seen in inflammatory monarthritides but also in many other conditions such as hemarthrosis and ligamentous strains. The duration of the complaint may provide a clue inasmuch as pain that has been present for weeks is unlikely to be a bacterial arthritis but could be mycobacterial or fungal infection.

If there is a moderate or larger effusion, the joint should be aspirated. Only arthrocentesis for culture can definitively rule out infection, the only disorder in which prompt identification is crucial. A single episode of bleeding in the joint (hemarthrosis) should clear within several days to 1 week and may be seen in association with trauma or pseudogout. Persistent blood after this point implies rebleeding; a coagulopathy or even a joint tumor should be considered.

Polyarthritis

Polyarthritis is synovitis of three or more joints and is distinct from polyarthralgia in which joint complaints are not associated with actual inflammation. Acute polyarthritis is a diagnostic dilemma that may be a feature of almost any systemic rheumatic disease, including some associated with high morbidity. Acute polyarthritis of less than 6 weeks' duration often cannot be diagnosed with any certainty and could be benign. A complete history, physical examination, and diagnostic evaluation are always necessary (Table 22-4).

The elements of the history particularly helpful in sorting out this presentation are the pattern of joint involvement, the temporal sequence, the course, the presence or absence of extraarticular symptoms or signs, and the functional consequences of the articular involvement.

The sequence of symptoms generally follow three major patterns: additive, migratory, and intermittent. In **additive arthritis,** new joints are added to previously involved joints. In **migratory arthritis,** an inflamed joint subsides as new ones become involved. In **intermittent arthritis,** inflammation is episodic with virtually no signs or symptoms between flare-ups.

When one pattern dominates the clinical presentation, a diagnosis may be suggested. For instance, an additive pattern is seen in patients with rheumatoid arthritis, systemic lupus erythematosus, and Still's disease; migratory arthralgia and arthritis occur typically in patients with disseminated gonococcal infection, acute rheumatic fever, and the arthritis associated with bacterial endocarditis and hepatitis.

Table 22-4 Selected Differential Diagnosis Suggestive History, and Findings in Common Rheumatic Conditions

Joint disease	Suggestive history	Most specific findings
Traumatic		
Fracture	Acute onset after significant trauma	Radiographs
Internal derangement (e.g., meniscal tear, loose body)	Acute onset, locking, giving way, often after trauma	MRI or arthroscopy
Tendinitis/bursitis	Localized pain, nighttime pain, worse with use, following overuse	Active motion more painful and limited than passive motion
Hemarthrosis	After trauma or with history of coagulopathy	Tests of coagulation, synovial fluid analysis
Inflammatory		
Rheumatoid arthritis	Chronic, symmetric polyarthralgia	Chronic, symmetric polyarthritis
Systemic lupus erythematosus	Multisystem inflammatory disease, especially skin and joints	Rash, oral ulcers, arthritis, pericardial or pleural rub, blood count/differential, RPR, ANA, urinalysis
Spondyloarthropathies		
Inflammatory bowel disease	Oligoarthralgia, back pain, chronic or episodic diarrhea	Oligoarthritis, sacroiliitis by x-ray film; endoscopic evidence for inflammatory bowel disease
Psoriatic arthritis	Oligoarthralgia, skin plaques, nail pitting	Oligoarthritis, especially of the DIPs, sacroiliitis by x-ray film, psoriasis, nail pitting
Ankylosing spondylitis	Oligoarthralgia, back pain that improves with exercise	Oligoarthritis, sacroiliitis by x-ray film
Reiter's disease	Oligoarthralgia, eye symptoms, dysuria, rash, history of chlamydia or dysenteric infection	Oligoarthritis, conjunctivitis, sterile urethritis, rash, sacroiliitis by x-ray film
Crystal-induced arthritis	Acute, episodic monarthritis	Synovial fluid analysis with polarizing microscopy; erosions or chondrocalcinosis on x-ray film
Infection		
Bacterial (nongonococcal)	Abrupt onset arthralgia, fever, systemic symptoms	Fever, CBC, synovial fluid analysis with Gram's stain, culture
Gonococcal	Abrupt onset migratory arthralgia in sexually active patient; vaginal or urethral discharge; rash	Fever, tenosynovitis, rash, urethral or cervical discharge, Gram's stain, culture (oral, rectal, genital)
Viral	Abrupt onset polyarthralgia of small joints; self-limited	Serology, liver function tests
Lyme disease	Tick bite or exposure, rash, polyarthralgia followed by monarthralgia	Serologic testing, synovial fluid testing (to rule out other causes of inflammatory monoarthritis)
Noninflammatory		
Osteoarthritis	No morning stiffness, use-related pain, night pain	Lack of inflammatory findings (e.g., no effusion), x-ray films
Avascular necrosis	Abrupt onset, predisposition (e.g., alcohol or steroid exposure)	X-ray films, MRI, or bone scan
Tumor	Chronic, unrelenting pain, history of malignant disease	X-ray films, bone scan

ANA, antinuclear antibody; CBC, complete blood count; DIP, distal interphalangeals; MRI, magnetic resonance imaging; RPR, rapid plasma reagin.

Intermittent arthritis is typically seen in crystal-induced disease and palindromic rheumatism (a variant of RA).

The specific joints involved and the pattern can narrow the diagnostic possibilities. For instance, RA would be the most likely diagnosis in the patient with a symmetric synovitis of the small joints of the hands, wrists (excluding the distal interphalangeal joints [DIPS]), elbows, knees, ankles, and feet. DIP involvement without synovitis usually is due to osteoarthritis. Asymmetric synovitis of knees and the ankle with backache suggests a spondyloarthropathy such as ankylosing spondylitis, Reiter's syndrome, psoriatic arthritis, or arthritis associated with inflammatory bowel disease.

NONARTICULAR RHEUMATISM

Polyarthralgia is a common but nonspecific complaint in women, with an extensive differential diagnosis (see box, below). Such complaints can be evaluated through the history, physical examination, and limited laboratory tests, particularly an ESR in patients older than 60 years of age. Gelling or morning stiffness longer than 30 minutes suggests inflammatory rheumatic diseases such as polymyalgia rheumatica, rheumatoid arthritis, or systemic lupus erythematosus. When symptoms are less than 6 weeks in duration, postviral arthralgias/myalgias are common diagnoses.

Myalgias—muscle pain and aching—often occur with arthralgias. This sensation differs from other sources of pain by being less intense, and it usually does not awaken the patient from sleep or prevent function. Common causes of myalgia include bacterial or viral infections and unusual or prolonged exertion. Weakness, malaise, and fatigue are nonspecific symptoms and are frequently used interchangeably. True weakness implies loss of power or endurance. Such patients have difficulty initiating and maintaining a functional activity that requires strength. A patient with weakness or decreased endurance of one extremity may have a myopathy, a neurologic lesion, muscle atrophy, or a disrupted musculoskeletal unit such as a torn tendon (e.g., rotator cuff tear) or torn muscle.

Some patients mention weakness when they have decreased stamina. This can be a symptom of any chronic disease probably related to deconditioning, toxic-metabolic effects (uremia, severe anemia), or myopathies such as polymyositis myasthenia gravis, or a variety of muscle-enzyme disorders. Patients frequently use the term *weakness* for malaise, asthenia, or nonspecific loss of well-being.

Patients without functional impairment and with normal findings on physical examination and laboratory evaluation usually have benign arthralgias that wax and wane; synovitis or impaired function rarely develop in such patients. Most of these patients are women, but no systematic study has been made of the epidemiology, course, or pathogenesis of the condition. The clinical impression is that its peak prevalence is in women of childbearing age and that its prevalence is more common and seems worse during the second part of the ovulatory cycle and postpartum. It may be a part of premenstrual syndrome. No specific treatment is reliably effective, but it is important to take the symptoms seriously and to legitimate the condition as real but benign. Antiinflammatory drugs seem to have an inconsistent effect; exogenous hormones have not been studied formally.

Arthritis has long been considered a condition that often begins at the time of menopause. One study reported the onset of RA at the time of menopause in 9.7% of approximately 250 cases (Fletcher, 1947). Diffuse aches, pains, and stiffness in the muscles and joints in the first 2 years after cessation of menstruation, without objective signs of synovitis or increase in acute-phase reactants, have been termed *menopausal arthralgias*. The same profile has been said to follow oophorectomy in women of childbearing age, with the symptoms controlled by estrogens. There are no epidemiologically valid studies to show that menopause is an etiologic factor or that hormonal replacement is specifically effective in putative menopausal arthralgias or arthritis. The best population-based evidence, in fact, suggests that joint pain is reported with about the same frequency in the following groups: approximately 20% in unselected premenopausal women, 12% in postmenopausal women before final menses, and 17% in postmenopausal women after final menses.

Fibromyalgia

When the patient has diffuse aches without a definable systemic, rheumatic, infectious, or endocrine disease, and the findings of laboratory evaluation are negative, fibrositis or fibromyalgia should be considered. Fibromyalgia is a distinct syndrome characterized by diffuse aches and pains that do not seem to correspond to specific anatomic structures and that lack physical findings other than characteristic tender points (Fig. 22-1). Sleep disturbance, fatigue, and depression are common, but its cause is not well understood. Deprivation of non–rapid eye movement (REM) sleep in healthy persons can result in generalized achiness. A number of metabolic disturbances involving estrogens, endorphins, and enkephalins have been suggested but not proved. Muscle biopsy specimens of tender points compared with those taken from nontender points in patients and healthy control subjects show reduced high-energy phosphate compounds. As with many unexplained illnesses, psychosomatic factors have been implicated.

The patient with fibromyalgia needs support and reassurance that nothing life-threatening exists. Often the issue for such patients is not a dreaded illness but validation of their symptoms. To provide reassurance, the clinician needs to be attentive to and concerned about that patient's complaints, as well as explain fibrositis and the theories about its cause, what to expect, and a treatment strategy. In controlled trials, aerobic exercise and tricyclic antidepressants for sleep disturbance (such as amitriptyline 25 to 50 mg) help improve symptoms, but long-term benefit may not always result. Some patients with fibrositis, as in patients with chronic fatigue syndrome (a potentially related condition), may be very sensitive to doses of amitriptyline (e.g., 10 to 12.5 mg/day) that would not normally be expected to be thera-

---

DIFFERENTIAL DIAGNOSIS OF POLYARTHRALGIA

Viral infection
Idiopathic benign arthralgia
Early rheumatic disease (e.g., RA, SLE)
Lyme disease
Medications
    Accutane
    Fluoride
    Drug-induced systemic lupus
      (especially procainamide, hydralazine)
    Enalapril
Steroid withdrawal
Fibromyalgia
Hypothyroidism
Hyperparathyroidism
Subacute bacterial endocarditis
Sarcoidosis
Metabolic bone disease (e.g., osteomalacia)

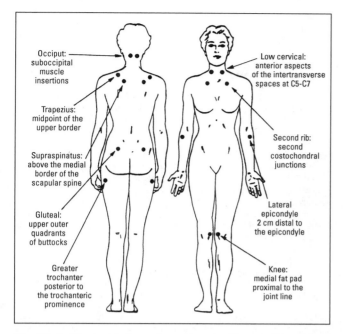

Fig. 22-1 Characteristic tender points in fibromyalgia. (From Schumacher HR, ed: *Primer on the rheumatic diseases,* Atlanta, Arthritis Foundation, 1993.)

peutic for depression. Cyclobenzaprine (Flexeril), 5 to 10 mg orally at night, is a muscle relaxant chemically related to the tricyclic antidepressants and is an alternative first-line option. Nonsteroidal antiinflammatory drugs and corticosteroid therapy rarely help.

In summary, a woman with polyarthralgias should be questioned about antecedent illness, prior episodes, arthritis, medications that can cause arthralgias/myalgias (see box, p. 165) symptoms from other organ systems, functional limitations, and mood. If these are normal and the examination shows no tender points, synovitis, or other abnormalities, benign arthralgia is the most likely diagnosis. If tender points can be identified, fibromyalgia is the diagnosis.

Raynaud's syndrome

Pain in the digits may be due to Raynaud's phenomenon, a reversible pallor caused by vasospasm of the vessels in the fingers and toes that is precipitated by cold or emotion. The reaction is episodic and may be accompanied by numbness or pain; it occurs only rarely in the nose, earlobe, or even tongue. It is classically described as a triphasic response with blanching white color, usually clearly demarcated from the rest of the digit, followed by cyanosis and then rubor as reperfusion takes place. Occasionally, edema accompanies reperfusion; in long-standing disease, sclerodactyly may develop. This disorder is much more common in women. A distinction is made between Raynaud's phenomenon, which occurs with or is an early manifestation of a connective tissue disease or another condition (secondary Raynaud's), and Raynaud's disease, which occurs as an isolated condition. The diagnosis must be made clinically, primarily based on the history, although cold challenge (e.g., running cool water over the hands) may be useful in select cases. The episodic

nature of symptoms and the development of sharply demarcated pallor are the most specific historic features.

Even in a referral practice rheumatic disease develops in only 5% of patients with Raynaud's phenomenon. Many rheumatic diseases may be associated with Raynaud's phenomenon (systemic sclerosis, limited scleroderma, SLE, mixed connective tissue disease, dermatomyositis, or RA), but the most important are scleroderma and related disorders.

The principal task for the primary care physician in evaluating Raynaud's phenomenon is to determine whether it is isolated (or primary) or associated with other diseases or exposures. The box below displays the differential diagnosis of secondary Raynaud's phenomenon. Most patients with the disease can be evaluated quite simply, and the pace of further evaluation depends on associated features (see Table 22-4). If Raynaud's phenomenon is present for several years without the development of another rheumatic disease, it is likely to remain an isolated problem.

Treatment of Raynaud's phenomenon begins with advice to avoid cigarette smoke, cold, and β-blockers and to wear

---

CONDITIONS ASSOCIATED WITH RAYNAUD'S PHENOMENON (SECONDARY RAYNAUD'S PHENOMENON)

Small vessel disease
Idiopathic
Systemic sclerosis (scleroderma)
Systemic lupus erythematosus
Rheumatoid arthritis
Dermatomyositis/polymyositis
Vasculitis
Vibration, chronic (e.g., jackhammers, chain saw)
Cold injury
Primary pulmonary hypertension

Large vessel disease
Arteriosclerosis
Thoracic outlet syndromes
Thromboangiitis obliterans

Intravascular (cyanosis without blanching)
Cryoglobulinemia
Cold agglutinins
Polycythemia

Drug or toxin associated
β-blockers
Ergots
Bleomycin
Cisplatin
Vincristine/vinblastine
Nicotine
Pseudoephedrine
Polyvinylchloride
Cocaine

Hormonal
Hypothyroidism
Estrogen/progesterone
Pheochromocytoma

REFERRAL CRITERIA

Undiagnosed synovitis
Failing function
Multisystem disease
Consideration of immunosuppressive, steroid, or disease-modifying agent, or intravenous colchicine
Diagnostic arthrocentesis/biopsy
Unresolved symptoms more than 6 weeks, especially if unresponsive to symptomatic or supportive therapy
Progressive symptoms or signs
Pregnancy in SLE, progressive systemic sclerosis

a hat, gloves or mittens, and a vest in the cold weather. Waving the involved arm can be helpful. Biofeedback if available may be beneficial. Calcium channel blockers, including nifedipine and diltiazem, have been used with success.

Patients with sclerodactyly or who are ill should have laboratory measurement of renal function, ANA, ESR, and CBC, as well as a urinalysis.

Any patient with Raynaud's phenomenon who has other organ involvement could have secondary Raynaud's phenomenon and should be referred to a rheumatologist. Raynaud's phenomenon with ischemic manifestations requires urgent referral and possible hospitalization.

INDICATIONS FOR REFERRAL TO A RHEUMATOLOGIST

The diagnosis and initial management of most musculoskeletal problems a primary care physician sees can be effectively undertaken in the office. Exceptions are situations in which greater experience and specialized knowledge are needed to ensure optimal outcome (see box, above). The primary care physician should refer these problems for another opinion but in most cases is still the best person to integrate and execute advice from the specialist.

BIBLIOGRAPHY

Arnett FC et al: The American Rheumatism Association 1987 revised criteria for the classification of rheumatoid arthritis, *Arthritis Rheum* 31:315, 1988.

Baker DG, Schumacher HR Jr: Acute monoarthritis, *N Engl J Med* 329:1013, 1993.

Clayburne G, Baker DG, Schumacher HR Jr: Estimated synovial fluid leukocyte numbers on wet drop preparations as a potential substitute for actual counts, *J Rheum* 19:60, 1992.

Coope J, Thomson JM, Poller L: Effects of "natural oestrogen" replacement therapy on menopausal symptoms and blood clotting, *Br Med J* 4:139, 1975.

Daltroy LH et al: Predictors and modifying factors of self-reported disability in the elderly: an analysis of discrepancies, in press, 1994.

Fitzgerald O et al: Prospective study of the evolution of Raynaud's phenomenon, *Am J Med* 84:718, 1988.

Fletcher E: *Medical disorders of the locomotive system including the rheumatoid diseases,* Baltimore, 1947, Williams & Wilkins.

Gerbarcht DD et al: Evolution of primary Raynaud's phenomenon (Raynaud's disease) to connective tissue disease, *Arthritis Rheum* 28:87, 1985.

Hawkins BR et al: Use of the B27 test in the diagnosis of ankylosing spondylitis: a statistical evaluation, *Arthritis Rheum* 24:743, 1981.

Hebert LA, Cosio FG, Neff JC: Diagnostic significance of hypocomplementemia, *Kidney Int* 39:811, 1991.

Hoppenfeld S: *Physical examination of the spine and extremities,* New York, 1976, Appleton-Century-Crofts.

Jennette JC, Falk RJ: Antineutrophil cytoplasmic autoantibodies associated disease: a review, *Am J Kidney Dis* 15:517, 1990.

Juby A, Johnston C, Davis P: Specificity, sensitivity and diagnostic predictive value of selected laboratory generated autoantibody profiles in patients with connective tissue diseases, *J Rheumatol* 18:354, 1991.

Katz JN et al: Differences between men and women undergoing major orthopaedic surgery for degenerative arthritis, *Arthritis Rheum* 37:687, 1994.

Lichtenstein MJ, Pincus T: Rheumatoid arthritis identified in population based cross-sectional studies: low prevalance of rheumatoid factor, *J Rheum* 18:989, 1991.

Litwin SD, Singer JM: Studies of the incidence and significance of antigamma globulin factors in the aging, *Arthritis Rheum* 8:538, 1965.

Maddison PJ, Provost TT, Reichlin M: Serologic findings in patients with "ANA-negative" systemic lupus erythematosus, *Medicine* 60:87, 1981.

McCarty GA: Autoantibodies and their relation to rheumatic diseases, *Med Clin North Am* 70:237, 1986.

Polley HF, Hunder GG: *Rheumatological interviewing and physical examination of the joints,* ed 2, Philadelphia, 1978, WB Saunders.

Richardson B, Epstein WV: Utility of the fluorescent antinuclear antibody test in a single patient, *Ann Intern Med* 95:333, 1981.

Schur PH: Inherited complement component abnormalities, *Annu Rev Med* 37:333, 1986.

Shmerling RH, Delbanco TL: The rheumatoid factor: an analysis of clinical utility, *Am J Med* 91:528, 1991.

Shmerling RH, Delbanco TL: How useful is the rheumatoid factor? Analysis of sensitivity, specificity, and predictive value, *Arch Intern Med* 152:2417, 1991.

Shmerling RH, Liang MH: General laboratory evaluation of rheumatic diseases. In Schumacher HR, editor: *Primer on the rheumatic diseases,* Atlanta, 1993, Arthritis Foundation.

Sox HC Jr, Liang MH: The erythrocyte sedimentation rate: guidelines for rational use, *Ann Intern Med* 104:515, 1986.

Thompson B, Hart SA, Durno D: Menopausal age and symptomatology in a general practice, *Johns Hopkins Biosoc Sci* 5:71, 1973.

Wolfe F, Cathey MA, Roberts FK: The latex test revisited: rheumatoid factor testing in 8,287 rheumatic disease patients, *Arthritis Rheum* 34:951, 1991.

Wood C: Menopausal myths, *Med J Austr* 1:496, 1979.

23 Osteoarthritis

Ronald J. Anderson

EPIDEMIOLOGY AND RISK FACTORS

Osteoarthritis is the one of the leading causes of morbidity in the female population. Although the disease clearly affects both sexes, the incidence of osteoarthritis of the knee in women is twice that seen in men. In the Framingham study the prevalence of knee osteoarthritis was 30% between ages 65 and 74 years. In addition to pain and loss of independence, osteoarthritis was responsible for 68 million work-loss days each year and nearly 4 million hospitalizations. Most of these hospitalizations were related to the performance of total joint arthroplasties. Various risk factors exist for the development of osteoarthritis, including obesity, repetitive trauma, female gender, several metabolic defects of cartilage metabolism, and genetic factors. This chapter deals with the diagnosis of osteoarthritis and addresses some of the key issues in treatment and rehabilitation.

PHYSIOLOGY

Critical to the understanding of osteoarthritis is the appreciation of several key points concerning the normal physiology and anatomy of the diarthrodial joint, its clinical and radiographic implications, and the pathophysiology of the disease process itself (see box, below).

Hyaline cartilage

Hyaline cartilage, which forms the articular surface of all diarthrodial joints, has an understructure consisting of arcades of collagen fibers encased in a matrix of proteoglycan. This provides an elastic, resilient surface that is nearly free of friction. Cartilage does not normally deteriorate with age, and degenerative joint disease should not be viewed as a normal accompaniment of aging. Unlike bone, however, cartilage lacks the ability, at least on a macroscopic level, to repair and reconstruct itself. Thus one should regard any lesion of cartilage on a clinical level as a permanent and irreversible step.

PREDISPOSING FACTORS FOR THE DEVELOPMENT OF OSTEOARTHRITIS

Previous mechanical trauma
Obesity
Metabolic abnormalities
  Acromegaly
  Hemachromatosis
  Wilson's disease
  Ochronosis
Genetic predisposition
Congenital dislocation of the hip
Slipped femoral epiphysis
Avascular necrosis
Intraarticular fracture

When cartilage loss does occur, it tends to develop initially in the region of the articular cartilage most exposed to weight bearing and stress. The subchondral and periarticular bone adjacent to areas of cartilage loss tends to buttress this region by local proliferation, resulting in the formation of subchondral and periarticular osteophytes.

PATHOPHYSIOLOGY AND DEFINITION OF OSTEOARTHRITIS

The term *osteoarthritis* is misleading because the suffix "itis" implies an inflammatory process. Most of the data suggest a degenerative rather than an inflammatory process. Pathologic examination, however, rarely demonstrates synovial inflammation, and the synovial fluid is characteristically free of inflammatory exudate. A leukocytosis of greater than 1000 cells/ml is seldom seen in the synovial fluid, and inflammatory mediators are found in low concentrations. Antiinflammatory agents are relatively ineffective in relieving symptoms and have not been shown to reverse the process. Although the precise mechanism responsible for producing pain in osteoarthritis is unclear, it appears that the symptoms are related to the mechanical opposition of two imperfect surfaces upon each other. The term *degenerative joint disease* or *osteoarthrosis* is often used as a synonym for osteoarthritis, implying the noninflammatory and degenerative nature of the process.

Cartilage loss in osteoarthritis is related either to localized trauma and mechanical stress or to these factors operating on cartilage that has an underlying metabolic or structural abnormality. The abnormalities can be divided into those associated with collagen structure and those related to an underlying biochemical abnormality of the cartilage matrix. Although various kindreds may be identified with an apparent propensity for the development of osteoarthritis, only recently has a specific abnormality of collagen formation been identified and genetically defined. Other abnormalities of collagen structure undoubtedly will be defined in the future, but the incidence of these syndromes would seem to be rare. Metabolic abnormalities of cartilage, which include acromegaly, hemachromatosis, Wilson's disease, and ochronosis, predispose the patient to premature degeneration of the cartilage. These conditions also are associated with the radiographic appearance of **chondrocalcinosis,** a clinically useful marker for abnormal cartilage and the resultant development of osteoarthritis. Chondrocalcinosis is associated with acute inflammatory attacks of **pseudogout,** in which calcium pyrophosphate crystals existing within lacunae in the articular cartilage enter the synovial fluid by an unknown mechanism and provoke an inflammatory response that clinically has the appearance of gout.

Only a small proportion of patients with osteoarthritis have a defined metabolic abnormality or genetic predisposition to arthritis. Most patients suffer cartilage loss related to "trauma" occurring in an "anatomically disadvantaged joint." Therefore, the joints affected are those involved with major weight bearing and stress, such as the metacarpocarpal joint at the base of the thumb, the hip, the knee, and the metacarpophalangeal (MCP) joint of the great toe. Prior injury to the cartilage of any joint such as occurs in congenital dislocation of the hip, slipped femoral epiphysis, avascular necrosis, intraarticular fracture, or any subtle asymmetry of the joint also creates a predisposition to mechanical wear and cartilage deterioration.

Osteophytes and osteoarthritis

Although x-ray study is the usual technique by which a diagnosis of osteoarthritis is made, it is helpful to remember that plain radiographs basically show only bone and not cartilage. Alterations in cartilage can be detected only by the rather insensitive method of demonstrating that bone margins are closer together. This will not pick up subtle changes in the articular surface. Radiologists also use the presence of osteophytes as a criterion for the diagnosis of osteoarthritis. The presence of osteophytes does not automatically follow the deterioration of cartilage, and it is absent in cartilage loss related to the destruction of cartilage by synovitis. In addition, the degree of osteophyte formation does not correlate well with the extent of cartilage loss in degenerative joint disease but is useful as a radiographic marker that the cartilage loss is not inflammatory in nature. Moreover, there are several clinical syndromes, such as **Heberden's nodes** and **diffuse idiopathic skeletal hyperostosis (DISH)** in which osteophyte formation is the dominant lesion and not directly related to the extent of primary cartilage loss.

DEGENERATIVE JOINT DISORDERS WITH A PREDILECTION FOR WOMEN
Heberden's nodes

Heberden's nodes is a hereditary disorder with a predilection for women in which a secondary spurt of bone growth occurs during the middle years of life and is localized to the distal interphalangeal joints of the hands. The condition is unrelated to osteoarthritis in other joints and is not an apparent risk factor for any other disorder. The symptoms are correlated with the phase of bone growth that usually persists for 1 to 2 years. Once the osteophyte is formed, the stiffness usually improves significantly although the rigidity and protuberance of bone persists. **Bouchard's nodes** is the term applied to the identical process when it occurs in the proximal interphalangeal joints.

Metacarpocarpal joint degeneration of the thumb

Metacarpocarpal (MCC) joint degeneration of the thumb is related to the hypermobility and resultant shear forces associated with ligamentous instability in the MCC joint of the thumb. Symptoms related to the degeneration of the MCC articulation of the thumb usually occur between the ages of 50 and 70 years. On physical examination, pain is produced by stressing the base of the metacarpal upon the triquetral bone. Often a high-pitched crepitus characteristic of cartilage loss may occur. X-ray films show cartilage loss when symptoms arise, and osteophytes will develop over the next few years. The natural course of the condition is symptomatic improvement as the development of osteophytes stabilizes the joint and reduces motion and therefore the

pain associated with it. The syndrome needs to be distinguished from **de Quervain's tendinitis** in which pain is produced by forced flexion at the MCP and ulnar deviation of the wrist, which causes tenderness and pain along the abductor pollicis longus (Finkelstein's test). (For more details on this syndrome see Chapter 24.)

Patellofemoral osteoarthritis

The same instability and mobility that occur in the MCC joint also occur in the female patellofemoral joint. This is related to an increased angle of the patellar groove of the female femur. This syndrome commonly occurs in younger women aged 15 to 35 years and is rare in middle-aged or elderly women, although knee radiographs in this older age-group frequently show degenerative changes in the patellofemoral joint. The symptoms do not correlate well with radiographic findings, which often are negative in the younger age-group. The pain is most often felt anteriorly and bilaterally. It is accentuated by use, particularly by walking downstairs. Pain that interferes with sleep is common and related to pivoting on the patella while switching from a prone to a supine position. On physical examination the pain can be reproduced by grinding the patella on the femur. Also, the maximal pain during range of motion occurs during the last 30 degrees of extension. The management of the syndrome is controversial, and surgical therapy is aimed at stabilizing the patella. Clinical observation has revealed, however, that the majority of patients will experience relief of symptoms over a period of several months to few years. The interventions for these patients include maintenance of strength and the use of benign analgesic and nonsteroidal antiinflammatory agents.

DIFFERENTIAL DIAGNOSIS

A physician's first concern on the presentation of probable osteoarthritis is to attempt to make another diagnosis. Osteoarthritis is a diagnosis of exclusion. Once again, the radiographic evidence of osteoarthritis should never be accepted as adequate evidence for the diagnosis. The clinical picture needs to be consistent with the diagnosis of osteoarthritis, and other readily treatable conditions need to be excluded. Frequently another condition, such as inflammatory arthritis, is superimposed on underlying osteoarthritis and is sufficient to precipitate symptoms in the affected joint. Another example is the generalized stiffness associated with **Parkinson's disease** and **myxedema.** These diseases, particularly in the elderly population, can be confused with osteoarthritis.

Local inflammatory disorders, **tendinitis** and **bursitis,** are prone to develop adjacent to joints whose leverage and anatomy are altered by degenerative changes. The most common syndrome is **anserine bursitis,** an inflammation of the anserine bursa located inferior and medial to the knee joint. The classic picture of this syndrome is the abrupt accentuation of knee pain, frequently with nocturnal pain, occurring in a patient with medial compartment osteoarthritis of the knee with its resultant bowlegged deformity. Exquisite tenderness over the anserine bursa is evident on physical examination. Erythema or swelling is seldom seen. The pain should respond to the local injection of 1 or 2 ml of 1% lidocaine (Xylocaine) mixed with 1 ml of a long-acting steroid such as methylprednisolone (Depo-Medrol), 40 mg/ml. Whenever doubt exists regarding the diagnosis, it is advisable to inject the tender area; the complications are minimal and the benefits may be significant and long-lasting.

The coexistent development of an inflammatory condition, most commonly **rheumatoid arthritis, gout, pseudogout,** and **polymyalgia rheumatica,** should always be excluded, at least on clinical grounds. Patients with these diseases often manifest mechanical symptoms but also have associated systemic malaise, physical findings of joint inflammation, a dramatic response to antiinflammatory therapy, and symptoms and deformities that occur in non–weight bearing joints such as the elbow, wrist, or MCP joint.

CLINICAL PRESENTATION

To reiterate, the diagnosis of osteoarthritis as the cause of the patient's symptoms should never be based solely on the radiologic demonstration of cartilage loss with associated osteophyte formation. Although radiographic evidence is required for the diagnosis of osteoarthritis, its presence should never be sufficient in itself to make the diagnosis. The physician should rely on other clinical criteria to ensure that the patient's symptoms are truly related to osteoarthritis. The criteria are as follows (see box, below).

History and symptom presentation

Mechanical symptoms. The cause of pain in osteoarthritis seems to evolve from the abrasive grinding of two imperfect surfaces, and symptoms therefore occur only when weight-bearing or similar mechanical stress occurs. In contrast, although an accentuation of symptoms occurs with use in patients with inflammatory joint disease, they also experience rest pain and stiffness. Rest pain and particularly nocturnal pain, defined as pain sufficient to interfere with sleep, is uncommon in osteoarthritis and seen only in the most advanced stages of the process when failure to consciously splint the joint during sleep allows surfaces totally devoid of cartilage to rub on each other and produce pain. The typical patient with degenerative joint disease of the knee has pain on walking and is asymptomatic at rest.

Gradual and progressive deteriorating course. Cartilage loss is irreversible with a gradual rate of change that becomes obvious only over months or years and not days or weeks. The latter pattern is more suggestive of inflammatory arthritis. An occasional exception to this rule occurs in osteoarthritis of the hip, which may infrequently follow an aggressively severe and rapid course of accentuated symptoms despite only gradual changes when monitored radio-

graphically or by physical examination. The reason for this presentation is unknown and seems more related to the observation that early osteoarthritis of the hip is often asymptomatic except for a characteristic difficulty in putting on shoes or socks. Because the pathologic changes of osteoarthritis are permanent, the clinical occurrence of a remission or significant improvement almost excludes degenerative joint disease as the diagnosis.

Failure to respond to antiinflammatory therapy. Because osteoarthritis is essentially a noninflammatory condition, its symptoms do not usually respond dramatically to the use of nonsteroidal and other antiinflammatory agents. Often acetaminophen is as effective. This may not be true, however, for degenerative joint disease of the hip in which some patients will experience significant symptomatic relief from the use of nonsteroidal antiinflammatory agents. The mechanism behind this unique situation is unknown. There is no evidence, however, that antiinflammatory therapy either reverses or prevents the progression of the changes to osteoarthritis.

Lack of inflammatory features. Joints involved with osteoarthritis do not exhibit significant synovitis or pannus formation. The presence of a large synovial effusion is rare, and the synovial fluid white cell count is low—in the range of under 1000 cells/ml. Symptomatic patterns of prolonged (more than 2 hours) morning stiffness, easy fatiguability, and generalized malaise, which are characteristic of systemic rheumatic diseases, are absent in osteoarthritis; their presence should lead the clinician to reassess the working diagnosis of osteoarthritis.

Patients with underlying osteoarthritis and articular chondrocalcinosis are prone to episodic attacks of inflammation related to pseudogout. (Joint aspiration and the diagnosis of pseudogout are detailed in the next section.)

Involvement only of mechanically stressed joints. In the absence of a unique trauma or injury such as intraarticular fracture, osteoarthritis develops only in weight-bearing or mechanically stressed joints, namely the MCC joint of the thumb (a fulcrum joint), the hip, the knee, and the MTP joint of the great toe. Presumably because of the springlike action of the tibiofibular-talar joint and the added resilience of the subtalar and intratarsal joints, osteoarthritis of the ankle is extremely rare and usually seen only after intraarticular fractures of the ankle or in persons with metabolic defects of the cartilage metabolism. Symptoms related to or the appearance of a deformity in a non–weight-bearing joint such as the elbow, wrist, or MCP joint are characteristic of an inflammatory joint disease in which any joint may be involved.

Physical examination

In addition to a complete physical examination, a thorough joint examination should be completed. Pertinent physical findings for the diagnosis of osteoarthritis are as follows.

High-pitched crepitus. The findings of high-pitched crepitus can be of help in the diagnosis. When a high-pitched palpable or audible crepitus is present upon manipulating the joint during the physical examination, it is specific for the absence of cartilage covering the articular surface and is indicative of bone grinding on bone. Although it is not specific for osteoarthritis, it suggests the diagnosis

---

SUMMARY OF CLINICAL PRESENTATION OF OSTEOARTHRITIS

Mechanical symptoms
Gradual and progressive deteriorating course
Lack of inflammatory features
Failure to respond to antiinflammatory therapy
Involvement of mechanically stressed joints only
High-pitched crepitus on physical examination
Radiographic or arthroscopic evidence of cartilage loss

because any process that destroys cartilage may be associated with this characteristic physical finding.

Quadriceps muscle weakness. Often degenerative changes of the knee joint are associated with profound quadriceps muscle weakness. Two physical findings are indicative of quadriceps muscle weakness. The first is instability on lateral stress. This can be demonstrated by having the patient hold the knee in full extension while the examiner applies lateral stress to the calf with the thigh held stable. Normally the tibia should not move on the femur. The other finding is the presence of an extensor lag. The patient is asked to extend the knee fully. The ability to further extend the knee by passive motion is abnormal.

Diagnostic tests

Joint aspiration. As mentioned before, generally the joint fluid in osteoarthritis either is not detectable on physical examination or is benign, with lack of inflammatory cells or crystals. Intraarticular calcium pyrophosphate crystals are identifiable within polymorphonuclear leukocytes in the synovial fluid aspirated from an affected joint of a patient with pseudogout. These crystals are difficult to identify by means of polarized light microscopy compared with the readily apparent urate crystals seen in attacks of gout; a period of 10 to 15 minutes of careful observation is required under polarized light until the examiner can say with certainty that calcium pyrophosphate crystals are not present.

Radiographic and arthroscopic evidence of cartilage loss

Plain films. Although x-ray examination is the usual technique by which a diagnosis of osteoarthritis is made, it is helpful to remember that plain radiographs basically show only bone and not cartilage and will not detect subtle alterations of the cartilage surface. Any joint that has deteriorated structurally to the point of producing symptoms should have at least some of the characteristic features of osteoarthritis on an x-ray film, especially joint space narrowing, which reflects cartilage loss and adjacent osteophyte formation. However, the radiographic appearance of osteoarthritis should never be accepted as adequate evidence that the patient's symptoms are related to osteoarthritis.

Magnetic resonance imaging (MRI). In recent years MRI has developed an increasingly larger role in the diagnosis of musculoskeletal disorders. Its major role has been in the more precise definition of lesions that are not apparent on plain films. This includes lesions such as meniscal derangements, soft tissue lesions such as synovial proliferation of neoplasms, and the early osseous changes associated with avascular necrosis. This later condition may have clinical manifestations for several weeks before the plain films show abnormal findings. Although all of these conditions may cause a predisposition to cartilage degeneration, by the time symptoms related to degenerative joint disease develop, the plain films will show characteristic changes.

Arthroscopic evidence. Arthroscopic examination, particularly of the knee, may be an even more sensitive technique for the early diagnosis of osteoarthritis, albeit not the most cost-effective. Several studies have compared arthroscopy with MRI or arthrography in defining early structural changes of the knee and meniscal derangements

and have suggested increased sensitivity with the use of arthroscopy. However, in view of the paucity of significant therapeutic interventions currently available, arthroscopy cannot be recommended as a routine early diagnostic procedure for this condition.

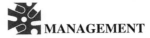

MANAGEMENT

Goals of management

The guiding principles in the management of osteoarthritis are as follows:
1. There is no evidence that either medical or surgical therapy can influence the course of the disorder.
2. The pathologic process appears to be irreversible, at least on a macroscopic level, and the lesion at best will remain stable but more likely will progress over the ensuing months to years.
3. Advances in orthopedic surgery over the past 25 years have provided patients with procedures for the reconstruction of damaged joints that not only relieve pain but also restore meaningful function. These procedures, although in a state of technical evolution, have been highly successful and have dramatically improved the quality of life for persons with these conditions.
4. The role of the nonorthopedist in the management of osteoarthritis is to initially and accurately diagnose the disorder, develop a program aimed at obtaining symptomatic relief and maintaining function, and, when indicated, orchestrate appropriate orthopedic intervention.

Choice of therapy

Pharmacologic therapy. The optimal pharmacologic agent for the treatment of osteoarthritis would be a substance to induce cartilage to regrow and repair itself. Such an agent does not exist. Acromegaly is the only condition in which cartilage is seen to increase quantitatively, but the cartilage formed is of poor quality and premature osteoarthritis develops.

The nonsteroidal antiinflammatory drugs (NSAIDs) are marketed for the treatment of both inflammatory arthritis and osteoarthritis. A recent study by Bradley et al. comparing acetaminophen with high- and low-dose ibuprofen in the treatment of osteoarthritis of the knee showed benefit from all agents but no significant difference among the three regimens. This result would be expected given the usual noninflammatory nature of knee osteoarthritis, and it is consistent with clinical experience. On the other hand, hip osteoarthritis for reasons that are still unclear may be symptomatically more responsive to the use of NSAIDs, particularly indomethacin, and a trial of these agents is worthwhile. There is no evidence, however, that NSAIDs alter the pathologic process or course of the disease. Therefore if complications from the use of nonsteroidal agents occur, such as gastritis or renal dysfunction, it seems best to avoid these medications and use acetaminophen for pain or consider other options. Because of the chronic nature of the pain, narcotic analgesics and muscle relaxants should be avoided.

Weight reduction. Obesity has been shown to be a risk factor in the development of osteoarthritis of the knee, and weight reduction in the asymptomatic obese woman does reduce the risk of developing symptomatic knee osteoarthritis. Whether weight reduction should be used as a universal therapy for osteoarthritis is controversial. In general the rate and degree of symptomatic relief achieved by weight reduction in the obese patient with osteoarthritis are equal to or exceeded by the rate of worsening caused by the natural progression of cartilage deterioration during the time period taken to lose the weight. Thus patients seldom perceive any symptomatic benefit from the tremendous effort involved in weight reduction, often feel frustrated and misled, and frequently respond inappropriately by rapidly regaining the lost weight. On the other hand, weight reduction significantly decreases the morbidity associated with reconstructive surgery and presumably will defer or delay the development of symptomatic osteoarthritis in currently unaffected joints. A reasonable practice would be to explain the benefits and options to the patient and strongly encourage weight reduction.

Weight bearing and exercise. Because osteoarthritis is a disease of weight-bearing joints, patients adjust their activities to remain comfortable. A patient should not be advised to avoid activity in hopes of "saving" the joints. Patients should maintain their present level of activity, including the optimal level of employment, aerobic exercise, and social and personal activities. If these activities become difficult to do, the patient might want to consider surgical options.

Use of external braces. The use of external braces is ineffective in most situations. Any brace rigid enough to provide stabilization will compress the soft tissue in a way that is detrimental to the patient. Soft elastic braces do not provide any real stability and create venous occlusion.

Physical therapy and rehabilitation. The obvious tendency is to avoid using a painful joint. Immobility will lead to both muscle atrophy and restricted motion related to soft tissue contracture. Motion also may be lost in osteoarthritis as a result of the stabilizing effect of periarticular osteophyte formation creating a "bony blockade." In certain joints such as the MCC joint at the base of the thumb, this immobility is beneficial, and with time much of the pain and disability disappears. In other joints such as the knee, immobility is deleterious. For a person to climb stairs and arise from a low chair, the knee should be able to move from 0 to 110 degrees. In addition, the muscular strength of the quadriceps lends stability to the knee, particularly in the flexed position.

The techniques of physical therapy are primarily of value when the goal is to add muscle strength or range of motion. Range of motion can be added either passively or actively. Restoring muscle strength requires active effort on the part of the patient.

The findings of quadriceps muscle weakness are an indication for an aggressive program of muscle strengthening, usually by means of quadriceps-setting exercise. Because at least some degree of thigh-muscle weakness exists in almost every patient with knee arthritis, these exercises may be routinely prescribed. Muscle strengthening can be achieved only by the patient's individual efforts. The therapist's role in obtaining this goal is that of an educator, and frequent visits to the therapist are not required after the patient has mastered the exercise routine. In the beginning of the process, the therapist may need to take an active role inasmuch as passive range of motion exercises may be needed. The use of other modalities such as local heat, massage, whirlpool, and ultrasound may be of preliminary value in manipulating the patient to increase passive range of motion. They have little role otherwise in the management of osteoarthritis.

Orthopedic interventions

Prophylactic procedures. There are few prophylactic procedures that will affect the development of osteoarthritis. **Arthroscopic débridement** of loose bodies may provide symptomatic relief from symptoms of internal derangement, but the clinical indications for the procedure are still unclear. Prior meniscectomy promotes the development of osteoarthritis in that specific knee. However, it is highly probable that the presence of a torn meniscus provides an intraarticular nidus and thus may accelerate the development of degenerative changes in that joint.

Tibial osteotomy should be considered for patients with **unicompartmental knee symptoms** and a **varus** (bowlegged) or **valgus** (knock-kneed) deformity. Unicompartmental knee osteoarthritis is a "self-fulfilling prophecy" in that the more the cartilage deteriorates in the medial compartment, the greater the bowlegged deformity and thus the greater the stress on that compartment, leading to a more rapid cartilage deterioration. In this situation, a tibial osteotomy consisting of the surgical removal of a triangular wedge of bone from the lateral aspect of the lateral upper tibia would correct the varus deformity and create a valgus deformity so that the patient will bear weight primarily on the healthy normal cartilage covering the lateral compartment of the knee. This procedure is indicated in relatively young persons (younger than 50 years old) who are physically active and wish to defer the more definitive procedure involved in a total joint replacement. The major disadvantage of the procedure is the need to use crutches for several months. Given that this procedure is performed in patients with "mild" disease, this group may be less eager to accept the long period on crutches.

Joint fusion. Fusion of osteoarthritis joints is seldom employed. Although considered a low-risk procedure, joint fusion requires a long period of immobility, and the resulting "long lever arm" produced by the fusion increases the stress on the adjacent joint and facilitates the development of osteoarthritis in that joint. It is the procedure of choice in unstable, painful interphalangeal joints of the hand and occasionally in the MCC joint of the thumb or the MTP joint of the great toe.

Total joint replacement. The definitive treatment for any destroyed joint is a total joint replacement. This is a **surface replacement arthroplasty** in which the destroyed articular surface is removed and replaced by a metallic prosthesis on one side and a plastic prosthesis on the other. The prosthesis is sometimes cemented to the bone.

General experience with joint replacement has been positive. The major complication has been infection in the prosthetic site, and the risk increases with each operation. It also should be assumed that the life expectancy of a total joint replacement is 5 to 15 years.

Once the clinician is certain that the symptoms arise from the mechanical lesion of osteoarthritis, the indication for an operation is based solely on the patient's symptoms of pain and dysfunction, surgical risk, and the anticipated result.

There is no reason to assume that an operation performed early is more successful than delayed surgery.

Pain is difficult to measure but may be defined as being severe enough to interfere with sleep. Function can be defined more quantitatively. Except in rare situations, pain sufficient to interfere with sleep in a major way is an indication for surgery irrespective of other problems. In considering an operation aimed at achieving a functional gain, it is critical to determine whether there is another factor such as angina, vascular or pulmonary insufficiency, or another marginal joint that is currently asymptomatic only because the patient is unable to stress herself past the limits set by the severity of symptoms arising from the one worst joint.

Finally, once convinced that osteoarthritis is the cause of the patient's symptoms, the clinician should never defer surgery with the expectation that the situation will spontaneously improve. If the diagnosis is correct, the symptoms will only increase in severity. The current critical issue in reconstructive joint surgery focuses on the longevity of the implants, with further research in progress.

BIBLIOGRAPHY

Bradley JD et al: Comparison of an anti-inflammatory dose of ibuprofen, and analgesic dose of ibuprofen, and acetaminophen in the treatment of patient with osteoarthritis of the knee, *N Engl J Med* 325:87, 1991.

Felson DT et al: Obesity and knee osteoarthritis: the Framingham study, *Ann Intern Med* 109:18, 1988.

Felson DT et al: Weight loss reduces the risk for symptomatic knee osteoarthritis in women: the Framingham study, *Ann Intern Med* 116:535, 1992.

Fischer SP et al: Accuracy of diagnoses from magnetic resonance imaging of the knee: a multi-center analysis of one thousand and fourteen patients, *J Bone Joint Surg [Am]* 73:2, 1991.

Gillies H, Seligson D: Precision in the diagnosis of meniscal lesions: a comparison of clinical evaluation, arthrography, and arthroscopy, *J Bone Joint Surg [Am]* 61:343, 1979.

Harris WH, Sledge CB: Total hip and total knee replacement, *N Engl J Med* 323:725, 1990.

Schumacher HR, editor: *Primer on the rheumatic diseases,* ed 10, Atlanta, 1993, Arthritis Foundation.

24 Regional Musculoskeletal Disorders

Jeffrey N. Katz

Regional musculoskeletal disorders are common and disabling, yet often underrecognized and inappropriately managed by clinicians because they fall between the cracks of rheumatology, orthopaedics, neurology, and physical medicine. The box on the following page lists a variety of regional musculoskeletal diseases by anatomic region and pathophysiologic mechanism. This chapter focuses on the most common of these disorders, particularly those seen frequently in females.

DISORDERS OF THE HANDS, WRISTS, AND ELBOWS
Epidemiology

Four frequently encountered upper extremity regional disorders are carpal tunnel syndrome, de Quervain's tenosynovitis, carpometacarpal osteoarthritis, and epicondylitis (see Table 24-1). Carpal tunnel syndrome has an annual incidence of 0.1% in the general population with the highest incidence in women in the sixth and seventh decades. In workers, there is no female predominance and the peak decade of onset is the 30s. Risk factors include medical conditions such as diabetes, amyloidosis, and hypothyroidism as well as forceful repetitive occupational hand movements. The incidence of de Quervain's tenosynovitis has not been studied; it is probably the most common upper extremity tendonitis seen in orthopedic and rheumatologic practices. In major clinical series 77% to 91% of patients with de Quervain's tenosynovitis are female. Activities that involve resisted extension of the thumb, excessive pinch, and excessive ulnar deviation of the wrist predispose to de Quervain's tenosynovitis. The problem is seen commonly among parents who lift their babies by the axillae.

The carpometacarpal (CMC) joint is one of the most common sites of osteoarthritis, with reported prevalence of 20% in males and 40% in females above 65 years old. Lateral epicondylitis, or tennis elbow, affects 1% to 3% of the population, with peak incidence between ages 40 and 60. There appears to be a female predominance with 60% to 70% female composition in reported series. It should be noted that work-related upper extremity disorders are the fastest growing source of disability in the American workplace, yet fewer than half of patients with these disorders fit neatly into any of the entities listed (see box, p. 173 and Table 24-1).

Pathophysiology

Carpal tunnel syndrome is caused by compression of the median nerve in the carpal tunnel, which is bounded posteriorly by the carpal bones and anteriorly by the transverse carpal ligament. Any process that increases pressure within the carpal tunnel can lead to median nerve compression and the symptoms of carpal tunnel syndrome, including inflammatory tenosynovitis (e.g., rheumatoid arthritis), infiltrative disorders such as amyloidosis, and generalized swelling as occurs in pregnancy or with use of birth control pills. Repeated forceful movements of the fingers, especially with

CHRONIC REGIONAL MUSCULOSKELETAL DISORDERS COMMONLY SEEN IN OFFICE PRACTICE

Upper extremity
Carpal tunnel syndrome
Trigger finger
Joint hyperextensibility
de Quervain's tenosynovitis
Osteoarthritis
Epicondylitis (lateral and medial)
Olecranon bursitis
Subacromial bursitis
Bicipital tendinitis
Nonspecific upper extremity pain

Neck and upper back
Cervical radiculopathy
Trapezius muscle spasm
Nonspecific neck pain

Lower back and pelvis
Mechanical back pain
Sciatica
Spinal stenosis

Knee
Anterior (patellofemoral) pain
Osteoarthritis
Anserine bursitis
Meniscal tear
Prepatellar bursitis

Foot and ankle
Plantar fasciitis
Achilles tendonitis
Osteoarthritis
Metatarsalgia

Table 24-1 Prevalence and key clinical findings in select upper extremity regional disorders

Disorder	Prevalence	% Female	Clinical Findings
Carpal tunnel syndrome	0.1%	>60%	See Table 24-2
de Quervain's tenosynovitis	NA	77%-91%	Finkelstein's maneuver, tenderness at radial styloid
Osteoarthritis	30% in patients >65 yr	66%	Tender joint line; pain with loading; radiographic changes
Lateral Epicondylitis	1%	60%-70%	Tenderness at lateral epicondyle; pain with wrist extension

NA, not available.

the wrist in flexion or extension, produces a low-grade tenosynovitis within the carpal canal leading to carpal tunnel syndrome.

de Quervain's tenosynovitis arises from inflammation of the abductor pollicis longus or extensor pollicis brevis. These tendons share a passage through a thick fibrous sheath at the distal radius. Inflammation generally results from repeated forceful thumb extension. Carpal metacarpal osteoarthritis arises from excessive load at the carpal metacarpal joint. Joint space narrowing occurs along with osteophyte formation and decreased motion. Lateral epicondylitis arises from inflammation at the origins of the wrist and finger extensors at the lateral humeral epicondyle; medial epicondylitis results from inflammation of the flexors at the medial epicondyle. Repeated forceful contraction of these muscle groups is proposed to cause small tears of the tendons, which is followed by an inflammatory response.

Clinical presentation

History and physical examination. Carpal tunnel syndrome is typically accompanied by numbness, tingling, and noctural symptoms in a characteristic dermatomal pattern involving the first three fingers. Percussion of the median nerve at the wrist—*Tinel's sign*—and prolonged wrist flexion—**Phalen's sign**—may produce paresthesias in the median nerve distribution. In advanced cases the physical examination may reveal sensory loss in the first three fingers and wasting of the thenar eminence. The sensitivity and specificity of these historical and physical findings are presented in Table 24-2. Nocturnal symptoms and Phalen's sign are quite sensitive, and sensory loss in the median nerve distribution is specific. The opinion of an experienced neurologist is more valuable than any of the diagnostic tests. The gold standard for the diagnosis of carpal tunnel syndrome is nerve conduction testing, which has a sensitivity of 90% to 92% and unknown specificity. A positive response to a therapeutic injection of corticosteroids into the carpal canal also has diagnostic value, although this has not been evaluated critically.

de Quervain's tenosynovitis patients usually complain of pain along the radial styloid that is exacerbated by movements of the thumb, particularly extension against resis-

Table 24-2 Diagnostic value of clinical findings in carpal tunnel syndrome

Finding	Sensitivity	Specificity	Positive predictive value with population prevalence 0.15	Positive predictive value with population prevalence 0.01
Nocturnal symptoms	0.77	0.28	0.16	0.87
Tinel's sign	0.60	0.67	0.25	0.91
Phalen's sign	0.75	0.47	0.20	0.91
Sensory loss	0.32	0.81	0.23	0.87
Hand symptom diagram	0.61	0.71	0.27	0.91
Neurologist's assessment	0.84	0.72	0.34	0.96

tance. Physical examination reveals marked tenderness over the radial styloid as well as a **positive Finkelstein's sign,** elicited by having the patient fold the thumb into the palm, curl the fingers around the thumb, and then deviate the wrist toward the ulnar side. This motion pulls on the thumb extensor tendons and is quite painful.

Carpometacarpal osteoarthritis, like other forms of osteoarthritis, is generally worse with use and better with rest. The joint margin is tender and radiographs reveal joint space narrowing and osteophyte formation. Lateral epicondylitis is characterized by pain at the lateral epicondyle that radiates up and down the arm. The lateral epicondyle is tender to palpation, and pain is exacerbated by resisted wrist extension. Medial epicondylitis is similarly characterized by pain in the medial epicondyle that is exacerbated by resisted wrist flexion. Radiographs are generally unrevealing.

Management

Carpal tunnel syndrome. Patients with carpal tunnel syndrome should be offered neutral wrist splints that can be worn at night and during the day unless they interfere with work activity. Underlying disorders such as inflammatory arthritis, diabetes mellitus, or hypothyroidism should be sought and treated. Although treatment of underlying inflammatory arthritis clearly improves secondary carpal tunnel syndrome, there are few data on whether optimizing glucose control in diabetics or thyroid hormone levels in patients with subclinical hypothyroidism improves carpal tunnel symptoms. Antiinflammatory medicines are typically of marginal value. Vitamin B_6 has been advocated on the basis of the supposition that carpal tunnel syndrome may arise from pyridoxine deficiency. However, there are few data supporting this contention or documenting the efficacy of pyridoxine therapy. Modification of work and recreational activities is critical. Corticosteroid injection into the carpal tunnel is safe and usually effective. In patients with intermittent symptoms and no evidence of sensory dysfunction, the combination of splinting and a carpal tunnel injection produces relief for at least a year in about 80%. However patients with constant symptoms or evidence of nerve dysfunction generally respond only transiently to injection, with recurrent symptoms developing in over 80%.

For patients unresponsive to conservative measures **carpal tunnel surgery** is generally safe and effective in 80% to 90%. The duration of conservative therapy will depend upon the patient's tolerance for ongoing symptoms. The transverse carpal ligament is incised under direct visualization. More recently **endoscopic carpal tunnel release** has been introduced; critical studies are in progress. Sensory function generally returns over a period of months after carpal tunnel release, although in cases of long-standing nerve compression sensory and motor function may not return completely. There is preliminary evidence that carpal tunnel release is much less effective in patients who are receiving Workers' Compensation. After carpal tunnel release patients frequently have tenderness for a few months at the incision and along the thenar and hypothenar eminences. Complications of carpal tunnel release occur in

less than 1% of cases and include reflex sympathetic dystrophy, infection, and transection of the superficial palmar branch of the median nerve.

de Quervain's tenosynovitis. The most important goal in the management of de Quervain's tenosynovitis is modification of activities that provoke symptoms. Antiinflammatory medications are useful, as is immobilization of the thumb with a splint. Injection of corticosteroids into the first dorsal compartment over the radial styloid is effective in 60% to 90% of cases. In over half of cases unresponsive to injections an aberrant separate sheath for the extensor pollicis brevis tendon is noted. Surgical release of the extensor tendon sheath is highly successful and can be done under local anesthesia.

Carpometacarpal osteoarthritis. Carpometacarpal osteoarthritis is generally treated by reducing load across the joint with activity modification and a splint that immobilizes the CMC joint. Injection of corticosteroids is also effective. Both **arthroplasty (joint replacement)** and **arthrodesis (joint fusion)** can be performed in refractory cases. More details on management of this condition can be found in Chapter 23.

Epicondylitis. Modification of activities and use of antiinflammatory medicines are the initial interventions for epicondylitis. Corticosteroid injections for lateral epicondylitis have up to 90% short-term success but frequent relapse. Commercially available forearm straps may be used to absorb force across the extensor tendons. Lateral release of the extensor aponeurosis rarely is performed.

LOWER BACK PAIN
Epidemiology

Back pain affects over 80% of Americans at some point in their lives and its direct and indirect costs exceed $20 billion annually. Low back pain can be categorized as (1) mechanical back pain syndromes that involve injury to musculoligamentous structure without nerve root involvement; (2) herniated disk syndromes with sciatica; and (3) lumbar spinal stenosis. Compression fractures (covered elsewhere in this text), tumors, infections, inflammatory back disease, and a few other diagnoses constitute the remainder. Mechanical back pain is the most common. It peaks in incidence in the third or fourth decade. Risk factors include smoking, lower socioeconomic status, and occupational activities that involve lifting or exposure to vibration. Men are generally affected more than women because of greater exposure to occupational risk factors. Mechanical back pain is also a common complication of the late months of pregnancy, presumably because the added weight and lordosis impose increased demand on the paraspinal muscles. Unfortunately low back pain in pregnancy appears to be associated with a higher risk of low back pain later in life. Documented herniated disk syndrome occurs in 1% to 2% of Americans with peak incidence in the fourth and fifth decades. There does not appear to be any male or female predominance. The incidence and prevalence of degenerative lumbar spinal stenosis are not known. Its recognition is rising because of greater suspicion among physicians and easier access to computed tomography (CT) scanning and magnetic resonance imaging. Lumbar spinal stenosis is more common in women, who constitute about 60% of most series.

Pathophysiology

The pathogenesis of mechanical back pain is debated and is likely heterogeneous. Age-related degenerative changes in the disks and apophyseal joints are ubiquitous and appear to play an important role. Equally important, particularly in younger patients, is the role of repetitive muscular and ligamentous strain. Myofascial pain is a frequent concomitant.

Lumbar disk herniation appears to result from repeated torsional and compressive stresses on the lumbar disks resulting in weakening of the annular fibers. The disk material generally protrudes posterolaterally into the spinal canal, impinging on the exiting nerve root. Degenerative lumbar spinal stenosis arises from compression of the cauda equina, or nerve roots within the spinal canal. Repeated loading of the spine leads to disk degeneration, loss of disk height, apophyseal joint osteoarthrosis with osteophyte formation, and attendant ligamentum flavum hypertrophy. The osteophytes, ligamentum flavum, and protruding disks all narrow the space available for the cauda equina and exiting nerve roots, resulting in a nerve compression lesion.

Clinical presentation

History and physical examination. The differential diagnosis of low back pain syndromes requires a careful history and physical examination. Table 24-3 lists some of the key clinical findings. Mechanical back pain is usually of a deep aching quality, generally perceived in the lower lumbar spine, and may radiate to the buttock and thighs. Paralumbar muscle spasm is frequent. Straight leg raising and the neurologic examination in the lower extremities yield negative findings. Radiographs are of little value in mechanical back pain, as the involved structures—ligaments, muscles, and tendons—are not visible radiographically.

Herniated lumbar disk syndromes characteristically produce sciatica, a lancinating pain radiating from the back to the buttock and along the posterior thigh and calf, usually into the foot. In over 90% of cases the vertebral levels involved are L4-5 or L5-S1. Numbness and paresthesia are also commonly perceived in a dermatomal pattern. On physical examination a positive straight leg raising test result is pain or paresthesia radiating down the leg. The sensitivity of the straight leg raising test is over 90%, specificity about 40%. The cross straight leg raising test, in which elevation of the asymptomatic leg produces sciatic pain in the symptomatic extremity, is much less sensitive (30%) but more specific (around 90%). The neuromuscular examination (sensory, strength, reflexes) is less sensitive and more specific than the ipsilateral straight leg raise.

Patients with spinal stenosis generally have insidious onset of aching pain that is worse with lumbar extension and improves with flexion, causing patients to stoop. Pain worsens with continued walking and improves with rest, often suggesting a diagnosis of vascular claudication. The pain is less circumscribed then in acute lumbar disk syndromes. It often is bilateral; radiates into the thighs, legs, and feet; involves more than one dermatome, and is accompanied by paresthesia and numbness. In addition, much of the pain is nondermatomal, arising from degenerative disease in the lower back. The physical examination generally reveals normal straight leg raising. Pain with lumbar extension is probably the most useful diagnostic clue to spinal stenosis. Vibratory sensation is lost early in the course of the disease, followed by pinprick sensation and motor loss in a polyradicular distribution. Sensitivity and specificity of physical examination findings in lumbar spinal stenosis have not been studied critically.

Diagnostic tests. Confirmation of a herniated disk requires a CT scan, myelogram, or magnetic resonance imaging (MRI) study. Up to 20% to 25% of asymptomatic individuals have disk herniations on CT scanning or MRI. MRI probably has superior sensitivity in detecting abnormalities of soft tissues including disks and neural structures, whereas CT produces better resolution of bony structures. MRI is certainly more expensive and available in fewer centers. Imaging tests are obtained far too frequently and in general should only be performed if an intervention requiring visualization of the anatomy is comtemplated, such as epidural steroid injection or surgery, or if tumor, infection, or other ominous lesions are to be excluded.

The diagnosis of spinal stenosis can be confirmed with an imaging procedure. CT scanning provides better definition of bony detail; MRI provides better visualization of the soft tissue abnormalities. Many clinicians still prefer to use a myelogram followed by CT for planning surgical therapy. The relative advantages and costs of these procedures have not been studied formally.

Differential diagnosis. It is important to distinguish mechanical back pain, disk syndromes, and spinal stenosis from more ominous causes of low back pain. Approximately 0.7% of patients with low back pain in primary care settings have malignant spinal neoplasms. These are generally metastatic. In women the most common tumor is breast carcinoma. Factors that raise the likelihood of cancer include age greater than 50, previous history of cancer, unexplained weight loss, and back pain that is not relieved by bed rest and not improved after a month of therapy. Unexplained weight loss and previous history of cancer have specificities greater than 0.90 and should prompt aggressive investigation for carcinoma. Patients with spinal infections also do

Table 24-3 Prevalence and key clinical findings in low back syndromes

Syndrome	Prevalence	% Female	Clinical findings
Mechanical LBP	>80%	50%	Use related, no neurologic deficits
Herniated disk	1%-2%	50%	Sciatica (dermatomal), root tension signs, dermatomal neurologic deficits
Degenerative spinal stenosis	NA	60%	Dermatomal and nondermatomal pain, pseudoclaudication, pain with extension, polyradicular neurologic deficits

not improve with conservative therapy and generally have systemic features.

Management

Overview. Management of low back pain syndromes requires an understanding of the natural history. Over 90% of patients with mechanical back pain improve after 1 month. Similarly over 90% of patients with sciatica are improved after 6 months and fewer than 5% go on to have surgery. Spinal stenosis, on the other hand, worsens insidiously as the underlying degenerative disease in the spine progresses.

Choice of therapy

Conservative therapy. The management of mechanical back pain and sciatica includes explanation of the excellent prognosis along with nontoxic interventions to accelerate the healing process and prevent future episodes. Antiinflammatory medicines and muscle relaxants are useful. Physical therapy is often prescribed to strengthen the abdominal flexor and lumbar extensor muscles and to stretch the muscles of the hip girdle. Structured physical therapy programs yield better results in acute and chronic back pain syndromes. Modalities including ultrasound and diathermy are less well studied. A recent trial of transelectrical nerve stimulation for chronic low back pain found it to be no more effective than a placebo.

Conservative therapy for degenerative lumbar spinal stenosis is much less effective than it is in mechanical or disk syndromes because of the poor natural history of disease. Antiinflammatory medicines may be useful, lumbar corsets are valuable though inconvenient, and exercises to increase abdominal strengthening are rational but have not been studied critically. Epidural steroid injections have a transient benefit.

Alternative therapies such as massage, acupuncture, and meditation are used commonly, with little scientific evaluation. Chiropractic manipulation is the best studied alternative therapy and leads to faster recovery in patients with acute low back pain. Traction has been used in sciatica but without scientific support. Epidural steroid injections provide substantial but transient (weeks to months) relief to many patients with nerve root compression. Invasive interventions and antiinflammatory drugs are relative (though not absolute) contraindications in pregnant women. Thus postural education, acetaminophen, physical medicine modalities, and alternative therapies assume a more prominent role in management.

Surgical intervention. Over 200,000 diskectomies are performed in the United States annually. The rate increased 60% from 1981 to 1987. Cauda equina syndrome, which occurs in less than 2% of disk prolapses, is an absolute indication for surgery. Rapid progression of muscle weakness occurs in less than 20% of patients and is also a strong indication for surgery. The other 75% to 80% of operated patients have less clear indications. In one randomized trial involving patients without absolute indications for surgery, 70% of operated patients compared with 33% of unoperated patients were completely satisfied with their status after 1 year. Ten years after diskectomy 63% of operated patients

were satisfied compared with 55% of unoperated patients. Women comprised 40% of patients in this study and had similar outcomes to men. Thus the long-term outlook is little changed by surgery although there appears to be short-term benefit.

An increase of literature on failed back surgery has stimulated attempts to improve patient selection. Favorable outcomes are associated with neurologic evidence of nerve root entrapment, positive root tension signs (such as straight leg raising), imaging studies showing lesions that correspond with physical examination abnormalities, and absence of adverse psychosocial indicators such as Workers' Compensation, litigation, depression, hysteria, or hypochondriasis. In one study by Herron and Turner, less than 25% of patients with the worst prognostic profiles had positive outcomes, compared with 100% of patients with the best prognostic profiles.

Unlike conservative therapy for lumbar spinal stenosis laminectomy appears to be successful in the short term in approximately 70% of patients. However, after 4-year follow-up observation 17% of patients in one study required a second operation and 30% continued to have severe pain. Worse outcomes were associated with more limited laminectomy as well as presence of comorbid conditions. Patients bothered primarily by leg pain preoperatively are more satisfied with surgery than patients bothered primarily by back pain, indicating that laminectomy effectively relieves nerve root compression but does not alleviate symptoms of progressive degenerative spine disease. Women undergoing laminectomy preoperatively appear to be more functionally limited than men, suggesting they are operated upon at a more advanced stage in the course of the disease. It is unclear whether this reflects preference for avoiding surgery or lack of access for women.

KNEE PAIN
Epidemiology

Knee pain is a common complaint, particularly in women. Four of the most frequently encountered entities are covered in this section: patellofemoral or anterior knee pain, anserine bursitis, meniscal tears, and osteoarthritis. Unfortunately prevalence data are not available for any of these conditions except osteoarthritis. Anterior knee pain is probably the most common cause of knee disability in patients under 40 years old. Surgical series include 60% to 90% women, indicating that women are affected much more frequently than men. Osteoarthritis of the knee is a leading cause of pain and disability in patients over 50 years old. Risk factors for osteoarthritis (OA) of the knee include older age, female gender, obesity, occupations involving repeated trauma to the knee, previous knee injury, and smoking. Radiographic OA is present in 27% of women aged 65 to 69 and 53% over age 80. Symptomatic OA occurs in 8% of women age 60 to 70 and 16% of those over 80. Men have slightly lower rates of radiographic OA and up to 50% lower rate of symptoms at each level of severity. Meniscal tears generally arise from trauma in younger patients, with males affected more frequently, and from trivial trauma or spontaneously in patients over 50 years old. More information can be found in Chapter 23. Degenerative meniscal tears often occur in older patients with degenerative arthritis of the knee and therefore are more common in females. Another lesion that often arises in association with degenerative arthritis of the knee is anserine bursitis, inflammation of the insertion of the medial hamstrings onto the tibia. This lesion is seen considerably more frequently in females than in males.

Pathophysiology

Patients with patellofemoral disorders generally have lateral deviation of the patella with respect to the distal femur, caused by excessive tension in the lateral supporting structures, particularly the lateral retinaculum. Continued tension upon the patella from a tight lateral retinaculum ultimately damages the patellofemoral joint, producing cartilage damage. This is a late finding, however, that generally occurs after patients have been symptomatic for years.

The primary insult in osteoarthritis appears to be mechanical load resulting from either acute trauma or repetitive injury. Morphologic changes in the articular cartilage include fragmentation with pitting, clefts, and ultimately ulceration of cartilage down to bone. Bony proliferation, in the form of osteophytes, accompanies the cartilage destruction (for a more detailed discussion refer to Chapter 23).

The **menisci** provide stability against rotational forces and cushion load applied across the joint. In young patients meniscal tears usually result from trauma. In older patients the menisci degenerate and are at risk for horizontal clevage tears. The medial two thirds of the meniscus is sparsely vascularized and heals poorly, whereas the outer third may heal spontaneously. Mechanical symptoms arise from the free flap of meniscus moving about the joint.

The **pes anserinus bursa** surrounds the medial hamstring tendons and allows them to glide smoothly over the bony prominence of the superior tibia. These tendons may become inflamed acutely from athletic activities or chronically from valgus stress as often occurs in patients with osteoarthritis.

Clinical presentation

History and physical examination. Anterior knee pain is perceived just behind the patella and is exacerbated by forceful knee flexion, such as occurs in kneeling or squatting. The physical examination often shows lateral tilting of the patella, tenderness at the insertion of the lateral retinaculum onto the patella, and pain with compression of the patellofemoral joint. Radiographs, including a patellar view, assess damage to the retropatella cartilage and alignment of the patellofemoral joint. (See Table 24-4.)

In osteoarthritis dull aching pain is perceived deep within the knee and increases with activity. In advanced cases pain occurs at night. The physical examination may show quadriceps atrophy and usually reveals joint line tenderness. Range of motion is normal until late in the disease, when bony crepitus may also be noted. Radiograph reveals sclerosis of the bony end-plates, followed by a narrowing of the joint space, formation of osteophytes, and subchondral cysts.

The signs and symptoms of meniscal tears are somewhat insensitive and nonspecific. For example, locking is present

Table 24-4 Key clinical findings in select regional disorders of the knee

Disorder*	% Female	Clinical findings
Anterior knee pain	80%	Pain with stairs, squat; tender lateral retinaculum; patellar tilt; patellofemoral compression, tenderness
Osteoarthritis	60%	Use-related pain; Joint line tenderness; radiograph: cartilage loss, osteophytes, sclerosis
Meniscal tears	40%	Mechanical symptoms, joint line tenderness McMurray's test
Anserine bursitis	80%	Tenderness at anserine bursa

*Prevalence unknown except for osteoarthritis.

in about 84% of patients with vertical tears but only 52% of patients with horizontal cleavage tears. Instability, or a feeling of giving way, is seen in 70% of patients with meniscal tears but also in about 60% of patients with other types of knee pain. Joint effusion is seen in about half of patients with meniscal tears. Joint line tenderness is observed in over two thirds of patients with meniscal tears but also is common in osteoarthritis. A positive McMurray's sign is elicited in about 60% of patients with meniscal tears and about 40% of patients with other lesions. **McMurray's test** involves flexion of the knee and concomitant internal or external rotation of the tibia. A positive response is a painful and palpable click as the knee goes through the arc of flexion.

The diagnosis of pes anserinus bursitis can be made on the physical examination without radiographic tests. Patients complain of pain along the medial aspect of the knee inferior to the medial joint line. Pain worsens with activities involving resisted knee flexion. The physical examination reveals exquisite tenderness at the pes anserinus bursa, located about 4 fingerbreadths below the medial joint line at the level of medial collateral ligament.

Diagnostic Tests. Arthrography has sensitivity over 90% and specificity of about 80% for meniscal tears. Arthroscopy is regarded as the gold standard for diagnosis of meniscal tears but is invasive. MRI is the best noninvasive method, with sensitivity over 90% for medial meniscal tears and 80% for lateral meniscal tears. Specificity is about 95% for lateral meniscal tears and 90% for medial meniscal tears.

Management

Over 80% of patients with significant anterior knee pain can be managed successfully with conservative therapy. The treatment program should consist initially of eliminating or modifying activities that produce symptoms, then progressive resistance exercises to strengthen the medial knee extensors, counterbalancing the tight lateral structures. Next a graduated running or other exercise protocol is instituted. A maintenance program of continued quadricep strengthening should be continued indefinitely. Adjunctive measures such as use of knee pads, patellar braces, and shoe orthotics can be tried if appropriate. In one study of 75 patients with severe anterior knee pain the program outlined here allowed 66% to return to unrestricted athletic activities after an average follow-up period of 1 year. Only 8% of these patients required surgical treatment. Patients unresponsive to the preceding measures who desire a high level of functional activity may be candidates for release of the lateral retinaculum. Surgery is successful in over 80% of carefully selected patients with anterior knee pain unresponsive to conservative therapy. However, patients without objective evidence of lateral patellar malalignment have success rates well below 50%.

Treatment of osteoarthritis of the knee begins with modification of activities. Antiinflammatory medications are superior to placebo although there is evidence that acetaminophen is as efficacious as antiinflammatory doses of ibuprofen. A cane can remove up to 30% of the load off the affected joint, resulting in considerable symptomatic relief. Intraarticular injections of steroids are effective in some patients, suggesting an inflammatory component. Intraarticular lavage with large volumes of fluid and arthroscopic debridement procedures have not been studied critically. Total knee arthroplasty is remarkably effective. Approximately 120,000 are performed annually in the United States at a direct cost of about $25,000 per case. Medical complications occur in 1% to 2% of patients. Prostheses ultimately loosen and require revision, seldom before about 12 years. In view of the need for revisions other procedures such as osteotomy should be attempted in younger patients. As mentioned about laminectomy for spinal stenosis, women have been noted to undergo knee arthroplasty for OA at a more advanced point in the course of functional decline than have men.

In patients with osteoarthritis of the knee it is important to diagnose and treat associated lesions that may be more amenable to therapy. Chief among these is pes anserinus bursitis, which is relieved predictably with a local injection of corticosteroid mixed with 1% lidocaine.

Meniscal tears are managed with decreased activity, antiinflammatory therapy, and simple observation. Conservative therapy appears to work in up to 25% of patients with severe symptoms, and an even higher proportion of all patients with meniscal tears.

Arthroscopic partial meniscectomy is the most commonly performed orthopedic procedure. It is indicated in patients with meniscal tears that have not responded to several months of conservative therapy. The operator removes the torn flap of meniscus, preserving as much meniscal tissue as possible. The success rate of arthroscopic partial meniscectomy in well-selected patients approaches 85%. The procedure is most successful in young patients with acute vertical tears and less successful in older patients with degenerative tears because meniscectomy itself does nothing to ameliorate the underlying osteoarthritis. Meniscal repair may be performed on lesions in the peripheral third of the meniscus, which is well vascularized.

Patients should be counseled carefully about the advantages and disadvantages of arthroscopic partial meniscectomy. Postoperative swelling and pain are common. Rehabilitation requires months of hard work. Patients with risk factors for poor outcomes (preoperative) including underlying osteoarthritis, Workers' Compensation, and poor functional status should be informed that their expected outcome is less favorable.

BIBLIOGRAPHY

Anderson BC, Mantley R, Brouns MC: Treatment of de Quervain's tenosynovitis with corticosteroids, *Arthritis Rheum* 34:793, 1991.

Anderson GBJ: The epidemiology of spinal disorders. In Frymoyer JW, editor: *The adult spine: principles and practice,* New York, 1991, Raven Press.

Binder A et al: Is therapeutic ultrasound effective in treating soft tissue lesions? *Br Med J* 290:512, 1985.

Bradley JD et al: Comparison of an anti-inflammatory dose of ibuprofen, an analgesic dose of ibuprofen, and acetaminophen in the treatment of patients with osteoarthritis of the knee, *N Engl J Med* 325:87, 1991.

Brown MS: The source of low back pain and sciatica, *Semin Arthritis Rheum* 18(suppl 2):67, 1989.

Chard MD, Hazelman BL: Tennis elbow: a reappraisal. *J Rheum* 28:186, 1989 (editorial).

DeHaven KE, Dolan WA, Mayer PJ: Chondromalacia in athletes, *Am J Sports Med* 7:5, 1979.

Deyo RA, Bigos SJ, Maravilla KR: Diagnostic imaging procedures for the lumbar spine, *Ann Intern Med* 111:865, 1989.

Deyo RA, Loeser JD, Bigos SJ: Herniated lumbar intervertebral disc, *Ann Intern Med* 112:598, 1990.

Deyo RA, Rainesville J, Kent DL: What can the history and physical examination tell us about low back pain? *JAMA* 268:760, 1992.

Deyo RA, Tsui-Wu Y-J: Descriptive epidemiology of low back pain and its related medical care in the United States, *Spine* 12:264, 1987.

Deyo RA et al: A controlled trial of transelectrical nerve stimulation (TENS) and exercise for chronic low back pain, *N Engl J Med* 322:1627, 1990.

Felson DT et al: The prevalence of knee osteoarthritis in the elderly, *Arthritis Rheum* 30:914, 1987.

Ferkel RD et al: Arthroscopic partial medial meniscectomy: an analysis of unsatisfactory results, *Arthroscopy* 1:44, 1985.

Franklin GM et al: Occupational carpal tunnel syndrome in Washington State, 1984-88, *Am J Public Health* 81:741, 1991.

Frymoyer JW: Back pain and sciatica, *N Engl J Med* 318:291, 1988.

Fulkerson JP, Shea KP: Current concepts review: disorders of patellofemoral alignment, *J Bone Joint Surg* 72A:1424, 1990.

Gelberman RH, Aronson D, Weismann MH: Carpal tunnel syndrome: results of a prospective trial of steroid injection and splinting, *J Bone Joint Surg* 62A:1181, 1980.

Glashon JL et al: Double blind assessment of the value of magnetic resonance imaging in the diagnosis of anterior cruciate and meniscal lesions, *J Bone Joint Surg* 71A:113, 1989.

Graves EJ: Detailed diagnoses and procedures: National Hospital Discharge Survey 1987: National Center for Health Statistics 1989; *Vital Health Stat* [13](100).

Herron LD, Turner J: Patient selection for lumbar laminectomy and discectomy with a revised objective rating system, *Clin Ortho* 199:145, 1985.

Katz JN: The assessment and management of low back pain: a critical review, *Arthritis Care Res* 6:104, 1993.

Katz JN et al: The carpal tunnel syndrome: diagnostic utility of the history and physical examination findings, *Ann Intern Med* 11:321, 1990.

Katz JN et al: The outcome of compressive laminectomy for degenerative lumbar spinal stenosis, *J Bone Joint Surg* 73A:809, 1991.

Katz JN et al: Predictors of functional outcomes after arthroscopic partial meniscectomy, *J Rheumatol* 19:1938, 1992.

Katz JN et al: Clinical correlates of patient satisfaction following laminectomy for degenerative lumbar spinal stenosis, *Spine* 1995 (in press).

Katz JN et al: Differences in functional status between men and women undergoing major orthopedic surgery for osteoarthritis, *Arthritis Rheum* 37:687, 1994.

Koes BW et al: Physiotherapy exercises and back pain: a blinded review. *Br Med J,* 1991.

Kulick MI et al: Long term analysis of patients having surgical treatment for carpal tunnel syndrome, *J Hand Surg* 11A:59, 1986.

Medical news and perspectives: symptoms may return after carpal tunnel syndrome, *JAMA* 265:1922, 1991.

Noble J, Erat K: In defense of meniscus: a prospective study of 200 meniscectomy patients, *J Bone Joint Surg* 62B:7, 1980.

Ridley MG et al: Outpatient lumbar epidural corticosteroid injection in the management of sciatica, *Br J Rheumatol* 27:295, 1988.

Shekelle PG et al: Spinal manipulation for low back pain, *Ann Intern Med* 117:590, 1992.

Silverstein BA, Fine LJ, Armstrong TJ: Occupational factors and carpal tunnel syndrome, *Am J Indust Med* 11:343, 1987.

Spengler DM: Degenerative stenosis of the lumbar spine, *J Bone Joint Surg* 69A:305, 1987.

Stevens JC et al: Carpal tunnel syndrome in Rochester, Minnesota, 1961-1980, *Mayo Clinic Proc,* 1988.

Survey of occupational injuries and illnesses, Washington, DC, US Bureau of Labor Statistics, November 14, 1990.

Van Saase JLCM et al: Epidemiology of osteoarthritis: Zoetermeer survey: Comparison of radiologic osteoarthritis in a Dutch population with that in ten other populations, *Ann Rheum Dis* 48:271, 1989.

Weber H: Lumbar disc herniation: a controlled prospective study with ten years observation, *Spine* 8:131, 1983.

Weisel SE et al: A study of computer-assisted tomography: I. The incidence of positive CAT scans in an asymptomatic group of patients, *Spine* 9:549, 1984.

Witt J, Pess G, Gelberman RH: Treatment of de Quervain's tenosynovitis: a prospective study of the results of injection of steroids and immobilization in a splint, *J Bone Joint Surg* 73A:219, 1991.

25 Rheumatoid Arthritis

Richard I. Sperling

EPIDEMIOLOGY

Rheumatoid arthritis (RA), a systemic, inflammatory disease of unknown etiology, has a prevalence of approximately 1% (range 0.3% to 2.0% in most populations) and a worldwide distribution. In general, 75% of patients with RA are women. However, erosive, seropositive RA is more equally distributed between men and women. The onset of RA may occur from adolescence to old age; however, the peak age of onset of RA is between the fourth and sixth decades. RA is characterized by a symmetric, polyarticular, inflammatory arthritis preferentially affecting distal, appendicular joints, particularly involving the small joints of the hands and the wrists. Involvement of axial joints, synovial-lined periarticular sites, and extraarticular manifestations, including constitutional symptoms, rheumatoid nodules, pleuritis, pericarditis, neuropathy, scleritis, and episcleritis, lymphadenopathy, splenomegaly, and arteritis occur as well.

PATHOPHYSIOLOGY

Although some reports have suggested viruses, antibody, and cellular immune responses to autoantigens in cartilage, and rheumatoid factor as etiologic agents in RA, the causative factor in RA is not defined. Nevertheless, genetic factors which predispose to RA have been determined. An increased risk of RA is found in first-degree relatives of patients with seropositive RA (3% to 5%) and twin studies have shown a 30% concordance for monozygous twins. The development and severity of RA have been linked with specific human leukocyte antigen (HLA)–DR specificities, especially the HLA-DR4 haplotype. The association of specific, disease-related HLA-DRB1 locus alleles (0101, 0401, 0404/0408, and 1402) with the presence of RA in 96% of 102 patients, and the correlation of DRB1 haplotype group

with severity of articular disease and the presence of extraarticular disease in one study, was impressive (Weyand et al., 1992). The association of the presence and severity of RA with specific alleles in the DR locus underscores the importance in the pathophysiology of RA of T lymphocytes and their ability to recognize antigens in the context of specific allelic variants of the class II major histocompatibility complex. Hypotheses on the localization of the disease primarily to joints have focused on in situ formation of immune complexes and local cellular hypersensitivity; either of these proposed mechanisms could initiate the inflammatory reaction and destruction of the joints in RA.

Although some researchers have attributed the increased incidence of RA in women to immunomodulatory effects of estrogen, no clear causative link between estrogens and RA has been established. Indeed, some studies have shown a protective or ameliorative effect of oral contraceptives on disease activity of RA. There are, however, several contradictory studies, and a metaanalysis of the effects of oral contraceptives on the risk of RA showed a small protective effect that was not statistically significant. Although pregnancy generally is associated with decreased activity of RA and a lower incidence of new cases, the postpartum period is associated with RA flare and an increased incidence of new cases of RA. A cohort study revealed no significant association between parity, age at birth of first child, or menopause and the incidence of RA. Replacement estrogen therapy in postmenopausal patients has not been shown to affect the risk for RA.

CLINICAL PRESENTATION

The diagnosis of RA remains a clinical diagnosis based on the presence of typical features in the history and physical examination and supported by the results of laboratory and radiographic tests. The American College of Rheumatology has devised revised classification criteria for RA for use in clinical research. Although the 1987 American College of Rheumatology criteria—especially in the diagnostic tree format—are useful guides for the diagnosis of RA (Fig. 25-1), the diagnosis for individual patients is best based on the judgment of an experienced clinician.

History

The onset of RA is insidious and slowly progressive in most patients; a subacute polyarthritis, with onset occurring over several weeks, is another common presentation. In occasional patients, however, the onset is acute (24 to 48 hours) and polyarticular and in others occasionally may begin as a palindromic rheumatism with episodes of a transient, migratory, monarticular or oligoarticular, inflammatory arthritis. The salient articular symptoms include a pronounced morn-

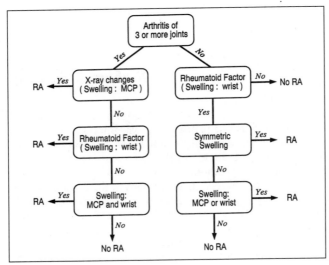

Fig. 25-1 Diagramatic representation of the 1987 classification tree criteria for rheumatoid arthritis. Parentheses indicate surrogate variables that may be substituted when another variable is not available. Definitions of criteria: (1) Arthritis of three or more joint areas: at least three joint areas simultaneously have had soft tissue swelling or fluid (not bony overgrowth alone) observed by a physician and present for 6 weeks or longer. The 14 possible joint areas are the right or left PIP, MCP, wrist, elbow, knee, ankle, and MTP joints. (2) Arthritis of hand joints (wrist, MCP, MCP or wrist, MCP and wrist): soft tissue swelling or fluid (not bony overgrowth alone) of the specified area observed by a physician and present for 6 weeks or longer. If two areas are specified, simultaneous involvement is required. (3) Symmetric swelling: simultaneous involvement of the same joint areas—as defined in (1)—on both sides of the body observed by a physician and present for 6 weeks. Bilateral involvement of any of the PIP, MCP, or MTP joints is acceptable without absolute symmetry. (4) Serum rheumatoid factor: demonstration of abnormal levels by any technique for which less than 5% of normal control subjects are seropositive. (5) X-ray changes of RA: radiographic changes typical of RA on posteroanterior hand and wrist radiographs, which must include erosions or unequivocal bony decalcification localized in or most marked adjacent to the involved joints. PIP, Proximal interphalangeal; MCP, metacarpophalangeal; MTP, metatarsophalangeal. (From Arnett FC et al: *Arthritis Rheum* 31:315, 1988.)

ing stiffness often lasting more than 1 hour, joint pain and tenderness, and joint swelling. RA is characterized by a symmetric, inflammatory polyarticular arthritis with a predilection for involvement of the proximal interphalangeal (PIP) and metacarpophalangeal (MCP) joints of the hands and the wrists. Distal interphalangeal (DIP) joints are rarely, if ever, involved. Elbows, shoulders; temporomandibular, acromioclavicular, and sternoclavicular joints; and hips, knees, ankles, and feet are frequently involved, although more often as the disease progresses. The cervical spine often is involved in RA; stiffness and pain are the most common symptoms, and neurologic symptoms are rare (see box, above).

Although symptoms wax and wane, especially early in the disease, **persistent swelling** and **pain of the joints** is a hallmark of RA. Patients frequently report constitutional symptoms such as fatigue, malaise, anorexia, and depression. Low-grade fevers occur occasionally in patients with polyarticular disease; however, high-grade fevers suggest infection or other febrile illnesses. Although patients occasionally report pain from rheumatoid nodules if they have ulcerated or become infected, rheumatoid nodules are generally asymptomatic. Symptoms of associated syndromes, including those of secondary Sjögren's syndrome, nerve entrapment such as carpal tunnel syndrome, and Raynaud's phenomenon are sometimes reported.

Physical examination

Articular manifestations. A thorough physical examination is warranted at the initial evaluation of a patient with RA (see box, below). **Joint swelling** is a cardinal feature of RA.

Swelling of the periarticular soft tissue, synovial thickening, and/or joint effusions may be observed. Early in the course of RA, swelling of the metacarpophalangeal (MCP) and wrist joints, as well as fusiform swelling of the proximal interphalangeal (PIP) joints, are most commonly noted; characteristically the swelling involves joint groups in a symmetric fashion. Although symptoms wax and wane, especially early in the disease, persistent swelling and pain of the joints is a hallmark of RA. If joint swelling is not present on the initial examination of a patient in whom RA is suspected, it is reasonable to reexamine the joints for swelling in a few days, early in the morning and after withdrawing nonsteroidal antiinflammatory drugs (NSAIDs) and corticosteroids (for patients receiving these therapies). The absence of joint swelling on repeated examination of a patient with symptoms calls into question the diagnosis of RA. Tenderness and warmth are generally present in involved joints, whereas erythema usually is less prominent than in gouty or septic arthritis. Pain on range of motion and limited range of motion usually are evident in the actively involved joints of patients with RA, even in the absence of permanent joint deformity. As the disease progresses, and usually after a minimum of 2 years of active synovitis, permanent joint deformities may occur. Typical deformities occurring in RA include **ulnar deviation** of the fingers at the MCP joints, **extensor subluxation** of the metacarpals at the MCP joints, **swan-neck deformities** (hyperextension of the PIP joint with flexion at the distal interphalangeal [DIP] joint), **boutonniere deformities** (flexion deformity of the PIP joint with extension at the DIP joint), **ankylosis** of the wrist and ankle, **hallux valgus** (bunion), **subluxation of the metatarsophalangeal** joints, and **flexion** (cock-up) deformities of the toes. Tenderness, muscle spasm, and limited rotation of the neck frequently are observed on examination of the neck; however, the presence of neurologic findings is rare.

Extraarticular manifestations. **Rheumatoid nodules,** the most common extraarticular manifestation of RA, are present in approximately 25% of patients, (see box, below). Nearly all of the patients with rheumatoid nodules are

EXTRAARTICULAR MANIFESTATIONS

Rheumatoid nodules
Rheumatoid vasculitis
Pleural disease
Pericardial effusion/pericarditis
Neurologic:
    Entrapment neuropathies
    Carpal tunnel syndrome
    Tarsal tunnel syndrome
    Cervical cord compression
    Mononeuritis multiplex
Eye:
    Xerophthalmia
    Keratoconjunctivitis sicca
    Episcleritis
    Scleritis
Anemia
Felty's syndrome
Still's disease

seropositive for rheumatoid factor and generally have more severe, erosive, and HLA-DR4–positive disease. These nodules are generally firm, nontender, round, or elliptic masses found in the subcutaneous or deeper tissues, with a predilection for the olecranon bursae, extensor surfaces of the forearms and hands, and the Achilles tendons. They are generally several millimeters in diameter but not uncommonly reach a few centimeters in diameter. Rheumatoid nodules also may occur in the pleura, lung, pericardium, myocardium, heart valves, meninges, and sclera (**scleromalacia perforans**). Histologically, rheumatoid nodules are indistinguishable from granuloma annulare and are essentially identical in appearance to the subcutaneous nodules occurring in systemic lupus erythematosis and rheumatic fever. Rheumatoid nodules are composed of a central area of fibrinoid necrosis surrounded by a middle zone of palisades of macrophages and an outer ring that consists chiefly of lymphocytes and plasmacytes.

In autopsy series, 10% to 25% of patients with RA have evidence of **rheumatoid vasculitis. Splinter hemorrhages** and **small digital infarcts** of the nail beds are the most common clinical manifestations of rheumatoid vasculitis. Other skin manifestations of rheumatoid vasculitis include **palpable purpura** (which on pathologic examination is a leukocytoclastic vasculitis) digital ulceration, and gangrene caused by distal arteritis. Less than 1% of patients with RA develop clinically significant arteritis. Clinically significant rheumatoid vasculitis generally develops only in patients with very active, long-standing RA and high-titer rheumatoid factor, although rheumatoid vasculitis can develop early in the RA course of patients with abrupt-onset, very active disease. In these patients, arterioles and venules, as well as small- and medium-sized arteries, may be involved in skin, nerves, and visceral organs, including intestines, heart, lung, cerebrum, kidney, liver, spleen, and pancreas. Full-blown involvement may mimic polyarteritis nodosa.

RA is associated with **pleurisy** with or without **pleural effusions,** rheumatoid nodules with (**Caplan's syndrome**) or without an associated pneumoconiosis and **pulmonary fibrosis.** Pleural disease in RA is usually asymptomatic. Typically the pleural fluid is exudative: protein and lactate dehydrogenase (LDH) levels usually are elevated, glucose levels are low, and white blood cell counts (polymorphonuclear or mononuclear predominant) are over 5000/mm^3. Low levels of total hemolytic complement, C3 and C4 relative to serum, and the presence of rheumatoid factor in the pleural fluid are common in RA, but in general these tests are not sensitive enough to be of much clinical value. The most common cardiac involvement in RA is an asymptomatic **pericardial effusion** observed on ultrasound examination or on autopsy. Symptomatic **pericarditis** is the most common symptomatic cardiac manifestation of RA; the course ranges from mild and self-limited to chronic pericarditis and pericardial constriction to fatal cardiac tamponade. Other cardiac manifestations include granulomatous involvement of the pericardium or myocardium with rheumatoid nodules and, rarely, aortitis and coronary arteritis.

Neurologic manifestations of RA include **entrapment neuropathies, cervical cord compression** and **mononeuritis multiplex. Carpal tunnel syndrome** (episodic burning pain, tingling, or numbness of the three middle fingers, and sometimes the thumb, relieved by shaking the hand) is a common finding in patients with RA. A positive **Tinel's sign** (symptoms elicited by digital pressure or percussion with a hammer over the palmar aspect of the wrist) or **Phalen's sign** (symptoms elicited by forced flexion of the wrist for 30 to 60 seconds) commonly is observed. Weakness (in thumb opposition and abduction) and atrophy of the muscles of the thenar eminence are seen in more severe and chronic cases. **Tarsal tunnel syndrome** (episodic burning pain, tingling, or numbness of the heel and medial aspect of the foot) caused by compression of the anterior tibial nerve, is another entrapment neuropathy commonly seen in RA. Wristdrop, footdrop, and patchy sensory loss in an extremity are findings related to mononeuritis multiplex seen in rheumatoid vasculitis. Although involvement of the cervical spine in RA is common, cervical spinal cord compression is distinctly rare. Atlantoaxial involvement with subluxation may result in weakness of the extremities, incontinence of the bowel or bladder, occasionally vertebral artery compression resulting in vertigo or syncope, and frank quadriplegia.

Eye involvement in RA is frequent. **Xerophthalmia** and **keratoconjunctivitis sicca** caused by Sjögren's syndrome are the most common ocular complications of RA. **Episcleritis,** which generally causes mild pain without affecting visual acuity, usually lasts only a few weeks. **Scleritis**, less common than episcleritis, usually is more painful and indolent but can affect visual acuity and lead to blindness. Thinning of the sclera can occur in prolonged attacks of scleritis, allowing the dark-blue color of the underlying choroid to show (**scleromalacia perforans**).

A mild normochromic normocytic **anemia** with low levels of both serum iron- and total iron-binding capacity is commonly observed and, in the absence of a concomitant iron-deficiency anemia as a result of blood loss, usually is unresponsive to iron supplementation. Other hematologic manifestations of RA include lymphadenopathy (25% or more), splenomegaly (5% to 10%), and Felty's syndrome. **Felty's syndrome** is defined by the triad of chronic RA, splenomegaly, and leukopenia and occurs predominantly in patients with long-standing erosive, high-titer seropositive, nodular disease. The leukopenia is a neutropenia that can be severe and can be associated with frequent infections with gram-positive organisms. The neutropenia in an individual patient may be attributed to maturation arrest, hypersplenism, or the presence of both conditions. Leg ulcers, lymphadenopathy, anemia, thrombocytopenia, and constitutional symptoms occur commonly in patients with Felty's syndrome.

Although less common than in children, **Still's disease** can occur in adults. Salient features of adult-onset Still's disease include quotidian fevers, an evanescent, salmon-colored macular rash usually occurring during fever spikes, serositis, and an inflammatory oligoarticular or polyarticular arthritis. The disease tends to be polycyclic with a polycyclic or chronic arthritis.

Diagnostic tests

Laboratory findings

Rheumatoid factor. Rheumatoid factor—antibodies reactive to the Fc domain of IgG—is present in approximately 80% of patients with RA. Rheumatoid factor also is associated with a number of other diseases, including many chronic infections and chronic inflammatory diseases (see box, below). Only 5% of the general population tests seropositive for rheumatoid factor; however, the frequency of positive test results for rheumatoid factor in healthy persons increases with age. Of healthy persons older than 65 years of age, 5% to 10% show seropositivity for rheumatoid factor, although in most of this group, rheumatoid factor titers are low. Therefore, a positive test result for rheumatoid factor alone does not establish the diagnosis of RA; however, it will help to establish the diagnosis in conjunction with an appropriate history and findings on physical examination. Rheumatoid factor status in patients with RA may be of prognostic significance; seronegative patients generally have less active articular disease and fewer extraarticular manifestations than do seropositive patients. Conversely, patients with RA who have high titers of rheumatoid factor generally have a more severe, erosive disease and a greater likelihood of having extraarticular manifestations of RA.

Hematology. Complete blood cell counts and differential diagnoses are generally normal in patients with RA except for the common findings of thrombocytosis and a mild normochromic, normocytic anemia associated with low levels of both serum iron- and total iron-binding capacity. Eosinophilia greater than 5% and neutropenia occasionally are observed. The erythrocyte sedimentation rate usually is greater than 30 mm at 1 hour.

Synovial fluid analysis. Synovial fluid analysis is useful to determine the presence of an inflammatory arthritis in distinction to typically noninflammatory conditions such as osteoarthritis, a traumatic or mechanical derangement. Nev-

---

CONDITIONS IN WHICH A POSITIVE RHEUMATOID FACTOR IS FREQUENTLY PRESENT

Rheumatologic diseases
Rheumatoid arthritis
Systemic lupus erythematosus
Sjögren's syndrome
Scleroderma
Polymyositis/dermatomyositis
Mixed cryoglobulinemia

Infectious diseases
Bacterial endocarditis
Tuberculosis
Syphilis
Viral hepatitis
Schistosomiasis
Leprosy
Kala azar

Noninfectious conditions
Healthy elderly persons
Chronic active hepatitis and cirrhosis of the liver
Diffuse interstitial pulmonary fibrosis and silicosis
Intravenous drug abuse
Sarcoidosis
Waldenström's macroglobulinemia

Modified from Zvaifler NJ. In Schumacher HR Jr, Klippel JH, Robinson DR, editors: *Primer on the rheumatic diseases,* ed 9, Atlanta, 1988, The Arthritis Foundation.

ertheless, the findings of synovial fluid analyses are not specific for RA and cannot distinguish RA from many of the other common inflammatory arthritides. In RA the synovial fluid of actively involved joints is characteristically exudative: protein levels generally are greater than 3 g/dl, white blood cell counts generally are in the range of 2000 to 20,000/mm^3, polymorphonuclear leukocytes generally, but not invariably, predominate (50% to 70%), and the glucose level is low to normal. Depending on the circumstances, synovial fluid analysis may be important to exclude the presence of other inflammatory arthritides. Examination for the presence of crystals may be important to exclude the possibility of gout or pseudogout—each can manifest as a polyarticular, inflammatory arthritis. Septic arthritis, including gonococcal arthritis, generally is monarticular or oligoarticular but can on rare occasions be polyarticular. If the diagnosis of a septic arthritis is considered, a Gram's stain and culture of synovial fluid are indicated. Synovial biopsy is almost never specific for RA but may be of value when performed as part of a clinical research protocol.

Radiographic evaluation. Radiographic findings are not specific for RA, although they may help differentiate RA from osteoarthritis or other inflammatory arthritides. Early in the course of the disease, radiographs generally demonstrate soft tissue swelling and/or effusion—findings that should be apparent on physical examination. Juxtaarticular osteopenia, which may be evident after 6 weeks of involvement, and bony erosions, which in a rare patient may be evident after 6 months of continuous synovitis but generally is not apparent until after 2 years of active synovitis, are suggestive of the diagnosis of RA. Radiographic evaluation is not often indicated in RA; the primary use is to evaluate disease progression in order to guide management with surgical options and with "remittive agents" (such as the antimalarials, gold salts, and methotrexate). Hand and wrist radiographs are commonly obtained for this purpose because they often demonstrate early juxtaarticular osteopenia and erosions and symmetry of the disease.

Differential diagnosis

The onset of RA is typically a polyarticular presentation with an insidious and gradual onset; however, a subacute or acute onset or onset as palindromic rheumatism with episodes of a transient, migratory, monarticular or oligoarticular, inflammatory arthritis is not unusual. Therefore the differential diagnosis of RA is broad and depends on the initial presentation of the individual patient. A definitive diagnosis of RA is difficult to make with accuracy early in the course of the disease. For example, in studies in which the diagnosis of RA was based on the less rigorous, 1958 ARA criteria for RA, "remission" was reported to be common during the first two years after diagnosis; however, this probably reflects a higher rate of remission in patients who were misdiagnosed.

The differential diagnosis of RA includes the other polyarticular inflammatory arthritides, osteoarthritis, those infectious and inflammatory arthritides that typically are monarticular, collagen-vascular diseases and other systemic inflammatory diseases, viral and chronic infections, lymphoproliferative diseases, amyloidosis, and fibromyalgia.

Osteoarthritis. A generalized osteoarthritis involving the small joints of the hand, as well as the major weight-bearing joints, may be difficult to distinguish from RA if joint swelling is present. In end-stage disease, osteoarthritis and RA can appear more similar; in late RA a secondary osteoarthritis may dominate the clinical picture, and in late osteoarthritis, joint swelling and even a mild synovitis may occur. The joint distribution in osteoarthritis and RA remain somewhat different and help differentiate these two arthritides. In RA, the MCP and PIP joints are most often and most actively involved joints of the hands and signs of inflammation are generally present, whereas in osteoarthritis involvement of the DIP joints and the joints of the thumb and bony enlargement (**Heberden's nodes** at the DIP joints and **Bouchard's nodes** at the PIP joints) are most commonly observed on physical examination. The presence of morning stiffness in and around the joints of duration greater than 1 hour (especially early in the disease), the presence of rheumatoid factor, elevation of the erythrocyte sedimentation rate, and the presence of characteristic radiographic findings help to distinguish RA from osteoarthritis. Because the management of RA and osteoarthritis differs considerably, it is important to distinguish these two common arthritides. For a more detailed discussion of osteoarthritis see Chapter 23.

Other rheumatic diseases. Other rheumatic diseases, including systemic lupus erythematosus, mixed connective tissue disease, dermatomyositis, polymyositis, and scleroderma, are associated with a symmetric, inflammatory polyarthritis or symptoms that suggest a symmetric, inflammatory polyarthritis. Demonstration of systemic symptoms or signs typical of the aforementioned diseases would suggest the appropriate alternative diagnosis to RA. Any of these diseases may evolve into RA over time. Polymyalgia rheumatica, vasculitides, and familial Mediterranean fever also may manifest with a symmetric, inflammatory polyarthritis or symptoms that suggest a symmetric, inflammatory polyarthritis. In polymyalgia rheumatica, synovitis and signs of an inflammatory arthritis are not often observed; in the other entities, the development over time of extraarticular signs and symptoms should indicate the appropriate diagnosis. Rheumatic fever is much less common now than it was previously. However, it should still be considered in the differential diagnosis of RA in adults inasmuch as the arthritis of rheumatic fever in adults often is additive (like RA), the carditis of rheumatic fever is less common, and the other manifestations of rheumatic fever are rare in adults compared with children.

Fibromyalgia. Although fibromyalgia (fibrositis) is not associated with arthritis or a serum rheumatoid factor, the **fibromyalgia syndrome** is not uncommonly confused with RA. The history of patients with fibromyalgia often is identical to that of patients with RA. Patients with fibromyalgia feel as stiff in the mornings, as fatigued, and as disabled as patients with RA. Often they also believe that their joints are swollen. The absence of physician-observed joint swelling on repeated visits and the presence of the extraarticular trigger points classic for the fibromyalgia syndrome lead to the correct diagnosis. Fibromyalgia often occurs in patients with RA or other rheumatic diseases (for more detailed discussion see Chapter 22).

Systemic inflammatory disease. Systemic inflammatory diseases can be confused with RA. **Inflammatory bowel disease** and **Whipple's disease** may occur with synovitis before the development of signs of bowel involvement;

however, the arthritis usually is an asymmetric, oligoarticular, and nonerosive arthritis of large joints and in inflammatory bowel disease may be associated with spondylitis and sacroiliitis. Although the acute arthritis associated with **sarcoidosis (Lofgren's syndrome)** is easily differentiated from RA by the presence of erythema nodosum and bilateral hilar adenopathy, chronic sarcoidosis may be more difficult to differentiate from RA inasmuch as chronic sarcoidosis can cause a polyarticular arthritis with significant involvement of the small joints of the hands and feet and with the radiographic appearance of an erosive arthritis as a result of periarticular bone cysts caused by granulomas. **Amyloidosis** can infiltrate the synovium and periarticular tissue, mimicking a polyarticular arthritis, and also can cause carpal tunnel syndrome. In patients receiving hemodialysis therapy, the presence of a polyarticular arthritis (because of gout or pseudogout) and carpal tunnel syndrome (caused by amyloidosis) may be difficult to distinguish from RA.

Bacterial septic arthritis. Bacterial septic arthritis, like the crystal-induced arthritides, generally is monarticular but occasionally may manifest as an oligoarticular or polyarticular arthritis. In addition, septic arthritis may be superimposed on RA. In the febrile patient, synovial fluid analysis and culture are indicated. **Lyme** arthritis, a late manifestation of Lyme disease, generally is an intermittent monarticular or oligoarticular arthritis that affects large joints such as the knees; however, in about 10% of patients, a chronic erosive polyarticular arthritis develops. In this latter group of patients, Lyme arthritis can be confused with RA. The diagnosis can be confirmed by serologic testing for Lyme disease. Some viral infections may cause a polyarthritis or polyarthralgias, including hepatitis B, parvovirus B19, rubella virus or live vaccine, Epstein-Barr virus, human immunodeficiency virus, and human T cell leukemia virus 1. Infectious endocarditis is associated with monarticular and, less commonly, an oligoarticular septic arthritis. Subacute bacterial endocarditis not infrequently is associated with polyarthralgias and a symmetric, inflammatory polyarthritis in which the culture and Gram's stain of synovial fluid are negative—attributed to circulating immune complexes. Because rheumatoid factor is present in the serum of up to 40% of patients with subacute bacterial endocarditis, there are circumstances when RA and endocarditis are difficult to distinguish. Although patients with active, polyarticular RA may have low-grade fevers, any patient with RA and fever and leukocytosis out of proportion to the degree of arthritis should have blood cultures and be examined carefully for septic arthritis and other sources of infection.

Crystal-induced arthritides. The crystal-induced arthritides—gout, calcium pyrophosphate deposition disease (pseudogout), and apatite/hydroxyapatite-induced periarthritis—generally manifest as acute, inflammatory monarthitis. The polyarticular presentation of these arthritides is more difficult to distinguish from RA. Calcium pyrophosphate deposition disease in particular occasionally appears as a symmetric, less acute, inflammatory polyarthritis termed *pseudorheumatoid arthritis*; patients with hyperparathyroidism, hypothyroidism, and hemochromatosis are at increased risk for calcium pyrophosphate deposition disease. Gout and less commonly apatite/hydroxyapatite disease also may manifest as polyarticular disease. Each of these arthritides may cause erosions. In apatite/hydroxyapatite disease, periarticular or tendon calcium deposits are observed radiographically, and the appropriate crystals generally will be observed on synovial fluid analysis. Distinguishing these arthritides from RA is necessary for appropriate management of the arthritis.

Other arthritides. Ankylosing spondylitis, psoriatic arthritis, Reiter's syndrome, undifferentiated spondyloarthritis, and reactive arthritis are all commonly associated with an inflammatory, polyarticular arthritis. Differentiating these disorders from RA in patients who manifest obvious appendicular disease and mild or minimal back pain may be problematic. The appendicular arthritis in these disorders tends to be asymmetric and involves the large joints or manifests as sausage digits. Evidence of sacroiliitis, the presence of inflammation at entheses—often resulting in pain at the insertion of the Achilles tendon or the heel, insertional tendinitis, or periarticular inflammation as evidenced by sausage digits—and extraarticular signs and symptoms characteristic for one of these disorders (such as a psoriatic rash, nail pitting, diarrhea, ocular or genitourinary symptoms) suggest one of the spondyloarthropathies as opposed to RA. Seronegativity for rheumatoid factor, a normal or minimally elevated erythrocyte sedimentation rate, and the frequent presence of HLA-B27 antigen helps to distinguish the spondyloarthropathies from RA. RA, psoriasis, and the spondyloarthropathies are not rare, and seropositive RA may coexist with psoriasis or with spondyloarthropathies. Because patients with the spondyloarthropathies are treated with NSAIDs and many of the same "remittive agents" as patients with RA, it is not critical to distinguish these disorders from RA early in the course of the disease.

Malignant disease. Malignant disease usually causes a monarticular arthritis through direct involvement in a joint, however, it also may occasionally mimic RA. Non-Hodgkin's lymphoma can cause a seronegative polyarticular arthritis in the absence of obvious lymphadenopathy or splenomegaly. A symmetric, nonerosive, seronegative arthritis is a frequent presentation of angioimmunoblastic lymphadenopathy, a rare entity that many consider a malignant disease.

Elderly-onset rheumatoid arthritis

Elderly-onset RA is usually defined as onset at age 60 or later. Elderly-onset RA probably reflects a spectrum of disease ranging from classic RA to polymyalgia rheumatica or a polymyalgia rheumatica-like illness with some evidence of synovitis. Patients with elderly-onset seropositive RA have a course similar to that of other patients with seropositive RA, and respond and tolerate therapy with gold compounds as well as the younger patients. Elderly-onset RA is commonly seronegative and includes patients with a disease resembling polymyalgia rheumatica with some evidence of synovitis. Patients with elderly-onset seronegative RA tend to have a more acute onset of disease, have more proximal, especially shoulder, involvement, are more likely to be seronegative, are less likely to have erosive disease, tend to respond very well to low-dose corticosteroids, and tend to have a better outcome than patients with younger onset of RA. Inclusion of these elderly patients in studies of elderly-onset RA have led to the overall conclusion that elderly-onset RA tends to have more benign disease with characteristics shaded towards those of elderly-onset seronegative RA.

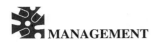
MANAGEMENT

Overview

In the 10% to 15% of patients with RA who have a monocyclic or mild intermittent course with prolonged periods of remission, management by a primary care practitioner with salicylates or other NSAIDs, as well as physical or occupational therapy or both, usually is appropriate. The management of most patients with RA who have chronic, progressive disease or intermittent but prolonged exacerbations of RA generally requires, in addition to NSAIDs, the use of other antirheumatic drugs that generally are administered by or in consultation with a rheumatologist, and a multidisciplinary approach involving a physiatrist, physical and occupational therapist, a nurse specialist, orthopedist, orthotics technician, and a psychiatrist. RA is usually a chronic, expensive, and disabling disease associated with a shortened life expectancy.

Nonpharmacologic treatment is an important component of the management of RA that often is neglected or underutilized by primary care physicians and therefore deserves emphasis. Patient education is a time-consuming yet important aspect of the treatment of RA, which often is neglected by generalist and specialist alike. Physical and occupational therapy usually is required during the course of treatment of RA to help reduce pain and inflammation and to restore and maintain range of motion and strength, as well as capacity for activities of daily living (ADL), including work activities. Surgical intervention sometimes is indicated relatively early in the disease to provide symptomatic relief (such as synovectomy for hand and wrist pain and release of the transverse carpal ligament for carpal tunnel syndrome) whereas later in the course of RA, surgical intervention is indicated for pain relief in joints with severe cartilage destruction.

Response to therapy should be evaluated with serial determinations of the number (and severity) of tender joints/painful joints on range of motion, the number (and severity) of swollen joints, the duration of morning stiffness, grip strength of the hands, the patient's and the physician's global assessment, and a functional assessment of the patient regarding ADL and occupation. Occasionally, evaluation of the erythrocyte sedimentation rate may be useful to evaluate present disease activity, and radiographs of hands, wrists, or other involved areas may be useful in evaluating the response to therapy or rate of disease progression, or both.

Choice of therapy

Nonpharmacologic therapy. Adequate patient compliance requires a high level of patient motivation and comprehension of regimen because treatment consists of multiple nonpharmacologic therapies and polypharmacy with drugs that are frequently ineffective, have many significant side effects, and require laboratory monitoring for toxicity. The way to achieve this is through patient education. Most patients with RA know little about the disease or its treatment, course, or outcome. Many patients have misconceptions regarding the disease, which can lead to poor compliance, intense anxiety, and depression. Patients need to understand that (1) RA is a chronic, usually lifelong disease, (2) although no cure exists, treatment generally controls the disease adequately enough that the patient will remain rea-

sonably functional, and (3) most of the treatments require weeks or months to produce a therapeutic effect and that several drugs may need to be tried before a drug that provides adequate control is found. Nurse specialists can help with patient education, in addition to coordinating care with allied health practitioners and social services, monitoring for drug toxicity, and administering injectable therapies. The national office and local chapters of the Arthritis Foundation are excellent resources for patients with RA and physicians caring for patients with RA. The Arthritis Foundation provides pamphlets regarding the course and treatments of RA, conducts self-help groups, and provides listings of rehabilitative services, appropriate exercise classes, and an information and referral service for patients with joint disease.

Rehabilitative medicine is an important part of the management of RA at all stages of the disease. Early in the course of the disease, consultation is appropriate for patient education regarding appropriate rest and exercise, assessment of function, joint protection, and gentle range of motion exercises. Splinting of actively inflamed joints may reduce synovitis and minimize the risk of joint trauma. Splinting of wrists is used in the treatment of carpal tunnel syndrome in patients with RA. Cervical collars may help relieve neck symptoms. Modalities such as the application of heat and cold, diathermy, and ultrasound also are useful for actively inflamed joints. Massage may aid in relieving muscle tension and pain, and traction may be used to reduce severe flexion contractures. When the arthritis is less active, strengthening, endurance, and aerobic exercises may be added to the regimen. Orthotics can aid in patient comfort, the redistribution of weight to less inflamed joints, and the provision of support and stabilization to joints. As joint deformity and impairments begin to limit ADL, occupational therapy can reassess function and recommend assistive devices and energy-conserving techniques.

Surgical intervention sometimes is indicated early in the course of RA. Tenosynovectomy and synovectomy of the wrist and hand for relief of pain and prevention of extensor tendon rupture and release of the transverse carpal ligament for carpal tunnel syndrome unresponsive to conservative therapy are perhaps the most common surgical interventions employed in early RA. Arthrodesis of wrists and ankles with active synovitis and limited motion is employed for pain relief and joint stabilization. In the rare instance of severe involvement by RA of the atlantoaxial joint with neurologic symptoms and radiographically demonstrated spinal cord compression, surgical stabilization of the cervical spine is indicated. Late in the course of RA, pain and loss of function caused by joint destruction may be surgically ameliorated by osteotomy or total arthroplasty. This is most successful for the hips and knees.

Pharmacologic therapy

Goals of therapy. Current concepts for the management of RA unfortunately are not based on well-controlled, well-designed, and well-executed, large, long-term, clinical trials of therapy because there is a wide spectrum of disease, because there is high variability of disease activity over time in an individual patient, because RA is a chronic disease in which maintenance of function and symptom control over the long term are the main goals, and because in most patients the disease cannot be adequately controlled by relatively constant therapy for a period of several years. The management of RA is based on a combination of (1) well-designed, controlled, and blinded short-term clinical trials, (2) cross-sectional, longer term longitudinal, and metaanalytic studies, and (3) case reports and clinician experience. The traditional paradigm for the treatment of RA was founded on using the least toxic therapies first and advancing to more risky therapies in patients whose disease was unresponsive. This paradigm has been presented as a "treatment pyramid"; over time the actual treatments within the levels of the pyramid have changed. At the base of the pyramid is patient education, rest, exercise, salicylates and other NSAIDs, and social services. The next level includes antimalarial agents, gold salts, and possibly sulfasalazine. The middle level includes methotrexate, penicillamine, and possibly azathioprine. The fourth level includes cytotoxic therapy and experimental drugs or procedures, and systemic corticosteroids occupy the apex. The sides of the pyramid are flanked by intraarticular therapy and surgery, which may be appropriate at any stage of the disease.

Current concepts for the management of RA are in a state of flux. Recently some experts have recommended "inverting" or scrambling the traditional "treatment pyramid" because some data have indicated that long-term therapy with salicylates and NSAIDs may be associated with more morbidity and mortality than usually suspected. The benefit-to-risk ratio for higher level therapies such as the antimalarials, methotrexate, and even gold possibly may be relatively more favorable than NSAIDs. These clinicians suggest that patients who would appear to be at higher risk for articular destruction in the long term—such as patients with persistent disease, an abrupt or severe polyarticular onset, high-titer rheumatoid factor, or extraarticular involvement—may benefit from early treatment with what traditionally might be considered aggressive therapy, that is, methotrexate or gold salts. Long-term longitudinal studies now being conducted and multicenter trials will help to clarify the optimal management of RA with the currently available treatments.

The goals of therapy for RA remain maintenance of reasonable function, pain control, and control of disease activity in the hopes of preventing or reducing joint destruction. Treatment of RA should be tailored to the individual patient because no one approach or scheme will work in all patients. Decisions regarding the management of RA should be made together by the physician and patient on the basis of the stage of the disease, prognostic factors, treatment history, and the presence of concomitant medical illnesses.

Choice of therapy

SALICYLATES AND NONSTEROIDAL ANTIINFLAMMATORY DRUGS. For patients with new onset or recently diagnosed disease, it is generally accepted that treatment with an NSAID is appropriate in the absence of obvious contraindications. **Aspirin** (acetylsalicylic acid) is the first choice of many rheumatologists. The advantages of aspirin are its long history of excellent efficacy, the ability to monitor serum salicylate levels to determine compliance and aid in dosing, and low cost. The frequency of gastrointestinal distress, the prolonged effect on platelet function, and the dosing intervals of most aspirin preparations (three to four times daily) are its main disadvantages. Gastrointestinal symptoms may be reduced by using buffered aspirin, enteric-coated aspirin, or zero-order release aspirin. The last also has the advantage of

twice-a-day dosing. **Nonacetylated salicylates** (diflunisal, salsalate, and choline magnesium trisalicylate) also offer twice-a-day dosing, cause less gastrointestinal distress, and do not have a prolonged inhibitory effect on platelets, but they are generally perceived as less effective than other NSAIDs. The antiinflammatory dosage of salicylates begins at 3 to 4 g daily in divided doses; the dosage may be raised gradually until limited by side effects. Doses of salicylates lower than 3 g daily will achieve only analgesia. In elderly persons, lower doses of aspirin may achieve therapeutic, antiinflammatory levels of salicylate in the serum; appropriate dosing in this group is best determined by serum salicylate levels. There are several classes of **nonsalicylate NSAIDs.** Although the NSAIDs differ somewhat in effect and toxicities, perhaps the main differences among them are their pharmacokinetics and the availability of sustained-release formulation for some NSAIDs. Piroxicam, oxaprozin, and nabumetone are taken daily; naproxen, sulindac, zero-order release aspirin, nonacetylated salicylates, and sustained-release indomethacin are taken twice daily, as is etodolac. The other NSAIDs have to be taken three or four times a day.

The main side effects of the NSAIDs (including salicylates) are gastritis and peptic erosions and ulceration, minor gastrointestinal symptoms (which do not correlate very well with the more serious lesions or with blood loss); tinnitus, headaches, and change in mental status; inhibition of platelet function possibly resulting in bleeding; chemical evidence of hepatic dysfunction and, rarely, significant hepatic dysfunction; renal insufficiency, especially in patients with underlying prerenal or renal disorders or receiving diuretic therapy; and allergic, bronchospastic, and hematologic side effects. The NSAIDs may block, at least in part, the antihypertensive effect of diuretics and increase the risk of bleeding in patients on anticoagulation therapy. Aspirin, and to a lesser extent other NSAIDs, (1) may displace phenytoin from albumin, transiently raising levels of the unbound drug, (2) may potentiate the effect of first-generation sulfonylureal oral hypoglycemic agents, (3) may potentiate the effect of warfarin both by inhibiting platelet function and by displacing warfarin from albumin, transiently raising levels of the unbound drug, and (4) may decrease the renal excretion of methotrexate, raising levels of methotrexate. (This effect generally is clinically significant only in patients receiving methotrexate for cancer chemotherapy and is not generally of clinical importance in patients on low-dose, weekly pulse methotrexate therapy for RA.)

In general, (1) the efficacy of NSAID therapy should be judged after a 4- to 6-week trial unless side effects are noted earlier; (2) the concomitant use of two or more NSAIDs should be avoided because of an increased risk of toxicity; and (3) if an NSAID is not tolerated or is ineffective, it may be preferable to try an NSAID from another class. It is appropriate to begin therapy with what has traditionally been considered a "second-line" antirheumatic drug in most patients with RA who have tried three or four NSAIDs without achievement of adequate control and tolerable side effects. In selected patients it may be appropriate to begin therapy with a second-line antirheumatic drug even sooner.

SLOW-ACTING ANTIRHEUMATIC DRUGS. Antirheumatic drugs such as the antimalarialagents, gold salts, sulfasalazine, methotrexate, penicillamine, azathioprine, and other immunosuppressive drugs are referred to as slow-acting antirheumatic drugs (SAARDs), disease-modifying antirheumatic drugs (DMARDs), and second-line antirheumatic drugs. The mechanism of action in RA of most of these drugs is unknown. There is some evidence that disease progression may be slowed or halted by most of the drugs in this class. Some of these drugs have similar toxicities. However, the characteristic that most unites this class of antirheumatic drugs is their slow or delayed onset of action; the delay in onset ranges from 6 weeks to 6 months.

The decision to start therapy with a SAARD is multifactorial. The presence of poor prognostic features (radiographic evidence of erosions, abrupt or very active polyarticular onset of disease, extraarticular disease, and high-titer rheumatoid factor), progressive or persistently active arthritis, disease unresponsive to NSAID therapy, progressive deformity or loss of function, and steroid dependency are factors that would favor starting SAARD therapy. An uncertain diagnosis, the lack of objective signs of active synovitis on physical examination, the lack of compliance with follow-up visits or laboratory monitoring for drug toxicity, and the absence of effective contraception in a woman of childbearing potential (for methotrexate, hydroxychloroquine, penicillamine, and the cytotoxic drugs) are factors that would favor the delay of SAARD therapy. NSAID therapy usually is continued when SAARD therapy is initiated, although if the disease responds dramatically to SAARD therapy, the NSAID may be tapered or discontinued. Most primary care physicians prefer to manage patients with RA who require SAARD therapy in consultation or concurrently with a rheumatologist. Table 25-1 delineates characteristics of the various SAARDs, including dosages, typical regimens for monitoring toxicity, typical lag times for a response, and indications and contraindications.

HYDROXYCHLOROQUINE. Hydroxychloroquine (Plaqueril) is the antimalarial agent most commonly used in RA. Although hydroxychloroquine generally is considered to be a less effective SAARD, it poses the fewest side effects and is the easiest SAARD to administer. Pigmentary retinopathy, the most worrisome side effect of hydroxychloroquine, is fortunately quite rare at the currently employed dosage ($\leq$400 mg/day or $\leq$6.5 mg/kg/day). Even more rarely, muscular weakness and congestive heart failure have been reported with hydroxychloroquine, usually early in the course of treatment. Patients receiving antimalarial therapy should have a baseline ophthalmologic examination, including a full retinal examination, and should be followed up with ophthalmologic visits every 6 months.

GOLD SALTS. Treatment with gold salts has been the mainstay of SAARD therapy for RA until recent years. Three preparations are available in the United States: two injectable gold salts, aurothioglucose and gold sodium thiomalate, and the oral preparation, auranofin. Auranofin has been shown to be effective in the treatment of RA but is generally considered to be less effective than the injectable preparations. Auranofin probably has fewer major side effects than the injectable gold salts, but it has a higher incidence of nuisance side effects, particularly diarrhea, nausea, and, rarely, vomiting. Aurothioglucose and gold sodium thiomalate are similar except that gold sodium thiomalate can cause flushing and faintness within a few minutes of administration (nitritoid reaction). The major toxicities of gold therapy are hematologic (leukopenia, agranulocytosis, anemia, and thrombocytopenia), renal (proteinuria, nephrotic syndrome, and membranous glomerular nephritis, which usually is reversible), and mucocutaneous (pruritus, psoriasiform rash, exfoliative dermatitis, and stomatitis). Injectable gold salt therapy usually begins with weekly intramuscular doses of 50 mg; many clinicians first give test doses of 10 and 25 mg separated by 1 week. A clinical response usually is observed after 3 to 6 months of treatment in patients who do respond to gold therapy. After a satisfactory response at a cumulative dose of 1 g, or a substantial, earlier response every other week, dosing is instituted. After several months, the dosing can be decreased to every third or every fourth week.

METHOTREXATE. Methotrexate has compared favorably with gold salt therapy in short-term, blinded trials, and metaanalysis indicates a relatively favorable risk-benefit ratio. Many rheumatologists use methotrexate early in the treatment of aggressive RA. Treatment usually starts at 7.5 mg weekly and can be advanced to a maximum of 15 mg weekly for oral methotrexate and up to 25 mg weekly for intramuscularly or subcutaneously administered methotrexate, if needed to control disease activity. Methotrexate generally is well-tolerated in patients without risk factors for methotrexate toxicity; patients with alcoholism, renal disease, folate deficiency, dehydration, and preexisting chronic liver disease are at increased risk for toxicity from low-dose methotrexate. Pulmonary fibrosis, hepatic fibrosis, and cirrhosis are rare but serious and possibly irreversible complications of methotrexate therapy. Bone marrow suppression is another important toxicity of methotrexate. Other, less severe, toxicities of methotrexate include rashes, stomatitis, nausea, vomiting, diarrhea, elevations in serum transaminases, and renal toxicity. Birth defects, oncogenesis, and infertility are potential major complications of methotrexate therapy, which, however, have not been clearly documented in patients with RA receiving low-dose, weekly methotrexate. Methotrexate is contraindicated during pregnancy, and women of childbearing potential must use appropriate birth-control methods. Patients receiving methotrexate therapy must be advised to abstain from alcohol consumption and sulfa antibiotics, which may increase methotrexate toxicity. Therapy with methotrexate usually is stopped during serious infections, perioperatively, and in men 3 months before and in women one menstrual cycle before attempting conception.

SULFASALAZINE. Sulfasalazine is widely used as a SAARD in the treatment of RA in both the United States and Europe, although sulfasalazine has not been approved by the FDA for use in RA. Sulfasalazine has a risk-benefit ratio that is nearly comparable with methotrexate and plaquenil, the SAARDs with the most favorable risk-benefit ratio. The minor but common side effects of sulfasalazine are nausea, vomiting, anorexia, headache, reversible oligospermia, rashes, fever, and hemolytic anemia. The major toxicities of sulfasalazine, which are quite rare, are similar to those of gold and methotrexate: bone marrow suppression, renal toxicity, hepatitis, and severe rashes (including exfoliative dermatitis, Stevens-Johnson syndrome, and toxic epidermal necrolysis). If possible it is best to stop sulfasalazine treatment during pregnancy; sulfasalazine is categorized by the FDA as pregnancy category B.

Table 25-1 Drugs for the treatment of rheumatoid arthritis

	Hydroxychloroquine	Gold compounds	Sulfasalazine	Methotrexate	Penicillamine	Azathioprine
Indications	Disease unresponsive to NSAIDs and physical medicine; seronegative or less aggressive disease than for gold or methotrexate as the first SAARD	Disease unresponsive or progressive on hydroxychloroquine regimen or disease responsive to NSAIDs and relatively more aggressive disease	Disease unresponsive or progressive on hydroxychloroquine regimen or disease unresponsive to NSAIDs and relatively more aggressive disease	Disease unresponsive or progressive on hydroxychloroquine regimen or disease unresponsive to NSAIDs and relatively more aggressive disease	Failure of gold and methotrexate	Failure of gold, methotrexate, and penicillamine
Relative contraindications	Preexisting macular disease	Proteinuria, renal disease	Allergy to sulfa antibiotics, sensitivity to salicylates; porphyria	Alcohol consumption; liver or renal disease	Proteinuria, renal disease	Renal or liver disease
Usual dosage	200-400 mg qd	10-mg test dose; week 2 start 50 mg IM q/wk, tapering to 50 mg q/mo, starting after 0.5-1 g auranofin 3 mg bid	2-4 g divided tid to qid	7.5-15 mg once weekly; can be in divided doses over 1 day	125-750 mg daily; start with 125 mg daily and advance by 125 mg/mo	50-150 mg/day; start with 50 mg qd and raise dose by 25 mg every other week
Maximal dosage	400 mg qd or 200 mg bid	50 mg q/wk	1 g qid	25 mg q/wk	750 mg daily	200 mg qd
Major and common toxicities	Gastrointestinal upset, pigmented macular degeneration and rashes	Rashes, oral ulcers, rare exfoliation, membranous glomerular nephritis, bone marrow suppression	Rashes (may rarely be severe), hepatitis, bone marrow suppression, renal toxicity	Rashes, oral ulcers; rarely pulmonary or hepatic fibrosis, or cirrhosis; bone marrow suppression	Rashes, oral ulcers, membranous glomerular nephritis, bone marrow suppression, and rarely autoimmune diseases	Gastrointestinal upset, rashes, and bone marrow suppression
Suggested monitoring	Ophthalmologic examinations at baseline and q6mo, including Amsler grids, color vision testing, and retinal examinations	CBC, differential and platelet count; urine dipstick before each injection	CBC, differential and platelet count, BUN, creatinine and liver function tests every 4-6 wk	CBC, differential, and platelet count; BUN, creatinine and liver function tests every 4-6 wk	CBC, differential, and platelet count; urine dipstick for protein every 2 wk; may lengthen interval to monthly at 6 mo	CBC, differential, and platelet count; before adjusting dosage and every month; liver function tests every month
Length of typical trial	3-6 mo	6 mo	6 mo	3 mo (many respond in the first month)	7-9 mo	3 mo
FDA category for pregnancy	No official category; not recommended in pregnancy	Category C	Category B	Category X	No official category; not recommended in pregnancy	Category D

Modified from Ruddy S, Roberts WN. In Kassirer JP, editor: *Current therapy in internal medicine*, ed 3, Philadelphia, 1991, BC Decker.
NSAIDs, nonsteroidal antiinflammatory agents; SAARD, slow-acting antirheumatic drugs; CBC, complete blood count; BUN, blood urea nitrogen.

PENICILLAMINE. Penicillamine is an effective therapy for RA, on a par with gold and sulfasalazine, but is more toxic than the aforementioned SAARDs. At present penicillamine is used less than in the past and mainly after failure of gold and methotrexate therapy. Dosing generally follows the "go low, go slow" regimen of 125 mg daily with monthly increments in daily dosage of 125 mg, using the minimum effective dosage, to a maximum of 750 mg daily.

CYTOTOXIC THERAPY. Cytotoxic therapy generally is indicated only in patients with vasculitis or in those who have progressive, active disease and were unresponsive to or intolerant of SAARDs. Of the cytotoxic drugs, only aza-thioprine has been approved by the FDA for the treatment of RA. The management of patients with RA who require cytotoxic therapy is best left to a rheumatologist.

Corticosteroids. Intraarticular administration of corticosteroids is a useful adjunct therapy for RA during flares in which only a few joints are predominantly involved and for the treatment of joints that are persistently active after systemic therapy has controlled disease activity in most other joints. Intraarticular and soft tissue injection of corticosteroids should be performed by trained physicians. The injections generally are well tolerated. Intraarticular corticosteroid injections to each joint should be limited to three or four per year. Postinjection flares may occur hours to a day after injection in a small number of patients. Serious complications are rare.

Because of the severe toxicity, the absence of disease modification by systemic corticosteroids, and the difficulty of weaning patients with RA from systemic corticosteroids, systemic corticosteroid therapy should be limited to only a few circumstances: the treatment of patients with rheumatoid vasculitis, women who are pregnant, patients who have begun therapy with a SAARD ("bridge therapy") or are already receiving optimal SAARD therapy—but require greater control to maintain performance at work or for basic ADL—and as the drug of last resort for pain control. Except for the treatment of rheumatoid vasculitis, the minimum dose necessary to maintain function and control pain should be prescribed.

Investigational and unapproved therapies. Cyclosporine has been shown in several controlled trials to be efficacious in the treatment of RA; however, renal insufficiency and hypertension that are only partially reversible are major problems, especially in patients receiving concomitant NSAID therapy. Cyclosporine therapy can be considered in patients with RA who are intolerant of or unresponsive to standard SAARDs. Dietary supplementation with fish oil–based supplements that contain eicosapentaenoic acid have shown some efficacy in several small, controlled clinical trials. Only minimal toxicity of the dietary supplementation with eicosapentaenoic acid–containing oils has been observed. Preliminary studies with dietary supplementation with oils that contain gamma linoleic acid (evening primrose oil and borage oil) have shown some promising results and minimal toxicity. A new and emerging area is "biologic" treatment. Therapies based on infusion of monoclonal antibodies directed at molecular determinants on cells of the immune system such as CD5 are in the early stages of development. Therapy based on retinoid compounds and other products with immunomodulatory properties also are in the early stages of investigation. Radiation synovectomy, produced by intraarticular injection of a short-lived radioactive compound, appears to be effective local therapy, based on studies from a few centers. Total nodal irradiation, plasmapheresis, and leukophoresis are treatments that showed some efficacy in some initial reports, but toxicity and/or lack of reproducible efficacy have dampened interest in these modalities. Pulse, high-dose methylprednisolone therapy maintains a small following but is risky and has not been demonstrated to have an acceptable benefit-risk profile in controlled studies.

PREGNANCY AND RHEUMATOID ARTHRITIS

Approximately 70% of patients with RA who become pregnant will experience significant improvement of the RA; however, in most of these patients, the disease will flare within 6 to 9 months postpartum. Patients with RA need to be counseled regarding the course of pregnancy in RA, the toxicities of antirheumatic therapy to the mother and fetus during pregnancy and to the infant of a nursing mother in the postpartum period, and the limitations in lifting and caring for the newborn (if any) related to the individual patient's handicaps. The FDA classification of the safety in pregnancy of the antirheumatic drugs ranges from categories B through X; none demonstrate proved safety. In general, NSAIDs and SAARDs are stopped during pregnancy, and symptoms may be controlled with acetaminophen and low-dose corticosteroids. Low-dose corticosteroids probably present the least additional risk during pregnancy, although all the antirheumatic drugs, including corticosteroids, present additional risks during pregnancy. In some circumstances the patient and the team of physicians will continue therapy with sulfasalazine or gold salts during pregnancy if it is believed that the benefits of the drug to the mother outweigh the potential risks to the mother and fetus. Usually, RA does not flare until several months after cessation of SAARD therapy (with the notable exception of methotrexate), and most patients experience at least a partial remission of RA during pregnancy. Patients with severe RA who require the more toxic SAARDs should be counseled as to whether pregnancy is inadvisable because of undue risks to the fetus if therapy is continued and risks to the mother if therapy is discontinued. It is advisable to restart antirheumatic therapy shortly after parturition because most patients with RA flare within 6 to 9 months postpartum. Since most of the antirheumatic drugs are secreted to some extent in the milk of nursing mothers and none of the antirheumatic drugs are approved by the FDA for nursing mothers, it is advisable for mothers with RA who are taking antirheumatic medications to abstain from nursing their newborn infants.

PROGNOSIS AND OUTCOME

Both the physician and the patient need to be aware of the great variability of the course of RA. Although statistical analyses of outcomes in RA based on clinical or radiographic features have been performed, the prognosis in any particular patient remains uncertain. However, with appropriate management and use of a multidisciplinary team approach, progression to a severely disabled or bedridden condition is uncommon.

BIBLIOGRAPHY

Arnett FC et al: The American Rheumatism Association 1987 revised criteria for the classification of rheumatoid arthritis, *Arthritis Rheum* 31:315, 1988.

Bennett JC: Rheumatoid arthritis: clinical features. In Schumacher HR Jr, Klippel JH, Robinson DR, editors: *Primer on the rheumatic diseases,* ed 9, Atlanta, 1988, The Arthritis Foundation.

Felson DT, Anderson JJ, Meenan RF: Use of short-term efficacy/toxicity tradeoffs to select second-line drugs in rheumatoid arthritis: a meta-analysis of published clinical trials, *Arthritis Rheum* 35:1117, 1992.

Hess EV: Rheumatoid arthritis: treatment. In Schumacher HR Jr, Klippel JH, Robinson DR, editors: *Primer on the rheumatic diseases,* ed 9, Atlanta, 1988, The Arthritis Foundation.

Kelley WN et al, editors: *Textbook of rheumatology,* ed 3, Philadelphia, 1989, WB Saunders.

McCarty DJ, Koopman WJ, editors: *Arthritis and allied conditions: a textbook of rheumatology,* ed 12, Philadelphia, 1993, Lea & Febiger.

Ruddy S, Roberts WN: Rheumatoid arthritis. In Kassirer JP, editor: *Current therapy in internal medicine,* ed 3, Philadelphia, 1991, BC Decker.

Weinblatt ME et al: Low-dose methotrexate compared with auranofin in adult rheumatoid arthritis: a thirty-six week, double-blind trial, *Arthritis Rheum* 33:330, 1990.

Weyand CM et al: The influence of HLA-DRB1 genes on disease severity in rheumatoid arthritis, *Ann Intern Med* 117:801, 1992.

Williams HJ et al: Comparison of auranofin, methotrexate and the combination of both in the treatment of rheumatoid arthritis, *Arthritis Rheum* 35:259, 1992.

Wilske KR, Healey LA: Remodeling the pyramid: a concept whose time has come, *J Rheumatol* 16:5, 1989.

Zvaifler NJ: Rheumatoid arthritis: epidemiology, etiology, rheumatoid factor, pathology, pathogenesis. In Schumacher HR Jr, Klippel JH, Robinson DR, editors: *Primer on the rheumatic diseases,* ed 9, Atlanta, 1988, The Arthritis Foundation.

26 Systemic Lupus Erythematosus

Patricia A. Fraser

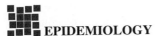

EPIDEMIOLOGY

Systemic lupus erythematosus (SLE, lupus) is an autoimmune systemic rheumatic disease of unknown etiology that preferentially afflicts women. Lupus is found worldwide. Very limited epidemiologic studies suggest that SLE may be less common in equatorial Africa. The prevalence of SLE varies among population groups. This is best exemplified by lupus statistics in the United States, where a several-fold variation in the prevalence of SLE exists, ranging from 140/100,000 in white women, 280/100,000 among Native Americans in Alaska, to 410/100,000 in African-American women. The prevalence estimates suggest a gradient of predisposition to SLE in several population groups in the United States. It is likely that this differential risk is due to several factors. Genetic factors that confer susceptibility to SLE may vary from one racial group to another. In addition, different levels of exposure to environmental factors that influence predisposition to lupus in a genetically susceptible population also may account for the observed differential risk of SLE. The prognosis for SLE in African-Americans is significantly worse than in white persons. Several studies suggest poorer prognosis is due to socioeconomic factors, including access to health care.

PATHOPHYSIOLOGY

Most symptoms of SLE are due to small vessel vasculitis and its associated vascular injury and vasocclusion. Multiple causes of the vasculitis are likely. The sequence of events has not been defined. Environmental stimuli such as exposures to microorganisms may initiate the disease process through the induction of T and B lymphocyte dysfunction in genetically susceptible persons. Autoantibodies are produced, some of which are capable of tissue injury through the formation of immune complexes. Immune complex disease has been clearly demonstrated in fetal cardiac tissue in neonatal lupus with congenital heart block, in a variety of cutaneous lupus lesions, and in the glomerulus, but it is also presumed to be present in the synovium, serosal surfaces, and the vasculature of the nervous system (brain and spinal cord). Cytokines exert direct and indirect influences on the acute inflammatory processes, and they also may contribute to the perpetuation of the chronic inflammatory state in SLE.

CLINICAL PRESENTATION
Criteria for classification

The 1982 revised criteria for the classification of SLE were developed as entry criteria for epidemiologic studies of SLE (see box, below). Clinical and laboratory manifestations are combined to define the spectrum of common signs and symptoms associated with SLE. These criteria permit comparisons among clinical studies in which patient selection is limited to those who have 4 of 11 criteria. The clinical diagnosis of SLE is not dependent on the number of criteria met. Rather, the diagnosis of SLE is framed by the clinical impression of the practitioner and the specific clinical manifestations.

History and symptom presentation

Fever and systemic lupus erythematosus. A temperature greater than 100° F often accompanies lupus flares. Lupus patients who are receiving systemic corticosteroids or immunosuppressive agents such as azathioprine (Imuran) and cyclophosphamide (cytoxan) are immunocompromised and at risk for opportunistic infections, as well as for serious sequelae of routine bacterial infections. Even if a lupus flare

---

CRITERIA FOR THE CLASSIFICATION OF SYSTEMIC LUPUS ERYTHEMATOSUS

Discoid rash
Malar rash
Antinuclear antibody
Photosensitivity
Oral ulcers
Arthritis
Serositis
Renal disorder
Neurologic disorder
Hematologic disorder
   Hemolytic anemia
   Leukopenia
   Lymphopenia
   Thrombocytopenia
Immunologic disorder
   (+)Le cell preparation
   Anti-DNA antibody
   Anti-Sm: biologic false-positive test for syphilis

Modified from Tan EM et al: *Arthritis Rheum*: 25:1271, 1982

is present, the febrile lupus patient should be evaluated and treated for infection.

Constitutional symptoms. In addition to fevers, lupus patients often report severe fatigue and loss of appetite.

Menses. Transient menstrual abnormalities in SLE most often are due to acute severe illness or rapid weight loss and systemic corticosteroid use. It is not known whether menarche is significantly delayed in childhood-onset SLE. Secondary amenorrhea and premature ovarian failure also may occur with daily or pulse (intravenous or monthly) cyclophosphamide therapy (see Chapter 29 for discussion on amenorrhea and premature ovarian failure).

Cutaneous manifestations. Disease-specific cutaneous symptoms of SLE may be acute, subacute, or chronic.

Acute cutaneous changes. The common acute cutaneous lupus eruptions include **malar erythema,** the so-called butterfly rash, and generalized facial and truncal erythema. Rarely, focal or diffuse acute bullous lesions develop in the setting of SLE.

Chronic cutaneous changes. Chronic cutaneous changes comprise most of the cutaneous symptoms in SLE patients. **Discoid lupus erythematosus (DLE)** is more common in men but frequently occurs in women. It may be localized to the face or scalp, or both, or may be generalized. Scarring hypopigmentation and/or hyperpigmentation, and permanent alopecia are complications of DLE and can be distressing to the patient. **Lupus profundus** or **lupus panniculitis** appears as painful, hyperesthetic, indurated truncal lesions.

Alopecia. Alopecia is a troublesome symptom for lupus patients because it dramatically affects body image. As stated before, DLE lesions often are accompanied by scarring and the alopecia associated with DLE usually is permanent. Transient alopecia also occurs with SLE. Patchy alopecia **(alopecia areata)** occurs in up to 10% of SLE patients whereas diffuse alopecia is even more common, with more than 50% of the patients affected. Alopecia correlates with disease activity (see also Chapter 7 for discussion of alopecia).

Photosensitivity. Photosensitivity is more common in SLE patients who have anti-RO autoantibodies.

Polyarthritis. Lupus arthritis is a **symmetric peripheral arthritis** that usually affects (in order of decreasing frequency) the small joints of the hands, the knees, and the small joints of the feet. Cricoarytenoid arthritis also occurs, and can manifest as persistent sore throat, hoarseness, or stridor.

The arthritis of SLE has been described as nondeforming. This is a relative misnomer because lupus patients rarely develop erosive joint disease but frequently develop deformities. In fact, chronic lupus arthritis may lead to joint deformities that are indistinguishable from those seen in RA, such as swan neck, boutonniere deformities, and ulnar drift (ulnar deviation of the metacarpophalangeal [MCP] joints). Reconstructive surgery is effective in reducing these deformities.

Recurrent tendon ruptures occur more commonly in SLE than in other systemic rheumatic diseases. The cause of this tendon disorder is unclear, but chronic steroid therapy has been implicated as one predisposing factor.

Acute monarticular arthritis in SLE requires urgent evaluation. The chronic lymphopenic state associated with SLE results in decreased natural immunity to microbial agents, which is compounded by corticosteroids and other immunosuppressive agents. Arthrocentesis of the affected joint (with simultaneous fluoroscopic examination of the hip joint), synovial fluid analysis (cell count, differential, Gram's stain, and polarized microscopic examination for crystals), and culture should be performed when the patient manifests acute monarticular arthritis even in the absence of fever (see Chapter 22 for a more detailed discussion). In the febrile patient, parenteral antibiotic coverage for *Staphylococcus aureus* should be continued until the joint fluid culture is negative for the organism.

Pleuropulmonary disease. **Pleurisy** is the most common pulmonary symptom of SLE. At least 50% of the patients will have either unilateral or bilateral pleural involvement at some time during the course of their disease. Frequently an afebrile patient reports pleuritic pain, but a pleural rub is inaudible and a chest film shows no effusion. It is important to consider other causes of the pleuritic chest pain such as pulmonary embolism. If there is no obvious cause, the practitioner generally treats the symptoms (see section on management) and then, if unsuccessful, the radiograph should be repeated. Often a pleural effusion will develop later in the course of disease. In the febrile patient with effusion and pulmonary infiltrate, diagnostic thoracentesis should be considered to exclude infection.

Parenchymal involvement is less common in SLE but may take the form of diffuse interstitial pneumonitis or acute focal, migratory infiltrates. Infectious processes must always be considered in this setting, even if the patient is afebrile. It may be necessary to consider bronchoscopy, bronchoalveolar lavage, and transbronchial or open lung biopsy to confirm the diagnosis. Diffuse interstitial pneumonitis often progresses to diffuse pulmonary fibrosis, with restrictive lung disease, pulmonary hypertension, and cor pulmonale even after appropriate treatment.

The "**shrinking lungs syndrome**" in SLE is distinct from diffuse interstitial pneumonitis. This syndrome is characterized by severe progressive dyspnea, restrictive lung disease, and an elevated diaphragm. There is uncertainty about the pathogenetic mechanisms leading to the shrinking lungs syndrome. Popular theories include alveolar microatelectasis and diaphragmatic weakness secondary to fibrosis.

Pulmonary hemorrhage also may complicate SLE. The prominent features of this presentation are variable amounts of hemoptysis, acute respiratory distress, diffuse pulmonary infiltrates, and a sudden drop in hematocrit.

Cardiac disease. **Pericarditis** is the most common cardiac manifestation of SLE. Massive pericardial effusions may occur and can be associated with echocardiographic evidence of impending cardiac tamponade. Serial echocardiographic imaging is an essential part of management. Management issues are discussed later in the chapter.

SLE may be complicated by **myocardial** (including hypertrophic cardiomyopathy), **valvular**, and **coronary artery disease.** Coronary artery disease is multifactorial, possibly related to the vasculopathy of SLE or the effects of steroid therapy (hypertension and hyperlipidemia). Management of these conditions is not disease specific, and standard interventions are used.

Serositis and other causes of abdominal pain. Frequently encountered causes of abdominal pain in SLE are listed in the box, below. Abdominal pain associated with **lupus serositis** is nonspecific and may even suggest an acute abdominal condition. Patients with lupus serositis are often febrile, with diffuse abdominal pain. Abdominal ultrasound examination may demonstrate a localized fluid collection consistent with lupus serositis. Because lupus serositis is a diagnosis of exclusion, it is often necessary to exclude acute abdominal and pelvic conditions by exploratory laparotomy, or laparascopy. If other causes for the symptoms have been excluded, treatment with steroids (prednisone 40 mg daily) may be considered.

Another cause of abdominal pain in SLE is **acute pancreatitis**. The mechanisms proposed for its occurrence in SLE include pancreatic vasculitis and steroids. Recurrent bouts of pancreatitis may develop, and they are treated with standard pancreatitis management.

Less common causes of abdominal pain in SLE include **mesenteric vasculitis** and **colonic perforation**. Mesenteric vasculitis may be associated with intermittent, sharp, or crampy abdominal pain and hematochezia. The symptoms of colonic perforation are nonspecific and intermittent. The cause of perforation is unclear but also may be vasculitic in origin.

Lupus nephritis. Predisposition to renal involvement in SLE varies among different ethnic groups and is associated with specific human leukocyte antigen (HLA) alleles. Renal disease is an important cause of morbidity and mortality in SLE. More than 70% of all SLE patients will have renal involvement sometime during the course of their illness. Ideally, potential therapies would be used early in the course of renal involvement to minimize permanent damage. It is important to assess whether the renal disease (usually manifested by elevated creatinine levels and abnormalities of the urinary sediment) is active or inactive before considering invasive studies or cytotoxic therapy. Renal biopsy should be considered if there is either an active urinary sediment (red blood cells and/or cellular casts) or significant proteinuria (>1 g/24 hr). Other indications for biopsy are abnormal renal function (abnormal serum creatinine level or creatinine clearance) of unknown duration and decrements in renal function observed by the practitioner in association with an active urinary sediment or proteinuria or consideration of cytotoxic drug therapy.

Neurologic syndromes. **Headache** is one of the most common neurologic symptoms in SLE. Some patients have classic migraine, but most do not but have symptoms that suggest a vascular component to the headache. Chronic headache is well tolerated and is not a major cause of disability.

Depression may be the most common neuropsychiatric manifestation of SLE, and it usually is multifactorial in origin. The chronic and acute symptoms of systemic illness such as SLE may induce reactive depression. Reactive depression also may result from disability caused by SLE. Alteration in physical appearance because of SLE (e.g.,

hyperpigmentation/hypopigmentation and the scarring of discoid rash, alopecia, and malar rash) or side effects of medications used to treat SLE (moon facies and generalized weight gain from systemic steroids) all may cause reactive depression.

It is difficult to distinguish between steroid-induced depression and that caused by central nervous system (CNS) SLE. MRI scanning can be helpful in identifying vasculitis.

Cognitive impairment in SLE may manifest as attention deficit and memory disorders that interfere with activities of daily living. For example, work capacity, shopping, banking, driving, and housekeeping may be impaired. Frequently, depressive symptoms are superimposed. Psychometric testing is helpful in identifying the contribution of depression to cognitive impairment. Imaging techniques such as single photon emission computed tomography (I-123 SPECT) scan may be useful in the evaluation of cognitive disorders in SLE.

Coma, seizure disorder, cranial and periheral neuropathies, myelopathy, stroke, movement disorders, and aseptic meningitis may occur in patients with SLE. The mechanisms for manifestations are unclear, but microangiopathy from immune complex disease or vascular thrombosis due to antiphospholipid antibodies is suspected. Variable success in localizing pathologic lesions has been obtained by use of diagnostic techniques, such as electroencephalography (EEG), magnetic resonance imaging (MRI), and lumbar puncture.

DIAGNOSTIC TESTS
Laboratory tests

Antinuclear antibody (ANA). Although many of the ANA patterns are highly specific for lupus, others are not. The spectrum of the pattern of ANA is important in differentiating the various connective tissue disorders but is always supplemental to the history, symptoms, and physical examination.

The fluorescence antinuclear antibody test is the screening test of choice for SLE. ANA is superior to the LE cell preparation in terms of sensitivity and ease of performance. ANA findings are positive in more than 90% of persons with SLE. Positive test reactions for ANA may show one of several different patterns of immunofluorescence, which assist the practitioner in choosing the necessary additional diagnostic studies to distinguish among the various systemic rheumatic diseases. Homogeneous and peripheral patterns correlate with antibodies to DNA and are most specific for SLE. A speckled pattern indicates antibodies directed toward extractable nuclear antigen (ENA). Antibodies to ENA may be further subdivided into four antibody types. Anti-Sm is commonly found in SLE. Anti-RNP also is commonly found in SLE but is seen in mixed connective tissue disease (MCTD) as well. Anti-Ro (SSA) and anti-La (SSB) are positive in SLE, Sjögren's syndrome, and rheumatoid arthritis. These two antibodies are important risk factors for neonatal lupus syndrome and should be measured in every pregnant lupus patient (pregnancy and lupus are discussed in greater length at the end of this chapter). The nucleolar pattern of ANA, which most often is seen in systemic sclerosis and related syndromes, generally suggests antibodies to Pm-Scl and RNA polymerase I but also may be seen in

---

CAUSES OF ABDOMINAL PAIN IN SYSTEMIC LUPUS ERYTHEMATOSUS	
Serositis	Mesenteric vasculitis
Acute pancreatitis	Colonic perforation

anti-RNP positivity. A centromeric pattern indicates antibodies to topoisomerase I, a marker of systemic sclerosis. Cytoplasmic staining, which occurs rarely in SLE, may be seen in primary biliary cirrhosis and autoimmune thyroiditis. Figure 26-1 summarizes the diagnostic tests and diagnoses that the patterns of ANA suggest.

Complete blood cell count (CBC). A CBC should be obtained in any patient for whom the diagnosis of SLE is considered. **Anemia** in lupus may be multifactorial. Hemolysis (positive Coombs' test reaction), iron deficiency (exacerbated by menses, poor iron intake, and chronic gastrointestinal bleeding from nonsteroidal antiinflammatory medications), pernicious anemia, and anemia of chronic disease may all contribute to the anemia of SLE. **Thrombocytopenia** and **leukopenia/lymphopenia** seen in SLE may be on an autoimmune basis, although specific antibodies may not be detected.

Creatinine level and urinalysis. Renal disease occurs in up to 70% of SLE patients and is an important cause of morbidity and mortality. Screening tests of renal function should include a serum creatinine and urinalysis (microscopic and chemical) specifically to ascertain the presence of hematuria cellular casts and proteinuria.

Other diagnostic tests

Serositis, specifically pleurisy, pericarditis, and peritonitis, may complicate early SLE. Chest pain should be evaluated with a chest film to exclude pleural or pericardial effusions. Abdominal ultrasound examination is useful in assessing focal peritoneal fluid collections caused by SLE.

The **antiphospholipid antibodies** cause a predisposition to adverse pregnancy outcomes and peripheral arterial, venous, and CNS thrombotic events in SLE. Screening for these antibodies should be limited to symptomatic individuals and should include a serologic test for syphilis Veneral Disease Research Laboratory [VDRL] or rapid plasma reagin [RPR], anticardiolipin antibody a Russel Viper venom (RVV) test, and an activated partial thromboplastin time (PTT). A summary of the initial laboratory work-up for probable SLE is shown in Table 26-1. A different panel of tests is needed to evaluate definite, active, inactive, and pregnant SLE patients.

DIFFERENTIAL DIAGNOSIS

Several clinical and laboratory features of SLE also occur in other rheumatic conditions. For this reason, it is sometimes difficult to distinguish SLE from other systemic rheumatic diseases (see box on the next page).

Rheumatoid arthritis

Symmetric, peripheral polyarthritis is a frequent initial presentation of SLE and may be indistinguishable from the arthritic manifestations of early rheumatoid arthritis (RA). Rheumatoid factor is present in most RA patients (more than 75%) and is uncommon in SLE. In contrast, ANA is present in more than 90% of persons with SLE but also may occur in up to 30% of those with RA. When present, anti-dsDNA antibodies are specific for active SLE. Similarly, **hypocomplementemia** is highly suggestive of active SLE but also can occur in RA in the setting of cutaneous or systemic vasculitis. Subcutaneous nodules are commonly found in rheumatoid factor–positive (seropositive) RA but are seen infrequently in SLE. Hand films, with posteroante-

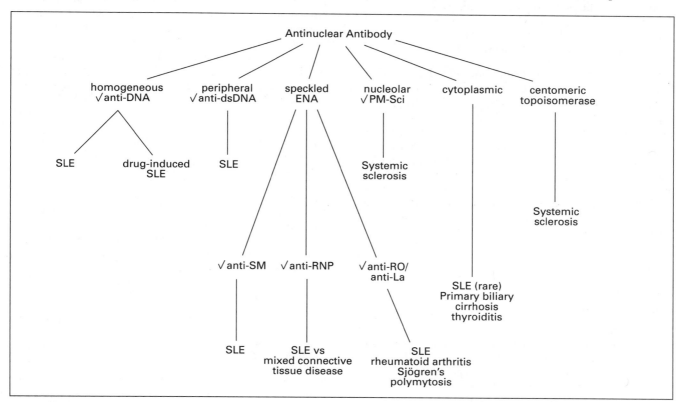

Fig. 26-1 Diagnostic tests and diagnoses to consider from ANA pattern.

Table 26-1 Initial laboratory work-up for probable systemic lupus erythematosus

Test	Probable SLE	Definite SLE	Active SLE	Inactive SLE	Pregnant SLE
ANA	Yes	No	No	No	No
CBC	Yes	Yes	Yes	Yes	Yes
Anti-DNA	No	Yes	Yes	Yes	Yes
Serum creatinine	Yes	Yes	Yes	Yes	Yes
Urinalysis	Yes	Yes	Yes	Yes	Yes
Ro/La	No*	No	No	No	Yes
Anticardiolipin	No	No	No	No	Yes
CH_{50}	No	Yes	Yes	Yes	Yes

*Ro/La testing would not be performed at the initial visit but might be undertaken subsequently if ANA results are negative and there is strong suspicion of SLE.

rior, lateral, and oblique views of both wrists and both hands, provide a useful comparison. Although **periarticular osteopenia** is present with RA and SLE polyarthritis, **marginal erosions** are specific for RA. (Chapter 25 covers rheumatoid arthritis in detail.)

Dermatomyositis

The proximal muscle weakness associated with early dermatomyositis may be subtle and overshadowed by the patient's more prominent complaints of symmetric, polyarthralgias, polyarthritis, and severe myalgias. The heliotrope rash of dermatomyositis affects the periorbital and malar areas, may be exacerbated by sun exposure, and can be confused with the butterfly rash of SLE. ANA is present in dermatomyositis and SLE. The speckled pattern of ANA is more common in dermatomyositis whereas homogeneous (diffuse) and peripheral ANA patterns are seen in SLE.

Systemic sclerosis (scleroderma) and mixed connective tissue disease

Raynaud's phenomenon (See Chapter 22) is a prominent feature of systemic sclerosis (SS) and mixed connective tissue disease (MCTD) but also occurs in SLE. ANA is present in all of these conditions. Speckled ANA is more likely to occur in SS and MCTD. Antibodies to nuclear precipitins may help to distinguish SLE from MCTD. Anti-RNP is more common in MCTD whereas anti-Sm is specific for SLE in white persons. Both anti-SM and anti-RNP occur more commonly in African-Americans, and distinction between these SLE and MCTD may not be possible on the basis of autoantibody profile in this ethnic group.

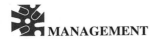 **MANAGEMENT**

Goals of management

Because there is currently no cure for SLE, therapeutic interventions focus on reducing the symptoms and organ dysfunction that affect lupus-related morbidity and mortality. Lupus disease activity may vary spontaneously, even with optimal therapy. Prophylactic measures for maintaining lupus remissions are very limited but for certain patients

may include sun avoidance or protection (suncreens) and hydroxychloroquine therapy.

Choice of therapy by organ system manifestation

Cutaneous manifestations. Malar rash may respond to topical corticosteroid creams or ointments. If possible, treatment with fluorinated corticosteroid preparations for facial lesions should be prescribed for a limited period to minimize the complications of fluorinated corticosteroid creams, namely atrophy, hypopigmentation/hyperpigmentation, and telangiectasias. Once the acute lesions respond to the fluorinated preparations, attempts should be made to switch to hydrocortisone cream. Steroid- and antimalarial-unresponsive bullous lesions that have neutrophils on biopsy may respond to dapsone. The use of **dapsone** is contraindicated in glucose-6-phosphate dehydrogenase (G6PD) deficiency. Starting dose is 25 to 50 mg/day. Weekly laboratory testing should include CBC, reticulocyte count, and lactic dehydrogenase (LDH) measurement. If laboratory parameters remain stable, the dose may be increased to 100 to 200 mg/day.

Combinations of therapies usually are required to treat chronic cutaneous symptoms. Regimens include **hydroxychloroquine** (Plaquenil) (400 mg/day) and/or topical and intradermal injections of corticosteroids into the active lesions. Hydroxychloroquine deposits in the retina and occasionally is associated with retinopathy. For this reason, baseline and serial (every 6 to 12 months) ophthalmologic evaluation is necessary. If there are baseline retinal abnormalities, the use of fluorescein angiography may be required. Refractory skin lesions sometimes are treated with combination antimalarial therapy (hydroxychloroquine and quinacrine (Atabrine). Atabrine does not cause retinopathy but does cause yellow-orange skin discoloration.

Lupus profundus may be refractory to conventional treatments. Combinations of therapies usually are required to treat these cutaneous symptoms. Regimens include antimalarial agents (hydroxychloroquine 200 to 400 mg/day) and topical and intralesional corticosteroids.

Alopecia often responds to systemic steroids as the other disease manifestations improve. Systemic steroids should not be used routinely to treat alopecia unless the alopecia is associated with some cutaneous form of SLE.

Sun avoidance and topical sunscreens are the best treatments for the associated photosensitivity. Sunscreens of skin protection factor (SPF) 2 to 15 protect against UVA whereas those with an SPF greater than 15 provide protection from UVB.

Lupus fatigue. Chronic fatigue that is severe enough to interfere with activities of daily living is common in SLE and may improve with a low-impact aerobic exercise program. (For a more detailed discussion on management of fatigue, see Chapter 70.)

Polyarthritis. Aspirin and nonsteroidal antiinflammatory drugs (NSAIDs) provide the first line of therapy. Hydroxychloroquine (Plaquenil), 200 mg twice daily, is used in combination with acetylsalicylic acid (ASA) or NSAIDs. As mentioned before, patients who are treated with hydroxychloroquine need baseline and quarterly to semiannual ophthalmologic examinations to monitor potential retinal toxicity from this medication. Short courses of low-dose prednisone (5 to 10 mg orally every morning) provide transient relief of joint complaints. Resting wrist and hand splints reduce inflammatory symptoms.

Pleuropulmonary disease. For those patients with pleurisy but no evidence of pleural effusion or pulmonary embolism, a brief course of steroids (prednisone 10 to 20 mg orally for 7 to 10 days) will generally control pleuritic symptoms. Sometimes combination therapy with NSAIDs (in particular, indomethacin 50 mg orally three times daily if tolerated) and transient narcotic analgesic use (codeine preparations for the first 3 days of symptoms) becomes necessary. For pleurisy that the clinician believes is caused by the lupus rather than infection, higher doses of steroids (prednisone 30 mg orally every morning often are needed for 4 to 6 weeks.

For parenchymal involvement, high-dose corticosteroids (prednisone 40 to 60 mg daily) are used in this setting with variable efficacy.

Uncontrolled studies on the shrinking lung syndrome suggest that treatment with prednisone 40 mg/day may be beneficial.

For pulmonary hemorrhage, treatment includes maintenance of respiratory function, reversal of coagulopathy if present, and the administration of high-dose steroids for presumed immune-complex disease.

Cardiac disease. For pericardial effusion with impending tamponade, the decision about invasive versus noninvasive treatment—that is, whether to rapidly decompress the pericardial sac by pericardiocentesis or pericardial window to prevent progression to tamponade or whether to treat with steroids—is a difficult one. High-dose steroids have been shown to improve symptoms and reduce fluid volumes within 48 to 72 hours. Clinically, however, if the patient's cardiac status is unstable, a more invasive approach may have to be pursued.

Myocorditis requires steroids in combination with standard therapies. Valvulitis and vegetations in the SLE patient may be due to acute or subacute bacterial endocarditis.

Pancreatitis. During an episode of pancreatitis, there is no known therapeutic benefit of adjusting the dose of steroids.

Lupus nephritis. Randomized control trials in severe lupus nephritis suggest that combinations of **cyclophosphamide** and **corticosteroids** (both given in daily oral dose vs. monthly intravenous injections) may be efficacious for the treatment of renal lesions within World Health Organization (WHO) guidelines. This regimen is limited to WHO classification grades III, IV, and V disease (segmental, proliferative, diffuse proliferative and membranous nephritis with either segmental or proliferative features, respectively) that show some degree of active inflammation (fibrinoid necrosis, crescent formation, hyaline thrombi, or subendothelial deposits). The "pulse" (monthly bolus schedule) cyclophosphamide regimen is more popular because it is better tolerated and equally effective as daily dosing sched-

ules. A randomized control trial of plasmapheresis plus cyclophosphamide and prednisone showed no additional benefit attributable to plasmapheresis (Lewis et al., 1992).

Neurologic syndromes. Depression may respond to combination treatment with antidepressants and long-term psychotherapy, informal group counseling, or support group participation. (See Chapter 67 for discussion of treatment for depression).

For CNS vasculitis, high-dose steroids (orally or intravenously administered) are used most often alone or in combination with cytotoxic drugs, although their benefit is unknown. Aseptic meningitis in SLE occasionally is associated with NSAID use (ibuprofen and other NSAIDs). Pleocytosis and meningeal signs rapidly improve with cessation of medication.

Corticosteroid use

Steroid preparations are used to treat almost all manifestations of SLE. The most serious side effects of corticosteroids are increased susceptibility to opportunistic infections and predisposition to osteoporosis and aseptic necrosis. Other side effects are associated diabetes, hypertension, and cataract formation. Prolonged use of systemic cortico-steroids is unavoidable in the treatment of renal and CNS SLE. The goal is to relieve symptoms related to SLE and to decrease long-term morbidity.

Daily prednisone dosages as low as 5 mg orally may alter mood and sleeping patterns. Emotional liability and insomnia develop within several days of initiating oral corticosteroid therapy and usually improve in 7 to 10 days. Severe depression and psychosis are more likely to occur at higher doses and may develop at any time during the course of steroid use. Acne, moon facies, and weight gain resolve when steroids are tapered or discontinued, but cataracts and purple striae are permanent sequelae. Calcium supplementation (1000 to 1500 mg elemental calcium on a daily basis) and vitamin D (calcitriol 0.25 mcg/day) are administered to minimize steroid-induced osteoporosis. Serial determinations of serum and 24-hour urinary calcium are necessary on this regimen.

Plaquenil therapy

Hydroxychloroquine affects disease activity. The mechanisms are unknown and do not appear to be only organ-specific. Generally the therapy is used when any of the symptoms of lupus appear with a twice-daily oral dose of 200 mg. Cessation of this medication may result in lupus flare. As mentioned before, the side effects include retinopathy; thus close ophthalmologic follow-up is necessary.

Immunization and chemoprophylaxis

Immunization with pneumococcal and *Haemophilus B* vaccine is an essential component of the management of the SLE patient who has undergone splenectomy. Similarly, pneumococcal vaccine is recommended in lupus patients with leukopenia and also in those receiving corticosteroid and other immunosuppressive therapies. Isoniazid (INH) is not routinely used in SLE patients who receive long-term steroids, but close screening for tuberculosis exposure is important.

Monitoring disease activity

Accurate assessment of disease activity is essential for appropriate decision making in caring for SLE patients. Several activity indexes have been developed to facilitate epidemiologic studies. These standardized measures are valuable tools but too time-consuming for use by the busy practitioner in following up SLE patients. Serial sedimentation rates are useful for monitoring disease activity in most lupus patients, whereas CH_{50} and anti-DNA antibody factors assist in monitoring many forms of lupus nephritis and some patients with pleuropericardial disease. CNS disease activity is difficult to assess and often requires serial cognitive and imaging studies.

PREGNANCY AND LUPUS

Overview

Outcomes of interest for SLE patients considering pregnancy are fertility, the influence of pregnancy on SLE, lupus effects on pregnancy, and the possible adverse fetal effects of maternal SLE (see box, below).

With the exception of the subset of SLE patients who experience severe lupus nephritis with chronic renal failure or who require cytotoxic drugs such as cyclophosphamide, fertility studies of SLE show no direct effects of the disease and no overall reduction in fertility.

Cohort analyses indicate that pregnancy causes mild exacerbations in SLE. Patients with SLE require clinical and laboratory monitoring of disease parameters (anti-DNA, CH_{50}, platelet count) on a biweekly to monthly basis during their pregnancies.

Preeclamptic toxemia (PET) is three times more common in SLE than in women with normal pregnancies. PET is more common in patients with any renal dysfunction and may explain the higher prevalence of this condition in SLE. The manifestations of preeclampsia may be indistinguishable from active lupus nephritis (Table 26-2), and simultaneous treatment for both lupus nephritis and preeclampsia often is necessary.

Fetal wastage (early and late fetal loss) is more common in SLE pregnancy. Fetal distress and late fetal loss are associated with antibodies to phospholipids (APL), which occur in 6.7% to 25% of SLE patients. APL can be detected by a biologically false-positive test for syphilis, by prolongation of the activated partial thromboplastin time (APTT), by tests of the lupus anticoagulant (LAC) (Russell viper venom), or by assays for IgG antibodies to cardiolipin (ACL). Pregnant SLE patients with ACL require close fetal observation (biophysical profiles weekly) throughout the third trimester. Preterm delivery is also more common in lupus pregnancies. Estimates of the frequencies of intrauterine growth retardation (IUGR) and low birth weight that are adjusted for known risk factors are not avail-

Table 26-2 Manifestations of lupus nephritis and preeclamptic toxemia

	Systemic lupus erythematosus	Preeclampsia
Hypertension	+	+
Proteinuria	+++	+
Edema	±	±
Oliguria	±	±
Thrombocytopenia	+	+
Uric acid	Normal to elevated	Elevated
Active sediment	+	−
Complement (CH_{50})	Low	Low
	Normal	Normal
	High	High

able for SLE so we cannot determine whether there is SLE-specific predisposition to these adverse pregnancy outcomes.

Neonatal lupus erythematosus (NLE) is a rare condition with transient cutaneous or hematologic manifestations or permanent congenital complete heart block (CCHB) (see box, below). The presence of maternal anti-Ro (SSA) or La (SSB) antibodies is a risk factor for NLE. There are no preventive therapies with proved efficacy, nor are there any known therapies to reverse CCHB.

SLE patients should have testing for antibodies Ro (SSA), antibodies La (SSB), anticardiolipin antibodies (IgG and IgM ACL), and APTT in early pregnancy. CCHB can occur as early as week 20. If anti-Ro or anti-La antibodies are present, fetal heart auscultation after the week 20 may detect the regular bradycardia of CCHB. If ACL or an abnormal APTT is detected, nonstress testing should be performed. SLE monitoring should include serial measurements of serum complement (CH_{50}) and platelet counts (see box, next page). Serum complement rises to supernormal levels in pregnancy. Normal, low, or decreasing levels during pregnancy suggest active or flaring disease but are not conclusive because normal or low-normal complement levels also may be associated with PET.

Drug therapy

During pregnancy. The most commonly used drugs in SLE include aspirin and NSAIDs, corticosteroids, antimalarial agents, and cyclophosphamide. If the patient can tolerate dose adjustment, NSAIDs are reduced or discontinued in early pregnancy to minimize maternal and fetal bleeding tendencies associated with the drugs and also to reduce the risks of delayed labor in the mother and premature closure of the ductus arteriosus in the fetus. Prednisone is the most commonly used corticosteroid preparation. Because it is metabolized by the placenta, only very small amounts are present in the fetal circulation and minimal—if any—fetal adrenal suppression is associated with it. The

---

PREGNANCY AND THE LUPUS PATIENT

Fertility in SLE
Impact of pregnancy on lupus
SLE effects on pregnancy
Fetal effects of SLE

FEATURES OF THE NEONATAL LUPUS SYNDROME

Skin lesions
Thrombocytopenia and/or hemolytic anemia
Congenital complete heart block (CCHB)

LABORATORY TESTS IN PREGNANT LUPUS PATIENT

Anti-Ro (SSA)
Anti-La (SSB)
  If positive, monitor fetal heart rate
Anticardiolipin (IgG/IgM)
  If positive, monitor fetal biophysical profile
Activated partial thromboplastin time
  If abnormal, monitor fetal biophysical profile
Baseline and serial complement (CH_{50}) levels
  Normal to low CH_{50} suggests active SLE, follow-up 2/mo
  Sudden decrease suggests SLE flare and/or PET, Rx specific
    symptoms
Baseline and serial platelet counts

---

dose of prednisone often is adjusted to compensate for the withdrawal or reduction of NSAIDs. Prophylactic use of prednisone is not recommended for patients with inactive lupus because no evidence exists of its benefit. In addition, prednisone causes fluid retention and hypertension, and these effects may increase the risk of pregnancy-induced hypertension, which is more common in SLE. Maintenance therapy with antimalarial agents sustains a stable course or remission in SLE. This clinical observation must be balanced against the finding in experimental animals of hydroxychloroquine (Plaquenil) deposition in fetal retinal tissue. The options are to discontinue hydroxychloroquine as soon as pregnancy is confirmed and to observe for possible flare of symptoms, or to maintain the medication throughout pregnancy if the patient is informed of the experimental data and the lack of known adverse effects on the fetus and she can accept this uncertainty. Cyclophosphamide should not be used in the first trimester because of its teratogenic potential.

During lactation. Most of the literature on drug use in lactation stems from case reports. Thus the absence of a case report of adverse effect on a nursing infant may reflect the low frequency of side effects or a truly "safe" drug. Aspirin and indomethacin should not be used. Ibuprofen (Motrin, Advil) and piroxicam (Feldene) have no reported side effects. Although hydroxychloroquine has no reported adverse effects, it may precipitate hemolysis in a G6PD-deficient infant and should be avoided during lactation. Prednisone has no reported adverse effects in nursing infants.

PROGNOSIS AND OUTCOME

Longitudinal studies suggest that at least 4% of SLE patients will experience serologic and clinical remission. Survival in SLE is influenced by age of onset, race, socioeconomic status, duration of disease, pattern of organ involvement, and the presence of IgM anticardiolipin antibodies. Cardiopulmonary, renal (especially the histology of the renal lesion), and CNS symptoms are all important predictors of survival. Overall 5-year survival in SLE approaches 90%, and 10-year survival is about 80%.

BIBLIOGRAPHY

Arnett FC et al: Increased frequencies of Sm and nRNP autoantibodies in American blacks compared to whites with systemic lupus erythematosus, *J Rheumatol* 15:1773, 1988.

Asherson RA et al: Hypertrophic cardiomyopathy in systemic lupus erythematosus and "lupus-like" disease: chance association? A report of two cases, *J Rheumatol* 19:1073, 1992.

Boyer GS, Templin DW, Lanier AP: Rheumatic diseases in Alaskan Indians of the southeast coast: high prevalence of rheumatoid arthritis and systemic lupus erythematosus, *J Rheumatol* 18:1477, 1991.

Bush TM, Shlotzhauer TL, Grove W: Serum complements: inappropriate use in patients with suspected rheumatic disease, *Arch Intern Med* 153:2363, 1993.

Buyon JP, Yaron M, Lockshin MD: First international conference on rheumatic disease in pregnancy, *Arthritis Rheum* 36:59, 1993.

Canadian Hydroxychloroquine Study Group: A randomized study of the effect of withdrawing hydroxychloroquine sulfate in systemic lupus erythematosus, *N Engl J Med* 324:150, 1991.

Committee on Drugs, 1992-1993: The transfer of drugs and other chemicals into human milk, *Pediatrics* 93:137, 1994.

Ellis SG, Verity A: Central nervous system involvement in systemic lupus erythematosus: a review of neuropathologic findings in 57 cases, 1955-1977, *Semin Arthritis Rheum* 8(3):212, 1979.

Franks AG: Nonspecific lesions, cutaneous LE management overview. III. Identifying dermatologic manifestations of lupus erythematosus, *J Musculoskel Med* 5(7):39, 1988.

Galve E et al: Prevalence, morphologic types, and evolution of cardiac valvular disease in systemic lupus erythematosus, *N Engl J Med* 319:817, 1988.

Ginzler EM: Clinical features and complications of systemic lupus erythematosus, and assessment of disease activity, *Curr Opin Rheumatol* 2:703, 1990.

Ginzler EM et al: Hypertension increases the risk of renal deterioration in systemic lupus erythematosus, *J Rheumatol* 20:1694, 1993.

Gladman DD: Prognosis of systemic lupus erythematosus and factors that affect it, *Curr Opin Rheumatol* 2:294, 1990.

Golbus J, McCune WJ: Neuropsychiatric lupus: clinical features, pathophysiology, diagnosis and treatment, *Intern Med* 8(9):141, 1987.

Gulko PS et al: Anticardiolipin antibodies in systemic lupus erythematosus: clinical correlates, HLA associations, and impact on survival, *J Rheumatol* 20:1684, 1993.

Heller CA, Schur PH: Serological and clinical remission in systemic lupus erythematosus, *J Rheumatol* 12:916, 1985.

Hochberg MC: Systemic lupus erythematosus, *Rheum Dis Clin North Am* 16:617, 1990.

Hochberg MC et al: Systemic lupus erythematosus: a review of clinico-laboratory features and immunogenetic markers in 150 patients with emphasis on demographic subsets, *Medicine* 64:285, 1985.

Jacobs L et al: Central nervous system lupus erythematosus: the value of magnetic resonance imaging, *J Rheumatol* 15:601, 1988.

Kaine JL, Kahl LE: Which laboratory tests are useful in diagnosing SLE? *J Musculoskel Med* 9(11): 15, 1992.

Lawrence RC et al: Estimates of the prevalence of selected arthritic and musculoskeletal disease in the United States, *J Rheumatol* 16:427, 1989.

Lewis EJ et al (Lupus Nephritis Collaborative Study Group): A controlled trial of plasmapheresis therapy in severe lupus nephritis, *N Engl J Med* 326:1373, 1992.

Liang MH et al: Reliability and validity of six systems for the clinical assessment of disease activity in systemic lupus erythematosus, *Arthritis Rheum* 32:1107, 1989.

Lockshin MD et al: Antibody to cardiolipin as a predictor of fetal distress or death in pregnant patients with systemic lupus erythematosus, *N Engl J Med* 313:152, 1985.

Lockshin MD et al: Neonatal lupus risk to newborns of mothers with systemic lupus erythematosus, *Arthritis Rheum* 31:697, 1988.

McLaughlin J et al: Kidney biopsy in systemic lupus erythematosus. II. Survival analyses according to biopsy results, *Arthritis Rheum* 34:1268, 1991.

Older SA, Boumpas DT, Austin HA: Management of lupus nephritis. I. *J Musculoskel Med* 8:35, 1991.

Older SA, Boumpas DT, Austin HA: Management of lupus nephritis, II. *J Musculoskel Med* 8:74, 1991.

Perez-Gutthann S, Petri M, Hochberg MC: Comparison of different methods of classifying patients with systemic lupus erythematosus, *J Rheumatol* 18:117, 1991.

Petri M, Howard D, Repke J: The frequency of lupus flare in pregnancy, *Arthritis Rheum* 34:1538, 1991.

Petri M et al: The frequency of lupus anticoagulant in systemic lupus erythematosus, *Ann Intern Med* 106:524, 1987.

Pillemer SR et al: Lupus nephritis: association between serology and renal biopsy measures, *J Rheumatol* 15:284, 1988.

Robb-Nicholson C et al: Effects of aerobic conditioning in lupus fatigue: a pilot study, *Br J Rheumatol* 28:500, 1989.

Rogers MP et al: I-123 iofetamine SPECT scan in systemic lupus erythematosus patients with cognitive and other minor neuropsychiatric symptoms: a pilot study, *Lupus* 1:215, 1992.

Rothfield NF: Distinguishing lupus from three other rheumatic diseases, *Diagnosis,* p. 51, Oct 1987.

Steigerwald JC: Pulmonary involvement in systemic lupus erythematosus, *Intern Med* 4:78, 1983.

Studenski S, Ward MM: Systemic lupus erythematosus in men: a multivariate analysis gender differences in clinical manifestations, *J Rheumatol* 17:220, 1990.

Tan EM et al: The 1982 revised criteria for the classification of systemic lupus erythematosus, *Arthritis Rheum* 25:1271, 1982.

Walz-Leblanc BAE et al: The "shrinking lungs syndrome" in systemic lupus erythematosus—improvement with corticosteroid therapy, *J Rheumatol* 19:1970, 1992.

Ward MM, Studenski S: Clinical manifestations of systemic lupus erythematosus: identification of racial and socieconomic influences, *Arch Inter Med* 150:849, 1990.

Watson RM et al: Neonatal lupus erythematosus: a clinical, serological and immunogenetic study with review of the literature, *Medicine* 63:362, 1984.

Werth VP et al: Incidence of alopecia areata in lupus erythematosus, *Arch Dermatol* 128:368, 1992.

Wilson WA, Hughes GRV: Rheumatic disease in Jamaica, *Ann Rheum Dis* 38:320, 1979.

Part Two

The Reproductive Cycle

Section I

GENERAL GYNECOLOGY

27 Contraception

Rapin Osathanondh, Michael R. Stelluto, and Karen J. Carlson

Preventing unwanted pregnancy is a multifactorial process. The willingness and ability to use contraception is influenced not only by the efficacy of the methods, but also by cost, availability, personality, life circumstances, and culture. Although the range of prescription and nonprescription contraceptive options is large, including hormonal methods, barrier methods, intrauterine devices, and sterilization, no method is ideal. It is a challenging and complex task to assist women in making choices that are appropriate for a particular stage of life and medical and social circumstances.

This chapter describes a framework for approaching the female patient who desires contraception, and outlines the physiology, effectiveness, benefits, and risks of available contraceptive methods.

EPIDEMIOLOGY

A woman's life expectancy is inversely proportional to the number of pregnancies she experiences. All contraceptive methods available in the United States are safer than carrying a pregnancy to term. Theoretically, the safest contraceptive practice for a monogamous woman is the diaphragm or condom, followed by early, legal abortion should one of those methods fail.

Effectiveness in prevention of pregnancy (Table 27-1) is a critical attribute of any contraceptive method, although it is only one of several factors that must be weighed in the selection of the optimal birth control method for an individual woman. Theoretic effectiveness rates reflect the ideal which can be achieved under ideal conditions. The actual or use effectiveness depends on many individual factors that introduce error.

APPROACH TO THE WOMAN WHO DESIRES CONTRACEPTION

Effective contraceptive management requires time for education and counseling. Because conflicting primary data about the sequelae of various methods has confused many women, education about risks and benefits is crucial to clarify what is known and what remains controversial. Counseling explores values and life circumstances, including marital status, partner(s), work or educational opportunity, home responsibilities, future childbearing plans, sexuality and body image, and the need for security versus the willingness to risk pregnancy or side effects.

Informed consent, in nontechnical terminology and in the woman's native language, should be obtained for any prescription method of contraception and before any invasive procedures. Informed consent recognizes that contraceptive interventions that involve hormones, devices, or surgery expose healthy people to known and unknown risks. Beyond delineating medicolegal and ethical responsibilities, informed consent provides useful information for assisting women in selecting a contraceptive method and in gaining the confidence to use it.

The screening history is directed toward the gynecologic and obstetric history, review of systems to establish potential contraindications and risk factors for complications, and personal history to elicit lifestyle preferences. Similarly, the screening physical examination and laboratory studies

Table 27-1 Effectiveness rates of contraceptive methods

Method	Theoretical effectiveness (%)	Use effectiveness (%)
Oral contraceptive pill		
Combination	99.9	97
Progestin only	99.5	97
Long-acting progestins		
Depo Provera	99.7	99.7
Norplant	99.96	99.96
Barrier methods		
Condoms	98	88
Diaphragm	94	82
Cervical cap	94	82
Vaginal sponge		
Nulliparous women	94	82
Parous women	91	72
Spermicides	97	79
Intrauterine device		
Copper T380	99.2	97
Progestasert	98	97
Sterilization		
Male	99.9	99.9
Female	99.8	99.6

Data from Trussel J et al: *Obstet Gynecol* 76:558, 1990.

uncover potential contraindications or risks for complications of chosen contraceptive methods.

HORMONAL METHODS
Oral contraceptive pill

There are two types of oral contraceptive pills (OCPs). **Combination** or combined pills contain a synthetic estrogen, ethinyl estradiol (or its methyl ester, mestranol) and a progestin, a progesterone-like steroid. Combination pills are packaged in 21-day or 28-day cycles; the last seven tablets in 28-day packs are hormonally inert and may contain iron. Monophasic pills contain the same amount of estrogen and progestin in the 21 hormonally active tablets. Efforts to lower the total exposure to steroids while mimicking the patterns of the physiologic menstrual cycle led to the marketing of multiphasic (biphasic and triphasic) pills. They contain 35 μg or less of estrogen in each active tablet, and varying amounts of progestin. The progestins have differing levels of androgenic and estrogenic activity. Table 27-2 shows the relative androgenic and estrogenic activity of combination pills containing 35 μg or less of estrogen.

Progestin-only pills, also called the "mini pill," contain a small dose of progestin and no estrogen.

Mechanism of action. Estrogens and progestins in low daily dosage synergistically prevent ovulation by inhibiting the midcycle surge of the gonadotropins-luteinizing hormone (LH) and follicle-stimulating hormone (FSH). This suppresses endogenous ovarian estrogen and progesterone production, which then inhibits endometrial proliferation. Bleeding occurs in response to progestin withdrawal, which mimics monthly menstrual periodicity.

Progestins decrease tubal function, diminish endometrial receptiveness to implantation, and render the cervix less permeable to penetration by sperm. Progestins alone can provide adequate contraceptive effects but do not totally suppress LH surges or ovarian estrogens, which accounts for their higher failure rate compared to combined pills. In addition, the irregular bleeding which is sometimes a side effect of progestin-only pills contributes to noncompliance.

Benefits. A principal benefit of the OCP is its very high effectiveness rate (97%-99%). Daily pill-taking is dissociated from the sexual act, which may make compliance easier for some women. The combination pill protects the user from ectopic pregnancy, reduces primary dysmenorrhea, and reduces the incidence of fibrocystic breast disease and functional ovarian cysts. Increased cycle regularity is another potential benefit of the combination pill. Use of the OCP is associated with a decreased risk of ovarian cancer and endometrial cancer, and there is some evidence of increased bone mineral density after several years of use.

Risks. Confusion about pill-associated morbidity and mortality stems from two major factors. First, studies conducted in the 1960s and 1970s were based on the use of pills with 50 μg or greater estrogen content. Lowering the amount of ethinyl estradiol in each tablet diminished many unwanted effects. Second, long-term sequelae of oral contraceptive use, particularly neoplasia, may take 20 to 30 years to manifest; the original cohort of users is just entering that period.

Cardiovascular disease incidence was increased in early studies of the OCP, which showed higher rates of myocardial infarction, stroke, and thromboembolic disease in current users of the pill. The mechanism of ischemic heart disease was thought to be thrombosis, not atherosclerosis, mediated through the estrogen component of the pill. In these early studies, which mostly involved pills containing greater than 50 μg of estrogen, risk was limited to current users; no studies have shown increased risk after cessation of the pill. In the early studies, higher rates of myocardial infarction were limited to women over 35 years of age with other risk factors such as smoking, hyperlipidemia, hypertension, or diabetes. Most recent studies of current users of lower-dose pills (35 μg of estrogen) have shown no increase in risk. Porter and colleagues reported on a cohort of 65,000 healthy women ages 15 to 44 (including smokers) among cases and controls; no myocardial infarctions occurred during six years of observation. A recent case-control study by Thorogood showed a slight increase in fatal myocardial infarction (risk ratio of 1.9) in women receiving low-dose

Table 27-2 Androgenic and estrogenic activity of progestins in combination oral contraceptive pills containing 35μg or less of estrogen

Level	Androgenic activity		Estrogenic activity	
High	Norgestrel Levonorgestrel	LoOvral Nordette, Levlen Triphasil, Trilevlen	Ethynodiol	Demulen 1/35
Middle	Norethindrone	Genora 1/35, OrthoNovum 1/35, Norinyl 1/35 Ortho 10/11 TriNorinyl Ortho 7/7/7 Modicon, Brevicon Ovcon 35		
	Norethindrone acetate	Loestrin 1/20 Loestrin 1.5/30		
Low	Ethynodiol Norgestimate Desogestrel	Demulen 1/35 Orthocyclen, Orthotricyclen Desogen, Orthocept	All other progestins	

pills. The risk of cardiovascular disease increases with age, and is heightened by smoking. Therefore current recommendations limit pill use beyond age 35 to nonsmokers.

Hypertension develops in about 5% of normotensive women after 3 months of OCP use. Up to 15% of women with preexisting hypertension demonstrate elevated blood pressure readings associated with pill use.

The pill is sometimes the cause of **lipid abnormalities.** Estrogens tend to increase high density lipoprotein (HDL) levels and decrease low density lipoprotein (LDL) levels; progestins generally have the opposite effect. The net effect is little or no change in total cholesterol, HDL, or LDL levels; triglycerides may increase, sometimes substantially.

Glucose intolerance is a consequence of the progestin component of the pill and occurs least with progestins having lower androgenic activity.

Studies since 1980 have shown no overall effect of oral contraceptives on **breast cancer** risk. However, some have shown a small increase in risk within subgroups, such as young nulliparous women who use OCPs for more than 8 years. Because such findings have been inconsistent, no recommendations for any change in current prescribing practices have been made. **Cervical dysplasia** is increased twofold in pill users, even after controlling for factors such as frequency and age at onset of intercourse. Cervical epithelial abnormalities associated with OCP use predispose to infection with human papillomavirus (HPV), human immunodeficiency virus (HIV), and chlamydia.

The risk of **gallbladder disease** is increased approximately twofold in OCP users. **Hepatic adenomas** are rare benign vascular tumors associated with the oral contraceptive pill.

Management issues. Most clinicians benefit from familiarity with a few of the many formulations of the oral contraceptive pill. When initiating OCP use, it is advisable to begin with a low dose (30-35 μg estrogen) pill. The choice of pill may be modified by a history of estrogen-sensitive symptoms (premenstrual breast tenderness, weight gain), for which a progestin with low estrogenic activity is best; or of hirsutism or acne, for which a progestin with low androgenic activity is preferred (see Table 27-2). Two progestins recently introduced in the United States, desogestrel (Desogen, Orthocept) and norgestimate (Ortho-Cyclen), have decreased androgenic activity and less effects on blood pressure and carbohydrate and lipid metabolism than older progestins.

Women over 40 who do not smoke are good candidates for the lowest dose estrogen pills (such as Lo-Estrin 1/20 with 20 μg of estrogen). Good cycle control and relief of vasomotor symptoms are potential benefits in this age group, although sometimes breakthrough bleeding occurs. A baseline mammogram and lipid profile should be obtained.

Postpartum women who desire oral contraceptives should be given the lowest estrogen preparations. Controversy exists regarding the appropriate commencement time. Manufacturers recommend delaying the start of OCP use until 4 to 6 weeks postpartum. However, most authorities feel that the benefits of an early start outweigh the risks because ovulation can occur as early as two weeks postpartum. Combination OCPs reduce the amount of breast milk. Breastfeeding women should consider a barrier method of contraception. Alternatively, progestin-only pills have long been used in lactating women, although the long-term effects on the baby are not known.

Women with diabetes should be discouraged from using the pill if they have elevated blood pressure, nephropathy, or retinopathy. **Hypertensive women** generally are not appropriate candidates for combination oral contraceptives. The progestin-only pill may be considered in some cases with careful monitoring of lipid levels.

Women with migraine headaches often experience an increase in the frequency or severity of headaches, particularly women with menstrual migraines. To avoid this problem, as well as the possible slight increase in risk for stroke, a progestin-only pill is a reasonable alternative.

The box below lists absolute and relative contraindications to OCP use.

Basic guidelines for pill use should be reviewed. The woman should begin the pill on the first day of her next menstrual period, which provides greater immediate effectiveness than the traditional Sunday start date. A backup method for the first cycle is generally recommended because common minor problems with side effects or forgetfulness may occur. If a woman forgets one pill, she should be advised to take her previous day's pill with her current one. If she forgets two consecutive pills, she should take two pills for two days and resume one pill daily for the remainder of the cycle; a barrier method should also be used. If the woman forgets three or more consecutive pills, she must be considered unprotected; the pill may not be an appropriate method for her.

A woman beginning the OCP should be evaluated after 3 cycles to review pill use, measure blood pressure, and assess the presence of any side effects (see box on the following page). Thereafter she should be seen annually to monitor for side effects.

Breakthrough bleeding is a common problem, occuring in approximately 15% of women beginning OCP use. If it has not resolved after the third cycle, the pill should be changed according to the timing of the bleeding. Late cycle bleeding responds to an increase in progestin, while early cycle bleeding is often a consequence of inadequate estrogen effect. Bleeding that develops after prolonged pill use may be related to inadequate estrogen, but should always be

---

CONTRAINDICATIONS TO ORAL CONTRACEPTIVE PILL USE

Absolute contraindications

History of cardiovascular disease or stroke
History of thromboembolic disease
Known coagulation disorder: protein C or S deficiency,
    antithrombin III deficiency
Severe liver disease
Known or suspected malignancy of breast or endometrium
Undiagnosed genital bleeding
Known or suspected pregnancy

Relative contraindications

Smoking	Migraine headaches
Hypertension	Seizure disorder
Diabetes	Sickle cell anemia
Hyperlipidemia	Uterine leiomyoma

SIDE EFFECTS OF ORAL CONTRACEPTIVE PILL USE

Estrogen-related	Progestin-related
Nausea	Increased appetite
Breast tenderness	Depression
Fluid retention	Fatigue
Weight gain	Decreased libido
Headaches	Acne
	Headaches

evaluated to rule out infection, neoplasia, and pregnancy (see Chapter 28).

Amenorrhea occurs after long-term pill use in 1% to 3% of women. When pregnancy has been ruled out, the woman can be reassured that it is safe to continue the OCP. If the absence of a menstrual period is bothersome to the woman, a change to a higher estrogen preparation is reasonable. Postpill amenorrhea is said to be present if the menstrual cycle does not resume six months after cessation of pill use. A full evaluation (see Chapter 29) is necessary.

Nausea is thought to be related to the estrogenic component of the pill. Taking the pill with the evening meal or at bedtime may help. If not, a change to a lower estrogen formula is appropriate.

Drug interactions with the oral contraceptive pill are listed in Appendix 6. The effect of the OCP on laboratory measures is outlined in Appendix 7.

Morning-after pill

Postcoital contraceptive methods using high-dose estrogens act by preventing implantation. In addition to high-dose estrogens, progestins alone, danazol, and RU 486 (a progestin antagonist) have been used for postcoital prevention of pregnancy.

The most popular postcoital treatment is the combination of a potent progestin with 50 μg of ethinyl estradiol (Ovral). The dosage is two tablets of Ovral followed by two more tablets 12 hours later. Therapy must be initiated within 72 hours of unprotected intercourse. Nausea and vomiting are common and an antiemetic should be prescribed. Withdrawal bleeding sometimes occurs. The failure rate is reported at less than 2 per 100 isolated courses of treatment. A careful menstrual history (and testing, when indicated) to exclude an existing pregnancy is essential.

Long-acting progestins

Progestins can be injected intramuscularly or subdermally to provide prolonged contraception for several months to up to five years. Two long-acting injectables are intramuscular medroxyprogesterone acetate (Depo-Provera) and subdermal levonorgestrel (Norplant). Both are highly effective, with failure rates of less than 1% per year (Table 27-1).

Mechanism of action. Long-acting progestins act by inhibiting ovulation and impairing sperm transport and implantation. After one injection of 150 mg. Depo-Provera remains measurable in the circulatory system for 8 to 9 months. Estradiol levels during Depo-Provera treatment are suppressed to the level in the early follicular phase of the normal cycle. Norplant provides a blood level of lev-

onorgestrel similar to that in a progestin-only pill or one-fourth to one-half of combination oral contraceptives.

Benefits. The principal benefits of the long-acting progestins are ease of compliance, high effectiveness, and avoidance of estrogen-related side effects.

Risks. Breakthrough bleeding is a common side effect. An average of 100 days of irregular bleeding occurs during the first year of Norplant use. Other side effects include weight gain, headaches, and occasionally androgenic effects. In several studies, discontinuation of Norplant was requested by 10% to 20% of its users because of side effects.

Prolonged use over years will result in mildly decreased bone density. Another problem is that resumption of fertility may not occur for a year or longer in some cases.

Management issues. Depo-Provera is administered by intramuscular injection of 150 mg every 3 months. The initial dose should be given during the first five days of menses and pregnancy should be excluded. A pregnancy test should also be performed if an interval greater than 14 weeks elapses between injections.

The insertion technique for the Norplant system involves placement of six polymeric silicone rods in a fan-shaped arrangement under the skin. It is a fairly simple technique but does require special training.

BARRIER METHODS
Condoms

The male condom is the most popular contraceptive method. The recent introduction of a female condom provides women with another option for protection from pregnancy and sexually transmitted diseases. Effectiveness rates are 85% to 95%; male condoms prelubricated with spermicide have an estimated effectiveness rate of 96%.

Mechanism of action. Male condoms cover the penis during coitus and serve as a reservoir to prevent the deposit of semen in the vagina. Female condoms consist of a polyurethane pouch held in place by an outer and an inner ring.

Benefits. Condoms are inexpensive, available without prescription, and free of systemic side effects. Condoms made of polyurethane or latex may be effective in preventing viral transmission.

Risks. Allergic reactions to latex are rare. Use of the female condom or male condoms made of polyurethane avoids such reactions.

Intravaginal devices

The **diaphragm** is a dome of latex rubber or polyurethane inserted in the vagina to cover the cervix. A spermicide containing nonoxynol-9 is applied at the time of insertion and before repeated intercourse. The diaphragm is sized according to the diameter of the circular rim; the 3 sizes in the middle range (65, 70, and 75 mm) will fit most women. The **cervical cap** is a rubber dome that fits tightly over the cervix and is also used with spermicide at the time of insertion. It is much smaller than the diaphragm, with a diameter of 22 to 35 mm. The **vaginal contraceptive sponge** is a one-size-fits-all disposable barrier made of polyurethane containing nonoxynol-9. The theoretic effectiveness rates of intravaginal devices range from 91% to 94% (see Table 27-1).

Mechanism of action. All intravaginal devices provide a mechanical barrier to sperm transport which is augmented by spermicide. See Appendix 9 for a diagram of the method for inserting the diaphragm and vaginal sponge.

Benefits. Intravaginal devices allow avoidance of systemic side effects while achieving fairly high effectiveness rates in motivated users. Nonoxynol-9 has microbicidal properties which reduce the risk of sexually transmitted diseases, including HIV, gonorrhea, and chlamydial infection.

Compared to the diaphragm, the cervical cap has the advantage of providing effective contraception while being left in place for one to two days without insertion of additional spermicide. The vaginal sponge will also remain fully effective for 24 hours of use.

Risks. The diaphragm can increase the risk of urinary tract infections because of urethral compression; this problem can sometimes be avoided by use of the wide-seal diaphragm. Use of the cervical cap has been associated with abnormal Pap test results in approximately 4% of users. Women using the cervical cap should have a Pap smear before fitting and another one 3 months later. Odor, discharge, and partner discomfort are occasional problems. Candida vaginitis is more common in users of the vaginal sponge.

Spermicides

Most vaginal spermicides contain nonoxynol-9, a detergent that immobilizes sperm. It is available as cream, jelly, aerosol foam, a foaming tablet, and film which dissolves into a gel. Because spermicides alone result in failure rates of over 20%, they are not generally recommended as the sole contraceptive method.

THE INTRAUTERINE DEVICE

The intrauterine device (IUD) represents a highly effective means of birth control for a select group of women. In the United States two kinds are available: the Copper T380 (effective up to 10 years) and the Progestasert (effective for one year). Both are small radiopaque plastic T-shaped rods.

Mechanism of action. The IUD prevents fertilization and implantation by several mechanisms, all of which are promptly reversible on removal of the device.

Benefits. The IUD has high effectiveness rates and long-term ease of use, without unwanted metabolic effects.

Risks. The chief complication of IUD use is pelvic infection, which may lead to tubal infertility. The risk appears to be highest within the first few months after insertion. Women at high risk for developing pelvic inflammatory disease (PID), including those with a prior history of PID or sexually transmitted disease, multiple sexual partners, and nulliparous women under age 25, should be discouraged from using the IUD. The IUD is most appropriate for parous women in a stable and mutually monogamous relationship.

A high incidence of ectopic pregnancy has been observed among women who conceive while using an IUD, particularly the progestin-containing IUD. Other problems include an increase in dysmenorrhea and menstrual bleeding.

Management issues. Dysmenorrhea and increased menstrual flow may improve with short-term intermittent use of a nonsteroidal antiinflammatory drug such as ibuprofen. If these problems persist or worsen, an alternative method should be used.

Actinomyces-positive Pap smears are occasionally found in women with IUDs. Although not common, true pelvic actinomycosis is a serious disease. In asymptomatic women, it is reasonable to treat with oral ampicillin for 2 weeks and repeat the Pap smear.

Women using an IUD should be instructed to immediately report any lower abdominal pain, unusual vaginal bleeding, dyspareunia, or vaginal discharge.

NATURAL METHODS

A variety of methods to prevent unwanted pregnancy are in common use, all of which have high failure rates. The **rhythm method** (periodic abstinence) involves avoidance of coitus during the woman's fertile period; the fertile period is estimated from the calendar, basal body temperature, or cervical mucus. Factors that limit this method's effectiveness are individual variations in cycle length, length of survival of sperm, and compliance. **Prolonged breastfeeding** is also unreliable because the resumption of ovulation may occur before the first menstrual period. **Withdrawal** of the penis before ejaculation fails because conception can occur from preejaculatory release of seminal fluid.

STERILIZATION

Sterilization permanently blocks or removes the male or female genital tracts so that fertilization will not occur. From a couple's standpoint, the safest and most effective method of permanently preventing pregnancy is male sterilization (vasectomy).

Permanency should be the main consideration for any individual who contemplates a surgical method of contraception. Reversal of sterilization requires major surgery and is successful in only two-thirds of women and one-third of men.

Vasectomy is an ambulatory surgical procedure to occlude a portion of the vas deferens. It requires local anesthesia and usually takes 15 minutes. Complications include hematomas and sperm leakage leading to granulomas. Semen analysis is required two months later, as it may take up to 20 ejaculations to become sperm-free; two negative ejaculations are considered proof of sterility. Long-term adverse effects of vasectomy have never been established. Recent reports of increased rates of prostate cancer have yet to be confirmed.

Tubal sterilization in the female can be performed by two routes: the vaginal approach through colpotomy or culdoscopy, and the abdominal approach through laparoscopy or minilaparotomy. Laparoscopy is the most commonly used method in the United States. It is usually performed under general endotracheal anesthesia as an ambulatory surgical procedure. The operative risk in a healthy woman is approximately 1 in 10,000. Recent reports of a reduction in risk of ovarian cancer following tubal ligation require confirmation.

BIBLIOGRAPHY

Archer DF: Reversible contraception for the woman over 35 years of age, *Curr Opin Obstet Gynecol* 4:891, 1992.

Baird DT, Glasier AF: Hormonal contraception, *N Engl J Med* 328:1543, 1993.

Chilvers CE, Smith SJ: The effect of patterns of oral contraceptive use on breast cancer risk in young women, The UK National Case Control Study Group, *Br J Cancer* 69:922, 1994.

Mishell DR: Contraception, *N Engl J Med* 320:777, 1989.

Mishell DR, Jr: Contraception, sterilization, and pregnancy termination. In Herbst et al, editors: *Comprehensive Gynecology,* ed 2, St Louis, 1992, Mosby-Year Book.

Osathanondh R: Conception control. In Ryan, Berkowitz, Barbieri, editors: *Kistner's Gynecology,* ed 6, St Louis, 1995, Mosby-Year Book.

Porter JB, Jick H, Walker AM: Mortality among oral contraceptive users, *Obstet Gynecol* 70:29, 1987.

Rushton L, Jones DR: Oral contraceptive use and breast cancer risk: a meta-analysis of variations with age at diagnosis, parity, and total duration of oral contraceptive use, *Br J Obstet Gynaecol* 99:239, 1992.

Thorogood M et al: Is oral contraceptive use still associated with an increased risk of fatal myocardial infarction? Report of a case control study, *Br J Obstet Gynaecol* 98:1245, 1991.

Thomas DB: Oral contraceptives and breast cancer: review of the epidemiologic literature, *Contraception* 43:597, 1991.

Trussel J et al: A guide to interpreting contraceptive efficacy studies, *Obstet Gynecol* 76:558, 1990.

28 Abnormal Vaginal Bleeding

Soheyla D. Gharib

In the course of caring for women, every primary care physician is confronted with questions from patients about alterations in patterns of menstruation. Whether it is irregular and unpredictable bleeding in an adolescent, midcycle bleeding in a mature woman, or spotting in a postmenopausal woman, unexpected changes in vaginal bleeding can be alarming for patients and can pose a diagnostic challenge for their physicians.

In approaching the woman with abnormal bleeding, the physician should pose the following questions:

Is the patient pregnant?

At what stage of the reproductive life cycle is the patient (adolescence, mature cycle, perimenopausal, or postmenopausal)?

Is the bleeding occurring in the setting of an ovulatory cycle?

What is the pattern of abnormal bleeding?

The answers to these qustions will direct the evaluation and determine whether the patient will need referral to a gynecologist.

NORMAL MENSTRUAL CYCLE

Menstruation is a bloody, vaginal discharge that occurs as the result of endometrial shedding after ovulation when fertilization has not occurred. Changes in the interval between menses, the duration of menses, or the amount of menstrual flow can cause women to visit their physicians. In the normal menstrual cycle there is a regularity to the interval of menstrual bleeding, usually between 24 and 35 days (only one sixth of cycles are exactly the lunar 28 days in length). The duration of normal, ovulatory menses is 3 to 7 days, with the average blood loss being 33 ml. More than 80 ml of blood loss is considered excessive. Inquiries about the number of pads or tampons used usually are made to assess the amount of blood loss—use of a pad or tampon per hour suggests unusually vigorous bleeding. Patients' estimates of blood loss, however, correlate poorly with measured blood loss.

The physiology of the menstrual cycle is reviewed in Chapter 29.

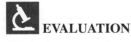 **EVALUATION**

Clinical presentation

History. The history, physical, and pelvic examinations take place in a focused fashion to determine the site of bleeding and its cause (see box at right). The pace of the evaluation is determined by the patient's complaints. The physician should seek to understand whether the bleeding is an annoyance, if it is interfering with the patient's life-style,

or if it is a dramatic change in the patient's baseline that is alarming to her.

The *age* of the patient can point the clinician in the proper direction to reach the appropriate diagnosis. In adolescent patients, acute menorrhagia is attributed usually to anovulation. In patients in their reproductive years, the cause of bleeding often is related to pregnancy. In perimenopausal patients the cause of excessive bleeding most likely is anovulation secondary to ovarian failure. Finally, in postmenopausal women, abnormal bleeding is usually, but not always, secondary to a neoplastic process.

The *timing, duration,* and *amount* of the vaginal bleeding should first be determined. As already noted, the particular pattern of bleeding abnormality may furnish clues about the underlying diagnosis. The interval of bleeding may be abnormal: increased (polymenorrhea), decreased (oligomenorrhea), or irregular (metrorrhagia); the duration may be increased (hypermenorrhea) or decreased (hypomenorrhea); or the amount may be altered—increased (menorrhagia) or decreased (hypomenorrhea) (Table 28-1).

It is important to establish whether the abnormal bleeding is occurring in a patient who usually has menstrual bleeding at regular intervals. If the patient has bleeding at regular intervals (24 to 35 days) with molimina (menstrual cramps, back pain, mood changes), it is likely that she has ovulatory cycles (see box on the following page). If the patient usually has ovulatory cycles and has had an isolated episode of abnormal bleeding, the most important diagnosis to consider is pregnancy. The patient should be asked the date of her last menstrual period, whether she has had unprotected

---

EVALUATION: KEY FACTORS IN THE HISTORY

Age
Timing, duration, and amount of menses
Pattern of abnormal menses
Last menstrual period
Pain associated with the bleeding
Evidence of ovulatory cycling
Past gynecologic surgical procedures
Contraceptive history
Other medical symptoms:
  Symptoms of hypothyroidism
  Symptoms for blood dyscrasias
Medication history:
  Oral contraceptives, Norplant, medroxyprogesterone
    (Depo-Provera)
  Coumadin, aspirin, nonsteroidal antiinflammatory drugs
  Postmenopausal hormonal therapy

Table 28-1 Definitions for the changes in menstrual flow

Parameter	Definition
Interval of bleeding	
Polymenorrhea	Increase in interval of bleeding
Oligomenorrhea	Decrease in interval
Metrorrhagia	Irregularity of interval
Duration of bleeding	
Hypermenorrhea	Increase in the duration of flow
Hypomenorrhea	Decrease in the duration of flow
Amount of bleeding	
Menorrhagia	Increased amount of bleeding
Hypomenorrhea	Decreased amount of bleeding

intercourse, and if the symptoms of pregnancy are present (amenorrhea, breast tenderness, anorexia, or nausea).

The patient's menstrual and gynecologic history, from the time of menarche to the present, should be taken carefully. If the patient has had irregular menses without molimina, a diagnosis of polycystic ovary syndrome is likely. A history of hirsutism makes this diagnosis even more likely. If the patient has always had heavy, prolonged menses, a coagulopathy may be present. Past gynecologic procedures may suggest a preexisting anatomic lesion (cervical carcinoma, fibroids, polyps) that may be causing the present episode of bleeding. Contraception use also can be associated with abnormal bleeding. Oral contraceptives can cause midcycle bleeding, and the most common complaint of patients who use intrauterine devices is prolonged menstrual bleeding.

The presence of *pain* during a bleeding episode can suggest a number of diagnoses. The most important diagnosis to consider is ectopic pregnancy. The classic presentation is vaginal bleeding with unilateral pelvic pain after an episode of amenorrhea, but the diagnosis can elude even the most experienced clinician because of the many variations of presentation (a detailed discussion on ectopic pregnancy appears in Chapter 49). Intermenstrual cramps with or without bleeding can occur in patients with endometrial polyps. Degenerating fibroids, endometritis, persistent corpus luteum, and adenomyosis (endometrial tissue in the myometrium, or endometriosis interna) also can be associated with varying degrees of pain.

The *past medical history* of the patient is important. A history of liver or renal disease may explain abnormal patterns of bleeding. In patients with chronic renal failure who are undergoing hemodialysis, menorrhagia may be observed (see Chapter 20). Hypothyroidism commonly is associated with prolonged, heavy menses. A careful drug history should be obtained because the use of certain medications (oral contraceptive pills, anticoagulants, aspirin, nonsteroidal antiinflammatory agents) commonly cause abnormal bleeding patterns.

Physical examination. A complete physical examination of any patient with abnormal bleeding is essential (see box, below). The patient's *body habitus* should be noted. Patients who are under the tenth percentile in body weight, whether because of anorexia nervosa/bulimia or chronic disease, may have oligomenorrhea because of hypothalamic dysfunction. Obese patients often have irregular, anovulatory bleeding because of increased circulating levels of estrogen as a result of conversion of androgens to estrogen in adipose tissue. The *pattern of hair distribution* should be checked because hirsutism can be associated with polycystic ovary syndrome, a cause of oligomenorrhea. The *skin* should be checked for petechiae and other findings that might suggest an abnormal clotting mechanism. *Breast examination* should include inspection and palpation for milky discharge. A thorough general physical examination should detect any signs of thyroid and liver disease.

A careful examination of the vagina and cervix may identify the source of the bleeding. Vaginal atrophy and cervical lesions (cervicitis, polyps, or carcinoma) can explain postcoital bleeding. Blood coming from the os confirms a higher source of the bleeding (uterus or fallopian tubes). Products of conception may be found in the vaginal vault or in the cervical os. Bimanual examination may identify uterine myomata, ovarian masses, or ectopic pregnancy. A rectal examination may reveal hemorrhoids that have been mistaken by the patient as vaginal bleeding. Rectovaginal examination also can detect nodules suggestive of endometriosis.

Differential diagnosis

One of the important goals in the evaluation of abnormal vaginal bleeding is to determine whether the bleeding is originating from the gynecologic tract. On rare occasions patients may mistake slight bleeding from the rectum or urethra for vaginal bleeding.

The findings of a careful history and physical examination should provide the clinician with adequate data on

---

EVIDENCE OF OVULATORY CYCLING

Regular menstrual intervals (24-35 days)
Moliminal symptoms
  Breast tenderness
  Fluid retention
  Menstrual cramps
  Back pain
  Mood changes
Midcycle cervical mucus
Increase in basal body temperature: 0.2°-0.6°
Luteal phase progesterone >3 ng/ml
Secretory changes on endometrial biopsy

EVALUATION OF ABNORMAL VAGINAL BLEEDING: KEY FACTORS IN THE PHYSICAL EXAMINATION

Body habitus
Hair distribution
Presence or absence of petechiae
Thyroid examination
Presence or absence of galactorrhea
Breast examination
Pelvic examination with speculum and bimanually
Rectovaginal examination

which to form a differential diagnosis and then proceed with an appropriate diagnostic evaluation.

There is a vast list of diagnoses that can cause abnormal vaginal bleeding, but a list is not always helpful in organizing an evaluation. A far more productive way to think about the differential diagnoses is to subdivide this cumbersome list into diagnoses that are likely to affect women at specific points in their reproductive life cycle (pregnancy vs. the nonpregnant state), and if not pregnant, ovulatory cycling and specific pattern of vaginal bleeding (see box, below). A list of differential diagnoses in terms of these parameters appears in Table 28-2. It is important to remember that certain diagnoses, notably trauma and neoplasia, may be the underlying cause of vaginal bleeding in any female patient, whether she is pregnant or not or whether she is premenopausal or postmenopausal.

Pregnancy. In a pregnant patient the two most common times of bleeding are in the first and third trimesters (see box, below right). Usually only patients in the first trimester will seek the care of a primary care physician. The causes of first-trimester bleeding include miscarriage ("missed," incomplete, or complete), ectopic pregnancy, and "implantation bleeding."

The most *important* of these diagnoses for the clinician is **ectopic pregnancy,** which is treatable but life-threatening if missed. The classic presentation of ectopic pregnancy is a history of amenorrhea followed by abnormal vaginal bleeding and unilateral pelvic pain. (For a detailed discussion regarding the diagnosis and management of ectopic pregnancy see Chapter 48.)

The most *common* cause of bleeding in the first trimester of pregnancy is miscarriage. An abortion is called *missed* when products of conception are retained after a fetal death has occurred. The patient's pregnancy test is positive and weeks of amenorrhea are followed by vaginal bleeding. Ultrasound examination may reveal an empty gestational sac or the presence of a fetus without a heartbeat. An incomplete abortion is defined as the expulsion of fetus or the placenta, or both. When the placenta, in whole or in part, is retained in the uterus, bleeding ensues to produce the profuse bleeding of incomplete abortion. A complete abortion is the complete expulsion of the products of gestation.

Implantation bleeding is a general phrase that applies to any bleeding that occurs in the first weeks of pregnancy. Implantation occurs approximately 6 days after conception (day 20 of the woman's menstrual cycle) and sometimes is associated with spotting, which may be mistaken for an early menstrual period. However, bleeding also can occur in the subsequent weeks of a viable, early pregnancy, and the cause of this bleeding is not known. It may be secondary to continued invasion of the trophoblast into the decidua.

**FACTORS AFFECTING ABNORMAL
VAGINAL BLEEDING**

Pregnancy status
Stage of reproductive life cycle
Presence of ovulatory cycling
Pattern of vaginal bleeding

Table 28-2 Differential diagnosis: abnormal vaginal bleeding

Factors	Diagnosis
General	Trauma
	Neoplasia
Specific to reproductive cycle	
Pregnancy	
First trimester	Miscarriage
	Ectopic implantation
Third trimester	Placenta previa
	Placental abruption
	Premature labor
Ovulatory cycles present	Shortened follicular luteal phase
	Anatomic lesion
	Endometrial polyps
	Cervical polyps
	Adenomyosis
	Fibroids
	Systemic disease
	Coagulopathies
	Intrauterine device
	Cervical cancer
	Sarcomas
	Pelvic inflammatory disease
Anovulatory cycles	Immature hypothalamic regulation
	Polycystic ovary syndrome
	Perimenopausal changes
	Endometrial hyperplasia
	Endometrial carcinoma
	Postmenopausal hormone replacement
	Dysfunctional uterine bleeding (no pelvic organ disease or systemic disorder)
	Endometriosis

Abnormal bleeding in early pregnancy is discussed in detail in Chapter 48.

Pregnant patients in the third trimester are less likely to see a primary care physician unless they are unaware that they are pregnant. Causes of third-trimester bleeding

---

**DIFFERENTIAL DIAGNOSIS OF ABNORMAL VAGINAL
BLEEDING IN PREGNANT WOMEN**

First trimester	**Third trimester**
Implantation bleeding	Placenta previa
Abortion	Placenta abruption
Threatened	Premature labor
Complete	Choriocarcinoma
Incomplete	
Missed	
Ectopic pregnancy	
Neoplasia	
Hydatidiform mole	
Cervix	

include placenta previa, placental abruption, and premature labor. Of course, pregnant patients also can have causes of bleeding that are unrelated to the pregnancy, such as neoplasia or trauma.

Ovulatory cycles. If clinical data suggest that a nonpregnant patient ovulates (see box, p. 208), abnormal bleeding should be considered evidence for an anatomic lesion or a systemic illness (liver or renal disease, a thyroid disorder, or a coagulopathy). Anatomic lesions may arise from the vagina (laceration, carcinoma, atrophy), cervix (polyps, carcinoma, or cervicitis), uterus (tumor, endometritis, ovulatory bleeding, myomata, or endometriosis), fallopian tubes (tumor), or the ovary (tumor or persistent corpus luteum). Patients who have ovulatory cycles also may have hormonal derangements that can lead to polymenorrhea (shortened follicular or luteal phases) (see Table 28-2).

Pattern of abnormal bleeding. The pattern of abnormal bleeding can give important clues to the diagnosis, especially in the woman with ovulatory cycles. The history usually reveals that the bleeding has changed in terms of its frequency, duration, or amount, or any combination of these characteristics (Table 28-3).

Polymenorrhea (cycle lengths of 16 to 22 days) can result from the shortening of the follicular or luteal phase. Luteal phase defects can occur in the setting of hypothy-

Table 28-3 Abnormal vaginal bleeding: pattern of bleeding for nonpregnant women

Bleeding pattern	Differential diagnosis
Ovulatory	
Polymenorrhea	Shortening follicular luteal phase
	Pelvic inflammatory disease
	Endometriosus
	Dysfunctional uterine bleeding
Menorrhagia	Endometrial polyps
	Adenomyosis
	Fibroids
	Intrauterine device
	Sarcoma
	Blood dyscrasias
	Systemic lupus erythematosus, hypothyroidism
	Persistent corpus luteum
	Dysfunctional uterine bleeding
Hypomenorrhea	Oral contraceptive pills
	Hyperthyroidism
	Renal failure
Metrorrhagia	Endometritis
	Polyps
	Physiologic
	Oral contraceptive pills
Anovulatory	
Oligomenorrhea	Hypothalamic dysfunction
	Chronic illness
	Stress
	Anorexia
	Polycystic ovary
Delayed menses with polymenorrhagia	Any anovulatory state

roidism or hyperprolactinemia. Decreased menstrual frequency, or **oligomenorrhea**, usually is the result of hypothalamic dysfunction. Stress, anxiety, starvation, chronic illness (such as renal failure), and anorexia nervosa can turn off the gonadotropin-releasing hormone (GnRH) pulse generator, so that the characteristic gonadotropin-pulsatile secretion is disrupted and menses may occur infrequently or cease altogether. Hypothalamic dysfunction also can occur idiopathically. In addition, there are peripheral causes of oligomenorrhea, including polycystic ovary and other hyperandrogenic disorders. Oligomenorrhea can be the result of oligoovulation or infrequent anovulatory bleeding (see Table 28-2).

Alterations in the duration of menses or in the amount of its flow suggest other diagnoses. Increased duration or flow, **menorrhagia,** is seen in blood dyscrasias, hypothyroidism, systemic lupus erythematosus, uterine fibroids, irregular menstrual shedding, and persistence of the corpus luteum. The blood dyscrasias that cause abnormal menstrual bleeding are usually platelet abnormalities and often are detected at menarche. Claessens and Cowell (1981) reported 59 cases of abnormal bleeding in adolescents and noted that 44 (77%) patients were anovulatory and 11 had bleeding disorders. Irregular menstrual shedding is characterized by prolonged menses that result from an unusually long desquamation phase. This diagnosis can be made only by endometrial biopsy or curettage on the fifth or sixth day of bleeding, which can reveal the simultaneous presence of secretory and proliferative endometrium. Persistent corpus luteum is a rare syndrome that can be mistaken for ectopic pregnancy. In both there is unilateral pain, adnexal mass, and abnormal bleeding. In persistent corpus luteum, however, the human chorionic gonadotropin–beta subunit (β-hCG) is negative. The problem is self-limited and may last only a week, but the bleeding is profuse.

Decreased duration or flow of menses (**hypomenorrhea**) occurs most commonly in patients who take oral contraceptive pills. The reduced estrogen content of most preparations causes the endometrium to be thinner than in ovulatory women, and thus there is less to shed. Hypomenorrhea also can be seen in patients with hyperthyroidism, renal failure, or tuberculous endometritis.

Irregular menstrual bleeding, or **metrorrhagia,** is a characteristic of endometritis. It also may be seen in patients with retained products of gestation or with endometrial cancer. Patients who report intermenstrual bleeding, especially postcoital bleeding, should be evaluated for cervical polyps and cervical carcinoma. Midcycle bleeding can be physiologic (bleeding at ovulation) or the result of oral contraceptive use. Usually, midcycle bleeding that occurs in patients who take oral contraceptive pills occurs only in the first three cycles.

Anovulatory cycles. If the patient has a history of anovulation (see box on the following page), her age will be an important factor in determining the likely diagnosis (see Table 28-2).

Adolescent girls and young women often have irregular, anovulatory bleeding as a result of hypothalamic immaturity. As already noted, even 5 years after menarche a substantial number of women (20%) still experience anovulatory menstrual cycles.

SIGNS AND SYMPTOMS OF ANOVULATORY CYCLES

Prolonged bleeding at irregular intervals after several
    months of amenorrhea
No increase in basal body temperature after time of
    ovulation
Luteal phase progesterone <3 ng/ml
Proliferative changes on endometrial biopsy

Anovulatory cycles also can be seen in more mature women, often a result of **polycystic ovary syndrome.** These patients often are amenorrheic or oligomenorrheic, obese, and hirsute and have enlarged ovaries, with elevated levels of ovarian (testosterone, androstanedione) or adrenal androgen (dehydroepiandrosterone). Polycystic ovary syndrome has been associated with a number of disorders, including hyperprolactinemia, hypothalamic dysfunction, and increased androgen production by the adrenal glands. Although the etiology of the syndrome is as yet unclear, it is thought that hyperinsulinism may play a role (see Chapter 12).

In perimenopausal women, cycles become anovulatory as the number and quality of remaining follicles diminish and estrogen production declines in spite of rising levels of follicle-stimulating hormone (FSH). The low levels of estrogen, in the absence of progesterone, produce a persistently secretory endometrium that will periodically shed when estradiol levels decline. Menses may be irregular for a period of months to years. When no viable ovarian follicles remain, menses stop and the woman enters the menopause.

In the postmenopausal woman, all bleeding should be considered secondary to neoplasia until proved otherwise. More benign causes of bleeding in this group of patients include obesity, trauma, and iatrogenic factors. Obese women may have enough circulating estrogen from the aromatization of adrenal androgens by fat cells to cause irregular bleeding from endometrial hyperplasia, which may be a precursor to endometrial carcinoma. The other important cause of vaginal bleeding in this age-group is atrophic vaginitis, which usually results from coital trauma.

Patients who are receiving hormone-replacement therapy may experience irregular bleeding during the initiation of exogenous hormonal therapy. There are two commonly used methods of administering estrogen-replacement therapy. In the first, oral conjugated estrogens, or oral or transdermal estradiol, are taken daily, and a progestational agent is taken for 10 to 12 days of the month (Fig. 28-1). Approximately 3 days after the progestational agent is stopped, withdrawal bleeding ensues. In the second method, estrogen is taken daily with a low daily dose of a progestational agent. With this method of hormonal replacement, there is very irregular, unpredictable bleeding for 3 to 4 months, after which most women become amenorrheic. If irregular bleeding persists after 4 months, a full evaluation to explore anatomic causes of bleeding should be pursued (see Chapter 36).

It is important to remember that patients with anovulatory cycles may still have anatomic causes of abnormal bleeding. Neoplasia and trauma should be considered in every patient with abnormal vaginal bleeding.

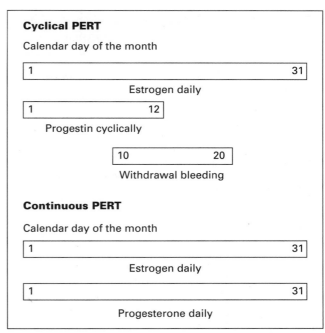

Fig. 28-1 Progestin-estrogen replacement therapy (PERT). From Matzen R and Lang R: *Clinical preventive medicine*, St. Louis 1993, Mosby.

Diagnostic tests

After the differential diagnosis is considered, the following ancillary tests may be necessary to confirm a suspected diagnosis or to make a diagnosis in cases that remain a mystery after the clinical evaluation (see box on the following page).

Determination of pregnancy. The first test that should be performed in all premenopausal patients is a pregnancy test. The urine pregnancy test, which can be completed easily in the office, has the advantage of providing immediate results. The sensitive enzyme-linked immunoassays for urine hCG are 99% accurate in diagnosing intrauterine pregnancy by the time of the first missed period. This test is not quantitative; the result is positive if the serum β-hCG level is greater than 25 mIU/ml. The serum β-hCG assay is more sensitive, detecting levels of β-hCG subunit as low as 5 mIU/ml. Levels below the limit of assay detection are never consistent with pregnancy. The serum assays are extremely sensitive and are capable of detecting "chemical" pregnancies, in which β-hCG is present in the serum but there is no evidence of a pregnancy on ultrasound examination. False-positive results can occur because of the cross-reactivity with luteinizing hormone. The specificity varies among assays and depends on the antibodies used.

Determination of ovulatory status. There are several methods of determining whether the patient is ovulating. First, and least expensive, the physician may ask the patient to fill out **basal body temperature charts.** The patient should record her temperature each morning before getting out of bed. Ovulation thermometers are available at most pharmacies, but digital thermometers also are accurate and are easier for patients to use. The patient makes note of days that bleeding occurred. When graphed against time in days, ovulatory cycles exhibit a biphasic curve, with higher temperatures present in the latter half of the cycle, or after ovu-

KEY DIAGNOSTIC TESTS FOR EVALUATION OF ABNORMAL VAGINAL BLEEDING

To determine pregnancy

Pregnancy test
Urine β-hCG
Serum β-hCG
Ultrasound (if clinically indicated)

To determine ovulation

Basal body temperature charts
Serum progesterone (obtained after ovulation during the luteal phase in cycle)
Endometrial biopsy (to evaluate for cancer or to establish anovulation)

Other tests

Pap smear
Cervical cultures for chlamydia/gonorrhea
Hematocrit value, red blood cell indexes, platelet count, PT/PTT

When clinically indicated

TSH, LFT
FSH (to confirm PCO, ovarian failure, or menopause)
Testosterone, DHEAS, follicular phase 17-hydroxyprogesterone (for suspected hirsuitism)
Prolactin (if galactorrhea)
DST (for suspected Cushing's syndrome)

PT, Prothrombin time; PTT, partial thromboplastin time; TSH, thyroid-stimulating hormone; LFT, liver function test; FSH, follicle-stimulating hormone; PCO, polycystic ovary; DHEAS, dehydroepiandrosterone sulfate; DST, dexamethasone suppression test.

---

lation. If the patient detects a rise in temperature, she can ascertain that ovulation did in fact occur by using a nonprescription **ovulation kit.** These kits use antibodies to luteinizing hormone (LH) to detect secreted LH during the LH surge.

Serum progesterone levels greater than 3 ng/ml also can be used to confirm that ovulation has occurred. In a normal cycle, peak progesterone secretion occurs on day 20, or about a week after ovulation. The blood test for progesterone should be timed so that it takes place after ovulation is thought to have occurred, using information either from the patient's symptoms or from the basal body temperature chart.

The definitive test to prove whether a patient has ovulated is the **endometrial biopsy.** The presence of a secretory endometrium at the start of menses definitively proves that ovulation has occurred. The pathologist dates the secretory endometrium based on the changes seen in a typical 28-day cycle. An endometrium that is reported to be more than 2 days out of phase with the actual cycle day of the biopsy is considered diagnostic of a luteal-phase defect.

Other diagnostic tests. Other laboratory tests that may be of value include the hematocrit value, red blood cell indexes, platelet count, prothrombin time (PT) and partial thromboplastin time (PTT), cervical cultures for chlamydia and gonorrhea, and a Pap smear. When indicated by the history or physical examination, liver function tests, thyroid function tests, and levels of progesteron, LH, FSH, estradiol, progesterone, and prolactin may be helpful. If the LH

value is more than twofold greater than that of FSH, the patient may have polycystic ovary syndrome. An FSH concentration that is greater than that of LH can be the earliest sign of ovarian failure.

If the patient is pregnant and is experiencing abnormal bleeding, an ultrasound examination should be performed, which can confirm an intrauterine pregnancy but cannot rule out ectopic pregnancy. Ultrasound findings also can provide information about whether a miscarriage is occurring. If the pregnancy is greater than 6 weeks' gestation, a fetal heartbeat should be detectable if the pregnancy is viable. If there is no heartbeat and the bleeding is occurring at about 6 weeks of gestation, the ultrasound should be repeated in a week to determine if there has been a missed abortion (see Chapter 48).

APPROACH TO THE PATIENT WITH ABNORMAL VAGINAL BLEEDING

Goals of management

The two goals in the management of abnormal uterine bleeding are to control the acute bleeding episode and to prevent recurrent episodes. For the woman with massive vaginal hemorrhaging and hypotension, the first step is to stabilize the patient's condition (see box, below). This includes a focused physical and pelvic examination in addition to establishing an intravenous access, obtaining blood for type and cross match, and completing initial hematologic studies (hematocrit, platelet estimate) and serum pregnancy test. After the cause is established, often suction curettage by a gynecologist will stop the bleeding unless the causative factor is a blood dyscrasia or a carcinoma.

If the bleeding is not severe, the first step is to determine if the patient with abnormal vaginal bleeding is pregnant. This can be accomplished by performing a simple urine test. Sometimes if the vaginal bleeding occurs within 2 to 10 days after a reported missed period, the urine test is negative for pregnancy. In this event, if the physician still suspects pregnancy (especially an ectopic pregnancy), a serum β-hCG level should be obtained. In fact, 1% to 2% of patients with ectopic pregnancies have serum β-hCG levels below 25 mIU/ml, and thus the urine pregnancy test would miss the diagnosis. Therefore, if results of the urine test are negative and the patient is complaining of unilateral abdominal

MANAGEMENT OF ACUTE VAGINAL HEMORRHAGE

Hemodynamic instability

IV access and fluid resuscitation and determine pregnancy
Blood type and crossmatching
Initial hematologic screen
Suction curettage

Hemodynamic stability and no pregnancy

Conjugated equine estrogen 25 mg IV q4h (maximum of 6 doses)
Estradiol/norgestrel oral contraceptive (2 pills of Ovral) 50 μg/0.5 mg pills bid for 3-5 days until bleeding stops; then remaining pills 1/day

pain with bleeding which would heighten the suspicion of ectopic pregnancy, a pelvic ultrasound examination should be performed. In addition, ultrasound examination is appropriate if there is no time to wait for results of the serum pregnancy tests. If the serum β-hCG level is greater than 2000 mIU/ml, ultrasound examination should show a gestational sac in an intrauterine pregnancy. If it does not, the patient will require immediate laparoscopy because the diagnosis of ectopic pregnancy cannot be ruled out (see Chapter 48).

The ultrasound findings are unlikely to be helpful if the serum β-hCG level is less than 2000 mIU/ml, because a gestational sac will not be present even if the pregnancy is intrauterine. In these early cases of pregnancy with bleeding, the stability of the patient's condition will dictate management. The patient whose condition is unstable (severe pain, hypotension, massive bleeding), should undergo laparoscopy on an emergent basis. If the serum β-hCG level is less than 2000 mIU/ml and the patient is clinically stable, she should be observed and the hCG level should be obtained again in 48 hours. If the hCG level fails to double and the patient continues to have bleeding and pain, laparoscopy should be performed.

As mentioned before, other causes of abnormal bleeding in patients with positive pregnancy test results include complete and incomplete abortion and molar pregnancy. In both molar pregnancy and abortion, serum β-hCG levels are higher than expected for a given gestational age. Because bleeding after complete abortion is usually minimal, continued bleeding usually indicates that gestational products have been retained. If bleeding does not resolve within 1 week, these patients should be evaluated by a gynecologist for possible dilation and curettage.

If the patient is not pregnant but is ovulating, she may have a systemic illness, a hormonal disruption of normal physiology, or an organic lesion. As mentioned before, the most common cause of abnormal bleeding in ovulatory patients, after pregnancy, is blood dyscrasia, the most common of which is von Willebrand's disease. Acute bleeding episodes in these patients are managed by administering factor VIII. Abnormal vaginal bleeding that occurs as the result of other systemic illnesses, such as chronic renal failure, systemic lupus erythematosus, liver disease, and thyroid disease, can be expected to improve by treating the underlying disease. When a systemic illness or blood dyscrasia cannot be detected in ovulatory patients, a thorough search for an anatomic lesion should be performed.

Finally, patients can have alterations in the frequency of menses but still have ovulatory cycles. Polymenorrhea that results from shortened follicular phase can occur in adolescence and usually will correct with time. Shortened luteal phases, or inadequate luteal phase, can be treated with natural progesterone suppositories beginning the day after ovulation. When an anatomic lesion is suspected, the patient should be referred to a gynecologist.

Anovulatory bleeding results from chronic unopposed estrogen stimulation of the endometrium. Management and treatment of dysfunctional uterine bleeding are discussed in Chapter 32. Management and treatment of abnormal bleeding associated with polycystic ovary syndrome is discussed in Chapter 28.

SUMMARY

Abnormal uterine bleeding is one of the most common problems that the primary care physician will face. The bleeding can be the result of a normal physiologic state, such as puberty, or it can signal serious, life-threatening illness. A complete understanding of the physiology of the normal menstrual cycle and the differential diagnoses for each phase in a woman's reproductive life will enable the physician to come to a correct diagnosis and appropriately manage the problem.

BIBLIOGRAPHY

Barbieri RL, Smith S, Ryan KJ: The role of hyperinsulinemia in the pathogenesis of ovarian hyperandrogenism, *Fertil Steril* 50:197, 1988.

Bayer SR, DeCherney AH: Clinical manifestations and treatment of dysfunctional uterine bleeding, *JAMA* 269:1823, 1993.

Chan WY, Hill JC: Menstrual prostaglandin levels in nondysmenorrhic and dysmenorrheic subjects, *Prostaglandins* 15:365, 1978.

Claessens EA, Cowell CA: Acute adolescent menorrhagia, *Am J Obstet Gynecol* 139:277, 1981.

Cowan BD, Morrison JC: Management of abnormal genital bleeding in girls and women, *N Engl J Med* 324:1710, 1991.

Emans SJ, Grace E, Goldstein DP: Oligomenorrhea in adolescent girls *J Pediatr* 97:815, 1980.

Fraser IS, McCarron G, Markham R: A preliminary study of factors influencing perception of menstrual blood loss volume, *Am J Obstet Gynecol* 149:788, 1984.

Fraser IS et al: Measured menstrual blood loss in women with menorrhagia associated with pelvic disease of coagulation disorder, *Obstet Gynecol* 68:630, 1986.

Givens JR et al: Dynamics of suppression and recovery of plasma FSH, LH, androstenedione, and testosterone in polycystic ovarian disease using an oral contraceptive, *J Clin Endocrinol Metab* 37:407, 1973.

Hallberg L et al: Menstrual blood loss: a population study, *Acta Obstet Gynecol Scand* 45:320, 1966.

Hamilton JV, Knab DR: Suction curettage: therapeutic effectiveness in dysfunctional uterine bleeding, *Obstet Gynecol* 45:47, 1975.

Keye WR: Dysfunctional uterine bleeding. In Glass R, editor: *Office gynecology,* Baltimore, 1988, Williams & Wilkins.

Long CA, Gast MJ: Menorrhagia, *Obstet Gynecol Clin N Amer* 17:343, 1990.

Matzen R and Lang R: *Clinical preventive medicine,* St. Louis, 1993, Mosby.

Mishell DR et al: Oral contraception for women in their 40s, *J Reprod Med* 35(suppl):447, 1990.

Sherman BM, Korenman SG: Hormonal characteristics of the human menstrual cycle throughout reproductive life, *J Clin Invest* 55:699, 1975.

Wentz AC: Abnormal uterine bleeding. In Jones HW, Wentz AC, Burnett LS, editors: *Novak's testbook of gynecology,* Baltimore, 1988, Williams & Wilkins.

Wilansky DL, Greisman B: Early hypothyroidism in patients with menorrhagia, *Am J Obstet Gynecol* 160:673, 1989.

Winter JSD, Fairman C: The development of cyclic pituitary-gonadal function in adolescent females, *J Clin Endocrinol Metab* 37:714, 1973.

29 Amenorrhea

Janet E. Hall

Normal menstrual cycles occur monthly, with the exception of pregnancy, from their onset in adolescence until the time of menopause, which occurs between the ages of 45 and 55 years. Studies of the duration of the menstrual cycle during the reproductive years in a large cohort of American women indicate that the median menstrual cycle length is 28 days, with a range between 25 and 35 days considered normal. Menstrual-cycle disturbances occur relatively infrequently, with estimates of amenorrhea ranging from 2% to 8% in large studies. However, both the delayed onset of menstrual function and subsequent menstrual-cycle abnormalities represent an important biologic marker of potential disease. A framework for the diagnosis and therapy of these disorders can best be constructed by combining a functional and anatomic approach using gonadotropin measurements to help locate the site of the primary abnormality. Key to this framework is an understanding of the physiology of normal reproductive cycles.

PHYSIOLOGY OF THE NORMAL MENSTRUAL CYCLE

The normal menstrual cycle requires precise integration of hormonal events involving the hypothalamus, pituitary gland, and ovaries, with the uterus acting as an end organ for ovarian steroid effects (Fig. 29-1). The reproductive system functions in a classic endocrine mode with hypothalamic stimulation of the pituitary via the releasing hormone, gonadotropin-releasing hormone (GnRH), which is also known as luteinizing hormone–releasing hormone (LHRH), resulting in pituitary secretion of the gonadotropins, luteinizing hormone (LH) and follicle-stimulating hormone (FSH). LH and FSH, in turn, stimulate ovarian follicular development and hormone secretion. Ovarian secretion of estradiol, progesterone, and probably inhibin restrains the secretion of LH and FSH through actions at both the hypothalamus through control of GnRH secretion and directly at the pituitary level. In addition to these negative feedback controls, the menstrual cycle is uniquely dependent on positive feedback to produce the preovulatory LH surge.

The normal menstrual cycle is generally divided into the follicular or preovulatory phase, which begins on the first day of menses, and the luteal phase, which begins with ovulation (Fig. 29-2). During the early follicular phase, FSH is responsible for recruitment of a cohort of follicles, one of which will achieve dominance and eventually ovulate. The increases in estrogen produced by the emerging follicles inhibit further FSH secretion to ensure that a single egg is ovulated each month. The dramatic rise in estrogen secretion that occurs late in the follicular phase stimulates the LH surge required for ovulation. In addition, estrogen has a proliferative effect on the lining of the uterus, resulting in thickening of the endometrium that can be monitored by ultrasound.

The luteal or postovulatory phase begins immediately after ovulation and is characterized by secretion of progesterone and estrogen by the corpus luteum. These hormones produce the secretory changes of the endometrium that are necessary for implantation. Progesterone is also responsible for the

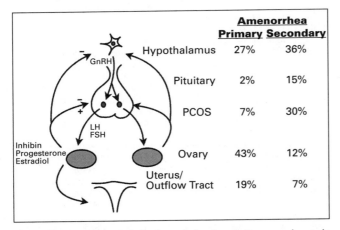

Fig. 29-1 Integration of the hypothalamic-pituitary-ovarian axis with the uterus as an end organ for estradiol and progesterone action. This schema is key to the evaluation of amenorrhea. The prevalence of a given cause of amenorrhea depends on whether amenorrhea is primary or secondary. FSH, follicle-stimulating hormone; LH, luteinizing hormone; GnRH, gonadotropin-releasing hormone; PCOS, polycystic ovary syndrome. (Modified from Hall JE, Crowley WF Jr. In DeGroot LJ, editor: *Endocrinology*, ed 3, Philadelphia, 1994, WB Saunders. Prevalence figures are derived from Reindollar [1981; 1986]).

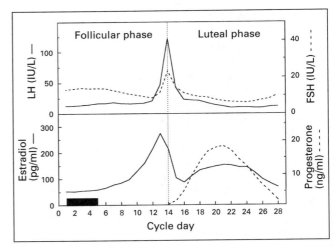

Fig. 29-2 Dynamic changes in mean LH, FSH, estradiol, and progesterone levels throughout the normal menstrual cycle based on daily blood samples in over 100 normal cycles emphasize the importance of anchoring a sample drawn for clinical indications to preceding and subsequent menses. Menses is indicated by the *solid box*. The *dotted line* indicates ovulation, which separates the follicular and luteal phases.

postovulatory rise in basal body temperature that can be used clinically as an indicator of ovulatory cycles. The luteal phase ends with menses, which results from removal of the hormonal support of the endometrium that accompanies the natural regression of the corpus luteum. If a pregnancy has been established, human chorionic gonadotropin (hCG), which is produced by the placenta, can prolong the function of the corpus luteum until placental production of progesterone and estrogen is adequate to sustain the pregnancy.

The length of the luteal phase is fairly constant among women (12 to 16 days) and therefore the major variability in cycle length is in follicular-phase duration. With age, both follicular-phase length and total cycle length decrease somewhat. At both ends of reproductive life, adolescence and perimenopause, there is an increased incidence of anovulatory cycles and erratic bleeding patterns.

DEFINITIONS

Amenorrhea refers to the absence of menses. It is termed *primary* in an adolescent or woman who has never menstruated. Normal menarche (the first menstrual period) occurs relatively late in the series of pubertal milestones that mark the onset of reproductive function. The appearance of pubic hair (adrenarche), breast development (thelarche), and the growth spurt all precede the first menstrual period, which occurs at 12.7 years on average, with the ages between 11 and 15 years constituting the 95% confidence limits. Amenorrhea is termed *secondary* in a woman who previously has had at least one episode of menstrual bleeding. *Oligomenorrhea* refers to infrequent or irregular menstrual bleeding, with cycle lengths generally in excess of 35 to 40 days.

DIFFERENTIAL DIAGNOSIS

When the physician is faced with a disorder of normal menstrual function, it is useful to employ a diagnostic evaluation that segregates the causes of menstrual dysfunction into uterine or outflow tract disorders versus ovulatory disorders and then to consider the expected gonadotropin profile to determine the cause of the ovulatory disorders (see Fig. 29-1 and Table 29-1). The distinction between primary and secondary amenorrhea is an important one because primary amenorrhea encompasses a more extensive differential diagnosis that includes congenital and genetic abnormalities. In addition, the relative frequency of presentation of disorders at each level of consideration is influenced by whether amenorrhea is primary or secondary (see Fig. 29-1). However, it is also important to remember that most processes commonly thought of in association with secondary amenorrhea also can produce primary amenorrhea. Oligomenorrhea is a manifestation of disordered ovulation; therefore the pathophysiologic considerations in the following discussion are the same for oligomenorrhea as for secondary amenorrhea.

Uterine or outflow tract disorders

Abnormalities at the level of the uterus or outflow tract account for a small but extremely important proportion of all patients with menstrual cycle disorders and are particularly important in the diagnosis of primary amenorrhea (see Fig. 29-1). Most patients with anatomic causes of primary amenorrhea have **müllerian agenesis** (congenital absence of the vagina and/or uterus), also known as Mayer-Rokitansky-Küster-Hauser syndrome. Less commonly, patients manifest other müllerian anomalies such as a transvaginal septum or an imperforate hymen, although they have otherwise normal pubertal developmental and normal levels of sex steroids and gonadotropins. Depending on the level of the anatomic obstruction, they may have cyclic abdominal pain and distention from blood within the obstructed uterus (hematocolpos).

Some of these patients are difficult to distinguish from the much smaller proportion of patients with primary amenorrhea who have androgen resistance, an X-linked dominant syndrome also known as **androgen resistance syndrome** or testicular feminization. These patients are genotypic males with one of a number of defects in the androgen receptor that leads to its inability to respond to testosterone. As such, there is failure to develop normal male external genitalia, a testosterone-dependent process, and thus normal female external genitalia develop. However, because the testes of these persons produce müllerian-inhibiting substance (MIS), the müllerian system regresses and they do not have a uterus or the proximal two-thirds of the vagina. Therefore the clinical presentation is primary amenorrhea in the presence of minimal body hair, good breast development, an absent uterus and a blind vagina. FSH levels are normal, but levels of LH, estradiol, and testosterone are elevated and a karyotype confirms the diagnosis. Because of the potential for malignant change, gonadectomy is recommended in these patients.

In patients with a history of uterine instrumentation, particularly in the setting of infection or pregnancy, amenorrhea, scant menstrual flow, or subsequent miscarriage, hysterosalpingography or hysteroscopy should be employed to search for uterine synechiae or scarring. These patients have normal levels of all reproductive hormones. This constellation of findings, known as **Asherman's syndrome,** accounts for approximately 7% of all cases of secondary amenorrhea.

Ovulatory disorders

A much larger proportion of patients with menstrual-cycle abnormalities includes those with ovulatory disorders. Measurement of gonadotropin levels is key to the further subdivision of these patients into those with ovarian failure (hypergonadotropic), abnormalities of the hypothalamus or pituitary (hypogonadotropic), or polycystic ovary syndrome (elevated LH to FSH ratio).

Hypergonadotropic disorders: ovarian failure. Females begin life at birth with approximately 2 million primary oocytes. However, as a result of a natural process of atresia, only 400,000 oocytes remain at the time of puberty, and despite ovulation of only 400 oocytes during the period of normal reproductive capability, ovarian failure occurs between the ages of 45 and 55 years. Factors that can advance the time of ovarian failure may be genetic (decreased initial complement of germ cells or accelerated atresia) or acquired (destruction of oocytes). An elevation of FSH greater than 2 SD above the normal follicular-phase range in a patient with amenorrhea and low levels of estrogen is virtually pathognomonic of ovarian failure. Levels of LH may be elevated, but FSH is a more sensitive marker of ovarian failure than is LH because of its greater sensitivity

Table 29-1 Differential diagnosis of amenorrhea

Site of abnormal function	Disorder	Primary or secondary amenorrhea	Gonadotropin levels	Estradiol levels	Clinical findings	Confirmatory tests
Uterus or outflow tract	Müllerian anomalies or agenesis	Primary	LH, FSH normal	Normal	May have cyclic pelvic pain	
	Testicular feminization	Primary	LH increased, FSH normal	Increased	Minimal body hair, good breast development, blind vagina	Elevated testosterone karyotype
	Uterine synechiae (Asherman's syndrome)	Secondary	LH, FSH normal	Normal	History of instrumentation or infection	Hysteroscopy or hysterosalpingogram
Ovary	Turner's syndrome (or mosaic)	Primary; sometimes secondary in mosaic form	FSH increased	Decreased	Short stature, webbed neck, shield chest, cardiac abnormalities and hypothyroidism (mosaics may be atypical)	Karyotype
	Premature ovarian failure	Secondary	FSH increased	Decreased	May have history of autoimmune disorder	
	Resistant ovary syndrome	Primary	FSH increased	Decreased		
Pituitary gland	Prolactinoma	Secondary	FSH, LH decreased or normal	Decreased	May have galactorrhea	Prolactin, cranial imaging
	Other tumors	Secondary	FSH, LH decreased or normal	Decreased	Signs of Cushing's syndrome or acromegaly	Urine free cortisol, growth hormone, cranial imaging
	Pituitary infarction	Secondary	FSH, LH decreased or normal	Decreased	Usually occurs postpartum	
Hypothalamus	Hypothalamic amenorrhea	Primary or secondary	FSH, LH decreased or normal	Decreased	Sometimes associated with stress, exercise, weight loss, chronic illness	
	Pituitary tumors	Primary or secondary	FSH, LH decreased or normal	Decreased	May manifest headache, visual symptoms	Cranial imaging
	Traumatic: head injury or irradiation	Secondary	FSH, LH decreased or normal	Decreased	History of head trauma or cranial irradiation	
Other	Polycystic ovarian syndrome	Secondary	Increased LH:FSH ratio	Decreased or normal	Signs of androgen excess	Testosterone, dehydroepiandrosterone sulfate, ultrasound

LH, luteinizing hormone; FSH, follicle-stimulating hormone.

to estrogen negative feedback. FSH also is more sensitive to the negative feedback effects of inhibin. Although the physiology of inhibin is still being elucidated, it is likely that a deficiency of inhibin plays a role in the selective rise in FSH with ovarian failure. Patients may have primary or secondary amenorrhea. In the latter case the clinical history often reveals the finding of hot flashes that cause nighttime

wakening. It is important to bear in mind that the course of ovarian failure may be one of waxing and waning, with reciprocal changes in estradiol and FSH levels occurring over several years.

Primary amenorrhea rarely can be associated with **ovarian agenesis,** but the most common cause of primary amenorrhea and the most common genetic cause of ovarian failure is **Turner's syndrome** (45 XO), in which primary amenorrhea is associated with the characteristic somatic features of short stature, webbed neck, shield chest, cubitus valgus, and multiple nevi, as well as cardiac and renal malformations and a predisposition to hypothyroidism. In these patients the ovarian failure results from a process of rapid atresia both in utero and after birth, and studies have documented a normal complement of germ cells early in gestation, suggesting that the second X chromosome is vital to the protection of the germ cells from accelerated atresia. Although patients with Turner's syndrome generally are of short stature and have primary amenorrhea, they may be of normal height or have secondary amenorrhea, or both. Many of these exceptions to the typical presentation of Turner's syndrome have been documented to be mosaics. Because some patients may have an XO/XY mosaic pattern, with a high potential for development of malignant changes in the gonad, it is important to obtain a karyotype on all patients with ovarian failure who are younger than 30 years old.

Premature ovarian failure is defined as menopause before the age of 40 years. It may result from accelerated atresia as in the aforementioned Turner's mosaic pattern and in women with an XX/XXX mosaic pattern. On the other hand, follicular destruction is the mechanism behind the ovarian failure associated with chemotherapy (particularly with the use of alkylating agents), radiation therapy, viral factors such as mumps oophoritis, and galactosemia. Autoimmune mechanisms are likely to be involved in a large subset of patients with premature ovarian failure. Premature ovarian failure has been associated with a number of autoimmune disorders, including the polyglandular failure syndromes in which autoimmune destruction is responsible for failure of a number of endocrine organs, for example, the adrenal gland, the pancreas, the parathyroid glands, and the thyroid. Other autoimmune associations include pernicious anemia, rheumatoid arthritis, systemic lupus, myasthenia gravis, vitiligo and premature gray hair.

It is likely that autoimmune mechanisms are also responsible for some of the reported cases of **resistant ovary syndrome** in which amenorrhea and elevated FSH levels occur in the presence of a large complement of ovarian follicles. Evidence exists for the presence of both antibodies to the ovarian FSH receptor and substances that compete for binding of FSH to its receptor. In addition, this syndrome could result from defects in the FSH receptor or defects in the FSH molecule as has been reported for LH. In both cases the presentation would be of primary amenorrhea.

Hypogonadotropic disorders. In patients with hypogonadotropic hypogonadism, the absence of cyclic gonadal function may be associated with gonadotropin levels, which often are normal or only slightly decreased in comparison with those of normal women in the follicular phase. Patients may have either primary or secondary amenorrhea. Although this clinical presentation is most commonly seen with a functional hypothalamic defect, it also may be a clue to a specific neuroanatomic lesion of the hypothalamus or pituitary.

Pituitary causes. Approximately 20% of cases of amenorrhea result from defects at the pituitary level with most of these being **prolactinomas**. Amenorrhea is often the earliest symptom of a prolactin-secreting microadenoma, and up to one third may manifest with galactorrhea. Other patients have infertility associated with a luteal-phase deficiency. The gonadotropin profile of these patients is identical to patients with hypothalamic amenorrhea; however, the prolactin level will be consistently elevated. Although the anatomic defect is clearly at the level of the pituitary in these patients, the cause of gonadotropin deficiency is not the inability of the pituitary to secrete gonadotropins but rather the increase in dopamine turnover as a result of increased prolactin secretion that, in turn, inhibits GnRH secretion. Cranial imaging is important to determine whether the prolactin-secreting tumor is a microadenoma or a macroadenoma and to rule out the rare occurrence of a large pituitary mass in which relatively mild degrees of hyperprolactinemia may result from stalk compression and interference with the normal inhibitory control of prolactin secretion by dopamine. Hyperprolactinemia is discussed in detail in Chapter 10.

Other **pituitary tumors** such as those secreting growth hormone, adrenocorticotropic hormone (ACTH), or gonadotropin subunits or those considered nonfunctional are rare causes of hypogonadotropic hypogonadism and generally are associated with other clinical or biochemical features that help to localize the site of the defect to the pituitary. **Pituitary infarction** has been associated with postpartum hemorrhage (Sheehan's syndrome) and occasionally occurs spontaneously in the perimenopausal age-groups. The degree of hypopituitarism in such patients is highly variable, as is the potential for recovery. **Lymphocytic hypophysitis,** an inflammatory infiltrate of the pituitary of unknown etiology, also has been reported in association with isolated gonadotropin deficiency, again primarily in the postpartum period. **Pituitary irradiation** and extensive **pituitary surgery** are uncommon causes of amenorrhea.

Hypothalamic causes. The most common group of patients in whom low levels of gonadotropins accompany low levels of estrogen is that in whom a structural neuroanatomic lesion cannot be found. The diagnosis given to such patients is **hypothalamic amenorrhea.** In some situations an antecedent cause can be found, but in most of such patients the pathophysiology is not understood. Studies in which the patterns of pulsatile secretion of LH have been compared with those of normal women matched for sex steroid levels have revealed an underlying spectrum of defects of pulsatile GnRH levels (Fig. 29-3). The most severe form of this GnRH abnormality is characterized by a complete lack of pulsatile secretion of GnRH, which manifests by extremely low levels of LH but FSH levels that are often within the normal range. This pattern is seen in patients with primary amenorrhea, often in the presence of anosmia (Kallmann's syndrome), in whom the defect in GnRH secretion is congenital and also in patients with anorexia nervosa. In fact, amenorrhea is part of the *Diagnostic and Statistical Manual of Mental Disorders* (DSM)–III criteria for the diagnosis of anorexia nervosa, and this disorder often is associated with the most profound suppression of gonadotropin and estrogen levels. Other endocrine abnormalities associated with anorexia nervosa include hypersecretion and decreased metabolism of cortisol, decreased adrenal androgen secretion, partial diabetes insipidus that is usually asymptomatic, elevated growth hormone levels with very low levels of somatomedin C, and thyroid function abnormalities compatible with the euthy-

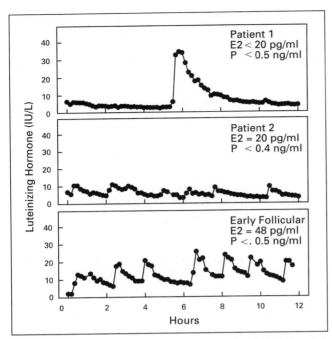

Fig. 29-3 Three representative patterns of pulsatile LH secretion in women with hypothalamic amenorrhea compared with the pattern seen in normal women in the early follicular phase (*lower panel*) emphasizing the range of values that are compatible with this diagnosis on single samples. (Modified from Crowley WF et al: *Rec Prog Horm Res* 41:473, 1985.)

roid sick syndrome. Of importance is that both the resumption of a normal weight and the amelioration of psychologic and behavioral traits are required for resumption of normal menses in these patients.

Other abnormalities of pulsatile GnRH secretion in patients with a hypothalamic cause of their menstrual cycle disturbance include patterns of low amplitude, slow frequency, and nighttime augmentation (Fig. 29-3), all of which are inadequate to sustain orderly folliculogenesis and ovulation. Patients in whom amenorrhea is clinically associated with exercise, weight loss, stress, and acute or chronic intercurrent illness (including other endocrine disorders such as hypothyroidism and hyperthyroidism, Cushing's syndrome, and diabetes) attest to the clinical consequences of environmental factors on control of hypothalamic coordination of the reproductive axis. The recent recognition of both the frequency of bulimia in young women of reproductive age and its association with a similar spectrum of hypogonadotropic menstrual cycle disorders indicates that this is a diagnosis that must be specifically excluded in women with amenorrhea. The recognition of this spectrum of defects in GnRH and therefore LH secretion is particularly relevant to the clinical picture inasmuch as it explains the variation in gonadotropin and estrogen levels encountered during random diagnostic testing in an individual patient, as well as the varying responses to different therapies that have been observed clinically.

In a small subset of patients, structural lesions of the hypothalamus interfere with the normal pattern of GnRH secretion and stimulation of gonadotropin secretion, result-

ing in hypogonadotropic amenorrhea. In most of such patients, a careful history provides specific clues that suggest a neuroanatomic lesion. **Craniopharyngiomas** are the most common of these abnormalities and usually occur with growth retardation, visual impairment, or headache. Other midline **central nervous system** (CNS) **tumors** such as germinomas, gliomas, meningiomas, and endodermal sinus tumors, as well as rare metastatic tumors, dermoid cysts, or teratomas, are found rarely and often are associated with headache and visual symptoms. **Histiocytosis X** and **infiltrative disorders** such as sarcoidosis and tuberculosis generally manifest with diabetes insipidus. **Head injuries** are a rare cause of hypogonadotropic hypogonadism, but **cranial irradiation** for CNS and head and neck tumors frequently is associated with abnormalities in gonadotropin secretion but normal pituitary responsiveness. The hypothalamus generally is more radiosensitive than is the pituitary, and therefore many of these patients have intact pituitary responsiveness to the hypothalamic-releasing factors.

Increased LH to FSH ratio. An increased ratio of LH/FSH typically is seen in patients with polycystic ovary syndrome (PCOS). The clinical presentation usually is oligomenorrhea, with its onset around the time of puberty in association with clinical or biochemical evidence of hyperandrogenism. However, patients may have amenorrhea or dysfunctional bleeding, and infertility is common. The diagnosis is made on clinical grounds (oligomenorrhea/amenorrhea plus signs of androgen excess), assuming that other causes of hyperandrogenism have been ruled out. Differentiation of patients with PCOS from those with hypothalamic amenorrhea is important because the management issues may be somewhat different. PCOS also is discussed in Chapter 9.

EVALUATION

The patient with primary amenorrhea should be evaluated if neither menarche nor breast development has occurred by age 14 years or in the absence of menarche by age 16 years, even in the presence of normal breast development. In addition, the girl with primary amenorrhea should be evaluated if menarche has not occurred within 3 years of the onset of breast development or if she also is under the third percentile for height by age 14 years.

Once menses have been established, it is not uncommon for normal women to skip an occasional menstrual period. Even this should prompt the clinician to rule out pregnancy in the patient who is sexually active, but a more thorough evaluation of amenorrhea should be reserved for those who have had 3 to 6 months of irregular or absent menses.

History and physical examination

A careful and directed clinical history can provide many clues to the underlying cause of the patient's menstrual cycle disorder (see box on the following page). Specific questions should focus on the developmental history, previous menstrual history, and elicitation of relevant localizing symptoms. From a developmental perspective, the pattern of growth and pubertal development is key, as well as parental height and a family history of pubertal delay, anosmia, or

HISTORY AND PHYSICAL EXAMINATION

History

Developmental history

Growth, pubertal development

Previous menstrual history

Last menstrual period
Sexual activity, use of contraception
Age, weight at menarche
Characteristics of previous cycles (regularity, duration, molimina)

Other events or illnesses

Stress, weight changes, anorectic behavior, medications, pregnancy, instrumentation)

Exercise patterns
Other symptoms

Androgenic symptoms (acne, oily skin, hirsutism)
Nausea, breast tenderness, weight gain
Galactorrhea or visual symptoms
Significant weight loss or gain
Hot flashes

Physical examination

General

Height, weight
Stigmata of Turner's syndrome

Skin

Axillary and pubic hair development
Acne, hirsutism, oiliness, acanthosis nigricans
Signs of weight loss, lanugo hair, carotenemia
Stigmata of Cushing's syndrome

Visual fields
Breasts

Breast development
Galactorrhea

Pelvic examination

Presence of normal external and internal genitalia
Vaginal atrophy
Ovarian and uterine enlargement

---

androgen-resistance syndromes. Menstrual history should include the age and weight at menarche, the characteristics of early and most recent cycles—including regularity and duration of menstrual interval and menstrual flow—the presence or absence of symptoms associated with ovulation (breast tenderness, mood changes, food cravings), and the date of the last menstrual period. The manner of onset of amenorrhea and associations with other events such as illness, stress, weight changes, exercise patterns, medications, pregnancy, and uterine instrumentation should be delineated. In addition, it is critical to determine whether the patient is sexually active and to discuss contraceptive practices. Relevant localizing symptoms include hot flashes, anorectic behaviors or attitudes, galactorrhea, headache or visual disturbances, significant weight changes, acne, hirsutism or

oily skin, symptoms of other endocrine dysfunction, systemic illness, and depression.

Physical examination should include height, weight, arm span, secondary sexual characteristics, evaluation for the stigmata of Turner's syndrome already noted, visual field defects, galactorrhea, signs of androgen excess, and clues to the presence of anorexia nervosa (such as lanugo hair or carotenemia). A pelvic examination is performed to determine the presence of normal external and internal genitalia.

Diagnostic tests

The initial evaluation of the amenorrheic patient includes a pregnancy test to rule out the most common cause of amenorrhea in women of reproductive age, an FSH level to rule out ovarian failure, and a prolactin level to help to determine whether further investigation for a neuroanatomic cause of hypogonadotropic hypogonadism is required (see box, below). Administration of medroxyprogesterone acetate (Provera) (10 mg for 5 days) provides an assessment of overall estrogen status. Any amount of bleeding within 10 days of stopping the medication is considered a positive result. Alternatively an estradiol level can be measured, and basal body temperature charting or an appropriately timed progesterone level helps to determine the ovulatory status of the patient.

Further evaluation is based on the history and physical examination findings and may include thyroid function tests, androgen levels, pelvic ultrasound, karyotype, and cranial imaging. Measurement of bone density is suggested only if it will help either the physician or the patient to determine a course of treatment.

Cranial imaging may be performed by use of computed tomography (CT) or magnetic resonance imaging (MRI) with attention to the hypothalamic-pituitary area and should be undertaken in any patient with a persistently elevated prolactin level, even if the elevation is only modest. In addition, cranial imaging should be employed for any patient with hypogonadotropic primary amenorrhea, as already outlined, and in patients with amenorrhea and headache, visual field

DIAGNOSTIC TESTING

First-order tests

Human chorionic gonadotropin–β subunit (β-hCG)
Follicle-stimulating hormone (FSH)
Prolactin

Second-order tests

Luteinizing hormone (LH)
Estradiol or progestin challenge
Progesterone or basal body temperatures

Other tests

Thyroid-stimulating hormone (TSH)
Androgens (dehydroepiandrosterone sulfate [DHEAS], free testosterone)
Pelvic ultrasound
Cranial imaging

defects, neurologic symptoms, diabetes insipidus, or evidence of pituitary hypofunction such as growth abnormalities.

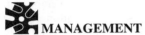

MANAGEMENT

The therapy for amenorrhea depends on both the diagnosis and the goals of the patient, in particular whether pregnancy is desired. In addition, long-term follow-up is important to evaluate the results of therapy if instituted, as well as to respond to the changing concerns of the patient. Although ongoing management of these patients is often complex and is best managed by a specialized endocrinologist or gynecologist, the primary care physician should be aware of the options available to the patients and the general therapeutic issues that are unique to each group of patients.

Uterine or outflow tract disorders

Surgical correction may be possible in some patients with congenital müllerian abnormalities, whereas most patients with Asherman's syndrome will be successfully cured with hysteroscopic lysis of synechiae and administration of estrogen. In patients with androgen-resistance syndromes, removal of the gonads is important because of risk of testicular malignant disease. The timing of removal of the gonads is controversial, with some investigators suggesting that this should be performed as soon as the diagnosis is made (often in conjunction with surgery for bilateral hernias) and others suggesting that there is some advantage in terms of normal breast development if removal is delayed until secondary sexual development is complete. Thereafter, estrogen replacement therapy is required for protection from osteoporosis, vaginal dryness, and possibly cardiovascular disease. Progestin replacement is not indicated in these patients.

Ovulatory disorders

Ovarian failure. In patients with ovarian failure, pregnancy is often not possible other than with the use of ovum donation, the results of which are extremely promising. Hormonal replacement with estrogen and a progestin are required for long-term management of symptoms (hot flashes and vaginal dryness) and for prevention of osteoporosis and possibly cardiovascular disease. Hormone-replacement therapy is discussed in detail in Chapter 36.

Prolactinomas. Bromocriptine, a dopamine agonist, is usually the treatment of choice for patients with a microprolactinoma and generally will restore normal ovulatory cycles. Transsphenoidal surgery and radiation also have been employed but usually are reserved for those patients with larger tumors. In patients who are interested in fertility, the ovulation-induction agents detailed in the next section for use in patients with hypothalamic amenorrhea also are appropriate if the patient is intolerant of bromocriptine or remains infertile or anovulatory despite its use. Management of prolactinomas is discussed in detail in Chapter 10.

Hypothalamic amenorrhea. In the patient with hypothalamic amenorrhea who is not interested in fertility, the major concerns are the long-term consequences of hypoestrogenism. There is ample evidence that many of these women have bone-density measurements that are below the normal range for their age, placing them at increased risk for osteo-

porotic fractures with age, and that even young amenorrheic athletes and ballet dancers have a high incidence of stress fractures. These same women are also at risk for inadequate calcium intake and should receive supplementation to a total intake of 1500 mg of elemental calcium per day, including that from dietary sources.

As a rule, estrogen replacement should be seriously considered in any patient who has been amenorrheic for more than 6 months, and it must be administered in association with a progestin. Oral contraceptives are often the most convenient form of estrogen replacement and also address the issue of contraception for any patient who is sexually active. In the patient who is resistant to consideration of estrogen replacement or in whom estrogen replacement is contraindicated, bone-density measurements may help to ensure that the appropriate decisions are made. Specific interventions and appropriate referral are required for patients with eating disorders.

For those patients who are interested in fertility, life-style changes with weight and exercise modification may be all that are necessary to restore ovulatory cycles. If these interventions are not successful, ovulation induction is generally highly successful. Before proceeding, however, it is necessary to rule out a significant male factor by performing a semen analysis. The simplest form of ovulation induction is oral therapy with clomiphene citrate, an estrogen antagonist. Although clomiphene citrate is often unsuccessful in this group of patients because of their inherently low estrogen level, a limited trial is generally worthwhile inasmuch as this form of therapy has relatively low risk and is convenient for the patient in comparison with other ovulation-induction methods. Pulsatile GnRH is probably the therapy of choice for those who fail to respond to clomiphene citrate; the risk for hyperstimulation and multiple gestation with this form of therapy is relatively low in comparison with exogenous gonadotropins, although both are highly successful methods of inducing ovulation. These forms of ovulation induction generally are managed in specialized endocrine or gynecology practices.

Polycystic ovary syndrome. In all patients with infertility who are overweight, weight loss is likely to be beneficial whether or not they are currently interested in fertility. For the patient with PCOS who is not interested in fertility, the main concerns are endometrial protection, management of androgenic effects, and contraception. The treatment of oligomenorrhea or amenorrhea in women with PCOS is discussed in Chapter 9.

In patients who are interested in fertility, estrogen-antagonist treatment (clomiphene citrate) is the therapy of first choice; it is successful in induction of ovulation in approximately 60% of patients. In patients with increased levels of adrenal androgens (dehydroepiandrosterone sulfate, [DHEAS]), the addition of dexamethasone to clomiphene may be of additional benefit. Exogenous gonadotropins also are highly successful although they present an increased risk of hyperstimulation and multiple gestation. In addition, pulsatile GnRH has been found to be effective in some patients although not all patients ovulate in response to this form of therapy. Overall, women with PCOS have a slightly increased rate of pregnancy loss with all forms of therapy in comparison with other anovulatory patients.

SUMMARY

Deviations from normal patterns of development and maintenance of regular menstrual cycles are important clues to the presence of an underlying pathologic condition. For the primary care physician it is important to have an understanding of what represents normal and when to initiate a diagnostic evaluation in such patients. The evaluation itself can be highly focused if attention is given to the general categories of uterine/outflow tract versus ovulatory disorders and the latter further delineated with consideration of the pattern of the gonadotropins (LH and FSH). Subsequent management depends on the underlying diagnosis. Although the care of many of these patients will be managed in consultation with an endocrinologist or gynecologist, the ongoing nature of many of the abnormalities dictate that the primary care physician remain intimately involved.

BIBLIOGRAPHY

Buttram VC Jr, Gibbons WE: Müllerian anomalies: a proposed classification (an analysis of 144 cases), *Fertil Steril* 32:40, 1979.

Crowley WF et al: The physiology of gonadotropin-releasing hormone (GnRH) secretion in men and women, *Recent Prog Horm Res* 41:473, 1985.

Dunaif A et al: *Current issues in endocrinology and metabolism—polycystic ovary syndrome,* Boston, 1992, Blackwell Scientific Publications.

Frisch RE, McArthur JW: Menstrual cycles: fatness as a determinant of minimum weight for height necessary for their maintenance or onset, *Science* 185:949, 1974.

Hall JE: Polycystic ovarian disease as a neuroendocrine disorder of the female reproductive axis, *Endocrinol Metab Clin North Am* 22:75, 1993.

Kallmann FJ, Schoenfeld WA, Barrora SE: The genetic aspects of primary eunuchoidism, *Am J Ment Defic* 48:203, 1944.

March CM, Israel R, March AD: Hysteroscopic management of intrauterine adhesions, *Am J Obstet Gynecol* 130:653, 1978.

Martin K et al: Management of ovulatory disorders with pulsatile gonadotropin-releasing hormone, *J Clin Endocrinol Metab* 71:1081A, 1990.

Reindollar RH, Byrd JR, McDonough PG: Delayed sexual development: a study of 252 patients, *Am J Obstet Gynecol* 140:371, 1981.

Reindollar RH et al: Adult-onset amenorrhea: a study of 262 patients, *Am J Obstet Gynecol* 155:531, 1986.

Sanborn CF, Martin BJ, Wagner WW: Is athletic amenorrhea specific to runners? *Am J Obstet Gynecol* 143:859, 1982.

Soules MR: Adolescent amenorrhea, *Pediatr Clin North Am* 34:1083, 1987.

Suh BY et al: Hypercortisolism in patients with functional hypothalamic amenorrhea, *J Clin Endocrinol Metab* 66:733, 1988.

Taylor AE et al: Ovarian failure, resistance and activation. In Adashi EY, Leung PCK, editors: *The ovary,* New York, 1993, Raven Press.

Villaneuva AL et al: Increased cortisol production in women runners, *J Clin Endocrinol Metab* 633:133, 1986.

Yen SSC, Jaffe RB: *Reproductive endocrinology,* Philadelphia, 1991, WB Saunders.

30 Benign Breast Disease and Breast Implants

Susan E. Bennett and Barbara L. Smith

Symptoms associated with benign breast disease are alarming to women and their clinicians primarily because breast carcinoma is in the differential diagnosis of all breast complaints. Most breast symptoms are not due to disease at all; rather they represent normal glandular response to fluctuating levels of ovarian hormones. When presented with a breast symptom, the examining clinician's first concern is whether there is a discrete palpable breast abnormality. If there is such an abnormality, further evaluation must be undertaken to exclude breast carcinoma, even if the likelihood of benign breast disease is great.

BREAST LUMPS
Differential diagnosis

Few physical signs evoke as much anxiety in the patient and physician as a palpable breast lump. The differential diagnoses are cyst, adenoma (most are fibroadenomas), abscess, galactocele, and fat necrosis as a result of breast trauma and carcinoma. In a premenopausal woman, a discrete breast lump is likely benign. Three quarters of all breast lumps in women 70 years of age and older are malignant.

The most common causes of benign breast lumps are cysts and fibroadenomas. Breast tissue *must* be stimulated by estrogen and progesterone to form cysts and fibroadeno-

mas. **Fibroadenomas,** solid benign tumors, tend to occur in younger women in the first decade after menarche. Although fibroadenomas can occur after menopause, the incidence is exceedingly low. **Cysts,** fluid-filled structures within glandular tissue, tend to occur in the more mature breast, after 35 years of age, but they are rare after menopause. Although cysts tend to feel fluctuant or soft on palpation, they can feel like solid masses. Fibroadenomas, which tend to have regular borders, to be freely movable, and to feel firm but not hard, can easily be confused with carcinoma. In the absence of signs of infection such as fever, local erythema, heat, and pain, a **breast abcess** can be promptly ruled out. If the patient is not lactating, a **galactocele** can be excluded from the diagnostic possibilities. Both abscess and galactocele must be managed by prompt referral to a breast surgeon. Breast lumps associated with **fat necrosis** usually follow significant trauma that women readily recall, but occult trauma is not uncommon.

Clinicians commonly believe they can predict whether a lump is cystic, benign, or malignant by its tactile characteristics. Surgeons in the Health Insurance Plan Study of screening for breast cancer were asked to document tactile characteristics of lumps before biopsy. Table 30-1 shows that a significant proportion of malignant tumors felt cystic or had otherwise benign characteristics. The Physician Insurers Association of America conducted an analysis of civil litigation as a result of delayed diagnosis of breast cancer and found that most cases involved self-discovered breast lumps in young women. In most cases, physicians were falsely reassured by negative results on mammograms and by their perception that the patients were not at risk because of their young age. Furthermore, the most common reason for delayed diagnosis was that physicians were unimpressed by the physical findings.

Physicians are hesitant to perform invasive testing on every breast lump regardless of the woman's age or risk factors. Experienced and skilled clinicians resist the temptation to practice defensive medicine at the expense of their patients' comfort and peace of mind, but if the existence of a discrete breast lump has been established, malignancy must be excluded. It is difficult to ascertain whether a lump is discrete, especially in young women. Accurate diagnosis of malignancy by physical examination alone is most difficult in younger women whose malignant tumors appear against a background of dense nodular breast tissue. For very young women, and in cases in which the examination results are uncertain, waiting one or two cycles before proceeding to biopsy for diagnosis is reasonable. If uncertainty about the examination remains after subsequent palpations, the patient should be referred to a breast surgeon for further evaluation.

Diagnostic tests

Mammography should always be included in the evaluation of a palpable breast lump but *not* to help the clinician decide whether to biopsy; a mammogram must be obtained to exclude occult, preclinical carcinoma. Exceptions to this rule are the following: pregnant or lactating women and those younger than 30 years of age if breast tissue is too dense for interpretation. A suggestive mammogram result in a patient with a palpable breast lump does not alter the course of management, which is to obtain a biopsy specimen; a negative or equivocal mammogram result cannot be trusted to exclude malignancy. Overall, 10% to 15% of cancers are not visible on mammography, and up to 58% of cancers in women younger than 50 years are not detected by mammography.

Although **ultrasound** examination can differentiate a solid mass from a cystic mass, **fine-needle aspiration** makes

the diagnosis earlier, with less expense, and also treats the cyst by removing the fluid. Most primary care physicians refer patients to surgeons for fine-needle aspiration.

An algorithm for the evaluation of a palpable breast mass is diagrammed in Fig. 30-1. In this algorithm all breast masses must undergo excisional biopsy with the exception of a cyst that disappears after aspiration together with negative results on a follow-up mammogram. Note that for solid masses, biopsy occurs whether results of mammogram or *cytologic* findings on fine-needle aspiration are positive or negative. The false-negative rate of fine-needle aspiration cytology is as high as 35% in some series; thus a negative result cannot justify avoiding biopsy.

Breast specialists sometimes choose to follow discrete lumps without intervention in women who have recurrent breast cysts or fibroadenomas. These patients must become partners in their own health care and must be fully informed about the risks of missing malignancy. All patients should be aware of the rationale behind the approach to breast lump management and should be encouraged to become partners in the decision to biopsy.

FIBROCYSTIC BREAST DISEASE

Does having a breast cyst mean that the patient has fibrocystic breast disease? Approximately 50% of women have palpable breast *lumpiness* characterized by fluctuating fibronodular breast changes. Many of these women believe they have fibrocystic breast disease when their true diagnosis is simply physiologic breast change in response to circulating ovarian hormones or exogenous hormones, such as oral contraceptives. These symptoms typically are intermittent and cyclic and usually are confined to the luteal phase of the menstrual cycle. Fibrocystic breast disease is a diagnosis that should be reserved for women in whom recurrent or multiple cysts form and who have localized, persistent nodular tissue or documented atypical hyperplasia. Benign breast lesions can be classified as nonproliferative, proliferative without atypia, and atypical hyperplasia. Autopsy series document that these lesions can be histologically detected in up to 90% of the female population. Only atypical hyperplasia increases the risk for breast cancer, as shown in Table 30-2. The course of women with atypical hyperplasia and those in whom multiple breast cysts form is best followed up by a breast surgeon.

MASTALGIA

Cyclic breast pain usually is bilateral but may be unilateral, predominantly in the upper outer quadrants, diffuse and dull, and it usually occurs in premenopausal women with a mean age of 33 to 35 years. Mastalgia that occurs after initiation of oral contraceptives or estrogen-replacement therapy usually subsides within the first three cycles.

Some women with mastalgia require biopsy to exclude malignancy if they have a persistent, localized area of nodularity. After malignancy has been excluded by a normal clinical examination and mammogram result, reassurance is the only treatment necessary for most patients. A small proportion of women will seek further treatment after reassurance that breast pain is a benign condition. Women seeking further treatment should keep a record of their symptoms and menses to determine whether their breast pain is cyclic or

Table 30-1 Clinical characteristics of breast lumps specified prior to biopsy* in the Health Insurance Plan Study of screening for breast cancer

Clinical attributes	% of 78 cancers†	% of 324 benign†
Single lump	92	91
Soft or cystic	37	61
Freely movable	63	84
Regular borders	43	68
<2 cm	27	66

Modified from Venet L et al: *Cancer* 28:1546, 1971.
* Includes cases with biopsy recommendation based on both clinical and radiologic findings.
† Biopsy result.

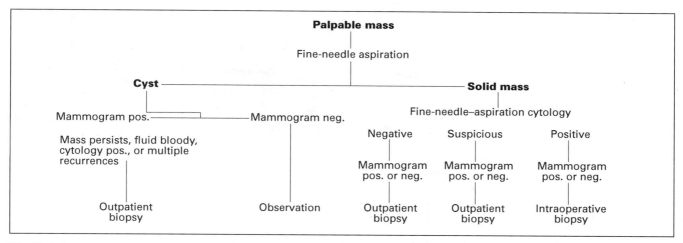

Fig. 30-1 Suggested management of palpable breast masses in women. (From Donegan WL: *N Engl J Med* 327:937, 1992.)

noncyclic. If pain is cyclic, hormonal therapy can be attempted under the care of a breast specialist. Such therapies include danazol, tamoxifen, and bromocriptine.

There is a prevalent notion that elimination of dietary caffeine results in improvement of mastalgia and fibronodular change. This has never been established by a controlled, prospective study. There is some evidence that a low-fat diet (fewer than 15% of calories from fat) can reduce cyclic breast pain.

For women with noncyclic pain, which tends to be a sharp, stabbing unilateral pain occurring in women in their 40s, hormonal manipulation is not usually necessary inasmuch as symptoms abate with menopause. Breast pain occurs rarely with **breast carcinoma,** manifesting as a symptom in only 6% of cases. Ductal obstruction as a result of neoplasm or inflammatory breast carcinoma can cause mastalgia. Inflammatory breast carcinoma also can cause erythema and heat of the skin overlying the malignant tumor; these findings along with breast pain mimic mastitis.

Mastitis is bacterial cellulitis of the breast, usually caused by nipple trauma during lactation and invariably associated with systemic signs and symptoms of infection such as chills, fever, and malaise. Breast pain is almost always present. In the absence of a palpable lump, empiric therapy with antibiotics directed against staphylococci (such as dicloxacillin or cephalexin) should be prescribed, and follow-up is necessary to ensure complete resolution. If a lump is palpable in association with mastitis, prompt surgical evaluation is necessary to rule out breast abscess and inflammatory carcinoma. Intramammary and axillary lymphadenopathy frequently accompany mastitis and can be confused with malignancy. Postpartum mastitis is discussed in detail in Chapter 64.

NIPPLE DISCHARGE

Nipple discharge associated with breast carcinoma is almost always spontaneous, unilateral, and bloody. In approximately 90% of cases, spontaneous bloody discharge is associated with an intraductal papilloma, papillomatosis, fibro-

Table 30-2 Summary of breast cancer risk related to histologic findings in benign breast biopsies

Histologic category	Relative risk*	95% confidence interval	p Value
Nonproliferative			
All patients	0.89	0.62-1.3	0.51
No family history	0.86	0.59-1.3	0.43
Family history†	1.2	0.43-3.1	0.78
Proliferative without atypia			
All patients	1.6	1.3-2.0	0.0001
No family history	1.5	1.2-1.9	0.0002
Family history†	2.1	1.2-3.7	0.0009
Atypical hyperplasia			
All patients	4.4	3.1-6.3	<0.0001
No family history	3.5	2.2-5.5	<0.0001
Family history†	8.9	4.8-17	<0.0001

From Schnitt SJ, Connolly JL. In Harris JR et al, editors: *Breast diseases,* ed 2, Philadelphia, 1991, JB Lippincott; modified from Dupont WD, Page DL: *N Engl J Med* 312:146, 1985.
* As compared with women from Atlanta (Third National Cancer Survey).
† History of breast cancer in a mother, sister, or daughter.

cystic breast disease, duct ectasia, or idiopathic causes. A safe principle to follow is to obtain a mammogram in all cases of unilateral nipple discharge, whether bloody or clear, followed by an appointment with a breast specialist. Patients should be reassured, however, about the likelihood of a benign process.

Bilateral serous nipple discharge can be expressed from the breasts of 50% to 80% of asymptomatic adult females. This physiologic nipple discharge must be differentiated from pathologic causes in a patient who reports nipple discharge. Physiologic discharge typically is nonspontaneous, bilateral, yellow to green, and arises from multiple ducts. Women should be reassured that such discharge is normal and results from nipple stimulation, repetitive nipple squeezing to check for discharge, or exogenous estrogen therapy.

Nonpuerperal lactation is called *galactorrhea* and is a clue to an underlying endocrine disorder. The most common cause of galactorrhea is continued nipple stimulation after weaning; in most cases, women are simply frequently expressing milk to determine whether lactation has ceased, and such nipple stimulation provokes ongoing prolactin secretion through oxytocin release. In patients who have not recently weaned, especially nulliparous women or those reporting *spontaneous* milky discharge, the clinician should order tests to detect a prolactinoma or hypothyroidism—that is, a serum prolactin level and a thyroid-stimulating hormone (TSH) assay. Imaging studies reveal evidence of pituitary adenoma in up to 20% of women with galactorrhea. Certain medications cause galactorrhea, primarily as a result of inhibiting dopamine synthesis and release. Among such pharmacologic agents are the phenothiazines, methyldopa, reserpine, antiemetics, tricyclic antidepressants, opiates, and verapamil. Less common causes include other central nervous system disease, hydatidiform moles, and certain carcinomas that synthesize prolactin or lactogen. Evaluation of galactorrhea is described in Chapter 10.

NIPPLE DERMATITIS

All skin abnormalities of the nipple must be evaluated by a breast specialist who will obtain a biopsy specimen to determine whether the patient has Paget's disease of the breast, a malignant condition resulting from extension of ductal carcinoma into the terminal nipple ducts and easily confused with eczema or nonspecific dermatitis. Figure 30-2 shows the appearance of this dermatologic carcinoma, which usually but not always is unilateral. Erosive nipple lesions are more suggestive of malignancy, but early Paget's disease can be quite subtle. (See also Plate 7 in the front feature section.)

BREAST IMPLANTS

It is estimated that more than 1 million women in the United States have silicone or saline breast implants in place, most of which were placed for cosmetic purposes. A smaller number of women have had implants placed as part of breast reconstruction after mastectomy.

Physical examination

For cosmetic breast augmentation, implants are now usually placed in the subpectoral position, that is, in a pocket created beneath the greater pectoral muscle. In this situation, all

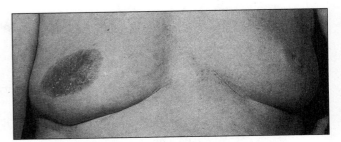

Fig. 30-2 Paget's disease of the breast. (From Skarin AT, editor: *Atlas of diagnostic oncology,* 1992, New York, Gower Medical Publishing.)

native breast tissue is pushed forward and remains accessible to physical examination. Implants also have been placed in the retromammary position, behind native breast tissue but superficial to the greater pectoral muscle. Because more prominent capsule formation and contraction often occur with an implant in this position, this technique is now used infrequently. In addition, inasmuch as the implant is within rather than behind the breast, some areas of breast tissue may be less accessible to physical examination.

When implants are placed as part of breast reconstruction after mastectomy, the implant is placed behind the greater pectoral muscle. In this position, there is little interference with detection of chest wall recurrences, because the tissue where recurrence is most likely to appear is in the superficial position. Implants also may be used in latissimus dorsi muscle flap reconstructions to add bulk for symmetry with the contralateral breast.

Mammography

With either subpectoral or retromammary implant positioning, native breast tissue may be significantly compressed, decreasing mammographic sensitivity. In addition, silicone-filled implants are radiopaque. Even with special techniques using multiple tangential views, it is estimated that a significant proportion of breast tissue is not well seen. Although saline implants are less radiodense, they still significantly obscure adjacent breast tissue on mammographic examination. Despite these limitations, it is still advisable for a woman with implants to undergo screening mammography and physical examination as appropriate for her age.

Complications

Capsule formation. All implants will have dense fibrous capsules form around them in a standard foreign-body reaction. Over time, there is a variable degree of contraction of this capsule, which tends to force the implant into a more hemispheric shape and may result in migration of the implant upward or laterally on the chest wall. In some cases discomfort may be associated with capsule formation and contracture. Severe contracture occurs in only a small fraction of implants placed. On physical examination, the capsule may result in a firm-to-hard breast texture but does not create masses or nodularity. All palpable masses in women with implants must be viewed as suspicious masses and followed up with biopsy.

Implant leak. It is not known with certainty how frequently breast implants leak. So-called gel bleed, the appearance of small silicone droplets outside the implant and within the body's fibrous capsule, is difficult to detect by physical examination or mammography. It is therefore not known how often such gel bleed occurs. In the past some implants were constructed with polyurethane foam coverings to reduce capsule formation. There is a variable degree of breakdown of this covering over time. Again, the extent and significance of this breakdown is not well known. Rupture of the implant's outer membrane with free leakage of silicone into the body's fibrous capsule may be detected by physical examination as a change in the shape of the augmented breast. The use of ultrasound or mammography also can detect the leak. Such gross ruptures require replacement of the implant.

The types and extent of medical problems created by degradation of polyurethane coverings, gel bleed, and gross silicone leakage are not well known. It has been suggested in anecdotes and case reports that these problems may be associated with certain autoimmune or collagen vascular diseases. No large prospective studies exist. This has become a medicolegal issue with a well-publicized jury award to a woman with breast implants and an autoimmune disorder. These events led in January 1992 to the Food and Drug Administration (FDA) placing a moratorium on the placement of silicone implants to allow a review of implant safety. It was not suggested, however, that implants currently in place be removed. This moratorium subsequently was modified to allow implant use for breast reconstruction after mastectomy or for cosmetic purposes in the setting of a scientifically conducted study, with registration of patients and appropriate informed consent.

The scientific and medicolegal issues surrounding silicone breast implants are still under active debate and investigation. In practice, however, medicolegal concerns have made most plastic surgeons unwilling to place silicone implants under any circumstances. Saline-filled implants are now used almost exclusively. These saline implants still use an outer silicone membrane to contain and shape the saline. In the past, saline implants had a significantly higher leak rate than did silicone implants, but this seems to be less frequent with current saline implants.

There continues to be a consensus that silicone implants currently in place need not be removed unless specific medical problems or complications develop.

Infections. Infection of breast implants is relatively uncommon and is estimated to occur in only a small percentage of women. Infections require removal of the implant and antibiotic therapy.

Breast cancer and implants

There is no evidence that either silicone or saline breast implants are carcinogenic or teratogenic. In a study of 3111 women with breast implants in place, no increase in the frequency of breast carcinomas was observed (Deapen et al., 1986). A very small increased risk of sarcomas was observed.

If breast carcinoma develops in a woman with implants in place, it has generally been recommended that she be treated with a mastectomy, with or without reconstruction. There is, however, increasing anecdotal experience of positive results with lumpectomy, axillary dissection, and radiation in these women. It is generally believed that with appropriate perioperative antibiotic coverage, the risk of infection with breast surgery in the presence of implants is only minimally increased. Skin necrosis is rarely a problem after surgery and radiation.

The main complication of radiation therapy in women with breast implants is increased capsule formation and contracture. This may result in increased firmness of the breast and potential migration of the implant. Follow-up for local recurrence after lumpectomy and radiation is made more difficult by the limitations of physical examination and mammography already discussed. These factors must be weighed by the woman and her physician in making a decision about breast cancer management.

BIBLIOGRAPHY

Byron MA, Venning VA, Mowat AG: Post mammoplasty human adjuvant disease, *Br J Rheumatol* 23:227, 1987.
Consensus Meeting: Is "fibrocystic disease" of the breast precancerous? *Arch Pathol Lab Med* 110:171, 1986.
Deapen DM et al: The relationship between breast cancer and augmentation mammoplasty: an epidemiological study, *Plast Reconstr Surg* 77:361, 1986.
Donegan WL: Diagnosis. In Donegan WL, Spratt JS Jr, editors: *Cancer of the breast,* ed 3, Philadelphia, 1988, WB Saunders.
Donegan WL: Evaluation of a palpable breast mass, *N Engl J Med* 327:937, 1992.
Goldsmith M: Image of perfection once the goal—now some women just seek damages, *JAMA* 267:2439, 1992.
Haagensen CD: *Diseases of the breast,* ed 3, Philadelphia, 1986, WB Saunders.
Kleinberg D, Noel G, Frantz A: Galactorrhea: a study of 235 cases, including 48 with pituitary tumors, *N Engl J Med* 296:589, 1977.
Kramer WM, Rush BF: Mammary duct proliferation in the elderly: a histopathologic study, *Cancer* 31:130, 1973.
Layfield LJ, Glasgow BJ, Cramer H: Fine-needle aspiration in the management of breast masses, *Pathol Annu* 24:23, 1989.
Love SM, Gelman RS, Silen W: Fibrocystic "disease" of the breast—a nondisease? *N Engl J Med* 307:1010, 1982.
Martin JE, Moskowitz M, Milbrath JR: Breast cancer missed by mammography, *AJR* 132:737, 1979.
Mclaughlin C, Coe J: A study of nipple discharge in the nonlactating breast, *Ann Surg* 157:810, 1963.
Sartorius O et al: Cytologic evaluation of breast fluid in the detection of breast disease, *J Natl Cancer Inst* 59:1073, 1977.
Smith BL: Fibroadenomas. In Harris JR et al, editors: *Breast diseases,* ed 2, Philadelphia, 1991, JB Lippincott.
Trombly ST: The breast cancer "epidemic," *Forum* 13(3):2-5, 1992.
Venet L et al: Adequacies and inadequacies of breast examinations by physicians in mass screening, *Cancer* 28:1546, 1971.
Weisman MH et al: Connective tissue disease following breast augmentation: a preliminary test of the human adjuvant hypothesis, *Plast Reconstr Surg* 82:626, 1988.
Wilson JD: Endocrine disorders of the breast. In Braunwald E et al, editors: *Harrison's principles of internal medicine,* ed 11, New York, 1987, McGraw-Hill.

31 Benign Vulvar Disorders

Harold Michlewitz

With the control of common gynecologic cancers, the field of gynecology has refocused attention on the vulva. Primary care physicians have assumed greater responsibility for identifying vulvar complaints. This chapter is designed to expand their familiarity with common benign vulvar disorders. Diagnosis and management of vulvovaginitis are discussed in Chapter 42 and herpes genitalis in Chapter 17.

Vulvar disorders can be categorized according to their predominant presenting characteristics (Table 31-1). These include vulvar masses, pruritus, and pain or irritation. A high index of suspicion for preinvasive carcinoma of the vulva is necessary whenever a vulvar complaint is evaluated. The clinical presentation of a preinvasive vulvar lesion may be a reddened or whitish, flattened, or slightly raised patch, often with hyperkeratosis. Biopsy is the only way to establish a diagnosis of benign disease. If any lesion is treated with topical agents without biopsy, it is important that the patient be reevaluated in 3 to 4 weeks and a biopsy performed if signs and symptoms have not remitted.

Table 31-1 Typical presentations of benign vulvar disorders

Predominant symptom	Causes	
	More common	Less common
Mass		
Cystic	Epidermal inclusion cyst	Inguinal hernia
	Bartholin's gland cyst	Pilonidal cyst
	Follicular cyst	Cysts of embryonic origin
		Hidradenoma
		Urethral diverticulum
Solid	Condyloma acuminatum	Seborrheic keratosis
	Acrochordon (skin tag)	Nevi
		Fibromas and lipomas
		Urethral caruncle
		Endometriosis
Pruritus	Infectious vulvitis (*Candida, Trichomonas*)	
	Bacterial vaginosis	
	Squamous hyperplasia	
	Lichen sclerosus	
	Contact dermatitis	
	Human papillomavirus	
Pain	Herpes genitalis	Dysesthetic vulvodynia
	Human papillomavirus	Pudendal neuralgia
	Lichen planus	
	Vulvar vestibulitis	

BENIGN VULVAR MASSES

Epidermal inclusion cyst

The most common subcutaneous vulvar lesion, the epidermal inclusion cyst, is a smooth, yellowish cyst that generally measures 5 to 15 mm in diameter. It usually is nontender and slow-growing. Multiple lesions may occur.

Differential diagnosis. Subcutaneous labial cystic masses must be distinguished from **inguinal hernias.** Rarely a **cyst of Nuck's canal** (a vestigial peritoneal sac passing through the inguinal canal) can manifest as a large, nontender cystic vulvar mass.

Management. Asymptomatic cysts can be managed by observation alone. If significant enlargement takes place under observation, or if the cyst causes discomfort, excision is needed. Aspiration of fluid should be avoided because of the likelihood of inoculating the cyst with bacteria, leading to abscess formation.

Bartholin's gland cysts

Bartholin's gland cysts are common vulvar lesions that arise in the labia minora in the greater vestibular gland, that is, Bartholin's gland. The swelling encountered is in the posterior labia minora and deep to the perineal body. A noninfected cyst usually is compressible and not tender. Secondary bacterial infection may occur in an obstructed Bartholin's gland duct, usually with mixed flora. Infection produces a fluctuant, extremely tender mass at the inferior margin of the labia minora. Swelling may extend superiorly under the labia majora. An abscess that ruptures subcutaneously will track superiorly toward the mons pubis or deep toward the ischiorectal fossa. In severe cases, necrotizing fasciitis may occur.

Differential diagnosis. Rarely, a **cutaneous fistula** from **Crohn's disease** may resemble a Bartholin's duct abscess. In a postmenopausal woman, a mass at the site of Bartholin's gland may arise from a **benign** or **malignant neoplasm.**

Management. Incision and drainage usually are required. This can be performed under no or local anesthesia (ethyl chloride spray or lidocaine [Xylocaine] injection). Maintaining drainage and disruption of septations are essential for satisfactory resolution. Antibiotics are used only if associated cellulitis is present. Chronic or recurrent Bartholin's gland abscess is best treated with marsupialization.

Folliculitis

Subcutaneous masses of the labia majora can represent infections at the base of the hair follicle. These tender lesions may vary from 5 mm up to several centimeters. These lesions or small abscesses may respond to warm compresses or sitz baths inasmuch as they become fluctuant and drain spontaneously. When large, they require incision and drainage.

Condyloma acuminatum

Condyloma acuminatum (an anogenital wart) is a benign growth caused by human papillomavirus (HPV). Spread can occur through sexual contact and, less frequently, through inadvertent touching of the genitals with wart-infested hands or during delivery. Condylomata often proliferate during pregnancy; rarely, significant bleeding or obstruction of the birth canal may require cesarean section. Laryngeal papilloma may be transmitted to the neonate.

An association between vulvar intraepithelial neoplasia and vulvar condylomata has been observed. The malignancy potential of HPV is discussed in detail in Chapter 77.

The moist vulvar environment, concomitant vaginal infections, pregnancy, and an immunocompromised state influence the quantity and location of genital warts. Inspection of the genitals by the naked eye—even careful inspection—may miss numerous condylomata. A magnifying glass or colposcope allows for more comprehensive detection of warts. The warts may be minute or grow to the size of 8 to 10 cm, interfering with the ability to sit or walk.

Management. Local treatment with topical agents such as tricholoroacetic acid (TCA) or podophyllum is the initial therapy for small lesions (less than 2 cm). TCA (50% to 80% solution) is a caustic agent applied directly to the lesions, which typically blanch within a few hours and slough within 2 to 4 days. Temporary intense burning usually occurs, but a local reaction of the surrounding skin is less common than with podophyllum.

Podophyllum (20% solution or 25% ointment) is applied similarly, but it must be washed off after 4 to 6 hours. A 0.5% podofilox cream, applied twice daily by the patient for 3 consecutive days each week, for up to 3 weeks, also has been effective. Topical podophyllum occasionally is associated with a severe local reaction and, rarely, with severe systemic toxicity. Podophyllum should not be used during pregnancy.

Complete healing usually occurs in 1 week. The patient should then be reexamined for persistent or new lesions requiring further applications. Regrowth of lesions may reflect inadequate treatment or resistance. Resistance demands histologic clarification of potential cancer before a long-term plan of local therapy is initiated.

For lesions greater than 2 cm, the patient should be referred for laser treatment or loop electrode excision. Laser treatment of extensive areas of warts is not without complications. Occasional residual perineal pain may be incapacitating and can lead to vulvar vestibulitis (see next section). The presence of micropapillations or areas that blanch with acetic acid application is insufficient cause to initiate laser therapy.

For persistent or recurrent warts, intralesional interferon injection may be effective, with a complete response rate of up to 60%. Intramuscularly administered interferon B from human fibroblasts is a successful and less painful therapy, although not yet available in the United States.

Examination and treatment of the sexual partner are advised to help stop the spread of infection in the general population. However, recurrence rates in women are similar regardless of whether the male partner is examined and treated.

VULVAR DYSTROPHIES

The vulvar dystrophies are nonneoplastic epithelial disorders of the vulvar skin and mucosa. Clinically they often appear as thickened or thinned white vulvar lesions. Biopsy is essential for diagnosis and determination of any malignancy potential.

Squamous hyperplasia

The cause of squamous hyperplastic lesions is unknown. They typically manifest with pruritus. On examination, the appearance is highly variable, ranging from a dusky-red vulva in mild cases to well-defined white patches, often with lichenification, fissures, and excoriations. The histopathologic findings are hyperkeratosis and epithelial thickening.

Lichen sclerosus

Lichen sclerosus (Fig. 31-1) is one of the most prominent of the white vulvar lesions. It usually appears in postmenopausal women, although it can occur at any age. The lesion also can be seen in locations outside the vulva. Although the skin appears atrophic, that appearance belies a truly active epithelium. There is increased cell turnover, epithelial thinning, and subjacent dermal inflammation. An autoimmune mechanism is postulated. (See also Plate 8 of the front feature section.)

Pruritus is a common symptom of lichen sclerosus. The typical lesion is white and initially can occur in an isolated area, evolving to encompass the entire vulva. The skin appears atrophic and glistening, and focal areas may be thickened or eroded. Focal ecchymosis also may be seen. The atrophic appearance is accompanied by progressive loss of the labia majora, labia minora, and fusion of the clitoral hood, which appears as marked introital narrowing (kraurosis).

Biopsy is required for diagnosis. Lichen sclerosus, which is associated with vulvar carcinomas, is present in the epithelium in about 10% of such cancers. The risk of future carcinoma developing in lichen sclerosus is approximately 1% to 5%.

Differential diagnosis. Vulvar lesions appear in a variety of forms; thus their pathologic characteristics cannot be distinguished solely by visual inspection. One must be ready to sample tissue by means of excisional or incisional biopsy to

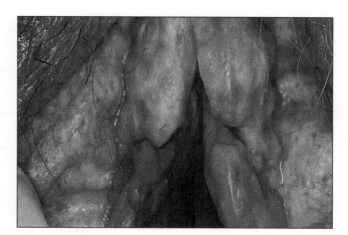

Fig. 31-1 Lichen sclerosus.

make the proper diagnosis. A biopsy specimen should be obtained from any white, ulcerated, nodular, fissured, or abnormal raised pigmented area.

Local anesthesia is achieved with use of lidocaine (Xylocaine) 1% or 2% by injection (with a 27- or 30-gauge needle), ethyl chloride spray, or topical anesthetic ointments. The lesion can be excised with either a scissors or scalpel. A Keyes punch biopsy also allows a core of tissue to be readily retrieved with use of forceps and a scissors to free the base of the tissue core. The biopsy specimen from an area of erosion or ulcer should include adjacent noneroded tissue to help make the diagnosis. Control of bleeding can be achieved with either Monsel's solution (a paste of ferrous subsulfate) or silver nitrate sticks. Larger biopsy sites may require sutures. In general, the wound will heal in 7 to 10 days and will require some local anesthetic application if significant pain is encountered.

The incidence of vulvar carcinoma is low, but this should not discourage biopsy when an undiagnosed lesion is encountered. Early identification of its pathology, even if benign, will allow for proper treatment.

Management. After diagnosis by biopsy, squamous hyperplasia is treated with topical steroids. A regimen of high-potency or medium-potency steroids (such as 0.01% triamcinolone acetonide or 0.025% to 0.01% fluocinolone acetonide), applied twice or three times daily for 4 to 6 weeks, generally is effective.

Mild steroid creams work well in the management of early lichen sclerosus. If the condition worsens or is advanced on presentation, 5% testosterone cream (in a Eucerin base) may alleviate symptoms. The cream is rubbed into the skin twice daily and may require up to a twice-weekly maintenance application. Clitoral hypertrophy may occur, but systemic androgen effects are unlikely. Recently, excellent results in refractory cases have been achieved with superpotent steroids such as clobetasol (Temovate). Short-treatment courses have not been associated with a systemic steroid effect.

Recurrence of lichen sclerosus is common. For this reason, and because of the increased risk for vulvar carcinoma, it is optimal for affected women to be followed up by physicians with a special interest in this condition.

OTHER VULVAR CONDITIONS

This section considers other common vulvar conditions that often are accompanied by pain or irritation.

Lichen planus

Lichen planus affects the mucosal surfaces of the vulva, especially the vestibule (Fig. 31-2). The cause of this condition is unknown. There is thickening of all layers of the epithelium, as well as hyperkeratosis and a subepithelial lymphocytic infiltrate. (See also Plate 9 of the front feature section.)

Clinically, painful erosive areas may be present and adhesions of opposite mucosal surfaces can cause marked stenosis of the introitus and vagina. Bleeding on contact and severe dyspareunia are characteristic of the lesion.

On physical examination, lichen planus appears as a white, raised lesion with a reticular, lacy pattern. The erosive variant has the appearance of a desquamation bordered

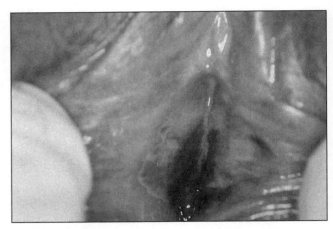

Fig. 31-2 Lichen planus after application of acetic acid.

by reticular white epithelium. The external labia may have the appearance of lichen sclerosus (see previous discussion), but the mucosal changes are quite characteristic. The condition can be associated with changes in other mucosal surfaces such as the vagina and particularly the gingivobuccal mucosa.

Management. High-potency topical steroids may control the condition. To reestablish the vaginal canal in severe cases of scarring, systemic steroids or reconstructive surgery may be required.

Vulvar pain syndromes

Women with vulvar pain syndrome (vulvodynia) experience varying levels of vulvar discomfort manifested as either burning, stinging, pain, dryness, irritation, or rawness. Pruritus is absent. Vulvodynia may have an organic cause, or it can occur with no apparent predisposing condition (dysesthetic or "essential" vulvodynia).

Common organic causes of vulvodynia include contact dermatitis, infection with yeast or trichomonal organisms, HPV, and herpes genitalis. Vulvar vestibulitis (see next section) represents a subset of vulvodynia.

In dysesthetic vulvodynia, constant vulvar burning, not localized to a specific focus, is a typical symptom. There is no pain related solely to touch or introital sexual intercourse. The pain does not radiate as it might in a pudendal neuralgia. It is also distinct from vulvar pain associated with sexual arousal (occlusion of the Bartholin's gland duct must be suspected in this circumstance). The pain pattern is reminiscent of a cutaneous distribution as seen in postherpetic neuralgia.

Treatment with low-dose antidepressants has been fairly effective for this condition, as for other neuropathic pain syndromes. A starting dosage of amitriptyline, 10 mg twice daily, can be increased every 2 to 3 weeks until pain is relieved. In McKay's series of patients with essential vulvodynia, the average dose required was 60 mg daily, and the average length of treatment was 7 months. For pain that is refractory to antidepressants, a computed tomography (CT) scan or magnetic resonance imaging (MRI) to exclude sacral tumors or nerve root cysts is advisable.

Women with essential vulvodynia may have histories of pain that date back decades. The disruption in their lives is significant enough to produce psychologic difficulties that need recognition.

Vulvar vestibulitis

The hallmarks of vulvar vestibulitis are (1) severe pain with touch or attempted vaginal entry, (2) focal areas of tenderness to light touch localized within the vulvar vestibule (the portion of the vulva that extends from the clitoris to the fourchette, visible on separating the labia minora), and (3) physical findings limited to vestibular erythema.

The etiology of vulvar vestibulitis has not been established. Mann's study of the variables associated with this condition found that recurrent candidiasis and previous condyloma acuminatum were more common in women with vulvar vestibulitis than in control subjects. Some investigators have theorized that a candidal or HPV infection may elicit an autoimmune response, leading to local inflammation. The histopathologic examination reveals a chronic inflammatory response without evidence of allergic phenomena or a hypersensitivity reaction.

Symptoms associated with vulvar vestibulitis include superficial dyspareunia, pain with any vulvar pressure, and persistent burning. Occasionally dysuria and frequency are present, and an association with interstitial cystitis has been observed by some investigators.

Patients in many instances have received therapy or have self-treated for "vaginitis" without the establishment of a proper diagnosis. The acute phase of common vaginitides will result in a vulvitis, but with appropriate treatment the condition is limited. Other inciting causes (irritants, topical therapeutic agents) may be identified. Only when symptoms persist for 6 months or more is the patient said to have chronic vulvar vestibulitis.

On physical examination the external vulva appears normal except for erythema of the vestibule. Rarely, shallow ulcers may be seen adjacent to the hymenal ring. The classic finding of vulvar vestibulitis is the elicitation of typical burning pain with gentle pressure from a cotton-tipped applicator on specific foci within the vestibule.

Management. Lack of understanding of the etiology of vulvar vestibulitis has hampered efforts to find effective treatment for this disorder. Most reported studies are case series, and there are few clinical trials. Topical or injectable steroids, estrogen, antibiotics, antifungal agents, and retinoid compounds appear to have no significant effect. Local destruction of tissue with either topical acids, cryotherapy, or laser treatment has had limited, if any, benefit, and concern has arisen that overzealous treatment with these modalities may lead to residual vulvar vestibulitis.

Solomons and colleagues reported an association between excessive urinary oxalate excretion and vulvar vestibulitis. A low-oxalate diet, coupled with calcium citrate tablets (200 mg calcium/950 mg citrate, two tablets three times daily) has been recommended. This regimen, which inhibits calcium oxalate–crystal formation, needs further study but appears to have little potential toxicity.

Recombinant interferon α2b, approved by the Food and Drug Administration (FDA) for treatment of condyloma acuminatum, has been effective for reducing or relieving symptoms in 50% to 80% of patients with vulvar vestibulitis. Recombinant interferon is administered by injection beneath the vulvar mucosa (0.5 mg to a single site, repeated every 2 to 3 days at different locations around the vestibule for a total of approximately 12 injections). Local pain and mild flulike symptoms may occur.

The most successful treatment for vulvar vestibulitis has been surgical excision of the vestibule and hymen, with significant improvement reported in 60% to 80% of women. The healing process can sometimes be slow and require several weeks for complete recovery. Sexual function has been reported to be restored to normal in more than 75% of patients.

Studies of the psychosexual aspects of vulvar vestibulitis suggest that the syndrome may result from an interaction of physiologic and psychologic factors. Psychiatric treatment as the sole modality is not appropriate until full evaluation by a physician knowledgeable in the area of vulvar vestibulitis is completed.

BIBLIOGRAPHY

Kaufman RH, Faro S: *Benign diseases of the vulva and vagina,* ed 4, St Louis, 1994, Mosby.

Krebs HB, Helmkamp BF: Treatment failure of genital condylomata acuminata in women: role of the male sexual partner, *Am J Obstet Gynecol* 165:337, 1991.

Mann MS et al: Vulvar vestibulitis: significant variables and treatment outcome, *Obstet Gynecol* 79:122, 1992.

Marinoff SC, Turner MLC: Vulvar vestibulitis syndrome: an overview, *Am J Obstet Gynecol* 165:1228, 1991.

McKay M: Dysesthetic ("essential") vulvodynia, *J Reprod Med* 38:9, 1993.

Solomons CC, Melmed MH, Heitler SM: Calcium citrate for vulvar vestibulitis, *J Reprod Med* 36:879, 1991.

Von Krogh G, Hellberg D: Self-treatment using a 0.5% podophyllotoxin cream of external genital condylomata acuminata in women, *Sex Transm Dis* 19:170, 1992.

32 Dysfunctional Uterine Bleeding

Raja A. Sayegh and Johnny T. Awwad

Dysfunctional uterine bleeding (DUB) is a diagnosis of exclusion that indicates excessive uterine bleeding in the absence of an organic uterine pathologic condition. The term *DUB* sometimes is used to denote noncyclic, anovulatory bleeding; in this chapter, menorrhagia (heavy menstrual bleeding) and idiopathic intermenstrual bleeding are considered as forms of DUB. The management of idiopathic postmenopausal bleeding also is addressed.

The pathophysiology of DUB is poorly understood, but most cases are believed to result from dyssynchronized sex steroid action on the endometrium. Although chronic anovulation at any age may be associated with DUB, most commonly it is observed at the extremes of reproductive age, perimenarche and perimenopause. Less frequently, DUB can occur in ovulatory cycles and manifest as menorrhagia, midcycle bleeding, or irregular menses.

The parameters of normal menstrual function are shown in the box below. The repetitiveness and constancy of any given set of parameters define normal menstrual function for each woman. Any perceived deviation from the usual interval, duration, or flow pattern often prompts a woman to seek medical attention.

GOALS OF MANAGEMENT

It is essential to rule out endocrinopathies, abnormal pregnancy, and an organic pathologic condition of the uterus and ovaries before making a diagnosis of DUB. Chapter 28 describes the evaluation of abnormal uterine bleeding.

Once a diagnosis of DUB is made, management is guided by consideration of the woman's age and the presence of ovulatory or anovulatory cycles (Table 32-1). The primary management goals are to alleviate excessive bleeding, to correct anemia if it exists, and to monitor response to treatment in order to detect the rare case of occult disease missed on the initial diagnostic evaluation.

ADOLESCENCE

The interval between menarche and the establishment of regular ovulatory cycles is variable and depends on the rate of maturation of the hypothalamic-pituitary-ovarian axis. During this period, acyclic ovarian activity prevails, and unopposed estrogen action on the endometrium may extend over several months. The proliferating endometrium reaches a critical height beyond which it cannot maintain its structural integrity. Fragmented endometrial shedding occurs, causing DUB that at times may be heavy and prolonged.

Choice of therapy

The choice of therapy for DUB in the adolescent is dictated by the severity and frequency of bleeding and the need for contraception. A large proportion of patients have a self-limited course with a few episodes of light to moderate bleeding that can be reliably managed until regular ovarian cycles are established. Others may have frequent, heavy, and painful episodes of bleeding, and iron-deficiency anemia may develop. In this case a regimen of hormonal therapy that prevents prolonged unopposed estrogen action and ensures regular menstrual shedding is used.

The **combination oral contraceptive pill** that contains a progestin along with 30 to 35 μg of ethinyl estradiol generally is the first choice of therapy. This provides predictable 28-day cycles, as well as reliable contraception. There is no evidence that maturation of the hypothalamic-pituitary-ovarian axis is delayed or adversely affected by oral contraceptives.

Another option is to simulate a luteal phase with **oral progestins.** A typical regimen is medroxyprogesterone acetate 10 mg daily, or its equivalent (see box on the following page), for 10 to 13 days. Patients completing the first course of treatment must be cautioned to expect a heavy episode of bleeding as a result of the shedding of a thick endometrial build-up. Nonsteroidal antiinflammatory drugs (NSAIDs) are helpful to control the discomfort that often coexists with such heavy flow. The course of progestins may be repeated in 6 weeks unless spontaneous menses occurs, signaling a remission of anovulation.

The clinician should recognize that concerns about future fertility are common in adolescent women with irregular bleeding. These concerns should be addressed directly, and the transient nature of this condition should be emphasized.

REPRODUCTIVE YEARS
Ovulatory dysfunctional uterine bleeding

It is estimated that 15% of women with DUB are ovulatory. The presence of molimina (breast tenderness, pelvic cramping, fullness, edema) and cycle regularity generally indicate the presence of ovulatory cycles. Basal body temperature charting over a 1- to 2-month period may be used to document ovulation. The postovulatory rise in progesterone causes a sustained elevation in basal body temperature of at least 0.5° C throughout the luteal phase. In equivocal situations, ovulation can be confirmed by measuring serum progesterone; a level greater than 3 ng/ml is indicative of ovulation. Results of an endometrial biopsy that demonstrate secretory changes also indicate ovulation and progesterone production.

Menorrhagia. Menorrhagia in the absence of any anatomic abnormality or systemic illness is considered to be a form of DUB caused by an imbalance between endome-

PARAMETERS OF NORMAL MENSTRUAL FUNCTION	
Cycle interval (days)	21-45
Duration of flow (days)	2-8
Blood loss/cycle (ml)	30-80

Table 32-1 Management of dysfunctional uterine bleeding

Bleeding pattern	Cause	Treatment
Ovulatory DUB		
Heavy menstrual bleeding	Imbalance in endometrial prostacyclins and prostaglandins	Nonsteroidal antiinflammatory drugs Combination oral contraceptive pill Progestin intrauterine device Endometrial ablation
Midcycle spotting	Periovulatory estrogen decline	None
Delayed menses	Persistent corpus luteum	None (rule out pregnancy)
Anovulatory DUB		
Irregular menses	Unopposed estrogen stimulation of endometrium	Combination oral contraceptive pill Cyclic progestins Endometrial ablation
Postmenopausal bleeding	Endometrial atrophy	Hormone replacement therapy Endometrial ablation

DUB, dysfunctional uterine bleeding.

trial prostacyclin and prostaglandin production. Although menstrual blood loss in excess of 80 ml is considered abnormal, there are no practical objective means to assess the severity of menstrual bleeding other than the presence of iron-deficiency anemia. Women's subjective reports of heavy bleeding and patterns of sanitary protection use correlate poorly with measured menstrual blood loss. The passing of blood clots is thought to indicate excessive menstrual bleeding. Another useful clinical criterion for gauging bleeding severity is whether bleeding repeatedly interferes with a woman's important daily activities. Menorrhagia should be treated when it produces iron-deficiency anemia or when it is bothersome to the woman's comfort.

Options for initial treatment of menorrhagia include prostaglandin synthetase inhibitors or the oral contraceptive pill. **Prostaglandin synthetase inhibitors** such as mefenamic acid, naproxen sodium, or ibuprofen may reduce blood loss up to 50%. The usual dose is 1 to 1.5 g daily of any of the aforementioned agents divided in two to three oral doses, started 1 day before the onset of menses. The main side effect of prostaglandin synthetase inhibitors is gastric irritation, which is less likely if medication is taken with food.

Estrogen-progestin combination oral contraceptives generally produce a reduction in menstrual flow and are particularly appropriate for initial treatment when contraception is needed. Another treatment option is a **levonorgestrel-impregnated intrauterine device** (IUD) that delivers the progestin locally and renders the endometrium atrophic, thus effectively reducing menstrual blood loss. The progestin-medicated IUD is an option for women desiring contracep-

tion who are not candidates for the oral contraceptive pill and have no contraindications to the IUD (see Chapter 27).

Iron replacement with ferrous sulfate or gluconate 300 mg two to three times a day should be given when iron-deficiency anemia is present.

Women whose menorrhagia is not controlled by medical therapy should be referred to a gynecologist for further management. Alternatives include **endometrial ablation, gonadotropin-releasing hormone (GnRH) agonists,** or **hysterectomy** (described in the next section).

Persistent corpus luteum. Another cause of DUB in ovulatory cycles is a persistent corpus luteum, or Halban's syndrome. In this instance the life span of the corpus luteum is longer than the usual 10 to 16 days, and menstrual withdrawal bleeding is delayed and unpredictable. The etiology of this condition is unknown, and the important differential diagnosis is pregnancy, which can be ruled out with a serum chorionic gonadotropin (β-hCG) level. The condition often is self-limited, and no treatment is necessary.

Midcycle spotting. Midcycle spotting that occurs in the periovulatory period is attributed to a transient physiologic decline in serum estradiol level after ovulation. Such bleeding may be associated with *mittelschmerz,* or acute midcycle abdominal pain. Midcycle spotting usually is self-limited and requires no intervention.

Anovulatory dysfunctional uterine bleeding

The pathophysiology of anovulatory DUB in the reproductive years is similar to that in the adolescent, namely prolonged, unopposed estrogen action on the endometrium and breakthrough bleeding. Anovulation in the reproductive years (approximately ages 16 to 44 years) may be idiopathic and self-limited, in which case it often is ascribed to central nervous system or hypothalamic dysfunction associated with stress, heavy exercise, or rapid weight changes. Up to 90% of women in the fifth decade of life experience increased variability in their menstrual cycles before the onset of menopause. A dwindling ovarian reserve, abnormal folliculogenesis, and altered hypothalamic feedback result in frequent anovulatory cycles and unopposed estrogen action on the endometrium. The menopausal transition may extend over several years and may be punctuated by episodes of DUB.

EQUIVALENT DAILY DOSES OF ORAL PROGESTINS FOR THE TREATMENT OF DYSFUNCTIONAL UTERINE BLEEDING

Medroxyprogesterone acetate	10 mg
Norethindrone acetate	0.7-1.0 mg
DL-norgestrel	150 μg
Micronized progesterone	300 mg

Idiopathic anovulation. Women with DUB caused by idiopathic anovulation may be treated with cyclic progestins or the combination oral contraceptive pill. The purpose of treatment is to provide predictable flow, to avoid heavy episodes of bleeding, and to prevent the increased risk of endometrial hyperplasia and cancer associated with prolonged unopposed estrogen action. Because spontaneous ovulation and conception can occur during cyclic progestin therapy, oral contraceptives may be preferred when contraception is needed.

In women of reproductive age, the **combination oral contraceptive** (30 to 35 μg of ethinyl estradiol or the equivalent) is appropriate for healthy nonsmoking women without contraindications to oral contraceptive pill use. (Use of the oral contraceptive pill is discussed in detail in Chapter 27.)

In perimenopausal women, **low-dose oral contraceptives** (containing 20 μg of ethinyl estradiol) have several advantages over cyclic progestins, including predictable cycle control, decrease in perimenopausal symptoms (such as mood swings, irritability, decreased libido, and hot flashes), reliable contraception, and, possibly, the prevention of accelerated bone mineral loss that is believed to start in the perimenopausal years. Most women complete the menopausal transition by age 50 to 52 years, at which time it is reasonable to switch to conventional postmenopausal hormone replacement therapy.

Cyclic progestin therapy is an alternative when the low-dose oral contraceptive pill is contraindicated, not tolerated, or not desired. A widely used regimen is oral medroxyprogesterone acetate, 10 mg daily for 10 to 13 days every 6 weeks to 3 months. One general rule is to start with a course of progestins every 8 weeks and to ask the patient to keep a record of the amount of withdrawal bleeding. Heavy bleeding indicates the need to shorten the interval; scant bleeding suggests that the interval may be increased. No bleeding, in the absence of pregnancy, indicates that the perimenopausal transition may have been completed and treatment can be stopped or replacement estrogen added.

Premature ovarian failure and polycystic ovary syndrome. **Oral contraceptives** are the preferred treatment of DUB in premature ovarian failure, in which estrogen deficiency is likely. The oral contraceptive pill (30 to 35 μg ethinyl estradiol or equivalent) is also the optimal choice for treatment in polycystic ovary syndrome because it suppresses ovarian androgen production and helps control the androgenic manifestations of the disorder.

Women with anovulatory DUB who do not respond to hormonal therapy should be further examined for an occult, focal, intrauterine pathologic condition (small submucous myomas, endometrial polyps, or focal endometrial hyperplasia or carcinoma) that could not be identified on initial investigation. Women older than 40 years of age who have already undergone endometrial biopsy before treatment should be referred for hysteroscopic examination or dilation and curettage. Small-caliber fiberoptic hysteroscopes can be introduced transcervically without anesthesia, making this a relatively easy office procedure. The procedure is preferably performed during nonbleeding intervals because visibility may be impaired otherwise. Focal lesions often require the use of operative hysteroscopy for resection and histologic evaluation. Women younger than 40 years of age whose bleeding is not controlled by hormonal therapy should undergo endometrial evaluation by endometrial biopsy, hysteroscopy, or dilation and curettage.

Endometrial ablation is a conservative surgical alternative for the treatment of DUB in women who have completed childbearing. This procedure uses laser or electrocautery under hysteroscopic guidance to destroy the endometrium. Its effectiveness for reducing or abolishing excessive bleeding is 80% to 90%. Bleeding can recur, however, and the long-term risks of the procedure are unknown. Because of the limited data on outcomes of endometrial ablation, its use usually is limited to women who have not responded to or cannot tolerate hormonal therapy or NSAIDs.

GnRH agonists may provide an alternative treatment for women who do not respond to the aforementioned therapies. GnRH agonists, delivered by the intramuscular, subcutaneous, or intranasal routes, produce a profound hypoestrogenic state within a few weeks of initiation. Endometrial atrophy and amenorrhea or oligomenorrhea occur. Use of GnRH agonists for DUB currently is limited by systemic complications of hypoestrogenemia (particularly decreased bone density), which occur after as little as 6 months of use. At present GnRH agonists are used primarily in women whose medical conditions preclude hormonal therapy (e.g., after liver transplantation). Long-term use may become feasible with "add-back" hormone-replacement therapy, which in early studies has appeared to maintain bone density while preventing recurrence of DUB. This treatment is considered investigational. **Hysterectomy** may be necessary for treatment of severe, functionally limiting menorrhagia that is refractory to conservative treatment in women who have completed childbearing.

Management of acute bleeding. Management of DUB that is severe and prolonged requires rapid control of bleeding and hemodynamic resuscitation as needed to restore effective circulation. Women with evidence of severe hypovolemia (orthostatic hypotension or tachycardia) or anemia (hematocrit less than 25%) require hospitalization. Outpatient management is appropriate if the woman has no signs of significant hypovolemia, can take medications orally, and is able to maintain close follow-up.

Initial treatment to control bleeding is either high-dose medroxyprogesterone acetate (30 mg/day in three divided dosages) or intramuscular injection of 150 mg depot medroxyprogesterone acetate. The latter preparation maintains endometrial atrophy for 2 to 3 months, providing adequate contraception and significant relief from anovulatory DUB, but it also can cause DUB through endometrial atrophy.

In some instances, patients who have been bleeding heavily for weeks do not respond to progesterone, possibly because of a denuded endometrial lining. High-dose estrogens can be added if bleeding has not diminished within 24 hours of initiating progestin therapy. A convenient form of adding estrogens is use of an oral contraceptive that contains 35 μg ethinyl estradiol; the dosage is one tablet every 4 to 6 hours given over 2 to 3 days. Although the mechanism of action of bolus estrogen is not very well understood, its effect is thought to be mediated via accelerated proliferation of the endometrial basal layer, which seals the bleeding vessels.

Once the acute bleeding is brought under control, long-term management should aim at restoring depleted iron stores with oral iron replacement and preventing recurrences by use of cyclic progestins or conventional doses of oral contraceptives. Failure to achieve tight cycle control in the ensuing months necessitates further evaluation, for example, endometrial biopsy, office hysteroscopy, or dilation and curettage.

If the acute episode is not controlled within 24 hours of hormonal therapy, hospital admission and surgical dilation and curettage are advisable, both for diagnostic value and immediate therapeutic effects. However, occult pathologic conditions such as polyps and submucous myomas may be missed with blind curettage. The use of continuous flow hysteroscopy provides a panoramic view of the uterine cavity and is an invaluable diagnostic and therapeutic adjunct to curettage when such focal endometrial abnormality is suspected. Hysteroscopically directed resections of endometrial lesions can be safely performed, with low morbidity and good outcome. In certain instances a lesser curettage may be performed on an ambulatory basis with a Karman suction apparatus and the patient under light sedation and with local cervical anesthesia. In extremely rare circumstances, when all conservative medical and surgical efforts have failed and life-saving measures are needed, a hysterectomy may be necessary.

POSTMENOPAUSAL YEARS

Menopause is associated with amenorrhea as a result of cessation of ovarian estrogen production and an inactive, atrophic endometrium. In some postmenopausal women, however, sufficient estrogen is produced from peripheral conversion of ovarian and adrenal androgens to stimulate the endometrial lining and cause resumption of bleeding. An endometrial biopsy that shows evidence of endometrial activity (proliferative endometrium, hyperplasia, or cancer) in postmenopausal women necessitates a thorough search for estrogen- or androgen-producing tumors of the ovary and adrenal gland. In the absence of such a pathologic condition, endometrial activity in postmenopausal women usually is caused by excessive peripheral production of estrogens, commonly observed in obese women who are at increased risk of developing endometrial hyperplasia and cancer. These women can be treated with cyclic progestins as already described.

Postmenopausal uterine bleeding in the absence of any endometrial activity is due mostly to endometrial atrophy, but focal uterine disease may coexist with atrophy and is best ruled out with hysteroscopic examination in the office. Treatment of atrophic DUB is not necessary unless bleeding is bothersome, recurrent, or severe. Treatment options include hormone replacement therapy, hysteroscopic endometrial ablation, or hysterectomy. Bleeding from an atrophic endometrium rarely is severe enough to warrant surgical intervention. However, postmenopausal women with certain chronic medical illnesses (e.g., renal failure and liver disease) may have coexistent coagulopathies that may predispose them to heavy bleeding from an atrophic endometrium. These women are appropriate candidates for endometrial ablation rather than hormonal therapy or hysterectomy.

SUMMARY

DUB is a common disorder of menstrual function that affects women of all age-groups. The diagnosis is one of exclusion, and it is important not to mistake benign and malignant disease for DUB. Hormonal therapy of DUB can be effective in a large proportion of patients and usually consists of cyclic withdrawal with a 10- to 15-day course of progestins or cycle control with oral contraceptives. Surgical treatment in the form of dilation and curettage, or even hysterectomy, may be needed in cases of heavy and nonresponsive bleeding. In selected patients such bleeding can be successfully treated with hysteroscopic procedures such as endometrial ablation and resection of polyps.

BIBLIOGRAPHY

Anderson JK, Rybo G: Levonorgestrel-releasing intrauterine device in treatment of menorrhagia, *Br J Obstet Gynaecol* 97:690, 1990.

Baird DT, Glasier AF: Menstrual bleeding patterns and contraception, *IPPF Med Bull* 254:1, 1991.

Baird DT, Glasier AF: Drug therapy: hormonal contraception, *N Engl J Med* 328:1543, 1993.

Barth JH et al: Spironolactone is an effective and well tolerated systemic antiandrogen therapy for hirsute women, *J Clin Endocrinol Metab* 68:966, 1989.

Berqkvist L et al: The risk of breast cancer after estrogen and estrogen-progestin replacement, *N Engl J Med* 321:293, 1989.

Blumenfeld Z et al: Gonadotropin-releasing hormone analogues for dysfunctional bleeding in women after liver transplantation: a new application, *Fertil Steril* 57:1121, 1992.

Brooks PG, Serden SP: Hysteroscopic findings after unsuccessful dilatation and curettage for abnormal uterine bleeding, *Am J Obstet Gynecol* 158:1354, 1988.

Chamberlain G et al: A comparative study of ethamsylate and mefenemic acid in dysfunctional uterine bleeding, *Br J Obstet Gynaecol* 98:707, 1991.

DeCherney AH et al: Endometrial ablation for intractable uterine bleeding: hysteroscopic resection, *Obstet Gynecol* 70:668, 1987.

DeVore GR, Owens O, Kase N: Use of intravenous Premarin in the treatment of dysfunctional uterine bleeding—a double blind randomized control study, *Obstet Gynecol* 59:285, 1982.

Dickey RP, Stone SC: Drugs that affect the breast and lactation, *Clin Obstet Gynecol* 18:95, 1975.

DiSaia PJ, Creasman WT: *Clinical gynecologic oncology,* ed 4, St Louis, 1993, Mosby.

Early Breast Cancer Trialists Collaborative Group: Systemic treatment of early breast cancer by hormonal, cytotoxic, or immune therapy, *Lancet* 39:1, 1992.

Field CS: Dysfunctional uterine bleeding, *Prim Care* 15:561, 1988.

Fortney JA: Oral contraceptives for older women, *IPPF Med Bull* 243:3, 1990.

Gimpelson RJ: Panoramic hysteroscopy with directed biopsies versus dilatation and curettage for accurate diagnosis, *J Reprod Med* 29:575, 1984.

Hall P et al: Control of menorrhagia by the cyclo-oxygenase inhibitors naproxen sodium and mefenamic acid, *Br J Obstet Gynaecol* 94:554, 1987.

Kleerekoper M et al: Henry Ford Hospital Osteoporosis Research Group: oral contraceptive use may protect against low bone mass, *Arch Intern Med* 151:1971, 1991.

Krettek JE et al: *Chlamydia trachomatis* in patients who used oral contraceptives and had intermenstrual spotting, *Obstet Gynecol* 81:728, 1993.

Lahti E et al: Endometrial changes in postmenopausal breast cancer patients receiving tamoxifen, *Obstet Gynecol* 81:660, 1993.

Leather AT, Sawas M, Studd JW: Endometrial histology and bleeding patterns after eight years of continuous combined estrogen and progestogen therapy in postmenopausal women, *Obstet Gynecol* 78:1008, 1991.

Lindsay R, Tohme J, Kanders B: The effect of oral contraceptives use on vertebral bone mass in pre- and postmenopausal women, *Contraception* 34:333, 1986.

Magos AL et al: Experience with the first 250 endometrial resections for menorrhagia, *Lancet* 337:1074, 1991.

Metcalf MG: Incidence of ovulatory cycles in women approaching the menopause, *J Biosci Sci* 11:39, 1979.

Metcalf MG, Livesey JH: Gonadotropin excretion in fertile women: effect of age and the onset of the menopausal transition, *J Endocrinol* 105:357, 1985.

Mishell DR Jr et al: Oral contraception for women in their 40s, *J Reprod Med* 35 (suppl) :447, 1990.

Moncayo J et al: Ovarian failure and autoimmunity, *J Clin Invest* 84:1857, 1990.

Rapaport E et al: Triglyceride, high density lipoprotein, and coronary heart disease, *JAMA* 269:505, 1993.

Rees M: Menorrhagia, *Br Med J* 294:759, 1987.

Serden SP, Brooks PG: Preoperative therapy in preparation for endometrial ablation, *J Reprod Med* 37:679, 1992.

Session DR, Kelly AC, Jewelewicz R: Current concepts in estrogen replacement therapy in the menopause, *Fertil Steril* 59:277, 1993.

Stadel SV et al: Oral contraceptives and perimenopausal breast cancer in nulliparous women, *Contraception* 38:287, 1988.

Steinberg KK et al: A meta-analysis of the effect of estrogen replacement therapy on the risk of breast cancer, *JAMA* 265:1985, 1991.

Thomas EJ, Okuda KJ, Thomas NM: The combination of a depot gonadotropin releasing hormone agonist and cyclical hormone replacement therapy for dysfunctional uterine bleeding, *Br J Obstet Gynaecol* 98:1155, 1991.

Whitehead MI, Hillard TC, Crook D: The role and use of progestogens, *Obstet Gynecol* 75:59S, 1990.

33 Endometriosis

Keith B. Isaacson

Endometriosis is defined as the presence of endometrial glands and stroma outside the endometrial cavity and uterine musculature. Because it is such a common condition, the primary care clinician must be familiar with the clinical manifestations, spectrum of treatment options, and prognosis of endometriosis; these topics are reviewed here. Chapter 38 discusses the differential diagnosis of pelvic pain, which includes consideration of endometriosis.

 EPIDEMIOLOGY

The prevalence of a disease is defined as the number of known cases at any given time. Because endometriosis is a disease that can be diagnosed only by direct visualization or biopsy, the reported prevalence of the disease is biased by the indication for surgical exploration. The prevalence of endometriosis has been reported to be 1% to 50% depending upon the indication for surgery. Fertile patients undergoing tubal ligation will have the lowest prevalence, and as may be expected, the highest prevalence (nearly 50%) is reported in women with pelvic pain and infertility. In a series from Baylor University, of 858 hysterectomies performed for indications other than those in which endometriosis was suspected, 8.3% had histologically confirmed endometriosis (Wheeler, 1989). However, nearly 40% of women undergoing laparoscopy for infertility have endometriosis.

The median age for the diagnosis of endometriosis is 29 years. Most endometriosis patients are in the reproductive age-group although a small population is postmenopausal. Endometriosis is diagnosed in similar proportions of white, African-American, Israeli, Afghani, Iranian, and Japanese women. Endometriosis crosses all socioeconomic barriers. The early data suggesting that the disease was more prevalent in women of higher socioeconomic status were flawed by not correcting for access to technologically advanced medical care.

CAUSES

The exact histogenesis of endometriosis is unknown. The most accepted theories include transplantation, lymphatic and vascular metastasis, and coelomic metaplasia.

The **transplantation theory,** or Sampson's theory, was proposed in 1927 and suggests that viable endometrial tissue is refluxed through the fallopian tubes at the time of menses and that this endometrial tissue is capable of implanting on surfaces within the peritoneum. This theory is supported by recent data from Halme et al. demonstrating that up to 90% of women have bloody peritoneal fluid at the time of menses and by others who have shown that endometrial cells within the menstrual effluent are capable of glandular formation. The ability of menstrual endometrium to implant has not been clearly demonstrated in the human. The major problem in Sampson's theory is that although more than 90% of women have retrograde menstruation, 90% of menstruating women do not develop endometriosis.

The transplantation theory for endometriosis is supported by the fact that endometriotic lesions often occur in the scars from cesarean sections and episiotomies. In addition, animal models demonstrate that endometrium can be surgically transplanted and that the transplanted material behaves similarly to spontaneous endometriosis. Although it has been proved that endometriosis can arise from surgical transplantation, this does not explain the development of spontaneous endometriosis.

The presence of extrapelvic endometriosis in the lung, brain, and lower extremities supports the theory that endometriosis can spread via hematogenous and lymphatic channels. Experimental demonstration that intravenous injection of homogenized endometrium results in pulmonary endometriosis in the rabbit also supports this concept.

The **coelomic metaplasia theory** proposes that endometriosis arises from metaplasia of totipotential mesothelial cells within the peritoneum. This concept implies that in the presence of certain stimuli—for example, infection, hormones, or menstrual effluent—these cells will differentiate into endometriotic cells. The reports of endometriosis in men often have been used to support this theory; however, all of these men were undergoing estrogen therapy and one cannot rule out that the endometriotic lesions arose from müllerian rests. Conclusive proof that peritoneal epithelium can undergo spontaneous or induced metaplasia is lacking.

In summary, there seems to be little doubt that two factors play a role in the development of endometriosis: retrograde menstruation and genetics. Any obstruction to menstrual outflow such as congenital absence of the cervix increases the likehood of the development of endometriosis. In addition, there has been no valid documentation of the presence of endometriosis before menarche. First-degree female relatives of women with endometriosis have a sevenfold increased risk of developing endometriosis. Most available data suggest a polygenic/multifactorial mode of inheritance; however, a dominant gene of low penetrance cannot be ruled out.

PATHOPHYSIOLOGY

There have been many well-described immune and nonimmune pathologic changes identified in women with endometriosis. These include increased peritoneal fluid volume, increased concentration of peritoneal macrophages, activation of macrophages, and the subsequent release of cytokines into the peritoneal fluid. The question remains as to how the presence of ectopic endometrium can lead to the development of these immunologic changes. One possibility involves an inherent alteration in the macrophages of patients with endometriosis that is responsible for the immunologic changes, as well as the implantation and proliferation of ectopic endometrium. However, women with endometriosis are not susceptible to other immunologically related diseases.

A second theory to explain how the presence of ectopic endometrium may yield the pathophysiologic changes seen in endometriosis hypothesizes that the active endometriotic glands and stroma may synthesize and secrete proteins that create these changes. Endometrial tissue produces prostaglandins and complement component–3 (C3) (Isaacson et al., 1989). This may be an important factor in the pathophysiology of endometriosis because C3, the most abundant protein in the complement system, plays an integral role in the classic and alternate complement cascade. Directly or indirectly, C3 can increase capillary permeability, stimulate fibroblasts leading to the formation of pelvic adhesions, and attract and activate peritoneal macrophages that then deposit monokines into the peritoneal environment.

It is well-known that the amount of endometriosis does not correlate with the degree of symptoms, including pelvic pain, dysmenorrhea, and infertility. Other than mechanical factors from pelvic adhesions that contribute to infertility, there are only limited in vivo data to explain the relationship of the various immunologic changes to symptomatology.

It is estimated that up to 50% of infertile women have endometriosis and that 30% to 50% of women with endometriosis are infertile. There are also data that suggest a lower fecundity rate in women undergoing donor insemination with laparoscopically proved mild endometriosis than in those without endometriosis. Several studies demonstrate, however, that women with mild endometriosis do not have improved fecundity rates with surgical or medical therapy over expectant management alone. Proposed mechanisms for endometriosis-associated infertility include pelvic adhesions and tubal obstruction, anovulation, luteal phase defects, luteinized unruptured follicle syndrome, spontaneous abortion, and embryo toxic effects from prostaglandins and peritoneal macrophages. Of these proposed mechanisms, only the presence of significant pelvic adhesions, which rarely lead to tubal blockage but may alter the tube's ability to capture an oocyte, has been clearly demonstrated to play a major role in endometriosis-related infertility.

Just as primary dysmenorrhea has been linked to elevated prostaglandin production from the myometrium, severe dysmenorrhea in patients with endometriosis may result from local prostaglandin production by the ectopic endometrium. Vernon et al. suggest that endometriotic lesions can be characterized by their prostaglandin production, which may explain why some patients with minimal disease experience intense pelvic pain whereas others with severe disease remain asymptomatic.

CLINICAL PRESENTATION
History and physical examination

The symptoms of endometriosis are varied and often depend on the organs involved (see box, below). The most common symptoms include dysmenorrhea, pelvic pain, dyspareunia, premenstrual spotting, and infertility. This is not surprising inasmuch as endometriotic lesions are found most commonly on the peritoneal surfaces of the cul-de-sac, the uterosacral ligaments, and the ovaries. When the bowel or bladder is deeply involved, cyclic dyschezia or hematuria may be the first presenting complaint. Patients rarely have catamenial hemoptysis, pleuritic chest pain, pneumothorax, incisional masses, footdrop, posthysterectomy vaginal bleeding, irritable bowel symptoms, and bowel obstruction. Endometriosis has been found in 10% to 40% of women with infertility, in up to 65% of women with chronic pelvic pain, and in more than half of women who have undergone laparoscopy for cyclic pain and dysmenorrhea.

Unfortunately, just as there is no specific symptom complex to aid in the diagnosis of endometriosis, there are no specific physical signs of the disease. Many patients with endometriosis have no abnormal findings on physical examination. However, there are certain findings that should create suspicion that endometriosis may be present. These findings include uterosacral and cul-de-sac nodularity and tenderness, adnexal mass or ovarian enlargement, rectoseptal mass, and a retroflexed uterus with limited mobility (see box on following page). Pigmented lesions in any site that

---

SYMPTOMS OF ENDOMETRIOSIS

More common

Dysmenorrhea
Dyspareunia
Infertility
Premenstrual spotting
Pelvic pain

Less common

Cyclic hematochezia or dyschezia
Cyclic hematuria or dysuria
Cyclic hemoptysis or pleuritic chest pain
Constipation, bowel obstruction, or irritable bowel symptoms
Posthysterectomy vaginal bleeding
Incisional masses
Footdrop or sciatic pain

PHYSICAL EXAMINATION FINDINGS

PHYSICAL EXAMINATION FINDINGS

Uterosacral and cul-de-sac nodularity and tenderness
Adnexal mass or ovarian enlargement
Rectovaginal septal mass
Retroflexed uterus with limited mobility

---

either enlarge or become symptomatic at the time of menses also may represent endometriosis.

Diagnostic tests

The diagnosis of endometriosis, unlike most other neoplasms, is made mostly by visual identification of endometriotic lesions at the time of surgery. Although many patients have various signs and symptoms that may raise the clinician's suspicions about the presence of the disease, the diagnosis can be made with certainty only at the time of surgery. Endometriosis is a benign disease and is usually not considered premalignant (although it has been suggested that 5% of ovarian endometrioid cancers may arise from prior endometriotic lesions). Thus, it is not necessary to perform surgery to make the diagnosis of endometriosis unless the patient's symptoms require surgical or medical intervention and therapy.

Endometriotic lesions have classically been characterized as "powder-burn lesions" that did not require histologic confirmation for the diagnosis. Today, however, we understand that many endometriotic lesions have an atypical appearance, including peritoneal implants that are white, red, brown, yellow, or clear and whose configuration may be polypoid, flat, or raised (see box, below). When atypical lesions are seen at surgery a biopsy specimen should be obtained for histologic confirmation of the diagnosis. Other lesions seen at surgery that suggest the presence of endometriosis include peritoneal pockets and adhesions, as well as subovarian adhesions. Because more than 50% of endometriotic lesions are clear or atypical, endometriosis remains an underdiagnosed condition even with the tremendous increase in the use of laparoscopy.

Imaging modalities such as ultrasound, computed tomography (CT), and magnetic resonance imaging (MRI) can provide information about the likelihood of endometriosis but have limited value in the diagnosis of the disease. The main role of ultrasound is defining whether a pelvic mass is cystic, solid, or mixed. Endometriotic cysts are homogeneous; their echogenic pattern is increased, and their

---

VISUAL APPEARANCE OF ENDOMETRIOSIS

Typical lesions

Black "powder-burn" lesions

Atypical lesions

White opacification
Red, brown, yellow, and clear vesicular lesions
Glandular excrescences
Petechial peritoneum
Circular peritoneal defects

---

appearance is similar to corpora lutea, dermoid cysts, or borderline ovarian carcinomas. CT and MRI scanning also detect cystic lesions, as well as fibrous lesions that may be present in the rectosigmoid wall, rectovaginal septum, and retroperitoneal space. Rarely does this additional information justify the added expense of the CT and MRI over a pelvic ultrasound examination.

It would be helpful if a blood test were available to aid in the diagnosis of endometriosis. Three substances currently being investigated include CA-125, placental protein 14 (PP-14), and antiendometrial antibodies. Assays for antiendometrial antibodies and PP-14 are available only in research laboratories and their clinical usefulness has not been determined. The CA-125 assay is commercially available. A great deal of work has been done by Pittaway et al. who have demonstrated that the sensitivity of the serum CA-125 assay ranges from 100% in women with endometriomata greater than 4 cm to 33% in women with dysmenorrhea. CA-125 levels correlate with the stage of endometriosis, and they are most useful when elevated levels are detected preoperatively with stage 3 and stage 4 disease. After medical or surgical therapy or both, the CA-125 levels likely will fall, and serial levels correlate well with the status of the disease.

MANAGEMENT

The treatment for endometriosis can include surgical or medical intervention, a combination of these two therapies, or expectant management. Because endometriosis generally is considered neither a premalignant nor progressive disease, it should be treated only because of symptoms that are not tolerated by the patient. The course of endometriosis is unpredictable. The probability of progression to moderate or severe disease in a woman with early-stage endometriosis, is 25% to 40%. Unfortunately, the inability to predict in which patients the disease will progress makes it imprudent to treat asymptomatic endometriosis for the purpose of preventing or delaying future sequelae. The clinician should not subject a patient to medical or surgical therapy if the patient's only concern is fertility in the distant future.

In developing a treatment plan for endometriosis there are several issues to consider: (1) Is the goal to provide pain relief or enhancement of fertility, or both? (2) Is medical therapy an option that will give equal or better results than surgery? and (3) What is the skill of the operating surgeon? Not many laparoscopists possess the expertise and talent to perform difficult techniques such as extensive adhesiolysis or laparoscopic bowel resections.

CHOICE OF THERAPY FOR PELVIC PAIN
Medical therapy

The rationale for hormonal therapy is supported by the dogma that steroid hormones are the major regulators of growth and function of endometriotic tissue. This theory has been supported by the clinical observation that endometriosis is rare before menarche and equally rare in menopausal and amenorrheic women. An additional supporting rationale for hormonal therapy is the observation that endometriosis improves with physiologic pregnancy and that early and frequent pregnancies seem to protect against the disease.

The current strategy for hormonal therapy for endometriosis is to create an acyclic, hypoestrogenic environment with or without increased serum androgens. Low estrogen levels create atrophy of the endometriotic lesions whereas the acyclic environment minimizes the chance of miniature menstruation within the implants and prevents reseeding via retrograde menstruation. High androgens and synthetic progestins also induce endometrial atrophy and interfere with follicular development, thereby lowering estrogen levels.

The currently available hormonal therapies for endometriosis include pseudopregnancy regimens, danazol, gestrinone, medroxyprogesterone acetate, and gonadotropin-releasing hormone agonists (Table 33-1).

In 1958, Kistner reported a series of 58 patients with endometriosis treated with a continuous **pseudopregnancy regimen,** 70% to 80% of whom experienced pain relief. This regimen produced a pseudodecidualized endometrium that contained inactive glandular epithelia with little potential for growth. Any low-dose oral contraceptive can be used if administered continuously for 15 weeks followed by 1 week of withdrawal. The progestins within the birth control pill have sufficient androgenic and progestational activity to block the activity of the coadministered estrogen that is present to minimize breakthrough uterine bleeding. No data are available to indicate a role for cyclic oral contraceptives in either the management or prevention of endometriosis.

The use of continuous oral contraceptives without a monthly withdrawal period is approximately 80% effective in relieving pelvic pain and dysmenorrhea. This treatment is associated with minimal side effects and can be taken for extended periods of time. It is for these reasons that this regimen is recommended as a first-line therapy in patients with early symptomatic disease who are not attempting conception.

The most common progestin-only therapy for endometriosis is orally administered **medroxyprogesterone acetate** (Provera) 30 mg daily for 3 to 6 months. Medroxyprogesterone acetate (MPA) also can be given intramuscularly in its depot form at a dose of 100 to 300 mg monthly. At this dose MPA will inhibit luteinizing hormone (LH) and follicle-stimulating hormone (FSH) secretion and lead to suppression of follicular activity and the creation of a hypoestrogenic acyclic environment. MPA also may have direct

effects on endometriotic tissue via binding to androgen and progestin receptors. This medication has been found to be 80% to 90% effective in relieving pelvic pain. It is not used more commonly because of the high rate of unacceptable side effects. More than 80% of women experience a 5- to 30-pound weight gain, and a high percentage suffer from breast tenderness, breakthrough bleeding, irritability, and depression.

Danazol was the first medication approved by the U.S. Food and Drug Administration for the treatment of endometriosis. It is the α-third isoxazole derivative of 17-α-ethinyl testosterone. The usual oral dosage is 400 to 800 mg daily in divided doses. Danazol acts on endometriosis via many mechanisms, including pituitary suppression of gonadotropin secretion, binding to steroid receptors in endometriotic implants, inhibition of ovarian and adrenal steroidogenesis, and alterations in steroid-binding proteins. Normally approximately 40% of testosterone is loosely bound to albumin, and 1% is free. In patients taking danazol, 80% of testosterone is bound to albumin and 2% is free as a result of the reduction in testosterone-binding globulin. Although this phenomenon is responsible for the 80% reduction in pelvic pain related to endometriosis, it also is responsible for the common side effects associated with danazol use. Studies have shown that more than 80% of women on a regimen of danazol complain of one or more of the following side effects: weight gain, edema, acne, breast atrophy, oily skin, hot flashes, muscle cramps, libido changes, and fatigue. Danazol also lowers the levels of high-density lipoprotein (HDL) cholesterol and raises those of low-density lipoprotein (LDL) cholesterol. It has no detrimental effect on bone density.

Gestrinone is a 19 nor-testosterone derivative manufactured in France. It was originally developed in the 1970s as a once-a-week contraceptive with an efficacy rate equivalent to established oral contraceptives. Its development was abandoned because of the high costs of phase 2 trials. This medication is similar to danazol in its binding to estrogen receptors, progestin receptors, and androgen receptors, as well as its effect on steroid-binding proteins. It does not, however, block steroidogenic enzymes or prostaglandin

Table 33-1 Hormonal therapy for endometriosis

Treatment	Dosage	Side effects
Pseudopregnancy	Any 21-day low-dose oral contraceptive, continuously, with 1 wk withdrawal every 15 wk	Breakthrough bleeding
Medroxyprogesterone acetate	30 mg qd for 3-6 mo	Weight gain, breast pain, bleeding, mood changes
Danazol	200-400 mg bid	Acne, hirsutism, weight gain, hot flashes, fatigue
Gonadotropin-releasing factor (GnRH) agonists	Leuprolide acetate 1 mg SC qd or depot form 3.75 IM monthly Nafarelin acetate 1 spray bid Goserelin acetate implant every 28 days	Hot flashes, irregular bleeding, headaches, depression, insomnia, vaginal dryness, weight loss

SC, subcutaneous.

synthesis. Gestrinone does not eliminate endometriotic implants but arrests glandular proliferation, thus producing a cellular progesterone withdrawal effect. Gestrinone generally is well tolerated at doses of less than 5 mg (twice weekly) or 2.5 mg (three times weekly); 95% of patients are asymptomatic on a regimen of 5 mg twice weekly, and all are amenorrheic at the completion of 2 months of therapy. Only 5% to 15% of patients discontinue therapy because of unwanted side effects. The most frequent side effects are increased appetite, acne, and vaginal discharge. Lipid profiles are not well-studied.

Gonadotropin-releasing hormone (GnRH) agonist administration is now the treatment of choice if the pain fails to respond to surgery, recurs after surgery, or does not respond to continuous oral contraceptives. The administration of a GnRH agonist produces a paradoxic fall in the pituitary secretion of bioactive LH and FSH, resulting in a hypogonadal state. The serum estradiol concentrations are similar to those seen in women after menopause. Unlike menopause, however, this hypogonadal state is reversible.

Currently, three GnRH agonist formulations have been approved by the FDA for gynecologic conditions; leuprolide acetate (Lupron), nafarelin acetate (Synarel), and goserelin acetate (Zoladex). Lupron may be given by daily subcutaneous injection or in a depot form requiring monthly intramuscular injections. Synarel is administered by nasal spray twice daily, and Zoladex is a 3.6-mg subdermal implant placed within the upper abdominal wall every 28 days.

While taking these medications, 95% of patients will experience hot flashes, 20% to 40% irregular bleeding, and 5% to 15% headache, depression, insomnia, vaginal dryness, weight loss or gain, hair loss, or edema. There have been rare reports of vaginal hemorrhage and allergic reactions. Of patients with pelvic pain from endometriosis 90% to 95% will experience pain relief from GnRH agonist therapy. In 1989 Franssen et al. reported a follow-up study of 42 women 6 months after cessation of GnRH agonist therapy and noted persistent relief of dysmenorrhea and dyspareunia in 58% and 88%, respectively, whereas pelvic pain returned to pretreatment scores in more than 90% of these patients.

Because of the risk of bone loss created by the hypoestrogenic state (which has been reported to be as great as 15% after 6 months of therapy when the lumbar vertebrae are measured by quantitative CT), GnRH agonist therapy can be given only for a 6-month treatment cycle. As already noted, however, the recurrence of pelvic pain is quite high after the discontinuation of therapy, and thus several investigators currently are evaluating the effectiveness of estrogen and progestin "add-back" therapy. The goal of add-back therapy is to titrate the estrogen to a level that provides protection from trabecular bone loss but ensures that the endometriosis will not be stimulated. Friedman and Hornstein recently reported on six patients with laparoscopically documented endometriosis who were treated with depot leuprolide 3.75 mg every 4 weeks for 24 months in addition to equine estrogen sulfate 0.625 mg and medroxyprogesterone 2.5 mg daily during months 3 to 24. These patients' pain remained improved during this course of therapy and for an additional 6 months after therapy. On follow-up laparoscopic examination the severity of endometriosis remained lower than pretreatment levels, and findings on dual x-ray absorptiometry showed no change in the lumbar spine during the 24-month period. Certainly more data are necessary to better evaluate "add-back" therapy.

Surgery

The same goal exists for the relief of pelvic pain as for the treatment of infertility: the destruction or excision of all endometriotic disease. This may be accomplished by excision of endometriotic tissue by means of laparoscopy or laparotomy. In refractory cases, hysterectomy with bilateral salpingo-oophorectomy may be performed to reduce formation of new lesions in women who do not wish to preserve fertility.

As Koninckx et al. have demonstrated, pelvic pain resulting from endometriosis is correlated with the amount of deeply penetrating disease. Consequently, the treatment of pain from endometriosis should consist of as much excision of the lesion as possible to a depth where normal underlying tissue is reached. Excision can be performed equally well with laser, electrosurgery, and sharp dissection. Sharp dissection has the added advantage of providing the pathologist with a specimen without thermal damage; however, hemostasis is easier to control with electrosurgical or laser excision.

In 12 studies that examined the effect of hysterectomy with bilateral salpingo-oophorectomy for relief of pain related to endometriosis, 345/390 (88%) of patients reported improvement, and 84% experienced pain relief with the removal of only one affected ovary. In studies of ablative techniques, approximately two thirds of patients experienced relief from electrocautery and 80% reported relief after laser therapy. A success rate of more than 85% also has been reported with excisional techniques; however, there are no controlled studies to validate these reports.

Using life-table analysis, Redwine evaluated the recurrence rate after laparoscopic excision and found it to be comparable to excision via laparotomy: approximately 20% within the first 5 years. If a patient has been diagnosed and surgically treated for pain related to endometriosis, and similar pain remains or recurs, a trial of medical therapy should then be offered.

CHOICE OF THERAPY FOR INFERTILITY
Medical therapy

There are no controlled data that demonstrate improvement in fertility rates with medical therapy.

Surgery

The objective of surgery for endometriosis-related infertility is to destroy or resect as much disease as possible without creating new adhesions that may affect ovum capture. The available methods include electrocautery, endocoagulation, laser vaporization, and excision. Unfortunately, almost all reports on the treatment of endometriosis-related infertility utilize crude pregnancy rates obtained by dividing the number of pregnancies by the number of patients treated. Obviously, the longer the follow-up period, the higher the pregnancy rate. A more useful statistic now employed is the monthly fecundity rate, defined as the rate of achieving pregnancy per ovulatory cycle.

The first reported use of **electrocautery** to treat endometriosis through the laparoscope was by Eward in 1978.

Since then at least seven additional studies have been published and the crude pregnancy rates for the treatment of minimal, mild, and moderate endometriosis with electrocautery are approximately 65%, 50%, and 35%, respectively. The pregnancy rate for severe endometriosis has been reported at 50% in a small number of patients. Overall, approximately 75% of patients who achieved pregnancy did so within the first 6 months. Murphy et al., using life table analysis, studied 72 patients with stages I and II endometriosis who underwent electrocoagulation and noted a 10% and 8% fecundity rate, respectively.

Endocoagulation has not been widely reported in the English literature. In one study by Mettler, Giesel, and Semm, 40 of 90 patients treated by endocoagulation became pregnant.

Overall, the use of the **laser therapy** has not improved the crude pregnancy rates over other methods of ablation. The overall crude pregnancy rates in the literature for stages I, II, III, and IV are 59%, 58%, 58%, and 64%, respectively. As with electrocoagulation, most of the pregnancies occurred within the first 6 months. In a large retrospective study by Olive and Martin, the monthly fecundity rates of stages I and II endometriosis treated with laser were comparable with those found with expectant management, danazol treatment, and conservative surgery. With stage III endometriosis the fecundity rate was 4.5% with laser treatment and 1.5% after danazol therapy.

In an overview of controlled trials in endometriosis-associated infertility, Hughes, Fedorkow, and Collins concluded that no medical therapy for endometriosis provided benefit for infertility. There was a treatment benefit in all laparoscopic surgery, including laser and electrosurgery, with an odds ratio (OR) of 2.67 (95% confidence interval [CI] 2.08-3.45) as well as with conservative surgery (OR of 1.67, 95% CI 1.27-2.10). There appears to be no benefit in adding danazol therapy to either laparoscopic surgery or conservative surgery via laparotomy.

PROGNOSIS

As with many problems associated with chronic pelvic pain and infertility, there is an absence of data from randomized controlled clinical trials to guide the therapy of endometriosis-related symptoms. However, as a result of improved training and the development of innovative surgical techniques and technology, physicians are making great strides in providing maximum therapeutic benefit while minimizing patient morbidity through operative laparoscopy.

On average, patients will obtain between 18 and 24 months of pain relief from surgery or suppressive medical therapy (i.e., danazol or GnRH agonist). Because of the risks and side effects of both forms of therapy, alternating medical and surgical therapy often is advised. With this approach, the patient will undergo laparoscopic examination to evaluate the pelvis and treat the disease about every 4 years and will be exposed to the side effects of the medical therapy every 4 years until menopause. The immediate goal is to significantly lengthen these treatment intervals with improved laparoscopic excisional techniques and innovative medical therapy.

BIBLIOGRAPHY

Cook AS, Rock JA: The role of laparoscopy in the treatment of endometriosis, *Fertil Steril* 55:663, 1991.

Eward RD: Cauterization of stages I and II endometriosis and the resulting pregnancy rate. In Phillips JM, editor: *Endoscopy in gynecology*, Downey, Calif, American Association of Gynecologic Laparoscopists.

Franssen AMHW et al: Endometriosis: treatment with gonadotropin-releasing hormone agonist buserelin, *Fertil Steril* 51:401, 1989.

Friedman AJ, Hornstein MD: Gonadotropin-releasing hormone agonist plus estrogen-progestin "add-back" therapy for endometriosis-related pelvic pain, *Fertil Steril* 60:236, 1993.

Halme J et al: Retrograde menstruation in healthy women and in patients with endometriosis, *Obstet Gynecol* 64:151, 1984.

Hughes EG, Fedorkow DM, Collins JA: A quantitative overview of controlled trials in endometriosis-associated infertility, *Fertil Steril* 59:963, 1993.

Isaacson KB et al: Production and secretion of complement component 3 by endometriotic tissue, *J Clin Endocrinol Metab* 69:1003, 1989.

Kistner RW: The use of newer progestins in the treatment of endometriosis, *Clin Obstet Gynecol* 9:271, 1958.

Koninckx PR et al: Suggestive evidence that pelvic endometriosis is a progressive disease whereas deeply infiltrating endometriosis is associated with pelvic pain, *Fertil Steril* 55:759, 1991.

Mettler L, Giesel H, Semm K: Treatment of female infertility due to tubal obstruction by operative laparoscopy, *J Reprod Med 18:265, 1979.*

Murphy AA et al: Laparoscopic cautery in the treatment of endometriosis-related infertility, *Fertil Steril* 55:246, 1991.

Olive DL, Martin DC: Treatment of endometriosis-associated infertility with CO$_2$ laser laparoscopy: the use of one and two-parameter exponential models, *Fertil Steril* 48:18, 1987.

Pittaway DE: CA-125 in women with endometriosis, *Obstet Gynecol Clin North Am* 16:227, 1989.

Redwine DB: Conservative laparoscopic excision of endometriosis by sharp dissection: life table analysis of reoperation and persistent or recurrent disease, *Fertil Steril* 56:628, 1991.

Vernon MW et al: Classification of endometriotic implants by morphologic appearance and capacity to synthesize prostaglandin F, *Fertil Steril* 46:801, 1986.

Wheeler JM: Epidemiology of endometriosis-associated infertility, *J Reprod Med* 34:41, 1989.

34 Incontinence and Genital Prolapse

David H. Nichols and Linda Brubaker

INCONTINENCE
Physiology

Urinary continence is basically the result of a synergistic balance between detrusor function and the urethral closure mechanism. The detrusor urinae, the muscle that contains and contracts the bladder, is primarily under parasympathetic control, with some beta-adrenergic innervation. The urethral closure mechanism consists of the internal sphincter, a smooth muscle under alpha-adrenergic control, and the external sphincter, which is under voluntary control.

Urinary function is regulated by a variety of neurologic, structural, and hormonal factors, all of which act to keep urethral pressure greater than intravesical pressure until voiding is desired. Urethral tone, which is related to elasticity, estrogen-influenced circulation, and smooth and voluntary muscle tone, affects the urethral closure mechanism and is, in turn, affected by detrusor contraction. When such a contraction occurs, regardless of whether it is voluntary or involuntary, the urethral sphincter mechanism relaxes and intraurethral pressure decreases. Then, with voluntary relaxation of intraurethral pressure or augmentation of intravesical pressure (i.e., detrusor contraction), or normally with both, voiding may ensue.

The lower urinary tract has two main functions: (1) filling and storage and (2) emptying. During filling and storage, the bladder should accommodate the increasing urine load. There should be appropriate compliance, allowing the bladder pressure to remain low despite the increasing volume. No phasic bladder contractions should occur and the bladder outlet should remain closed during moments of increased intraabdominal pressure. During the emptying phase, the urethra should relax, followed within moments by a detrusor contraction that is of adequate strength and duration to void to completion.

These two main functions require the integrity of complex neurologic processes. Diseases that affect cortical, spinal, or local neuronal pathways frequently cause disorders in the function of the lower urinary tract. Even when neurologic control is totally intact, structural or motor considerations can affect voiding. Continence requires that sudden increases in abdominal pressure surround and are transmitted to both the bladder and the proximal urethra in a way that preserves the internal pressure relationship of one to the other. The urethrovesical angle should be stable and should not change involuntarily. The urethral sphincter mechanism must be competent, as evidenced by adequate urethral tone. If one of these factors fails, another may compensate for it; if two or more factors fail, however, the woman is likely to develop identifiable incontinence. (See box, below.)

Causes of incontinence

Stress incontinence. Circumstances that chronically increase intraabdominal pressure, such as coughing or sneezing, wearing tight abdominal support, and heavy lifting, may reduce the effective difference between intraurethral and intravesical pressure and lead to urinary stress incontinence. In response to brief increases in intraabdominal pressure, the woman experiences a brief involuntary loss of urine. The loss ceases if the woman voluntarily contracts the muscles of the pelvis, increasing the resting urethral tone and pressure. If levator tone is poor, these muscles cannot be relied on to stop the involuntary loss.

Any abnormal position of the bladder neck and proximal urethra wherein they, unlike the bladder, are not exposed to sudden changes in intraabdominal pressure may lead to stress incontinence. Rotational descent of the bladder neck, as well as the presence of any coincident cystocele, may be evident on physical examination.

Detrusor hyperactivity. The normal bladder should accommodate an increasing volume of urine while maintaining a low intravesical pressure. There should be no contractions, except as the woman voluntarily initiates voiding. Approximately 10% of all women show some evidence of involuntary detrusor hyperactivity, but this is clinically significant only when intraurethral closure pressure drops

---

INTERNATIONAL CONTINENCE SOCIETY NOMENCLATURE FOR INCONTINENCE

Overflow incontinence: involuntary loss of urine associated with overdistension of the bladder

Genuine stress incontinence: involuntary loss of urine occurring when, in the absence of a detrusor contraction, the intravesical pressure exceeds the maximum urethral pressure

Reflex incontinence: loss of urine due to detrusor hyperreflexia and/or involuntary urethral relaxation in the absence of the sensation usually associated with the desire to micturate (only seen in patients with neuropathic bladder/urethral disorders)

Detrusor instability: a detrusor that is shown objectively to contract, spontaneously or on provocation, during the filling phase while the patient is attempting to inhibit micturition

Detrusor hyperreflexia: overactivity due to disturbance of the nervous control mechanisms. There must be objective evidence of a relevant neurological disorder

Detrusor-sphincter dyssynergia (DSD): the presence of a detrusor contraction concurrent with an involuntary contraction of the urethral and/or periurethral striated muscle (in the adult, this is a feature of a neurologic disorder)

From Abrams P et al: *Neurol Urodynam* 7:403, 1988.

below intravesical pressure as a result of structural weakness, poor tone, or sacral reflex activity. Transient detrusor hyperactivity also occurs with lower urinary tract infections.

When phasic detrusor contractions cause urinary incontinence, this is called *detrusor instability*. In the presence of a relevant neurologic disease, this is termed *detrusor hyperreflexia*. The prevalence of this disorder increases with aging, but it is not a normal finding at any age.

Symptoms of detrusor hyperactivity often include urgency and nocturia. Physical examination may in some cases show a delayed loss of urine after precipitating maneuvers or a loss of urine with bladder filling to critical capacity.

Combined or mixed incontinence (detrusor hyperactivity with coexisting stress incontinence). Combined or mixed incontinence is quite common, constituting approximately one third or more of all cases of incontinence. Either form of incontinence may predominate, and it is this form of incontinence that should receive the primary treatment.

Overflow incontinence. When the bladder is sufficiently full and the intravesical pressure exceeds intraurethral pressure without a detrusor contraction, overflow incontinence occurs. It may occur when there is either an anatomic or a neurologic obstruction to the urinary outlet, when detrusor inadequacy produces bladder hypotonia (as a result of coincident neuropathy, such as multiple sclerosis, diabetes, or herniated low intervertebral disk, or because of the use of muscle relaxants) or when there is a vesical sensory impairment as a result of diabetes or multiple sclerosis.

Overflow incontinence may occur in the woman with a very large cystocele, particularly in an elderly woman, in whom detrusor tone has been effectively diminished and the bladder has become decompensated. Intravesical pressure rises sufficiently to exceed intraurethral pressure only when the volume of urine in the bladder has reached a critical level, and urine is mechanically forced through the urethra even without a detrusor contraction. There is always a high residual urine volume, which may predispose the patient with this condition to chronic infection.

Extraurethral causes. Conditions such as a congenital ectopic ureter that opens into the vagina or a urinary fistula at any site (ureter, bladder, or urethra) are extrinsic causes of incontinence. The patient usually complains of a constant dribble or loss of urine with no sense of urgency or warning. The leakage may be associated with a change in position, however, such as standing up from the supine position. A history of past pelvic surgery or radiation therapy is often present in patients with urinary fistula.

Functional incontinence exists when there is little or no abnormality in the lower urinary tract, but physical immobility or limitations prevent timely voiding. This is particularly common in institutionalized settings. Simple modifications of the external environment may dramatically assist these patients. Modifications may include bedside commodes, female urinals, timed toileting, and adjusting medication doses to coincide with the patient's schedule.

Evaluation

The depth to which the clinician should evaluate incontinence depends on the clarity of the symptom complex and the degree of disability perceived by the woman and those around her. The percentage of women with some disorder of urinary incontinence is approximately 5% to 10% and increases with age. It is difficult to standardize the degree of disability caused by urinary incontinence in women of any age, however, because the disability depends on the woman's perception of it. A degree of incontinence that is acceptable to one woman may be unacceptable to another.

History. The history focuses first on the pattern of incontinence, aiming to distinguish stress, urge, and overflow incontinence. Table 34-1 outlines the differential diagnosis

Table 34-1 Differential diagnosis of stress incontinence versus detrusor instability

	Stress incontinence	Detrusor instability
Typical symptoms	Urine loss with physical stress; Urgency, frequency, urge incontinence usually absent	Urgency, frequency (day and night), painless incontinence
Timing of leakage	At instant of physical stress	Lag of several seconds between stress and leakage
Volume of urine lost	Variable but limited	Large volume of urine over several seconds
Effect of bladder volume	Occurs even soon after voiding	More likely when bladder moderately full
Effect of position	Only in upright position; never at night in bed	Occurs in any position, often triggered by change in position
Precipitating factors	Coughing, sneezing, laughing, vigorous activity	Walking, running, or hearing running water often triggers incontinence, whereas coughing, laughing, sneezing generally do not
Voluntary control of stream	Can usually stop stream while in act of normal voiding	Difficult to stop stream during normal voiding
Associated disorders	No associated psychosomatic disorder	Underlying generalized anxiety or depressive state often present
Natural history	No spontaneous remissions or exacerbations, although progressive increase may occur with time	Often spontaneous remissions and exacerbations in relation to changes in life situation
History of bladder disorders	In general, no history of functional disorders of bladder control, except for transient symptoms related to pregnancy	Often history of voiding and bladder difficulties, including childhood enuresis

Modified from Green TH: *Am J Obstet Gynecol* 122:368, 1975.

of stress incontinence versus detrusor instability according to history. Urge incontinence typically occurs as spontaneous loss of urine without any urge or specific precipitating activity. The extent of disability can be measured by whether the patient loses urine both day and night; whether she must always wear wetness protection; whether she loses urine daily or only in connection with an occasional respiratory infection; and whether the woman, sensing an involuntary loss of urine, can willfully stop the stream.

A careful search for precipitating factors is important inasmuch as new or worsened incontinence often is due to problems outside the urinary tract that are amenable to intervention. A detailed medication history is often revealing. Many commonly used drugs have a secondary effect on urinary function. For example, beta blockers may induce bladder hypertonia, terbutaline may stimulate beta receptors and cause bladder hypotonia, and alpha blockers (such as prazosin) may cause genuine stress incontinence by decreasing the urethral tone and pressure. Persons who are hypertensive or who have been taking diuretics for a long time may experience nocturia from the rapid production of urine. In many persons, caffeine intake is related to detrusor hyperactivity, as well as to increased diuresis.

Physical examination. The physical examination (see box, below) includes a pelvic examination to detect atrophy and prolapse and to assess the woman's ability to isolate and contract the pubococcygeus. During a rectal examination, the clinician assesses perineal sensation and the bulbocavernosus reflex ("anal wink"), sphincter tone and control, and the presence of any fecal impaction. A targeted general examination includes screening of mental status and of neurologic function in the lower extremities.

To assess the effects of gravity on perineal support, it is useful to perform a preliminary pelvic examination when the woman's bladder is full, first while she is in the recumbent position and again while she is standing. The patient is asked to bear down and cough; if there is any loss of urine, its volume and the interval between the cough and the loss should be noted. The physician also should determine whether the patient can voluntarily stop the stream immediately or only after a few seconds. As noted earlier, detrusor instability typically is associated with a delayed loss of urine a few seconds after a precipitating stimulus with delayed

control of the stream, whereas stress incontinence is characterized by an immediate spurt of urine with immediate cessation of the stream if pubococcygeal strength is sufficient.

After the patient voids, the physician should quickly and gently repeat the examination, noting whether the bladder is palpable. When there is any suspicion of urinary retention, catheterization will determine the amount of residual urine present.

Diagnostic tests. A urinalysis and urine culture should be obtained to exclude infection. Screening for metabolic disorders that can precipitate incontinence is accomplished by obtaining levels of serum glucose, calcium, blood urea nitrogen, and creatinine.

A simple form of cystometry can be performed in the office. The first step is to catheterize the patient; any difficulty in introducing the catheter suggests that a urethral stricture may be contributing to the patient's problem. The clinician then attaches the glass or plastic tip of a 50-ml Asepto syringe to the original catheter and holds it just above the level of the pubis. Instilling the bladder with 50-ml increments of sterile saline solution, the clinician notes the volume at the patient's first urge to void. To determine the patient's bladder capacity, the clinician continues the instillation of saline until the patient feels that she can hold no more. Normal results are a residual volume of less than 50 ml, a first desire to void between 150 and 200 ml, and a bladder capacity between 400 and 500 ml.

As the bladder fills, the physician should closely watch the level of the fluid in the barrel of the syringe. This level rises if the procedure stimulates or provokes a detrusor contraction; thus an elevated level suggests some detrusor instability. The clinician must be cautious in interpreting this finding, however, because any straining, coughing, or talking on the part of the patient may increase intraabdominal pressure and cause a rise in the saline level.

The clinician then removes all but 250 ml of the saline solution, along with the catheter. After 1 or 2 minutes, the patient is asked to cough, first in a supine and then in a standing position. Any loss of urine, both without and with support from the examiner's fingers on the anterior vaginal wall, is noted while supine or standing. The patient is then asked to stand on her toes and come down hard on her heels (heel jounce) so that the examiner can determine whether this provokes a detrusor contraction with resultant urine loss.

Finally, the patient is asked to void, and the urine volume is recorded. The time during which urine is passed is roughly measured. Provided that the volume of urine voided is at least 200 ml, the rate of voiding is significant. A flow of at least 20 ml/sec rules out any obstruction of the outlet. An average flow of consistently less than 15 ml/sec strongly suggests outflow obstruction, and the patient should be referred for further evaluation. Values between 15 and 20 ml/sec should be interpreted in the light of other clinical data.

Management

The history and physical findings may strongly suggest a diagnosis or at least make it possible to establish a working plan for further evaluation. If there is evidence of urinary infection or vaginal atrophy, the first step is to treat this condition and plan to evaluate the response to treatment in several weeks. (See Chapters 18 and 42 for details of treatment.)

PHYSICAL EXAMINATION IN THE EVALUATION OF INCONTINENCE

General
 Screening mental status
 Neurologic examination of lower extremities

Pelvic
 Vaginal atrophy
 Prolapse of bladder, rectum, or uterus
 Pubococcygeus tone and control

Rectal
 Perineal sensation
 Bulbocavernosus reflex ("anal wink")
 Fecal impaction

Stress incontinence. If there has been an obvious loss of pubococcygeal tone, the woman should start a program of **isometric pubococcygeal contractions** (Kegel exercises). The program should consist of 15 voluntary contractions in a row, 3 seconds long each, six times daily. It is helpful to have the woman isolate the appropriate muscle during the pelvic examination. Kegel exercises must be continued indefinitely. For some women, use of weighted vaginal cones can significantly improve pubococcygeal muscle control (Femina Vaginal Cones, available from Dacomed Corporation).

Medications that increase the barrier capability of the bladder neck may be used in conjunction with Kegel exercises. These drugs include the **alpha-stimulating agents** phenylpropanolamine, pseudoephedrine, and imipramine (Table 34-2). **Estrogen,** either topically or systemically, can reduce stress incontinence by increasing the barrier capability of the urethra.

If significant anatomic prolapse is present, or if there is an inadequate response to the preceding treatment, referral to a gynecologist or urologist is appropriate.

Detrusor hyperactivity. The woman with detrusor hyperactivity should remove all caffeine from her diet and limit evening fluids. A particularly helpful technique is **bladder training** to increase voluntary control over detrusor activity. Bladder training involves voiding during waking hours at predetermined intervals (e.g., every hour), regardless of desire. There is no voiding whatsoever in between these intervals. After the woman has established some control with this schedule, she can progressively lengthen the interval between voids by small increments. She should keep a record of her progress for periodic review and should be given strong encouragement. This long-term retraining system is the single most important measure in efforts to obtain relief from symptoms.

Urge incontinence related to detrusor hyperactivity may respond to medications that increase the reservoir capability of the bladder (see Table 34-2). A trial of **anticholinergic or antispasmodic medications** is appropriate if neither significant postvoid residual nor contraindications (particularly glaucoma) are present. **Calcium antagonists** such as nifedipine and **tricyclic antidepressants** (which have both anticholinergic and alpha-stimulating properties) also may be effective.

When anticholinergic or antispasmodic drugs are prescribed the dosage should start low and be titrated upward to maximize effectiveness until side effects develop. These include dry mouth, urinary retention, and sometimes heat intolerance. The woman should be warned to report any symptoms of urinary retention. Constipation should be avoided.

If bladder retraining and medications are ineffective or poorly tolerated, referral for further evaluation, including sophisticated cystometry, is warranted. Transvaginal (or transanal) electrical stimulation is another option for treatment of detrusor instability. Although the mechanism of action remains unclear, approximately 60% of women experience significant improvement after a course of electrical stimulation.

Overflow incontinence. Eliminating any precipitating causes is the first step. These include medications (anticholinergic or alpha-stimulating drugs) and fecal impaction. If symptoms do not improve after treatment of the apparent precipitants, referral is necessary to exclude obstruction.

A variety of palliative measures may be employed, usually under the direction of a urologist or urogynecologist. These include a trial of medications to relax the bladder outlet (**alpha blockers** such as phenoxybenzamine, prazosin, or terazosin), **augmented voiding** (using double voids, Credé's or Valsalva's maneuver), and **intermittent clean catheterization** by the patient or a caregiver. An indwelling urinary catheter rarely is needed.

Indications for referral

Most patients seen by primary care physicians can be diagnosed and treated after these simple tests. The average primary care office does not need sophisticated urodynamic equipment. Instead each community should have a center that provides thorough urodynamic testing for those patients who have complex conditions that are difficult to diagnose and treat effectively or whose response to a treatment regimen is unclear.

Patients who should proceed to additional testing include those with an uncertain diagnosis, unsuccessful prior surgery, abnormal voiding, significant genital prolapse, relevant neurologic disease, and patients who do not improve with conservative therapy.

Ideally, a urodynamic evaluation in a referral center should be performed before any surgical procedure is undertaken for urinary stress incontinence. Any evidence of detrusor instability should be treated and stabilized medically before any surgery.

Most clinical series to date have studied white women. There is evidence that black women may have different symptoms and different conditions causing their incontinence. Until further data are available, black women should undergo extensive testing before surgery for incontinence.

Many options are available for the evaluation and treatment of women affected by genitourinary problems. Physi-

Table 34-2 Medical therapy for incontinence

Drug	Dose (mg)	Timing
Anticholinergic agents		
Propantheline bromide (Pro Banthine)	7.5-30	qd-tid
Methantheline bromide (Banthine)	50	bid
Antispasmodics		
Dicyclomine hydrochloride (Bentyl)	10-30	tid-qid
Oxybutynin chloride (Ditropan)	2.5-10	bid-tid
Flavoxate hydrochloride (Urispas)	100-400	tid-qid
Hyoscyamine sulfate (Donnatal, Levsin)	0.125-0.375	tid-qid qid
Calcium antagonists		
Nifedipine (Procardia)	10-20	qd-bid
Tricyclic antidepressants		
Imipramine hydrochloride (Tofranil)	10-25	bid-qid
Doxepin hydrochloride (Sinequan)	25-75	tid
Sympathomimetics		
Pseudoephedrine	30-60	bid-tid
Phenylpropanolamine hydrochloride (Ornade, Entex, Hycomine)	25-75	bid-tid

cians providing care to these patients have a valuable opportunity to improve the quality of life for these women. A stepwise evaluation approach is appropriate. Only rarely is the causative factor a life-threatening disorder such as cancer or serious neurologic disease. Therefore initial management should integrate simple nonsurgical techniques, including muscle strengthening, bladder retraining, fluid management, and judicious use of medications. Patients who do not show significant improvement, however, should proceed to additional evaluation and consideration of more invasive treatment, including medical and definitive surgical correction.

GENITAL PROLAPSE

In its simplest form, genital prolapse can be considered a downward displacement of any of the pelvic organs from their normal position either singly or in any combination. Such changes are generally most evident when the woman is standing, grow worse as the day lengthens, and are to a large extent relieved by lying down, because gravity no longer pulls the tissues downward. The condition may involve descent of the uterus, descent and elongation of the uterine cervix, prolapse of the vaginal vault, dropping of the bladder (cystocele), development of a peritoneal hernia between the vagina and rectum (enterocele), and a bulging of the rectum into the vagina with consequent increase in the size of the rectal reservoir (rectocele). To this may be added the presence of a perineal defect, most likely a result of stretching from childbirth. These descents occur in varying degrees but are at their maximum when there is total eversion of the vault of the vagina and the uterus has descended to a point where it is outside of the pelvis bringing with it the vagina, bladder, and rectum (procidentia).

Causes

The causes of genital prolapse are grouped into three categories: congenital defect, trauma, and the effects of aging.

Congenital defect includes an inherited lack of connective tissue strength of the pelvic organs and their support, which can be a defect intrinsic within the supporting tissues themselves or the consequence of a defective nerve supply as might be seen in some cases of spina bifida.

Trauma is the second cause, and it may be the consequence of damage resulting from labor and delivery in which the neuromuscular and connective tissues were stretched beyond their limits of elasticity, with permanent damage. Prolapse also may develop in women who experience massive sustained increases in intraabdominal pressure. This is seen in occupations that require heavy lifting but more commonly is a consequence of obstetric trauma. Chronic increases in intraabdominal pressure also can be brought about by wearing of tight corsets and girdles, as well as the result of chronic obstructive respiratory disease.

Aging produces damage to the pelvic support because the tissues replicate themselves less readily. Most of the pelvic supporting tissues are estrogen-dependent, and decreases in estrogen after the menopause weaken such dependent tissues and effectively diminish their blood supply.

In each woman any combination of these causes may be present. Very often the phenomenon of prolapse can be identified as a family characteristic, affecting siblings, parents, grandparents, and other female relatives.

Evaluation

History. The symptoms of genital prolapse are largely the consequence of the pull of gravity on these organs when the patient is standing. They include a feeling of pelvic heaviness, a feeling of bearing down, the presence of a mass, or a backache that most likely is absent when the patient first arises but grows progressively more severe throughout the day.

Specific questions should be asked about urinary and rectal function, including frequency, pain, disability, and incontinence. Some patients with severe degrees of prolapse profess to be completely asymptomatic.

Physical examination. Pelvic examination should aim to identify all sites of damage, first by inspection of the tissues and asking the patient to strain or bear down. Then, by manual examination, the clinician should identify the size, shape, and position of the uterus and vaginal vault and whether these tissues descend when the patient strains. The supporting tissues of the vagina and its adjacent organs roughly can be divided into two groups: the upper suspensory tissues (broad ligament, round ligaments, cardinal and uterosacral ligaments), and the lower supportive structures, including the pelvic diaphragm, levator ani muscle, urogenital diaphragm, and perineum. It is important for the clinician to identify the primary site of damage. One method of determining the primary site is for the physician, with the patient in the lithotomy position, to replace the prolapsed organs within the pelvis, then ask the patient to bear down and see which tissues appear first. If the cervix or vaginal vault appears first, followed by the cystocele and rectocele, one may conclude that the primary site of damage is to the upper suspensory system, whereas if the cystocele and rectocele appear first, followed by the cervix or vaginal vault, one may generally interpret this to mean that the primary site of damage is in the lower supporting tissues. The length of the cervix should be determined to ascertain if an elongation has developed, and an assessment should be made of the height of the uterine fundus at its normal position or in descent. The strength of voluntary contraction of the pubococcygeal muscles and the external anal sphincter should be noted, as well as the presence and degree of cystocele, paravaginal defect, enterocele, vaginal vault prolapse, rectocele, and perineal defect. Inspection of the rectum should identify any mucosal or rectal prolapse that is present along with the presence of any hemorrhoids.

At the conclusion of the bimanual examination, the patient should be asked to stand, with one foot on the shelf at the end of the examining table, and examined while she is bearing down as in Valsalva's maneuver, the examiner having placed a thumb in the vagina that will identify any prolapse of the vault and any cystocele that may be present and inserted a finger in the rectum to identify any rectocele, along with any perineal defect. By spreading the thumb and forefinger and asking the patient to strain, the examiner can feel an enterocele—if one is present—as a bowel-filled sac coming down between the thumb and forefinger. The examiner should ask the patient to voluntarily contract her pubococcygeal muscles, noting their strength, as well as that of the external anal sphincter, and ask the patient to cough, noting any urinary incontinence.

Management

The effective treatment of genital prolapse must embrace three goals: (1) the relief of symptoms, (2) the restoration of normal anatomic relationships in the pelvis, and (3) the return of normal function. Effective medical and surgical methods for achieving these goals exist.

The medical treatment includes topical or systemic estrogen-replacement therapy for the postmenopausal woman. For women in whom surgery is not desired or feasible, very often the tissues can be adequately supported by an intravaginal pessary. Although many pessaries are available, most patients can be helped with the ring, inflatable, Gellhorn, or doughnut pessary. The woman should be fitted with the largest size with which she is comfortable and that will permit the physician to painlessly insert the examining fingertip around the rim of the pessary to determine that intravaginal pressure is not excessive. The patient is then asked to stand and strain to determine her comfort and her ability to retain the pessary. She returns in a few days for reinspection to make sure that the pessary has not slipped since its insertion and then returns bimonthly for removal of the pessary and inspection of the vagina, followed by reinsertion. Surveillance of the pessary is important because a neglected pessary can cause serious erosion.

If the woman is interested, she can be taught to remove the pessary herself at bedtime and to replace it on arising in the morning, sparing the vaginal surface the trauma of around-the-clock pressure. She should be told that the pessary is fundamentally a foreign body and to expect some increase in vaginal discharge.

Over time, a pessary may no longer be adequate because of either worsening prolapse or worsening urinary incontinence. Patients should be referred for surgical consultation if they desire definitive surgical correction, are unable to retain a pessary, or have unacceptable stress incontinence despite pessary correction of the prolapse. Surgical counseling should review the indications for surgery, cure rates for each component (incontinence and prolapse), risks, complications, and perioperative course. Rarely is there a need for an urgent decision regarding surgical correction of these problems.

BIBLIOGRAPHY

Abrams P et al: Standardisation of terminology of lower urinary tract function, *Neurourol Urodynam* 7:403, 1988.

Bent AE et al: Transvaginal electrical stimulation in the treatment of genuine stress incontinence and detrusor instability, *Int Urogynecol J* 4:9, 1993.

Bergman A, Bhatia NN: Urodynamic appraisal of the Marshall-Marchetti test in women with stress urinary incontinence, *Urology* 24:458, 1987.

Bump RC: Racial comparisons and contrasts in urinary incontinence and pelvic organ prolapse, *Obstet Gynecol* 81:421, 1993.

Cammu H et al: Pelvic physiotherapy in genuine stress incontinence, *Urology* 38:332, 1991.

Dwyer PL, Teele JS: Prazosin: a neglected cause of genuine stress incontinence, *Obstet Gynecol* 79:117, 1992.

Fantl JA et al: Postmenopausal urinary incontinence: comparison between non–estrogen-supplemented and estrogen-supplemented women, *Obstet Gynecol* 71:823, 1988.

Green TH: Urinary stress incontinence: differential diagnosis, pathophysiology, and management, *Am J Obstet Gynecol* 122:368, 1975.

Hu T et al: A clinical trial of a behavioral therapy to reduce urinary incontinence in nursing homes: outcomes and implications, *JAMA* 261:2656, 1989.

Kinn A-C, Lindskog M: Estrogens and phenylpropanolamine in combination for stress urinary incontinence in postmenopausal women, *Urology* 32:273, 1988.

Krane RJ, Siroky MB, editors: *Clinical neuro-urology,* ed 2, Boston, 1991, Little, Brown & Co.

Kulseng-Hanssen S, Kristoffersen M: Urethral pressure variations in women with and without neurourological symptoms, *Neurourol Urodynam* 6:299, 1987.

Moore KH et al: Oxybutynin hydrochloride (3 mg) in the treatment of women with idiopathic detrusor instability, *Br J Urol* 66:479, 1990.

Murakami S et al: Strategies for asymptomatic microscopic hematuria: a prospective study of 1,034 patients, *J Urol* 144:99, 1990.

Nichols DH: *Reoperative gynecologic surgery,* St Louis, 1991, Mosby.

Nichols DH, Randall CL: *Vaginal surgery,* ed 3, Baltimore, 1989, Williams & Wilkins.

Torrens M, Morrison JFB, editors: *The physiology of the lower urinary tract,* New York, 1987, Springer-Verlag.

Turner-Warwick R, Whiteside CG, editors: *The urologic clinics of North America,* vol 6 (No 1), Philadelphia, 1979, WB Saunders.

35 Infertility

Robin A. Fischer and Veronica A. Ravnikar

The purpose of this chapter is to provide an overview of the basic infertility evaluation and the treatment options for specific infertility problems. The tasks in the primary setting include counseling of women (and their partners) who have concerns about fertility, initial assessment of infertility, and referral for specialist care. Infertility is becoming increasingly common, and for most couples the associated stress and anxiety are considerable. It is important for the primary care physician to be familiar with the basic evaluation of and treatments for infertility in order to provide support to the patient, as well as appropriate medical care.

DEFINITION

The operational definition of *infertility* is failure to achieve a pregnancy after at least 1 year of regular sexual intercourse without contraception. The condition is considered primary if the woman has never been pregnant, and secondary when there have been one or more conceptions.

The *incidence* of infertility is defined as the number of new infertile couples who start a consultation within a given period (usually 1 year) and in a given place, in proportion to the total number of women of procreational age at the beginning of the same period. The incidence of infertility in married couples in the United States is 10% to 20%.

Fecundibility is defined as the probability of a couple's conceiving during a menstrual cycle. In normal couples, this probability is estimated at 15% to 20% per month, with a cumulative chance of pregnancy in about 90% of healthy couples after 1 year.

RISK FACTORS FOR INFERTILITY

A number of factors may affect the risk of infertility in women and in men. Fertility rates decline with **increasing age** (Fig. 35-1). This is independent of a decrease in sexual activity with advancing age. The infertility risk for a woman aged 35 to 44 years old is twice the risk of a woman aged 30 to 34 years. An age-related decline in fertility is present, but less marked, in males.

Tobacco and illicit drug use (for example, marijuana, narcotics, and cocaine) has been found to affect both female and male fertility. Tobacco may alter tubal physiologic characteristics and transport, result in follicle and oocyte destruction, and impair sperm density, motility, and morphologic features. Ways in which illicit drugs affect fertility include changing libido, causing sexual dysfunction, and altering luteinizing hormone (LH) and follicle-stimulating hormone (FSH) secretion, with resulting abnormalities in ovulation and menstrual function.

Extremes of exercise activity and **dietary restrictions** affect fertility in women by causing ovulatory dysfunction.

Specific **occupational** and **environmental exposures** are now being recognized as factors affecting fertility for both men and women. Occupational hazards affecting fertility in women are discussed in detail in Chapter 79.

APPROACH TO THE PATIENT WITH FERTILITY CONCERNS

Because of increasing awareness of infertility, women often consult the primary care clinician about fertility concerns. Some women are concerned about the risk of infertility related to coexisting conditions (for example, a history of sexually transmitted disease) and others have a fertility evaluation after attempting pregnancy unsuccessfully for a very limited number of cycles. There is sometimes concern about the risks of infertility associated with delaying childbearing.

The primary care clinician can provide useful information about the effect of age on fertility, fecundity, and factors known to affect fertility. Awareness of these facts can help a woman to have realistic expectations for pregnancy and can reduce anxiety and its effects on the couple's relationship.

EVALUATION

In general, a woman needs a basic infertility investigation if she has been trying to conceive for at least 1 year without success. In some instances it is appropriate to initiate a fertility evaluation after 6-months, for example in couples over 30 years of age.

The major factors associated with infertility include central or ovulatory disorders, male factor, mucus or cervical factor, endometrial factor, uterine anatomic factors, tubal factor, and peritoneal factor (see box on following page). Although initial screening (particularly for central or ovulatory disorders) can be undertaken by the primary care physician, referral to an infertility specialist is usually required.

History and physical examination

Both partners should be present for the initial evaluation of infertility, which begins with a history and physical examination. This chapter focuses primarily on evaluation of the

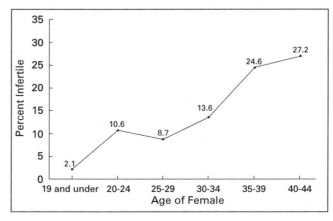

Fig. 35-1   Infertility related to age in the female. (Modified from Mosher WD: *Am Demographics* 9:42, 1987.)

MAJOR FACTORS ASSOCIATED WITH INFERTILITY

Male factors, 40%

Decreased production of spermatozoa
   Varicocele
   Testicular failure
   Endocrine disorders
   Cryptorchidism
   Stress, smoking, heat, systemic infections
Ductal obstruction
   Epididymis, postinfection
   Congenital absence of vas deferens
   Postvasectomy
   Ejaculatory duct, postinfection
Failure to deliver into vagina
   Ejaculatory disturbances
   Hypospadias
   Sexual problems (i.e., impotence)
Abnormal semen
   Volume problems
   Necrospermia and agglutination
   High viscosity

Ovulation factors, 20%

   Anovulation
   Inadequate corpus luteum
   Amenorrhea with low estrogen production

Tubal obstruction or dysfunction, 20%

   Pelvic inflammatory disease, tuberculosis,
     puerperal infection
   Congenital abnormalities
   Endometriosis
   Peritonitis (ruptured appendix or viscus,
     surgery)

Cervical and uterine factors, 10%

   Myomata, polyps, developmental
     abnormality or endometrial
     cavity, synechiae
   Abnormalities of cervix
     Obstruction (surgical, new growths)
     Destroyed endocervical glands
       (surgical, infections)

Unexplained (can account for up to 20% of all infertility)

Modified from Romney et al: *Gynecology and Obstetrics: the healthcare of women*, ed 2, New York, 1981, McGraw Hill.

THE HISTORY IN THE EVALUATION OF INFERTILITY

Nature and duration of infertility

   How long couple has been trying to conceive
   Any previous children for either partner
   Any prior infertility evaluation

General medical history for both partners

Past surgical history for both partners

   Pelvic or abdominal surgery in female

Past gynecologic history

   Menstrual history: age of menarche, cycle interval,
     duration, flow
   Presence of molimina, pelvic pain, abnormal bleeding
   Past birth control methods
   History of pelvic inflammatory disease
   History of abnormal Papanicolaou test results and any
     treatment
   DES exposure in utero
   Other gynecologic problems (e.g., fibroids, endome-
     triosis)
   Coital history (frequency, use of lubricants, sexual
     difficulties)

Past obstetric history

Social history of both partners

   Alcohol, tobacco, and drug use
   Occupational exposures
   Stress
   Eating disorders
   Exercise patterns and frequency

Family history

   Endocrine disorders

Endocrine review of systems

   Hirsutism, acne
   Galactorrhea
   Weight loss and gain
   Tiredness, weakness

Medication use by both partners

DES, diethylstilbestrol.

female, while reviewing briefly the assessment of male factor infertility. The box, above right, outlines the relevant history for the evaluation of infertility.

Physical examination in the female focuses on assessment for endocrine and reproductive tract disorders, including hirsutism and other signs of androgen excess, galactorrhea, and signs of hypothyroidism or hyperthyroidism (see Chapters 9, 10, and 12). A pelvic examination is performed to look for evidence of endometriosis, uterine fibroids, adnexal masses, cervicitis or other cervical abnormalities, and congenital anomalies.

Diagnostic tests

Diagnostic tests are guided by the history and physical examination and performed in a stepwise fashion. The ini-

tial evaluation includes simultaneous analysis of the female and male.

Disorders of ovulation may be suggested on the basis of the history and physical examination. Initial assessment of ovulation can be made by basal body temperature measurements or a single luteal-phase progesterone level. Serum thyroid-stimulating hormone (TSH) and prolactin levels will screen for thyroid disorders and hyperprolactinemia, common causes of ovulatory dysfunction.

Procedures performed during the initial evaluation of infertility include a semen analysis, postcoital test, endometrial biopsy, and hysterosalpingogram. After this outpatient evaluation is completed, laparoscopy and hysteroscopy are performed. Generally laparoscopy and hysteroscopy are the last diagnostic procedures to be done; these procedures may be performed earlier in women with a known history of tubal disease or symptoms suggestive of endometriosis.

Semen analysis. An abnormality in the semen analysis result defines male factor infertility. Male factor accounts for 40% of infertility in the United States. Examination of semen should be an early diagnostic step, if not the first step. If the semen analysis finding is abnormal, it should be repeated. (This is done to confirm a persistent semen problem.) If the semen analysis result is again abnormal the male partner should be referred for urologic consultation. Invasive diagnostic testing of the female partner may be deferred until evaluation of the male partner is completed.

The semen sample is obtained by masturbating into a clean plastic or glass container. If the male is unable to obtain a specimen in this fashion, silicone condoms with an attached pouch may be used to collect a specimen through intercourse. Latex condoms are spermicidal and so cannot be used. The specimen must be kept warm (body temperature is best) and should be delivered within approximately 1 to 2 hours after collection. The couple can be instructed to place the specimen under an armpit or against the body during transport. Abstinence from sexual activity for 2 to 3 days before semen analysis is generally recommended, as increased ejaculatory frequency reduces the volume and sperm count on semen analysis. However, if the couple usually has intercourse daily, abstinence may provide an analysis of a semen sample that is different from what is usually deposited in the female reproductive tract.

World Health Organization (WHO) criteria are generally used for evaluation (see Table 35-1). Volume, count, motility, and morphologic characteristics are the basic semen parameters evaluated. A laboratory accustomed to semen analysis should be used.

One must keep in mind that semen samples vary and that couples can conceive despite an abnormal semen analysis finding. Abnormal semen analysis results can occur from failure to collect the entire specimen, temperature effect during transportation, interval from collection until evaluation, abnormal hormone levels, genetic or congenital abnormalities, drug and occupational exposures, infections (including extragenital infections), and surgical procedures. It is important to confirm an abnormal semen analysis result with a second evaluation. This provides evidence of a per-

sistent semen problem and usually rules out a problem with collection and transport. If the male had been ill around the time of the first semen analysis, one might consider waiting 2 to 3 months to repeat the test to ensure there is no persistent effect of that illness. A new sperm maturation cycle takes approximately 70 to 90 days.

Postcoital test (PCT, PK, or Simms-Huhner test). Cervical factor accounts for 5% to 10% of infertility. The PCT provides information about cervical mucus, coital adequacy, and sperm/cervical mucus interaction. Athough this test is still part of the basic outpatient infertility evaluation, its role has been the subject of debate because of concerns about unreliability and limited correlation with chance of pregnancy.

The timing of the PCT is important. It must be performed before or at the LH surge, when estrogen levels peak. The couple is asked to have intercourse 2 to 12 hours before an office examination. The optimal time to perform the test after intercourse has not been defined. It has been reported that sperm number starts to decrease after 8 hours. It has also been reported that complement-dependent reactions that immobilize sperm take 8 to 10 hours to occur and, therefore, the PCT is best performed at least 8 hours after intercourse.

To obtain the specimen, position the woman in the dorsal lithotomy position. Place a speculum and obtain cervical mucus with a polyp forceps, Kelly clamp, or a 14-gauge or 16-gauge angiocath attached to a tuberculin syringe. It is not necessary to obtain mucus from a specific area of the cervical canal, as mucus quality and sperm density are well distributed throughout the canal. One first observes quantity and quality of the cervical mucus. Estrogen stimulates secretion of clear, stringy mucus from the cervical glands. Copious amounts of clear cervical mucus are expected if the PCT is appropriately timed. If the PCT is performed too early in the menstrual cycle one observes a small amount of clear cervical mucus that is not yet watery. Shortly after ovulation progesterone production counters estrogen's effect on cervical mucus. The mucus becomes thick, viscous, and cellular (indicated by presence of white opacities on gross visualization).

Depending on the mechanism of collection, spinnbarkeit should be evaluated by allowing the mucus to fall slowly onto a microscope slide from the tuberculin syringe or stretching it between the two arms of the polyp forceps or Kelly clamp. The mucus should be stretched 8 to 10 cm or more (spinnbarkeit) in the periovulatory period. When well-estrogenized mucus is allowed to dry on the microscope slide, a fern pattern should be seen. All these parameters indicate adequacy of the cervical mucus and appropriate timing of the test. Coital adequacy and sperm/mucus interaction are assessed in the PCT by the number of motile sperm seen per microscope high-power field (hpf). A total of 1 to 20 motile sperm/hpf has been considered adequate. Absence of sperm on PCT should prompt a review of the couple's coital technique.

Endometrial biopsy. Ovulation disorders account for approximately 20% of infertility. The endometrial biopsy is performed to confirm ovulation and evaluate the adequacy of the endometrial response to progesterone production in the luteal phase. Inadequacy of an endometrial response or luteal phase defect (LPD) accounts for 3% to 14% of infertility. Progesterone's effect on the endometrium is evaluated by an office endometrial sampling late in the luteal

Table 35-1 World Health Organization (WHO) criteria used for semen evaluation

Volume	2 ml or more
pH	7.2-7.8
Sperm concentration	20×10^6 spermatozoa/ml or more
Total sperm count	40×10^6 spermatozoa or more
Motility	50% or more with forward progression or 25% or more with rapid linear progression within 60 min after collection
Morphologic characteristics	50% or more with normal morphologic features

Modified from *WHO laboratory manual for the examination of human semen and semen-cervical mucus interaction,* New York, 1987, Cambridge University Press.

phase (postovulation day 10-12). If vaginal bleeding has begun, the endometrial biopsy should be rescheduled.

The endometrial sampling is usually performed with a small suction curette (pipelle). This procedure is done in the office and produces a few minutes of moderately intense uterine cramping. The tissue should be obtained from the uterine fundus, as tissue from the poorly vascularized lower uterine segment is frequently "out-of-phase" (lagging behind expected histologic maturation). Risk of interruption of pregnancy with the endometrial biopsy appears to be theoretic ($\leq$2% if the implantation site is directly biopsied).

The histologic endometrial dating criteria were well established by Noyes and colleagues in 1950. First the histologic features should document ovulation; the endometrium should have changed from proliferative to secretory. Second the endometrium should be dated. If the endometrial histologic dating lags behind actual endometrial day by more than 2 days on at least two endometrial samplings, the woman is considered to have LPD. The actual postovulation day may be calculated by (1) onset of menses, (2) day of follicular rupture (as documented by ultrasound), or (3) urine luteinizing hormone (LH) testing.

LPD is thought to cause infertility because maturation of the endometrium is delayed. The endometrium is not ready to accept the fertilized ovum when it reaches the uterine cavity. Causes of LPD include inadequate progesterone production by the corpus luteum, hyperprolactinemia, thyroid disease, exercise, chronic disease, use of certain medications (e.g., medications that increase serum prolactin level such as metoclopramide and many of the antipsychotic drugs). Clomiphene citrate (when used in ovulatory women) can be associated with development of LPD. It is thought that clomiphene citrate interferes with development of sex steroid receptors in the endometrium, causing delayed maturation.

Endometrial biopsy is the most reliable method of evaluating the luteal phase; less sensitive indirect tests are basal body temperature measurements of luteal temperature elevation (more than 11 days) and a midluteal progesterone serum level. Since serum progesterone levels vary with meal consumption and activity level, a single luteal serum progesterone level may confirm that ovulation has occurred, but most likely is not a good marker of LPD.

Hysterosalpingogram (HSG). Tubal factor accounts for 30% to 50% of infertility. One half of all patients found to have tubal damage or adhesions have no identifiable risk factors. The HSG assesses fallopian tube patency, as well as outlining uterine cavity anatomic characteristics; it does not diagnose peritubal or pelvic adhesions. The procedure has a 75% correlation with operative findings at laparoscopy.

This radiographic procedure is performed early in the follicular phase, after menstrual flow has ceased. The test is done in the follicular phase to be sure the patient is not pregnant and to obtain a clear outline of the uterine cavity. The endometrium is thinnest in the early follicular phase. A nonsteroidal antiinflammatory drug given 30 minutes to 2 hours before the procedure will minimize abdominal cramping. The procedure involves injection of radiopaque dye through the cervix into the uterus and tubes, under fluoroscopic guidance.

Complications of HSG are pelvic infection, pain, vaginal bleeding, uterine perforation, and intravascular injection of dye. Pelvic infection occurs in less than 1% of all women having this procedure, and in approximately 3.5% of women who have risk factors (such as history of pelvic infection, ectopic pregnancy, tubal surgery, or ruptured appendix). Oil-soluble and water-soluble contrast are available. Oil-soluble dye has been associated with oil embolization and death. If one knows the patient has patent fallopian tubes, risk of intravasation of the dye is minimal. Oil-soluble contrast media cause less discomfort, produce sharper contrast on radiographic films, and may be therapeutic in some cases of infertility. Water-soluble dye (e.g., Renografin or Sinografin) is usually used for diagnostic HSG.

Laparoscopy/hysteroscopy. Laparoscopy/hysteroscopy is the final diagnostic procedure. When it is performed after a negative outpatient infertility evaluation, 50% of patients have some form of peritoneal factor (e.g., endometriosis or pelvic adhesions) identified at the time of laparoscopy. The procedure is usually postponed for 6 months if the findings of the outpatient infertility evaluation are negative. Exceptions are advancing maternal age, high clinical probability of endometriosis, long history of infertility, or high patient anxiety.

The procedure is usually done in an ambulatory surgery setting, under general anesthesia, and takes approximately 1 to 2 hours. It should be carried out by an infertility specialist who is able to treat peritoneal factors found during surgery, using methods that include laser vaporization, cautery, and excisional biopsy.

Unexplained infertility. If an outpatient infertility evaluation has been completed, a laparoscopy/hysteroscopy has been performed, and all test results are normal, the diagnosis is unexplained infertility. Unexplained infertility accounts for up to 20% of all infertility cases. Additional tests such as microbial testing, immunologic testing (for example, antisperm antibodies), and periovulatory ultrasound monitoring (to look for abnormalities such as luteinized unruptured follicle syndrome) may be performed under the guidance of an infertility specialist.

MANAGEMENT

Abnormal semen analysis result. The male partner should be referred to a urologist with an interest in infertility. If the semen quality cannot be improved, the couple should be referred to an infertility specialist. Treatment options include washed intrauterine insemination (IUI) of the female partner with the partner's sperm, donor insemination, and in vitro fertilization (IVF). Insemination involves concentrating the motile fraction of sperm by one of many separation techniques and injecting them directly into the upper uterine cavity. At certain IVF centers methods are now available to inject sperm directly under the zona pellucida of an oocyte or directly into the oocyte's cytoplasm. This technique is reserved for couples with specific types of male factor infertility such as severe oligoasthenospermia, or couples with less than 20% fertilization during two standard IVF cycles.

Abnormal PCT result. Intrauterine insemination (IUI) is the most common form of treatment. Intrauterine inseminations bypass the cervical mucus and therefore prevent immobilization of sperm in the lower reproductive tract. Timing of the insemination is critical: IUI ideally is performed just after ovulation has occurred. Sperm must be present in the upper reproductive tract when the oocyte has been released from the ovarian follicle and is present in the distal fallopian tube (ovulation) and still is capable of being fertilized (12 to 24 hours after ovulation).

Abnormal endometrial biopsy result. Initial ovulation induction with low-dose clomiphene citrate is appropriate in most cases of anovulation (50 mg once daily, cycle day 5-9). If pregnancy does not occur within 3 months of therapy during which ovulation is documented by basal body temperature chart or mid–luteal phase progesterone level, patients should be referred to an infertility specialist for optimal management. Higher-dose clomiphene citrate therapy usually includes ultrasound follicular monitoring. If a patient does not respond or becomes resistant to clomiphene citrate therapy, or for the initial treatment of certain causes of anovulation, ovulation induction therapy with human menopausal gonadotropin (HMG-[Pergonal]) is undertaken. This therapy requires the expertise of an infertility specialist. Patients must be educated about the risks and benefits of this therapy (e.g., 30% to 40% chance of multiple gestation and hyperstimulation syndrome), as well as techniques in mixing and injecting of Pergonal. Injection of medication takes place in the evening, so partners are taught how to mix and give an intramuscular injection. Patients must be monitored closely during therapy with frequent ultrasound and serum hormone levels.

Treatment for LPD (documented on two or more endometrial biopsy results) should be undertaken by an infertility specialist. For minor discrepancies, usually progesterone vaginal suppository treatment is initiated (25 or 50 mg per vagina, bid). For larger discrepancies clomiphene citrate therapy is usually prescribed. Repeat endometrial biopsy is mandatory to ensure that therapy has adequately corrected the endometrial defect.

Abnormal HSG result. The infertility specialist will define the exact uterine or tubal abnormality and help the couple decide whether surgical correction or IVF therapy is more appropriate. Therapy decisions include emotional and financial concerns of the couple, as well as consideration of the relative effectiveness of each therapy.

Abnormal laparoscopy/hysteroscopy result. Therapy (under the supervision of the infertility specialist) is guided by the severity of endometriosis. Superovulation/IUI therapy is used to treat infertility caused by minimal and mild cases of endometriosis, with or without surgical removal of endometriosis implants. For more severe cases of endometriosis therapy is surgical correction with or without postoperative medical suppressive therapy. If conception has not occurred by 6 months to 2 years after surgery, infertile couples with any stage of endometriosis are usually referred for IVF therapy. Superovulation drugs used to treat infertility patients with mild and minimal cases of endometriosis may induce growth of endometriosis implants. Endometriosis patients must understand this before initiating superovulation therapy.

It is important to remember that many of these tests and therapies are expensive, stressful, and time-consuming. Adoption should always be considered as an alternative to therapy. Counseling and support are often essential for the couple experiencing infertility. Many couples find group sessions helpful; community resources, such as RESOLVE (a national organization for infertile couples), can be used in addition to services provided through the infertility center. Couples must also be reminded they still have a small chance of spontaneous conception without undergoing any form of infertility therapy.

BIBLIOGRAPHY

Blackwell RE: The infertility workup and diagnosis, *J Reprod Med* 34:81, 1989.

Green BB et al: Exercise as a risk factor for infertility with ovulatory dysfunction, *Am J Public Health* 76:1432, 1986.

Jaffe SB, Jewelewicz R: The basic infertility investigation, *Fertil Steril* 56:599, 1991.

Mosher WD: Infertility trends among US couples: 1965-1976, *Fam Plann Perspect* 14:22, 1982.

Mosher WD: Infertility: why business is booming, *Am Demographics* 9:42, 1987.

Noyes RW, Hertig AT, Rock J: Dating of the endometrial biopsy, *Fertil Steril* 1:3, 1950.

Paul M: *Occupational and environmental reproductive hazards: a guide for clinicians,* Baltimore, 1993, Williams & Wilkins.

Paul M, Himmelstein J: Reproductive hazards in the workplace: what the practitioner needs to know about chemical exposures, *Obstet Gynecol* 71:921, 1988.

Phipps WR et al: The association between smoking and female infertility as influenced by cause of the infertility, *Fertil Steril* 48:377, 1987.

Romney et al: *Gynecology and Obstetrics: the health care of women,* ed 2, New York, 1981, McGraw Hill.

Smith CG, Asch RH: Drug abuse and reproduction, *Fertil Steril* 48:355, 1987.

Soules MR, Spadoni LR: Oil versus aqueous media for hysterosalpingography: a continuing debate based on many opinions and few facts, *Fertil Steril* 38:1, 1982.

Speroff L, Glass RH, Kase NE: *Clinical gynecologic endocrinology and infertility,* ed 4, Baltimore, 1989, Williams & Wilkins.

Stillman RJ, Rosenberg MJ, Sachs BP: Smoking and reproduction, *Fertil Steril* 46:545, 1986.

Thonneau P, Spira A: Prevalence of infertility: international data and problems of measurement, *Eur J Obstet Gynecol Reprod Biol* 38:43, 1990.

Tietze C: Reproductive span and rate of reproduction among Hutterite women, *Fertil Steril* 8:89, 1957.

Warren MP: Effects of undernutrition on reproductive function in the human, *Endocr Rev* 4:363, 1983.

Wentz AC et al: Cycle of conception endometrial biopsy, *Fertil Steril* 46:196, 1986.

WHO laboratory manual for the examination of human semen and semencervical mucus interaction, New York, Cambridge University Press, 1987.

36 Menopause and Estrogen Replacement Therapy

Kathryn A. Martin

Menopause is an important time of transition in a woman's life. Life expectancy for women has gradually increased and is now estimated to be approximately 78 years. Therefore, for most women up to one third of one's total life span occurs after the menopause. This aging of the population has raised many important questions about the public health impact of menopause.

Because of the explosion of information about menopause now available to women, many women discuss questions and concerns about menopause with their primary physicians. Others will experience symptoms related to menopause. Although estrogen replacement was historically used short-term to treat symptoms of the menopause, the current emphasis is on long-term use of estrogen to prevent both osteoporosis and coronary artery disease (CAD). However, there are many unresolved issues about the risks and benefits of hormone replacement therapy.

EPIDEMIOLOGY

The average age of menopause in recent epidemiologic studies is approximately 51, although the range considered to be normal is quite wide, as menopause can occur in normal women anytime between the ages of 42 and 58. The only factor identified as a predictor of age at menopause is smoking history: women who smoke undergo menopause approximately 2 years earlier than nonsmokers.

PHYSIOLOGY

Although menopause is defined clinically as permanent cessation of menses, the neuroendocrine and ovarian changes leading up to the menopause occur over a 5- to 10-year period referred to as the perimenopausal transition. The groundwork for menopause begins in utero, and by the sixth month of fetal life the human ovary contains approximately 6 to 7 million oocytes. However, after this peak a degenerative process known as follicular atresia occurs until there are no remaining oocytes at the time of menopause. Fewer than 1% of oocytes are lost via ovulation; the remainder are lost via atresia, a process that is poorly understood.

Endocrine changes seen during menopause include changes in ovarian sex steroid biosynthesis and pituitary gonadotropin secretion. The premenopausal ovary contains three functioning compartments—the stroma, follicle, and corpus luteum. After menopause, however, the only remaining functional compartment is the stroma, the site of androgen production. Although testosterone production rates and levels do not change significantly after menopause, androstenedione levels do decrease by approximately 50%. The postmenopausal ovary appears to make little or no estrogen, and circulating estrogen in postmenopausal women is derived primarily from peripheral conversion of androstenedione to estrone.

The earliest endocrine finding during the perimenopausal transition is a selective rise in serum follicle-stimulating hormone (FSH), which is often seen in women over 40 with ovulatory cycles. This is thought to be due primarily to a decrease in serum estradiol secretion across the cycle, although a decrease in other ovarian hormones such as inhibin may also play a role.

CLINICAL PRESENTATION

The earliest clinical finding during the perimenopausal transition is a **decrease in cycle length.** It has been demonstrated that ovulatory women over 40 have a mean cycle length of 25 days compared to 30 days in 18- to 30-year-old control subjects, whereas 45-year-old women have a mean cycle length of only 23 days. Although most women initially experience these short cycles, many then have long, anovulatory cycles that may be interspersed with shorter, ovulatory cycles. The reasons for this waxing and waning of ovarian activity are unclear but may reflect a difference in the responsiveness of the remaining oocytes, or a difference in the types of FSH the pituitary secretes during the perimenopausal transition.

The **vasomotor flush** is the most common clinical finding of the menopause. Approximately 75% of women having a natural menopause experience flushes, and as many as 90% of women who have surgical menopause. There are two components to a flush. The hot flash describes the subjective feeling of warmth that proceeds any physiologically measurable change. The hot flush is the physiologically measurable change and is characterized by visible redness in the chest, neck, and face, usually followed by sweating in the same distribution. Nocturnal hot flushes are more common than daytime hot flushes, and sleep deprivation is a common result. Studies have demonstrated nocturnal flushes with corresponding waking episodes, using skin temperature and electroencephalographic (EEG) recordings. This is clinically relevant as many of these women experience insomnia-related symptoms such as fatigue, irritability, and depression. It has been demonstrated that estrogen treatment of these symptomatic women results in improved sleep latency and an increased percentage of rapid eye movement (REM) sleep.

Genitourinary atrophy is another common phenomenon as the vagina and the outer third of the urethra are estrogen-responsive tissues. Therefore, patients often experience vaginal dryness, dyspareunia, and urinary symptoms that mimic urinary tract infection. All of these symptoms are responsive to estrogen.

In addition to these immediate consequences menopause affects a woman's risk for other chronic diseases, chiefly **osteoporosis** and **ischemic heart disease.** The increased risk of osteoporosis is clearly related to accelerated decrease in bone mass per unit volume during the years following menopause. The effect of menopause on coronary risk is less straightforward. When age and smoking are taken into account there is no difference in heart disease risk between naturally premenopausal and postmenopausal women. However, bilateral oophorectomy in premenopausal women does increase the risk of heart disease, even though natural menopause does not.

APPROACH TO THE WOMAN AT MENOPAUSE

Counseling

The proliferation of information in recent years has helped many women become more knowledgeable about menopause. However, the negative tone of much of this information, coupled with cultural stereotypes, has fostered fears and worries about menopause in some women. It is important for the primary care physician to be able to counsel patients about what to expect at menopause. Some perimenopausal women with concerns may be reluctant to voice their worries. Counseling about what to expect as a woman approaches menopause should be part of routine primary care for women in their 40s.

The primary care clinician can provide information about the epidemiologic and physiologic characteristics of menopause and guidelines for what is normal and when symptoms should prompt medical attention (see box, below). It is important to acknowledge the cultural emphasis on negative aspects of menopause and provide a more balanced view of the positive physical, emotional, and social aspects. The authority of the clinician's role can be helpful in countering negative expectations, which may influence a woman's experience of menopause.

Menopause is a convenient time for examining health maintenance and prevention measures. Fluctuations in the rate of change in serum cholesterol levels around menopause may make more frequent screening desirable. Nutrition should be reviewed to ensure that a woman is receiving 1000 to 1500 mg of calcium daily. A regular weight-bearing

---

COUNSELING THE PERIMENOPAUSAL WOMAN

Epidemiology of menopause
    Average age is 51; 1-2 years earlier in smokers
    Typical changes in cycles before menopause
        Shortening cycle length
        Skipped menstrual periods
        Occasional heavy menstrual periods

What to expect at menopause
    Symptoms related to menopause significant for a *minority* of women
    Great variation among individual women in the experience of menopause

When to seek medical attention
    Vaginal bleeding more frequently than every 21 days
    Heavy bleeding or bleeding lasting more than 7 days
    Bothersome hot flashes, insomnia, or other symptoms
    After 6 to 12 months of amenorrhea

---

exercise program is important for women at midlife, both for osteoporosis prevention and for maintenance of appropriate body weight.

A discussion of hormonal replacement therapy (HRT) should generally be initiated with every menopausal woman. Because of the widespread interest in HRT, the clinician can anticipate that a perimenopausal woman will have questions about its use for symptom relief or prevention, even if its use is not appropriate in her case.

Hormone replacement therapy

Pharmacology. The relative potency of estrogens in hormone replacement therapy is much less than in the oral contraceptive pill. Most low-dose oral contraceptives currently contain 35 μg of ethinyl estradiol, a dose equivalent to approximately seven times what is used for menopausal replacement. However, estrogen replacement doses are more physiologic and in general restore follicular phase levels of estrogen. Therefore, when considering the risks and benefits of hormone replacement therapy one cannot necessarily extrapolate from the oral contraceptive literature because of the large difference in estrogen dose.

The exogenous estrogens that are used clinically have striking variability in potency. All oral preparations are metabolized in the liver, with potential effects on liver protein synthesis, including renin substrate, clotting factors, and hepatic lipase. In contrast transdermal preparations avoid this first-pass hepatic metabolism. With regard to potency, the synthetic estrogens (ethinyl estradiol) are the most potent estrogens available. Conjugated estrogens are the next most potent; natural estrogens, estradiol and estropipate, are the least potent.

Progestins are synthetic compounds with progesteronelike activity, most of which have mild androgenic properties. Medroxyprogesterone acetate is the progestin used most commonly after menopause. In addition there are progestins derived from testosterone, referred to as 19-nor-testosterones, that are used in oral contraceptives. In general testosterone derivatives tend to be more potent and androgenic and are infrequently used for postmenopausal replacement.

Risks and benefits. When making a risk/benefit analysis of hormone replacement therapy the risk of coronary artery disease (CAD) is the most important factor, as death of ischemic heart disease is four to five times more common than death of breast and endometrial cancer combined. Therefore a very small change in risk could result in a profound change in morbidity and mortality rates.

The increased risk of **endometrial hyperplasia** and **carcinoma** with estrogen use has been well documented (see box on the following page). Endometrial cancer risk has been studied in users versus nonusers of estrogen. It has been found that short-term users (less than 1 year of use) appear to have no increased risk in cancer, while the long-term users have a fivefold increase in risk. Similar results have been confirmed in many other studies as well.

It is known that addition of a progestin dramatically reduces the risk of endometrial cancer. Although dose and type of progestin are obviously important, there are data suggesting that the duration of progestin exposure is equally important. The incidence of hyperplasia with unopposed estrogen in one study was 18% to 32%, with a decrease to

RISKS OF HORMONE REPLACEMENT THERAPY

Estrogen
  Gallbladder disease
  Endometrial hyperplasia and cancer
  Breast cancer (risk unresolved)

Progestins
  Adverse effect on serum lipid levels
  Effect on breast cancer unknown
  Effect on coronary artery disease unknown

3% to 4% if a progestin is added for 7 days, and a further reduction to 0% for 12 to 13 days of progestin (Whitehead, Hilliard, and Crook, 1990). The current trend in clinical practice is to give a low dose of medroxyprogesterone acetate (5 mg) for 12 to 13 days.

The association of hormone replacement with **breast cancer** remains controversial. Many studies in the past decade have attempted to examine the risk of estrogen and breast cancer, with conflicting results. A recent study examining a large cohort of Swedish women demonstrated an increased risk of breast cancer in long-term users of estrogen (>9 years). In addition an increased risk was seen after only 6 years in combined estrogen-progestin users. However, the number of subjects in this group was small, and the difference was not statistically significant (Bergkvist et al., 1989). The Nurses' Health Study, a mail survey of over 120,000 women, found a small increased risk of breast cancer in any current user of estrogen (regardless of duration of use) when compared to that of past users, suggesting that estrogen has a more acute effect. Both of the groups discussed have also reported that the survival rate in the estrogen-related breast cancers was better. This finding does not appear to be simply a function of early diagnosis because tumor size, estrogen receptor status, and presence of nodes were no different in the estrogen and nonestrogen breast cancer cases in the Nurses' Health Study, suggesting that the biologic characteristics of these breast cancers may be different.

One metaanalysis of the relation of estrogen to breast cancer suggests that there is no increased risk of breast cancer in postmenopausal women on estrogen, while another analysis found that for long-term use of estrogen, the relative risk of breast cancer was approximately 1.3 when compared to that of nonusers. In addition this analysis found that women with a family history of breast cancer are at particularly high risk when estrogen replacement is used. Other analyses have not found this association with family history. Although it is possible that estrogen use may be associated with an increase in breast cancer risk with long-term use (>10 to 15 years), the question has been difficult to answer because few women have thus far been on long-term estrogen. As long-term hormone replacement has become more common in recent years, this question should be readdressed in the future.

Prevention of **osteoporosis** with estrogen is well established (see box at right). Many studies have demonstrated that estrogen prevents bone loss, whereas a steady rate of bone loss is seen in untreated women. If estrogen is discontinued at any point bone loss resumes. The dose required to prevent bone loss is conjugated estrogen 0.625 mg or its equivalent. Progestins appear to have a synergistic effect with estrogen on bone in preliminary studies, although the dose required to produce this effect is quite high.

There is epidemiologic evidence that estrogen replacement therapy reduces the risk of **coronary artery disease.** When considering the epidemiologic data on cardiovascular risk it is important to note that nearly all studies have looked at the effect of unopposed estrogen, as it is only recently that physicians have begun routinely to add progestins. Therefore, until recently there were no large studies looking at the combined effect of estrogens and progestins. In addition there are few available data from randomized clinical trials, only observational data. In a review of the available epidemiologic studies, 12 case control studies are described, 11 of which found a reduced risk of CAD in estrogen users versus nonusers. There are 13 prospective cohort studies, of which all but one found a reduced risk. When this group reanalyzed their data, they did indeed find a protective effect of estrogen in women aged 50 to 60. There are several cross-sectional angiographic studies, representing perhaps the strongest evidence to date that estrogen is cardioprotective. All studies looked at women who were hospitalized for cardiac catheterization, and all three found that women who were on estrogen had half the risk of severely stenotic lesions at the time of catheterization. Stroke risk appears to be unchanged in many studies. A recent reassuring population study (Falkeborn et al., 1992) suggests that risk of myocardial infarction appears to be comparable in women on combined hormones versus those on unopposed estrogen, suggesting that progestins may not have the negative impact that was initially feared.

The mechanism of estrogen's cardioprotective effect is not firmly established. Although it was initially believed that the protective effect of estrogen was due exclusively to lipid levels, it is now thought that only 30% to 50% of the beneficial effects can be explained by lipid level changes. The observation that both estrogen and progesterone receptors are present in vessel walls suggests that more direct mechanisms may play a role as well.

Sex steroids have well-known effects on **serum lipid levels**. At all ages after puberty women have higher high-density lipoprotein (HDL) levels and HDL-2 levels, and lower low-density lipoprotein (LDL) levels than men of the same age. Estrogen tends to cause an improvement in lipid profiles, whereas progestins cause a worsening. Studies of estrogen replacement in postmenopausal women have con-

BENEFITS OF HORMONE REPLACEMENT THERAPY

Estrogen
  Symptomatic relief
  Osteoporosis
  Coronary artery disease

Progestins
  Prevention of estrogen-induced endometrial cancer
  Possible synergistic effect with estrogen on bone

sistently shown increases of HDL and HDL-2 of approximately 12% and 25% when unopposed estrogen is used, with a decrease in LDL of approximately 12%. Progestins appear to negate some of the beneficial effect of estrogen. The testosterone derivatives appear to have more of an impact than medroxyprogesterone acetate; natural progesterone has the least impact. Oral preparations of natural progesterone are currently not approved by the Food and Drug Administration, and somnolence is a particularly bothersome side effect of this preparation. The optimal type, dose, and duration of progestin to minimize lipid effects are currently not known. Although there has been concern that the addition of progestins might negate the protective effect of estrogen on CAD, there are recent reassuring data from a population study that metabolic risk factors for CAD, including HDL and HDL-2 levels, are comparable in women taking combined estrogen-progestin regimens and those using unopposed estrogen.

Conjugated estrogen, 0.625 mg, has not been associated with increases in **blood pressure** with short-term use. It has been demonstrated that a natural estrogen, estropipate, may be associated with a mild blood pressure lowering effect when compared to conjugated estrogens, where no effect on blood pressure was seen. In this study the findings were the same in women with mild hypertension on antihypertensives, suggesting that replacement doses of estrogen appear to be safe, even in women with mild hypertension.

The risk of **gallbladder disease** appears to be slightly increased, but the associated morbidity and mortality rates are minimal. The effects of estrogen on **glucose tolerance** are dose-related, and replacement doses of estrogen have not been associated with abnormal glucose tolerance test results in postmenopausal women. Estrogen's effects on the **coagulation system** include an increase in clotting factors and thromboembolic events when high doses of estrogen are used. However, changes in clotting factors have not been consistently seen in postmenopausal women on replacement doses of estrogen. Clinically there appears to be no increased risk of deep venous thromboses or other thromboembolic events with estrogen replacement therapy.

Estrogen is very effective for relief of **vasomotor flushes** and **genitourinary atrophy**.

Choice of therapy. Indications for hormone replacement therapy are summarized in Table 36-1. There are currently three categories of hormone replacement regimens: unopposed estrogen, cyclic estrogen plus progestin, and continuous estrogen plus progestin.

Unopposed estrogen is indicated for women who have undergone hysterectomy, as there is currently no known role for adding a progestin other than to prevent the increased risk of estrogen-induced endometrial cancer. If unopposed estrogen is used in women with an intact uterus, routine endometrial sampling is essential. Bleeding patterns in women on unopposed estrogen are unpredictable, as these women may experience regular withdrawal bleeding, irregular bleeding, or amenorrhea. The pattern of bleeding does not predict endometrial histologic characteristics in this group. The standard unopposed estrogen regimen is conjugated equine estrogens (Premarin) 0.625 mg daily on days 1 to 25 of the calendar month (Table 36-2). There is evidence that the risk of endometrial cancer associated with uninter-

rupted use of estrogens is no different from that with regimens incorporating a 1-week interruption.

Cyclic use of combined estrogen and progestin is recommended for most postmenopausal women with an intact uterus. The most popular regimen in the United States has been conjugated estrogen 0.625 mg given daily (or days 1 to 25 of the calendar month) with 10 mg of medroxyprogesterone acetate for 12 consecutive days each month. However, the recent trend has been to decrease the dose of progestin, to minimize metabolic effects, while maximizing endometrial protection. Examples of these regimens are shown in Table 36-2.

One of the major drawbacks of the cyclic regimens is that 85% to 90% of women have monthly withdrawal bleeding. In an effort to avoid menses there has been recent emphasis on the use of **continuous combined estrogen and progestin regimens.** In the United States, continuous conjugated estrogen 0.625 mg is given with daily medroxyprogesterone acetate 2.5 mg (see Table 36-2). Although many studies now suggest that these regimens are protective of the endometrium, a beneficial effect on lipid profiles has not been firmly established. Of women using continuous combined regimens, 30% to 50% experience irregular bleeding that can last up to the sixth month of therapy. However, most women eventually have amenorrhea. The irregular bleeding seems to be more of a problem in perimenopausal women, and less of a problem in older postmenopausal women, who presumably have an atrophic endometrium before starting therapy.

Use of vaginal estrogen is an alternative regimen in women with symptomatic genitourinary atrophy who are not candidates for systemic estrogens. A commonly used regimen is conjugated equine estrogen (Premarin) cream, one half to one applicator daily for 3 weeks, followed by one half applicator once or twice weekly. A serum estradiol level greater than 30 pg/ml on this regimen warrants endometrial monitoring as for unopposed oral estrogens.

Contraindications to postmenopausal estrogen use (see box on the following page) include a history of estrogen-dependent neoplasia (breast and endometrial cancer) or active liver disease. Although a history of thromboembolic event has previously been considered to be an absolute contraindication to estrogen use, recent data do not support this notion. Estrogen use may be reasonable if the previous thromboembolic event did not occur in the setting of high-dose estrogen (i.e., oral contraceptives or pregnancy). In this instance transdermal estrogens should be considered, because of the lack of first-pass hepatic metabolism.

Monitoring. (See Table 36-3.) When assessing response to treatment in a symptomatic patient, there is no reliable parameter to follow aside from symptom relief. It takes up to 3 to 4 weeks for patients to have complete relief of hot flushes. Therefore, there is no role for increasing the dose before that time. Measuring serum FSH levels in general is not a useful way to monitor estrogen replacement, as extremely high doses of estrogen are necessary to suppress the FSH level into the premenopausal range. Estradiol level measurements are also not helpful in most instances, although persistent hot flushes with a serum estradiol level less than 20 pg/ml may suggest noncompliance. However, persistent flushes with an estradiol level greater than 150 pg/ml suggest another cause of the flushes.

Table 36-1 Indications for hormone replacement therapy

Indications	Rationale	Treatment	Onset	Duration	Other
Menopausal symptoms	Symptom relief	Systemic conjugated estrogens 0.625 mg* daily with appropriate progestin cycling; titrate estrogen dose to symptom relief	When symptoms become bothersome to patient during perimenopause or after menopause	6 months to several years	Taper estrogen over 6 to 12 months when discontinuing use; slower taper if symptoms recur
Genitourinary atrophy	Symptom relief or prevention of postmenopausal recurrent urinary tract infections	Systemic conjugated estrogens 0.3 mg daily with appropriate progestin cycling; or vaginal conjugated estrogens $\frac{1}{4}$ to 1 applicator daily to weekly	When symptoms become bothersome to patient	Indefinitely	Progestins warranted with long-term vaginal estrogen use if serum estradiol level >30 pg/ml
Prevention of osteoporosis and coronary artery disease	Risk reduction	Systemic conjugated estrogens 0.625 mg* daily with appropriate progestin cycling	Ideally within 6 to 12 months of menopause; preferably within 5 years of menopause	Uncertain; at least 8 years to produce significant reduction in osteoporosis risk	Cardiovascular effects of transdermal estrogens less well established
Treatment of osteoporosis	Prevention of future fractures	Systemic conjugated estrogens 0.625 mg* daily with appropriate progestin cycling	At diagnosis of osteoporotic fracture	Indefinite	Ensure adequate calcium and vitamin D intake
Treatment of premature menopause	Treatment of any symptoms; prevention of premature osteoporosis and coronary artery disease	Systemic conjugated estrogens 0.625 mg* daily with appropriate progestin cycling	At diagnosis	At least until expected age of menopause; generally at least 5 to 8 years beyond expected menopause	

*Equivalent doses of estrogen: oral conjugated estrogens (Premarin) 0.625 mg daily; oral estradiol-17β (Estrace) 2 mg daily; transdermal estradiol-17β (Estraderm) 0.050 mg twice weekly.

Pelvic and breast examinations as well as mammography should be performed at baseline and at yearly intervals during hormone replacement therapy. Endometrial biopsies should be performed before treatment and annually while on treatment for those on unopposed estrogen because of the known increased risk of endometrial hyperplasia and carcinoma. It is now agreed that pretreatment biopsy is not necessary for women on combined hormone regimens as these regimens have not been associated with an increased risk of endometrial cancer. The American College of Obstetricians and Gynecologists (ACOG) recently recommended that for the cyclic regimens biopsy should be performed if bleeding begins before the sixth day of progestin. For those on continuous regimens, biopsy recommendations are somewhat vague. However, most would agree that biopsy should be performed for heavy or prolonged bleeding, or bleeding that persists beyond the sixth month of therapy.

Table 36-2 Types of hormonal replacement regimens

	Dose	Duration (days)
Cyclic unopposed estrogens:		
Conjugated estrogens	0.625 mg	Daily or 1-25
Cyclic estrogens with progestins:		
Conjugated estrogen	0.625 mg	Daily or 1-25
Medroxyprogesterone acetate	10 mg	16-25
Conjugated estrogen	0.625 mg	Daily
Medroxyprogesterone acetate	5 mg	1-12
Continuous combined estrogen and progestin:		
Conjugated estrogen	0.625 mg	Daily
Medroxyprogesterone acetate	2.5-5 mg	Daily

CONTRAINDICATIONS TO HORMONE REPLACEMENT THERAPY

Absolute contraindications
 Known or suspected breast or uterine cancer
 Active liver disease
 Active thrombophlebitis or thromboembolic disorders

Relative contraindications
 Chronic hepatic dysfunction
 Family history of breast cancer

Table 36-3 Indications for endometrial biopsy

	Pretreatment	During treatment
Unopposed estrogen	Yes	Yearly
Cyclic estrogen and progestin	No	Irregular bleeding (before day 6 of progestin)
Continuous estrogen and progestin	No	Heavy or prolonged bleeding
		Bleeding >6 months

Alternatives to hormone replacement therapy for menopausal symptoms

Some women with menopausal symptoms are unable to have estrogen replacement because of other conditions—most commonly, breast cancer. Others prefer to use nonhormonal means of coping with symptoms such as hot flashes that may be bothersome but are self-limited.

A variety of **nonpharmacologic methods** of minimizing hot flashes are in common use, but have been little studied. Some of these methods involve avoidance of factors thought to precipitate hot flashes, including stress, hot weather or warm rooms, hot drinks, alcohol, caffeine, and spicy foods. Paced deep breathing, biofeedback, and other relaxation techniques have been helpful to some women.

Alternative drug therapies for hot flashes when estrogen is not suitable include clonidine (0.1 mg twice daily), medroxyprogesterone acetate (Provera) 10 mg daily, and β-blockers. Vaginal lubricants (such as Replens) are helpful for some women with symptomatic genitourinary atrophy.

SUMMARY

Menopause is a time when many women can benefit from examining their health habits and considering the available interventions for prevention of chronic disease. Although some women seek medical attention for symptoms related to menopause, the majority adapt well to this transition. The clinician should counsel all premenopausal women about what to expect at menopause and should review preventive measures, including the use of hormone replacement therapy.

Cost-benefit analyses of long-term postmenopausal estrogen use overwhelmingly support it because of the protective effect against osteoporosis and CAD. For women with an intact uterus, routine addition of progestins is recommended to prevent the estrogen-induced increase in endometrial cancer. It is possible that long-term use of estrogen is associated with a modest increase in breast cancer risk, but the effect of progestins on breast cancer risk remains unclear. Although it is not known what impact progestins will have on CAD risk, recent data suggest that progestins may not have the negative impact that was initially feared. Definitive studies on risk of breast cancer and prospective trials on cardiovascular risk with combined estrogen-progestin regimens will be essential to answer these important questions.

BIBLIOGRAPHY

ACOG Technical Bulletin 166:1, 1992.

Bergkvist L et al: Prognosis after breast cancer diagnosis in women exposed to estrogen and estrogen-progestogen replacement therapy, *Am J Epidemiol* 130:221, 1989.

Bergkvist L et al: The risk of breast cancer after estrogen and estrogen-progestin replacement, *N Engl J Med* 321:293, 1989.

Colditz G et al: Prospective study of estrogen replacement therapy and risk of breast cancer in postmenopausal women, *JAMA* 264:2648, 1990.

Devor M et al: Estrogen replacement therapy and the risk of venous thrombosis, *Am J Med* 92:275, 1992.

Dupont WD et al: Menopausal estrogen replacement therapy and breast cancer, *Arch Intern Med* 151:67, 1991.

Erlik Y et al: Association of waking episodes with menopausal hot flashes, *JAMA* 245:1741, 1981.

Falkeborn M et al: The risk of acute myocardial infarction after oestrogen and oestrogen-progestogen replacement, *Br J Obstet Gynaecol* 99:821, 1992.

Gallagher J, Kable W, Goldgar D: Effect of progestin therapy on cortical therapy on cortical and trabecular bone: comparison with estrogen, *Am J Med* 90:171, 1991.

Gordon T: Menopause and coronary heart disease, *Ann Intern Med* 89:157, 1978.

Grodin J et al: Source of estrogen production in postmenopausal women, *J Clin Endocrinol Metab* 36:207, 1973.

Hammar M et al: Climacteric symptoms in an unselected sample of Swedish women, *Maturitas* 6:345, 1984.

Lobo RA: Effects of hormonal replacement on lipids and lipoproteins in postmenopausal women, *J Clin Endocrinol Metab* 73:925, 1991.

Nabulsi AA et al: Association of hormone-replacement therapy with various cardiovascular risk factors in postmenopausal women, *N Engl J Med* 328:1069, 1993.

Notelovitz M et al: Combination estrogen and progestogen replacement therapy does not adversely affect coagulation, *Obstet Gynecol* 62:596, 1983.

Ottoson UB: Subfractions of high-density lipoprotein cholesterol during estrogen replacement therapy: a comparison between progesterone and natural progesterone, *Am J Obstet Gynecol* 151:746, 1985.

Richardson S et al: Follicular depletion during the menopausal transition; evidence for accelerated loss and ultimate exhaustion, *J Clin Endocrinol Metab* 65:231, 1987.

Schiff I et al: Effects of estrogens on sleep and psychological state of hypogonadal women, *JAMA* 242:2405, 1979.

Shapiro S et al: Risk of localized and widespread endometrial cancer in relation to recent and discontinued use of conjugated estrogens, *N Engl J Med* 313:969, 1985.

Sherman B et al: The menopausal transition: analysis of LH, FSH, estradiol, and progesterone concentrations during menstrual cycles of older women, *J Clin Endocrinol Metab* 42:629, 1976.

Stampfer MJ, Colditz GA: Estrogen replacement therapy and coronary heart disease: a quantitative assessment of the epidemiologic evidence, *Prev Med* 20:47, 1991.

Steinberg KK et al: A meta-analysis of the effect of estrogen replacement therapy on the risk of breast cancer, *JAMA* 265:1985, 1991.

Thom M: Effect of hormone replacement therapy on glucose tolerance in postmenopausal women, *Br J Obstet Gynecol* 84:776, 1977.

Weinstein L, Bewtra C, Gallagher J: Evaluation of a continuous combined low-dose regimen of estrogen-progestin for treatment of the menopausal patient, *Am J Obstet Gynecol* 162:1534, 1990.

Whitehead M, Hilliard T, Crook D: The role and use of progestogens, *Obstet Gynecol* 75:59S, 1990.

Wren BG et al: The effect of type and dose of oestrogen on the blood pressure of postmenopausal women, *Maturitas* 5:135, 1983.

37 Pelvic Masses

Karen J. Carlson and Isaac Schiff

Evaluation of a pelvic mass by the primary care physician is required when an asymptomatic mass is detected during a routine pelvic examination or when a woman bothered by pelvic pain or other symptoms is found to have a mass on examination or imaging study. In either case the initial diagnostic priorities are to identify disorders that require urgent intervention (e.g., ectopic pregnancy) and to determine whether a malignant condition is present. The diagnostic approach is based on clinical data and noninvasive imaging studies, particularly the use of ultrasonography.

This chapter outlines the approach to evaluation of a pelvic mass by the primary care clinician. Evaluation of pelvic pain, sometimes accompanied by a pelvic mass, is discussed in detail in Chapter 38.

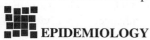

EPIDEMIOLOGY

Pelvic masses may arise from the uterus, ovaries, fallopian tubes, bowel, peritoneum, or urinary tract (see box, below). The prevalence of benign and malignant masses varies according to age and menopausal status. In women of reproductive age, one of the most common causes of an adnexal mass is a **functional ovarian cyst.** Such cysts may arise from the corpus luteum or follicle. A dominant follicle often measures close to 2 cm in diameter before ovulation. Functional ovarian cysts generally regress during the course of one or more menstrual cycles. Aside from use of the oral contraceptive pill, which is clearly protective, other factors affecting risk have not been defined.

Other disorders that may commonly manifest as a pelvic mass in the premenopausal woman include leiomyomas, endometriomas, and cystadenomas. **Ovarian cystadenomas** are benign epithelial tumors that have been reported to undergo malignant transformation. Women with a family history of ovarian cancer have been found to have a higher prevalence of serous cystadenomas than do women without such a history. The probability of malignant transformation is unknown.

In postmenopausal women, **ovarian cancer** is a more common cause of a pelvic mass. In published case series of postmenopausal women with adnexal masses who have undergone laparotomy, the prevalence of ovarian cancer has ranged from 30% to 60%. The annual incidence of ovarian cancer increases with age from approximately 20 per 100,000 in women younger than 50 years of age to 40 per 100,000 in women older than 50 years of age. The mean age at clinical presentation of ovarian cancer is 59 years.

Knowledge of risk factors for ovarian cancer is important in assessing the likelihood of malignancy from clinical data (Table 37-1). The strongest risk factor for ovarian cancer identified to date is familial evidence of the disease. There are two types of familial patterns: (1) hereditary ovarian cancer syndromes and (2) a family history of ovarian cancer in isolated female relatives without evidence of a hereditary pattern. Most women with familial evidence of ovarian cancer fall into the latter group, which carries a modestly increased risk. Other factors consistently shown to modify risk include parity and oral contraceptive pill use, which decrease risk by approximately one half.

DIFFERENTIAL DIAGNOSIS OF PELVIC MASSES

Benign

Ovarian

Simple cyst (follicle or corpus luteum)
Hemorrhagic cyst
Cystadenoma
Endometrioma
Teratoma
Other benign tumors: papilloma, fibroma

Nonovarian

Leiomyoma
Paraovarian cyst
Hydrosalpinx
Tuboovarian abscess
Ectopic pregnancy
Intrauterine pregnancy
Diverticulitis
Appendiceal abscess
Peritoneal inclusion cyst

Malignant

Ovarian

Epithelial ovarian carcinoma
Germ cell tumors of the ovary
Borderline tumors

Nonovarian

Leiomyosarcoma
Endometrial cancer
Carcinoma of fallopian tube
Colorectal carcinoma

Table 37-1 Risk factors for ovarian cancer

Factor	Relative risk
Age >50 yr	2
Familial ovarian cancer syndrome	Unknown; up to 50% lifetime risk
One first- or second-degree relative with ovarian cancer	3
Two or three relatives with ovarian cancer	5
Oral contraceptive pill use	0.65
Pregnancy	0.5

Modified from Carlson KJ, Skates SJ, Singer DE: *Ann Intern Med* 121:124, 1994.

The **postmenopausal enlarged ovary** is encountered with increasing frequency as use of diagnostic ultrasonography has expanded. The traditional teaching has been that a palpable ovary in a postmenopausal woman indicates a pathologic condition and requires further evaluation. However, it is now appreciated that the postmenopausal ovary is not totally quiescent and that benign ovarian cysts do occur in postmenopausal women.

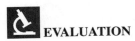 EVALUATION

History

The history focuses on assessment of reproductive factors, symptoms, and (particularly when the mass is adnexal) risk factors for ovarian cancer (see box, below). The possibility of ectopic pregnancy in a woman of reproductive age must always be considered. A careful menstrual history is essential, including the date of the last and previous menstrual periods, sexual history, and use of contraception. Risk factors for pelvic inflammatory disease, such as previous sexually transmitted disease and multiple sexual partners, also should be determined. The diagnosis of ectopic pregnancy and pelvic infection is discussed in more detail in Chapter 38.

Age and menopausal status are key elements of the history in assessing the likelihood of ovarian cancer. Symptoms of pelvic pain or discomfort, abnormal vaginal bleeding, and gastrointestinal problems should be sought. The relationship of the symptoms to the menstrual cycle (in premenopausal women) and other precipitating factors may provide useful clues. Women with ovarian cancer may experience abdominal swelling or bloating, nonspecific gastrointestinal complaints, and loss of appetite or weight loss.

Physical examination

Differentiation of uterine enlargement and adnexal masses is the first step in the physical examination. Uterine enlargement is caused most commonly by uterine leiomyomas, adenomyosis, or intrauterine pregnancy. The characteristics of the pelvic mass should be noted, as well as the presence of other abnormalities (such as cervical or uterine tenderness, cervical discharge, or bleeding).

Diagnostic tests

Pelvic ultrasonography is the single most important test in the evaluation of a pelvic mass. Ultrasound can differentiate a uterine from an adnexal mass, determine ovarian size and morphology, localize an ectopic pregnancy, identify extraovarian disease, and provide a preliminary assessment of the likelihood of malignancy in an ovarian mass. In addition to transabdominal ultrasonography, transvaginal sonography with use of an intravaginal probe is now widely available. Although direct comparisons are lacking, it is likely that transvaginal sonography offers enhanced sensitivity and specificity.

The sensitivity of pelvic ultrasonography for diagnosis of ovarian cancer in published series ranges from 80% to 90%; specificity varies widely, from 40% to 90%. Several scoring systems having been developed to predict malignancy according to the characteristics of ovarian masses. Although there is no universally accepted system for classification according to the likelihood of malignancy, existing systems generally incorporate some combination of ovarian size, inner wall structure, wall thickness, presence of septations, and echogenicity (Table 37-2).

Other imaging studies are sometimes appropriate. **Color-flow Doppler** techniques to detect tumor neovascularization have been studied in efforts to improve the specificity of ultrasound. **Magnetic resonance imaging** may prove valuable in the diagnosis of adenomyosis as the cause of uterine enlargement. Computed tomography is generally of less value than ultrasound in the evaluation of pelvic masses.

The use of other diagnostic tests in the initial evaluation should be guided by the results of the history and physical examination. In any woman of reproductive age with even a remote possibility of pregnancy, a urine or serum pregnancy test should be obtained. A complete blood count with differential and an erythrocyte sedimentation rate are useful in assessing the possibility of hemorrhage (as from a ruptured ectopic pregnancy) or infection.

The **CA125 radioimmunoassay** (CA125) is an important aid in the diagnosis of adnexal masses. CA125 is an antigenic determinant on a glycoprotein that is expressed by tissues derived from coelomic epithelium. It is shed in the blood stream by malignant cells arising from coelomic epithelium, and it is elevated in approximately 80% of ovarian cancers and advanced endometrial cancers, as well as in some pancreatic cancers and other solid tumors. It also is elevated in women with certain benign gynecologic conditions, including endometriosis, uterine leiomyoma, pelvic inflammatory disease, early pregnancy, and benign ovarian cysts. Serum levels have been shown to fluctuate during the menstrual cycle. The normal level generally is set at less than 35 U/ml.

EVALUATION OF PELVIC MASS

History

Reproductive factors

Menopausal status
Menstrual history
Sexual history: risk for pregnancy, pelvic inflammatory disease (PID)
Contraceptive use

Symptoms

Pelvic pain or discomfort
Bleeding
Gastrointestinal or urinary symptoms
Systemic symptoms: fever, weight loss, anorexia

Physical examination

Vital signs
Pelvic mass: size, shape, consistency, mobility, tenderness
Cervical, uterine tenderness; cervical discharge; bleeding
Abdominal and rectal examination

Diagnostic tests

Complete blood count, differential
Urine or serum beta-human chorionic gonadotropin (β-hCG)
Erythrocyte sedimentation rate (ESR)
Serum CA125 radioimmunoassay
Pelvic ultrasound

Table 37-2 Ultrasonographic features of an ovarian mass* and probability of malignancy

Feature	Probability of malignancy	
	Low	High
Inner wall	Smooth	Papillary
Wall thickness	Thin (<3 mm)	Thick (>3 mm)
Septations	None	Multiple
Echogenicity	Cystic (lucent)	Solid (echogenic)

*Normal ovarian volume: 7.5 cm³; enlarged ovary: >10 cm³.

In premenopausal women a serum CA125 level can aid in differentiating a cystic adnexal mass from an endometrioma, providing support for expectant management of an adnexal cyst. Pittaway and colleagues showed that a serum CA125 level less than 20 U/ml reliably identified nonendometriotic cysts from all cysts 4 cm or more in diameter. Because functional ovarian cysts are so common in premenopausal women, a reasonable approach would be to obtain a serum CA125 level if the ultrasonographic appearance of an adnexal mass was equivocal or if a benign-appearing cyst (particularly if larger than 4 cm) did not resolve during the course of one or two menstrual cycles.

In postmenopausal women, in whom the probability of ovarian cancer is considerably greater, a serum CA125 level should be obtained at the outset of the evaluation. On the basis of the published operating characteristics of serum CA125 (sensitivity 80%, specificity greater than 95%) in postmenopausal women with adnexal masses, obtaining an abnormal serum CA125 result shifts the estimated probability of malignancy from approximately 40% to more than 80%.

APPROACH TO THE PATIENT WITH A PELVIC MASS

The approach to the woman with a pelvic mass is guided by the patient's age and reproductive status, presenting complaints, and the results of history and physical examination. If the clinical findings are not suggestive of a process that requires urgent intervention (e.g., ectopic pregnancy, ovarian torsion, tuboovarian or appendiceal abscess), the first step generally is to obtain an ultrasonogram of the pelvis (Fig. 37-1).

For a premenopausal woman with an ultrasound finding that indicates a small simple cyst, it is appropriate for the primary care physician to repeat the physical and ultrasound examination in 1 to 3 months to assess resolution. When the cyst persists, a trial of the oral contraceptive pill may promote resolution and prevent recurrence. A serum CA125 level may help differentiate an endometrioma from a benign cyst. Additional research is needed to define the optimal use of the CA125 assay in this setting.

In a postmenopausal woman with a small cyst that has benign ultrasonographic characteristics, a serum CA125 level should be obtained and gynecologic consultation arranged.

When a simple cyst is greater than 6 to 8 cm in diameter, the chance of cyst rupture increases. In this situation, referral to a gynecologist for consideration of laparoscopy is appropriate. Functional cysts can be treated by puncture and biopsy or by laparoscopic cystectomy. If there are any equivocal ultrasonographic findings, a serum CA125 level and gynecology referral are indicated. Finally, if the ultrasound finding suggests malignancy, or if the serum CA125 is elevated in a postmenopausal woman, referral to a gynecologic oncologist is necessary.

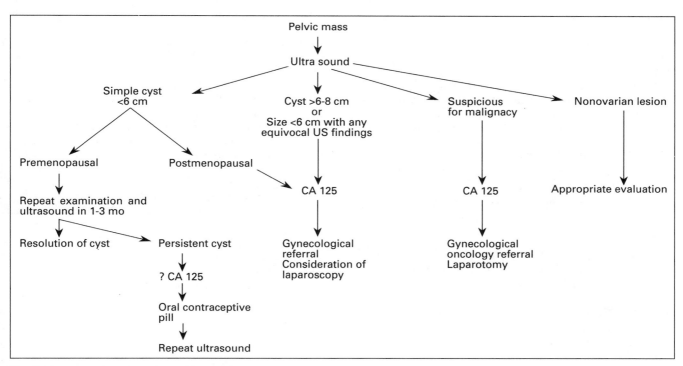

Fig. 37-1 Approach to the patient with a pelvic mass.

BIBLIOGRAPHY

Carlson KJ, Skates SJ, Singer DE: Screening for ovarian cancer, *Ann Intern Med* 121:124, 1994.

Finkler NJ et al: Comparison of serum CA125, clinical impression, and ultrasound in the preoperative evaluation of ovarian masses, *Obstet Gynecol* 72:659, 1988.

Herrman JR, Locher GW, Goldhirsch A: Sonographic patterns of ovarian tumors: prediction of malignancy, *Obstet Gynecol* 69:777, 1987.

Kerlikowske K, Brown JS, Grady DG: Should women with familial ovarian cancer undergo prophylactic oophorectomy? *Obstet Gynecol* 80:700, 1992.

Luxman D et al: The postmenopausal adnexal mass: correlation between ultrasonic and pathologic findings, *Obstet Gynecol* 77:726, 1991.

Malkasian GD Jr et al: Preoperative evaluation of serum CA 125 levels in premenopausal and postmenopausal patients with pelvic masses: discrimination of benign from malignant disease, *Am J Obstet Gynecol* 159:341, 1988.

Parker WH, Berek JS: Management of the adnexal mass by operative laparoscopy, *Clin Obstet Gynecol* 36:413, 1993.

Pittaway DE, Fayex JA, Douglas JW: Serum CA 125 in the evaluation of benign adnexal cysts, *Am J Obstet Gynecol* 157:1426, 1987.

Whittemore AS, Harris R, Itnyre J: Characteristics relating to ovarian cancer risk: collaborative analysis of twelve U.S. case-control studies. II. Invasive epithelial ovarian cancers in white women, *Am J Epidemiol* 136:1184, 1992.

38 Pelvic Pain

Kathleen F. Thurmond

Pelvic pain is a common problem in the primary care of women. In recent years there has been an explosion of scientific knowledge and technology allowing early diagnosis of acute pelvic pain. However, there is a surprising dearth of clinical research on the causes of and treatments for chronic pelvic pain.

The problem of pelvic pain presents challenges in both diagnosis and treatment. The challenge in diagnosing pelvic pain is to identify causes that, inadequately treated, may lead to serious short-term sequelae (internal hemorrhage and fulminant infection) or long-term complications (chiefly infertility). The management of chronic pelvic pain, in view of the uncertainty about the cause of this complex problem and sparse scientific evidence to guide treatment, presents an equally challenging clinical task.

The evaluation of pelvic pain begins with differentiating acute and chronic pelvic pain. This chapter addresses the evaluation of acute and chronic pelvic pain and the management of chronic (idiopathic) pelvic pain and dysmenorrhea.

ACUTE PELVIC PAIN

Acute pelvic pain is pain that has been present for hours or days; in some cases pain may develop over the course of a few weeks. Causes of acute pelvic pain are listed in the box at right.

Differential diagnosis

Ectopic pregnancy. An ectopic pregnancy is a pregnancy that implants in a location other than the endometrial cavity of the uterus. Most ectopic pregnancies are located in the tube (tubal pregnancy), within the ovarian cortex (ovarian pregnancy), between the leaves of the broad ligament (ligamentous pregnancy), or within the abdominal cavity (abdominal pregnancy). An ectopic pregnancy and an intrauterine pregnancy can coexist, although this condition is very rare.

The incidence of ectopic pregnancy has been increasing over the past three decades. This increase may be related to

the increasing number of women who have had pelvic inflammatory disease, tubal ligation, an intrauterine device (IUD), prior surgery to treat infertility, a previous ectopic pregnancy, or reversal of a tubal ligation.

Spontaneous abortion. An early abortion is loss of a pregnancy before the completion of 22 gestational weeks. About 10% of all pregnancies over 6 menstrual weeks spontaneously abort; earlier pregnancy losses are even more common.

Adnexal cyst or mass. Adnexal cysts or masses may cause acute pelvic pain if their location results in stretching of tissue or pressure on adjacent organs, if rapid growth occurs, or if rupture or torsion occurs.

Pelvic inflammatory disease. Pelvic inflammatory disease (PID), the commonly used term for active infection or chronic inflammation of the endometrium, tubes, or ovaries (with or without a pelvic abscess), is a frequent cause of acute pelvic pain. The pathogens most frequently implicated in PID are *Neisseria gonorrhoeae, Chlamydia trachomatis,* anaerobic and facultative anaerobic bacteria (particularly *Bacteroides* spp., *Escherichia coli,* and groups B and D *Streptococcus* spp.). It is not clear whether genital

---

CAUSES OF ACUTE PELVIC PAIN

More common
  Ectopic pregnancy
  Spontaneous, incomplete, or threatened abortion
  Adnexal mass or cyst
  Pelvic inflammatory disease
  Appendicitis
  Urinary tract infection

Less common
  Degenerating fibroid
  Ureteral obstruction
  Intestinal obstruction
  Diverticulitis

mycoplasma is a pathogen implicated in PID. Risk factors for PID include multiple sexual partners, previous gonorrhea, and use of the intrauterine contraceptive device.

Appendicitis. Appendicitis must always be considered as a potential cause of pelvic pain. Appendicitis reaches its maximum incidence in the second and third decades of life. The female to male ratio is about two to three until after age 25, when the incidence begins to equalize between the sexes.

Chronic appendicitis is seen in a small number of patients in whom the attack of acute appendicitis subsides spontaneously, followed by recurrent, usually milder attacks of right lower quadrant pain. If it is erroneously diagnosed as pelvic inflammatory disease, the antibiotic course may result in temporary improvement.

Urinary tract disorders. Lower urinary tract infection and urethritis can cause acute suprapubic pressure, pain, or a pulling sensation that intensifies with urination. Other common symptoms are dysuria, frequency, urgency, and hesitancy. Evaluation and management of acute dysuria are discussed in Chapter 18.

Evaluation

The first task in evaluating a woman with acute pelvic pain is to assess whether a potentially life-threatening condition, such as internal hemorrhage caused by a ruptured ectopic pregnancy or septic shock related to a ruptured ovarian abscess or septic abortion, is present. Signs of significant hypovolemia, hypotension, or peritonitis should prompt immediate referral to a gynecologist for emergency laparotomy or laparoscopy.

When there is no immediate evidence of a life-threatening condition the evaluation of acute pelvic pain focuses on rapid assessment for potentially serious conditions. These include ectopic pregnancy, pelvic inflammatory disease, appendicitis, and rupture or torsion of an ovarian cyst. (See Table 38-1.)

History. An **ectopic pregnancy** must be ruled out in any woman of reproductive age who has pelvic pain or abnormal vaginal bleeding. Pain and abnormal bleeding are sometimes, but not always, present in ectopic pregnancy. Pain is caused by localized bleeding, which occurs when the trophoblast invades blood vessels and the serosa is stretched. Pelvic pain may be dull or sharp, localized or diffuse.

Many patients with ectopic pregnancy have some abnormal bleeding; however, the absence of bleeding does not rule out ectopic pregnancy. When taking a menstrual history, it is important to determine the last menstrual period (LMP) and to confirm that it was normal in flow, length, and onset. The same information should be obtained about the previous menstrual period (PMP). Otherwise, aberrant bleeding that occurred any time up to 4 weeks before the evaluation may be erroneously considered a normal LMP.

Spontaneous abortion may produce pelvic pain (typically uterine cramping) and abnormal vaginal bleeding as the products of conception are expelled. A threatened abortion is characterized by light bleeding and mild cramping without evidence of passed tissue; the cervical os remains closed.

Pain from an **adnexal mass** or cyst is usually lateralized, unless the involved adnexa is in the midline, in which case mid-lower abdominal pain may be present.

PID typically causes diffuse lower abdominal pain, which may be more severe on one side if there is a unilateral tuboovarian abscess. Increased vaginal discharge, fever, chills, nausea, and vomiting may be present.

In **appendicitis** the typical sequence of symptoms is pain in the epigastrium or around the umbilicus, followed by anorexia, nausea, and sometimes vomiting. Although the pain typically localizes to the right lower quadrant, it may remain diffuse. Approximately 45% of patients experience atypical pain.

Physical examination. Physical findings in **ectopic pregnancy** span the spectrum from an entirely normal examination to hypotension with obvious peritoneal signs. On pelvic examination there may be blood in the vagina with or without cervical motion tenderness. Adnexal tenderness may be present, with or without a mass, on the side of the ectopic pregnancy or on the side of the corpus luteum, which may be contralateral to the pregnancy.

Depending on gestational age and stage of abortion the physical examination in **spontaneous abortion** can reveal an enlarged uterus, an adnexal mass associated with a corpus luteum cyst, and evidence of uterine bleeding with an open or closed cervical os.

In **PID** the abdominal examination typically reveals diffuse lower abdominal tenderness. Peritonitis, if present, can result in rebound and guarding. Right upper quadrant pain or tenderness suggests that perihepatic inflammation is present (Fitz-Hugh–Curtis syndrome). Pelvic examination often indicates increased vaginal discharge, cervical motion tenderness, and bilateral adnexal tenderness. A palpable mass should alert the clinician to a possible tuboovarian abscess.

Appendicitis may manifest without fever, even when rupture has occurred. There is either diffuse or right lower quadrant tenderness, sometimes with guarding or rebound. Rectal examination may elicit right lower quadrant tenderness, and occasionally a right lower quadrant mass is palpable. Some manifestations of appendicitis may be difficult to distinguish from PID, especially when the woman has diffuse abdominal pain and pelvic examination reveals cervical motion tenderness and diffuse pelvic tenderness.

Diagnostic tests. The basic laboratory evaluation of pelvic pain includes a complete blood count with differential, sedimentation rate, serum or urine pregnancy test, and urinalysis.

In **ectopic pregnancy** and **spontaneous abortion** the hematocrit and hemoglobin may be normal, or low if significant bleeding has occurred. Leukocytosis and an elevated erythrocyte sedimentation rate (ESR) are present in more severe cases of PID but may be lacking in mild cases. Although the white blood count is most often elevated in appendicitis, it is estimated that 30% of patients have a normal white blood count. However, there is usually a left shift in the differential, even when the total white blood count is not elevated.

When an ectopic pregnancy exists, the serum β-hCG is always >10 mlU/ml; human chorionic gonoadotropin (hCG) is also elevated in spontaneous abortion. Serum β-hCG levels should double about every 2 days in a normal pregnancy. In an ectopic pregnancy the level of serum β-hCG is often less than what would be expected for a normal pregnancy at the same gestational age.

A single serum progesterone level is useful in the diagnosis of suspected ectopic pregnancy and spontaneous abor-

Table 38-1 Evaluation of acute pelvic pain

Cause	History	Physical examination	Diagnostic tests*
Ectopic pregnancy	Nonspecific pelvic pain with or without abnormal vaginal bleeding	Normal or low blood pressure; orthostatic hypotension Normal pulse or tachycardia; orthostatic tachycardia Blood in vagina Adnexal tenderness Peritoneal signs	Hct and Hb normal or low Serum β-hCG >10 mlU/ml Serum progesterone level ≤25 ng/ml Ultrasound showing empty uterus and possibly adnexal mass or cyst
Spontaneous abortion	Cramping pelvic pain, abnormal vaginal bleeding	Enlarged uterus Cervical os open or closed Blood or tissue in cervix or vagina	Serum β-hCG >10 mlU/ml Serum progesterone ≤25 ng/ml Ultrasound showing intrauterine pregnancy or tissue
Adnexal mass or cyst	Unilateral pelvic pain	Unilateral mass or fullness Adnexal tenderness	Ultrasound showing mass
Pelvic inflammatory disease	Diffuse pelvic pain; may be lateralized if tuboovarian abscess present Vaginal discharge	Normal or elevated temperature Vaginal or cervical discharge Diffuse pelvic and/or cervical motion tenderness Adnexal mass (tuboovarian abscess)	Normal or increased WBC Normal or increased ESR Increased polys in cervical secretions Ultrasound may show tuboovarian abscess
Appendicitis	Epigastric or periumbilical pain localizing to right lower quadrant Diffuse abdominal pain Anorexia, nausea, vomiting	Normal or elevated temperature Right lower quadrant tenderness and/or mass	Normal or increased WBC Left shift in differential cell count

Hct, hematocrit; Hb, hemoglobin; β-hCG, beta-human chorionic gonodotropin; WBC, white blood cell count; ESR, erythrocyte sedimentation rate; polys, polymorphonuclear leukocytes.

tion, particularly when the date of the LMP is uncertain. Progesterone is produced by the corpus luteum in a viable intrauterine pregnancy. When the β-hCG finding is positive, a single progesterone level can be used to exclude ectopic pregnancy (when the level is appropriately high) and to identify nonviable pregnancies (when the level is inappropriately low). A serum progesterone level ≥25 ng/ml has over 97% sensitivity for exclusion of ectopic pregnancy. A level ≤5 ng/ml identifies nonviable pregnancy with 100% specificity. Levels between 5 and 25 ng/ml indicate the need for ultrasonography to determine viability.

When PID is suspected, cervical cultures for gonorrhea and culture or antigen detection test for chlamydia should be obtained. The utility of mycoplasma cultures in the initial evaluation of acute pelvic pain has not been established. A wet mount of cervical secretions classically shows more than one polymorphonuclear leukocyte for each epithelial cell, or more than 30/1000 × microscopic field.

Pelvic ultrasonography is one of the most useful diagnostic tests in the evaluation of acute pelvic pain. A pelvic ultrasound should be performed if ectopic pregnancy is suggested. Ultrasonography may be unable to determine whether an intrauterine pregnancy exists before 5 weeks' gestation or when the β-hCG level is less than 2000 mlU/ml. In suspect-

ed spontaneous abortion, ultrasonography should be performed; it may show an intrauterine pregnancy or some pregnancy tissue in the uterus or vagina. Dilation and curettage would be necessary if there were residual pregnancy tissue or a nonviable pregnancy. If the cause of acute pelvic pain is unclear after the history and physical examination, ultrasonography is the next step in diagnosis. The result may be abnormal in appendicitis if there is a markedly enlarged appendix or appendiceal abscess, or in PID if there is a tuboovarian abscess. Pelvic ultrasonography should be performed when adnexal mass is detected or suspected (see Chapter 37).

Management

Ectopic pregnancy. If a woman has a positive pregnancy test result, an ultrasound without evidence of an intrauterine pregnancy, and pelvic pain, referral to a gynecologist is necessary. Laparoscopy with surgical removal of the ectopic pregnancy has been the standard approach. Laparotomy may be necessary in certain situations. In some cases medical therapy with systemic methotrexate is an alternative to conservative surgical management.

Because a woman's risk of ectopic pregnancy is increased by its initial occurrence, it is important to instruct her to seek medical attention early in any future pregnancy for serial serum β-hCG titers and appropriately timed ultrasonography. Early diagnosis permits conservative surgical management of ectopic pregnancy.

Spontaneous abortion. Management of threatened, incomplete, and complete abortion is discussed in Chapter 48.

Adnexal mass. Further evaluation and management of an adnexal mass are discussed in Chapter 37.

PID. Outpatient treatment for PID is appropriate when the woman can take oral medication, is available for follow-up evaluation, and has no signs of severe infection. A combination regimen with broad coverage of the typical pathogens in PID is ceftriaxone 250 mg intramuscularly (IM) (or cefoxitin sodium 2.0 g IM with probenecid 1.0 g orally), followed by doxycycline 100 mg bid for 14 days. Initial therapy can be modified, depending on the results of culture (see Chapter 17 for management of specific sexually transmitted diseases). The patient should be reassessed after 48 to 72 hours of outpatient antibiotic therapy, and sexual partners should be examined and treated for sexually transmitted diseases.

Admission for intravenous antibiotics is needed when there is evidence of a tuboovarian abscess, when nausea or vomiting precludes use of oral antibiotics, in pregnancy, or when there are signs of a severe infection.

Appendicitis. A woman with suspected appendicitis should be referred for laparoscopy or laparotomy, depending on the certainty of the diagnosis.

CHRONIC PELVIC PAIN

The term *chronic pelvic pain* has been used to denote the symptom of recurrent pelvic discomfort and also as a specific diagnosis (characterized by pelvic pain present for at least 6 months with no evidence of an organic cause after thorough evaluation, including laparoscopy). Conditions causing pelvic pain that is persistent or recurrent over months to years are listed in the box at right.

Causes

Dysmenorrhea. Primary dysmenorrhea is cyclic uterine pain that occurs before or during menses in the absence of any significant pelvic abnormality. It is thought to be caused by prostaglandins produced by the endometrium. Secondary dysmenorrhea may be caused by endometriosis, adenomyosis, and fibroids (if clots large enough to produce cramps are passed). Hematometrium, a collection of menstrual blood distending the endometrial cavity in the presence of cervical stenosis, is a rare cause of secondary dysmenorrhea.

Endometriosis. Endometriosis is a condition in which endometrial tissue implants in extrauterine locations, such as the pelvic peritoneum, uterine ligaments, ovaries, tubes, cervix, bowel, bladder, and rarely more distant sites. Endometriosis is discussed in detail in Chapter 33.

Adenomyosis. Adenomyosis is the presence of endometrial tissue ectopically located within the myometrium. Adenomyosis is common, occurring in over 50% of uteruses in some series, but often asymptomatic.

Adhesions. Adhesions, or scar tissue, are thought to cause pelvic pain by producing abnormal adherence between adjacent organs. Adhesions are more common when there has been prior pelvic infection or surgery. The mechanism for pain related to adhesions is unclear. The prevalence of adhesions (15% to 20%) is similar in women with no history of pelvic pain undergoing laparoscopy for infertility and those undergoing laparoscopy for pelvic pain. Laparoscopic lysis of adhesions has been reported to reduce symptoms in 40% to 75% of cases.

Fibroids. Fibroids (leiomyomas), benign fibromuscular growths within the uterus, are thought to cause chronic pelvic pain by pressure on adjacent organs or, in the case of degenerating fibroids, by outgrowing their blood supply. Fibroids are discussed in detail in Chapter 41.

Pelvic pain after gynecologic surgery. Retained ovary syndrome is a syndrome of recurrent adnexal pain after hysterectomy. The incidence of it is unknown. Pelvic adhesions, follicular cysts, and hemorrhagic corpus luteum cysts within the retained ovaries are among the suggested explanations. The only known treatment is oophorectomy.

Studies of late sequelae of tubal ligation have found chronic pelvic pain in a small number of women after tubal ligation. The mechanism is unclear; torsion of the ovary and ischemia have been proposed as possible causes.

Pelvic congestion. The role of pelvic congestion in chronic pelvic pain is controversial. The theory that pelvic congestion related to pelvic venous varicosities can cause chronic pelvic pain has been extensively researched at a single British center. In these studies varicosities have been seen on venography or transvaginal ultrasonography, and improvement in symptoms has been demonstrated in randomized trials of high-dose medroxyprogesterone acetate.

Other causes. A report of the multidisciplinary evaluation of chronic pelvic pain in women with negative laparoscopy findings (Reiter and Gambone, 1991) indicates that **myofascial pain syndrome** can be a cause of pelvic pain, along with **irritable bowel syndrome** and other gastrointestinal disorders, chronic **pelvic infection**, and urinary tract disorders.

Evaluation

A woman with chronic pelvic pain can also have an acute cause of pelvic pain. Once the causes of acute pain (described

---

CAUSES OF CHRONIC PELVIC PAIN

Gynecologic disorders
   Primary dysmenorrhea
   Endometriosis
   Adenomyosis
   Adhesions
   Fibroids
   Retained ovary syndrome posthysterectomy
   Previous tubal ligation
   Chronic pelvic infection

Musculoskeletal disorders
   Myofascial pain syndrome

Gastrointestinal disorders
   Irritable bowel syndrome
   Inflammatory bowel disease

Urinary tract disorders
   Interstitial cystitis
   Nonbacterial urethritis

---

previously) have been ruled out, the evaluation of chronic pelvic pain can proceed in a stepwise fashion (see Table 38-2).

History. In addition to characterizing the symptom of pain, gynecologic history (pelvic infections, IUD use or tubal ligation, pelvic or abdominal surgery), and any other gynecologic symptoms (such as irregular or excessive vaginal bleeding), the history should also address other organ systems that may be responsible for pelvic pain. Associated gastrointestinal symptoms such as diarrhea, constipation, and more generalized abdominal discomfort should be sought. Urinary symptoms such as dysuria, urgency, and frequency (with a negative urine culture result) may suggest interstitial cystitis or nonbacterial urethritis. Low back pain, unilateral or bilateral leg pain, or coccygeal pain may suggest a musculoskeletal process.

The woman's general health, nutritional status, and exercise habits should be assessed. The clinician should inquire about unrelated somatic symptoms and the extent of any past evaluation; such symptoms have been reported more frequently in women with chronic pelvic pain.

A careful exploration of psychosocial factors is essential. The prevalence of childhood sexual abuse in women with chronic pelvic pain has been reported at 20% to 60%, and of childhood physical abuse at 40%. Women with chronic pelvic pain have also been found to have a higher number of sexual partners than women having routine care. The clinician should be alert to the presence of depression (see Chapter 67) or a somatization disorder (see Chapter 74). Indications for referral are shown in the box on the following page.

Endometriosis may cause cyclic pelvic pain, which may not be relieved by nonsteroidal antiinflammatory drugs (NSAIDs) or oral contraceptives. If adhesions or an endometrioma has developed, pelvic pain can occur throughout the menstrual cycle. The pain may be unilateral or diffuse. Dyspareunia may be present if there are significant uterosacral ligament implants, adhesions, or an endometrioma.

The clinical presentation of **adenomyosis** has not been well described, but progressively worsening dysmenorrhea and menorrhagia are thought to be typical symptoms.

Pain attributed to **adhesions** can occur without provocation, or with activities that put tension on the adhesions, such as intercourse, exercise, defecation, ovulation, or filling or emptying of the bladder. The nature of the pain is nonspecific.

Physical examination. The pelvic examination result in endometriosis may be normal or may reveal diffuse or localized tenderness. The classic finding of nodularity on rectovaginal examination may be absent. A pelvic mass suggests the presence of an endometrioma. In adenomyosis the uterus is typically diffusely enlarged (though not generally above 12 weeks' gestational size) and soft. Adhesions may produce no abnormality on examination. Fibroids are typically palpable as a bulky enlarged uterus, or a midline or adnexal mass, but may not be detectable on examination.

Diagnostic testing. Initial laboratory testing includes a complete blood count with differential, urinalysis, and (when sexually transmitted disease is possible), antigen detection test or culture for chlamydia and culture for gonorrhea, and

Table 38-2 Evaluation of chronic pelvic pain

Cause	History	Physical examination	Diagnostic tests
Primary dysmenorrhea	Cyclic uterine cramping	Normal pelvic examination finding	None
Endometriosis	Cyclic or constant pelvic pain, unilateral or diffuse Dyspareunia Premenstrual spotting	Pelvic examination result may be normal Adnexal tenderness or mass Tender nodules on rectovaginal examination Uterus with limited mobility	Ultrasound may show endometrioma; often produces normal findings Laparoscopy required for definitive diagnosis
Adenomyosis	Progressively worsening cyclic cramping Heavy menstrual bleeding	Mildly enlarged, soft uterus	Sometimes detectable by MRI
Adhesions	Previous pelvic or abdominal surgery Nonspecific pain, sometimes related to specific activities	Often normal Diffuse or localized tenderness	Requires laparoscopy for definitive diagnosis
Chronic pelvic infection	Risk factors for PID Localized or diffuse noncyclic pain	Normal or elevated temperature Diffuse pelvic tenderness Adnexal tenderness or mass Cervical motion tenderness	Normal or increased WBC, ESR Culture or antigen detection test for *Chlamydia* spp.; mycoplasma and gonococcal cultures
Fibroids	Heavy menstrual bleeding Cyclic or constant pelvic pressure or pain	Uterine enlargement Adnexal or midline mass Pelvic examination result may be normal	Hct/Hb result normal or decreased Ultrasound showing single or multiple myomas
Idiopathic	Unilateral or diffuse cyclic or noncyclic pain	Diffuse or localized pelvic tenderness, no masses	Diagnosed by exclusion of other causes

MRI, magnetic resonance imaging; PID, pelvic inflammatory disease; WBC, white blood cell count; ESR, erythrocyte sedimentation rate; Hct, hematocrit; Hb, hemoglobin.

Acute pelvic pain

Signs of intraabdominal hemorrhage or peritonitis
Known or suspected ectopic pregnancy
Spontaneous, incomplete, or threatened abortion
Pelvic inflammatory disease with tuboovarian abscess
Suspected appendicitis

Chronic pelvic pain

Dysmenorrhea refractory to NSAIDs and/or oral
    contraceptive pill or with suspected endometriosis
Consideration of laparoscopy when diagnosis uncertain
    after initial evaluation
Symptomatic uterine fibroids
Idiopathic chronic pelvic pain, for multidisciplinary
    management

NSAIDs, nonsteroidal antiinflammatory drugs.

microscopic examination of cervical secretions. Mycoplasma cultures may be appropriate in cases of suspected chronic pelvic infection and in the evaluation of dysmenorrhea.

Pelvic ultrasonography should be performed to detect fibroids and to rule out a pelvic mass as the cause of pain. Magnetic resonance imaging (MRI) may prove useful in diagnosing adenomyosis. Use of unselected radiographic studies such as barium enema and intravenous pyelography has been shown to have limited value. Barium enema or colonoscopy should be reserved for evaluation of gastrointestinal symptoms when the diagnosis of irritable bowel syndrome is uncertain.

The standard approach to evaluation of chronic pelvic pain that is undiagnosed after the initial evaluation is laparoscopy. Laparoscopy has been shown to identify pelvic abnormality in 60% to 80% of women with chronic pelvic pain, compared to 30% of those undergoing tubal ligation. An alternative approach, supported by a single randomized trial (Peters et al., 1991), limits use of laparoscopy in the context of a multidisciplinary evaluation that includes psychologic, nutritional, and physical therapy assessments. In this setting laparoscopy was found to have an unimportant role in diagnosis and treatment.

Management

Dysmenorrhea. Initial treatment for dysmenorrhea is **nonsteroidal antiinflammatory drugs (NSAIDs)**. The effectiveness of NSAIDs for relieving primary dysmenorrhea is approximately 70%. There are no data on the relative efficacy of different NSAIDs for this condition. Commonly used regimens include naproxen sodium 375 to 750 mg bid, ibuprofen 200 to 800 mg qid, and mefenamic acid 250 to 500 mg bid. Effectiveness is greater when medications are started 1 day in advance of expected onset of pain. The oral **contraceptive pill** is also effective for dysmenorrhea. It acts to reduce endometrial prostaglandin production by decreasing the amount of endometrium that is built up in each cycle.

Pain that is not relieved by trials of multiple NSAIDs or the oral contraceptive pill warrants consideration of laparoscopy to rule out endometriosis.

Idiopathic chronic pelvic pain. The clinician should approach treatment of idiopathic chronic pelvic pain by appreciating that the causes of pain are complex, and that scientific data to guide therapy are limited. Principles for treatment of any chronic pain syndrome are applicable here. These include (1) the establishment of an ongoing relationship and contacts between clinician and patient, independent of the presence of pain symptoms; (2) an empathic attitude in the clinician and validation of the woman's experience of pain; (3) a focus on learning to adapt to pain symptoms, including use of relaxation techniques and exercise; (4) an expressed willingness of the clinician to reopen a diagnostic evaluation when new evidence warrants.

The high prevalence of a history of sexual and physical abuse in women with chronic pelvic pain highlights the importance of psychosocial factors as causes of this pain syndrome. The clinician must become comfortable in inquiring in a sensitive way about a history of abuse.

A multidisciplinary approach to chronic pelvic pain is most effective. A randomized trial of multidisciplinary treatment showed that attention to somatic, psychologic, nutritional, environmental, and physical conditioning factors (with selective use of laparoscopy) was more effective at 1 year than standard care that emphasized medications and laparoscopy. Provision of specialized care in a multidisciplinary setting may reduce the stigma associated with psychologic evaluation and treatment and enhance a woman's ability to address the nonsomatic aspects of her condition. Although multidisciplinary units are not widely available, these findings suggest that treatment of chronic pelvic pain by individual clinicians should include psychologic evaluation (and therapy when indicated), referral for physical therapy (if therapists are experienced in treatment of chronic pelvic pain), and nutritional assessment.

Medical therapy of chronic pelvic pain is reasonable as one component of management. Treatment typically is initiated with NSAIDs or (particularly when cyclic pain is present) the oral contraceptive pill. Use of narcotic analgesics should be avoided because of the high risk of dependency. Limited data on the effectiveness of antidepressant treatments suggest that nortriptyline (and probably other antidepressants) may be beneficial.

Surgical treatment for chronic pelvic pain has included hysterectomy with or without bilateral salpingooophorectomy. Studies have shown that 5% to 20% of women undergoing hysterectomy for idiopathic chronic pelvic pain report persistent pain more than a year after surgery. Consideration of hysterectomy should take place only after more conservative medical therapy has failed, and after thorough psychologic evaluation has ruled out a somatization disorder, a posttraumatic disorder, or depression.

BIBLIOGRAPHY

Andolsek KM: Ectopic pregnancy: classic vs. common presentation, *J Fam Pract* 5:481, 1987.
Beral V: An epidemiological study of recent trends in ectopic pregnancy, *Br J Obstet Gynaecol* 82:775, 1975.
Braunstein GD et al: Subclinical spontaneous abortion, *Obstet Gynecol* 50:41, 1977.
Carson SA, Buster JE: Ectopic pregnancy, *N Engl J Med* 329:1174, 1993.
Check JH, Weiss RM, Lurie D: Analysis of serum human chorionic gonadotropin levels in normal singleton, multiple and abnormal pregnancies, *Hum Reprod* 7:2176, 1992.

Farquhar CM et al: A randomized controlled trial of medroxyprogesterone acetate and psychotherapy for the treatment of pelvic congestion, *Br J Obstet Gynaecol* 96:1153, 1989.

Harris WJ, Daniell JF, Baxter JW: Prior cesarean section a risk factor for adenomyosis? *J Reprod Med* 30:173, 1985.

Lewis FM et al: Appendicitis: a critical review of diagnosis and treatment in 1000 cases, *Arch Surg* 110:677, 1975.

Noer T: Decreasing incidence of acute appendicitis, *Acta Chir Scand* 41:431, 1975.

Nyberg DA et al: Early gestation: correlation of hCG levels and sonographic indentification, *Am J Roentgenol* 144:951, 1985.

Peters A et al: A randomized clinical trial to compare two different approaches in women with chronic pelvic pain, *Obstet Gynecol* 77:740, 1991.

Reiter RC, Gambone JC: Nongynecologic somatic pathology in women with chronic pelvic pain and negative laparoscopy, *J Reprod Med* 36:253, 1991.

Rocker I: *Pelvic pain in women: diagnosis and management,* London, 1990, Springer-Verlag.

Saferins S et al: Long-term sequelae of acute pelvic inflammatory disease, *Am J Obstet Gynecol* 166:1300, 1992.

Scott GR et al: Infection with *Chlamydia trachomatis* and *Neisseria gonorrhoea* in women with lower abdominal pain admitted to a gynaecology unit, *Br J Obstet Gynaecol* 96:473, 1989.

Walker E et al: Relationship of chronic pelvic pain to psychiatric diagnosis and childhood sexual abuse, Am J Psychiatry 145:1, 1988.

39 Premenstrual Syndrome

Karen J. Carlson and Kathleen Hubbs Ulman

DEFINITION

In recent years the term *premenstrual syndrome* (PMS) has come to be used in everyday parlance to refer to a variety of unpleasant symptoms associated with the menstrual cycle. The diagnostic criteria and nomenclature for premenstrual syndrome are often unclear to both physicians and patients. The appropriate definition of premenstrual syndrome depends on the context in which the diagnosis is being considered.

A research definition of PMS was initially proposed through the National Institute for Mental Health. This definition stipulates that all subjects diagnosed as having PMS demonstrate a 30% increase in average symptom severity for the 5 days before menstruation when compared with the average of the 5 days after menstruation.

The *Diagnostic and Statistical Manual of Mental Disorders (DSM-IV)* includes "premenstrual dysphoric disorder" in the category of research criteria needing further study (see box, right). "Premenstrual dysphoric disorder" is not yet a clinical psychiatric diagnosis. *DSM-IV* suggests that "depressive disorder not otherwise specified" be used when symptoms severely interfere with a woman's everyday functioning and that the term *premenstrual syndrome* be used to describe less severe symptoms.

A useful definition for clinical practice is "The cyclic occurrence of changes in mood, somatic functioning, and behavior that are of sufficient severity to interfere with some aspects of life and which appear with a consistent and predictable relationship to menses" (Rubinow et al., 1984). The best way to determine the timing and severity of symptoms in relation to the menstrual cycle is to obtain from the patient a prospective recording of daily symptoms over several cycles.

EPIDEMIOLOGY

Large population-based studies indicate that approximately 1% to 5% of women experience serious premenstrual symptoms. Ramcharan's cross-sectional survey found such symptoms were markedly increased in women who were between 26 and 35 years of age, had cycle lengths from 25 to 28 days, and reported experiencing stressful life events in the preceding year. Other research has identified additional factors associated with severe premenstrual symptoms, including having a history of family or personal depression, having a history of migraines or postpartum depression, having several children, and having a high intake of alcohol and chocolate.

Premenstrual syndrome historically has been associated with psychologic problems, at times in ways that demean

---

DIAGNOSTIC CRITERIA FOR PREMENSTRUAL DYSPHORIC DISORDER

Symptoms occur cyclically and occurred in most cycles during the past year

At least five of the following are present (including at least one of the first four):

Markedly depressed mood, feelings of hopelessness, or self-deprecating thoughts

Marked anxiety, tension

Marked affective lability

Persistent and marked anger or irritability or increased interpersonal conflicts

Decreased interest in usual activities

Subjective sense of difficulty concentrating

Lethargy, easy fatigability, or marked lack of energy

Marked change in appetite, overeating, or food cravings

Hypersomnia or insomnia

Physical symptoms, such as breast pain, bloating, headaches

Symptoms are serious enough to interfere with activities and relationships

Symptoms are not an exacerbation of an underlying disorder

Symptoms are confirmed by prospective daily ratings during two cycles

Modified from *Diagnostic and statistical manual of mental disorders*, ed 4, Washington DC, 1994, American Psychiatric Association.

women with premenstrual symptoms, depicting them as neurotic or manipulative. Although the association of PMS with neurotic and personality problems is unfounded, often underlying psychiatric illness is exacerbated in the premenstrual phase of the cycle. Psychotic symptoms and the frequency of panic attacks can increase premenstrually. In primary care, the most relevant association with psychiatric illness is the strong relationship between PMS and a lifetime diagnosis of affective illness.

CAUSES

Although many factors have been considered as causative agents, the existing data on the cause of PMS are inconclusive. Rubinow and colleagues established that there are no differences in daily levels over the menstrual cycle of progesterone, estradiol, follicle-stimulating hormone (FSH), luteinizing hormone (LH), testosterone-binding globulin, dehydroepiandrosterone sulfate (DHEA-S), dihydrotestosterone, prolactin, and cortisol between women with and without PMS. The most promising research indicates that premenstrual symptoms may be associated with changes in circadian rhythms, decreases in the neurotransmitter serotonin, or sensitivity to endorphins. These mechanisms may be affected indirectly by changes in gonadal hormones. The complexity of this relationship is indicated by the findings that ovulation suppression with gonadotropin-releasing hormone (GnRH) analogs will abolish premenstrual symptoms, yet Schmidt demonstrated that artificially induced menses are associated with PMS even when the peripheral endocrine profile is that of the follicular phase.

Rubinow has proposed a promising model for PMS that takes into account the complexity of existing data. He suggests that PMS may reflect an underlying susceptibility to changes in behavior and mood when triggered by an unknown biologic stimulus premenstrually. This underlying susceptibility may be caused by (1) antecedent events (for example prior sexual abuse, recent stress, or compromised psychologic functioning) or (2) a biologic condition such as hypothyroidism.

 EVALUATION

The goals of the initial evaluation are to clarify the nature and timing of the premenstrual symptoms, to determine whether an underlying medical or psychiatric illness is present, and to enlist the woman's active participation in evaluation and treatment to enhance her sense of control.

History and physical examination

The history should collect information about the nature, timing, and severity of symptoms and the woman's perception of their relationship to the menstrual cycle (see box, right). Variability in the intensity of symptoms over time and changes in symptom patterns during the course of reproductive life are commonly seen. A detailed psychiatric history is important to determine whether an underlying or exacerbating condition is present. Understanding the context of the woman's current life as well as the significance of menstrual events in the woman's family and culture is essential to formulating an effective approach to treatment.

The physical examination focuses on identifying any underlying systemic disorders that may mimic PMS (for example, hypothyroidism) or any anatomic causes of symptoms (such as endometriosis, fibroids, or other gynecologic disorders that may contribute to pelvic pain).

Diagnostic tests

Prospective daily symptom recording is essential for diagnosis. Some women incorrectly attribute symptom changes to the menstrual cycle and others are unaware of a relationship between specific symptoms and the menstrual cycle. Women with severe PMS are less likely to report their symptoms incorrectly than women with mild to moderate symptoms. Because of underlying biologic variability in the menstrual cycle, it is necessary to record symptoms for a minimum of two cycles to discern the symptom pattern. Several instruments are available for formally recording symptoms.

Laboratory tests are of little value in the diagnosis of PMS, except to rule out other disorders such as hypothyroidism or anemia.

 MANAGEMENT

When the diagnosis of PMS has been established through careful assessment of prospective symptom records and exclusion of other medical or psychiatric disorders, a spectrum of treatment approaches should be considered. These include changes in life-style, psychoeducational groups and other techniques for coping with stress, vitamin supplements, and medical therapy directed at specific symptoms or constellations of symptoms.

Diet and exercise

The first level of intervention for women with PMS involves modification of diet and exercise habits and development of effective techniques for coping with stress. The rationale underlying these interventions derives from epidemiologic studies of factors associated with PMS, rather than from randomized trials; however, they have little risk

---

EVALUATION OF PREMENSTRUAL SYMPTOMS

History
  Nature, timing, and severity of symptoms
  Symptom course over time; precipitating events
  Effect of symptoms on daily functioning
  Psychiatric history
  Family history of psychiatric illness
  Personal history of psychiatric illness
  Alcohol and drug use
  Social history
  Diet and exercise habits

Physical examination
  General examination
  Pelvic examination

Diagnostic tests
  Daily symptom recording for minimum of two cycles
  Selective laboratory tests: TSH, CBC

TSH, thyroid-stimulating hormone; CBC, complete blood count.

or cost, and clinical experience supports their beneficial effects for some women.

Women with PMS consume significantly more caffeine and concentrated sweets than control subjects. Improvement in PMS symptoms has been observed after consumption of evening meals high in carbohydrates during the luteal phase; the mechanism may be alterations in serotonin level. Evidence from a randomized trial indicates that a strict low-fat diet (<15% calories from fat) reduces cyclic breast pain. Finally, moliminal symptoms have been observed to diminish after sedentary women begin a regular exercise program. The recommended interventions based on these observations are outlined in the box below.

Psychosocial interventions

An important adjunct to modifications in diet and exercise is the development of techniques for actively coping with premenstrual symptoms and with stress in general. This can be accomplished most effectively through meeting with an individual counselor or participating in a time-limited psychoeducational group.

These psychosocial interventions should focus on (1) the development of an awareness of the relationships among external stress, internal responses, and behavior; (2) the development of an active problem-solving attitude toward the symptoms; and (3) the implementation of behavior changes and coping strategies that diminish the symptoms. Individual or group interventions such as these will provide a supportive setting in which to diagnose as well as to treat PMS. Through the use of prospective symptom recording and discussion, a woman has the opportunity to determine the relationships among her menstrual cycle, external events, internal psychologic states, her behavior, and premenstrual symptoms. In addition the individual therapist or group leader can provide education about life-style changes and support to help each woman implement these changes.

When available, time-limited psychoeducational groups are preferable to individual counseling sessions. In addition to the benefits of education and discussion previously listed, group meetings provide the unique opportunity for women with PMS to meet and work with other women who share similar experiences. This shared experience promotes group cohesiveness and reduces the sense of shame and isolation many women experience. Over time many group members derive a sense of hope and energy from the group process that helps them to take an active role in developing new behavior and techniques to diminish their premenstrual symptoms and to decrease the overall stress in their lives.

If a psychoeducational group is offered, the group leader should be experienced in group psychotherapy. Each member should have at least one pregroup interview to review her complaints and determine suitability for the group. All women who complain of PMS and who are not psychotic or paranoid can be included. Each member should be willing to make a commitment to attend all 12 sessions. At the time of the interview the patient can be asked to start charting her symptoms daily so that she will go to the first meeting of the group with some data about the relationship between her symptoms and her menstrual cycle.

A group meeting for 12 weeks' duration works well. It allows time for each woman to go through several menstrual cycles while in the group and time for the members to establish some comfort with each other. In order to include time for both diagnosis and treatment, each meeting can be divided roughly into thirds. At the start of each meeting members can be given time to relate the status of their symptoms for the past week, discuss the ways they reacted to their symptoms, and outline and readjust goals for the upcoming week. The group leader can then spend some time (about one half hour) presenting some educational material. Areas that are useful to cover are the physiologic characteristics of the menstrual cycle, questionnaires that assess areas of stress, methods of relaxation and stress management, nutrition, and behavioral management of stress at home and work. In addition the leader should save time each week (about one half hour) to allow for unstructured discussion of feelings regarding PMS. Many women who have felt out of control premenstrually may never have discussed the extent of their symptoms with anyone. This time allows the group to develop a sense of commonality that will reduce shame and isolation and increase the likelihood that the members will implement behavioral changes.

Vitamin and mineral supplements

Several vitamin and mineral supplements have been evaluated as treatments for PMS in randomized controlled trials. The rationale for the potential effectiveness of some vitamins is clear; vitamin B_6, for example, is a cofactor in serotonin metabolism and has been shown in controlled studies to alleviate depression associated with use of the oral contraceptive pill. Although the number of trials of vitamin and mineral supplements is limited and the biologic mechanism of action is uncertain for some, in general these supplements are associated with minimal risk and cost and may be offered to the woman whose symptoms do not respond to the interventions discussed (see box, left).

Choice of therapy

In critically evaluating the evidence for effectiveness of medical therapy for PMS, it is important to bear in mind the factors that complicate interpretation of research on this subject. Consensus on the definition of PMS for research purposes has evolved only in recent years, and many studies differ in their definitions of PMS and their methods for

---

INITIAL INTERVENTIONS FOR WOMEN WITH PREMENSTRUAL SYNDROME

Life-style modifications

  Frequent small meals
  Adequate protein and complex carbohydrates
  Elimination of concentrated sweets, caffeine, and alcohol
  Regular aerobic exercise for 20 to 45 minutes, at least
    3 times weekly
  Stress management

Vitamin and mineral supplements

  Calcium 1000 mg qd
  Vitamin B_6 50-200 mg qd
  Vitamin E 150-300 IU qd
  Magnesium 200 mg qd during the luteal phase

measuring symptoms. The duration of therapy is rarely more than two or three cycles. The large placebo effect observed in many studies of PMS virtually requires that clinical decisions about the effectiveness of treatment be based on randomized trials, particularly when those treatments are associated with potential adverse effects or significant costs.

Studies of treatments for PMS include symptom-specific therapy; hormonal therapy, generally involving ovarian suppression; and psychotropic medications. The evidence for the effectiveness of each of these forms of treatment, derived from published randomized controlled trials, is summarized in the following sections, and clinical recommendations for their use are presented in Table 39-1.

Symptom-specific therapy. For symptoms of bloating and edema, **spironolactone** taken during the luteal phase is effective. Other diuretics have not been studied but probably are equally effective.

Cyclic breast pain is reduced by **bromocriptine,** which may be used in low doses during the luteal phase. Evidence to support a benefit from vitamin E is lacking, although it is widely used clinically and has little apparent toxicity.

The effectiveness of **nonsteroidal antiinflammatory drugs** for cyclic pelvic pain is well known. Some evidence for a beneficial effect of these agents on fatigue, mood swings, and headache also exists.

Hormonal therapy. The results of studies of **progesterone** for premenstrual syndrome are conflicting. Published studies have used varying forms and dosages of progestins. If a trial of progesterone is undertaken, the patient should understand the limited evidence for effectiveness and the possibility of exacerbating premenstrual symptoms.

Other hormone interventions based on ovulation suppression have shown more consistent evidence for effectiveness, but their use is limited by short- and long-term side effects. **GnRH analogs** have generally reduced both physical and psychologic symptoms; however, use for more than 6 months is precluded by their negative effects on bone density. Studies of "add-back" therapy with replacement-level doses of estrogen and progestin, designed to minimize long-term risks of GnRH analogs, appear promising. The high cost of GnRH analogs further limits their use.

Danazol, which also results in ovulation suppression and eventual amenorrhea, alleviates a range of premenstrual symptoms but is often associated with bothersome side effects, including hirsutism, acne, and hot flashes. The **oral contraceptive pill** affects only a limited number of premenstrual symptoms; a trial may be appropriate in women who also need contraception.

Psychotropic agents. Studies demonstrating a consistent benefit from **fluoxetine** (Prozac) support the hypothesis that some premenstrual symptoms may be mediated through alterations in the neurotransmitter serotonin. **D-fenfluramine,** which also acts by affecting serotonin levels, has been shown to alleviate depression and reduce premenstrual calorie, fat, and carbohydrate consumption in women with PMS, but is not currently available in the United States.

Studies of **alprazolam** indicate that both anxiety and depression, as well as somatic symptoms, are reduced with use of the agent during the luteal phase or throughout the cycle. The potential for dependency is minimized by con-

Table 39-1 Medical therapy for premenstrual syndrome

Symptom-directed treatment	Treatment alternatives
Fluid retention	Spironolactone 50-100 mg qd, luteal phase
	Hydrochlorothiazide 25-50 mg qd, luteal phase
Breast pain	Bromocriptine 2.5-5 mg qd, luteal phase
Pelvic pain	Any nonsteroidal antiinflammatory drug
Irritability	Atenolol 50 mg qd
Treatment of multiple symptoms	Fluoxetine 10-20 mg qd
	Alprazolam 0.25-1 mg tid, luteal phase
Hormonal therapy	Combination oral contraceptive pill
	Danazol 200-400 mg qd or in luteal phase (not effective for contraception)
	Transdermal estradiol 0.1 mg 2 ×/wk (or equivalent) with medroxyprogesterone 2.5-5 mg qd luteal phase
	GnRH analogs
	Leuprolide acetate 3.75-7.5 mg IM monthly
	Nafarelin acetate nasal spray 200 μg bid-tid
	Begin first dose at start of menses; limit use to 6 months
	With estrogen/progestin "add-back": Conjugated estrogens 0.625 mg qd Medroxyprogesterone 5 mg day 1-12

fining use to the luteal phase. Limited evidence supports the use of **atenolol** for irritability, particularly in women also bothered by premenstrual migraine.

Parry has investigated innovative approaches to reducing premenstrual symptoms through alterations in circadian rhythms. Controlled trials have demonstrated improvements in depression with **bright light treatments** throughout the cycle or **late sleep deprivation** (awakening at 2 a.m.) at symptom onset. These approaches need further study but may be offered to women with prominent affective symptoms who wish to avoid pharmacologic therapy.

Treatment options for women with clear evidence of PMS who do not respond to more conservative measures are listed in Table 39-1. If the patient and physician believe that further treatment is indicated, the patient should understand that the current state of medical knowledge about PMS is limited and that predicting response to treatment is difficult.

Hysterectomy with bilateral oophorectomy is a drastic measure for which there is some limited evidence of effectiveness for relief of premenstrual symptoms. Surgery should be considered only if the diagnosis has been prospectively established and confirmed, underlying psychiatric disorders have been ruled out through formal psychiatric evaluation, symptoms have not responded to multiple trials of medical and behavioral therapy, and symptoms substantially affect quality of life.

BIBLIOGRAPHY

Deeny M, Hawthorn R, Hart DM: Low dose danazol in the treatment of the premenstrual syndrome, *Postgrad Med J* 67:450, 1991.

Doll H et al: Pyridoxine (vitamin B$_6$) and the premenstrual syndrome: a randomized controlled trial, *J R Coll Gen Pract* 39:364, 1989.

Endicott J et al: Affective disorder and premenstrual depression. In Osofsky HJ, Blumenthal SJ, editors: *Premenstrual syndrome: current findings and future directions,* Washington DC, 1985, American Psychiatric Press.

Graham CA, Sherwin BS: A prospective treatment study of premenstrual symptoms using a triphasic oral contraceptive, *J Psychosom Res* 36:257, 1992.

Hellberg D, Claesson B, Nilsson B: Premenstrual tension: a placebo-controlled efficacy study with spironolactone and medroxyprogesterone acetate, *Int J Gynecol Obstet* 34:243, 1991.

Mortola JF, Girton L, Fischer U: Successful treatment of severe premenstrual syndrome by combined use of gonadotropin-releasing hormone agonist and estrogen/progestin, *J Clin Endocrinol Metab* 71:252A 1991.

Parry BL et al: Light therapy of late luteal phase dysphoric disorder: an extended study, *Am J Psychiatry* 150:1417, 1993.

Ramcharan S et al: The epidemiology of premenstrual syndrome in a population-bsed sample of 2650 urban women: attributable risk and risk factors, *J Clin Epidemiol* 45:377, 1992.

Rausch JL et al: Atenolol treatment of late luteal phase dysphoric disorder, *J Affect Disord* 15:141, 1988.

Rubinow DR: The premenstrual syndrome: new views, *JAMA* 268:1908, 1992.

Rubinow DR et al: Prospective assessment of menstrually related mood disorders, *Am J Psychiatry* 141:684, 1984.

Schmidt PJ et al: Lack of effect of induced menses on symptoms in women with premenstrual syndrome, *N Engl J Med* 324:1174, 1991.

Singer S, Schiff I: Modern management of premenstrual syndrome, New York, 1993, Norton.

Thys-Jacobs S et al: Calcium supplementation in premenstrual syndrome: a randomized crossover trial, *J Gen Intern Med* 4:183, 1989.

Watson NR et al: Treatment of severe premenstrual syndrome with oestradiol patches and cyclical oral norethisterone, *Lancet* 2:730, 1989.

Wood SH et al: Treatment of premenstrual syndrome with fluoxetine: a double-blind, placebo-controlled crossover study, *Obstet Gynecol* 80:339, 1992.

40 Sexual Dysfunction

Linda Shafer

In our society not only is sexual fulfillment important to people, it is closely linked to emotional and physical well-being. Although the exact incidence of sexual dysfunction in the general population is unknown, in a recent survey sexual difficulties ranked fourth among the top problems facing U.S. families, after rapid social changes, child and spouse abuse, and money.

It has been estimated that approximately 15% of medical outpatients consult primary care physicians for sexual complaints. However, it has been clearly demonstrated that the incidence of sexual problems treated in any medical office is directly associated with those clinicians who routinely take a sexual history. Since discussions of sexuality still cause shame and embarrassment for many people, the presentation of sexual problems may take on many covert forms. These include somatic symptoms that have no medical cause, including headaches, low back pain, generalized pelvic pain, and vulvar pruritis. Clinicians skilled in taking a sexual history who can carry out basic types of sexual counseling can provide a valuable service for their patients.

The first part of this chapter discusses the causes of sexual dysfunction, evaluation, and approach to treatment from the perspective of heterosexual relationships. The second section addresses what is known of sexual dysfunction in lesbian relationships.

FEMALE SEXUAL DISORDERS
Hypoactive sexual desire disorder (low libido)

The condition of hypoactive sexual desire disorder has been defined as persistently deficient or absent sexual fantasies and desire for sexual activity. The incidence of this problem in patients with a sexual disorder has increased from about 37% in the 1970s to about 50% in the 1980s. Recent data indicate that the number of men with complaints of low desire is higher than the number of women.

Sexual aversion disorder

Sexual aversion disorder has been defined as a persistent or recurrent extreme aversion to and avoidance of all or almost all genital sexual contact with a sexual partner. The exact incidence of this disorder is unknown, but it is one of the more common sexual disorders presenting for treatment. Primary sexual aversion seems more prevalent in men and secondary more common in women. The syndrome is associated with phobic avoidance of sexual activity or even thought of sexual activity. Of patients with sexual phobias and aversions, 25% meet the criteria for panic disorder. Most people with this disorder respond fairly naturally to sex, if they can get past the high anxiety associated with the initial dread. Typically the frequency of intercourse is only once or twice a year.

General unresponsiveness (excitement phase disorder)

General unresponsiveness is defined as a persistent or recurrent partial or complete failure to attain or maintain the lubrication swelling response of sexual excitement until the completion of the sexual activity. Although the exact incidence of this problem is unknown, it is believed to be a common disorder. The disorder is often linked to problems with sexual desire and painful intercourse.

Orgasmic dysfunction (orgasm phase disorder)

Orgasmic dysfunction is defined as a persistent or recurrent delay in or absence of orgasm despite a normal desire and excitement phase. Some women find it difficult to reach orgasm during intercourse but can do so with direct clitoral contact. This is usually a normal variant of response and does not justify the diagnosis of orgasmic dysfunction. Claims that stimulation of an area in the anterior wall of the vagina, called the "G spot" (Grafenberg spot), will trigger female orgasm and ejaculation have never been substantiated.

Anorgasmia in all of its forms represents the largest category of female sexual dysfunction. The incidence runs from about 5% to 8% of women who are totally unable to achieve orgasm to 30% to 40% of women who are unable to achieve orgasm without clitoral stimulation or during intercourse alone. The capacity for orgasm increases with experience. It is important to evaluate the partner, who may have premature ejaculation contributing to the female anorgasmia.

Vaginismus (sexual pain disorder)

Vaginismus is defined as recurrent or persistent involuntary spasm of the musculature of the outer third of the vagina (pubococcygeus muscles) that makes sexual intercourse impossible, difficult, or painful. Although the exact frequency of vaginismus is not known, it probably accounts for less than 10% of female sexual disorders. Because there is a high incidence of pelvic abnormality associated with this condition, a careful gynecologic examination is warranted and is the only definitive way to make the diagnosis. Secondary impotence in the male partner may develop. Vaginismus is the sexual disorder most often found in long-term unconsummated marriages.

Dyspareunia (sexual pain disorder)

Dyspareunia is defined as a recurrent or persistent genital pain before, during, or after sexual intercourse. The overall prevalence of dyspareunia in the general population is about 20%, but there are varied reports from a low of 4% to a high of 40%. The incidence of the problem increases with aging.

CAUSES OF SEXUAL DYSFUNCTION

The vast majority of sexual problems are caused by a multitude of factors, often a combination of biologic and psychogenic. Thus it is important to evaluate each individual carefully for organic and psychogenic contributions, so that proper treatment can be prescribed.

Table 40-1 lists some of the more common medical and surgical conditions that can cause sexual difficulties.

Table 40-2 provides a list of some drugs that are either known to affect the female sexual response or believed to cause female sexual dysfunction, on the basis of studies done on males.

There are many **psychogenic** issues leading to sexual problems, ranging from superficial causes such as anxiety over performance or fears of "letting go" to more deep seated issues in which sex is unconsciously equated with danger. There are no rigid correlations between certain background factors and dysfunctional syndromes. However, most sexual disorders can be related to prior experiences that place an individual at risk of having a sexual disorder. These may include negative family attitudes about sex, inadequate information or education about sex, and past traumatic sexual experiences such as rape or incest. There is usually an acute precipitant that will actually trigger the problem, causing the patient to seek help. Examples of such precipitating causes are childbirth, marital infidelity, a depression or other psychiatric problem, or a sexual problem in the partner. Moreover, there may be maintaining factors that prevent the problem from being solved such as ongoing communication issues, lack of cooperation, financial problems, and lack of foreplay. Sometimes there may be latent homosexuality underlying the complaint.

 EVALUATION

A brief **sexual history** should be a required part of every medical evaluation, both for its positive clinical value and for its moral and legal implications during this current acquired immunodeficiency syndrome (AIDS) crisis. It can be done most easily in conjunction with the gynecologic and menstrual review in women. In this way sexual concerns can be comfortably addressed in the context of routine history taking, especially if the physician displays an open non-judgmental attitude. Helpful screening questions include,

Table 40-1 Medical and surgical conditions causing female sexual problems

Disorder	Sexual impairment
Endocrine	
Diabetes; thyroid, adrenal, pituitary glands	Reduced vaginal lubrication, vaginal infection (diabetes)
Vascular	
Sickle-cell anemia	Decreased arousal and orgasm
Cardiac: MI, angina	Fear of death, decreased frequency
Neurologic	
Spinal cord damage	Decreased arousal, orgasm, and
Multiple sclerosis	genital lubrication
Gynecologic	
Vaginitis, PID, endometriosis, uterine prolapse, fibroids	Vaginismus, dyspareunia Decreased arousal and desire
Renal	
Renal failure	Decreased arousal and desire
(on dialysis)	Electrolyte and hormone imbalance
Musculoskeletal	
Arthritis	Chronic pain, limited motion
Sjögren's syndrome	Decreased lubrication
Surgery	
Gynecologic—oophorectomy, episiotomy	Decreased estrogen levels and lubrication Tightness of vaginal opening
Other—mastectomy, colostomy	Self-esteem issues, fears of discomfort

MI, myocardial infarction; PID, pelvic inflammatory disease.

Table 40-2 Medications that affect female sexuality

Drug	Side effect
Antihypertensives	
Methyldopa, reserpine, clonidine, propranolol, spironolactone	Decreased libido, anorgasmia
Anticholinergics	
Propantheline, methantheline	Decreased lubrication
Hormones	
Estrogen, progesterone, steroids, androgen	Decreased libido (variable) Increased libido
Psychotropics	
Sedatives—alcohol, barbiturates	Higher dose—sexual problems
Anxiolytics—diazepam, alprazolam	Anorgasmia
Antipsychotics—thioridazine	Anorgasmia
Antidepressants	
MAO inhibitors— phenelzine	Anorgasmia
Tricyclics—imipramine, clomipramine	Anorgasmia
Atypical—fluoxetine, trazodone	Anorgasmia Decreased libido (variable)
Lithium	Decreased libido
Opiates	
Morphine, codeine, methadone	Anorgasmia, decreased libido
Miscellaneous	
Phenytoin, indomethacin, clofibrate, cimetidine, carbamazepine	Decreased libido

MAO, monoamine oxidase.

"Have there been any changes in your sex life?" and "Would you like to change anything about your sexual functioning?"

If a sexual problem is uncovered, it should be discussed in detail, just as any problem would be, including elicitation of precipitating factors, duration, and severity. Careful history taking sometimes helps distinguish an organic cause from a psychogenic one. Moreover, a sexual history helps delineate which further diagnostic tests are indicated and helps determine the treatment approaches that will be needed. Keep in mind that failure to take a sexual history and educate the patient about risk factors for human immunodeficiency virus (HIV) infection and safe sex practices may leave the physician open to charges of negligence.

There are few **diagnostic tests** that are indicated in female sexual disorders beyond the physical examination, which should include a thorough gynecologic examination. In cases of vaginal dryness, an estrogen level and a microscopic study of vaginal smears may be done, especially in perimenopausal women, to determine whether ovarian failure has begun. For dyspareunia, a complete blood count (CBC), sedimentation rate, and cervical culture should be done to rule out pelvic inflammatory disease, especially if the pain is greatest on deep penetration. A Papanicolaou's smear should be done to rule out malignancy. Pelvic ultrasonography may help define a suspected pelvic mass, and referral for laparoscopy may help make the diagnosis of endometriosis, adhesions, or an adnexal mass. For complaints of low sexual desire in females, no laboratory testing is indicated unless there is a history of menstrual irregularity or galactorrhea or an organic cause is clinically suggested. Then serum testosterone, prolactin, follicle-stimulating hormone (FSH), and luteinizing hormone (LH) may be ordered.

More sophisticated diagnostic testing has also been developed, primarily for male sexual disorders, leading to the overall conclusion that sexual problems once thought to be psychogenic in origin have been found to have an organic basis. More psychophysiologic research into women's sexual problems needs to be done.

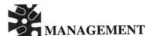

MANAGEMENT

Often the primary care physician is the first person to be consulted about a sexual complaint. Because there are many levels of intervention that may be helpful to patients, even physicians without formal training in sex therapy may enable patients to deal effectively with sexual problems. Physicians can help patients by giving permission and reassurance, providing information, and correcting misinformation. If this is insufficient, specific suggestions can be given to the patient and the partner. These encompass the behavioral techniques used in sex therapy. Although there are specific techniques used to treat particular kinds of dysfunctions some general principles of behavior therapy include increasing communication between partners, decreasing performance anxiety or "spectatoring" by changing the goal of the sexual activity away from emphasis on orgasm and more toward giving pleasure and feeling good, relieving the pressure to perform at any sexual encounter, and encouraging sexual experimentation. A trial of this kind of therapy is certainly reasonable where there is no evidence of more serious underlying psychopathologic condition or organic disease.

INDICATIONS FOR REFERRAL

Behavior therapy often leads to improvement in sexual functioning without the need for referral. If the condition does not improve this may be a sign that the patient needs more intensive therapy. A consultation with a mental health expert trained in sex and marital therapy may be indicated. Often a direct referral to a specialist may be indicated for patients known to have chronic psychologic issues, who experience gender confusion, or who have never had a period of satisfactory functioning.

SPECIFIC TREATMENT TECHNIQUES
Hypoactive sexual disorder

Positive sexual experiences help increase sexual desire, although most cases require some insight into background influences.

1. Sensate focus exercises (nondemand pleasuring techniques) to enhance enjoyment without pressure.
2. Use of erotic material.
3. Masturbation training with fantasy to help individuals become aware of conditions necessary for a positive sexual experience.

Sexual aversion disorder

1. Same as for hypoactive sexual desire (i.e., systematic desensitization with sensate focus exercises).
2. Where phobic/panic-type symptoms are displayed the addition of antipanic medication (tricyclic antidepressants such as imipramine, or benzodiazepines such as alprazolam) may be helpful when used for 3 or 4 months.

General unresponsiveness

Because general unresponsiveness usually results from a more severe psychopathologic condition, it usually requires referral for treatment.

1. Supplemental use of lubrication, such as water-soluble lubricant jelly or saliva, can be suggested for vaginal dryness.
2. Postmenopausal women with atrophic vaginal mucosa may benefit from topical estrogen cream given intermittently.

Orgasmic dysfunction

Totally anorgastic

1. Education and encouragement of self-exploration, including masturbation and use of fantasy material.
2. Kegel vaginal exercises to increase frequency of orgasm (contraction of pubococcygeus muscles).

Anorgastic with partner

1. Sensate focus exercises (from nongenital stimulation to genital stimulation).
2. Intercourse and orgasm prohibited at this time to take away performance pressure.
3. Use of back protected position (male in seated position with female between his legs with back against his chest) to allow the female to control the stimulation and eliminate self-consciousness).
4. Pelvic thrusting explored in nondemanding way, beginning with female superior position, followed by lateral position that allows for mutual freedom of movement.

Anorgastic during intercourse

1. Use of "bridge technique," in which clitoris is stimulated manually or with a vibrator after insertion of the penis into the vagina.

Vaginismus

1. Demonstrate to woman (and her partner) that the condition is involuntary and not willfully contrived, typically shown by inserting a gloved finger into the vagina, which has involuntary spasm.
2. Encourage the woman to insert larger and larger objects into the vagina in a gradual step-by-step fashion. Use of one finger, then several, to approximate the penis.
3. Use of Hegar graduated vaginal dilators to control dilation without pain. Syringe containers of different sizes make good alternative dilators.
4. In female superior position woman uses erect penis as her dilator to insert gradually into vagina, in conjunction with extravaginal lubricant (KY jelly).
5. Kegel vaginal exercises to develop sense of control.

Dyspareunia

1. Treat underlying gynecologic problem first.
2. If accompanying vaginismus, use previously mentioned techniques.
3. Treat insufficient lubrication as described.

PROGNOSIS

The prognosis with treatment for any sexual disorder is highly dependent on several factors: (1) the nature of the dysfunction, (2) the individual psychopathologic condition, and (3) the nature of the couple's relationship. Any organic factors that are present play a part in the ultimate diagnosis.

Hypoactive sexual desire

Usually a complexity of factors is involved, making hypoactive sexual desire difficult to treat. There have not been adequate follow-up studies done to show whether treatment gains are maintained.

Sexual aversion

When related to panic attacks, the prognosis for sexual aversion with the adjunctive use of antipanic medication is excellent. Otherwise, the prognosis is similar to that of hypoactive sexual desire.

General unresponsiveness

Estrogen deficiency states can be easily diagnosed and treated. When hormone levels are normal, short-term techniques are of limited benefit, usually because of the presence of deeper intrapsychic conflict.

Orgasmic dysfunction

The totally anorgasmic woman has an excellent prognosis with sex therapy. Of these women 90% have their symptoms relieved. In cases of secondary anorgasmia the prognosis depends on the nature of the couple's relationship and other situational factors. If the criterion for success is regular coital orgasm, the success rate is between 30% and 50%. If a more modest goal is to experience orgasm during heterosexual activity, a success rate of 70% to 80% is achieved.

Vaginismus

The prognosis is excellent with a reported cure rate of ≥95% using behavior modification treatment.

Dyspareunia

The prognosis is variable, depending on the organic factors involved and the ability to treat them.

SEXUAL DYSFUNCTION IN LESBIANS

On the basis of available studies the percentage of gay men and lesbians in the general population is somewhere between 2% and 10%. The clinician should expect to encounter some lesbian patients and be prepared to deal with their sexual complaints.

As a group lesbian couples have not been well researched. However, studies show that, like heterosexual women, lesbians value relationships highly. Single lesbians have less sex and fewer partners than do gay men. Lesbians are more sexually responsive and more satisfied with the sex they do have than are heterosexual women.

Lesbians have not been reported to have significant rates of orgasmic dysfunction, dyspareunia, or vaginismus, probably because of sexual technique. There is less emphasis on genital organs and orgasm and more on sensuality. However, lesbians do have low rates of sex within long-term committed relationships and often consult the clinician with a complaint of low sexual desire. Often they prefer nongenital physical contact (hugging, etc.) to genital sex. In one study half of the couples with a low frequency of genital sex were dissatisfied, leading to one partner's having an affair and the resulting dissolution of the relationship. Lesbian women tend to equate sexual attraction with love, moving from one relationship to another. They are not comfortable with sex outside the context of a relationship. Such relationships, which are not given much time to develop and lack the opportunity for the couple to explore their compatibility, have a high failure rate.

SAFE SEX FOR AIDS PREVENTION

Lack of knowledge of safe sex practices can contribute to the spread of AIDS. There should be an active attempt to eroticize safe sex behavior including holding, hugging, massage, mutual masturbation, use of vibrators, and dry kissing. The physician should be prepared to discuss the advantages of long-term relationships, the use of condoms, and spermicides containing nonoxynol-9 in minimizing the AIDS risk. Patients in high-risk groups such as intravenous drug users and those at above-average risk with multiple partners should be encouraged to modify their behavior.

BIBLIOGRAPHY

Abramowicz M, editor: Drugs that cause sexual dysfunction: an update, *Med Lett Drugs Ther* 34:876, 1992.

Barnes AB: Medical evaluation of dyspareunia and other female sexual dysfunction. In Goroll AH et al, editors: *Primary care medicine,* ed 2, Philadelphia, 1987, JB Lippincott.

Croft HA: Managing common sexual problems, *Postgrad Med* 60(3):200, 60(4):193, 60(5):186, 60(6):164, 1976.

Hawton K, Oppenheimer C: Sexual problems. In McPherson A, editor: *Women's problems in general practice,* ed 2, Oxford, 1988, Oxford University Press.

Heiman JR et al: The treatment of sexual function. In Gurman AS, Knishkern DP, editors: *Handbook of family therapy,* New York, 1981, Brunner/Mazel.

Hodge RH et al: Sexual function of women taking antihypertensive agents, *J Gen Intern Med* 6(4):290, 1991.

Jani NN, Wise TN: Antidepressants and inhibited female orgasm: a literature review, *J Sex Marital Ther* 14(4):279, 1988.

Kaplan HS: *The evaluation of sexual disorders,* New York, 1983, Brunner/Mazel.

Leiblum SR: The sexual difficulties of women, *J Med Assoc Ga* 81(5):221, 1992.

Leiblum SR, Rosen RC: *Principles and practice of sex therapy, update for the 1990's,* ed 2, New York, 1989, Guilford Press.

McCabe MP, Delaney SM: An evaluation of therapeutic programs for the treatment of secondary inorgasmia in women, *Arch Sex Behav* 21(1):69, 1992.

Nadelson C: Sexual dysfunction and treatment of sexual dysfunction. In Lazare A, editor: *Outpatient psychiatry,* Baltimore, 1979, Williams & Wilkins.

Nichols M: Lesbian relationships: implications for the study of sexuality and gender. In McWhirter DP et al, editors, *Homosexuality/heterosexuality,* New York, 1990, Oxford University Press.

Reiss JP et al: Prolactin and sexual dysfunction in women, *J Sex Marital Ther* 15(3):177, 1989.

Segraves RT: Psychiatric drugs and inhibited female orgasm, *J Sex Marital Ther* 14(3):202, 1988.

Shafer LC: Approach to the patient with sexual dysfunction, In Goroll AH et al, editors: *Primary care medicine* ed 2, Philadelphia, 1987, JB Lippincott.

Shafer LC: Sexual disorders. In Hyman SE, Jenike MA, editors: *Manual of clinical problems in psychiatry,* Boston, 1990, Little, Brown.

Shafer LC: The denial of the risk of AIDS in heterosexuals coming for treatment of sexual disorders. In Rutan JS, editor: *Psychotherapy for the 1990s,* New York, 1992, Guilford Press.

Shen WW, Lindbergh SS: Inhibited female orgasm resulting from psychotropic drugs, *J Reprod Med* 35(1):11, 1990.

Spector IP, Carey MP: Incidence and prevalence of the sexual dysfunctions: a critical review of the empirical literature, *Arch Sex Behav* 19(4):389, 1990.

Wincze JP, Carey MP: *Sexual dysfunction,* New York, 1991, Guilford Press.

RESOURCES

Patients have many questions and concerns about sexuality and may benefit from and find reassurance from the following suggested self-help books:

Barbach LG: *For yourself: the fulfillment of female sexuality,* New York, 1975, Doubleday.

Barbach LG: *For each other: sharing sexual intimacy,* New York, 1981, Doubleday.

Heiman J, LoPiccolo J: *Becoming orgasmic: a sexual growth program for women,* New York, 1988, Prentice-Hall.

Kaplan HS: *The real truth about women and AIDS: how to eliminate the risks without giving up love and sex,* New York, 1987, Simon & Schuster.

41 Uterine Fibroids

Andrew J. Friedman

EPIDEMIOLOGY AND RISK FACTORS

Uterine fibroids, otherwise known as myomas, fibromyomas, myofibromas, or leiomyomas, are the most common pelvic tumors in women. It is estimated that 20% to 25% of women in the reproductive years will have fibroids that are clinically recognizable, although 40% of women will have myomas noted at autopsy. In one study where gross hysterectomy specimens were serially sectioned at 2-mm intervals, leiomyomas were detected in 77% of uteruses, with several myomas noted in 84% of these cases. In this study there was no difference in the incidence of leiomyomas in premenopausal and postmenopausal women.

Uterine myomas most commonly are diagnosed in women between the ages of 30 and 50 years. These neoplasms are extremely rare before age 20. It has been suggested that uterine myomas are three to nine times more common in African-American women than in Caucasians, although additional epidemiologic studies are needed to assess the impact of race on the risk of developing these tumors. In addition the presumption that these tumors occur more frequently within families, suggesting a genetic mode of inheritance, remains untested.

PATHOPHYSIOLOGY

Uterine myomas are benign neoplasms composed of smooth muscle cells and extracellular matrix (ECM). ECM consists primarily of collagen, proteoglycan, and fibronectin. The relative amounts of smooth muscle and ECM vary among fibroids, but most tumors are composed primarily of noncellular elements.

Fibroids generally are classified by their location within the uterus (Fig. 41-1). Subserosal myomas are found near the external or serosal surface of the uterus and produce a noticeable distortion of the external uterine contour. These tumors usually are easily palpated on bimanual examination, especially when they are large. Intramural leiomyomas are located within the myometrium. Submucosal myomas are located near the endometrium and project into the uterine cavity. Most tumors span more than a single anatomic location. For example, a subserosal fibroid may have a significant intramural component. Only small intramural fibroids and those that are pedunculated in subserosal and submucosal locations may be classified as purely one fibroid subtype.

Uterine leiomyomas are believed to be clonal tumors resulting from somatic mutations. Cytogenetic studies and analyses of X-linked glucose-6-phosphate dehydrogenase isoforms support the concept of leiomyomas as monoclonal tumors. The factor(s) responsible for the neoplastic transformation of myometrial cells are not known.

There is a growing body of evidence to suggest that an estrogenic milieu is necessary for the expression of this mutation and for the subsequent growth of these tumors.

Uterine fibroids are not seen in prepubertal girls, and myoma regression is noted in women after menopause. In addition, a number of in vitro experiments suggest that the intramyoma environment is relatively hyperestrogenic compared with adjacent myometrium. Treatment of women with gonadotropin-releasing hormone agonist (GnRH-a) will result in profound hypoestrogenemia, which, in turn, will lead to significant reductions in uterine and myoma size. It is not clear whether estrogen exerts its effects on these tumors directly or through growth factors such as epidermal growth factor (EGF), insulin-like growth factor-I (IGF-I), or platelet-derived growth factor (PDGF). Finally, the role of other hormones such as progesterone, prolactin, and growth hormone in the pathogenesis of myomas is unclear.

Uterine myomas undergo malignant degeneration to become leiomyosarcomas in 0.13% to 0.29% of cases. Leiomyosarcomas are not steroid sensitive and are characterized by a high mitotic index and cellular pleomorphism. These malignancies are rarely seen before age 40. The incidence of leiomyosarcomas increases with advancing age.

APPROACH TO THE PATIENT WITH SUSPECTED FIBROIDS

History and symptoms

It is estimated that 20% to 50% of women with clinically recognizable fibroids have symptoms caused by these tumors. The presence of symptoms is dependent upon the number, size, and location of these tumors. Approximately 30% of women with leiomyomas have excessive uterine bleeding (i.e., menorrhagia, hypermenorrhagia), which is most common in women with intramural or submucous tumors. Another 30% of women with leiomyomas have noncyclic pelvic pain produced by direct pressure on adjacent pelvic structures or acute myoma degeneration. Pelvic pressure, urinary frequency, and, rarely, constipation may

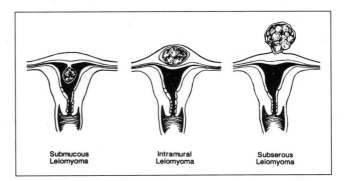

Fig. 41-1 Leiomyomas classified according to their location in the uterus. (From Muto M, Friedman AJ: The uterine corpus. In Ryan KJ, Berkowitz RS, Barbieri RL, editors: *Kistner's gynecology: principles and practice*, ed 6, St Louis, 1995, Mosby.)

result when subserosal or intramural tumors enlarge and press on adjacent pelvic organs. Reproductive dysfunction (e.g., infertility; spontaneous pregnancy loss; problems during pregnancy, labor, and delivery) is rarely caused by fibroids. Although myomas are present in 5% to 10% of infertile women, only 2% to 3% of infertile women have no other identifiable cause of infertility. Spontaneous pregnancy loss, abruption, and premature labor may be more common when the placenta implants on or near a submucous or intramural myoma.

It commonly is assumed that fibroids enlarge during pregnancy under the influence of increased circulating levels of estrogens. However, when serial sonographic measurements of fibroids are performed throughout pregnancy, some tumors are noted to grow, some remain unchanged, and some actually decrease in size. In general, if fibroids increase in size during pregnancy, most of the growth occurs in the first trimester. Occasionally rapid growth of fibroids during pregnancy may lead to acute degeneration of the tumor(s). When this occurs the woman often experiences severe pain and tenderness upon palpation of the fibroid and she may require narcotics for analgesia. Occasionally fibroid degeneration may precipitate premature labor.

Physical examination and differential diagnosis

Uterine fibroids are usually first suspected at the bimanual examination that reveals an enlarged, often irregular uterus. The presence of symptoms associated with leiomyomas will add to the clinician's level of confidence about the diagnosis. Other gynecologic and nongynecologic disorders may give rise to an enlarged pelvic mass and to symptoms often attributed to myomas (see box, below).

DIFFERENTIAL DIAGNOSIS OF AN ENLARGED PELVIC MASS AND EXCESSIVE MENSTRUAL FLOW

Enlarged pelvic mass

Benign

Pregnancy
Uterine myoma
Adenomyosis
Ovarian cyst/benign neoplasm/endometrioma
Hydrosalpinx
Diverticulitis
Pelvic abcess

Malignant

Uterine sarcoma
Ovarian carcinoma
Tubal carcinoma
Gastrointestinal carcinoma

Excessive menstrual flow

Uterine myoma
Adenomyosis
Coagulopathy (i.e., von Willebrand's disease, leukemia)
Aplastic anemia
Uterine malignancy
Cervical carcinoma
Dysfunctional uterine bleeding

Diagnostic tests

Pelvic ultrasonography will confirm that the enlarged pelvic mass is of uterine origin and may allow discrete tumors to be visualized within the uterus, thus further supporting the presumed diagnosis of uterine myomas. **Magnetic resonance imaging** (MRI) will provide better resolution of the tumors as well as an improved ability to assess the ovaries, but it is rarely necessary, as ultrasonography usually provides adequate images and is far less expensive. Pelvic ultrasonography is unable to differentiate between a benign tumor (e.g., myoma) and a malignant tumor (e.g., leiomyosarcoma). If the clinical presentation suggests the possibility of a uterine malignancy (e.g., rapidly enlarging uterus and abnormal uterine bleeding in a postmenopausal woman) the physician should attempt to obtain a tissue specimen for further diagnosis. An outpatient endometrial biopsy or dilation and curettage may suffice to diagnose the cause of abnormal uterine bleeding; occasionally hysteroscopy with a directed biopsy is useful. A total abdominal hysterectomy plus bilateral salpingo-oophorectomy is appropriate treatment for a rapidly enlarging uterine mass in a postmenopausal woman.

Management

Goals of management. The treatment options for women with uterine myomas have expanded over the last 10 to 20 years. In the past it was recommended that most women with symptomatic myomas or uterine size ≥12 gestational weeks regardless of symptoms have hysterectomies; myomectomy, or removal of the tumor(s) with uterine reconstruction, was recommended only in women below age 40 who were interested in future childbearing. Clearly the acute relief of myoma-related symptoms, correction of anemia, and ruling out of uterine malignancy are the main goals of surgical or medical treatment. But first the physician must decide whether medical or surgical treatment is necessary.

The presence of an enlarged pelvic mass that is not growing rapidly and is causing minor or no symptoms may not warrant treatment. Often the patient's quality of life is not impaired and the likelihood that the pelvic mass is malignant is so remote that close observation rather than intervention may be preferable. In cases where intervention is necessary to treat moderate to severe myoma-related symptoms, the patient's goals of treatment should be explored in detail before embarking on a particular therapy. For some women preservation of the uterus for future childbearing or for nonreproductive reasons may be so important that they are willing to risk tumor recurrence or continued myoma-related symptoms. Others may wish to eradicate symptoms permanently and are less concerned about organ preservation. In order to decide the best way to proceed, the treatment goals of the physician and patient must be fully understood and discussed.

Choice of therapy

Observation. The patient with an enlarged uterus that is not growing or slowly growing and is causing minor or no symptoms may be treated by close observation in many cases. A repeat outpatient visit is advisable 3 to 4 months after the original discovery of uterine myomas to assess whether the uterus and tumors have enlarged and symptoms have worsened. If there is no rapid increase of uterine size or symptoms, office visits may be made twice annually. In these cases annual pelvic ultrasonography is often helpful for measurement of the uterus and myomas and assessment of ovarian size and architecture, which may not be possible at the bimanual examination. If the severity of myoma-related symptoms worsens or the physician's suspicion of malignancy increases, surgical intervention may be recommended.

As has been noted, malignant degeneration of a myoma is a rare event, occurring in 0.13% to 0.29% of women. Controversy exists as to whether myomas degenerate into sarcomas or whether sarcomas arise spontaneously. The incidence of uterine sarcomas increases with each decade of life; they may grow rapidly or slowly and may range in size at diagnosis from less than 6 gestational weeks to more than 20 weeks. Abnormal uterine bleeding may occur in women with leiomyosarcomas. However, endometrial biopsy or uterine curettage, which reliably leads to the diagnosis of endometrial adenocarcinoma, rarely yields the diagnosis of leiomyosarcoma. For these reasons the correct preoperative diagnosis of leiomyosarcoma is uncommon. The presence of an enlarging uterus with or without abnormal uterine bleeding in a postmenopausal woman should be viewed with great concern and a tissue diagnosis should be obtained as rapidly as possible.

Surgical management

HYSTERECTOMY. Hysterectomy is the only treatment of uterine myomas that guarantees a cure of the condition. Uterine myomas constitute the single largest diagnostic category of all hysterectomies performed in the United States, accounting for 27%, or 175,000 procedures annually. Hysterectomy is most commonly performed for uterine myomas in women between the ages of 35 and 54 years; 44% of all hysterectomies performed in women in this age range are done for myomas. Removal of the ovaries at hysterectomy is recommended only for perimenopausal or postmenopausal women and for those with ovarian abnormalities. If the ovaries are removed, estrogen replacement therapy should be considered unless contraindicated. Although there is a widespread fear among women that hysterectomy will lead to decreased libido and sexual responsiveness, there are no adequate studies to address this issue. This concern must be explored by the physician to aid the patient in her decision about appropriate surgical treatment. Hysterectomy must be viewed as a major surgical procedure requiring 4 to 8 weeks for full recovery. The most common postoperative complication is febrile morbidity, present in up to 32% of women. Transfusion with homologous blood is necessary in approximately 5% to 10% of cases but, with a greater emphasis on preoperative blood donation and a greater willingness of physicians not to use transfusion for women with low hematocrits who are asymptomatic, this rate is declining. Serious postoperative complications, such as unplanned surgical procedures and pulmonary emboli, occur in <1% of women. Mortality rate of hysterectomy done for all causes is 0.1% but is clearly much lower when malignant diagnoses are excluded.

MYOMECTOMY. Uterine myomectomy—surgical removal of myomas with subsequent uterine reconstruction—may be performed if the woman wishes to preserve her uterus for any reason. Approximately 18,000 myomectomies are performed annually in the United States, although this number is likely to increase as more women are delaying childbearing and are requesting preservation of the uterus. Myomectomies are most commonly performed through laparotomy, but endoscopic myomectomies can be performed at hysteroscopy and laparoscopy in selected cases. Indications for hysteroscopic myomectomy include submucous myomas that cause excessive uterine bleeding or reproductive dysfunction; the indications for laparoscopic myomectomy are less clear and are evolving. Myomectomies are usually successful in alleviating preoperative symptoms. In a large retrospective series (Buttram and Reiter, 1981), 81% of women with menorrhagia had a significant decrease in menstrual flow after myomectomy. In addition, most women who have symptoms attributable to an enlarged pelvic mass experience resolution of these complaints after myomectomy. Although these results are encouraging, there is some difficulty interpreting the efficacy of myomectomy by these retrospective clinical studies, which have many inherent biases.

The morbidity associated with myomectomy is similar to that of hysterectomy, but febrile morbidity is more common after myomectomy. The risk of recurrence of myomas is another major concern. Although the risk of clinically recognizable recurrent myomas after myomectomy has been estimated to be 15% (with two thirds of these women requiring additional surgical therapy), recent studies using ultrasound to document small myomas demonstrate recurrence rates from 25% to 90%. The risk of recurrence is correlated positively with the numbers of myomas resected and is not correlated with myoma size. In addition, recurrence rates increase with time since myomectomy.

PREGNANCY AND MYOMECTOMY. A critical question for women with fibroids who are contemplating pregnancy is whether to undergo myomectomy before attempting conception. Myomectomy is often performed to preserve reproductive potential, yet only about 40% of women conceive after this operation. Postoperative adhesion formation involving the fallopian tubes or ovaries, or both, may render a woman infertile. A woman must be counseled about these risks before selecting a surgical treatment plan. Cesarean section is often recommended in women who conceive after myomectomy in which the uterine cavity was entered or extensive myometrial dissection was performed. Although the risk of uterine rupture during spontaneous labor in women who have previously undergone myomectomy is ≤1%, this recommendation is still made because of the potential catastrophic consequences to the mother and her baby, especially if rupture occurs outside a hospital setting.

There are also risks of not removing myomas in women who wish to conceive. It is estimated that 10% to 15% of women with infertility have myomas and that myomas are the primary cause of infertility in 2% to 3% of all infertile women. Women with myomas who conceive are at higher risk of having a spontaneous pregnancy loss than those without myomas. The incidence of spontaneous pregnancy losses in a large series of women undergoing myomectomy decreased from 41% preoperatively to 19% after this procedure. During pregnancy, myomas may undergo carneous degeneration that may lead to severe pelvic pain, often requiring narcotics and hospitalization, and premature labor. The risk of placental abruption is significantly higher in women in whom the myoma is subjacent to the placenta.

The risk of operative delivery is significantly greater in women with myomas as a result of higher rates of dystocia, dysfunctional labor, and malpresentation of the fetus compared to those of women without fibroids. Finally women with myomas have a greater likelihood of experiencing a postpartum hemorrhage than those without tumors. In the absence of data from clinical trials, generalized treatment recommendations cannot be made about when preconception myomectomy is prudent.

During pregnancy it is generally recommended to avoid surgical treatment of symptomatic or asymptomatic uterine fibroids. Uterine blood flow is greatly increased during pregnancy and myomectomy may result in significant blood loss, uterine irritability, premature labor, or infection, and may jeopardize the fetus. In rare cases pedunculated subserosal fibroids with thin pedicles may undergo torsion leading to severe, unrelenting abdominal pain. In these cases myomectomy may be performed safely during pregnancy.

Medical management. Currently there are no medical treatments that are approved by the U.S. Food and Drug Administration for the treatment of uterine fibroids. The general strategy behind the medical management of myomas consists of hormonal treatment directed at temporarily decreasing myoma and uterine size and menstrual blood flow. Myomas (and myometrium) are hormone-sensitive tissues that decrease in volume by 40% to 60% after estrogen withdrawal during treatment with a GnRH-a for 3 to 6 months or after menopause. Treatment with a GnRH-a will also result in amenorrhea in two thirds of women; the majority of the remaining women experience light irregular spotting. The decrease in menstrual bleeding results in dramatic improvements in hemoglobin concentrations and hematocrits in women with menorrhagia-associated anemia. Once GnRH-a treatment is discontinued uterine and myoma regrowth with return of pretreatment symptoms are usually noted within 3 to 6 months.

By dramatically decreasing bioactive gonadotropin secretion by the pituitary, GnRH-a therapy results in a hypogonadal state with side effects similar to those that follow acute estrogen withdrawal and menopause. Vasomotor flushes occur in approximately 90% of women; 25% to 40% experience insomnia and symptoms of vaginal atrophy. GnRH-a therapy for 6 months will also induce an average decrease in lumbar trabecular bone density of 6%, which is only partially reversible by discontinuation of GnRH-a treatment. For these reasons GnRH-a treatment is usually limited to 3 months as preoperative therapy to restore hemoglobin concentrations to normal; to decrease myoma and uterine size, which may facilitate a surgical procedure; and to create an atrophic endometrium, which will facilitate hysteroscopic surgery. Commonly used doses of GnRH-a are shown in Table 41-1. Other hormonal treatments such as synthetic androgens (e.g., danazol), progestins (e.g., medroxyprogesterone acetate), or a combination of an estrogen and a progestin (i.e., low-dose oral contraceptives) may control excessive menstrual blood loss but will not reliably decrease uterine or myoma size. Use of oral iron supplements (e.g., ferrous gluconate 324 mg or ferrous sulfate 325 mg one to three times daily) may help to increase hemoglobin concentrations in women with menorrhagia-associated anemia. Use of nonsteroidal antiinflammatory drugs will often alleviate

Table 41-1 Commonly used GnRH-a in clinical practice*

Dose	Trade name	Pharmaceutical company
Leuprolide acetate 3.75 mg IM q4wk	Lupron depot	TAP Pharmaceuticals Inc., Deerfield, Illinois
Nafarelin acetate 1-2 whiffs (200-400 μg) intranasally twice each day	Synarel	Syntex Laboratories, Palo Alto, California
Goserelin acetate 3.6 mg SC q4wk	Zoladex depot	Stuart Pharmaceuticals, Wilmington, Delaware

*First dose usually administered cycle days 1-3 or in the middle to late luteal phase if the patient is known not to be pregnant.

pain but will not reliably decrease bleeding or other myoma-related symptoms.

PROGNOSIS AND CONCLUDING REMARKS

In general the prognosis for a woman with myomas depends upon many factors: size, number, and location of tumors; severity of symptoms; and choice of treatment. Hysterectomy is the only guaranteed cure for myomas. In women with multiple myomas the risk of tumor recurrence after myomectomy is significant, and additional treatment may be necessary. Medical treatment with GnRH-a is highly successful in temporarily controlling symptoms produced by an enlarged pelvic mass and excessive uterine bleeding, although treatment is generally limited to less than 6 months. Finally, close observation may be prudent in the case of a slow-growing or nongrowing uterus causing minor symptoms or no symptoms in a woman who wishes to avoid surgical treatment.

BIBLIOGRAPHY

Bachmann GA: Hysterectomy: a critical review, *J Reprod Med* 35:839, 1990.

Burton CA, Grimes DA, March CM: Surgical management of leiomyomata during pregnancy, *Obstet Gynecol* 74:707, 1989.

Buttram VC Jr, Reiter RC: Uterine leiomyomata: etiology, symptomatology, and management, *Fertil Steril* 36:433, 1981.

Chandrasekhar Y et al: Insulin-like growth factor I and II binding in human myometrium and leiomyomas, *Am J Obstet Gynecol* 166:64, 1992.

Cramer SF, Patel D: The frequency of uterine leiomyomas, *Am J Clin Pathol* 94:435, 1990.

Dawood MY, Lewis V, Ramos J: Cortical and trabecular bone mineral content in women with endometriosis: effect of gonadotropin-releasing hormone agonist and danazol, *Fertil Steril* 52:21, 1989.

Dicker RC et al: Complications of abdominal and vaginal hysterectomy among women of reproductive age in the United States, *Am J Obstet Gynecol* 144:841, 1982.

Droegemueller W et al, editors: *Comprehensive gynecology*. St Louis, 1987, Mosby.

Friedman AJ et al: Treatment of leiomyomata uteri with leuprolide acetate depot: a double-blind, placebo-controlled, multicenter study, *Obstet Gynecol* 77:720, 1991.

Friedman AJ et al: Recurrence of myomas after myomectomy in women pretreated with leuprolide acetate depot or placebo, *Fertil Steril* 58:205, 1992.

Friedman AJ, Haas ST: Should uterine size be an indication for surgical intervention in women with myomas? *Am J Obstet Gynecol* 168:751, 1993.

Leibsohn S et al: Leiomyosarcoma in a series of hysterectomies performed for presumed uterine leiomyomas, *Am J Obstet Gynecol* 162:968, 1990.

Lev-Toaff AS et al: Leiomyomas in pregnancy: sonographic study, *Radiology* 164:375, 1987.

Mendoza AE, et al: Increased platelet-derived growth factor A-chain expression in human uterine smooth muscle cells during the physiologic hypertrophy of pregnancy, *Proc Natl Acad Sci USA* 87:2177, 1990.

Muto M, Friedman AJ: The uterine corpus, I Ryan KJ, Berkowitz RS, Barbieri RL, editors: *Kistner's gynecology:Principles and Practice,* ed 6, St. Louis, 1995, Mosby.

National Center for Health Statistics: Hysterectomies in the United States 1965-1984, National Health Survey Series 13 No 91, Lanham, Maryland; 1987, OHHS Publication No 88-1753, U.S. Department of Health, Education and Welfare, Public Health Service.

Norris HJ, Zaloudek W: Mesnechymal tumors of the uterus. In Blaustein A, editor: *Pathology of the female genital tract,* New York, 1977, Springer-Verlag.

Reiter RC, Wagner PL, Gambone JC: Routine hysterectomy for large asymptomatic uterine leiomyomata: a reappraisal, *Obstet Gynecol* 79:481, 1992.

Thomas EJ, Okuda KJ, Thomas NM: The combination of a depot gonadotrophin releasing hormone agonist and cyclical hormone replacement therapy for dysfunctional uterine bleeding, *Br J Obstet Gynaecol* 98:1155, 1991.

Townsend DE et al: Unicellular histogenesis of uterine leiomyomas as determined by electrophoresis of glucose-6-phosphate dehydrogenase, *Am J Obstet Gynecol* 107:1168, 1970.

Vardi JR, Tovell HM: Leiomyosarcoma of the uterus: a clinocopathologic study, *Obstet Gynecol* 56:428, 1980.

Yeh J, Rein M, Nowak R: Presence of messenger ribonucleic acid for epidermal growth factor (EGF) and EGF receptor demonstrable in monolayer cell cultures of myometria and leiomyomata, *Fertil Steril* 56:997, 1991.

Zawin M et al: High-field MRI and US evaluation of the pelvis in women with leiomyomas, *Magn Reson Imag* 8:371, 1990.

42 Vaginitis

May M. Wakamatsu

Complaints of vaginitis constitute a significant proportion of office visits to adult primary care health care providers. Recent advances in understanding disease mechanisms have refined diagnostic criteria of specific vaginal disorders. Nonetheless diagnosis and management of vaginitis, particularly recurrent or chronic vaginitis, can be frustrating and time consuming for the patient and the clinician.

Diagnosis may be difficult because the three most common vaginal disorders, bacterial vaginosis, candida vaginitis, and trichomonas vaginitis, have overlapping symptoms. Although there are "classic" symptoms and signs for each, the vaginitis may be atypical or asymptomatic.

Moreover, as vaginitis is generally not considered a serious medical problem, the diagnosis may be inaccurate because it is based on the patient's symptoms and gross examination of the vaginal discharge. Other times the initial vaginitis is diagnosed correctly, but subsequent complaints are treated as recurrences of that disorder. When treatment fails, patients are labelled as having "chronic yeast infections" or "recurrent bacterial vaginosis" without a sound basis. Ultimately both the patient and the health care provider's practice suffer.

The diagnosis of vaginitis may also be hampered by incomplete understanding of normal vaginal physiologic characteristics. Some patients believe that any discharge is abnormal; Godley (1985) demonstrated that 4 to 6 cm^2 of daily discharge is normal. Similarly, patients may notice a relative increase in vaginal discharge during and after ovulation or after discontinuation of oral contraceptives and interpret it as vaginitis. Fluctuating hormone levels during the menstrual cycle and higher endogenous estrogen levels than those associated with oral contraceptives may produce relative increases in vaginal discharge.

Educating patients about the characteristics and differences of normal and abnormal vaginal discharge can offer significant relief to the patient and prevent unnecessary phone calls and visits to the health care provider. Diagnosis may require repeated evaluations to develop a picture of the clinical problem. It is best not to presume a diagnosis but to insist that the patient seek proper evaluation, particularly in cases of treatment failure. As our understanding of the causes and pathogenesis of vaginitis and vaginosis increases, it is important to use that information methodically to diagnose and treat vaginal disorders.

This chapter will consider and contrast normal vaginal physiologic characteristics and flora with the characteristics of the vaginal disorders most diagnosed. The diagnosis and treatment of bacterial vaginosis, candida vaginitis, trichomonas vaginitis, atrophic vaginitis, and cytolytic vaginosis will be highlighted.

THE NORMAL VAGINA

It is important to understand that the vaginal milieu is a delicate ecosystem that is easily unbalanced by insult. The normal pH of 3.8 to 4.2 is thought to be the first line of defense against pathogenic bacteria, fungi, and protozoa and helps to maintain cornification of the vaginal epithelium. The acidic pH is predominantly maintained by the metabolism of glycogen to lactic acid in the vagina. This is accomplished primarily by the lactobacilli present in a normal vagina, but other bacteria probably contribute as well.

Besides lactobacilli, the normal vagina contains a variety of aerobic and anaerobic bacteria (Table 42-1). The types and numbers of the different bacteria are not static and have been demonstrated to fluctuate throughout a menstrual cycle. Although most of these bacteria in a normal vaginal

Table 42-1 Bacterial vaginal flora among asymptomatic women without vaginitis

Organism	Range of recovery (%)
Facultative organisms	
Gram-positive rods	
Lactobacilli	50-75
Diphtheroids	40
Gram-positive cocci	
Staphylococcus epidermidis	40-55
Staphylococcus aureus	0-5
β-Hemolytic streptococci	20
Group D streptococci	35-55
Gram-negative organisms	
Escherichia coli	10-30
Klebsiella spp.	10
Other organisms	2-10
Anaerobic organisms	
Peptococcus spp	5-65
Peptostreptococcus spp.	25-35
Bacteroides spp.	20-40
Bacteroides fragilis	5-15
Fusobacterium spp.	5-25
Clostridium spp.	5-20
Eubacterium spp.	5-35
Veillonella spp.	10-30

From Eschenbach DA: *Clin Obstet Gynecol* 26:187, 1983.

environment are nonpathogenic, if vaginal defenses are weakened these same endogenous bacteria can participate in pelvic inflammatory disease, amnionitis during pregnancy, or vaginitis. Alteration of the normal flora may also result in the proliferation of opportunistic fungi.

Normal vaginal discharge may appear clear or white, or even flocculent, but is odorless and does not cause pruritus or irritation. Asymptomatic women average 1.6 g of discharge every 8 hours.

The tools to distinguish normal vaginal discharge from abnormal and to make the diagnosis of a vaginal disorder are not expensive or complex. Most diagnoses can be made by examining the patient, testing the pH, and examining a wet preparation of the vaginal secretions; occasionally culturing the discharge is necessary (Table 42-2). It is important to keep in mind that malignancies of the fallopian tube, uterus, cervix, and vagina can also cause abnormal discharge. Unusual causes such as sigmoid-utero fistulas secondary to diverticular disease or appendiceal-fallopian tube fistulas secondary to appendicitis have been reported.

BACTERIAL VAGINOSIS

Bacterial vaginosis is currently the most common cause of vaginitis in the United States. The incidence ranges from 15% in private practice settings to 65% in sexually transmitted disease clinics.

Previously, bacterial vaginosis was known as "nonspecific vaginitis," as it was essentially a diagnosis of exclusion. It was believed that the condition was associated with a specific bacteria whose name changed taxonomically over time: *Hemophilus vaginitis, Corynebacterium vaginitis,* and *Gardnerella vaginitis.* However, now it is understood that bacterial vaginosis is not caused by a single bacterium, but by multiple types of bacteria, thus giving rise to the new name, bacterial vaginosis.

Pathophysiology

It is now accepted that bacterial vaginosis is caused by the overgrowth of many different types of anaerobic bacteria, including *Peptostreptococcus, Bacteroides,* and *Mobiluncus* species. These anaerobes produce aminopeptidase, which breaks down peptides to amino acids and decarboxylases and then to amines. These amines, putrescine, cadaverine, and trimethylamine, produce the characteristic "fishy" odor of bacterial vaginosis, particularly upon alkalinization of vaginal secretions. The numerous bacteria cling to the

Table 42-2 Differential diagnosis of vaginitis

	Symptoms	Volume of discharge	Appearance of discharge	Wet mount	pH	Culture
Normal vagina	None	4-6 cm³/day	Clear, white	Squamous epithelial cells	<4.5	Normal vaginal flora
Bacterial Vaginosis	Asymptomatic, irritation	Increased	Homogenous, gray	NS: clue cells KOH: amine odor	>4.5	Nondiagnostic
Candida Vaginitis	Pruritus, burning	Usually increased	Cottage cheese-like, white	KOH: pseudohyphae	4-5	90% sensitive
Trichomonas Vaginitis	Pruritus	Increased	Frothy, green or gray	NS: trichomonads, increased polys	>4.5	95% sensitive
Atrophic Vaginitis	Irritation, pruritus, dyspareunia	None or increased	Watery, yellow or green	Increased polys	>4.5	Normal vaginal flora
Cytolytic Vaginosis	Burning, irritation, dyspareunia	Increased	Clumpy, white	Cytolysis of squamous epithelial cells	>4.5	Nondiagnostic

NS, normal saline solution; KOH, potassium hydroxide 10% solution; polys, polymorphonuclear leukocytes.

epithelial cell surfaces, producing the "clue cell" on a normal saline solution wet mount preparation. Concomitant with the overgrowth of anaerobic bacteria is a decrease of the normal, "protective" lactobacilli.

Risk factors for development of bacterial vaginosis are undetermined. Thomason (1991) reviewed the literature and identified two probable risk factors: the presence of an intrauterine device and the number of different sexual partners during the month prior to diagnosis. Possible risk factors for bacterial vaginosis, such as age, lifetime number of sexual partners, abnormal Papanicolaou smears, and diaphragm use, were not consistently associated with bacterial vaginosis. Evidence for sexual transmission includes decreased incidence of bacterial vaginosis in monogamous couples, coital transmission of bacteria associated with bacterial vaginosis, and acquisition of new bacterial strains in women in whom bacterial vaginosis develops. Evidence against sexual transmission includes the demonstration that bacterial vaginosis does occur in virgins and that treatment of the partners of sexually active women in general is not beneficial.

History and physical examination

Patients will most often complain of an increased, malodorous vaginal discharge. Less frequently vulvovaginal irritation will also be present. However, up to 50% of patients can be asymptomatic even though the findings of bacterial vaginosis can be demonstrated. Classically the discharge is gray.

Diagnostic tests

Diagnosis can be made when three of the following four findings are present: increased vaginal discharge; pH >4.5; "clue cells" (epithelial cells heavily stippled with bacteria that obscure the cell border) (Fig. 42-1); or release of an amine odor with KOH 10% solution. The most sensitive and specific sign is the clue cell, but this finding is dependent on the skill of the examiner. Clue cell presence is usually determined by examining a normal saline solution wet mount preparation.

Cultures generally are not helpful in diagnosis as the associated bacteria can be found in women who do not have bacterial vaginosis.

Gram's stain can be used to aid in the diagnosis of bacterial vaginosis as clue cells can be recognized and the dominance or nondominance of lactobacilli can be determined.

Management

The standard treatment for bacterial vaginosis is metronidazole 500 mg orally twice daily for 7 days. This therapy yields an 80% to 90% cure rate. Previously the literature has not supported shorter-duration treatment regimens. However, a recent metaanalysis of oral metronidazole therapies supports the use of a 2 g single-dose regimen. Further randomized, placebo-controlled studies need to be conducted before recommendations can be changed.

As oral metronidazole is not tolerated by all patients and is relatively contraindicated in the first trimester of pregnancy, other therapies have been investigated. Clindamycin 300 mg orally twice daily for 7 days has been shown to be as effective as metronidazole orally. However, a course of clindamycin is more expensive than a course of metronidazole. Currently the Center for Disease Control recommends clindamycin as the second therapy of choice.

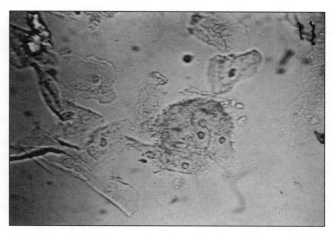

Fig. 42-1 Clue cells characteristic of bacterial vaginosis, squamous epithelial cells whose borders are obscured by bacteria.

More recent studies have concentrated on topical therapies for bacterial vaginosis in hopes of decreasing the incidence of side effects of oral therapy. Clindamycin 2% intravaginal cream has recently been approved to treat bacterial vaginosis. Studies show that clindamycin 2% cream 5 g intravaginally once daily for 7 days yields 94% to 97% cure rates. Metronidazole 0.75% intravaginal gel (5 g intravaginally twice daily for 5 days) has demonstrated a cure rate of 87% with a recurrence rate of 15%; similar cure rates have been achieved with metronidazole intravaginal tablets or sponges.

Ampicillin has been used to treat bacterial vaginosis; however, it yields a 50% to 60% cure rate. Given the efficacy of clindamycin and its safety in the pregnant patient, ampicillin is rarely used (see Table 42-3).

CANDIDA VAGINITIS

Candida vaginitis is the second most common vaginitis in the United States with an estimated 1.3 million cases annually. The incidence of candida vaginitis doubled from 1980 to 1990. Many health care providers are familiar with patients with recurrent or chronic candida vaginitis necessitating frequent visits for evaluation and treatment. These patients often have dyspareunia, which may significantly disrupt their personal lives, and their constant symptoms are a reminder that they are not "normal." Although candida vaginitis is not life-threatening, recurrent candida is frustrating for the patient and clinician and can consume health care resources.

Pathophysiology

Candida vaginitis is caused by the growth of the fungus *Candida* in the vagina. Most commonly *Candida albicans* is the causative fungal species, but over the past 20 years the incidence of non-*Candida albicans* species vaginitis has been increasing. Currently 20% of candida vaginitis may be non-*Candida albicans*. The clinical significance is that the symptoms may not be classic and some species may be slightly more resistant to the standard anticandidal treatments.

The familiar signs and symptoms, erythema, edema, burning, and pruritus, are probably a result of the alcohol that is produced by the fungal metabolism of sugar. Any condition

Table 42-3 Treatment of vaginitis

Bacterial vaginosis	Metronidazole 500 mg PO bid for 7 days Metronidazole 0.75% gel intravaginally bid for 5 days Clindamycin 300 mg PO bid for 7 days Clindamycin 2% cream intravaginally qd for 7 days
Candida vaginitis	Miconazole 2% cream intravaginally qd for 3-7 days Miconazole 200-mg vaginal suppositories qd for 3 days Clotrimazole 1% cream intravaginally qd for 3-7 days Butoconazole 2% cream intravaginally qd for 3-6 days Tioconazole 6.5% cream intravaginally as a single dose Terconazole 0.8% cream intravaginally qd for 3 days Terconazole 80-mg vaginal suppositories qd for 3 days Terconazole 0.4% cream intravaginally qd for 7 days
Chronic suppression	Ketoconazole 400 mg qd for 5 days monthly or 100 mg qd Fluconazole 150 qd once a month Clotrimazole 500-mg suppositories once weekly
Trichomonas vaginitis	Metronidazole 2 g PO as single dose, or 250 mg tid for 7 days
Atrophic vaginitis	Estradiol cream 0.25 mg (1/4 applicator) intravaginally twice weekly (or equivalent) Oral conjugated estrogens 0.3-0.625 mg qd (with progestin cycling when appropriate) or equivalent
Cytolytic vaginosis	Sodium bicarbonate douche (30-60 g/L warm water) 2-3 times weekly, then 1-2 times weekly as needed

that raises the sugar substrate availability may be a risk factor, such as diabetes and pregnancy. Other risk factors include conditions in which depressed cellular immunity is present, such as regimens of steroids or immunosuppressive agents. Any alteration of the normal vaginal flora, such as occurs with antibiotic treatment, often results in especially difficult to treat vaginal candidiasis. It is unclear whether oral contraceptives are really a risk factor as the literature both supports their role and shows no association. Occlusive clothing has traditionally been suspected of creating a more favorable climate for candida growth, and one study (Heidrich, Berg, and Bergman, 1984) has demonstrated a significant association between pantyhose use and candida vaginitis. Sexual transmissibility of candida vaginitis has been difficult to determine as well. Bisschop and Merkus (1986) demonstrated no effect of treating the male partner of female patients with candida vaginitis. However, these patients did not have a history of recurrent candidiasis, the male partners were not cultured for *candida* spp., and follow-up observation was only 4 weeks. Conversely, Horowitz and colleagues (1987) studied 33 couples in which the female patient had a history of recurrent candida vaginitis and were able to demonstrate a decrease in recurrence rate after the partner was treated. *Candida* spp. were cultured more frequently from the oral cavities and ejaculates of male partners of the female study group. There was no difference in the rectal cultures of male partners in the study versus those of the control group. After treatment 31 of 33 patients followed for 1 year had no recurrent candida vaginitis.

Chronic or recurrent candida vaginitis. The pathophysilogic characteristics of chronic or recurrent candida vaginitis in women without obvious risk factors such as diabetes or immunosuppression are highly debated. Traditional theories include the hypothesis that the intestinal tract acts as a reservoir from which the vagina can be reseeded; the "vaginal relapse theory," in which yeast colonies are so low

after treatment that the patients are culture-negative, but candida is still present and can then multiply and become symptomatic later; and the theory of sexual transmission of candida. More recently it has been suspected that some women may have a localized vaginal allergic response to candida that results in decreased cellular immunity, which then predisposes them to recurrent symptoms and infections.

History and physical examination

Classically candida vaginitis manifests a cottage cheese-like white discharge and pruritus. However, it can also exhibit no apparent increase of vaginal discharge, and patients may complain of "burning" instead of pruritus. These latter symptoms may be more characteristic of non-*candida albicans* candidal infections.

On examination the vulva and vagina may be erythematous, edematous, and covered with a characteristic discharge. Fissuring of the vulva may occur if the infection has been present for a longer duration.

Diagnostic tests

Diagnosis can be made by the presence of pseudohyphae or spores on examination of a KOH 10% solution wet mount preparation (see Plate 10 of the front feature section); however, the sensitivity of wet mounts is only 50%. Cultures are 90% sensitive and thus are a more reliable method to make the diagnosis. Cultures also offer the opportunity to determine the species in cases of recurrent or chronic candida vaginitis.

Management

Currently there are many therapeutic choices available. Choice of therapy should be determined by the patient's preference, history, severity of disease, and presence of risk factors.

For mild, nonrecurrent candida vaginitis in a patient without additional risk factors such as immunosuppression, the over-the-counter clotrimazole and miconazole creams are easily available and effective with a greater than 85% cure rate. In addition, creams are probably preferable to suppositories when candida vulvitis is also present.

If a patient has simple candida vaginitis with symptoms of short duration, single-dose therapies that may result in better compliance can be offered. However, the cure rate, 70%, may be slightly lower than that of longer-duration therapies. If the patient has been treated with antibiotics, has a long duration of symptoms, or complains of severe symptoms, one should consider the 3- or 7-day therapies. Cure rates do not significantly differ among the intravaginal imidazoles: clotrimazole, miconazole, butoconazole, and tioconazole. Most cure rates are above 85%.

The newer triazole, terconazole, offers the theoretic advantages of being more specific for the fungal cytochrome P-450, having less tendency to induce its own metabolism, and having increased contact with the fungal membrane. However, studies have shown either little or no increase in cure rate for terconazole when compared to that of the imidazoles. Terconazole may offer an advantage in treating non-*Candida albicans* species, such as *C. glabrata* and *C. torulopsis*. With its greater specificity for the fungal cytochrome P-450, one would expect adverse reactions to occur less often; however, clinically terconazole does not seem to be significantly different.

Oral therapy has been used for chronic or recurrent candida vaginitis, theoretically decreasing reseeding rates from the "intestinal reservoir." Previously ketoconazole has been used as the oral agent of choice, but a review of studies comparing the newer oral triazole, fluconazole 150 or 200 mg once, to standard intravaginal therapies and to ketoconzole shows that fluconazole is as effective as ketoconazole and has fewer adverse effects. Fluconazole is well absorbed given orally, has a lower risk of hepatotoxicity, and has a long half-life of approximately 25 hours. However, the risk of adverse effects from fluconazole therapy is still higher than that of local intravaginal therapy, so it should probably be reserved for chronic or recurrent cases.

Itraconazole has variable oral absorption and a higher risk of hepatotoxicity and therefore does not appear to offer an advantage over fluconazole.

Recurrent or chronic candida vaginitis can be successfully suppressed with intermittent intravaginal or oral antifungals. For chronic suppression oral therapy is usually preferred by the patient because of convenience. Ketoconazole 400 mg daily for 5 days monthly or 100 mg daily can reduce recurrence rates. Fluconazole may become the oral drug of choice for suppression. Fluconazole 150 mg orally once a month reduces recurrence rates by 50%.

Local therapy in the form of clotrimazole 500-mg suppositories has been used monthly and weekly for suppression. Monthly regimens have not shown to be effective, but weekly treatment may reduce recurrence rates similar to regimens using daily ketoconazole. When choosing therapy, the convenience of oral therapy, which may result in better patient compliance, must be weighed against the higher risks of oral therapy when compared to local therapy. Patients should participate in determining their suppressive therapy.

It is unclear from the literature whether treating the partner of patients with recurrent candida vaginitis will reduce recurrence rates. However, if other risk factors are ruled out

and other treatment regimens have failed to reduce recurrence rates, it is worth a trial. As Horowitz and colleagues (1987) demonstrated it is important to identify the reservoirs of candida in the partner and direct treatment accordingly. When this was done, recurrence rates were reduced.

Finally, hyposensitization may be considered when treating difficult, recurrent candida. A small trial of 10 women (Rosedale and Browne, 1979) with a history of recurrent candida vaginitis were hyposensitized to candida; the result was a decrease in the recurrence rate from every 5 months to every 15 months, and when an infection occurred the symptoms were reported as less severe and more amenable to treatment. However, as there is little literature on hyposensitization as a form of treatment it should be reserved for the difficult, recurrent cases in which other treatment modalities have been tried.

TRICHOMONAS VAGINITIS

Trichomonas vaginitis is the third most common vaginitis in the United States. Its incidence is actually decreasing, probably largely as a result of the effectiveness of metronidazole.

Pathophysiology

Trichomonas vaginitis is caused by the infection of the flagellated protozoan *Trichomonas vaginalis*. It is a sexually transmitted disease. There have been scattered reports documenting the viability of trichomonads on potential infective surfaces, such as toilet seats. However, whether actual transmission can occur via these surfaces remains conjectural.

History and physical examination

Most patients complain of vaginal and vulvar pruritus and an increased vaginal discharge. The discharge may be green, copious, and frothy. Edema and erythema of the vulva and particularly of the vagina may be present. The "strawberry" cervix is a classic finding resulting from punctate mucosal hemorrhages of the cervix.

Diagnostic tests

Diagnosis can be made by several methods. The normal saline solution wet mount preparation is most commonly used. (See Plate 11 of the front feature section.) This method is inexpensive, is convenient, and gives immediate results. However, a normal saline solution wet mount preparation has a wide range of sensitivity, 45% to 95%, because it is dependent on the experience of the microscopist. If the motile, flagellated trichomonads are identified, wet mount diagnosis is 100% specific.

Diagnosis by culture of trichomonas is more sensitive than that of the wet mount, 92% to 95%. Additionally, susceptibility testing can be performed if necessary. However, cultures are more costly and results are not available for several days, delaying treatment. Culture should be considered if the wet mount preparation finding is negative and trichomonas vaginitis is suspected.

Trichomonads can be found incidentally on Papanicolaou's smear in asymptomatic patients undergoing routine examination. It is debated whether asymptomatic trichomonads should be treated, although most clinicians favor treatment, as its risks are not great.

Several new diagnostic tests are not yet available for clinical use but probably will be in the near future. A direct immunofluorescence assay has been developed, but it is still only available in research settings. It is more sensitive than the wet mount, but less sensitive than a culture, 80% to 90%. The specificity is lower than that of both the wet mount and culture, 99%. A monoclonal-based enzyme-linked immuno-assay may become available, with the advantages of an in-office test with greater sensitivity than that of the wet mount. A latex agglutination test may also offer higher sensitivity than the wet mount, but the reliability has not yet been established.

Management

Because trichomoniasis is a multifocal infection of the vaginal epithelium, Skene's glands, Bartholin's gland, and urethra systemic treatment is necessary for cure. The standard therapy is metronidazole 2 g orally in a single dose. An alternative therapy for patients who have experienced significant nausea with the single-dose regimen is metronidazole 250 mg orally three times a day for 7 days. Both regimens usually yield cure rates of over 90%.

The incidence of trichomonas infection in the male partner has not been well defined. In an unpublished study in which only the male urethra was examined, 8% of the male contacts of infected women had positive results. The yield may have been higher if prostatic and seminal secretions had been examined. Up to 24% of women will be reinfected if their partners are not treated, so treatment of the male partner is recommended even when he is asymptomatic.

Resistant and recurrent trichomonas vaginitis. Resistance to metronidazole is uncommon although reports in the literature of cases have been increasing since 1982. Most metronidazole-resistant cases can be cured with larger doses of metronidazole as resistance is relative. If failure of initial therapy occurs the course should be repeated (with concomitant treatment of the partner). If the infection is persistent 2 to 4 g daily for 5 to 14 days can be given; however, with higher doses of longer duration the incidence and severity of adverse effects increase. These include nausea and vomiting, a metallic taste, glossitis, stomatitis, urticaria, vertigo, and, rarely, convulsive seizures and peripheral neuropathy that is reversible but may last months. Severely resistant cases should be managed in conjunction with susceptibility testing and in consultation with a specialist experienced in treating resistant cases.

 VAGINITIS IN PREGNANCY

Metronidazole is relatively contraindicated in pregnancy particularly in the first trimester because of its potential teratogenic effects. Clotrimazole intravaginally can be used during pregnancy for symptomatic relief. Cure rates are generally less than 60%. Saline solution 20% douches have been reported anecdotally to relieve symptoms as well. Povidone-iodine douches should not be used in pregnancy because absorption of the iodine may result in neonatal hypothyroidism. Acidification of the vagina through either vaginal jelly (Aci-Jel) or acetic acid washes would probably be safe, but efficacy and safety have not been documented.

ATROPHIC VAGINITIS

Atrophic vaginitis primarily affects postmenopausal women but may occur in any woman who is in a low estrogenic state (i.e., women who are breastfeeding or using oral contraceptives). As women now live one third of their lives after menopause and expect to continue to have fulfilling sexual lives, vaginal atrophy has become a significant disorder that can affect quality of living.

Pathophysiology

Atrophic vaginitis is the result of estrogen deprivation of the estrogen-dependent tissues of the genital tract. The most common cause is the postmenopausal state. Because the atrophic changes occur very gradually women often do not notice any symptoms until 5 to 10 years after menopause. Without estrogen the vulvar and vaginal epithelium become very thin, sensitive, and nonlubricated. Other hypoestrogenic states that may cause atrophic vaginitis include breastfeeding , oral contraceptive use, and gonadotropin-releasing hormone (GnRH) agonists for endometriosis.

History and physical examination

Women with atrophic vaginitis often complain of dyspareunia, which may be mild or severe relative to the amount of atrophy present. They may complain of "feeling dry" and uncomfortable even if not sexually active. Pruritis is another common symptom. Less often "postmenopausal bleeding" may send the patient to the physician's office. The site of bleeding may not be obvious, necessitating an endometrial biopsy to rule out endometrial cancer. Occasionally patients complain of a watery discharge along with some of the symptoms mentioned.

Diagnosis can usually be made by examination. The vulvar and vaginal epithelium appear less pink, thinner, and dryer, and vaginal rugae are absent.

Diagnostic tests

In patients who have complaints consistent with atrophy but have more subtle changes that are difficult to see, a vaginal Papanicolaou's test for a maturation index can be done. The *maturation index* is the percentage of basal, intermediate, and superficial cells present in the smear. In atrophy there is an increasing dominance of basal and intermediate cells. This test may be useful in women with vaginitis complaints who are using oral contraceptives or are breastfeeding when the diagnosis is uncertain.

It is important to rule out other causes that may have similar manifestations. The vulvar dystrophies, lichen sclerosus and squamous cell hyperplasia, may have a similar clinical picture. Diagnosis can be made by biopsy of the affected epithelium (see Chapter 31).

Management

Estrogen replacement is the treatment of choice for atrophic vaginitis. Estrogen administered either orally or locally results in maturation of the vaginal epithelium. If systemic hormone replacement therapy is not indicated, excellent response can be achieved by using estradiol cream 0.25 mg (or the equivalent dose in any of the other estrogen vaginal cream preparations) intravaginally twice a week. This dose has been demonstrated to have a minimal systemic effect. Some women can achieve a satisfactory response on a once-a-week regimen.

In patients for whom estrogen is contraindicated, for example women with a history of breast cancer, treatment alternatives are often ineffective. Vaginal lubricating agents can relieve vaginal dryness and dyspareunia secondary to vaginal dryness. Acidifying agents may help decrease the risk of infection by maintaining the vaginal pH in the normal acidic range (<4.5) and may help to cornify the epithelium, thus possibly lessening epithelial sensitivity. Many over-the-counter products that combine lubricating and acidifying properties are available. For patients who have mild symptoms, for example those who are recently postmenopausal, using oral contraceptives, or breastfeeding, a lubricating agent may be satisfactory. Generally, however, patients with moderate to severe atrophy are not satisfied with these agents as their effect on maturation of the epithelium, the underlying problem, is negligible.

CYTOLYTIC VAGINOSIS

Another vaginosis from which other types of vaginitis should be differentiated is cytolytic vaginosis. This vaginosis was previously known as Doderlein's cytolysis but more recently has been further characterized by Cibley and Cibley (1991). It is a condition that is often misdiagnosed as other vaginal infections, particularly recurrent candida. The typical patient is a woman referred for "recurrent candida" that has not been alleviated by multiple therapies.

Pathophysiology

The pathogenesis of cytolytic vaginosis is unclear. It is hypothesized that overgrowth of vaginal *Lactobacillus* spp. results in an environment that is too acidic and produces the symptoms. However, further studies are needed to elucidate the cause.

History and physical examination

Symptoms may be very similar to those of candida vaginitis, including pruritus, vulvar dysuria, dyspareunia, and a clumpy white discharge. The "typical" patient may have "a shopping bag full of partially used medications" that have failed. Some women may note that their symptoms occur or worsen during the luteal phase of the menstrual cycle.

Diagnostic tests

The current diagnostic criteria are absence of trichomonas vaginitis, candida vaginitis, or bacterial vaginosis; increased vaginal discharge, which is usually white, frothy, or cheesy; a pH between 3.5 and 4.5 and an increased number of lactobacilli on a normal saline solution wet mount preparation; evidence of cytolosis; and few polymorphonuclear cells. Culture would not be helpful as it would only reveal "normal vaginal flora."

Management

The recommended treatment of cytolytic vaginosis is douching with a sodium bicarbonate solution, 30 to 60 g of sodium bicarbonate in 1 L of warm water two to three times per week and then once or twice a week as needed. In patients who experience cyclic symptoms, prophylactic sodium bicarbonate douches 1 to 2 days before anticipated symptoms are recommended.

OTHER VAGINAL DISORDERS

There are other less common causes of vaginitis, some of which are controversial and others that are rarely seen in the United States. For a full discussion of these disorders, the reader is referred to Kaufman and Faro (1994).

Normal vaginal flora contains a fluctuating variety of aerobic and anaerobic bacteria. Bacteria that are potential pathogens in other parts of the body may be harmless in the vagina. However, it may be possible that overgrowth of certain types of bacteria such as *Streptococcus pyogenes* or *Escherichia coli* may result in vaginitis. It is important to rule out any other possible causes before treatment as this hypothesized cause is controversial and remains unconfirmed.

Amoebic vaginal infections are extremely rare in the United States, but if the patient has recently returned from a country where amoebiasis is prevalent and complains of a malodorous, serosanguinous, or bloody discharge with necrotic tissue fragments and vaginal ulcers, amoebiasis should be ruled out.

Retained foreign bodies, such as forgotten tampons, diaphragms, or contraceptive sponges, or the use of pessaries usually cause a malodorous, profuse, watery discharge. The discharge may be bloody because of vaginal erosions or fissures caused by pressure necrosis from the foreign body. Removal of the foreign body usually results in prompt resolution of symptoms. Management of discharge secondary to pessary use involves using intravaginal estrogen cream and acidifying agents and ruling out other causes of vaginitis.

Psychosomatic vaginitis is rarely encountered in a routine practice and is uncommon even at referral centers. Patients may have a chronic history of symptoms and multiple treatments without resolution and complain of dyspareunia resulting in abstinence. When they are examined repeatedly no pathologic findings can be demonstrated. There may be a background of psychologic problems that may not always be apparent at the beginning of the investigation. These patients must be differentiated from those with vulvar vestibulitis as some of the symptoms are similar. Patients with psychosomatic vaginitis will respond to psychotherapy and not to any nerve blocks or topical anesthetics, to which vestibulitis patients usually respond temporarily.

BIBLIOGRAPHY

Andres FJ et al: Clindamycin vaginal cream versus oral metronidazole in the treatment of bacterial vaginosis: a prospective double-blind clinical trial, *South Med J* 85(11):1077, 1992.

Bisschop MPJM, Merkus JMWM: Co-treatment of the male partner in vaginal candidosis: a double-blind randomized control study, *Br J Obstet Gynaecol* 93:79, 1986.

Cibley LJ, Cibley LJ: Cytolytic vaginosis, *Am J Obstet Gynecol* 165:1245, 1991.

Ernest JM: Topical antifungal agents, *Obstet Gynecol Clin North Am* 19(3):587, 1992.

Eschenbach DA: Vaginal infections, *Clin Obstet Gynecol* 26:187, 1983.

Eschenbach DA et al: Diagnosis and clinical manifestations of bacterial vaginosis, *Am J Obstet Gynecol* 158(4):819, 1988.

Godley MJ: Quantitation of vaginal discharge in healthy volunteers, *Br J Obstet Gynaecol* 92:739, 1985.

Greaves WL et al: Clindamycin versus metronidazole in the treatment of bacterial vaginosis, *Obstet Gynecol* 72(5):799, 1988.

Heidrich FE, Berg AP, Bergman JJ: Clothing factors and vaginitis, *J Fam Pract* 19(4):491, 1984.

Hillier S et al: Efficacy of intravaginal 0.75% metronidazole gel for the treatment of bacterial vaginosis, *Obstet Gynecol* 81:963, 1993.

Horowitz BJ, Edelstein SW, Lippman L: Sexual transmission of candida, *Obstet Gynecol* 69(6):883, 1987.

Kaufman RH, Faro S, editors: *Benign diseases of the vulva and vagina,* ed 4, St. Louis, 1994, Mosby.

Livengood CH, Thomason JL, Hill GB: Bacterial vaginosis: treatment with topical intravaginal clindamycin phosphate, *Obstet Gynecol* 76(1):118, 1990.

Lossick JG, Kent HL: Trichomoniasis: trends in diagnosis and management, *Am J Obstet Gynecol* 165:1217, 1991.

Lugo-Miro VI, Green M, Mazur L: Comparison of different metronidazole therapeutic regimens for bacterial vaginosis, *JAMA* 268 (1):92, 1992.

Mettler L, Olsen PG: Long-term treatment of atrophic vaginitis with low-dose oestradiol vaginal tablets, *Maturitas* 14:23, 1991.

Patel HS, Peters MD, Smith CL: Is there a role for fluconazole in the treatment of vulvovaginal candidiasis? *Ann Pharmacother* 26:350, 1992.

Rosedale N, Browne K: Hyposensitization in the management of recurring vaginal candidiasis, *Ann Allergy* 43:250, 1979.

Slavin MB et al: Single dose oral fluconazole vs. intravaginal tercanazole in treatment of candida vaginitis: comparison of pilot study, *J Fla Med Assoc* 79(10):693, 1992.

Sobel JD: Pathogenesis and treatment of recurrent vulvovaginal candidiasis, *Clin Infect Dis* 14(suppl l):448, 1992.

Thomason JL: Clinical evaluation of terconazole: United States experience, *J Reprod Med* 34(8):597, 1989.

Thomason JL, Gelbart SM, Scaglione NJ: Current review with indications for asymptomatic therapy, *Am J Obstet Gynecol* 1665:1210, 1991.

43 Abortion

Martha Ellen Katz and Rapin Osathanondh

Approximately 1.6 million therapeutic abortions have been reported in the United States each year since 1980. In addition, unreported menstrual extraction procedures are performed routinely that remove products of conception. At current rates, almost 50% of women have had at least one abortion by the time they reach 45 years of age. Both the lack of an ideal contraceptive method and the imperfect use of the available ones make abortion a valuable option for the resultant unintended or unwanted pregnancies.

This chapter outlines the evaluation, referral, and follow-up care of women who request abortions. It focuses on the most common procedure, first-trimester abortion by dilation and suction evacuation. The chapter also describes pharmacotherapeutic agents that soften the cervix and expel the products of conception, which are used as adjuncts and potential alternatives to surgical abortion. Termination of pregnancy by spontaneous abortion, also called miscarriage, is reviewed in Chapter 49. Recent advances in medical abortion and changes in health care financing and primary care practice have motivated internists and family physicians to obtain knowledge about abortion and thus provide women with more comprehensive care.

Although this chapter focuses on the medical aspects of induced abortion, current political controversies constrain the ability to obtain this service. The lack of universal public funding for induced abortion, harassment and violence against providers and patients at abortion facilities, as well as the dearth of abortion providers, limit access to abortion procedures. In the United States 84% of the counties have no known abortion provider. In 30 states laws, regulations, or constitutional amendments endorse public financial coverage only for induced abortion only for health reasons. Many of these states include cases of rape and incest; some states only include cases of life endangerment.

Abortion procedures differ by the trimester in which the procedure is performed. The gestational age is based on the onset of the last menstrual period (LMP) and thus 2 weeks earlier than the actual time of fertilization and age of the embryo. First-trimester abortions represent 95% of the total and are performed from weeks 5 or 6 to week 13; second-trimester procedures, fewer than 5% of the total, are performed between weeks 13 through 24. Fewer than 1% of therapeutic abortions are performed after week 20, and a few after week 24, usually for severe fetal anomalies or lethal maternal diseases.

There are two major types of therapeutic abortions: suction evacuation and labor induction. Minor methods involve the use of pharmacotherapeutic agents and ultrasound-guided procedures.

Ninety-nine percent of abortions, all first-trimester and most second-trimester, employ the suction evacuation technique. From week 6 or 7 of gestation through week 22, dilation is necessary to open the internal cervical os before suction. Consequently, this procedure is called *dilation and evacuation (D&E.)*. Between weeks 5 and 7, suction evacuation may be accomplished without cervical dilation; this is called *menstrual extraction, menstrual regulation,* or *mini-abortion.* Only 1% of all abortion procedures and 7% of second-trimester pregnancy terminations are performed by inducing labor.

EPIDEMIOLOGY

Although it might be inferred that some women use abortion in place of contraception, the relationship between contraception and abortion is a dynamic one. When populations are learning to control their fertility, such as in the United States between 1880 and 1900—and now among the young or unmarried—the use of contraception and the use of abortion rise concomitantly. With the subsequent falling birth rate, however, abortion levels tend to peak. Thereafter, when contraceptives are available and abortion laws are liberalized, the rate of contraceptive use continues to rise and abortion rates fall. Easy access to both contraception and abortion lowers the abortion rate but, because of unavoidable contraceptive failures, the need for abortion never is eliminated.

An accurate report of the illegal abortion rate is almost impossible to obtain. Although currently insignificant in the United States, most societies have a range of drugs, herbs, and procedures used by women on themselves and by unlicensed persons to end an unwanted pregnancy or to bring on a delayed menses. With the repeal of restrictive abortion laws in the 1970s it has been postulated in New York, England, and Wales that the total number of abortions did not change greatly. Rather, previously illegal operations were transferred into the legal sector.

Induced abortion today is a safe procedure. The number of maternal deaths declined more than 20-fold since abortion was legalized. Abortion is safe when compared with pregnancy. In 1985 only six deaths occurred (1/200,000 legal abortions) whereas maternal mortality was 20/200,000 births, and the rate of death from ectopic pregnancy was 1/2,000 cases. The mortality risk of childbearing approaches the risk of an abortion at 20 weeks' gestation.

PROCEDURES
Suction evacuation

Dilation and evacuation. In D&E, tapered metal rods of increasing diameter are inserted through and just beyond the internal cervical os to dilate it. After the dilation, a transparent plastic suction cannula appropriate for the gestational size is inserted into the uterine cavity. It is then attached to an electric or hydrostatic pump that produces adequate vacuum pressure for aspirating the pregnancy tissue into a container such as a gauze bag or a syringe. This vacuum aspiration causes the uterus to contract when it is empty, which feels like strong menstrual cramps. The surgeon then grossly inspects the aspirated products of conception (POC) to ensure completion of the procedure. Microscopic examination of the specimen may be useful clinically and is required in many states. The POC typically consist of chorionic villi, gestational sac, and decidua (hypertrophic gestational endometrium). A product of 9 week's gestation is only 1 cm long; that of 10 week's gestation has recognizable parts. An incomplete procedure implies removal of only the decidua and/or a fragment of the total chorionic villi.

Surgical abortion is a 5- to 15-minute procedure and can be performed in one visit. The woman recuperates for about 1 hour and can then be discharged home. At home she may participate in activities as tolerated and must refrain from intercourse, swimming, bathing, and vaginal insertions (i.e., tampons) for 2 weeks.

Menstrual extraction. Menstrual extraction, also known as *menstrual regulation, vacuum aspiration, miniabortion,* or *minisuction,* may be performed up to 7 weeks from the patient's LMP. The term *menstrual extraction* refers to the fact that the procedure may be performed at or before the time of the expected menses. It commonly is performed without cervical dilation because the soft and flexible 3- or 4-mm diameter plastic suction cannula can be inserted carefully into a gravid uterus without stretching the cervical canal. A self-locking or bulb syringe, or a small electric or hydrostatic pump, provides suction. These office procedures may be associated with a high failure rate because they are done early in pregnancy when it is difficult to visualize the complete POC.

Labor induction

Labor induction may be required for pregnancy termination beyond 15 to 18 weeks of gestation. The cervix is first prepared with osmotic dilators (see next section). On the following day, uterine contractions are induced by a variety of oral, intravaginal, intraamniotic, or intravenous pharmacotherapeutic protocols. One method instills 1.5 mg of 15-methyl-prostaglandin $F_2\alpha$ (carboprost tromethamine) into the amniotic fluid, followed immediately by 64 to 100 ml of 23.4% saline. The intraamniotic injection, similar to diagnostic amniocentesis, produces fewer side effects than the extraamniotic route. Myometrial contractions begin within an hour. If the cervical effacement reaches 90% and the last dose of prostaglandin was administered at least 2 hours previously, a high-dose intravenous oxytocin infusion is started. Induction to delivery time averages 8 hours, but the patient is allowed to labor until her cervix and lower uterine segment are favorable for instrumental extraction of the fetus. After delivery of the placenta, uterine exploration and sharp curettage should be routinely performed to remove the remaining decidual tissue and to complete the procedure. Most patients undergoing prostaglandin-induced abortion are discharged the same day.

Agents for softening the cervix

Gas-sterilized, osmotic, mechanical cervical dilators (laminaria, Lamicel, and Dilapan) (Fig. 43-1) gently swell and dilate the cervix hours before the abortion procedure. When used instead of metal dilators, they are inserted in the cervical canal at least 2 to 4 hours before first-trimester D&E and overnight for second-trimester procedures. As they slowly dilate the cervix, they may produce moderate, crampy pain. At the time of the procedure, the enlarged and softened dilators are removed. This pretreatment decreases the incidence of cervical laceration, cervico-vaginal fistula, uterine perforation, and excessive hemorrhage in D&E procedures, and shortens the induction-to-delivery time in labor-induction procedures. The primary risk of laminaria is infection caused by leaving them in place more than 48 hours.

Several varieties of osmotic dilators are available. Laminaria tents are 6-cm dried stems of seaweed in diameter sizes of 2 to 6 mm. They swell to three or four times their original width. In addition to their mechanical action, the use of laminaria is associated with increasing blood levels of prostaglandin metabolites and also may enhance the effectiveness of prostaglandin-induced labor. A synthetic dilator, Lamicel, is made of a dried polyvinyl alcohol sponge stick saturated with magnesium sulfate. Some magnesium is absorbed into the systemic circulation, but blood magnesium levels have not exceeded 4 mg/dl. Dilapan, a synthetic polymer similar to a soft contact lens, swells quickly and may be more uncomfortable than other dilators.

In addition to osmotic devices, intracervical or vaginal prostaglandin E_2 and other prostaglandin derivatives have been used successfully to soften the closed cervix.

Pharmacotherapeutic methods

Various agents are available that disrupt chorionic villi or promote cervical softening and uterine contractions. They are used in conjunction with oral or vaginal prostaglandins or surgical methods to terminate pregnancy. Although currently no U.S. Food and Drug Administration (FDA) approved pharmacotherapeutic agents are available to terminate a normal pregnancy, drugs approved for other indications are now being used for this purpose.

Agents that disrupt chorionic villi. Three different types of agents disrupt chorionic villi: progesterone receptor blockers, of which mifepristone is the prototype; inhibitors of progesterone biosynthesis, such as aminoglutethimide, epostane, and trilostane; and inhibitors of folate reductase, such as the antimetabolite methotrexate. Mifepristone represents the greatest advance as well as greatest current controversy.

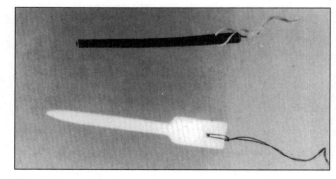

Fig. 43-1 Laminaria tent (*dark*) shown in comparison with synthetic dilator (Lamicel) (*white*). (From Ryan KJ, Barbieri R, Berkowitz R, editors: *Kistner's gynecology: principles and practice,* ed 6, St Louis, 1995, Mosby.)

Mifepristone. Mifepristone, an antiprogesterone derivative of norethindrone (a 19-nor steroid), was synthesized by the Roussel Uclaf pharmaceutical company in 1981. It has been approved for use in China, England, France, and Sweden as an abortifacient in the first 7 weeks of pregnancy. It also has been used as a morning-after pill and in the treatment of Cushing's syndrome. Under the aegis of the Population Council, a private agency that has obtained the patent rights to the drug, mifepristone is undergoing clinical trials in the United States as an oral abortifacient in conjunction with misoprostol, a methyl analog of prostaglandin E_1, for pregnancy termination up to 9 weeks' gestation.

MECHANISM OF ACTION. Mifepristone works primarily, but not exclusively, by blocking the effects of progesterone. It displaces progesterone from its receptors on the secretory endometrium, causing the chorionic villi to detach and, consequently, blood levels of progesterone and human chorionic gonadotropin to fall. Endogenous prostaglandins are stimulated, and the uterine myometrium becomes more sensitive to them. Mifepristone induces a fivefold increase in myometrial sensitivity to exogenous prostaglandins between 30 and 60 hours after oral administration. The cervix softens and opens, and 24 to 36 hours after a 600-mg dose, uterine contractions begin. Mifepristone acts at many sites on the hypothalamic-hypophyseal-ovarian-endometrial axis but appears to have no direct effect on the production of ovarian progesterone.

EFFICACY AND SAFETY. In earlier trials, after a single oral 600-mg dose of mifepristone, 80% of patients completely expelled the gestational products. The remaining cases required D&C for retained POC. Now, more successful protocols add a single dose of oral prostaglandin, misoprostol, 2 days after the mifepristone, which acts synergistically to induce uterine cramping and bleeding and potentiates the expulsion of pregnancy products. Women are asked to collect expelled tissue at home. The recovery rate of POC varies among different clinical trials. Overall, the success rate with the two-drug regimen approaches 97%, with greater success at earlier gestational ages. Up to 5% of patients require uterine suction evacuation or D&C, and fewer than 1% may lose enough blood to require transfusion. The misoprostol may cause mild systemic side effects (nausea, vomiting, or diarrhea). No cases of fetal abnormalities related to mifepristone have yet been documented among the few cases of continuing pregnancy, although significant concentrations of the drug have been shown to cross the placenta. The effects on the developing fetus still are unknown. Because progesterone opposes the effects of endogenous estrogens, it is possible, but not known whether repeated blockade of progesterone receptors would eventually lead to any estrogen-related disorders.

Mifepristone, so far, has not been shown to be reliable as a once-a-month contraceptive pill. Nor has it been shown to be beneficial, in limited, unpublished clinical trials, for terminating ectopic tubal pregnancy. Mifepristone reduces the size of certain brain tumors and also reduces intraocular pressure. In addition, the drug appears to alleviate the symptoms of endometriosis and leiomyoma uteri. Beyond the action of mifepristone on the female reproductive tract, the drug also binds to glucocorticoid receptors, thereby antagonizing the actions of cortisol and inducing compensatory rises of adrenocorticotropic hormone (ACTH).

Concurrent with a controversy about marketing mifepristone to increase abortion access in the United States, enthusiasm for the drug is tempered by several concerns. The method may not allow for routine examinatio of POC; the cost will be high for multiple visits, medications, and sonography; and long-term safety data are as yet unavailable.

Inhibitors of progesterone biosynthesis. Aminoglutethimide, epostane, and trilostane inhibit progesterone biosynthesis by blocking steroidogenic enzymes. High doses (epostane 800 mg/day for a week, for instance) usually are required for pregnancy termination up to 7 weeks. Inhibitors of progesterone biosynthesis are only moderately effective abortifacients and do not appear as promising as the progesterone receptor blockers. In addition to adrenocortical suppression, these drugs may depress the central nervous system and activate hepatic microsomal enzymes. Long-term effects on menstruation or ovulation have not been demonstrated.

Methotrexate. Inhibitors of folate reductase, such as the antimetabolite methotrexate, have been used in a single oral dose to terminate normal intrauterine pregnancy, but to date they appear more valuable in the pharmacotherapy of small ectopic pregnancies. Methotrexate is known to destroy abnormal or ectopic trophoblastic cells in contrast to mifepristone, which may be more effective in terminating early intrauterine pregnancies than ectopic ones. Methotrexate appears to potentiate the uterotonic effect of misoprostol in first trimester–induced abortions. However, use of methotrexate as an abortifacient is controversial because long-term risk, particularly its effects on hepatic and bone-marrow stem cells, is unknown. If hepatic enzymes rise, they usually return to normal after the drug is withdrawn. A fatal, idiosyncratic reaction has been documented when methotrexate is administered with nonsteroidal antiinflammatory drugs.

Uterotonic agents. Prostaglandins, oxytocin, and intra-amniotic hypertonic solutions cause contraction of the gravid uterus. They are used singly or in combination for inducing labor and delivery in therapeutic abortions. Prostaglandins and oxytocin are naturally occurring compounds that have been synthesized for use in pharmacologic doses.

Prostaglandins. Prostaglandins that induce contractions of the gravid uterus include the prostaglandin E_1 methyl analog, misoprostol; prostaglandin E_2, dinoprostone, and its synthetic derivatives such as meteneprost potassium; and 15-methyl-prostaglandin $F_2\alpha$ (carboprost tromethamine). Side effects vary among the different compounds, but each carries risks. Cardiovascular complications of certain prostaglandins can be life-threatening.

Prostaglandin E_1 methyl analog (misoprostol) is approved in the United States for the treatment of peptic ulcer disease. It also causes contractions of the gravid uterus at doses of 200 mg or higher by the oral or intravaginal route. It has been widely used for pregnancy termination in Africa and in South America because it is less expensive than other prostaglandins. If administered in unmonitored circumstances, it may result in congenital malformations of the brain, skin, and bones if the abortion is unsuccessful and the pregnancy continues, as well as hemorrhage and infection in the pregnant woman.

Recent reports in the United States of a combination of oral methotrexate and intravaginal misoprostol to terminate pregnancies at less than 10 weeks' gestation resulted in complete abortion in 90% of the cases. While this may eventually prove to be a safe option for medical abortion, at this time larger and more long-term studies are needed to determine efficacy and safety (Creinin and Vittinghoff, 1994).

Prostaglandin E_2 (dinoprostone), a vaginal suppository wax or gel, has been approved by the FDA for labor induction for fetal demise up to 28 weeks of pregnancy. The recommended dosage of 5 to 20 mg is readily absorbed through the vaginal mucosa into the systemic circulation. Prostaglandin E_2 stimulates the smooth muscle of the gravid uterus and, in some cases, those in the intestine and milk ducts. By stimulating the gastrointestinal tract and disturbing the body's thermoregulatory center, it may cause nausea, vomiting, diarrhea, and fever. Unlike prostaglandin $F_2\alpha$, prostaglandin E_2 dilates the bronchial and vascular smooth muscle when large doses are used. Thus for patients with active asthma or compromised cardiopulmonary status, prostaglandin E_2 is preferred.

15-Methyl-prostaglandin $F_2\alpha$ (carboprost tromethamine) is used in combination with hypertonic saline for intraamniotic abortion. This drug was approved by the FDA for treatment of postpartum hemorrhage by intramuscular injection. The injection-to-abortion time for second-trimester pregnancies averages 8 hours if used after laminaria preparation of the cervix. Untoward effects may include cardiac arrhythmia, bronchoconstriction, pulmonary hypertension, increased intrapulmonary shunting, and arterial oxygen desaturation. When 1.5 mg of 15-methyl-prostaglandin $F_2\alpha$ and 64 to 100 ml of 23% saline are administered via the intraamniotic route, there are minimal or no systemic effects when compared with the use of prostaglandin E_2 vaginal suppositories. However, accidental leakage of a large amount of 15-methyl-prostaglandin $F_2\alpha$ into the systemic circulation may result in cardiopulmonary complications.

Oxytocin. Endogenous oxytocin, a neurohypophysial octapeptide hormone, is released by suckling and, it is believed from animal data, by cervical dilation. It has been synthesized for clinical use for the induction of labor near term. Unlike prostaglandins, successful oxytocin-induced uterine contractions require an adequate number of oxytocin receptors. Oxytocin and prostaglandins work synergistically: the uterine muscle become more sensitive to prostaglandins with advancing gestational weeks and prostaglandins themselves may induce an increase in the number of oxytocin receptors. However, when these two drugs are administered concomitantly to induce labor, the combination may be too potent. Uterine rupture has been reported after simultaneous intraamniotic injection of prostaglandin $F_2\alpha$ or 15-methyl-prostaglandin $F_2\alpha$ with intravenously administered oxytocin.

Hypertonic solutions. Hypertonic solutions such as 23.4% saline, 30% or 40% hyperosmolar urea, and antiseptic acridine orange, when injected into the amniotic sac, induce a cascade of events leading to prostaglandin release in local tissues. Effective uterine contractions occur within several hours. However, if too large or too concentrated a volume of saline solution is accidently injected into the uterine circulation, life-threatening disseminated intravascular coagulation, intravascular hemolysis, or hypernatremia can occur.

ANESTHESIA AND ANALGESIA

Parenteral and local drugs given before surgical abortion allow the woman to be comfortable and to hold still inasmuch as movement increases the risk of trauma and uterine perforation by sharp instruments. Local (paracervical) anesthesia with or without intravenous (IV) conscious sedation is preferable to general anesthesia because blood loss and uterine perforation are significantly reduced. Recently, most complications from legal abortion in the United States are drug-related. Toxic reactions and overdosage occur with efforts to medicate the patient with vasopressors to reduce uterine bleeding and with barbiturates to relieve anxiety. A specially trained nurse, counselor, family member, or friend who accompanies the woman before and during the procedure can help relax the patient with emotional support, deep breathing, and verbal distraction.

Women generally are instructed to take nothing by mouth for 6 hours before the procedure to prevent aspiration of gastric contents in the event that a complication should require general anesthesia. Although no special indications support the use of general anesthesia for the procedure, a woman may request it. It is safer and preferable, however, to refer a frightened woman to a highly skilled operator who can complete the abortion procedure quickly with the use of local anesthesia and IV sedation.

Paracervical local anesthesia

Most D&Es up to 12 weeks can be performed with paracervical local anesthesia only. Chloroprocaine, an ester anesthetic, or lidocaine, an amide anesthetic, may be used. Chloroprocaine is more expensive but has a wider safety margin than does lidocaine. Acute drug reactions occur if a toxic dose is erroneously administered, if the anesthetic is too rapidly absorbed into the highly vascular gravid tissue, or if the operator inadvertently injects the anesthetic into the maternal circulation. The nervous system may become excited or depressed; similarly the cardiorespiratory system may react with myocardial depression, arrhythmias, hypotension, or even cardiac or respiratory arrest.

Intravenous sedation

IV sedation with short-acting benzodiazepines and opioids reduces anxiety, produces retrograde amnesia, and blunts discomfort. At our institution we use midazolam, not exceeding 2 mg, plus fentanyl, not exceeding 100 μg. Midazolam may prevent a rare syndrome of chest wall stiffness caused by IV injection of an opioid such as fentanyl. High doses of the latter drug may lead to a dose-related respiratory depression. Antidotes to midazolam (flumazenil) and of the opioid (naloxone) should be readily available. Excitement, dizziness, tachycardia, and hypotension, as well as nausea, vomiting, and respiratory depression, have been known to occur as a result of these agents. Some of these reactions may be potentiated by the increase in vagal tone that can accompany manipulation of the cervix. Occasionally 25 mg of diphenhydramine may be required for its mild anticholinergic effects.

PROPHYLAXIS
Antimicrobial

A therapeutic abortion is a clean but not necessarily sterile procedure. Only the portion of instruments entering the uterine cavity are kept sterile. Opening the cervical os exposes the endometrium to organisms in the perivaginal area. Organisms responsible for endomyometritis include aerobic and anaerobic gram-negative bacilli, aerobic streptococci, anaerobic gram-positive cocci, and mycoplasmas. Controversy surrounds the value of screening for genital pathogens before the procedure or treating with prophylactic antibiotics before, or afterward, or both because most clinical trials are uncontrolled or lack inadequate statistical power. Those who recommend screening point out that it is more cost-effective than universal prophylaxis. Without treatment, as many as 63% of women whose preoperative screening for chlamydia organisms were positive later become infected. Advocates of perioperative prophylactic treatment reason that compliance is best with IV doses. Those who recommend routinely treating patients intraoperatively or postoperatively note that in high-prevalence populations (greater than 10%), this course is cost-effective. Others are concerned about the overuse of broad-spectrum antibiotics in the absence of a specific organism to treat.

Although only some studies suggest that routine prophylactic antibiotics reduce the risk of infection after abortion, most agree that antimicrobial prophylaxis decreases the incidence of infection in women at high-risk. By literature review, we have a large at-risk population: those with fetal death, placenta previa, tattoo, Asherman's syndrome, an intrauterine device, an orthopedic or a cardiac prosthesis, or cervical cytologic findings of trichomonads or koilocytosis. We also treat women with a history of multiple abortions, pelvic inflammatory disease, sexually transmitted disease, tubal pregnancy, intravenous drug use, or multiple male partners, as well as adolescents, diabetics with vascular complications, HIV-positive women, women with sickle cell trait or disease or chronic hepatitis, and women in correctional institutions. In addition, we also prescribe antibiotics after excessive blood loss during the procedure if myometrial injury is suspected, or if a procedure takes longer than 20 minutes (see box, below).

Preoperative prophylaxis against bacterial endocarditis is recommended not only for patients with valvular heart disease or septal defects but also for intravenous drug users.

RECOMMENDED ANTIBIOTIC PROPHYLAXIS FOR THERAPEUTIC ABORTIONS

Doxycycline 100 mg bid + metronidazole* 500 mg bid × 5 days
Ampicillin 2 g + gentamicin 100 mg + clindamycin 900 mg or metronidazole 500 mg[1]*[†]
Doxycycline 100 mg 1 hour before the procedure and 200 mg one-half hour afterward[‡]
Metronidazole 400 mg 1 hour before and 4 and 8 hours afterward[§]
Aqueous penicillin G 1 million units IV, or doxycycline 100 mg PO before the procedure, 200 mg afterward; second trimester, cefazolin 1 g IV[//]

---

*Use metronidazole if a malodorous vaginal discharge suggests nonspecific vaginosis or if trichamonads are present.
[†]Centers for Disease Control: Morbidity and Mortality Weekly Reports, vol 42, 1993.
[‡]Levallois P, Rioux JE: *Am J Obstet Gynecol* 158:100, 1988.
[§]Heisterberg 1, Petersen K: *Obstet Gynecol* 65:371, 1985.
[//]*Met Lett Drugs Ther* 35:906, 1992.

RH sensitization

To prevent Rh isoimmunization, anti–D immune globulin such as RhoGAM or MICRhoGAM should be administered within 72 hours to all Rh-negative, Du-negative women who are undergoing induced abortion. Approximately 4% of these women would otherwise become sensitized after therapeutic abortion beyond 7 weeks' gestation. This incidence increases with advancing gestational age. The standard dose for first-trimester abortions is 50-μg anti–D immune globulin and 300 μg for procedures after week 13.

During medical abortion with mefepristone and prostaglandin or during menstrual extraction abortion, fetomaternal hemorrhage occurs, but less so than with dilated surgical procedures. Nevertheless, it is a safe and inexpensive practice to administer anti–D immune globulin to all women with Rh or Du negativity at or before the time of menstrual extraction or at the time of oral prostaglandin dose after mifepristone treatment.

COMPLICATIONS
Abortion facilities

Almost all D&E procedures can be safely accomplished in an outpatient facility. Mortality has been found to be equivalent in hospital and licensed outpatient settings. Patients with medical or technical complications should be referred to the most experienced hospital center with ancillary and emergency services and a surgeon with particular expertise. Candidates for specialty referral include women with uterine anomalies or leiomyoma restricting easy access to the uterus, severe cardiac or pulmonary disease, coagulopathies, or mental diseases that prevent cooperation. Previous cesarean section or other pelvic surgery may not be a contraindication to outpatient first-trimester abortion. Second-trimester pregnancies also can be safely terminated in an outpatient setting, with preoperative dilation with osmotic dilators and an experienced physician. Although the potential for major complications is small, licensed outpatient facilities are required to have available pulse oximetry, resuscitative and ultrasound equipment, and appropriate drugs, as well as ease and expediency in transporting patients to a hospital. Blood products should be available wherever second-trimester abortions are performed.

Intraoperative ultrasound guidance has been advocated by several authors to minimize complications. This guidance is beneficial if performed by experienced ultrasonographers, particularly in cases of anatomic abnormalities or in multifetal pregnancy reduction. Routine guidance, as advertised by some facilities, may even be harmful if performed by inexperienced sonographers.

Risk

The two most important determinants of mortality and morbidity as a result of abortion are the gestational age and the operator's experience. It has been shown repeatedly that the safest induced abortions are performed between weeks 7 and 12. Morbidity and mortality rates of first-trimester abortions are approximately one tenth those of later abortions. Increased risks of uterine trauma and hemorrhage occur in procedures performed by inexperienced physicians. The type of operation and method of cervical dilation, age of the patient, type of anesthesia, obstetric history, and body habitus also contribute to the risk of complications (see box on the following page).

FACTORS THAT DECREASE RISK OF UTERINE PERFORATION IN DILATION AND EVACUATION ABORTION

7 to 12 weeks' gestation
Use of laminaria
Patient older than 17 years of age (all gestational ages)
Use of local anesthesia
History of a prior abortion
Nulliparous patient
Patient not obese
Performed by attending physician
No cesarean scars

Common and rare complications

Complications occur in 0.11% of all abortions. The most common complications are retained tissue; and mild infection (Table 43-1).

Catastrophic and rare complications that occur in the perioperative period include laceration of uterine vessels, with subsequent expanding hematoma and hypovolemia, and undetected uterine perforation leading to generalized peritonitis from bowel injury. These problems may be fatal and require prompt surgical exploration and treatment.

Several other rare complications are primarily associated with second-trimester D&E and labor-induction procedures. Hematometra (the postabortal or redo syndrome) is characterized by dark, clotted blood in the uterus. Also, especially following a fetal demise, an unusual respiratory embarrassment associated with forceful uterine contractions may occur, causing transient coughing and bronchospasm. Amniotic fluid embolism is another rare complication of second-trimester abortion. It may occur after the disruption of the placental bed with surgical instruments and resultant leakage of a large volume of amniotic fluid into the uterine circulation. It usually is associated with cardiopulmonary collapse and disseminated intravascular coagulopathy.

APPROACH TO THE WOMAN CONSIDERING AN ABORTION

The goal of treatment for a woman who requests a pregnancy termination is to confirm the diagnosis of intrauterine pregnancy, estimate the age of the conceptus, support the decision for abortion, inform the patient of the appropriate type of termination, and perform or refer her for abortion. Afterward, medical follow-up and evaluation should include determining a usable form of contraception. When a woman seeks care for a suspected pregnancy, confirmation of the pregnancy and decision making about the potential outcome may proceed simultaneously.

Counseling

Counseling plays a critical role in the development of quality abortion services. Factors that may be explored in the decision to terminate or to continue a pregnancy include number of children, nature of the relationship with the father, and, in the case of adolescents, nature of the relationship with parents, emotional or financial ability to care for a child, medical risks, toxin or environmental exposures,

Table 43-1 Complications of first-trimester abortion

Complication	Ratio
Serious	
Incomplete	1:3,617
Sepsis	1:4,722
Uterine perforation	1:10,625
Vaginal bleeding	1:14,166
Inability to complete	1:28,333
Ectopic pregnancy	1:42,500
TOTAL	1:1405
Minor	
Mild infection	1:216
Repeat procedure, same day	1:553
Repeat procedure, subsequently	1:596
Cervical stenosis	1:6,071
Cervical tear	1:9,444
Underestimation of gestational age	1:15,454
Seizure	1:25,086
TOTAL	1:118

Modified from Hakim-Elahi E, Tovell HM, Burnhill MS: *Obstet Gynecol* 76:929, 1990.

and career or educational plans. Religious, moral, and political considerations also influence the decision. Medical risks associated with carrying a pregnancy to term and with abortion should be reviewed. Family or professional support should be assessed. Screening for psychiatric illness, substance use, and abusive relationships will help determine if additional support is needed. Carrying the pregnancy to term or adoption should be presented as options.

Once the decision to terminate a pregnancy is made, guidance about the anticipated medical and emotional experience prepares the woman for the procedure. Sometimes an unplanned pregnancy precipitates a life crisis with relationships or career plans. If the woman feels ambivalent, her anxieties may be relieved if the provider describes the decision as complex but not wrong and offers empathic, nonjudgmental listening. Preabortion counseling should differentiate ambivalence from confusion. Although some ambivalence is common, most women resolve their conflicts soon after the procedure, particularly if they have support.

A woman also may choose to terminate a second-trimester pregnancy for fetal structural defects or for chromosomal or metabolic abnormalities detected by amniocentesis. These pregnancies are likely to be at 15 weeks' gestation or more and are likely to be cared for already by an obstetrician.

History and physical examination

A directed history and a physical examination are required to confirm the diagnosis of intrauterine pregnancy and to estimate the gestational age. Findings also determine reproductive problems, elicit underlying disease, and uncover conditions that create risks for the abortion procedure or analgesia (see box on the following page). Estimation of gestational age may be made by a combination of the date of the LMP, the timing of intercourse, symptoms of pregnancy, and results of the abdominal and pelvic examination. The history and physical findings may be corroborated with

HISTORY AND PHYSICAL EXAMINATION BEFORE ABORTION

History
Age
Gravidity and parity:
  Prior spontaneous or elective abortions
  Prior ectopic pregnancies
Obstetric outcomes:
  Method of delivery/cesarean section
  Complications

Gynecologic history
Pelvic inflammatory disease
Sexually transmitted disease
Abnormal Pap smear
Fibroids
Congenital anomalies
DES exposure
Pelvic surgery
Menarche, interval, last normal menstrual period and duration
Reproductive history:
  Contraceptive history
  Number and sexual history of partners
  Frequency of intercourse
Future childbearing plans
Medical history:
  Diabetes
  Hepatitis
  Heart disease/rheumatic heart disease/heart murmur
  Hypertension
  Neurologic problems/seizures
  Phlebitis/thromboembolic disease
  Hematologic disorders
  Thyroid disorders/endocrine problems
  Asthma
  Urinary disorders/kidney problems
  Psychiatric or social problems, including family
    violence/abuse
Allergies
Medication
Surgery
Blood transfusions
Habits:
  Alcohol/drug use
  Smoking—packs per day
Family history

Current symptoms and duration
Breast tenderness
Nausea
Bleeding/spotting
Pain

Physical examination
Blood pressure
Pulse
Height/weight
Head/eyes/ear/nose/throat
Skin
Thyroid
Breasts and axilla
Heart
Lungs
Abdomen
Genitalia/pelvic

DES, diethyl stilbestrol.

ultrasound examination and, in problematic cases, quantitative serum human chorionic gonadotropin (hCG) levels.

The probability of error in establishing the LMP is highest in women who become pregnant postpartum or after discontinuing oral contraceptives, because the interval between the birth or stopping the oral hormones and ovulation is highly variable. Other causes for error in the LMP occur when vaginal bleeding or spotting follows implantation of the blastocyst, which may be misinterpreted as a menstrual period, especially when menses are irregular. According to World Health Organization (WHO) studies, one in five adolescents reports uncertainty of LMP, and ultrasound examination in the first-trimester is only accurate within 1 week. Preoperative ultrasound imaging successfully identifies 100% of cases past the first trimester despite the LMP and a bimanual examination that place the patient at 12 weeks or less. The probability of error in the bimanual examination increases with parity, obesity, fibroids, and prior pelvic surgery. Accuracy in the estimation of fetal age is important inasmuch as pregnancies before and after week 7, week 13, or week 18 may be handled differently.

Diagnostic tests

A positive result of a urine or serum test for hCG confirms the pregnancy. Nonprescription and commonly used laboratory qualitative urine tests show positivity at 4 to 5 weeks from the LMP. Current commercial tests are highly sensitive.

Serum quantitative pregnancy tests measure the level of total hCG using antibody against its β-subunit. hCG is detectable in the maternal circulation about 6 to 9 days after ovulation, or approximately 3 weeks from LMP. A single quantitative serum test result may give a crude estimate of gestational age. hCG levels are high in patients carrying multiple or molar pregnancies and are low in those with missed abortion, complete abortion, or ectopic pregnancy.

If a discrepancy is found between the LMP and uterine size by bimanual examination, the use of ultrasound is indicated. Women who have been taking oral contraceptives or who have recently delivered a child may be in an earlier period of pregnancy than their LMP would suggest. Such women may require ultrasound examination to confirm their pregnancy dating.

If the uterus feels small for the LMP, if there is pain, or if an adnexal mass is palpated, or if a quantative serum hCG level does not correspond to the clinical findings, an extrauterine (ectopic) pregnancy must be suspected and a transvaginal ultrasound scan obtained. If copious vaginal bleeding or clots have been expelled and abdominal pain is present, particularly if the cervical os if found to be open, a spontaneous or incomplete miscarriage can be ruled out by use of ultrasound as well. If the suspicion of ectopic pregnancy or incomplete miscarriage is low, quantative hCG levels should be obtained serially at appropriate intervals (Table 43-2). Serum levels of hCG double approximately every 2 days only during the first month of gestation. The doubling time varies greatly with the age of gestation as well as with the individual. Because standards differ, the same laboratory should be used for serial tests.

Nearly all women who want to terminate their pregnancy in the first trimester are good candidates for an outpatient procedure under local anesthesia. The patient may elect IV sedation to augment local paracervical block. Clinicians

Table 43-2 Pregnancy dating by ultrasound and quantative serum human chorionic gonadotropin

Measure by gestational sac (age/LMP diameter)	Serum hCG (Second system of units) 2nd International Reference Preparation (2nd IRP)	Transabdominal sonographic scanning	Transvaginal sonographic scanning
	0-180 mIU/ml	No sac	No sac
	500-1000 mIU/ml		Gestational sac usually seen
	≥1000 mIU/ml	•	Gestational sac consistently seen
5-1/2 wks	≥3600 mIU/ml		Yolk sac
	≥5400 mIU/ml		Embryo
4-6 wks	1800-10,000 mIU/ml	Gestational sac only	
5-6 wks	≥10,000 mIU/ml	Embryo	
5-7 wks		Cardiac activity	Cardiac activity
5-10 wks		Yolk sac	
5-16 wks		Amnion separate from chorion	Amnion separate from chorion
Up to 15 wks		Corpus luteum cyst	Corpus luteum cyst

Courtesy Peter M. Doubilet, MD, PhD, Boston, Mass.

should counsel against procedures at abortion facilities that seem to advocate general anesthesia for all patients.

Second-trimester abortion procedures up to 22 weeks may be performed by specially trained operators at certain outpatient sites. Women who require late second-trimester procedures should undergo ultrasound imaging to accurately size the pregnancy. If the biparietal diameter is greater than 50 to 55 mm, the woman generally is referred to a facility that performs labor-induction procedures.

Preoperative diagnostic and screening tests are listed in the box below.

Patients may have personal requests, such as having a companion in the procedure room, which is permitted in many facilities. Some women are curious about the size and the form of the POC. Those who may wish to see them at the time of the procedure should be encouraged to ask the surgeon.

Future contraception should be discussed at the time of preoperative counseling. Medroxy progesterone acetate (Deproprovera) or insertion of a levonorgestrel implant (Norplant) after the procedure can be offered.

Informed consent

In many states written informed consent is required before performing the abortion. Review of the information that describes the procedure and potential adverse outcomes provides an opportunity to answer questions and to prepare the patient regarding what to expect. In all but 13 states, adolescents need parental consent or notification for abortion procedures. In certain circumstances, a judicial waiver can bypass the **parental notification** requirements. Specific consent is required if the POC will be used for medical research.

Referral

Referral by the primary care physician to the clinician who performs the abortion should include the results of the physical examination and pregnancy test(s), the ultrasound scan if obtained, and the estimated period of amenorrhea. The referral should indicate any need for antibiotic, cardiac, or Rh prophylaxis, results of screening tests for infection, prior reactions to anesthetic agents, underlying diseases, allergies, and medications.

Patients with medical problems and those on long-term drug therapy

Patients with stable, well-controlled diabetes (no ketoacidosis or recent insulin adjustments) can undergo an abortion in an outpatient setting. If the woman is fasting all morning, it is recommended that she take half her normal insulin or oral hypoglycemic dose on the day of the procedure. Perioperative monitoring of glucose determines therapy afterward. Diabetic women should have an intravenous line in place and be well hydrated. Women with brittle diabetes and those with renal or vascular complications should have a hospital-based procedure and should receive antibiotic prophylaxis.

Patients with mild or moderate hypertension can undergo an abortion in an outpatient setting. If medicated, the woman should take her usual dose the morning of the procedure. Oxytocin is the drug of choice if bleeding occurs as a result of uterine atony. Ergotalkaloids (such as methylergonovine maleate (Methergine) or ergotrate maleate (Ergotrate) should not be used. Serum potassium levels should be obtained preoperatively in the event of surgical complications that require general anesthesia. For the woman with uncontrolled hypertension, an elective abortion should be deferred until the blood pressure is treated.

DIAGNOSTIC TESTS

Human chorionic gonadotropin (hCG)
Hematocrit
Blood type (ABO and Rh) and antibodies
Platelets
Gonorrhea culture*
Chlamydia assay*
Hepatitis B*
Rapid plasma reagin (RPR)*
Human immunodeficiency virus (HIV)*
Pap smear*
Rubella†

---

*For screening or if clinically indicated.
†For screening.

Patients with symptomatic cardiac disease and those with artificial heart valves, previous myocardial infarction, coronary heart disease, or history of bacterial endocarditis should undergo abortion procedures in a hospital setting. Intraoperative and postoperative cardiac monitoring may be required. Women with valvular heart disease or septal defects require antibiotic prophylaxis against bacterial endocarditis and may undergo an outpatient abortion if they are free of symptoms.

Women with severe or active asthma are most safely cared for in a hospital facility. Preoperative glucocorticoids and/or diphenylhydramine may be used for prophylaxis. Sympathomimetic agents are contraindicated because they can confound the accurate assessment of cardiopulmonary status.

Women with hemorrhagic disorders or conditions that alter blood clotting, such as uremia or lupus erythematosus, should undergo abortion procedures in a hospital facility.

A woman with a well-controlled seizure disorder may undergo an outpatient abortion. If she is on a daily medication regimen the woman should take her usual morning dose with a small amount of water. If the woman has a history of poorly controlled seizures, she should be referred for abortion at a facility where endotracheal intubation is available.

Disease secondary to HIV does not contraindicate an outpatient abortion. Platelet function and bleeding tendency should be assessed before the procedure. Women receiving nucleoside or oncolytic therapy may continue their use if hematologic parameters are stable. Antibiotic prophylaxis is recommended for HIV-positive women.

For mentally incompetent or psychiatric patients, complete control with neuropsychiatric medications is vital before they enter the abortion facility. This can be accomplished once the decision to terminate the pregnancy is certain, and thus the effects of the medication on the fetus are inconsequential. A consent form signed by the legal guardian or authority is required. These women should be accompanied by their guardian on all visits.

Vaginitis with trichomonads or bacterial vaginosis should be treated before and after the abortion with metronidazole. Candidiasis may be treated before the procedure or after the follow-up visit.

Women taking aspirin or aspirin-containing drugs should discontinue their use for 7 days before surgery. Women taking long-term nonsteroidal antiinflammatory medications should temporarily discontinue the drug 3 days before the surgical procedure.

Women taking warfarin (Coumadin) should discontinue it 2 days before the procedure or convert to heparin anticoagulation on the two preceding nights, depending on the clinical situation. Generally, for patients with a mechanical valve, heparin is preferred.

AFTER THE PROCEDURE

After the procedure, the woman is discharged from the center with instructions.

The postabortion visit

The routine postabortion visit may be scheduled 2 to 3 weeks after the procedure to detect complications, give emotional support, and answer questions about birth control and return to sexual activity (see box, above right).

THE POSTABORTION VISIT

Information from the abortion provider

Estimated gestational age after the procedure
Results of laboratory testing, usually including hematocrit level
Type of anesthesia or sedation used
Rh and anti D–immuneglobulins if administered
Discharge medications (antibiotics, ergot alkaloids)
Type of contraceptive anticipated or prescribed
Pathology report

History

Symptoms of pregnancy
Pain, bleeding, fever
Medications taken after discharge
Emotional status and support

Physical examination

Temperature, pulse, blood pressure
Abdomen
Genital/pelvic

Laboratory

Quantitative hCG (routine for menstrual extractions only)

Counseling/education/prescription

Emotional support
Contraceptive method

Iron may have been prescribed if bleeding during the procedure was excessive or if the patient had a low preoperative hematocrit level. Iron supplementation at some sites is routine for a hemotocrit value less than 32%. Unfortunately, this may complicate the diagnosis of a non–iron deficiency anemia. If bleeding during the procedure was excessive as a result of an atonic uterus, a short course of an oral ergot alkaloid may have been prescribed.

Bleeding and pain should have ceased by the postoperative visit. The physical examination will determine if there is fever, if the uterus has involuted, and if pelvic tenderness is present, which might indicate endoparametritis. The serum hCG should be undetectable at 4 weeks after a first-trimester abortion and 2 weeks after a second-trimester abortion although it is not routinely checked (Fig. 43-2).

For menstrual extraction procedures, some authorities recommend obtaining a routine postoperative hCG level to rule out retained POC. Most retained POC will be expelled spontaneously, but 1% to 2% of menstrual extraction procedures fail, resulting in the continuation of an intrauterine pregnancy.

Most women experience relief in the weeks after an abortion, but some feel emotionally labile. Even if the woman had positive feelings about the decision to terminate the pregnancy, she may experience some self-doubt and recrimination. Some women have grief reactions that resolve; few have prolonged grief. Adolescents are particularly prone to adverse psychologic reactions. Postpartum depression, especially after a second-trimester abortion, may have hormonal components, but this is not proved. Nevertheless, if distress is prolonged or severe, the woman should be referred for professional counseling or psychiatric evaluation.

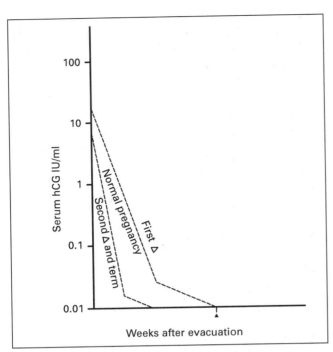

Fig. 43-2 Disappearance of human chorionic gonadotropin after termination of normal pregnancy. (From Osathanondh R: *Current problems in obstetrics and gynecology*, Chicago, 1980, Year Book Medical Publishers.)

The postabortion visit should include establishing a realistic, usable form of contraception. An unplanned pregnancy and the abortion experience may help a woman to become more consistent and assertive with partners in the use of contraception (see Chapter 27). A new prescription of oral contraceptives may be started on the Sunday after the procedure. Pills low in estrogen should be used for women in whom a relatively hypercoagulable state is suspected after pregnancy termination (see box, below).

RISK FACTORS FOR BLOOD-CLOTTING ABNORMALITIES

Activated clotting

Malignant disease or occult malignancy
Obesity
Oral contraceptive use
Intravenous drug use
Repetitive pregnancy loss (antiphospholipid antibodies)
Chronic abruptio placentae
Early fetal demise

Depressed clotting

Mild/occult von Willebrand's disease
Aspirin or nonsteroidal antiinflammatory drug use
Red wine three or more times a day
HIV
Uremia
Acute abruptio placentae
Late fetal demise

Evaluation of complications

Emergencies. Patients with persistent fever of 38° C (100.4° F), with bleeding that soaks one pad every 1 to 2 hours or that increases over 2 days, or with severe persistent pain, require evaluation for infection, perforation, retained POC, or ectopic pregnancy. Furthermore, if the microscopic examination of suctioned uterine contents reports neither villi nor implantation site, the patient must be evaluated for complete miscarriage or ectopic pregnancy.

The most common cause of unusually heavy postabortal bleeding is retained POC. This occurs in 0.2 to 0.6% of cases and may be diagnosed by ultrasound scan. Most excessive bleeding occurs within 1 week, although it occasionally occurs several weeks after the procedure. Severe pain, pelvic tenderness, or bleeding may suggest an infection or inflammation. Bleeding from infection and inflammation because of a subinvoluted uterus usually is modest if there are no retained POC. Fever and uterine tenderness are the most common signs of postabortal endometritis (0.5% of abortion complications present with uterine tenderness), which may require uterine reaspiration and antibiotic treatment. If reevacuation is indicated, only experienced surgeons should perform the second procedure because the risk of perforating the necrotic or inflamed uterine wall is greater than in the first procedure. Patients with fevers above 38° C (100.4° F) and signs of peritoneal irritation require hospitalization to be observed for acute abdominal signs and to receive intravenous antibiotics against anaerobes, gonorrhea, and chlamydia. Outpatient treatment with doxycycline, 100 mg twice daily for 7 to 14 days, should be reserved for patients whose signs and symptoms are confined to the empty uterus.

Dysfunctional uterine bleeding after abortion without signs or symptoms of retained POC or infection (no fever, closed cervix, nontender uterus) may be treated with three cycles of oral contraceptives. Curettage rarely is necessary unless bleeding is significant or symptomatic of acute blood loss. A slowly expanding broad-ligament hematoma requires immediate attention from an experienced gynecologic surgeon.

Most thromboembolic complications are diagnosed within 1 or 2 weeks after the abortion. (See box at left for conditions that activate or depress blood clotting.)

Ectopic pregnancy occurs in 0.5% to 1% of all pregnancies. From 1972 to 1985, the rate of ectopic pregnancy concurrent with induced abortion was 1.36/1000 abortions. Early clinical presentation may include pain, bleeding, and an adnexal mass. Late presentation is hypotension and shock. The use of transvaginal ultrasound is the procedure of choice to rule out an early ectopic pregnancy. In general, transvaginal sonography allows closer observation of the pelvic organs and has better resolution than does a transabdominal ultrasound scan. The former can visualize a smaller, one-half week earlier yolk sac and embryo at lower levels of hCG. Transabdominal scan may be performed routinely after the transvaginal route. Alternatively, if the transvaginal scan demonstrates a lower uterine–segment fibroid or raises the question of a higher pelvic mass, then the use of abdominal ultrasound is indicated. The diagnosis is certain if the ultrasound scan shows an embryo outside the uterine cavity. If ultrasound results show an intrauterine pregnancy, the likelihood of ectopic is less than 1:8000.

Likewise, this probability is low if there is a clearly demonstrated simple ovarian cyst. The probability is high in the absence of intrauterine pregnancy and the presence of a complex adnexal mass and/or free fluid.

Hematometra may occur 1 or 2 days after a D&E. The tense, tender, and globular uterus contains dark liquid and clotted blood. The patient usually shows facial signs of distress, as well sweating and tachycardia, but vaginal bleeding is not excessive. Referral for treatment by repeat suction evacuation of the uterine cavity is the recommended treatment. Although the cause of this problem is unknown at this time, we prescribe an ergot alkaloid and antibiotic drug in such cases for prophylaxis.

Late complications. Delayed complications of induced abortion include different degrees of postabortal infection from endoparametritis to pelvic septic thrombophlebitis and thromboembolic events. Infection usually is associated with retained POC. Common symptoms are crampy pain with prolonged vaginal bleeding and low-grade fever. The uterus is tender, slightly enlarged, and boggy. High-resolution ultrasound imaging with a full bladder may confirm or exclude the diagnosis of retained POC. Treatment consists of intravenously administered antibiotics and an ergot, and repeated uterine evacuation may be required. Patients with a continuing pregnancy or retained POC infrequently have an unrecognized positional, anatomic, or congenital uterine anomaly. Such patients should undergo a repeat D&E under ultrasound guidance.

Postabortal amenorrhea, usually without pain, may be related to a poorly understood complication called *Asherman's syndrome.* Destruction and scarification of the endometrium with adhesions and synechiae characterize the syndrome. It is a rare condition and may be related to a genetic propensity coupled with an as yet unrecognized endometrial infection. Hysteroscopic surgery is required to confirm the diagnosis and constitutes part of the various treatments.

Long-term sequelae

Long-term sequelae of repeat first-trimester abortions by vacuum aspiration are not associated with any subsequent adverse consequences on fertility, pregnancies, or the risk of ectopic pregnancy. Evidence from the 1970s suggested that two or more induced abortions increase the risk of subsequent first- and second-trimester spontaneous abortion, prematurity, and low-birth-weight infants. With current, more gentle surgical techniques and with better training of operators, these findings have been disputed. A rare long-term complication, related to Asherman's syndrome, may be caused by undiagnosed infection, hematometra, or genetic predisposition. A recent case-control study has demonstrated an increased risk of developing breast cancer in women who had an induced abortion (Daling et al., 1994). However, these results are preliminary and will remain inconclusive until larger studies with better control for reporting bias are done. Only large prospective or retrospective studies undertaken during the 1990s will allow conclusions about the long-term sequelae of appropriately performed second-trimester abortions.

REPEATED REQUESTS FOR ABORTION

It is widely believed that women who repeatedly request abortions are noncompliant or substitute abortion for contraception. During the 1980s, approximately 1.2 million live births per year occurred because of mistimed or unwanted pregnancies, many despite the use of contraception. Among one sample of abortion patients, 51% were using a method of contraception during the month in which they conceived. Studies examining the rate of abortion relative to the use of contraceptives indicate that contraceptive failure constitutes the major cause of repeat abortion.

Two general populations of women who select abortions have been identified. The first group has access to contraception. These women tend to use abortion as an adjunct to other family planning methods to postpone first births or to prevent late or higher parity order offspring, usually after the second child. Another group does not have easy access to contraception. These women use abortion to prevent late pregnancies or to increase birth spacing, usually after four or more children. The first group tends to rely on abortion for contraceptive failures, whereas the second group, which is still struggling to control its fertility, uses contraceptives intermittently and therefore depends on abortion instead of contraception to terminate unwanted or mistimed births.

SELECTIVE REDUCTION OF MULTIFETAL PREGNANCY

Successful in vitro fertilization, gamete intrafallopian transfer, and aggressive pharmacotherapy of infertility have led to an increase in gestations with three or more fetuses. To decrease the risk of premature birth, procedures to reduce multiple fetuses to twins have been performed with increasing success. At present, the most popular method is ultrasound-guided transabdominal injection of potassium chloride at the end of the first trimester. Selective reduction procedures also have been performed in the second trimester for termination of a defective twin. The risk of losing some or all of the fetuses varies at different gestational ages and increases with advanced maternal age. Maternal complications include bleeding, infection, leakage of amniotic fluid, and the need for a repeat procedure. Rarely, the patient may need to undergo D&E or hysterectomy.

SUMMARY

Therapeutic abortion is widely practiced as an adjunct to contraception. Surgical abortion in the first trimester between 7 and 12 weeks from the LMP is a safe operation when performed by an experienced provider with the patient under local anesthesia. Second-trimester procedures carry an added risk of hemorrhage and trauma but are still safer than carrying a pregnancy to term. Few women require hospital-based procedures. The postabortion visit returns the patient to the primary care setting to detect complications, assess emotional status, and establish a reliable method of contraception. Common complications include infection and bleeding as a result of retained POC. Late second-trimester abortions usually are accomplished by labor induction. Indications include fetal malformations or demise, as well as chromosomal or structural abnormalities, or rarely, the need to save the mother's life. Such procedures are managed by the obstetrician. The recent use of an oral abortion pill, mifepristone, in several countries has expanded therapeutic alternatives for early first-trimester pregnancy termination. However, cost, multiple visits even if in the privacy of a physician's office, the inability to routinely examine the POC, and lack of long-term safety data may continue to make surgical D&E the procedure of choice. New pharmacotherapeutic agents can, however, become useful adjuncts to make surgical abortions safer and more expedient. The initial evaluation, referral, and follow-up of surgical, therapeutic abortions by internists and family physicians and the imminent availability of medical abortion provide an opportunity to make these reproductive services integral to primary care medicine.

BIBLIOGRAPHY

Atrash HK, Cheek TG, Hogue CJR: Legal abortion mortality and general anesthesia, *Am J Obstet Gynecol* 158:420, 1988.

Atrash HK, Lawson HW, Smith JC: Legal abortion in the US: trends and mortality, *Contemp Ob/Gyn* 35:58, 1990.

Birgerson L et al: Termination of early human pregnancy with epostane, *Contraception* 35:111, 1987.

Buehler JW et al: The risk of serious complications from induced abortion: do personal characteristics make a difference? *Am J Obstet Gynecol* 153:14, 1985.

Creinin MD, Vittinghoff E: Methatrexate and misoprostol vs. misoprostol alone for early abortion, *JAMA* 272:15, 1994.

Daling JR et al: Ectopic pregnancy in relation to previous induced abortion, *JAMA 253:1005, 1985.*

Daling JR et al: Risk of breast cancer among young women: relationship to induced abortion, *J Natl Canc Inst* 86:1585, 1994.

Darj E, Stralin EB, Nilsson S: The prophylactic effect of doxycycline on postoperative infection rate after first trimester abortion, *Obstet Gynecol* 70:755, 1987.

Darney PD, Sweet RL: Routine intraoperative ultrasonography for second trimester abortion reduces incidence of uterine perforation, *J Ultrasound Med* 8:71, 1989.

Forrest JD, Henshaw SK: Providing controversial health care: abortion services since 1973, *Women's Health Institute* 152, 1993.

Freedman MA et al: Comparison of complication rates in first trimester abortions performed by physician assistants and physicians, *Am J Public Health* 76:550, 1986.

Freeman EW: Abortion: subjective attitudes and feelings, *Fam Plann Perspect* 10:150, 1978.

Grimes DA, Cates W Jr, Selik RM: Abortion facilities and the risk of death, *Fam Plann Perspect* 13:30, 1981.

Hakim-Elahi E, Tovell HMM, Burnhill MS: Complications of first-trimester abortion: a report of 170,000 cases, *Obstet Gynecol* 76:129, 1990.

Henshaw SK, Silverman J: The characteristics and prior contraceptive use of U.S. abortion patients, *Fam Plann Perspect* 20:158, 1988.

Henshaw SK, Van Vort J: Abortion services in the United States, 1991 and 1992, *Fam Plann Perspect* 26:100, 1994.

Henshaw SK, Van Vort J, editors: *The abortion fact book,* New York, 1992, Alan Guttmacher Institute.

Hogue CJR, Cates W Jr, Tietze C: The effects of induced abortion on subsequent reproduction, *Epidemiol Rev* 4:66, 1982.

Hogue CJR: Impact of abortion on subsequent fecundity, *Clin Obstet Gynecol* 13:95, 1986.

Hornstein M et al: Ultrasound guidance for selected dilatation and evacuation procedures, *J Reprod Med* 31:947, 1986.

Houang ET: Antibiotic prophylaxis in hysterectomy and induced abortion, *Drugs* 41:19, 1991.

Kleinman RL, editor: *Family planning handbook for doctors,* London, 1988, International Planned Parenthood Federation.

Koonin LM, Smith JC, Ramick M: Abortion surveillance—United States, 1990, *MMWR* 42:SS-6, 1993.

Landy U: Abortion counselling—a new component of medical care, *Clin Obstet Gynecol* 13:33, 1986.

Landy U, Lewit S: Administrative, counselling and medical practices in National Abortion Federation facilities, *Fam Plann Perspect* 14:257, 1982.

Lawson H, Atrash HK, Safflas A: Ectopic pregnancy surveillance—United States, 1970-1989, *MMWR* 42:SS6, 1989.

Levin A et al: Induced abortions and the risk of spontaneous abortion, *Am J Public Health* 1978 (abstract).

Mackay HT, Schulz KF, Grimes DA: Safety of local versus general anesthesia for second-trimester dilatation and evacuation abortion, *Obstet Gynecol* 66:661, 1985.

National Abortion Federation: *Summary of annual complication statistics, 1992,* Washington, DC, 1993, The Federation.

Osathanondh R: *Conception control.* In Ryan KJ, Barbieri R, Berkowitz R, editors: Kistner's gynecology, ed 6, St Louis, 1994, Mosby.

Osathanondh R: Endocrine tests in obstetrics and gynecology, Part I. *Current problems in obstetrics and gynecology,* Chicago, 1980, Year Book Medical Publishers.

Peterson WF et al: Second-trimester abortion by dilatation and evacuation: an analysis of 11,747 cases, *Obstet Gynecol* 62:185, 1983.

Potts M, Diggory P, Peel J: *Abortion,* Cambridge, 1977, Cambridge University Press.

Rosenberg L: Induced abortion and breast cancer: more scientific data are needed, *J Natl Canc Inst* 86:1569, 1994.

Smith N et al: Screening for chlamydia infection, *Lancet* 342:687, 1993 (letter).

Steinhoff PG et al: Women who obtain repeat abortions: a study based on record linkage, *Fam Plann Perspect* 11:30, 1979.

Stockley IH: Methotrexate-NSAID interactions, *Drug Intell Clin Pharm* 21:546, 1987.

Stotland NL: The myth of the abortion trauma syndrome, *JAMA* 268:2078, 1992.

Stubblefield PG, Grimes DA: Septic abortion, *N Engl J Med* 331:310, 1994.

Stubblefield PG et al: Fertility after induced abortion: a prospective follow-up study, *Obstet Gynecol* 62:186, 1984.

Whitfield CR: Future challenges in the management of rhesus disease. In Studd, J, editor: *Progress in obstetrics and gynecology,* ed 3, Edinburgh, 1982, Churchill Livingstone.

Williams L, Pratt WF: Wanted and unwanted childbearing in the United States 1973-88, Hyatsville, Md, 1990, National Center for Health Statistics.

44 Hysterectomy

Karen J. Carlson

In recent years, hysterectomy has come under scrutiny because of concerns about its appropriateness, as well as efforts to reduce the costs of medical care. Widespread variations in hysterectomy rates in the United States and among industrialized countries are clearly documented. These variations appear to be attributable primarily to physicians' uncertainty about the appropriate use of hysterectomy. This uncertainty is thought to stem from difficulties in diagnosis, lack of information on the outcomes of hysterectomy and alternative treatments, and disparities between physicians' judgments and patients' preferences for treatment.

Approximately 590,000 hysterectomies are performed annually in the United States, making hysterectomy the most frequently performed nonobstetric major surgery. Attempts to determine how many hysterectomies are truly necessary have been based on expert judgment applied retrospectively through medical record review. Using such methods, Bernstein and colleagues found that approximately 15% of hysterectomies performed in a group of seven health care systems were judged inappropriate. Determining whether a hysterectomy is "appropriate" is a complex clinical judgment and is limited by the lack of controlled clinical research on hysterectomy outcomes. Nonetheless, because of the concern about appropriateness of hysterectomy during the past two decades, many women considering hysterectomy seek more than one professional opinion to be sure that surgery is the best choice for them.

The primary care physician often is called on to advise women about the appropriate indications for hysterectomy, the experience of surgery and recovery, and the effectiveness and adverse effects of the procedure. This chapter provides an overview of the indications for hysterectomy and what is known of its effects on health and quality of life. Because 90% of hysterectomies are performed for benign conditions, the focus here is primarily on surgery performed for nonmalignant disorders. A detailed discussion of the role of hysterectomy and alternative treatments in the management of specific disorders is found in the chapters on uterine fibroids (Chapter 41), dysfunctional uterine bleeding (Chapter 32), pelvic pain (Chapter 38), prolapse (Chapter 34), and gynecologic cancers (Chapter 65).

INDICATIONS FOR HYSTERECTOMY

Common indications for hysterectomy are listed the in box at right, and represent conditions about which there is relatively little controversy concerning the appropriateness of hysterectomy. More controversial indications for hysterectomy include sterilization, dysmenorrhea, premenstrual syndrome, lesser degrees of uterine prolapse, and low-grade cervical intraepithelial neoplasia. Also controversial is the role of hysterectomy when more than one condition is present, each of which would not alone constitute an appropriate indication.

The most common indications for hysterectomy in women of reproductive age are conditions that interfere with a woman's quality of life but that are not life-threatening: symptomatic uterine fibroids, dysfunctional uterine bleeding, chronic (idiopathic) pelvic pain, and endometriosis. These diagnoses account for the majority of hysterectomies performed in the United States. For each of these conditions, hysterectomy can be highly effective in relieving symptoms and improving quality of life. However, a range of medical

INDICATIONS FOR HYSTERECTOMY

Uterine leiomyomas
Symptomatic leiomyomas
Asymptomatic leiomyomas that produce significant anemia or ureteral compression
Rapidly enlarging leiomyomas

Dysfunctional uterine bleeding
Chronic excessive bleeding refractory to medical therapy or endometrial ablation
Acute bleeding refractory to estrogen therapy and dilation and curettage

Chronic pelvic pain
Functionally disabling pain refractory to medical management—after thorough evaluation and trial of conservative treatment

Endometriosis
Symptomatic endometriosis refractory to medical or conservative surgical therapy
Symptomatic adenomyosis

Genital prolapse
Symptomatic third-degree uterine prolapse

Pelvic inflammatory disease
Persistent or recurrent severe infection

Endometrial hyperplasia
Symptomatic (with bleeding), if fertility not desired
Persistent hyperplasia after progestin therapy
Atypical hyperplasia, if fertility not desired

Malignant disease
Recurrent or refractory high-grade cervical intraepithelial neoplasia
Invasive cervical carcinoma
Endometrial, ovarian, and tubal carcinoma; uterine sarcoma

Obstetric indications
Massive postpartum hemorrhage
Septic endometritis with pyometra

and surgical alternatives exist that can be similarly effective for many women (see box, below). Thus a woman who wishes to retain her uterus often has options for treatment that may allow her to manage the condition until menopause, at which time most of the aforementioned conditions no longer cause symptoms.

LONG-TERM EFFECTS
Quality of life

Evidence from the Maine Women's Health Study, a prospective study of hysterectomy outcomes, indicates that hysterectomy is highly effective for relief of symptoms associated with common benign uterine conditions and that symptom relief is associated with a marked improvement in quality of life. Particularly for women who experience moderate or severe symptoms (including bleeding, pelvic pain, urinary symptoms, and fatigue) related to benign uterine conditions, hysterectomy is likely to result in an overall improvement in measures of general health, mental health, and activity. Ongoing prospective studies of hysterectomy outcomes should help identify subgroups of women at risk for less favorable outcomes after hysterectomy.

Psychologic and sexual function

Concern about the potential of hysterectomy to cause depression or other psychiatric problems stems from early retrospective studies that showed a higher rate of psychiatric disorders among women who had undergone hysterectomy. More rigorous prospective studies have demonstrated that the prevalence of psychiatric disorders has been higher in women undergoing hysterectomy than in the general population. There is no evidence that the operation itself leads to depression or greater psychologic distress. The risk of poor psychologic outcomes generally has been limited to women with preoperative psychiatric disorders. In women whose symptoms were severe enough to impair their quality of life, the Maine Women's Health Study showed that hysterectomy was associated with a significant improvement in indexes of mental health 1 year after surgery. New problems with depression and anxiety were reported in 8% and 6%, respectively, of women who reported no such problems before hysterectomy.

Several small prospective studies of sexual function after hysterectomy report improvement or no change in most women, with worsening of sexual function in about 20%. In the Maine Women's Health Study, there was a significant overall improvement in sexual function 1 year after hysterectomy. In women whose conditions were not associated with a preoperative impairment in sexual function, 1% reported new problems with enjoyment of sex after surgery, and 7% reported new problems with interest in sex.

A resurgence of interest in supracervical hysterectomy has occurred in recent years. The cervix and uterine corpus are known to play a role in orgasm. A single prospective study by Kilkku and colleagues comparing supracervical and total abdominal hysterectomy showed that supracervical hysterectomy was less often associated with a negative effect on orgasm, although there were no differences in other measures of sexual function. Helstrom et al. prospectively studied sexual function after supracervical hysterectomy and reported that about 20% of women reported deterioration of sexual function. At present, there is insufficient evidence to justify the routine performance of hysterectomy with cervical preservation.

Cardiovascular disease

Data from the Framingham Study (Gordon et al., 1978) and the Nurses' Health Study (Colditz et al., 1987) consistently point to an increase in the risk of coronary heart disease in premenopausal women who have undergone hysterectomy with bilateral salpingoophorectomy and have never taken estrogen-replacement therapy. The Nurses' Health Study provides the best evidence that hysterectomy with preservation of one or both ovaries is not associated with an increased risk of heart disease. However, smaller studies, including the Framingham Study, have reported modest increases in cardiovascular disease risk after hysterectomy alone, and premature ovarian failure has been documented as a consequence of hysterectomy.

The evidence for an overall decrease in cardiovascular risk when hysterectomy is followed by estrogen-replacement therapy is strong. It has not been proved, however, that hysterectomy without estrogen-replacement therapy in premenopausal women has no effect on cardiovascular risk.

Other problems after hysterectomy

Several other long-term adverse effects of hysterectomy have been reported, including urinary symptoms, constipation, fatigue, and the retained ovary syndrome (a little-understood syndrome of pelvic pain after hysterectomy). In the Maine Women's Health Study, the most common new problems 1 year after hysterectomy were weight gain, which

---

> ### ALTERNATIVES TO HYSTERECTOMY FOR SELECTED CONDITIONS
>
> **Uterine leiomyomas**
>   Hormonal therapy (progestins, oral contraceptives, gonadotropin-releasing hormone [GnRH] analogs)
>   Nonsteroidal antiinflammatory drugs
>   Myomectomy (abdominal or hysteroscopic)
>
> **Dysfunctional uterine bleeding**
>   Hormonal therapy (progestins, oral contraceptives, danazol, GnRH analogs)
>   Nonsteroidal antiinflammatory drugs
>   Endometrial ablation
>
> **Chronic pelvic pain and dysmenorrhea**
>   Nonsteroidal antiinflammatory drugs
>   Hormonal therapy (including oral contraceptives)
>   Laparoscopic uterosacral nerve ablation
>
> **Endometriosis**
>   Hormonal therapy (GnRH analogs, danazol, estrogen-progestin combinations)
>   Laparoscopic surgery
>
> **Genital prolapse**
>   Pessary
>   Repair of cystocele or rectocele without concurrent hysterectomy

Table 44-1 Complications of hysterectomy

Complication	No. (%)
Mortality*	0.1
Infection	
Febrile morbidity	15-25
Wound infection	<5
Pelvic infection	<10
Urinary tract infection	<10
Bleeding leading to transfusion	2-10
Reoperation	<1
Bladder injury	<1

*Mortality as a result of hysterectomy performed for nonmalignant, nonobstetric indications.

occurred in 12% of women who reported no problems with their weight before surgery, and hot flashes, which occurred in 13%, largely associated with bilateral oophorectomy. Other new problems reported included urinary symptoms in 4% and constipation in 6%.

COMPLICATIONS OF HYSTERECTOMY

The mortality rate of hysterectomy for nonmalignant conditions in published series is approximately 1/1000. The mortality risk increases with age and is threefold higher when the indication is associated with pregnancy. The most common perioperative complications include infection (e.g., febrile morbidity and urinary tract, pelvic, and wound infections), bleeding, and damage to other organs (Table 44-1).

The route of hysterectomy influences the complication rate, the recuperation process, and the cost of surgery. Abdominal hysterectomies generally are associated with higher rates of complications and a longer recovery period (Tables 44-1 and 44-2). Newer surgical approaches, including laparoscopically assisted vaginal hysterectomy, may increase the number of hysterectomies that can be performed by the vaginal route. Adequate data on the outcomes and costs of these procedures are not yet available.

HYSTERECTOMY AND OOPHORECTOMY

Elective bilateral oophorectomy sometimes is performed at the time of hysterectomy to reduce the future risk of ovarian cancer. The lifetime risk of ovarian, uterine, and cervical cancer is summarized in Table 44-3. (See Chapter 78 for more detailed estimates of ovarian cancer risk.) The benefit of oophorectomy is the reduction of this risk to near zero.

Counterposed to this potential benefit are the potential adverse effects of premature loss of ovarian hormone production. Bilateral oophorectomy in premenopausal women is clearly a risk factor for the development of cardiovascular disease. The increase in risk appears to be offset completely by estrogen-replacement therapy. Other potential adverse

Table 44-2 Recovery from hysterectomy

	Recovery at home (wk)	Return to normal activity (wk)
Abdominal hysterectomy	1-3	6-8
Vaginal hysterectomy	1-2	4-6

Table 44-3 Lifetime probability of uterine, cervical, and ovarian cancer for a 50-year-old woman

Site	Probability of cancer (%)	Probability of death from cancer (%)
Uterus	2.4	0.2
Cervix	0.6	0.3
Ovary	1.2	0.8

From Carlson KJ, Nichols DH, Schiff I: *N Engl J Med* 328:856, 1993.

effects of oophorectomy are vasomotor symptoms (also generally correctable by estrogen replacement) and, for some women, diminished libido. The latter effect is mediated by loss of ovarian androgens.

Although there are no universally accepted guidelines for elective oophorectomy at the time of hysterectomy, ovarian conservation at the time of hysterectomy generally is recommended for premenopausal women younger than 45 years of age, and oophorectomy is recommended for women older than 50 years of age. For women 45 to 50 years of age, the decision should be individualized on the basis of the patient's menopausal status, risk of ovarian cancer, and ability to take estrogen-replacement therapy.

COUNSELING THE WOMAN CONSIDERING HYSTERECTOMY

In considering whether to have a hysterectomy for a nonmalignant condition, a woman must evaluate the expected effectiveness of the procedure and of any alternatives; the likelihood of experiencing an immediate complication of surgery; and the likelihood of any long-term adverse effects (see box, below). Equally important considerations are the woman's attitudes toward loss of fertility, the feasibility of a

---

COUNSELING THE WOMAN CONSIDERING HYSTERECTOMY

Reproductive factors
  Fertility desires
  Proximity to menopause

Severity of symptoms
  Effect on quality of life
  Other physiologic effects (e.g., anemia)

Experience with other treatments
  Medical therapy: effectiveness, side effects
  Limited surgery (e.g., myomectomy, endometrial ablation, laparoscopic surgery)

Impact of potential adverse effects of hysterectomy
  Sexual function (e.g., degree of present impairment related to condition, potential impact of any change after hysterectomy)
  Attitudes regarding operative mortality risk
  Attitudes toward hormone-replacement therapy

Social impact of hysterectomy
  Recuperation time
  Attitudes of partner

hospital stay and recuperation period, concern about future cancer risk, and potential impact of hysterectomy on sexuality and self-image. In women with a prior history of psychiatric illness, careful attention to the psychologic impact of hysterectomy and loss of fertility is warranted. The primary care physician, together with the obstetrician-gynecologist, can help the woman to consider each of these factors to ensure that she is a fully informed partner in the decision-making process.

REFERENCES

Bernstein SJ et al: The appropriateness of hysterectomy: a comparison of care in seven health plans, *JAMA* 269:2398, 1993.

Carlson KJ, Miller BA, Fowler FJ: The Maine Women's Health Study. I. Outcomes of hysterectomy, *Obstet Gynecol* 83:556, 1994.

Carlson KJ, Miller BA, Fowler FJ: The Maine Women's Health Study. II. Outcomes of nonsurgical management of leiomyomas, abnormal bleeding, and chronic pelvic pain, *Obstet Gynecol* 83:566, 1994.

Carlson KJ, Nichols DH, Schiff I: Indications for hysterectomy, *N Engl J Med* 328:856, 1993.

Colditz GA et al: Menopause and the risk of coronary artery disease in women, *N Engl J Med* 316:1105, 1987.

Coppen A et al: Hysterectomy, hormones, and behavior: a prospective study, *Lancet* 1:126, 1981.

Gath D, Cooper P, Day A: Hysterectomy and psychiatric disorder. I. Levels of psychiatric morbidity before and after hysterectomy, *Br J Psychiatry* 140:335, 1982.

Gordon T et al: Menopause and coronary heart disease: The Framingham Study, *Ann Intern Med* 89:157, 1978.

Helstrom L et al: Sexuality after hysterectomy: a factor analysis of women's sexual lives before and after subtotal hysterectomy, *Obstet Gynecol* 81:357, 1993.

Kilkku P et al: Supravaginal uterine amputation vs. hysterectomy: effects on libido and orgasm, *Acta Obstet Gynecol Scand* 62:147, 1983.

Ryan MM, Dennerstein L, Pepperall R: Psychological aspects of hysterectomy: a prospective study, *Br J Psychiatry* 154:516, 1989.

Siddle N, Sarrel P, Whitehead M: The effect of hysterectomy on the age at ovarian failure: identification of a subgroup of women with premature loss of ovarian function and literature review, *Fertil Steril* 47:94, 1987.

Section II

OBSTETRICS
Preconception

45 Pregnancy in the Older Woman

Linda J. Heffner

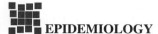
EPIDEMIOLOGY

Deliveries by older women have risen dramatically in the United States over the last 20 years, with a 440% increase in first births to women over 30 years of age since 1970. The large numbers are expected to continue through at least the year 2010 when the youngest of the baby boomers reach menopause. Although the absolute numbers of women aged 30 to 44 has increased by 60% since 1970, the decision to delay childbearing until after the age of 30 has largely been responsible for the increase.

In 1950 the term *elderly primigravida* was first used to describe a woman whose first birth occurs after her 35th birthday. In a landmark paper Waters and colleagues first queried the notion that pregnancy is a perilous journey, fraught with maternal and fetal risk, for the older parturient. Unfortunately for many older women contemplating bearing their first child, the notion that delayed childbearing is blatantly risky, even for healthy women, was widespread. Careful review of the literature on pregnancy outcome among older gravidas indicates that it can be quite good when the true risks are understood and managed. In this chapter each purported risk will be examined critically. Recommendations for addressing the real risks will conclude the discussion.

INFERTILITY

Actual fertility rates, defined as number of live births per 1000 women of the same age, have been increasing since the 1970s for women aged 30 to 39 as a result of the demographic characteristics of delayed childbearing. More accurately it is *fecundity,* or the ability of a couple to establish a pregnancy within a year, that appears to decline with age. This age-related decline in fecundity combined with the clinical definition of infertility (the inability of a couple to conceive despite 1 year of effort) results in a threefold increase in infertility rates in women over age 35 compared to women aged 20 to 29.

Because fecundity can be influenced by deliberate fertility control it is necessary to study populations seeking pregnancies in order to evaluate the impact of age on fecundity. These populations can also suffer from conditions limiting fertility that may or may not be independent of age.

Nonetheless, most studies do demonstrate a decline in fecundity with advancing maternal age that appears largely to be the result of a decline in oocyte quality. A decline in endometrial responsiveness to steroid hormones leading to implantation problems, earlier thought to be a major factor in age-related reproductive failure, has not been documented. No age-related decline in fertility rates was found in women in their 40s undergoing in vitro fertilization with oocytes donated by younger women.

MISCARRIAGE

Miscarriage (spontaneous abortion in the first half of pregnancy) is a common event, occuring in at least 15% of recognized pregnancies. Over 50% of first trimester miscarriages are chromosomally abnormal. It is not surprising, therefore, that the miscarriage rate rises as the risk of chromosomal abnormalities rises with maternal age. Numerous studies have confirmed this finding; however, an increase in first trimester spontaneous abortions of chromosomally normal (euploid) conceptions appears to occur in women over 35. Unfortunately, gravidity, pregnancy order, and number of prior miscarriages, which affect miscarriage rates, were not adjusted for in this study. In a study of 3500 female British physicians miscarriage rates increased with gravidity at the younger ages and decreased with pregnancy order with increasing age (Roman and Alberman, 1980). This would argue against an age effect on euploid miscarriage. The investigators noted that the interval leading up to a miscarriage tended to be longer than that leading up to a live birth, suggesting that women whose first pregnancy miscarries may be older because of a more difficult time conceiving. An alternative explanation is that pregnancies preceded by a long interval are more likely to miscarry because the women are older. A progressive increase in spontaneous losses also occurs with increasing numbers of previous miscarriages to the point where women with three or more previous miscarriages suffer a threefold increase in the age-adjusted incidence of miscarriage.

Thus older women do have a clearly increased risk of aneuploid miscarriage and may have an increased risk of euploid miscarriage that probably results either from a nonchromosomal decline in oocyte quality or from enrichment by a population of recurrent spontaneous abortors who age as they continue to miscarry.

CHROMOSOMAL ABNORMALITIES

Chromosomal abnormalities in the conceptuses of older women are probably the best documented and most widely recognized risk of delayed childbearing. Karyotypes supporting the increased risk of aneuploidy come from multiple sources: miscarriages, induced abortions, midtrimester amniocenteses, liveborn infants, and stillbirths. All indicate a steadily increasing risk of chromosomal abnormalities throughout a woman's lifetime such that by the time she is 45 years old she carries a 1:21 risk of an aneuploid fetus at delivery. Table 45-1 is an example of a risk chart used for genetic counseling of older women; the age entered for an individual woman is her age on her due date. The biologic basis for the increase in chromosomal abnormalities with increasing age is thought to be related to the fact that oocytes reach metaphase of meiosis I at about 5 months post conception and remain aligned upon the metaphase plate throughout a woman's reproductive life until the oocyte is stimulated to divide just before ovulation. Over time the risk of nondisjunction, or the failure of the chromosomes to divide equally, increases.

Table 45-1 Age-specific risks for chromosomal abnormalities in liveborn infants

Maternal age at delivery	Risk of Down syndrome	Risk of any chromosomal abnormality*
20	1/1667	1/526
22	1/1429	1/500
24	1/1250	1/476
26	1/1176	1/476
27	1/1111	1/455
28	1/1053	1/435
29	1/1000	1/417
30	1/952	1/385
31	1/909	1/385
32	1/769	1/322
33	1/602	1/286
34	1/485	1/238
35	1/378	1/192
36	1/289	1/156
37	1/224	1/127
38	1/173	1/102
39	1/136	1/83
40	1/106	1/66
41	1/82	1/53
42	1/63	1/42
43	1/49	1/33
44	1/38	1/26
45	1/30	1/21
46	1/23	1/16
47	1/18	1/13
48	1/14	1/10
49	1/11	1/8

Data modified from the maternal age-specific rates derived by Hook EB, Cross PK, Schreinemachers DM: *JAMA* 249:2034, 1983, and Hook EB: *Obstet Gynecol* 58:282, 1981.
*Excludes 46,XXX for ages 20-32 because data are not available.

CONGENITAL MALFORMATIONS

Although earlier evidence suggested an increased risk of nonchromosomal congenital malformations among the off-spring of older mothers more recent investigations have not confirmed this finding. In the largest earlier study facial clefts, cardiac malformations, anorectal defects, and hypospadias were reported in a larger proportion of firstborn infants of mothers over 40 years of age than in those of younger mothers (Hay and Barbano, 1972). The major limitation of this study, conducted from 1961 to 1966, is that chromosomal evaluation of the abnormal children was not possible. Although the investigators did exclude those infants with clinically apparent Down syndrome, which is associated with cardiac defects, this genetic disorder may not be clinically apparent at birth. Several trisomies, as well as other chromosomal abnormalities, also can be associated with cardiac defects and facial clefts.

Recently 26,859 live-born children in British Columbia were surveyed for birth defects not associated with chromosomal abnormalities, single gene defects, maternal diabetes, alcoholism, or teratogen exposure (Baird, Sadovnick, and Yee, 1991). No increase in any of 43 birth defect categories was found for older mothers.

LOW BIRTH WEIGHT

The incidence of low birth weight (<2500 g) has been repeatedly shown to be higher in older than younger gravidas; however low birth weight can result from either prematurity or decreased intrauterine growth. The causes and long-term consequences of these two sources of low birth weight are quite different. Unfortunately two thirds of the studies addressing maternal age and birth weight fail to distinguish between the two types of small infants. The remaining few are used to assess the risk of prematurity and inadequate fetal growth.

The risk of having a premature infant does not appear to increase substantially with advanced maternal age. Several studies have shown a modest increase in risk of premature delivery among primigravid women older than 35 years of age, others found either a decreased risk of prematurity or no difference when compared to younger control subjects.

Low birth weight resulting from inadequate intrauterine growth has been even less well studied than prematurity, but the rate would appear to be increased with maternal age. A group of 127 Canadian women delivering after the age of 40 were found to have an 11% incidence of small-for-dates infants compared to 2% in the women under 25 (Morrison, 1975). In a larger study of pregnancy outcomes in 4463 Swedish women aged 35 to 39 years rates of low birth weight term infants were increased in the primigravid patients (Forman, Merik, and Berendes, 1984). Among well-educated, mostly white women in New York City over age 35, a 5% incidence of small-for-dates infants did not differ from that of the younger control subjects (Berkowitz et al., 1990). Hypertension, which is a risk factor for low birth weight, has an increased incidence in older mothers (see later discussion), suggesting that the proportion of hypertensive women in the study population may influence the incidence of small-for-gestational-age infants. Cigarette smoking, a type of environmental exposure that can diminish intrauterine growth, has a more profound effect in older mothers. In light of the high proportion of studies that have reported an increase in births of low birth weight infants and the minimal change in the prematurity rate, more attention to fetal growth as a pregnancy outcome in older gravidas is warranted.

PERINATAL MORTALITY

Perinatal mortality is the sum of two components, fetal deaths in the second half of pregnancy (stillbirths) and neonatal deaths. Almost all large, controlled studies have shown an increased perinatal mortality rate with advancing maternal age such that women in their late 30s have a twofold risk that increases to a fourfold risk by age 45. The increase is essentially limited to stillbirths.

There are several explanations for the increased stillbirth rates in older mothers. First, older women have an increased incidence of medical complications, especially hypertension and diabetes, which can cause abnormal fetal growth and predispose to antenatal asphyxia and intrauterine death (see the section on Medical Complications). In older black women with hypertension, perinatal mortality rate was substantially higher than that attributable to either age or hypertension alone. Healthy older gravidas experienced minimal, if any, increases in perinatal loss. Second, older women are at increased risk for fetal chromosomal abnormalities and chromosomally abnormal fetuses are at increased risk for fetal death in utero. Most studies of perinatal outcome among older women do not control for the increased prevalence of chromosomally abnormal fetuses in that population.

Recently the safety of allowing older women to carry their pregnancies past the 42nd week of gestation (postdates) has been investigated in a small number of pregnancies. Although there was no indication of antepartum fetal compromise before arrival on the labor suite, significantly more low 1-minute Apgar scores, intrapartum decelerations, and cesarean deliveries occurred in the women over age 35. Five-minute Apgar scores of neonatal intensive care admissions did not differ between the older and younger parturients. Interestingly, in a much larger Swedish study of older gravidas significantly fewer women over age 35 delivered at or after the 40th week of gestation compared to the 20 to 24-year-old control population. Further investigation into the sensitivity and specificity of antepartum fetal surveillance at term in the older gravida is necessary.

MEDICAL COMPLICATIONS
Hypertension

In most studies of hypertension in pregnancy chronic hypertension, pregnancy-induced hypertension, and preeclampsia are all grouped together. All hypertensive disorders appear to be increased in older gravidas. All but two small studies of pregnant women over age 35 have shown at least a twofold elevation in risk for hypertensive complications for the older women regardless of parity. In the two largest studies, of 36,482 and 41,798 women, preeclampsia rates in women over 40 were double those in women under 30 (Kane, 1967; Tysoe, 1970). Very significant increases in the frequency of all hypertensive disorders from 2.7% between ages 20 and 30 to 9.6% over age 40 have been reported. Since preeclampsia is more common in first pregnancies the overall increase in hypertension with age is sustained by multiparas with chronic hypertension. In the latter study the increase in hypertensive complications was associated with maternal obesity. Most importantly in the studies that have examined perinatal outcome in light of maternal medical complications excess fetal deaths did not occur in the normotensive, normal weight older gravidas.

Diabetes

Like that of hypertension, the prevalence of diabetes mellitus increases with advancing age. The incidence of gestational diabetes rises from a low of 0.3% to 1.7% in younger women to 1.0% to 4.1% in nulliparous women over 35. Again obesity and parity are additive risk factors. Although insulin-dependent diabetes antedating pregnancy is associated with increased rates of perinatal morbidity and mortality, it is unclear whether gestational diabetes is associated with increased fetal risk in older mothers. Gestational diabetes is associated with increased risk of large infants, which may predispose to more difficult labors and the risk of birth injury. Infants with birth weight over 4000 g are found in higher proportions among older gravidas; parity, obesity, and diabetes appear to account for most, but not all, of the excess.

OBSTETRIC COMPLICATIONS
Abnormal bleeding

Bleeding in the third trimester can result from either placenta previa or placental abruption; such bleeding appears to occur about twice as frequently in older primigravidas. Women of any age who are hypertensive during pregnancy are at increased risk for a placental abruption; no measure of the independent contribution of maternal age is available. Postpartum hemorrhage in older women appears to be largely restricted to the multiparous patient.

Delivery difficulties

Every study since 1963 reporting the incidence of cesarean section in women 35 years or older compared to those in their 20s has shown an increase of at least 70% in the older gravidas. Some of the increase may result from a decreased ability of the fetuses of older mothers to tolerate labor; however the strong positive association between cesarean section and maternal age persists after adjustment for induction of labor, epidural anesthesia, meconium staining of the amniotic fluid, and fetal distress. In one study, advanced maternal age was the stated reason that 31% of the older women had primary cesarean section. It is not certain whether these higher cesarean section rates result from physiologic changes or from physician beliefs that somehow the infants of older women are more "precious" than those of younger women.

Maternal death

Maternal death rates increase with maternal age, largely as a result of obstetric complications of high parity and of indirect deaths resulting from underlying medical problems. Fortunately unlike fetal death, maternal death is a very rare complication of pregnancy, which had dropped to less than 8/100,000 live births by the mid-1980s compared to perinatal mortality, which has averaged 18/1000 total births over the period 1982 to 1992. Maternal death rates among women aged 35 and older are double those of 25-year-olds and quadruple by age 45. Nonwhite race is a more significant risk for maternal death than age, beginning at age 20. Healthy women over 35 who desire a baby should not be concerned about having a greater risk of dying than their younger counterparts because of the rarity of maternal death.

COUNSELING THE OLDER GRAVIDA

In older women with preexisting medical conditions counseling should be individualized to the specific medical problems encountered. Hypertension is among the most commonly encountered medical problems. These women carry a disproportionate amount of the risk for an adverse pregnancy outcome. This is largely manifested as higher perinatal morbidity and mortality rates from low birth weight that result from either prematurity or poor intrauterine growth. Maternal health is infrequently directly affected.

For the healthy, motivated woman who delays childbearing until after age 35 the likelihood of a good outcome is high with careful attention to the areas of greatest risk. The following specific points are useful in counseling older gravidas about delayed childbearing.

First, a delay in successful establishment of a pregnancy may result from the modest decline in fecundity with advancing maternal age. The presence of the "biologic reproductive clock" may be felt acutely by these women. It is generally recommended that older couples who have been trying unsuccessfully for 6 months to establish a pregnancy seek the advice of a medical professional. Although many will delay the start of complete infertility testing until a full year has passed, several simple tests of sperm quality and ovulatory capacity can be performed early.

Second, the risk of chromosomal abnormalities clearly increases with advancing maternal age. Fetal karyotyping after amniocentesis or chorionic villus sampling should be offered to all women age 35 and over. It is important in counseling not to equate use of prenatal diagnosis with willingness to undergo pregnancy termination for positive results as this is not the only option available to couples with chromosomally abnormal fetuses. Adoptive families are available for children born with chromosomal abnormalities if the biologic parents feel they would not be able to raise the child themselves but do not wish to terminate the pregnancy.

Third, all women age 35 and above should be screened for gestational diabetes by using a 50-g oral glucose challenge. A plasma glucose value greater than 140 mg/dl should be followed up with a diagnostic 3-hour glucose tolerance test. If the woman is obese a screen should be performed at the initial prenatal visit and again at 24 to 28 weeks of gestation even if the initial screen finding is negative. Normal-weight women should be screened at 24 to 28 weeks of gestation.

Liberal use of ultrasound and antepartum testing is appropriate if obstetric complications develop or abnormal fetal growth is suspected. Cigarette smoking should be discouraged; fetal growth should be carefully followed in older women who continue to smoke. There is no information on the usefulness of routine antepartum surveillance in preventing stillbirth in healthy older women with normally grown fetuses. Intrapartum electronic fetal monitoring in labor is reasonable for all older women.

Finally the need for genetic counseling, glucose screening, and careful surveillance and treatment for obstetric compli-

cations in all older women is likely to mean more interaction with the health care system than some women anticipate. Anxiety and disappointment later in pregnancy can be minimized if women are counseled about the expected content of their prenatal care and are prepared for this in advance.

BIBLIOGRAPHY

Atrash HK et al: Maternal mortality in the United States, 1979-1986, *Obstet Gynecol* 76:1055, 1990.

Baird PA, Sadovnick AD, Yee IML: Maternal age and birth defects: a population study, *Lancet* 337:527, 1991.

Berkowitz GS et al: Delayed childbearing and the outcome of pregnancy, *N Engl J Med* 322:659, 1990.

Cnattinguis S et al: Smoking, maternal age, and fetal growth, *Obstet Gynecol* 66:449, 1985.

Federation CECOS, Schwartz D, Mayaux MJ: Female fecundity as a function of age, *N Engl J Med* 306:404, 1982.

Forman MR, Meirik O, Berendes HW: Delayed childbearing in Sweden, *JAMA* 252:3135, 1984.

Grimes DA, Gross GK: Pregnancy outcomes in black women aged 35 and older, *Obstet Gynecol* 58:614, 1981.

Hansen JP: Older maternal age and pregnancy outcome: a review of the literature, *Obstet Gynecol Surv* 41:726, 1986.

Harlop S, Shiono PH, Ramcharan S: A life table of spontaneous abortions and the effect of age, parity, and other variables. In Porter IH, Hook EB, editors: *Embryonic and fetal death*, New York, 1980, Academic Press.

Hay S, Barbano H: Independent effects of maternal age and birth order on the incidence of selected congenital malformations, *Teratology* 6:271, 1972.

Hook EB, Cross PK, Schreinemachers DM: Chromosomal abnormality rates at amniocentesis and in live-born infants, *JAMA* 249:2034, 1983.

Hook EB: Rates of chromosomal abnormalities at different maternal ages, *Obstet Gynecol* 58:282, 1981.

Kajii T et al: Anatomic and chromosomal anomalies in 639 spontaneous abortuses, *Hum Genet* 55:87, 1980.

Kajonoia P, Widholm: Pregnancy and delivery in women aged 40 and over, *Obstet Gynecol* 51:47, 1978.

Kane SH: Advancing age and the primigravida, *Obstet Gynecol* 29:409, 1967.

Kirz DS, Dorchester W, Freeman RK: Advanced maternal age: the mature gravida, *Am J Obstet Gynecol* 152:7, 1985.

Lehman DK, Chism J: Pregnancy outcome in medically complicated and uncomplicated patients aged 40 years or older, *Am J Obstet Gynecol* 157:738, 1987.

Machin GA: Chromosome abnormality and perinatal death, *Lancet* 1(874):549, 1974.

Martel M et al: Maternal age and primary cesarean section rates: a multivariate analysis, *Am J Obstet Gynecol* 156:305, 1987.

Morrison I: The elderly primigravida, *Am J Obstet Gynecol* 121:465, 1975.

Navot D et al: Poor oocyte quality rather than implantation failure as a cause of age-related decline in female fertility, *Lancet* 337:1375, 1991.

Postponed childbearing—United States, 1970-1987, *JAMA* 263:360, 1990.

Roman E, Alberman E: Spontaneous abortion, gravidity, pregnancy order, age and pregnancy interval. In Porter IH, Hook EB, editors: *Embryonic and fetal death*, New York, 1980, Academic Press.

Sauer MV, Paulson RJ, Lobo RA: Reversing the natural decline in human fertility, *JAMA* 268:1275, 1992.

Shapiro H, Lyons E: Late maternal age and postdate pregnancy, *Am J Obstet Gynecol* 160:909, 1989.

Spellacy WN, Miller SJ, Winegar A: Pregnancy after 40 years of age, *Obstet Gynecol* 68:452, 1986.

Stein Z et al: Maternal age and spontaneous abortion. In Porter IH, Hook EB, editors: *Embryonic and fetal death*, New York, 1980, Academic Press.

Stovall DW et al: The effect of age on female fecundity, *Obstet Gynecol* 77:33, 1991.

Tuck SM, Yudkin PL, Turnbull AC: Pregnancy outcome in elderly primigravidae with and without a history of infertility, *Br J Obstet Gynecol* 95:230, 1988.

Tysoe FW: Effect of age on the outcome of pregnancy, *Trans Pac Coast Obstet Gynecol Soc* 38:8, 1970.

Waters EG, Wager HP: Pregnancy and labor experiences of elderly primigravidas, *Am J Obstet Gynecol* 59:296, 1950.

46 Preconception Counseling and Nutrition

Stephanie A. Eisenstat

Good prenatal care may reduce the risk for obstetric complications and result in improved pregnancy outcome. Although not all causes of low birth weight, infant mortality, and obstetric complications can be prevented, risk for certain birth defects can be markedly decreased if women of reproductive age receive preconception counseling as well as prenatal care. Supplementation of folate before conception can decrease the risk of fetal neural tube defects. Abstinence from alcohol can prevent fetal alcohol syndrome, and cessation of smoking can decrease the risk of intrauterine growth retardation. Cocaine use has been associated with congenital anomalies and birth complications. Prevention needs to start before the woman becomes pregnant.

It is important for the primary care clinician to discuss ways to improve pregnancy outcome with all women of reproductive age who may become pregnant. The effort at risk reduction before and during pregnancy involves collaboration between the obstetrician-gynecologist and primary care clinician and should be a continuous process that occurs at each visit for routine preventive care and, it is hoped, before and during pregnancy.

The essential components of preconception care in the primary care setting encompass risk assessment, health promotion, and intervention. Specific areas for preconception counseling are outlined in the box at right. This chapter summarizes aspects of preconception counseling in nutrition, substance abuse, alcoholism, and smoking. Other components of preconception care include the identification and treatment of women at risk for adverse psychologic outcomes (see Chapter 63), domestic violence (see Chapter 68), for preventable infectious diseases such as HIV (see Chapter 16), hepatitis, rubella, and toxoplasmosis (see Chapter 50), and for medical conditions such as hypertension and diabetes (see Chapters 53 and 54). The key recommendations for preconception counseling are summarized in Table 46-1.

NUTRITION AND VITAMIN SUPPLEMENTATION

The nutritional status of a woman has an impact on maternal and fetal health throughout pregnancy. Women who are underweight before conception have a higher risk of low-birth-weight infants (Kim et al., 1992). The first trimester is the time when critical development of the fetus occurs, normal development depends partially on adequate maternal nutrition. An accurate assessment of a woman's nutritional status is important in identifying women at risk.

Nutritional assessment

History. The first goal is to assess whether the woman is adhering to a balanced diet. The basic food groups and components of a healthy diet are covered in Chapter 71. Dietary practices that potentially carry additional risk to the fetus include pica (ingestion of nonnutritional substances, most commonly dirt or clay), bulimia and anorexia, specific dietary restrictions, vegetarianism, vitamin and mineral supplemen-

tation, and lactose intolerance. Each of these clinical situations affects the woman's ability to maintain an adequately balanced diet and is an indication for further nutritional counseling and more active monitoring during pregnancy.

Physical examination. Expected weight for height can be estimated by use of standard charts as appear in Appendix II. Although these estimates consist of averages, they serve as a baseline as the practitioner sets goals with the patient. If a woman falls above or below the range for ideal body weight, alteration in dietary patterns may be warranted. If the clinician has a concern about the patient, more intensive evaluation by a nutritional expert should be arranged.

Diagnostic tests. Iron deficiency anemia is common among menstruating women. As the iron demands of pregnancy increase, it is also common to develop iron deficiency anemia during the pregnancy even if it has not previously existed. It is still unclear if anemia during pregnancy is correlated with poor

---

PRECONCEPTION COUNSELING BY THE PRIMARY CARE CLINICIAN

Risk assessment

Individual and social conditions:
 Age, nutritional status, education, housing, economic status
Adverse health behaviors:
 Smoking, alcohol, and illicit drug abuse
Medical conditions:
 Medical disorders, immune status, medications, genetic illness, infection, prior obstetric history
Psychologic conditions:
 Readiness for pregnancy, stress, depression, anxiety
Identifying violence in the home
Environmental conditions:
 Workplace, toxic chemical exposure, radiation exposure
Access to health care:
 Family planning, prenatal care, primary medical care

Health promotion

Promotion of healthy behavior:
 Nutrition, cessation of adverse health behaviors, safe sex practices
HIV counseling
Counseling on social service resources
Promotion of prenatal care

Interventions

Treatment of medical conditions
Referral for treatment programs for alcohol and substance abuse
Smoking-cessation programs
Rubella and hepatitis immunization
Social service referrals and resources
Resources for domestic violence
Nutritional counseling and family planning services

Modified from Jack B, Culpepper L: *JAMA* 264:1147, 1990.

Table 46-1 Summary of recommendations for preconception counseling

Area for prevention	Potential adverse events	Recommendation
Nutrition	LBW, IUGR	Balanced diet with increased protein and iron
Folate supplementation	Neural tube defects	For women with prior history of neural tube defect–affected pregnancy: 0.4 mg folate or higher based on recommendation of physician
		For women contemplating pregnancy: 0.4 mg folate 1 mo before conception through 6 weeks' gestation
		For all women of reproductive age: dietary guidelines
Ingestion of caffeinated products	SAB, IUGR, microcephaly	Less than 2-3 cups per day
Adverse health behaviors		
Alcohol	Fetal alcohol syndrome, SAB Increased risk of abruption	There is no safe level; advise to limit drinking and attempt to quit
Smoking	LBW, IUGR, SAB, cleft palate, cardiovascular and urogenital malformations Increased risk of placental abnormalities	Smoking cessation including nicotine gum/patch if not pregnant
Illicit drugs	Urogenital malformations IUGR, LBW, placental abnormalities Neurobehavioral abnormalities	Drug rehabilitation and detoxification
Domestic violence and psychologic risk	Fetal fractures, premature labor	Resources and social service assessment
Infectious disease		
Rubella	Congenital rubella	Screening and immunization if necessary (before pregnancy)
Hepatitis	Fulminant hepatitis	Screening for hepatitis B (HBsAg), with vaccination for seronegative patients at high risk
Sexually transmitted diseases	Transmission to infant	Screening and intervention based on symptoms and risk profile
HIV	Transmission to infant	Education on HIV transmission; testing after informed consent Education on safe sex practices
Medical conditions		
Diabetes	Macrosomia, preeclampsia	For diabetic women, optimal control of glucose and normalization of hemoglobin A_{1C}
	Congenital malformations	For women without prior history of diabetes, screening based on symptoms before pregnancy; oral GTT after 24-28 weeks' gestation

LBW, low birth weight; IUGR, intrauterine growth retardation; SAB, spontaneous abortion; HBsAg, hepatitis B surface antigen; GTT, glucose tolerance test.

birth outcome (e.g., preterm birth, low birth weight, and increased perinatal mortality) as some observational studies have suggested or if supplementation with iron makes a difference in fetal outcome. Although routine screening for anemia in the nonpregnant female is not recommended by the U.S. Preventive Health Services Task Force, assessment for iron stores is recommended at the first prenatal visit and if clinically suspected should be assessed in the preconception period as well. The status of iron stores is also a good measure for overall nutritional status. Screening for iron deficiency anemia usually is measured by the hematocrit level. If the level is low (less than 36% to 38% for women), iron studies (iron and total iron-binding capacity [TIBC]) can be ordered to identify iron deficiency anemia. If the test results are equivocal, iron stores can be measured by use of ferritin. For more detailed discussion on iron deficiency anemia, detection, and treatment see Chapter 15.

General nutritional requirements during pregnancy

The recommended daily allowance (RDA) for the pregnant woman, developed by various government research groups, provides the clinician with guidelines on basic nutritional requirements (Table 46-2). Protein is important in the development of fetal tissue, especially brain tissue. The RDA of protein in pregnancy is 60 g/day. Amino acids must be ingested in adequate but not excessive amounts. Large doses of aspartame (Nutrasweet or Equal), which contains commercially produced L-aspartate and L-phenylalanine, have been found to cause hypothalamic neuronal destruction in rats but have not been shown to be teratogenic in human beings (Council Report, 1985). It generally is recommended that pregnant women use the substance in moderation.

The effects of various vitamin and mineral deficiencies and excesses are summarized in Table 46-3.

Folate supplementation to decrease risk of neural tube defects

Epidemiology. Recent evidence has shown that supplementation of the water-soluble vitamin folate is particularly important in preventing neural tube defects. Each year more than 6000 infants are born with a neural tube defect, most

Table 46-2 Recommended daily dietary allowances

Nutrient (unit)	Adult woman*	
	Nonpregnant	Pregnant
Protein (g)	46-50	60
Carbohydrates (g)	100	250
Vitamins		
A	4000 IU	4000 IU
D	200 IU	400 IU
E	15 IU	15 IU
K (μg)	65	—
Folic acid (μg)	180	400
Thiamine (B$_1$) (mg/day)	1.1	1.5
Riboflavin (B$_2$) (mg/day)	1.3	1.6
Niacin (mg niacin equivalent)	15	17
Pyridoxine (B$_6$) (mg/day)	1.6	2.2
Cyanocobalamin (B$_{12}$) (μg/day)	2.0	2.2
Pantothenic acid (mg)	10	4-7
Ascorbic acid (vitamin C) (mg/day)	60	70
Minerals		
Calcium (mg/day)	1200	1200
Phosphorus (mg/day)	1200	1200
Magnesium (mg/day)	400	300
Iron (mg/day)	15	30
Zinc (mg/day)	12	15
Iodine (μg/day)	150	175
Selenium (μg/day)	—	65
Copper (mg/day)	2	1.5-3.0

Modified from National Research Council: *Recommended dietary allowances,* ed 10, Washington, DC, 1989, National Academy Press.
*U.S. RDA (National Nutrition Consortium): *Nutrition labeling: how it can work for you,* Bethesda, Md, 1975, The Consortium.

commonly spina bifida. The recurrence rate in the subsequent pregnancies is estimated at 2% to 10%.

The RDA for pregnant adult women is 0.4 mg (400 μg) folate. However, the Food and Drug Administration (FDA) advises an RDA of 0.8 mg folate. Most multivitamins contain 0.4 mg. Prenatal vitamins contain 0.8 mg folate. Most women consume an average 0.2 mg folate in the usual diet, which is less than both the RDA and the FDA-RDA for the pregnant woman.

Retrospective studies and randomized controlled trials clearly support folate supplementation. In one randomized controlled trial, women who had a previous pregnancy resulting in a fetus with a neural tube defect were followed from before conception through 6 weeks' gestation (Laurence et al., 1981). They received high-dose folate (4 mg) daily 1 month before conception through 6 weeks' gestation. This intervention was associated with a 60% reduction in risk for neural tube defects. These results were corroborated in a multicenter study by the Medical Research Council Vitamin Study Research Group (1991) using a similar intervention that documented a 70% reduction in risk for neural tube defect.

Two nonrandomized intervention studies (Smithells et al., 1983; Vergel et al., 1990) also were completed in a similar population (women with a prior history of neural tube defect–affected pregnancy) using supplementation with 5 mg folate. These studies also demonstrated that folate supplementation decreased the recurrence rate for subsequent pregnancies (85% reduction in risk).

Based on all of these results, the Centers for Disease Control (1991) issued new recommendations for women who had a previous pregnancy resulting in an infant with neural tube defect: to consume 4 mg folate at least 1 month before conception and to continue for the first 3 months of pregnancy.

A recent carefully controlled randomized double-blind study was conducted that involved healthy women contemplating pregnancy who did not have a history of neural tube defect–affected pregnancy (Czeizel and Dudas, 1992). Supplementation with 0.8mg (800 μg) folate (a dose seen in most prenatal vitamins), along with supplemental vitamins and minerals and trace elements, was begun 1 month before conception through 6 weeks of gestation. The control group received only trace elements. The group that received the folate supplementation experienced close to one half the rate of neural tube defects.

The CDC extrapolated from these data and issued updated guidelines in 1992 with the following recommendations.

All women of childbearing age in the United States who are capable of becoming pregnant should consume 0.4 mg (400 μg) of folic acid per day for the purpose of reducing their risk of having a pregnancy affected with spina bifida or other neural tube defects. Because the effects of high intakes are not well known but include complicating the diagnosis of vitamin B$_{12}$ deficiency, care should be taken to keep total folate consumption at less than 1 mg per day, except under the supervision of a physician. Women who have had a prior neural tube defect–affected pregnancy are a high risk of having a subsequent affected pregnancy. When these women are planning to become pregnant, they should consult their physician for advice because they may recommend the high dose (4 mg) as used in most of the studies.

The effect of folate deficiency is particularly pronounced in women with twin pregnancies, in those taking anticonvulsants, and in those with hemoglobinopathies inasmuch as the need for folate is increased in these situations.

Because almost 50% of all pregnancies are unplanned and it is estimated that most women do not obtain the minimum daily requirements of folate in their diet alone, the CDC also has considered recommending that the FDA advise supplementation of flour so that all women are guaranteed minimal intake of folate. There is still controversy regarding the optimal dose of folate.

In support of this effort, a controlled study of mothers in North America whose infants had neural tube defects as compared with mothers of children with other malformations has demonstrated that ingestion of 0.4 mg folate reduced the risk by almost 60% in the cohort of women from 1988-1991 and that 0.4 mg should be the recommended amount to protect all women contemplating pregnancy (Werler, Shapiro, and Mitchell, 1993).

Counseling. The data clearly support the recommendation that women with a history of neural tube defect–affected pregnancy should take supplemental folate. The lowest dose of 0.4 mg 1 month before conception to 6 weeks of gestation is probably adequate, but 0.8 mg (prenatal vitamins) is the dose usually recommended. The CDC recommends that such women consult their physicians because higher doses may be indicated. There is also good evidence that clinicians should be advising all women who are con-

Table 46-3 Effect of nutrient, vitamin, and mineral excess and deficiency during pregnancy

Nutrient	Excess	Deficiency
Protein	For aspartame, data inconclusive in humans	Poor fetal growth and development in humans
Vitamins		
Fat-soluble		
A	Malformation of urinary tract, first trimester CNS/liver damage Skin changes	—
D	Hypercalcemia Supravalvular aortic stenosis Cranial/facial abnormalities in first trimester (elfin facies), growth retardation	—
E	—	High rate of CNS and skeletal defects and spontaneous abortion in rats
K	Skeletal abnormalities in rats	—
Water-soluble		
Folic acid	Masks B_{12} deficiency	Increased risk of neural tube defects and spontaneous abortion
Thiamine (B_1)	—	Severe fetal abnormalities and infant beriberi
Riboflavin	—	—
Niacin	—	—
Pyridoxine (B_6)	Neuropathy in mother	Hypoplasia of thymus and spleen; diminished neonatal immunocompetence in animals; mental retardation in humans
Cyanocobalamin	—	Megaloblastic anemia, coma, hyperpigmentation
Pantothenic acid	—	—
Ascorbic acid	—	Congenital scurvy, spontaneous abortion and premature births
Minerals		
Iron	—	Anemia Increased risk of premature delivery in some observational studies
Calcium	—	Neonatal hypocalcemia Abnormal fetal bone development and mineralization ? Increased preeclampsia
Zinc	In rats, fetal loss and growth retardation	Congenital lesions Low levels associated with pregnancy-induced hypertension
Chromium		Low levels associated with glucose intolerance
Iodine	Congenital goiter Hypothyroidism Mental retardation	Cretinism
Copper	—	In rats, increased congenital malformations

Modified from Hollingsworth DR, Resnik R: *Medical counseling before pregnancy,* New York, 1988, Churchill Livingstone.

templating pregnancy (and possibly even all women of reproductive age) to follow the same supplementation guidelines. This can be provided in the form of one prenatal vitamin per day (0.8 mg), but a nonprescription multivitamin that usually contains 0.4 mg is probably adequate. Because many pregnancies are unplanned, a daily multivitamin is recommended if the woman does not have adequate intake from the diet alone. At present, the American College of Obstetricians and Gynecologists is not advising all women of reproductive years to supplement their diet with folate because of lack of prospective data.

The only potential risk of folate supplementation is masking B_{12} deficiency with doses higher than 1.0 mg per day.

Caffeine

Data on the risks to the fetus from caffeine ingestion during pregnancy remain inconclusive.

Caffeine consumption increases circulating catecholamines, which is thought to be a possible mechanism for causing birth defects. Animal studies have demonstrated an increased incidence of skeletal defects in offspring of rats fed extremely high amounts of caffeine (equivalent to more than 50 cups of coffee per day) (Spiller, 1984). With lower intake of caffeine (4, 8, and 28 cups per day), no birth defects occurred in the pregnant rats' offspring.

Results from human studies have been inconsistent. In a prospective study of more than 400 pregnant women, moderate caffeine intake (less than 3 cups per day) was not associated with an increased risk for spontaneous abortion, intrauterine growth retardation, or microcephaly. However, more than 3 cups per day did appear to increase the risk for intrauterine growth retardation although the outcome events were small (Hatch and Bracken, 1993; Mills et al., 1993). However, in a case-controlled study of caffeine consumption among 331 women who suffered fetal loss, there was a significantly increased risk for spontaneous abortion with consumption of only 1 to 2 cups per day; high consumption (more than 3 cups) further increased the risk (Infante-Rivard et al., 1993).

There are no standard recommendations at this time regarding caffeine intake, but prudent intake (less than 2 cups of coffee, tea, or cola drinks per day) probably should be advised.

SUBSTANCE ABUSE
Alcohol

Epidemiology. Alcohol intake during pregnancy occurs commonly. According to the National Household Survey on Drug Abuse (1990), 73% of women between 12 and 34 years of age expose their fetuses to alcohol at some time during pregnancy.

Effects of alcohol on conception and pregnancy. Alcohol has profoundly negative effects on the fetus. Alcohol abuse during pregnancy is the third leading cause of mental retardation. Alcohol-related effects (see box, below) include physical effects, as well as risk of intrauterine death, prenatal and postnatal growth retardation, low birth weight, central nervous system abnormalities, and behavior deficits (Streissguth et al., 1980). A relationship between alcohol consumption and the development of the fetal alcohol syndrome has clearly been established. Fetal alcohol syndrome is defined as prenatal or postnatal growth retardation (less than 10th percentile in body weight, length, and head cir-

cumference), two or three characteristic facial abnormalities (microcephaly, microphthalmia, underdeveloped philtrum, thin upper lip, maxillary hypoplasia, and central nervous system dysfunctions (such as neurologic abnormalities, mental deficiency, and developmental delays) (Jones and Smith, 1973; Jones et al., 1973; Hanson, Jones, and Smith, 1976; Rosett, 1980) (see box, below). An increased incidence of fetal alcohol syndrome has been found in women who have consumed more than four drinks per day (Hanson, Streissguth, and Smith, 1978). It is not clear whether less than that amount also is associated with increased risk.

Mental retardation, hyperactivity, and developmental delays have all been reported in children of mothers who consume large amounts of alcohol. However, controlled studies on the long-term consequences of maternal alcohol ingestion during pregnancy are few. One study suggested that moderate drinking (one drink per day during pregnancy) was associated with attention deficit disorder in the children of moderate drinkers as compared with occasional drinkers and nondrinkers (Landersman-Dwyer, Ragozin, and Little, 1981). Alcohol consumption is associated with an increased risk of spontaneous abortion in the first trimester and an increased risk of abruptio placentae.

Although there is agreement that heavy drinking is detrimental, there is no agreement about the effects of lower levels of alcohol consumption. Evidence exists that the risk is markedly decreased if a woman stops drinking alcohol during pregnancy (Rosett et al., 1983). It appears that the timing of alcohol consumption is important, with the greatest negative impact being at the time of conception through the first month of pregnancy (Ernhart et al., 1985; Ernhart et al., 1987).

Counseling. It is important that the clinician who counsels a woman before conception obtains a clear history of alcohol consumption. Methods for obtaining an accurate history of alcohol intake are described in Chapter 66. It is clear that heavy ingestion is detrimental to the developing fetus and that cessation of alcohol intake, especially early in the pregnancy, can decrease the risk of fetal anomalies.

No level of alcohol consumption has been proved to be safe. For this reason many clinicians recommend complete abstinence. Explaining what is known of the effects of alco-

---

ALCOHOL-RELATED PHYSICAL PROBLEMS ASSOCIATED WITH PRENATAL ALCOHOL EXPOSURE

Dysmorphic features
Characteristic facial features, low-set ears, palmar creases

Intraoral deformities
Cleft palate, malocclusions, poor dental alignment

Hearing
Chronic otitis media, permanent hearing loss

Vision
Eyeground malformations, optic nerve hypoplasia, strabismus, ptosis, nystagmus, myopia

Cardiac
Heart murmurs, patent ductus arteriosus

Skeletal malformations
Congenital hip dislocation, scoliosis, bilateral halluces

Genitourinary
Hydronephrosis, labial hypoplasia

Growth retardation
Microcephaly, weight/height (less than 10% normal), failure to thrive

Immune system deficits
T cell loss, allergies

Modified from Coles C: *Clin Obstet Gynecol* 36:255, 1993.

FETAL ALCOHOL SYNDROME

Prenatal or postnatal growth retardation

Facial features (at least 2 or 3 abnormalities)
Absent philtrum
Thinned upper vermilion
Hypoplastic midface
Low nasal bridge
Epicanthal fold
Shortened palpebral fissure
Low-set ears
Microcephaly

Central nervous system dysfunction
Neurologic abnormalities
Mental deficiency
Developmental delays

Modified from Jones and Smith: *Lancet* 2:999, 1973.

hol use on pregnancy outcome is important. In women with identified alcohol abuse, referral for treatment before conception and maintaining close follow-up throughout pregnancy can prevent the development of major birth anomalies and obstetric complications.

Smoking

Epidemiology. In the United States 26% of women are smokers, most of whom are of reproductive age. Maternal smoking is a major preventable cause of low birth weight and perinatal mortality. Studies have shown that as many as 40% of infants born with low birth weight can be attributed to maternal smoking. Smoking also is associated with infertility, menstrual disorders, spontaneous abortions, ectopic pregnancies, placental irregularities, and increased childhood morbidity (Cefalo and Moos, 1995) (see box, below).

According to data from the National Health Interview Survey, completed by the U.S. Department of Health and Human Services, 1989, 32% of women were found to be smokers before pregnancy and 21% quit during the pregnancy. In other studies almost 70% of women who stopped smoking during their pregnancies resumed after completing the pregnancy (Fingerhut, Kleinman, and Kendrick, 1990; Mullen, Quinn, and Ershoff, 1990), and 25% of all women continue to smoke during pregnancy (Floyd et al., 1991).

Pathophysiology. The pathophysiology of the negative effects include exposure to nicotine and various by-products and additives in the cigarettes, such as polycyclic aromatic hydrocarbons and carbon monoxide. Nicotine causes vasoconstriction and vasospasm, hydrocarbons interfere with maternal fetal transport, and the carbon monoxide displaces the oxygen. Not only are there direct effects on the fetus but the adequacy of the placenta is affected by abnormal microcirculation.

Effects of smoking on conception and pregnancy. Review of the data on the effect of smoking on fertility has clearly demonstrated that fertility is adversely affected by

smoking and the effect is worse in women who smoke more than 16 cigarettes per day (Stillman, Rosenberg, and Sachs, 1986). A delay in conception for women who smoke is three times more likely than for nonsmokers, and it can take smokers more than 1 year to conceive (Baird and Wilcox, 1985). There is also a reported increased risk in ectopic pregnancy (Rosenberg, 1986). After cessation of smoking, the risk for infertility is the same as for nonsmokers.

Although the data are inconsistent, some studies have found an increased incidence of birth defects, including cleft palate (Fedrick, Alberman, and Goldstein, 1971) and cardiovascular and urogenital abnormalities (Himmelberger, Brown, and Cohen, 1978) in infants of mothers who smoke during pregnancy.

Many studies have shown that intrauterine growth retardation and low birth weight are causally related to smoking and are dose-dependent, with heavy smokers being at increased risk for low-birth-weight infants as compared with occasional smokers. There is also an increase in risk for spontaneous abortion, and the risk increases with heavier smoking patterns. Preterm birth (less than 37 weeks' gestation) has been shown to be more common in smokers, especially in those who consume more than one pack per day (Shiono, Klebanoff, and Rhoads, 1986), and placental complications, including placenta previa, abruptio placentae, and vaginal bleeding, also are more prevalent (Meyer, Jonas, and Tonascia, 1976; Shiono, Klebanoff, and Rhoads, 1986). Long-term consequences of increased respiratory infections in the infant and a link between smoking and sudden infant death syndrome exist as well.

Counseling. Counseling women on cessation of smoking is important especially if the women is contemplating pregnancy. Chapter 73 discusses in detail methods for approaching smoking cessation. If the women is pregnant, behavioral methods usually are most appropriate inasmuch as nicotine gum is contraindicated in pregnancy. The safety of the nicotine patch, which provides a lower, continuous release of nicotine, has not been established for pregnant women.

Cocaine use

Epidemiology. Prevalence of cocaine use among pregnant women is difficult to estimate. Approximately 5% of women of reproductive age reported cocaine ingestion in the 1990 National Household Survey on Drug Abuse. It is estimated that anywhere from 3% to 17% of pregnant women use cocaine (Slutsker, 1992; Volpe, 1992).

Pathophysiology. Cocaine has potent effects on both the peripheral and central nervous systems. The mechanism of the deleterious effects of maternal cocaine ingestion on the fetus have been outlined by Volpe (1992). In the mother, increased peripheral catecholamine production results in vasoconstriction, uterine contraction, and decreased placental flow. Fetal effects also are mediated by placental transfer of catecholamines, decreased nutrients, and decreased oxygen transfer, leading to focal cerebral ischemia and decreased cerebral blood flow. These factors result in severe interruption in the development of the fetal nervous system and increased risk of obstetric complications.

Effects of cocaine on conception and pregnancy (see box on the following page). Conflicting data exist on the effects of cocaine use during early pregnancy. Effects of

---

EFFECTS OF SMOKING ON CONCEPTION AND PREGNANCY

Fertility
  Delay in conception
  Risk of tubal pregnancy

Birth defects
  Cleft palate
  Cardiovascular and urogenital abnormalities

Obstetric complications
  Intrauterine growth retardation
  Low birth weight
  Spontaneous abortion
  Placenta previa
  Abruptio placentae
  Vaginal bleeding

Long-term consequences
  Increased respiratory infections
  Sudden infant death syndrome

**EFFECTS OF COCAINE ON
CONCEPTION AND PREGNANCY**

Birth defects

Congenital urogenital malformations

Obstetric complications

Intrauterine growth retardation
Low birth weight
Spontaneous abortion
Placental abruption
Abnormal labor
Premature rupture of membranes

Other effects on fetus

Behavioral abnormalities
Sudden infant death syndrome
Necrotizing enterocolitis
Cerebrovascular accidents
Long-term neurodevelopmental problems

Comorbidities

Malnutrition
Sexually transmitted diseases
Hepatitis B
HIV
Other addictions

---

cocaine use reported in some studies include an increased rate of spontaneous abortion, retardation in fetal growth, and congenital anomalies, particularly in the genitourinary tract. In addition, intrauterine exposure to cocaine significantly affects human brain development (Table 46-4).

Later in pregnancy, there appear to be higher rates of placental abruption, abnormal labor, and premature rupture of membranes (Slutsker, 1992; Volpe, 1992). Other effects on the fetus include an increase in sudden infant death syndrome, necrotizing enterocolitis, and cerebrovascular accidents.

Table 46-4 Disturbances in human brain development reported after intrauterine exposure to cocaine

Event	Peak gestational period	Abnormality
Neural tube formation	3-4 wk	Myelomeningocele Encephalocele
Prosencephalic development	2-3 mo	Agenesis of corpus callosum; agenesis of septum pellucidum; septooptic dysplasia
Neuronal proliferation	3-4 mo	Microcephaly
Neuronal migration	3-5 mo	Schizencephaly, neuronal heterotopias
Neuronal differentiation	5 mo-postnatal	Abnormal cortical neuronal cytodifferentiation (preliminary)
Myelination	After birth	None

Modified from Volpe J: *N Engl J Med* 327:399, 1992.

Severe long-term effects also have been demonstrated, including behavioral problems as children are followed into their school years (Little et al., 1989; Zuckerman et al., 1989).

The direct effects of cocaine for any user regardless of pregnancy include myocardial ischemia, cerebrovascular accidents, subarachnoid hemorrhage, hypertension, seizures, intestinal ischemia, pulmonary edema, and sudden death (Volpe, 1992). Associated comorbidities that result in a riskier pregnancy include malnutrition; increased rate of sexually transmitted diseases, hepatitis B, and HIV; and other drug addictions.

Counseling. Chapter 66 reviews methods for identifying cases of substance abuse. Referral and treatment before pregnancy are important but often are unavailable because of limited resources and programs. When a woman becomes pregnant, intervention becomes even more difficult because many programs do not accept pregnant women. A list of available resources appears in Appendix X.

DOMESTIC ABUSE

Domestic abuse increases during pregnancy and is associated with complications late in pregnancy such as abruptio placentae and premature rupture of membranes. It is important to elicit a history of domestic abuse during all routine visits and provide appropriate preventive intervention. This topic is covered in detail in Chapter 68.

DIABETES AND HYPERTENSION

Preconception counseling has clearly been shown to improve a pregnancy outcome in a woman with diabetes (see box, below). The incidence of congenital malformations in infants of diabetic women is 6% to 10%. Common malformations include ventricular septal defects, neural tube defects, and caudal regression syndrome. Macrosomia increases the risk for birth trauma and the need for cesarean section. In addition, the risk is increased for preeclampsia, susceptibility to urinary tract infections and pyelonephritis, and progression of preexisting diabetic nephropathy and retinopathy. Multiple studies have demonstrated that monitoring and control of glucose before conception and during early pregnancy result in a decrease in the likelihood of more serious malformations (Mills, Baker, and Goldman, 1979) and early pregnancy complications (Mills et al., 1988;

**EFFECTS OF DIABETES ON
CONCEPTION AND PREGNANCY**

Birth defects

Ventricular septal defects
Neural tube defects
Caudal regression syndrome

Other fetal effects

Macrosomia

Obstetric complications

Preeclampsia
Urinary tract infections
Premature labor

Kitzmiller et al., 1991). The incidence of major congenital fetal defects is clearly correlated with hemoglobin A_{1C} measurements during early pregnancy (Miller et al., 1988). Control of the glucose throughout pregnancy is correlated with improved pregnancy outcomes, including a decrease in risk of fetal macrosomia, premature labor, and stillbirth (Hollingsworth, 1984; Frankel, Dooley, and Metzger, 1985; Coustan, 1988; Hollingsworth and Resnik, 1988). Chapter 53 covers diabetes during pregnancy in detail.

BIBLIOGRAPHY

General

Burrow G, Ferris T: *Medical complications during pregnancy,* Philadelphia, 1988, WB Saunders.

Cefalo R, Moos M: *Preconception health care: a practical guide,* ed 2, St Louis, 1995, Mosby.

Hollingsworth D, Resnik R: *Medical counseling before pregnancy,* New York, 1988, Churchill Livingstone.

Jack B, Culpepper L: Preconception care risk reduction and health promotion in preparation for pregnancy, *JAMA* 264:1147, 1990.

Queenan J, Hobbins J: *Protocols for high risk pregnancies,* ed 2, Oradell, NJ, 1987, Medical Economics Books.

Nutrition

American College of Obstetricians and Gynecologists: *Nutrition in pregnancy* (ACOG Tech Bull 179), Washington, DC, 1993, The College.

Council Report: Aspartame: review of safety issues, *JAMA* 254:400, 1985.

Kim I et al: Pregnancy nutrition surveillance system—United States 1979-1980, *MMWR* 41 (SS-7):25, 1992.

National Research Council: Recommended dietary allowances, ed 10, Washington, DC, 1989, National Academy Press.

Nelson J et al: *Mayo Clinic diet manual: a handbook of nutrition practices,* St Louis, 1994, Mosby.

US Preventive Health Services Task Force (policy statement): Routine iron supplementation during pregnancy, *JAMA* 270:2846, 1993.

Folate supplementation

Bower C, Stanley FJ: Dietary folate as a risk factor for neural tube defects: evidence from a case-control study in Western Australia, *Med J Aust* 150:613, 1989.

Centers for Disease Control: Use of folic acid for prevention of spina bifida and other neural tube defects 1983-1991, *MMWR* 40:513, 1991.

Centers for Disease Control: Recommendations for the use of folic acid to reduce the number of cases of spina bifida and other neural tube defects, *MMWR* 41(RR-14):1, 1992.

Czeizel A, Dudas I: Prevention of the first occurrence of neural tube defects by periconceptual vitamin supplementation, *N Engl J Med* 327:1832, 1992.

Laurence KM et al: Double blind randomized controlled trial of folate treatment before conception to prevent recurrence of neural tube defects, *Br Med J* 282:1509, 1981.

Medical Research Council Vitamin Study Research Group: Prevention of neural tube defects: results of the Medical Research Council vitamin study, *Lancet* 338:131, 1991.

Mills JL et al: The absence of a relation between the periconceptional use of vitamins and neural tube defects, *N Engl J Med* 321:430, 1989.

Milunsky A et al: Multivitamin folic acid supplementation in early pregnancy reduces the prevalence of neural tube defects, *JAMA* 262:2847, 1989.

Mulinare J et al: Periconceptional use of multivitamins and the occurrence of neural tube defects, *JAMA* 260:3141, 1988.

Oakley G: Folic acid–preventable spina bifida and anencephaly, *JAMA* 269:1292, 1993.

Rosenberg I: Folic acid and neural tube defects—time for action? *N Engl J Med* 327:1875, 1992.

Smithells RW et al: Further experiences of vitamin supplementation for the prevention of neural tube defect recurrences, *Lancet* 1:1027, 1983.

Subcommittee on Dietary Intake and Nutrient Supplements During Pregnancy: *Nutrition during pregnancy,* Washington, DC, 1990, National Academy Press.

Vergel RG et al: Primary prevention of neural tube defects with folic acid supplementation: Cuban experience, *Prenat Diagn* 10:149, 1990.

Werler M, Shapiro S, Mitchell A: Periconceptional folic acid exposure and risk of occurrent neural tube defects, *JAMA* 269:1257, 1993.

Caffeine

Eskenazi B: Caffeine during pregnancy: grounds for concern? *JAMA* 270:2973, 1993.

Grimm VE, Freider B: Prenatal caffeine causes long-lasting behavioral and neurochemical changes, *Int J Neurosci* 41:15, 1988.

Hatch EE, Bracken MB: Caffeine use during pregnancy: what is safe? *JAMA* 270:47, 1993.

Infante-Rivard C et al: Fetal loss associated with caffeine intake before and during pregnancy, *JAMA* 270:2940, 1993.

Mills JL et al: Moderate caffeine use and the risk of spontaneous abortion and intrauterine growth retardation, *JAMA* 269:593, 1993.

Spiller J, editor: *The methylxanthine beverages and foods: chemistry, consumption and health effects,* New York, 1984, Alan Liss.

Watkinson B, Fried PA: Maternal caffeine use before, during and after pregnancy and effects upon offspring, *Neurobehav Toxicol Teratol* 7:9, 1985.

Substance abuse

Alcohol

Abel EL: *Fetal alcohol syndrome and fetal alcohol effects,* New York, 1984, Plenum Press.

Alcohol and the fetus—is zero the only option? *Lancet* 1:682, 1983.

Coles C: Impact of prenatal alcohol exposure on the newborn and the child, *Clin Obstet Gynecol* 36:255, 1993.

Council on Scientific Affairs: Fetal effects of maternal alcohol use, *JAMA* 249:2517, 1983.

Day N, Cottreau C, Richardson G: The epidemiology of alcohol, marijuana and cocaine use among women of childbearing age and pregnant women, *Clin Obstet Gynecol* 36:232, 1993.

Ernhart C et al: Alcohol-related birth defects: syndromal anomalies, intrauterine growth retardation, and neonatal behavioral assessment, *Alcoholism: Clin Exp Res* 9:447, 1985.

Ernhart C et al: Alcohol teratogenicity in the human: a detailed assessment of specificity, critical period and threshold, *Am J Obstet Gynecol* 156:33, 1987.

Hanson JW, Jones K, Smith D: Fetal alcohol syndrome, *JAMA* 235:1458, 1976.

Hanson JW, Streissguth AP, Smith DW: The effects of moderate alcohol consumption during pregnancy on fetal growth and morphogenesis, *Pediatrics* 92:457, 1978.

Harlap S, Shiono PH: Alcohol, smoking and the incidence of spontaneous abortions in the first and second trimester, *Lancet* 2:173, 1980.

Jones KL, Smith DW: Recognition of the fetal alcohol syndrome in early infancy, *Lancet* 2:999, 1973.

Jones KL et al: Pattern of malformation in offspring of chronic alcoholic mothers, *Lancet* 1:1267, 1973.

Kaufman MH: Ethanol induced chromosomal abnormalities at conception, *Nature* 302:258, 1983.

Kline J et al: Drinking during pregnancy and spontaneous abortion, *Lancet* 2:176, 1980.

Landesman-Dwyer S, Ragozin AS, Little RE: Behavioral correlates of prenatal alcohol exposure: a four year follow-up study, *Neurobehav Toxicol Teratol* 3:187, 1981.

Marbury MC et al: The association of alcohol consumption with outcome of pregnancy, *Am J Public Health* 73:1165, 1983.

National Institute on Drug Abuse: *National household survey on drug abuse: 1990 population estimates,* US Public Health Service Pub No ADM 91-1732, Washington, DC, 1991, US Government Printing Office.

Ouellette E et al: Adverse effects on offspring of maternal alcohol abuse during pregnancy, *N Engl J Med* 297:528, 1977.

Rosett HL: A clinical perspective of the fetal alcohol syndrome, *Alcoholism: Clin Exp Res* 4:119, 1980.

Rosett HL, Weiner L: *Alcohol and the fetus: a clinical perspective,* New York, 1984, Oxford University Press.

Rosett HL et al: Patterns of alcohol consumption and fetal development, *Obstet Gynecol* 61:539, 1983.

Streissguth AP, Clarren SK, Jones KL: Natural history of the fetal alcohol syndrome: a 10 year follow-up of eleven patients, *Lancet* 2:85, 1985.

Streissguth AP et al: Teratogenic effects of alcohol in humans and laboratory animals, *Science* 209:353, 1980.

Streissguth AP et al: Fetal alcohol syndrome in adolescents and adults, *JAMA* 265:1961, 1991.

Smoking

Baird DD, Wilcox AJ: Cigarette smoking associated with delayed conception, *JAMA* 253:2979, 1985.

Fedrick J, Alberman ED, Goldstein H: Possible teratogenic effect of cigarette smoking, *Nature* 231:529, 1971.

Fingerhut LA, Kleinman JC, Kendrick JS: Smoking before, during and after pregnancy, *Am J Public Health* 80:541, 1990.

Floyd RL et al: Smoking during pregnancy: prevalence, effects, and intervention strategies, *Birth* 18:48, 1991.

Himmelberger DU, Brown BW, Cohen EN: Cigarette smoking during pregnancy and the occurrence of spontaneous abortion and congenital abnormalities, *Am J Epidemiol* 108:470, 1978.

Meyer MB, Jonas BS, Tonascia JA: Perinatal events associated with maternal smoking during pregnancy, *Am J Epidemiol* 103:464, 1976.

Mullen PD, Quinn VP, Ershoff DH: Maintenance of nonsmoking postpartum by women who stopped smoking during pregnancy, *Public Health Briefs* 80:992, 1990.

Nieberg et al: The fetal tobacco syndrome, *JAMA* 253:2998, 1985.

Rosenberg MJ: *Smoking and reproductive health,* St Louis, 1987, Mosby.

Shiono P, Klebanoff M, Rhoads G: Smoking and drinking during pregnancy, *JAMA* 255:82, 1986.

Stillman R, Rosenberg M, Sachs B: Smoking and reproduction, *Fertil Steril* 46:545, 1986.

US Department of Health and Human Services: *The health consequences of smoking for women: a report of the surgeon general,* DHHS Pub No CDC89-8411, Washington, DC, 1989, US Government Printing Office.

Cocaine

Allen P, Sandler M: Critical components of obstetric management of chemically dependent women, *Clin Obstet Gynecol* 36:347, 1993.

Baciewicz G: The process of addiction, *Clin Obstet Gynecol* 36:223, 1993.

Chasnoff I: Drugs, *Alcohol, pregnancy and parenting,* Boston, 1988, Kluwer Academic Publishers.

Chasnoff I et al: Cocaine use in pregnancy, *N Engl J Med* 313:666, 1985.

Chasnoff I et al: Temporal patterns of cocaine use in pregnancy, *JAMA* 261:174, 1989.

Chavez G, Mulinare J, Coredero J: Maternal cocaine use during early pregnancy as a risk factor for congenital abnormalities, *JAMA* 262:795, 1989.

Cregler L, Mark H: Medical complications of cocaine, *N Engl J Med* 315:1495, 1986.

Dicke J, Verges D, Polakoski K: Cocaine inhibits alanine uptake by human placental microvillous membrane vesicles, *Am J Obstet Gynecol* 169:515, 1993.

Gillogley K et al: The perinatal impact of cocaine, amphetamine, and opiate use detected by universal intrapartum screening, *Am J Obstet Gynecol* 163:1535, 1990.

Glantz JC, Woods J: Cocaine, heroin and phencyclidine: obstetric perspectives, *Clin Obstet Gynecol* 36:279, 1993.

Little B et al: Cocaine abuse during pregnancy: maternal and fetal implications, *Obstet Gynecol* 73:157, 1989.

MacGregor S et al: Cocaine use during pregnancy: adverse perinatal outcome, *Am J Obstet Gynecol* 157:686, 1987.

MacGregor S et al: Cocaine abuse during pregnancy: correlation between prenatal care and perinatal outcome, *Obstet Gynecol* 74:882, 1989.

Mayes L et al: The problem of prenatal cocaine exposure: a rush to judgment, *JAMA* 267:406, 1992.

Ryan L, Ehrlich S, Finnegan L: Cocaine abuse in pregnancy: effects on the fetus and newborn, *Neurotoxicol Teratol* 9:295, 1987.

Slutsker L: Risks associated with cocaine use during pregnancy, *Obstet Gynecol* 79:778, 1992.

Smith C, Asch R: Drug abuse and reproduction, *Fertil Steril* 48:355, 1987.

Vega W et al: A prevalence and magnitude of perinatal substance exposures in California, *N Engl J Med* 329:850, 1993.

Volpe J: Effect of cocaine use on the fetus, *N Engl J Med* 327:399, 1992.

Warner E: Cocaine abuse, *Ann Intern Med* 119:226, 1993.

Zuckerman B et al: Effects of maternal marijuana and cocaine use on fetal growth, *N Engl J Med* 320:762, 1989.

Diabetes

Coustan D: Pregnancy in diabetic women, *N Engl J Med* 319:1663, 1988.

Frankel N, Dooley S, Metzger B: Care of the pregnant woman with insulin dependent diabetes mellitus, *N Engl J Med* 313:96, 1985.

Hollingsworth D: *Pregnancy, diabetes and birth: management guide,* Baltimore, 1984, Williams & Wilkins.

Hollingsworth D, Resnik R: *Medical counseling before pregnancy,* New York, 1988, Churchill Livingstone.

Kitzmiller J et al: Preconception care of diabetes: glycemic control prevents congenital abnormalities, *JAMA* 265:731, 1991.

Miller E et al: Elevated maternal HbA_{1C} in early pregnancy and major congenital anomalies in infants of diabetic mothers, *N Engl J Med* 304:1331, 1981.

Mills JL, Baker L, Goldman AS: Malformations in infants of diabetic mothers occur before the seventh gestational week, *Diabetes* 28:292, 1979.

Mills JL et al: Incidence of spontaneous abortion among normal women and insulin dependent diabetic women whose pregnancies were identified within 21 days of conception, *N Engl J Med* 319:1617, 1988.

HIV prevention and pregnancy

American College of Obstetricians and Gynecologists (ACOG): Special medical report: ACOG issues report on HIV infection in women, *Am Fam Physician,* 46:579, 1992.

47 Amniocentesis and Prenatal Genetics

Louise Wilkins-Haug

During the past 20 years prenatal genetics has evolved from a field of specialized testing into an integral component of routine obstetric care. Greater use of antepartum genetic testing has resulted from two major advances—first, improved screening to identify those women with increased risk; second, advancements in the techniques for diagnosing genetic disorders.

SCREENING
Chromosome abnormalities

A positive correlation between the frequency of chromosomally abnormal fetuses and maternal age is well recognized. Though women at all ages are at risk for an infant with Down syndrome (trisomy 21), at age 25 the risk is 1/890 pregnancies, increasing to a risk of 1/250 at 35 years and 1/90 at 40 years of age (Hook, Cross, and Regal, 1984). In 1966 amniocyte culture provided a means for examining fetal chromosomes. Amniocentesis, the removal of a small quantity of amniotic fluid containing fetal cells, can provide a karyotype of the fetus during the second trimester but is associated with approximately a 1/300 risk of miscarriage. Thus only women with a risk of having an affected fetus equal to or greater than the risk of complication from the procedure (1/300) have been offered amniocentesis. Traditionally, a maternal age of 35 years or greater at delivery (risk of trisomy 21 = 1/250) has been the screening parameter, used to identify women at sufficient risk to justify offering an invasive diagnostic test such as amniocentesis.

Maternal age as a screening parameter, however, has limitations. On average 5% to 7% of pregnant women are 35 years or older at delivery and thus have a "positive" maternal age screen for trisomy 21. However, only 20% of Down syndrome infants are born to women over 35 years of age. Furthermore, although acceptance of amniocentesis may vary on the basis of cultural and religious beliefs, by some reports acceptance of amniocentesis in women 35 or older may be as low as 50%, in part as a result of the risk associated with the procedure.

Maternal serum α-fetoprotein. Additional screening programs have been developed to identify women, other than those older than 35 at delivery, who are at an increased risk for a chromosomally abnormal fetus. Quantification of maternal serum α-fetoprotein (MSAFP) level, which is produced by the fetal liver, has shown lower levels to occur in fetuses with chromosomal abnormalities (Merkatz et al., 1984). As MSAFP quantification is now routinely offered for neural tube defect screening (see later discussion), the concomitant use of low MSAFP for trisomy 21 screening is also frequently performed. However, prospective studies of MSAFP screening for trisomy 21 in women less than age 35

at delivery have shown that a positive screen detects only 20% of affected fetuses.

Human chorionic gonadotropin and unconjugated estriol. In the past 5 years MSAFP screening for trisomy 21 risk has been expanded in many centers with the addition of other pregnancy hormones including human chorionic gonadotropin (hCG) and unconjugated estriol (UE3) determinations. In pregnancies with a trisomy 21 fetus hCG levels are higher than expected and estriol levels are lower. For an individual maternal blood sample the likelihood that the fetus has trisomy 21 can be calculated on the basis of the results of a triple panel (AFP, hCG, and estriol). This likelihood ratio in combination with the maternal age yields a new risk for trisomy 21 in any individual women (Wald et al., 1988). A triple panel risk for a trisomy 21 fetus of greater than 1/250 is considered a positive result. Approximately 7% of women below the age of 35 have a positive serum panel result. Women with a positive serum panel finding then have ultrasound confirmation of gestational age as the results of the three assays vary greatly with gestational week. In general only 3% of the originally screened population will continue to have positive serum triple panel findings after correction by ultrasound for inaccurate gestational age. Prospective studies have shown that in women <35 years at delivery, a positive triple assay serum screen can detect from 39% to 58% of Down syndrome fetuses (Table 47-1).

Screening for neural tube defects

Determination of maternal serum α-fetoprotein level at 16 to 18 weeks' gestation was established in the late 1970s for neural tube defect (NTD) screening. Elevated MSAFP levels (>2.5 MoM [multiple of the median]) lead to the detection of approximately 80% of infants with NTDs and 90% of those with anencephaly. In an average obstetric population approximately 3% of patients have an elevated MSAFP level. Generally half of these positive screen results can be explained by ultrasound findings such as twins, demise, or erroneous gestational age. Among the remainder, however, 1 in 15 will have an infant with a NTD. However, in many centers improved ultrasound resolution is now being considered in the counseling of patients with an elevated MSAFP level. Nadel and colleagues have reported less than a 1/1000 (0.01% to 0.15%) chance of an affected fetus given a normal targeted ultrasound finding and a MSAFP 2.0 to 3.5 MoMs. According to these authors, with MSAFP values up to 3.5 MoMs and an informative, high-resolution ultrasound, the risk of amniocentesis is greater than the chance of missing a NTD.

Population-specific disease screening

Tay-Sachs disease. Tay-Sachs disease is a degenerative neurologic condition caused by a deficiency of hexosamin-

Table 47-1 Prospective studies of maternal serum screening panels for trisomy 21 (Down syndrome)

Author	N	Initial result positive screen	Positive result after US	Detection of trisomy 21	PPV
Haddow et al. (1992)	25,207	6.6%	3.8%	58%	2.6%
Wald et al. (1992)	11,993	4.9%	3.3%	39%	1.7%
Phillips et al. (1992)	9,530	7.0%	3.2%	57%	1.9%

US, ultrasound; PPV, positive predictive value at amniocentesis.

idase A. The disorder first appears in infancy with signs of progressive neurologic damage, including blindness, deafness, seizures, and spasticity, with eventual demise in childhood. Tay-Sachs disease is inherited as an autosomal recessive trait with the gene most prevalent in the Ashkenazic Jewish population. Approximately 1 in 22 Ashkenazic Jewish individuals carry the gene for Tay-Sachs disease. Ninety percent of the Jewish population in the United States is estimated to have Ashkenazic background. Descendants of French Canadians also have an increased prevalence of the Tay-Sachs gene. Carrier detection can be accurately accomplished by detection of decreased serum hexosaminidase A levels, and prenatal diagnosis is undertaken with enzyme assay of cultured amniocytes.

Sickle-cell disease. Sickle hemoglobin results from a point mutation in the gene producing the β chain of hemoglobin A (a tetramer of two α and two β chains). Persons with two copies of the **sickle-cell gene (SS)** have a chronic hemolytic anemia that can be symptomatic with painful crises, a lowered resistance to infection, jaundice, and leg ulcers. Approximately 1 in 10 persons of African black ancestry carries one copy of the sickle-cell gene. Hispanic individuals as well as persons from the Middle East, Mediterranean, and parts of India also have a higher frequency of the sickle-cell gene than other populations. Couples in which both partners are carriers of the sickle-cell gene have a 25% chance of an affected child. Prenatal diagnosis from chorionic villus sampling (CVS) or amniocentesis can be offered to couples at risk.

Another variant, **hemoglobin C,** is also prevalent among African blacks. Like the mutation producing sickle-cell hemoglobin the genetic defect producing hemoglobin C is located in the β chain. However, unlike sickle-cell disease, hemoglobin C in the homozygous state results in a mild anemia without associated painful crises. More common than homozygotic CC disease, however, is hemoglobin SC. Occurring in approximately 1/1250 black Americans, SC disease can result in a chronic anemia. Couples in which one partner is a carrier of hemoglobin C and the other of hemoglobin S are at risk for a child with SC hemoglobin.

A "sickle dex" provides detection of the carrier status for only the sickle-cell gene and may fail to detect other potentially significant hemoglobinopathies (such as hemoglobin C varients). Hemoglobin electrophoresis is recommended for complete analysis of persons at risk.

Thalassemias. The major hemoglobin component of adult blood, hemoglobin A (Hb A), is a tetramer of two α and two β hemoglobin chains. The thalassemias are hemoglobin disorders characterized by decreased numbers of structurally normal α or β chains. β-**thalassemia** with decreased or absent β chain production can result from more than 30 molecular defects and is inherited as an autosomal recessive disorder. Persons homozygotic for the β-thalassemia gene have Cooley's anemia, or β-thalassemia major. Affected individuals become symptomatic at about 3 months of age when the switch from fetal hemoglobin (Hb F) to adult hemoglobin (Hb A) normally occurs. Deficient β chain production is reflected by a decrease in hemoglobin A (2 α/2 β, an increased level of A2 (2 α/2 δ chains), and an increased hemoglobin F (2 α/2 γ chains). A chronic anemia results and affected individuals are transfusion-dependent with problems secondary to transfusion-related iron overload.

The homozygotic state for α-**thalassemia** results in a four-gene deletion producing a fetus with Bart's hydrops fetalis. With α chains deficient the fetus is unable to produce fetal hemoglobin (2 α/2 γ) or any adult hemoglobin. Only Bart's hemoglobin (4 γ), which has a higher oxygen affinity and thus a lower release of oxygen to fetal tissue resulting in hypoxia, is produced. The affected fetus has high output failure, hydrops, and stillbirth. If a three-gene deletion is present, non–transfusion-dependent anemia, thalassemia intermedia, occurs. Two gene deletions produce α-thalassemia minor with a mild anemia often confused with iron deficiency anemia because of its microcytic, hypochromic nature.

Screening for the thalassemias should be offered to persons from high-risk populations (Table 47-2). Effective screening can be accomplished with a mean corpuscular volume (MCV) followed by a hemoglobin electrophoresis if needed (Fig. 47-1). Prenatal diagnosis for the thalassemias is now available through CVS or amniocentesis.

Cystic fibrosis. Cystic fibrosis (CF) is the most common autosomal recessive disorder among the white population. Approximately 1 in 25 Caucasians is a carrier of the CF gene though persons of other ethnic distributions can also be carriers (Hispanics 1/45, African-Americans 1/60, Asians 1/150). Affected individuals have a median life expectancy of 28 years. The disease is characterized by pancreatic insufficiency, respiratory infections, and inspissation of bronchial secretions. In persons with cystic fibrosis, an abnormal protein, the cystic fibrosis transmembrane regulator (CFTR) has been isolated and sequenced. The most common mutation producing an altered CFTR occurs at position 508 (δ 508). Among Caucasians, δ 508 is involved in 70% of the cases of CF. An additional 15% can be accounted for by an array of other mutations. In the remaining 15% a specific mutation cannot be identified.

Table 47-2 Diseases with increased prevalence in specific populations

Disease	Populations at increased risk	Carrier test
Tay-Sachs disease	Ashkenazic Jewish French Canadians	Serum hexosaminidase A
Sickle-cell disease	Black African Mediterranean (Greek, Italian) Arabic, Indian, Pakistani Caribbean (Cuban, Puerto Rican, Haitian) Hispanic, Central American	Sickle dex for hemoglobin S Hemoglobin electrophoresis for variants
Thalassemia	Mediterranean (Greek, Italian) Southeast Asian (Vietnamese, Laotian, Cambodian, Filipino) Southern Chinese North African Pakistanian, Indian	Hematocrit and MCV

MCV, mean corpuscular volume.

Carrier screening for cystic fibrosis has now become technically possible. In most centers approximately 85% of the cystic fibrosis mutations can be detected by analyzing an array of possible deoxyribonucleic acid (DNA) mutations. At this time, Caucasians undergoing carrier screening should understand that approximately 15% of the mutations causing CF have not been identified. Practically, this implies that couples in which one partner is identified as a carrier and the other as a noncarrier (but with a 15% chance of an undetected mutation) have a risk of 1/666 for an affected offspring. Though it is a relatively small risk, in these cases prenatal diagnosis would not be able to differentiate carrier from affected fetuses. This contrasts to the situation in which two individuals with identified CF mutations, most commonly δ 508, have a 1/4 (25%) risk of an affected fetus and for whom prenatal diagnosis, either CVS or amniocentesis, can accurately identify affected fetuses.

PRENATAL DIAGNOSIS OF GENETIC DISEASES
Overview

A diagnostic study of a fetus at risk for a genetic disorder is commonly undertaken because one of the screening tests described yields a positive result. The most frequent indication for both amniocentesis and chorionic villus sampling has traditionally been maternal age $\geq$35, years at delivery. Recently, with the increased use of maternal serum panels for trisomy 21 risk assessment in women less than 35, a positive serum screen has become the second most frequent indication. In contrast, an increased MSAFP is now accounting for fewer and fewer amniocenteses as ultrasound resolution improves. Heterozygotic couples identified as a result of population-specific screening (Tay-Sachs disease, sickle-cell disease, thalassemia, cystic fibrosis) or a positive family history represent a small fraction of the invasive prenatal genetic studies of the fetus.

An increasingly common indication for diagnostic studies of the fetus has emerged with improvements in ultrasound resolution. A fetus with multiple malformations has a significant risk of being chromosomally abnormal. Specific collections of findings as well as some isolated malformations are associated with a higher rate of chromosomal abnormality. In addition, with improved resolution

more subtle alterations in fetal structure can be detected. Although minor alterations, such as choroid plexus cysts and mild hydronephrosis, may be normal variants and disappear in follow-up ultrasounds, such findings also may occur with increased frequency in chromosomally abnormal fetuses. Whether to offer amniocentesis for chromosome evaluation of every fetus with such minor alterations has been a continuing debate. In recent studies when choroid plexus cysts were identified in an otherwise structurally normal fetus, the chance of a chromosome abnormality may be equal to or less than the risk of the diagnostic test. On the other hand, a collection of seemingly innocent ultrasound findings in the same fetus can denote an increased risk for chromosomal abnormality. Alterations of femur length, humeral length, renal pelvis size, and nuchal fold thickness have all been shown to be associated with an increased risk for trisomy 21 (Benacerraf et al., 1992). As an indication for diagnostic studies of the fetus the role of ultrasound is currently expanding beyond the isolated identification of major malformations to an integrated picture of the fetus.

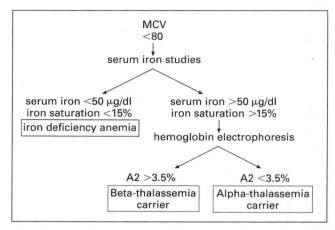

Fig. 47-1 Screening for thalassemias using MCV (mean corpuscular volume).

Diagnostic technologies

Chorionic villus sampling. CVS was first attempted in 1973 in women scheduled for pregnancy termination (Kullander and Sandahl, 1973). Ultrasound guidance of CVS did not occur until the early 1980s. The procedure involves obtaining a sample of placental tissue via a catheter placed transcervically or transabdominally. The trophoblastic tissue obtained can be prepared for chromosome analysis or DNA studies. However, amniotic fluid components such as α-fetoprotein or acetylcholinesterase cannot be evaluated. Performed at 9 to 12 completed weeks of gestation, CVS provides the earliest detection of a genetically abnormal fetus. Additionally, in cases of third-trimester pregnancies with fetal anomalies in which amniotic fluid is not available (such as oligohydramnios) or in which a fetal blood sampling is not possible, CVS for karyotype analysis has been employed with minimal risk to the fetus (Holzgreve, Miny, and Schloo, 1990).

Karyotype analysis from a chorionic villus sample can be obtained from a direct preparation of the rapidly dividing cytotrophoblasts in 2 days. Most centers, however, now elect also to analyze the results of cultured trophoblasts; analysis may take an additional 10 to 14 days. In approximately 2% of CVS samples a *mosaic,* a combination of karyotypically normal and abnormal cells, is identified. As the CVS reflects the chromosomal makeup of the placenta, amniocentesis to provide further information concerning the karyotype of the fetus is warranted. Although only a third of CVS mosaicisms are confirmed in the fetus, karyotypically abnormal cell lines confined to the placenta (confined placental mosaicism [CPM]) have been associated with an increased rate of pregnancy loss and fetal growth retardation.

In two large collaborative studies of the safety of transcervical CVS, the rate of pregnancy loss was noted to be 0.6% and 0.8% higher after CVS than after amniocentesis; in neither study were these numbers significant (Canadian Collaborative Trial, 1989; Medical Research Council European Trial, 1991). Likewise the safety of transabdominal CVS appears to be comparable to that of transcervical procedures. Complications include bleeding, rupture of membranes, and infection that may lead to pregnancy loss.

A possible association of limb reduction defects and oromandibular malformations with CVS sampling was first reported in 1991 (Firth et al., 1991). Subsequent reports have both supported and refuted an increased incidence of such birth defects in association with CVS. Proposed mechanisms of action include possible vasoconstrictive events in the fetus as a result of the CVS procedure.

Amniocentesis. Amniocentesis involves the removal of amniotic fluid from around the developing fetus. Fetal cells in the fluid can be analyzed for either chromosomal complement or specific DNA studies. Traditionally amniocentesis has been performed at 16 to 20 weeks. At this gestational age the amount of fluid removed (20 cc) is only 1/10 of the total volume. In most centers, pregnancy loss after a second-trimester amniocentesis has been approximately 1 in 300.

Early amniocentesis, performed at 10 to 14 weeks, is now available. Technically the procedure is the same as standard amniocentesis, though incomplete fusion of the amnion and chorion at the earlier gestational ages can occasionally hamper needle insertion. Cell culture failure and growth rates are not significantly different than those of 16- to 20-week amniotic fluid cultures. With the earlier procedures, less fluid is removed though the relative proportion to the total amniotic fluid volume is greater. Although initial studies suggested a minimal increase in fetal loss as compared to that in standard amniocentesis, other studies have not detected a significant difference; a randomized study remains to be published.

Karyotype analysis of amniotic fluid cell cultures typically requires 2 weeks to obtain sufficient cells for evaluation. The application of molecular cytogenetics to amniocentesis has provided a means of obtaining results in 24 to 48 hours. With traditional karyotype analysis dividing cells are required in order for the chromosomes to be sufficiently condensed to facilitate recognition. However, fluorescent in situ hybridization (FISH) using tagged segments of DNA allows determination of the chromosomal makeup of a nondividing cell. With FISH probes, the number of copies of a specific chromosome can be visually detected in the undivided interphase cell. A recent clinical study has shown that in 526 amniocenteses, FISH analysis detected all 21 fetuses with a chromosomal abnormality involving chromosomes 13, 18, 21, X, or Y (Klinger et al., 1992).

Percutaneous umbilical blood sampling. In the early 1980s ultrasound replaced fetoscopy as the method used in guiding percutaneous umbilical blood sampling (PUBS). Performed from approximately 18 weeks until term, PUBS provides access to the fetus for diagnostic studies of a peripheral blood sample (cytogenetic, hematologic, immunologic, DNA) as well as for treatment (transfusions). In some centers PUBS has been proposed for acid/base and lactate evaluations in growth-retarded fetuses. An anterior placenta facilitates obtaining the specimen from close to the insertion site of the cord into the placenta. Immobilization of the fetus with pancurarium is not needed for the short period required to obtain a fetal blood sample. The procedure has approximately a 1% to 2% risk of fetal loss. Other complications leading to preterm delivery can occur in another 5% (Daffos, Capella, and Forestier, 1985). Fetal bradycardias, the majority of which resolve without incident, occur. Damage to the umbilical cord with laceration or hematoma formation has been reported but is a relatively rare complication.

Preimplantation biopsy. Removing an individual cell early in gestation without subsequent harm to the developing fetus is possible at the four-cell stage in the mouse and at the eight-cell stage in the human (Wilton, Shaw, and Trounson, 1989). In women at risk for X-linked recessive disorders, identification of Y chromosome DNA in a single cell biopsy specimen from an embryo prepared for in vitro fertilization has allowed for the transfer of only XX-containing embryos (Handyside et al., 1990). In situations where a diagnosis of a molecular defect is desired, trophectoderm biopsy, opening the zona pellucida of the blastocyst, allows a greater quantity of cells (10 to 30) to be obtained. In humans, however, difficulties remain in successful recovery of the blastocyst stage from the uterus. DNA study of the second polar body in humans has been another approach to preimplantation diagnosis. Produced during meiosis II, the second polar body contains basically the same genetic material as the ovum and is extruded into the zona pellucida. For a woman who is a carrier for a specific disorder, polymerase chain reaction (PCR) analysis of the polar body will discern whether the mutant allele is present in the polar body and thus also present in the oocyte. Only oocytes with a normal allele, by analysis of the polar body, would be used for the fertilization. Such a technique has been used in couples at risk for CF, α-1-antitrypsin, and hemophilia (Verlinsky et al., 1990).

Fetal cells in maternal blood. Whether by CVS, amniocentesis, PUBS, or preimplantation biopsy, accurate diagnosis of genetic diseases in the fetus has traditionally relied on invasive tests associated with risk to the pregnancy. The ability to obtain fetal DNA through noninvasive studies has been an area of continued research since the late 1970s. Although small numbers of fetal cells are known to be present in the maternal circulation in all pregnancies, their use for diagnostic studies has previously been precluded by an inability to accurately identify and separate fetal from maternal cells as well as perform studies on extremely small quantities of DNA. During the 1980s, however, advances in molecular genetics rekindled interest in the detection of fetal cells in the maternal circulation. Use of PCR can now facilitate the identification of minute quantities of DNA. In addition improvements in the ability to sort fetal cells on the basis of cell surface markers of fetal red blood cells have now been described. Fetal cells sorted from a maternal blood sample can also be studied with the FISH technique and chromosomally abnormal fetuses detected. While still a technically difficult procedure, FISH analysis of fetal cells obtained from a maternal blood sample has identified at least one fetus with trisomy 18 (Price et al., 1991).

SUMMARY

Prenatal genetics has far-reaching implications for the routine obstetric practice. Advances in screening for either chromosomal or genetic diseases will eventually allow more directed use of invasive prenatal diagnostic studies. Women can now be screened for their risk of having a fetus with a chromosome abnormality by maternal age as well as by serum markers. Even for the woman over the age of 35 at delivery attempts to refine her risk for trisomy 21 through a combination of serum screening and ultrasound evaluation are being explored. Maternal serum α fetoprotein screening for neural tube defects continues; in some centers a detailed ultrasound examination is used to modify a high MSAFP result further, reducing the numbers of women undergoing amniocentesis. Many women are at risk for specific genetic disorders because of their racial or ethnic background and can be offered population-specific screening to ascertain their carrier status.

Currently, most prenatal diagnostic studies of the fetus are performed in the first or second trimester by CVS, early amniocentesis, or traditional amniocentesis. However, these studies are all associated with some increased risk of pregnancy loss. Research to improve the detection of genetic or chromosomal disease in the fetus through noninvasive studies, such as analysis of a maternal blood sample, is being actively pursued. In addition, preimplantation diagnosis in conjunction with in vitro fertilization may allow couples with a substantial risk for a genetically abnormal fetus to avoid diagnosis of an affected fetus entirely.

As advances in screening as well as diagnostic technologies become available prenatal genetics will continue to impact the routine obstetric practice. Recognition of women who could benefit from screening as well as the new diagnostic technologies will become increasingly important for all health care providers.

BIBLIOGRAPHY

Benacerraf BR et al: Sonographic scoring index for prenatal detection of chromosomal abnormalities, *J Ultrasound Med* 11(9):449, 1992.

Bianchi DW et al: Isolation of fetal DNA from nucleated erythrocytes in maternal blood, *Proc Natl Acad Sci USA* 87(9):3279, 1990.

Daffos F, Capella PM, Forestier F: Fetal blood sampling during pregnancy with use of a needle guided by ultrasound: a study of 606 consecutive cases, *Am J Obstet Gynecol* 153(6):655, 1985.

Djalali M et al: Introduction of early amniocentesis to routine prenatal diagnosis, *Prenat Diagn* 12(8):661, 1992.

Firth HV et al: Limb abnormalities and chorion villus sampling, *Lancet* 338(8758):51, 1991 (letter).

Firth HV et al: Severe limb abnormalities after chorion villus sampling at 56-66 days' gestation, *Lancet* 337(8744):762, 1991.

Haddow JE et al: Prenatal screening for Down's syndrome with use of maternal serum markers, *N Engl J Med* 327(9):588, 1992.

Handyside AH et al: Pregnancies from biopsied human preimplantation embryos sexed by Y-specific DNA amplification, *Nature* 344(6268):768, 1990.

Henry GP, Miller WA: Early amniocentesis, *J Reprod Med* 37(5):396, 1992.

Herzenberg LA et al: Fetal cells in the blood of pregnant women: detection and enrichment by fluorescence-activated cell sorting, *Proc Natl Acad Sci USA* 76(3):1453, 1979.

Holzgreve W, Miny P, Schloo R: 'Late CVS' international registry compilation of data from 24 centres, *Prenat Diagn* 10(3):159, 1990.

Hook EB, Cross PK, Regal RR: The frequency of 47,+ 21,47,+ 18, and 47, +13 at the uppermost extremes of maternal ages: results on 56,094 fetuses studied prenatally and comparisons with data on livebirths, *Hum Genet* 68(3):211, 1984.

Kalousek DK et al: Confirmation of CVS mosaicism in term placentae and high frequency of intrauterine growth retardation association with confined placental mosaicism, *Prenat Diagn* 11(10):743, 1991.

Klinger K et al: Rapid detection of chromosome aneuploidies in uncultured amniocytes by using fluorescence in situ hybridization (FISH), *Am J Hum Genet* 51(1):55, 1992.

Kullander S, Sandahl B: Fetal chromosome analysis after transcervical placental biopsies during early pregnancy, *Acta Obstet Gynecol Scand* 52(4):355, 1973.

Medical Research Council European Trial of Chorion Villus Sampling: MRC working party on the evaluation of chorion villus sampling, *Lancet* 337(8756):1491, 1991.

Merkatz IR et al: An association between low maternal serum alpha-fetoprotein and fetal chromosomal abnormalities, *Am J Obstet Gynecol* 148(7):886, 1984.

Multicentre randomised clinical trial of chorion villus sampling and amniocentesis: First report: Canadian Collaborative CVS-Amniocentesis Clinical Trial Group, *Lancet* 1(8628):1, 1989.

Nadel AS et al: Isolated choroid plexus cysts in the second-trimester fetus: is amniocentesis really indicated? *Radiology* 185(2):545, 1992.

Nadel AS et al: Absence of need for amniocentesis in patients with elevated levels of maternal serum alpha-fetoprotein and normal ultrasonographic examinations, *N Engl J Med* 323(9):557, 1990.

Ng IS et al: Methods for analysis of multiple cystic fibrosis mutations, *Hum Genet* 87(5):613, 1991.

Penso CA et al: Early amniocentesis: report of 407 cases with neonatal follow-up, *Obstet Gynecol* 76(6):1032, 1990.

Phillips OP et al: Maternal serum screening for fetal Down syndrome in women less than 35 years of age using alpha-fetoprotein, hCG, and unconjugated estriol: a prospective 2-year study, *Obstet Gynecol* 80:353, 1992.

Price JO et al: Prenatal diagnosis with fetal cells isolated from maternal blood by multiparameter flow cytometry, *Am J Obstet Gynecol* 165:1731, 1991.

Riordan JR et al: Identification of the cystic fibrosis gene: cloning and characterization of complementary DNA, *Science* 245(4922):1066, 1989.

Rommens JM et al: Identification of the cystic fibrosis gene: chromosome walking and jumping, *Science* 245(4922):1059, 1989.

Tabor A et al: Randomised controlled trial of genetic amniocentesis in 4606 low-risk women, *Lancet* 1(8493):1287, 1986.

Verlinsky Y et al: Analysis of the first polar body: preconception genetic diagnosis, *Hum Reprod* 5(7):826, 1990.

Wald NJ et al: Maternal serum-alpha-fetoprotein measurement in antenatal screening for anencephaly and spina bifida in early pregnancy: report of U.K. collaborative study on alpha-fetoprotein in relation to neural-tube defects, *Lancet* 1(8026):1323, 1977.

Wald NJ et al: Maternal serum screening for Down's syndrome in early pregnancy, *Br Med J* 297(6653):883, 1988.

Wald NJ et al: Antenatal maternal serum screening for Down's syndrome: results of a demonstration project *Br Med J* 305(6850):391, 1992.

Wilton LJ, Shaw JM, Trounson AO: Successful single-cell biopsy and cryopreservation of preimplantation mouse embryos, *Fertil Steril* 51(3):513, 1989.

48 Early Pregnancy Disorders: Hyperemesis and Vaginal Bleeding

Craig L. Best and Joseph A. Hill

Pregnancy can be a joyous experience for couples desiring children. The most common problems in early pregnancy, hyperemesis, vaginal bleeding, and abortion, not only disrupt this experience but may also be life-threatening. Understanding the pathophysiologic mechanisms involved in these disorders will enable women's health care providers to diagnose and manage these conditions effectively.

HYPEREMESIS GRAVIDARUM

Hyperemesis gravidarum is a pathologic state of pernicious nausea and vomiting during pregnancy with resultant dehydration, ketosis, electrolyte imbalance, inadequate caloric intake, and poor weight gain or even weight loss.

Epidemiology and risk factors

It is estimated that between 30% and 90% of pregnant women experience symptoms of nausea and vomiting during their pregnancy; 0.5% to 2% have symptoms severe enough to be considered hyperemetic. The incidence of hyperemesis is reported to be higher in developed countries. Selection bias may be a factor in the reported differences between groups of people. However, it is becoming increasingly clear that different life-styles and stress factors play an important role in the development of this condition.

Several risk factors for hyperemesis gravidarum have been proposed, although the cause of the disorder remains poorly understood. Younger age, first pregnancy, high body weight, previous history of hyperemesis gravidarum, and single marital status are all associated with an increased risk of hyperemesis. Racial and socioeconomic factors may also play a role as hyperemesis is more common in Caucasians of high socioeconomic status. The psychologic profile of many hyperemesis patients is that of a young, unmarried, immature, and dependent pregnant woman. These individuals are often ambivalent about their pregnancy. Identified hormonal risk factors include increased serum estradiol and the β subunit of human chorionic gonadotropin (β-hCG) levels. This may explain the association between hyperemesis gravidarum and pregnancies with multiple gestations or hydatidiform mole. More thorough analysis comparing hyperemetics with age- and gestation-matched control subjects has determined that serum estradiol levels and not β-hCG levels are related to hyperemesis gravidarum. Although most pregnant women can tolerate pregnancy levels of serum estradiol with only occasional episodes of nausea and vomiting, some women have lower tolerance secondary to psychologic and perhaps physiologic differences that may lead to a cycle of uncontrolled nausea and vomiting. In most cases the symptoms either abate or markedly improve after 12 to 14 weeks of pregnancy, but up to 20% will continue to have significant symptoms throughout gestation.

Pathophysiology

Attempts to pinpoint the pathophysiology of this disorder have been limited. Current knowledge is primarily based on retrospective studies that have examined the psychologic profile of affected women. A review of the literature suggests that hormone (estradiol and perhaps others) levels accentuated by pregnancy act on the emetic centers of the brain to produce nausea and vomiting. Women of a particular emotional state during their pregnancy have a lower threshold for symptoms, suggesting a psychosomatic component. However, it remains a matter of speculation whether the mind-set of these individuals directly contributes to the condition or whether it is the lack or the excess of some factor that either prevents or predisposes to disease development. It is also unclear why some women have hyperemesis whereas others of similar emotional and hormonal profile do not. More studies are needed before definitive statements can be made.

Differential diagnosis

Many women experience nausea and vomiting after 6 to 10 weeks of amenorrhea. A pregnancy test should be obtained regardless of the frequency of symptoms. Once pregnancy is determined, the clinician should make an attempt to determine whether the patient is having normal pregnancy-related symptoms of nausea and vomiting or hyperemesis. This is often determined by frequency of symptoms. If the patient requires hospitalization or intensive outpatient management to prevent dehydration and electrolyte imbalances in the absence of other medical conditions that may cause her symptoms, she has hyperemesis gravidarum. It is sometimes difficult to quantify vomiting since any amount is distressing. The clinician must therefore rely on history and physical examination along with appropriate laboratory testing to determine the need for medical intervention and possible hospitalization. Associated medical or pregnancy-related conditions must also be ruled out in order to determine treatment options. The box below lists the findings in the history, physical examination, and laboratory assessment that suggest the diagnosis of hyperemesis. Other associated medical and pregnancy-related conditions are also listed.

Management

Outpatient therapy. Outpatient therapy should be reserved for patients with mild dehydration and with only minor electrolyte abnormalities. Furthermore, these patients should be able to tolerate clear fluids and small quantities of bland food. The goal of therapy is to correct mild dehydration and to initiate antiemetic therapy that will raise the threshold for nausea and vomiting. The patient may be started on any of the standard antiemetics, such as prochlorperazine (Compazine, 5 to 10 mg PO qid, or 25 mg PR q12h), trimethobenzamide (Tigan, 250 mg PO qid, or 200 mg PR q6-8h), promethazine (Phenergan, 25 to 50 mg PO/PR q4-6h), or metoclopramide (Reglan, 10 mg PO 1h AC and qhs). Both oral and rectal suppository forms of one of these medications should be given. If one medication does not successfully relieve symptoms, often another medication will. The safety of these antiemetics as demonstrated by controlled trials in humans is lacking. Thus caution should be used and antiemetic medication use limited to cases of unrelenting symptoms. Most of the antiemetics are category C drugs as defined by the Food and Drug Administration with the exception of Reglan, a category B drug. Category C medications have been shown to be harmful in animals but

appropriately controlled human studies are lacking. In other cases there are no prospective controlled studies in animals or humans. However, with all the medication discussed, retrospective reviews have failed to show teratogenicity directly linked to these medications in humans. Thus they are used in cases of severe nausea and vomiting by primary care providers of pregnant women. As with any medication used during pregnancy, caution dictates that use be limited to individuals who do not respond to more conservative dietary measures. These drugs do cross the placenta at least at term, but most studies have shown the drugs to be safe. In addition to antiemetics, patients should be instructed to eat small frequent meals of bland foods rich in carbohydrates. It is helpful to consult a social worker or psychologist for evaluation of underlying emotional factors that may be contributing to disease severity. Psychotherapeutic techniques such as stimulus control, imagery conditioning, and hypnosis have been tried with reported success, as have acupressure and acupuncture, but studies of these therapies have been of insufficient sample size, poorly controlled, and confounded by questionable diagnosis and other treatments. Patients should be instructed to keep a chart of symptoms and daily weight with frequent follow-up visits.

Inpatient therapy. Patients admitted to the hospital for hyperemesis gravidarum often are dehydrated and have electrolyte imbalance. Furthermore, they may be unable to tolerate any food or even liquids. Therapy should be directed toward restoring fluid and electrolyte balance. Intravenous therapy with dextrose and half normal saline solution with supplemental potassium chloride as indicated by serum electrolyte levels is standard. Antiemetic agents are given intravenously or as rectal suppositories. Oral food intake may begin once fluid and electrolyte balances have been restored, and symptoms of nausea have ceased. Oral intake should begin slowly, starting with liquids and then advancing to solid bland food taken as small frequent meals. Initially, patient isolation from visitors and avoidance of other hospital stimulation such as television may be required on an individualized basis. Patient evaluation by social services or psychiatry may disclose underlying stress factors that may be managed by support aimed at relieving environmental stress. Tranquilizers may be necessary to treat anxiety states. Individuals admitted for hyperemesis gravidarum should be evaluated by a dietitian to determine their nutritional status and assist in recommending enteral or total parenteral nutrition needs, especially in those patients who do not respond to more conservative management and exhibit continued weight loss. Even patients who respond quickly to medical therapy often have frequent relapses and need a dietary management plan to optimize their nutritional status during pregnancy.

Daily weight measurement is the best guide for following therapeutic efficacy. Serum electrolyte levels and vital signs are also important treatment outcome variables.

Pregnancy outcome

The effect of hyperemesis on pregnancy outcome is dependent on the amount of weight loss. Early reports stressed favorable pregnancy outcomes in hyperemetic women because of the reduced risk of early pregnancy loss. This association, however, may be secondary to selection bias in

---

DIAGNOSTIC EVALUATION OF THE EXPECTED HYPEREMETIC PATIENT

History: Young primigravida, single parent, ambivalent about pregnancy, Caucasian, high socioeconomic class, dependent personality
Physical: Postural vital signs, dry mucus membranes, poor skin turgor, in severe cases hepatocellular jaundice, generally clear lungs, nontender abdomen and no costovertebral angle tenderness, normal uterine size for gestational age but may be enlarged secondary to multiple gestation or molar pregnancy
Laboratory: Serum-positive pregnancy test (β-hCG), hypokalemia, hyponatremia, hypochloremia, metabolic alkalosis, elevated blood urea nitrogen (BUN) and creatinine, urine ketosis and elevated specific gravity of urine
Other differential diagnoses:
   Medical conditions: gallbladder disease, hepatitis, pancreatitis, gastroenteritis, appendicitis, pyelonephritis
Pregnancy conditions: molar pregnancy, twin gestation

which pregnancies with sustained levels of estrogen and perhaps β-hCG may be more prone to hyperemesis. More recent studies have shown an increased risk of low birth weight and growth retardation in pregnant patients whose weight loss during pregnancy is >5% or whose symptoms are severe.

VAGINAL BLEEDING IN EARLY PREGNANCY

Women of reproductive age experiencing vaginal bleeding other than at the time of expected menses should be considered to have a pregnancy-related problem until proved otherwise. First-trimester vaginal bleeding occurs in up to 50% of pregnancies. Roughly 50% of these pregnancies result in a spontaneous abortion, especially if the bleeding is heavy and associated with cramping. Although vaginal bleeding other than menses is most likely the direct result of pregnancy, other conditions should be considered.

Differential diagnosis

The possible causes of vaginal bleeding in early pregnancy can be divided into those causative factors that are solely pregnancy-related and those that are pregnancy-associated (not caused by pregnancy but occurring during pregnancy) as listed in Table 48-1.

History and physical examination. A thorough history will often enable the clinician to arrive at the proper diagnosis for vaginal bleeding related to pregnancy (Table 48-2). Determining the date of the last menstrual period is important as implantation bleeding occurs around cycle day 21, whereas ectopic pregnancies usually do not become symptomatic until 6 to 8 weeks' gestation. Vaginal bleeding tends to become heavy in the case of spontaneous abortion, whereas ectopic pregnancies are usually characterized by spotting or no bleeding. Passage of tissue suggests spontaneous abortion; however, passage of decidual tissue with heavier bleeding may occur in ectopic pregnancies, mimicking spontaneous abortion. Presence of pain in a women who is pregnant with vaginal bleeding suggests either imminent abortion or ectopic pregnancy.

Spontaneous abortion most commonly results in lower abdominal cramping associated with vaginal bleeding. In ectopic gestations the pain may be described as cramping but more commonly is sharp and constant, often culminating in peritoneal signs resulting from the accumulation of blood in the abdomen and pelvis. Hemorrhage may also

Table 48-1 Causes of first trimester vaginal bleeding

Pregnancy-related	Pregnancy-associated
Implantation bleeding	Vulvitis
Abortion	Vaginitis
Ectopic pregnancy	Cervicitis
Molar pregnancy	Carcinoma of vagina, cervix
	Foreign body
	Polyp
	Thrombocytopenia
	Von Willeband's disease
	Anticoagulant therapy
	Disseminated intravascular coagulation

result in shoulder pain and Cullen's sign (periumbilical bruising). Therefore pelvic pain associated with vaginal bleeding during pregnancy should be considered to indicate an ectopic pregnancy until proved otherwise as shown in the diagnostic algorithm (Fig. 48-1).

Physical examination in women with vaginal bleeding in early pregnancy should always be performed especially if there is any associated with pain or risk factors for ectopic pregnancy. Risk factors for ectopic pregnancy include prior ectopic pregnancy, pelvic inflammatory disease, pelvic adhesions, prior ruptured appendix, prior tubal surgery, contraceptive failures with intrauterine device (IUD) or oral contraceptives, prior tubal ligation, diethylstilbestrol (DES) exposure, and history of recurrent abortion.

Diagnostic tests. A quantitative pregnancy test (β-hCG) should be performed on all women of reproductive age with abnormal vaginal bleeding. This test determines whether women are having bleeding during pregnancy but does not distinguish whether it is a direct result of the pregnancy.

Diagnosis of ectopic pregnancy. Often the diagnosis of an ectopic pregnancy is uncertain in cases of bleeding in early pregnancy (before 4 weeks' gestation). This is largely because it is often difficult to determine whether an intrauterine pregnancy exists by ultrasound assessment before 5 weeks' gestation or when the β-hCG level is less than 2000 mIU/ml unless done by experienced hands using a vaginal probe ultrasound. In cases of a ruptured corpus luteal cyst during pregnancy spotting associated with pain may mimic an ectopic pregnancy. Furthermore, free fluid in the posterior cul-de-sac may be seen on ultrasound after the release of the cyst fluid, which in appearance is ultrasonically indistinguishable from fluid seen in the cul-de-sac after a ruptured or unruptured but bleeding ectopic pregnancy. In such cases culdocentesis may be helpful.

CULDOCENTESIS. A culdocentesis involves placing a needle into the posterior cul-de-sac during speculum examination and withdrawing fluid into a syringe. Results are divided into three categories: (1) positive: nonclotting blood with a hematocrit greater than 10; (2) negative: clear fluid or blood-stained fluid with a hematocrit less than 10; (3) nondiagnostic: no fluid return. Although culdocentesis in some cases may be helpful, sophisticated ultrasound techniques with quantitative serum β-hCG level determinations have largely replaced it as a diagnostic modality. A positive culdocentesis finding together with a positive pregnancy test result is 99% predictive of an ectopic pregnancy. A false-positive culdocentesis result may occur in cases of ruptured and bleeding corpus luteum cysts.

SERIAL QUANTITATIVE β-hCG TITERS. Serial quantitative β-hCG titers can be helpful in these cases to determine whether a pregnancy is abnormal. If the β-hCG titer does not rise by 66% to 100% after 48 hours then an abnormal pregnancy (ectopic or potential abortion) may be present. A quantitative β-hCG titer >2000 mIU/ml warrants an ultrasound examination to look for an intrauterine pregnancy. If no intrauterine pregnancy is seen (gestational sac), this is strongly suggestive of an ectopic gestation.

Diagnosis of molar pregnancy. Abnormally high β-hCG titers associated with vaginal bleeding may be the result of molar pregnancy, although multiple gestation is also likely. Molar gestations have a characteristic ultrasound appear-

Table 48-2 Diagnosis and treatment of pregnancy-related first trimester vaginal bleeding

Diagnosis	Symptoms	Laboratory evaluation	Treatment
Implantation bleeding	Spotting or light bleeding lasts 1-3 days usually between cycle days 21 and 28	Urine hCG result may be negative; serum hCG usually <50 IU	Observation; may consider a repeat quantitative hCG
Abortion	May start as spotting but will progress to heavier bleeding; cramping pain common when abortion imminent; dizziness if excessive blood loss; passage of tissue; usually occurs at 4-8 wk gestation	hCG may not rise appropriately or may fall before abortion; intrauterine pregnancy seen on ultrasound finding but may not have normal heartbeat; low HCT	Observe early: if passes whole fetus and bleeding stops, observe; if passes small amount of tissue or bleeding continues, consider D&C
Ectopic pregnancy	Usually spotting but some have heavier bleeding and some do not have any vaginal bleeding; sharp constant pain ± peritoneal signs at rupture; pain usually present at 6 to 8 wk gestation; dizziness, nausea, vomiting, shock; shoulder pain; Cullen's sign	Inappropriate rise in hCG; low HCT; no intrauterine pregnancy or tubal pregnancy on ultrasound with β-hCG level >2000 mIU/ml; no chorionic villi on D&C; positive culdocentesis	Observation if β-hCG titers falling; methotrexate if small and not ruptured; surgery an option in most cases
Molar pregnancy	Spotting or heavy bleeding, usually occurs in late first trimester or early second trimester; uterine size >dates; usually no pain; if bleeding heavy may have cramping; pass grape-like tissue	Characteristic findings on ultrasound of fluid lakes in homogeneous tissue, no gestational sac; markedly elevated hCG level; hyperthyroid; elevated BP early in pregnancy	D&C; chemotherapy in some; strict follow-up evaluation after treatment; avoid pregnancy for 1 year

hCG, human chorionic gonadotropin; HCT, hematocrit; D&C, dilation and curettage; BP, blood pressure.

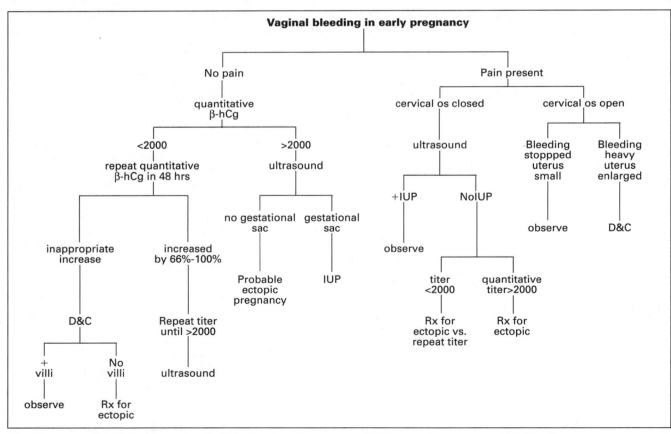

Fig. 48-1 Algorithm for diagnosis of vaginal bleeding in early pregnancy. IUP, intrauterine pregnancy; β-hCG, β-human chorionic gonadotropin; D&C, dilation and curettage.

ance as homogeneous material with some lucent fluid lakes of "grapelike" structures. The uterus may also be large for gestational age.

Management

Overview. Management of vaginal bleeding during pregnancy is determined by its cause. Infection is treated with appropriate antibiotics, taking into consideration preparations that should be avoided in early pregnancy, including tetracycline, metronidazole, and sulfa/trimethoprim. Polyps and other benign lesions located on the cervix should be managed after pregnancy if the bleeding is not profuse so as not to disrupt the pregnancy. Premalignant cervical lesions (dysplasia) should be evaluated by colposcopic examination during pregnancy. If there is a question of invasive cancer of the cervix, a biopsy should be performed. These lesions, particularly in pregnancy, should be handled by a competent gynecologic oncologist who is specifically trained to recognize the severity of the dysplasia and is able to make appropriate judgments about the need for a cervical biopsy during pregnancy. Clotting disorders rarely surface during pregnancy unless there is an initiating event such as spontaneous abortion. In such cases severe hemorrhage may occur. Appropriate blood product replacement to correct hematologic aberrations should proceed dilation and curettage (D&C) to prevent excessive bleeding.

Choice of therapy

Methotrexate therapy. Ectopic pregnancy may be managed with medical treatment or surgery. Medical management with methotrexate can be an alternative to surgery in carefully selected individuals. Methotrexate is indicated in cases of proven, presumed, or persistent ectopic pregnancy. Exclusion criteria for methotrexate include (1) evidence of hemoperitoneum or impending rupture; (2) a tubal mass greater than 3 cm or fetal heart activity; (3) β-hCG level greater than 6000 mIU/ml; (4) hepatic, renal, or hematologic abnormalities; (5) coexisting intrauterine pregnancy; and (6) poor follow-up. Methotrexate (1 mg/kg) may be administered in a single dose given intramuscularly over the course of 1 week on days 1, 3, 5, and 7. Calcium leucovorin 0.1 mg/kg PO should be taken on days 2, 4, 6, and 8 to reduce the gastrointestinal and dermatologic side effects of methotrexate. Methotrexate may also cause liver damage as reflected in elevated liver function test findings and result in varying degrees of bone marrow suppression. The reported incidence of methotrexate side effects is less than 5% and most cases are mild. Outpatient treatment should be monitored with daily β-hCG titers and repeat liver and renal function tests after 1 week. Patients may be treated in the hospital over a shorter period with intravenous methotrexate (100 mg/M^2 IV over 30 minutes, then 200 mg/M^2 IV over 12 hours). Calcium leucovorin 15 mg PO should be taken every 12 hours for four doses beginning 12 hours after the methotrexate infusion is completed. Follow-up evaluation consists of weekly β-hCG titers till less than assay. A repeat methotrexate dose may be given for slow decline or plateaus in β-hCG levels. In our practice methotrexate is more than 90% effective. Subsequent reproductive function may be better after methotrexate than surgery, although direct comparison studies are lacking. Methotrexate has also been injected directly into the ectopic site at laparoscopy or under ultrasound guidance.

Surgical therapy. Surgical therapy of ectopic pregnancy is the gold standard. Refined surgical techniques using laparoscopic equipment have made surgery a relatively simple, safe, and effective treatment. In cases of suspected ectopic pregnancy laparoscopy is an effective tool to confirm the diagnosis. In some cases of very early ectopic pregnancy tubal distension may be minimal and the ectopic site difficult to visualize. D&C at the time of laparoscopy will rule out an intrauterine pregnancy and support the diagnosis of ectopic pregnancy. If localization of the ectopic site is difficult, methotrexate may be used. Large or ruptured ectopic gestations most commonly require surgical intervention. The fallopian tube should be removed if it is damaged, if the patient has had many repeat ectopic gestations, or if a future pregnancy is not desired. It has been recommended to remove both fallopian tubes in patients who will require in vitro fertilization to conceive. Patients with unruptured ectopic gestations with otherwise healthy appearing fallopian tubes should have conservative surgery: a linear salpingostomy. After surgery β-hCG titers should be followed on a weekly basis until the result is negative. Plateaus or increases in β-hCG after surgery may be treated with methotrexate or repeat surgery.

Treatment of molar pregnancy. Molar pregnancy is managed by D&C. In cases of invasive, persistent, or metastatic mole, methotrexate alone or in combination with other chemotherapeutic agents is indicated.

BIBLIOGRAPHY

Boyce RA: Enteral nutrition in hyperemesis gravidarum: a new development, *J Am Diet Assoc* 92:733, 1993.

Brown CD, Smith BK; *Drugs in pregnancy and lactation,* ed 3, Baltimore, 1990, Williams & Wilkins.

Chin RKH, Lao TT: Low birth weight and hyperemesis gravidarum, *Eur J Obstet Gynecol Reprod Biol* 28:179, 1988.

Depue RH et al: Hyperemesis gravidarum in relation to estradiol levels, pregnancy outcome, and other maternal factors: a seroepidemiologic study, *Am J Obstet Gynecol* 156:1137, 1987.

Gross S, Librach C, Cecutti A: Maternal weight loss associated with hyperemesis gravidarum: a predictor of fetal outcome, *Am J Obstet Gynecol* 160:906, 1989.

Kadar N, DeVare G, Romero R: Discriminatory hCG zone: its use in the sonographic evaluation for ectopic pregnancy, *Obstet Gynecol* 58:156, 1981.

Kadar N, Freedman M, Zackar M: Further observation on the doubling time of human chorionic gonadotropin in early asymptomatic pregnancy, *Fertil Steril* 34:783, 1980.

Key TC: Gastrointestinal diseases: Creasy RK, Resnik R, editors: In *Maternal fetal medicine: principles and practice,* Philadelphia, 1989, WB Saunders.

Kijima E et al: The treatment of unruptured tubal pregnancy with intratubal methotrexate injection under laparoscopic control, *Obstet Gynecol* 75:723, 1990.

Long MD, Simone SS, Tucker JJ: Outpatient treatment of hyperemesis gravidarum with stimulus control and imagery procedures, *J Behav Ther Exp Psychiatry* 17:105, 1986.

Menard A et al: Treatment of unruptured tubal pregnancy by local injection of methotrexate under transvaginal sonographic control, *Fertil Steril* 54:47, 1990.

Milkovich L, Vanden Berg CJ: An evaluation of the teratogenicity of certain antinauseant drugs, *Am J Obstet Gynecol* 125:244, 1976.

Moya F, Thorndike V: Passage of drugs accross the placenta, *Am J Obstet Gynecol* 84:1778, 1962.

Nyberg DA et al: Early gestation: correlation of hCG levels and sonographic identification, *AJF* 144:951, 1985.

Stovall TG, Ling FW, Buster JE: Reproductive performance after methotrexate treatment of ectopic pregnancy, *Am J Obstet Gynecol* 162:1620, 1990.

Stovall TG, Ling FW, Gray LA: Methotrexate treatment of unruptured ectopic pregnancy: a report of 100 cases, *Obstet Gynecol* 77:749, 1991.

Stovall TG, Ling FW, Gray LA: Single dose methotrexate for treatment of ectopic pregnancy, *Obstet Gynecol* 77:754, 1991.

Tuomivaara L, Kauppila A: Radical or conservative surgery for ectopic pregnancy? A follow-up study of fertility of 323 patients, *Fertil Steril* 50:580, 1988.

Weckstein LN: Clinical diagnosis of ectopic pregnancy, *Clin Obstet Gynecol* 30:236, 1987.

Weigel RM, Weigel MM: Nausea and vomiting of early pregnancy and pregnancy outcome: a meta-analytical review, *Br J Obstet Gynaecol* 96:1312, 1989.

49 Early Pregnancy Disorders: Miscarriage and Recurrent Spontaneous Abortion

Joseph A. Hill and Craig L. Best

EPIDEMIOLOGY AND DEFINITION OF ABORTION

In approximately 70% of human conceptions fetal viability is not achieved, and an estimated 50% are lost before the first missed menses. The actual rate of pregnancy loss after implantation may be as high as 31%. *Spontaneous abortion,* defined as the loss of a clinically recognized (blood test or ultrasound) pregnancy before 20 weeks' gestation, occurs in 10% to 15% of all clinically established pregnancies. Approximately 60% of pregnancy losses before 8 weeks' gestation are chromosomally abnormal; trisomies are the most common abnormality. However, the most common single abnormality is monosomy X (45X). Spontaneous abortions are subdivided into threatened abortion, inevitable abortion, incomplete abortion, complete abortion, missed abortion, and recurrent abortion. *Threatened abortion* is a viable clinical pregnancy accompanied by vaginal bleeding. *Inevitable abortion* occurs during pregnancy in the presence of a dilated internal cervical os or in cases of ruptured membranes. In an *incomplete abortion* some but not all fetal-placental tissue has passed through the internal cervical os; in a *complete abortion* all fetal-placental tissue has been spontaneously passed through the internal cervical os. A *missed abortion* is a pregnancy in which the fetus is no longer viable in the absence of vaginal bleeding. Symptoms of pregnancy (nausea, breast tenderness) may or may not be present at the time of pregnancy loss. Pelvic examination and ultrasound assessment will usually lead to the proper diagnosis.

DEFINITION OF RECURRENT ABORTION

Recurrent abortion has been traditionally defined as the occurrence of three or more clinically recognized pregnancy losses before 20 weeks' gestation and occurs in approximately 1 in 300 pregnancies. Clinical investigation of pregnancy loss, however, should be initiated after two spontaneous abortions, especially when the women is older than 35 years, the couple has had difficulty conceiving, or when fetal heart activity had been identified on a prior ultrasound examination. It is important to understand the calculated risks for recurrent abortion, which are based on epidemiologic surveys, especially when reviewing the literature on potential success rates with various therapies. These surveys indicate that after one spontaneous abortion the recurrence risk is 24%; after two, 30%; after three, 35%; and after four consecutive clinical losses, approximately 40% (Warburton and Fraser, 1963; Alberman, 1988).

CAUSES

Chromosomal abnormalities

Parental chromosomal abnormalities remain the only uncontested cause of recurrent abortion and occur in approximately 5% of couples seeking evaluation (see box on the following page). Other associations with recurrent pregnancy loss have been made, including müllerian or anatomic anomalies (10%), endocrinologic abnormalities (17%), infections (5%), and autoimmunity (3%). The potential cause in the majority of cases, however, remains unexplained (60%) after a thorough conventional evaluation (see box on the following page).

The most common inborn parental chromosomal abnormality contributing to recurrent abortion is balanced translocation. Pericentric chromosomal inversion and sex chromosome mosaicism have also been associated with recurrent abortion. Other genetic causes of abortion include multifactorial inheritance of autosomal recessive genes and X-linked disorders.

Congenital and acquired anatomic causes

Anatomic causes can be divided into both congenital and acquired lesions. Congenital anomalies include incomplete müllerian fusion or septum resorption defects, diethylstilbestrol (DES) exposure, and uterine artery anomalies. Women with a septate uterus may have a 62% risk for spontaneous abortion. Second trimester losses are most commonly seen; however, first trimester abortions may be caused if the embryo implants on the intrauterine septum as the endometrium overlying a septum is poorly developed and blood supply to this area is often limited. Therefore abnormal placentation may occur, potentially culminating in an abortion. DES exposure in utero can lead to uterine devel-

POTENTIAL CAUSES OF RECURRENT ABORTION

Parental chromosomal abnormalities
Congenital anatomic abnormalities
   Incomplete müllerian fusions or septum resorption
   defects
   DES exposure
   Uterine artery abnormalities
Acquired anatomic abnormalities
   Uterine synechiae (adhesions)
   Uterine fibroids
   Endometriosis
Endocrinologic abnormalities
   Luteul phase insufficiency
   Hypothyroidism
   Diabetes mellitus
Maternal infections
   Cervical mycoplasma, ureaplasma, and chlamydia
Other causes
   Heavy metal and chemical exposures
   Chronic medical illness
   Thrombocytosis
Immunologic phenomena
   Allogenic immunity
   Autoimmunity

DES, diethylstilbestrol.

INVESTIGATIVE MEASURES POTENTIALLY USEFUL IN THE EVALUATION OF RECURRENT SPONTANEOUS ABORTION

Parental peripheral blood karyotypes
Hysterosalpingogram
Luteal phase endometrial biopsy
Thyroid function studies (TSH, T_4)
Anticardiolipin antibody
Antiphosphatidylserine antibody
Lupus anticoagulant (aPTT, Russell's viper venom time)
Antisperm antibodies
Cervical cultures

TSH, thyroid-stimulating hormone; T_4, thyroxine; aPTT, activated partial thromboplastin time.

opmental anomalies, most commonly hypoplasia, causing both first and second trimester abortions. DES exposed women also have a predisposition to development of incompetent cervix and premature labor. Isolated cases of uterine artery anomalies have been reportedly associated with recurrent abortion, most likely caused by compromised blood flow to the implanting blastocyst and developing placenta. Acquired anatomic lesions potentially predisposing to recurrent abortion include uterine synechiae (adhesions), submucous or intramural leiomyomata (fibroids), and endometriosis. These associations with abortion are tenuous, but theoretic mechanisms that may be involved include interference with blood supply, as in the case of adhesions and fibroids, and immunologic phenomena that may be involved in cases of endometriosis.

Endocrinologic abnormalities

Endocrinologic abnormalities associated with recurrent abortion include luteal phase insufficiency, thyroid disorders, and diabetes mellitus. The early maintenance of pregnancy is dependent upon progesterone production by the corpus luteum until the placenta takes over progesterone production between 7 and 9 weeks of gestation. Spontaneous abortion could ensue if (1) the corpus luteum fails to produce sufficient quantities of progesterone, (2) progesterone delivery to the uterus is compromised, or (3) progesterone use within endometrial/decidual tissue is disordered. Thyroid disorders—most commonly hypothyroidism—have also been associated with recurrent abortion, most likely because of ovulation disorders that lead to corpus luteum insufficiency. The mechanism of abortion in women with diabetes mellitus is unclear but may be due to compromised blood flow to the developing conceptus, especially in cases of advanced disease. Elevated hemoglobin A_{1C} levels in

peripheral blood before conception have also been associated with pregnancy failure.

Maternal infections

Maternal infections have been tenuously associated with recurrent abortion. The most commonly reported association between infection and pregnancy loss has been cervical colonization with mycoplasma, ureaplasma, and chlamydia. Causal mechanisms are poorly described but one theoretic possibility may involve immunologic activation.

Other causes

Other poorly established associations include environmental factors such as exposure to heavy metal toxicity, carbon tetrachloride, and trichloroethylene benzene; drugs such as folic acid antagonists, nicotine, ethanol, and inhalation anesthetic agents; ionizing radiation; and chronic medical illnesses such as cardiac and renal diseases or any other disorder that compromises uterine blood supply. Thrombocytosis (platelet counts greater than 1 million) has also been associated with recurrent abortion, presumably as a result of clotting and occlusion of the placental vasculature. It is important to reassure patients that exposure to video display terminals and microwave ovens does not cause abortion.

Immunologic phenomena

Immunologic phenomena involving allogeneic immunity and autoimmunity have also been associated with reproductive failure. The immune system is a complex integrated system that has evolved to protect the individual from nonself tissue. The immune system can be simplistically divided into the humoral immune system, which is mediated by antibody secreting plasma cells derived from B-lymphocytes, and the cellular immune system, which is mediated by cytokines secreted by activated macrophages, T-lymphocytes, and natural killer cells.

There have been four humoral immune mechanisms implicated in recurrent abortion (see box on the following page).

Antiphospholipid antibodies. Antiphospholipid antibodies are immunoglobulin G (IgG) or IgM directed against negatively charged phospholipid most commonly to cardiolipin and phosphatidylserine. They are also characterized

---

IMMUNE MECHANISMS IMPLICATED IN RECURRENT SPONTANEOUS ABORTION

Humoral
    Antiphospholipid antibodies
    Antisperm antibodies
    Antitrophoblast antibodies
    Blocking antibody deficiency (TLX)

Cellular
    Suppressor cell and factor deficiency
    Major histocompatibility antigen expression
    Cytokine, growth factor, and oncogene deficiency
    Cytokine-mediated immunodystrophism
      (embryotoxic factors)

TLX, trophoblast lymphocyte cross-reading antibodies.

by prolonged phospholipid-dependent coagulation tests in vitro and thrombosis in vivo. The basic hypothesis of how antiphospholipid antibodies mediate abortion is that they cause platelet adhesion within placental vessels through increased thromboxane and decreased prostacycline synthesis. Antisperm and antitrophoblast antibodies have been proposed but no longer appear to be valid mechanisms mediating abortion, except on theoretic grounds.

Blocking antibody deficiency. The blocking antibody deficiency hypothesis has received a lot of attention, especially in the lay press, promoted by entrepreneurs and caring practitioners alike. This hypothesis is based on three suppositions: (1) there is an antifetal, maternal cell-mediated immune response that develops in all pregnancies that must be blocked; (2) blocking factors (presumably antibodies) that prevent antifetal maternal cellular immunity develop in all pregnancies; and (3) in the absence of blocking antibodies abortion occurs. There remains, however, no direct pathologic evidence that immunologic abortion occurs, and it is well established that pregnancy maintenance is not dependent on an intact immune system since agammaglobulinemic mice and women can successfully reproduce. Further evidence against the blocking antibody deficiency hypothesis as a cause of recurrent abortion comes from studies indicating that as many as 40% of women who have had a successful pregnancy do not make blocking antibodies. Therefore, blocking antibody deficiency is unlikely to be a cause of abortion. Parental sharing of human leukocyte antigen (HLA) haplotypes or TLX antigens was originally proposed to cause blocking antibody deficiency, as measured by hyporesponsiveness in mixed lymphocyte cultures. It is now known that HLA compatibility is not necessarily associated with recurrent abortion, as many couples who share HLA haplotypes have successful pregnancies. Similarly, animal studies also do not support this theory since inbred animal strains having identical H-2 (HLA equivalent) haplotypes can be successfully bred for generations. Mixed lymphocyte culture (MLC) reactivities have been proposed but are no longer considered to be predictive of abortion as many fertile couples have hyporesponsive MLC reactivities and many couples with recurrent abortion are hyperresponsive. The concept that TLX is involved in abortion also appears unlikely because TLX is now known to be identical to CD46, which is a membrane-associated cofactor protein complement receptor. CD46 is found on trophoblasts and many other cell types including spermatozoa and lymphocytes. The proposed function of CD46 on trophoblast is to bind complement, thus preventing complement-mediated attack of the developing placenta.

Cellular immune mechanisms. There have been four cellular immune mechanisms implicated in recurrent abortion. Suppressor immune cell and factor deficiency has been reported in the decidua of mice and women at the time of fetal reabsorption or spontaneous abortion. Macrophage activation and function have also been reported to be enhanced in decidual tissues during spontaneous abortion. Cause versus effect mechanisms for these observations, however, have not been addressed. Major histocompatibility (MHC) antigen expression is usually absent on syncytiotrophoblast except for a unique truncated form of class I known as HLA-G. MHC antigens, however, have been expressed in vitro using the T-cell cytokine γ-interferon (γ-IFN). Expression of MHC antigens on trophoblast could mediate abortion by enhancing cytotoxic T-cell attack. Recent data, however, indicate that MHC antigens are not expressed on aborted tissues from women experiencing either their first miscarriage or their fourth or subsequent miscarriage. Therefore this theory too appears unlikely as a cause of spontaneous abortion. Certain cytokines, growth factors, and oncogenes, specifically the colony-stimulating factors, and c-fms, have been proposed to facilitate trophoblast growth and function. The absence of these same factors has been proposed to be involved in trophoblast growth and function failure.

Cytokine-mediated immunodystrophism. Recently another new hypothesis has been proposed: cytokine-mediated immunodystrophism. This hypothesis states that in susceptible women trophoblast and sperm can act as an antigen, activating immune cells residing in reproductive tissues to produce factors that are toxic to the developing conceptus (embryotoxic factors). Recent work has shown that one of the factors responsible for embryotoxicity is the T-helper cytokine γ-INF. Generation of these embryotoxic factors during pregnancy has been recently shown to predict subsequent abortion (Ecker, Laufer, and Hill, 1993).

Evaluation of women with history of recurrent abortion

History. Diagnostic evaluation of couples experiencing recurrent abortion should begin with a general history: medical, surgical, genetic, and psychologic. A description and sequence of all prior pregnancies are important as is whether histologic and karyotypic assessment of prior abortions was performed. The practitioner should also ask about chronic illnesses, uterine instrumentation, infection, DES exposure, and exposure to drugs, radiation, and possible environmental pollutants.

Physical examination. A general physical examination of the woman should look for signs of metabolic illness. On pelvic examination the examiner should look for signs of infection, DES exposure, or previous cervical laceration, on bimanual examination for irregularity of the size, shape, and contour of the uterus.

Diagnostic testing. Potentially useful laboratory measurements include (1) peripheral blood karyotype of both partners; (2) hysterosalpingogram followed by hysteroscopy and laparoscopy, if indicated; (3) luteal phase endometrial biopsy, ideally 10 days after the luteinizing hormone (LH) surge or after cycle day 24 of an idealized 28-day cycle (if the biopsy is out of phase by more than 2 days according to established criteria then repeat assessment in a subsequent cycle is required to make the diagnosis of luteal phase insufficiency; in cases of an abnormal biopsy result, a serum prolactin and androgen profile should also be determined); (4) thyroid function tests (TSH, free T_4); (5) anticardiolipin antibody and antiphosphatidylserine antibody; (6) lupus anticoagulant (a partial thromboplastin time [PTT] or Russell viper venom time); and, as a last resort, (7) a cervical culture for mycoplasma, ureaplasma, and chlamydia. Investigative measures that are of no benefit in the evaluation of recurrent spontaneous abortion and should only be obtained under a study protocol at no charge to the couple include (1) antinuclear antibodies, (2) antipaternal cytotoxic antibodies, (3) parental HLA profiles, and (4) mixed lymphocyte culture reactivities. Further work is needed before suppressor cell/factor determinations, cytokine, oncogene, and growth factor measurements or embryotoxic factor assessment can be clinically justified and available.

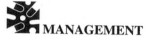

MANAGEMENT

Overview

Therapy should include appropriate measures for the individual known groups. For individuals with recurrent abortion of unknown cause it as follows: Antibiotic therapy is indicated only if findings on the cervical culture warrant treatment, normalization of ovulation, and synchronization of ovulation and sperm deposition. Early diagnosis and close monitoring during the first trimester may also be therapeutic. Serial human chorionic gonadotropin determinations for the β subunit (β-hCG) should be performed after the first period is missed. Ultrasound assessment should be performed to confirm an intrauterine pregnancy once the β-hCG attains 1000 to 5000 mIU/ml or 5 to 6 weeks' gestation, because women with recurrent spontaneous abortion have a 2% to 4% risk of ectopic gestation. A repeat pelvic ultrasound to confirm fetal viability should be performed every 2 weeks through the first trimester or past the point in gestation where the individual's abortions have previously occurred to help alleviate the couple's anxiety and to allow intervention for karyotype assessment should fetal demise occur.

Immunotherapy

Rarely, immunotherapy may be considered but only under a scientific protocol where the couple is not charged for experimental immunologic testing and therapy. Immunotherapy involving either immunostimulation or immunosuppression (see box, above right) has been proposed, however, all two often with little rationale or substantive data in support of therapeutic efficacy.

Immunostimulating therapies. Immunostimulating therapies have most commonly involved leukocyte immunization. Despite the many hundreds of women who have received either paternal or third-party leukocytes, only three reports have been published claiming to be randomized,

---

IMMUNOTHERAPIES PROPOSED FOR RECURRENT SPONTANEOUS ABORTION

Immunostimulation

    Leukocyte transfusions
    Trophoblast vesicle fluid transfusions
    Immunoglobulin transfusions
    Seminal plasma suppositories

Immunosuppression

    Corticosteroids
    Aspirin
    Heparin
    Progesterone
    Pentoxifylline
    Cyclosporin A
    Nifedipine

---

double-blinded, and placebo-controlled. A metaanalysis of these published reports indicates a relative risk of 1.0, suggesting lack of efficacy over placebo. Indeed a survey of the peer-reviewed medical literature of various immunostimulating therapies for recurrent abortion that included at least 20 patients per treatment group indicates no therapeutic benefit of any of the proposed therapies over unstimulated control therapy (Table 49-1). Leukocyte immunization also has potential risks, including anaphylaxis, serum sickness, sensitization, inability to receive donor organs later, graft versus host disease, intrauterine growth retardation, and infectious diseases (human immunodeficiency virus [HIV], cytomegalovirus [CMV], hepatitis, toxoplasmosis).

Immunosuppressive therapies. Immunosuppressive therapies have also been proposed for recurrent abortion believed caused by maternal immune hyperresponsiveness. Most remain untested in randomized, double-blind, placebo-controlled trials and therefore cannot be recommended. Evidence, however, does indicate that aspirin (80 mg/day) and heparin (10,000 units bid) may be efficacious in preventing abortion and other malobstetric outcomes associated with maternal antiphospholipid antibody production.

Safe and effective treatment modalities are needed for couples who are experiencing recurrent abortion. The rationale

Table 49-1 Summary of peer-reviewed literature on the efficacy of immunostimulating therapies and control therapy with at least 20 patients enrolled per group

Treatment	Number of patients	% Pregnancy success
Paternal leukocyte immunization	822	73
Third-party leukocyte immunization	79	75
Trophoblast membrane infusion	79	57
Intravenous immunoglobulin	69	68
Seminal plasma suppositories	44	55
Autologous leukocyte immunization	101	60
Intralipid infusion	20	70
Psychotherapy	135	85
Saline solution alone	32	67
No treatment	304	58

Table 49-2 Prognosis for live birth

Cause	% Success
Genetic (chromosomal)	30-60
Anatomic	60-70
Endocrinologic	90
Unknown (other)	30-90

for therapy, however, must be scientifically well founded and more innocuous than the disease. Practicing physicians should refrain from using or recommending immunotherapy for their patients with recurrent abortion until the rationale for such therapy has been proved and the safety and efficacy of potential regimens have been scientifically tested in double-blind, randomized, appropriately controlled trials.

PROGNOSIS FOR LIVE BIRTH

The prognosis for a subsequent live birth (Table 49-2) in couples with a history of recurrent abortion is not necessarily dismal. Most chromosomally abnormal pregnancies abort before achieving fetal cardiac activity. Recent evidence suggests that once fetal cardiac activity has been ultrasonically detected between 5 and 6 weeks' gestation, the risk of subsequent loss is approximately 23%. Although this is significantly higher than the 4% incidence in the general population, knowledge that a 77% chance of fetal viability exists once fetal cardiac activity has been detected can be tremendously reassuring to the couple who has experienced multiple miscarriages and helps establish a more realistic prognosis for pregnancy success.

SUMMARY

In conclusion, the diagnosis of early pregnancy disorders depends on an accurate assessment of the patient's history, physical examination, and appropriate laboratory tests. Understanding the potential pathophysiologic mechanisms involved in each diagnosis as outlined in this chapter will enable women's health care providers to manage the most commonly encountered disorders of early pregnancy effectively.

BIBLIOGRAPHY

Alberman E: The epidemiology of repeated abortion. In: Sharp F, editor: *Early pregnancy loss: mechanisms and treatment*, New York, 1988, Springer-Verlag.

Boue J, Boue A, Lasar P: Retrospective and prospective epidemiologic studies of 1,500 karyotyped spontaneous abortions, *Teratol* 11:11, 1975.

Ecker JL, Laufer MR, Hill JA: Measurement of embryotoxic factors is predictive of pregnancy outcome in women with a history of recurrent abortion, *Obstet Gynecol* 81:84, 1993.

Hill JA: Immunological contributions to recurrent pregnancy loss, *Bailliere Clin Obstet Gynecol* 6:489, 1992.

Hill JA: Sporadic and recurrent spontaneous abortion, *Curr Prob Obstet Gynecol Fertil* 17:113, 1994.

Hill JA et al: Evidence of embryo and trophoblast toxic cellular immune response(s) in women with recurrent spontaneous abortion, *Am J Obstet Gynecol* 166:1044, 1992.

Laufer MR, Ecker JL, Hill JA: Pregnancy outcome following ultrasound documented fetal cardiac activity in women with a history of multiple spontaneous abortions, *J Soc Gynecol Invest*, 1994.

Triplett DA: Obstetrical implications of anti phospholipid antibodies, *Bailliere Clin Obstet Gynecol* 6:507, 1992.

Warburton D, Fraser FC: Spontaneous abortion rate in man: data from reproductive histories collected in a medical genetics unit, *Am J Hum Genet* 16:1, 1963.

Wilcox AJ et al: Incidence of early loss of pregnancy, *N Engl J Med* 319:189, 1988.

50 Infectious Exposure and Immunization During Pregnancy

Stephanie A. Eisenstat

A number of infectious diseases in the pregnant woman can have devastating consequences for the fetus. To evaluate and counsel pregnant women who have been exposed to or have contracted specific infections the primary care clinician needs to be familiar with the effects of these diseases. Although there are vast observational data, controversy remains regarding screening for most of these infectious diseases; thus standard protocols have been difficult to implement. This chapter reviews the major issues in identification and prevention of the more common infectious diseases during pregnancy that have serious consequences for the fetus. Human immunodeficiency virus (HIV) infection and pregnancy is discussed in Chapter 16.

PATHOPHYSIOLOGY
Fetal immunity

The fetal immune system is immature until after 20 weeks' gestation. Because of the lack of maturity across all cell lines, there is a decrease in function in the T cell–mediated processes (delayed hypersensitivity, T-cell help for B cell differentiation, and cytokine production) and in B-cell line function (resulting in poorly functioning neutrophils and an inability to produce antibodies to bacterial polysaccharides). The fetus is able to produce IgM. Other cells such as natural killer (NK) cells are present but immature and not completely functional.

SCREENING DURING PREGNANCY

Screening for certain infectious diseases during pregnancy is an important part of routine prenatal care. The most common infections that have adverse fetal outcome are toxoplasmosis, rubella, cytomegalovirus, and herpes simplex viruses (TORCH). In some diseases, such as hepatitis, early identification in the mother followed by immunoprophylaxis of the newborn can prevent severe neonatal morbidity. Routine serologic screening to detect a variety of infections has been advocated by some during both the preconception and the early prenatal periods. Serologic diagnosis is based on the demonstration of a significant rise in antibody titer against the specific causative infectious agent. Many clinicians obtain prepregnancy antibody measurements to improve the ability to detect an antibody rise should primary infection occur during pregnancy. However, the sensitivity of the serologic tests and the cost effectiveness of routine screening have been controversial. The U.S. Preventive Health Services Task Force, after reviewing the data regarding the efficacy of certain screening interventions in pregnancy, concluded that serologic testing for rubella antibodies should be performed in *all* pregnant and nonpregnant women of reproductive age who are unclear about their immune status. Blood tests for hepatitis B surface antigen also should be performed at the time of the first prenatal visit and repeated during the third trimester for women at high risk for contracting Hepatitis B. Routine screening for toxoplasmosis and cytomegalovirus was not reviewed by the U.S. Preventive Health Services Task Force. A proposal for systematic screening was developed by Wilson and Remington (1980) and McCabe and Remington (1988) but has remained difficult and controversial to implement because of lack of quality control, difficulty in diagnosing the affected fetus, and lack of therapy of proved efficacy. Other infections for which routine screening during pregnancy has been advocated include syphilis, chlamydia, and gonorrhea in high-risk populations.

HERPES SIMPLEX VIRUS

Some sexually transmitted diseases can have significant effects on the fetus. It is well-known that infection with herpes simplex virus (HSV) (usually type 2, occassionally type 1) contracted from passage through an infected birth canal can result in severe disseminated herpes infection in the neonate, including central nervous system infection leading to mental retardation or death. It is estimated that one in five pregnant women has had HSV-2 infection, and the incidence of neonatal infection from herpes virus may be as high as 1 in 20,000 live births. The spectrum of genital herpes infection includes primary infection, recurrent infection (with or without symptoms), and asymptomatic viral shedding without clinical disease. Studies have shown that the risk of contracting herpes by the fetus is higher (more than 50%) if the mother has an active primary herpes infection than if she has recurrent infection (less than 5%). Transmission rates are lowest for women with asymptomatic viral shedding. Most cases of neonatal herpes result from contact with mothers who have asymptomatic viral shedding at the time of delivery.

The risk for the development of the more severe consequences of herpes in the newborn relates directly to the extent of viral shedding at the time of delivery. Thus the standard recommendation is cesarean delivery when examination at the time of rupture of membranes and labor reveals herpes lesions (primary or secondary). Although screening for herpes can be helpful in the mother with recurrent infection, routine screening cultures have demonstrated poor predictive value for identifying the patient who will be shedding at delivery. For this reason, and because the transmission rates are low for women without a history of recurrent disease, routine viral cultures are not currently recommended.

For primary herpes infection during pregnancy, treatment with acyclovir is recommended to prevent severe disease in the mother. Because these infections are associated with high rates of viral shedding and reactivation, some groups advocate weekly cervical cultures. If viral shedding continues at the time of labor (assumed by the presence of genital lesions or persistent seropositive surveillance cultures in the pregnant woman with primary herpes infection), delivery by cesarean section may be indicated in this subgroup. Treatment for herpes infection is the same for pregnant women as for nonpregnant women and is reviewed in Chapter 17. Prevention of herpes infection is important during pregnancy. Sexual contact with infected partners should be avoided, and patients should be counseled about safe sex practices.

SYPHILIS

Congenital syphilis, caused by the organism *Treponema pallidum,* is on the rise in the United States with an incidence of 1 in 10,000 live births. Congenital infection includes hepatosplenomegaly, jaundice, hemolysis, and lymphadenopathy. If untreated, there is also an increased risk of miscarriage, stillbirth, and premature delivery.

Regardless of sexual history, all pregnant women should be routinely screened for syphilis with a nontreponemal antibody test: Venereal Disease Research Laboratories (VDRL) or rapid plasma reagin (RPR). Screening should be performed as early as possible, preferably at the first prenatal visit. On the basis of the risk profile, screening may need to be repeated during the second and third trimesters of pregnancy and near the time of delivery.

In the case of a pregnant woman who shows evidence of clinical disease or has been exposed to an infected partner but whose VDRL or RPR test results are negative, the recommendation is to treat for primary syphilis and repeat the VDRL or RPR in 3 to 6 weeks because of the high likelihood of fetal infection (Dorfman and Glaser, 1990). The standard treatment protocols for the nonpregnant woman (see Chapter 17) should be used for the pregnant woman with the exception of the alternative treatment for the penicillin-allergic patient. In the nonpregnant woman erythromycin is the drug of choice for the patient with penicillin allergy but, because of the high failure rates, the current recommendation is to conduct skin testing to the major and minor penicillin determinants; in cases of positivity the pregnant patient should undergo desensitization to penicillin. This usually is performed in a controlled setting in consultation with an allergist. Close follow-up is mandatory with monthly syphilis serologic screening throughout pregnancy. Because eradication of the infection is paramount, retreatment should be implemented if there is not a fourfold decrease in the nontreponemal titer over a 3-month period in a patient whose initial test results were found to be positive. It is important for partners to be treated.

CHLAMYDIA AND GONORRHEA

Infection with *Chlamydia trachomatis* and *Neisseria gonorrhoeae* is associated with a number of sequelae for the fetus as well as the pregnant woman: increased risk for cervicitis, endometritis, peritonitis, perihepatitis, and disseminated infection and an associated risk for prematurity, premature rupture of membranes, intrauterine growth retardation, and chorioamnionitis. Neonatal infection with gonorrhea can result in eye (ophthalmia neonatorum), scalp, and disseminated infection. Multiple studies have estimated the prevalence of asymptomatic infection during pregnancy at 2% to 5%. Many clinicians recommend screening for both chlamydia and gonorrhea during early pregnancy and repeated screening in patients at high risk of contracting the infections. Treatment for gonorrhea is the same as in the nonpregnant woman. Alternatives to the tetracycline medications that are used for treatment of chlamydia but are contraindicated during pregnancy include erythromycin and amoxicillin, but high relapse rates exist. For a detailed discussion of the treatment of gonorrhea and chlamydial infection see Chapter 17.

CYTOMEGALOVIRUS

Cytomegalovirus (CMV) is a herpes virus infection that in adults generally causes no symptoms or manifests a syndrome similar to mononucleosis. Because CMV is endemic, many women have preexisting immunity although the actual percentage of pregnant women who are immune is difficult to determine. Approximately 2% of susceptible women develop asymptomatic primary CMV infection during pregnancy; 40% of the infants of these mothers develop infection (Stagno, 1985). The consequences for these infants can be devastating, including stillbirth, deafness, neurologic complications, developmental learning disabilities, and multiple physical defects, with an incidence of 1% in all newborns whose test results are positive, 10% of whom are seriously affected. In a study by Stagno et al. (1982), the rate of transmission of CMV from mother to fetus was almost 50% in the pregnant woman with primary CMV infection; 20% of those infants demonstrated obvious clinical disease at birth. Most of the infants who developed complications later in childhood had visible disease at the time of delivery. Infants of mothers with primary infection are at greater risk for congenital CMV infection although earlier studies by Stagno et al. (1977) demonstrated that infants of mothers who are immune can still contact CMV infection, with a 0.5% to 1% incidence of congenital infection caused by recurrent CMV in the mother and a less than 1% chance of clinically apparent disease at birth. A later prospective study of 3700 women by Stagno et al. (1982) demonstrated that immunity in woman who had CMV infection before pregnancy partially protected her baby and that congenital CMV occurred less frequently with less severe consequences than in offspring of women with primary CMV infection during pregnancy.

Because there is no effective drug intervention and the actual risk of infection to the fetus is low, routine screening has been advocated (Hunter et al., 1983). Unfortunately the methods for confirming primary infection in the fetus of the infected mother at present are inaccurate. Therefore there are no recommendations for universal screening for infants. Recommendations for prevention for high-risk women (i.e., day-care centers) include good hand-washing and hygienic measures (Stagno, 1995). There has been much discussion in the medical community concerning the development of a CMV vaccination as the ideal method for prevention. Counseling the woman who is currently infected is difficult. Demonstration of fetal infection often can be made by amniocentesis or umbilical blood sampling. How to use that information is more problematic because many fetal infections do not lead to long-term sequelae.

HEPATITIS

Hepatitis B virus (HBV) is a growing public concern. Data from the Centers for Disease Control (CDC) estimate that 22,000 infants are born annually to women with chronic HBV. Acute HBV occurs in 1 to 2 per 1000 pregnancies. The incidence of acute HBV in the newborn population is rising. Women at highest risk for contracting HBV include those with a history of intravenous drug use, history of multiple sexual partners, employment in health care, or household contact with HBV. If the mother contracts the disease early in the pregnancy, the rate of vertical transmission to the infant is 10% but rises to 50% to 60% if contracted during the third trimester (Snydman, 1985). Multiple studies have shown that women who are chronic carriers, with positive hepatitis B surface antigen (HBsAg) only or positive HBsAg and hepatitis Be antigen (HBeAg) have a 12% to 25% and 70% to 90% neonatal infection rate, respectively (Remington and Klein, 1995). Infants with neonatal hepatitis are at highest risk for becoming chronic carriers of hepatitis.

At present the American College of Obstetricians and Gynecologists (ACOG) and other groups recommend screening all pregnant women for HBsAg during the first prenatal visit to identify those infants who will need intervention for the prevention of perinatal HBV infection. If the woman is in a high-risk group, the test should be repeated during the third trimester and at the time of delivery. Testing for HBeAg can be helpful in assessing the degree of infectivity and risk, but the intervention with immunoprophylaxis is the same regardless of the presence of the e antigen. All infants of mothers who have active or chronic hepatitis should receive 0.5 ml of hepatitis B immune globulin during the first 12 hours of life. They should then be immunized with hepatitis B vaccine (Heptavax-B) during the first week of life, 1 month later, and a final dose at 6 months of age, which is now standard practice for all newborn infants.

Hepatitis C (HCV) is the current name for one of the parenterally transmitted non-A non-B hepatitides. The actual incidence of HCV infection during pregnancy and fetal transmission rate is unknown. Women at highest risk for contracting HCV are those with a history of multiple blood transfusions, personal use of intravenous illicit drugs, or intimate contact with a partner with a history of risk factors for HCV. The ability to identify HCV has improved recently with new methods for identification of the virus in the blood. Recent studies by Ohto et al. (1994) have shown that HCV is vertically transmitted and that the risk of transmission is correlated with high titers of HCV RNA in the mothers. Further research is necessary before standard recommendations regarding screening for HCV can be made.

PARVOVIRUS B19

Parvovirus B19, which causes mild systemic symptoms and distinct facial rash in children and susceptible adults (erythema infectiosum or fifth disease), can result in nonimmune fetal hydrops and death in infected infants. The greated risk to the fetus occurs during the first 20 weeks of pregnancy (Hall, 1994), which coincides with the major development of erythroid precursors. A prospective study from the Public Health Laboratory of Great Britain followed up 190 pregnant women who were identified as having recent parvovirus infection (IgM antibody positivity). Approximately 82% delivered healthy infants, and 30 (15%) fetal deaths were reported in this study. There have been no reported cases of congenital anomalies in live births after in utero exposure to parvovirus. The fetal risk during pregnancy from maternal exposure is low, and most women have been exposed before pregnancy.

Routine screening for parvovirus B19 is not recommended, but if infection is suspected, IgM and IgG antibodies for parvovirus can be obtained. Newer methods using B19 DNA–specific polymerase chain reaction tests are being developed for future use. The recommendation at this time is follow-up of pregnant women with serial ultrasound examinations to reveal any signs of fetal anemia or impending hydrops and if the initial IgM antibody test results are positive, to repeat determinations of alpha-fetoprotein (Remington and Klein, 1995).

RUBELLA

Most pregnant women are protected against contracting rubella because of their own childhood vaccination. According to reports from CDC, during the years 1988-1990 there was an increase in the number of reported cases of congenital rubella caused by lack of immunization of younger women. Consequences consist of an increase in congenital rubella syndrome, which includes intrauterine growth retardation (IUGR), prematurity, and increased risk for spontaneous abortion and stillbirth, as well as severe neurologic, ophthalmalogic, and cardiac complications. Not all sequelae manifest at birth. Hearing loss and other central nervous system problems have been identified years after in utero exposure. The greatest risk to the infant is exposure during the first trimester. The risk of *congenital rubella infection* in fetuses born to mothers with rubella has been found to be 90% before 11 weeks' gestation, 25% if infected during weeks 23 to 26, and 67% after 31 weeks (Miller, Cradock-Watson, and Pollack, 1982). Before 11 weeks' gestation the incidence of *birth defects* in infected infants approaches 100%.

It is recommended that all women of reproductive age be screened for rubella antibodies and if seronegative receive immunization. If rubella infection is suspected in the pregnant woman, the clinician should obtain acute and convalescent antibody titers 10 to 14 days apart that reveal a greater than or equal to fourfold rise between the two titers. The presence of rubella-specific IgM antibody also is diagnostic of acute infection but needs to be obtained within 7 days after the onset of the rubella rash. If an acute infection is documented—especially if earlier than 13 weeks' gestation—the patient needs to discuss options with the obstetrician or primary care clinician. There is a role for high-dose immune globulin for those women who are unable to termi-

nate their pregnancy, but the efficacy and protective effect for the fetus are unpredictible (Remington, 1995). Inasmuch as rubella is a live attenuated virus, it should not be administered during pregnancy or within 3 months of a planned pregnancy. Because as many as 50% of women will have unplanned pregnancy and there exists a theoretic risk of the fetus contracting congenital rubella from a vaccine (the CDC has no reported cases of the fetus developing congenital rubella syndrome after maternal vaccination during pregnancy), it is important to administer the vaccine at the time of menstruation if the woman is not taking an oral contraceptive pill. (For a detailed discussion on management of acute rubella disease during pregnancy see Remington and Klein, 1995.)

VARICELLA-ZOSTER VIRUS

Most women have been infected with chickenpox as children because of its high communicability and thus are immune to the development of infection with primary varicella infection during pregnancy. The incidence of chickenpox during pregnancy is estimated at 1.3 to 7 cases per 10,000 pregnancies (Sison and Sever, 1993). There is a small chance of reactivation of the virus resulting in clinical varicella-zoster virus (VZV) in the pregnant woman. Should primary varicella infection (chickenpox) develop, some studies have shown a greater risk for the development of severe maternal complications such as varicella pneumonia.

The effect on the fetus depends on the timing of the infection during pregnancy. Although infection before 20 weeks of gestation can result in severe congenital varicella syndrome (skin lesions, limb paresis, chorioretinitis, and limb hypoplasia), the actual incidence was rare (less than 1% to 2%) in a recent prospective study of more than 3000 infected pregnant women (Enders et al., 1994). The greatest risk posed to the fetus is the mother's infection with primary varicella during the later part of the pregnancy, especially around the time of delivery. Consequences in the fetus of maternal infection at this time include neonatal VZV and disseminated varicella. The risk for disseminated varicella infection is 30% when the mother develops the chickenpox rash between the period 5 days before and 2 days after delivery. Although disseminated varicella is associated with severe neonatal morbidity and mortality, it may be prevented by use of the VZV immune globulin (Sison and Sever, 1993). If the maternal infection occurs after delivery, the infant is at risk for developing chickenpox. Although this disease is usually mild, there is a small increase in risk for a severe case of chickenpox in the newborn.

Diagnosis of chickenpox is usually straightforward because of the classic presentation of the rash, but if the diagnosis is in question, varicella-specific IgM antibodies can be helpful in diagnosing recent infection and varicella-specific IgG for assessing long-term immunity. The IgM test will not show positivity for at least several days after the onset of the rash. If a pregnant woman has been exposed to varicella but is seronegative, she should receive varicella-zoster immune globulin (VZIG) intramuscularly in a dose of 0.125 ml/kg. After that period the mother will have mounted her immune response and passed her antibodies to the fetus. Infants born to mothers who have contracted chickenpox in the period between 5 days before and 2 days after delivery should receive VZIG to decrease the risk of disseminated varicella.

GROUP B STREPTOCOCCAL INFECTION

Group B *Streptococcus* (GBS) is present in the vaginal and rectal areas of 15% to 40% of pregnant women. Although clinical disease in women is uncommon, the newborn can suffer consequences from contact with an infected maternal birth canal, including meningitis, neurologic complications, and death. Of the neonates born to women who are carriers of GBS, colonization occurs in 40% to 73%, but clinical disease develops in only 1 in 50 infants born to women in whom colonization has occurred. Neonatal sepsis from GSB develops in approximately 1 in 1000 infants, with a 50% mortality rate. The risk of neonatal disease is increased for those fetuses born to mothers who have preterm delivery, multiple gestations, prolonged rupture of membranes, heavy colonization of GBS, and low maternal levels of circulating antibodies to GBS.

In 1992 ACOG recommended that routine cultures of the urine, the outer third of the vagina, and the rectum be obtained in the pregnant women with a history of a *previous child* with GBS infection or in a pregnant woman with risk factors such as preterm labor, preterm premature rupture of membranes, prolonged rupture of membrane, or fever during delivery. Studies of treatment of this subgroup of women with positive cultures have demonstrated a significant reduction in vertical transmission of GBS and neonatal mortality from group B streptococcal sepsis. Even though carriage of GBS is common in women (especially in those with the aforementioned risk factors), the carrier status often changes spontaneously during pregnancy. Thus screening cultures are not always reliable, even in women at high risk. Cultures negative for GBS are not uncommon for many women who may in fact show GBS colonization. ACOG, in recent considerations of the prevention of neonatal GBS infection, proposed that empiric treatment be initiated without culturing in pregnant women with any of the aforementioned risk factors. The American Academy of Pediatrics' committees on infectious diseases in the fetus and newborn have recommended that screening with vaginal and anorectal cultures occur for *all* pregnant women between 26 and 28 weeks of gestation. If surveillance cultures are positive for GBS near the time of delivery and if the woman has risk factors at the time of labor (preterm labor, preterm premature rupture of membranes, prolonged rupture of membranes, or maternal fever during labor), intravenous penicillin (or erythromycin if the patient is allergic to penicillin) should be administered. ACOG concurs with the treatment recommendations but does not yet advocate routine screening with cultures.

TOXOPLASMOSIS

Toxoplasma gondii is a protozoan infection to which most adults have been exposed as children and have antibody protection. The cat is the predominant host for *Toxoplasma gondii*. When adults contract toxoplasma infection, it usually is asymptomatic or associated with mild constitutional symptoms and lymphadenopathy except in the immunocompromised host. The actual prevalence of seropositive pregnant women varies depending on the geographic area and mode of exposure to the sources of *Toxoplasma gondii*: cats or raw meat. Primary infection during pregnancy can be detrimental to the fetus, resulting in seizures, hydrocephaly, microcephaly, and jaundice. Approximately 4100 of 4.1 million infants born each year in the United States have congenital toxoplasma infection (Remington and Klein, 1995). The more severe cases of toxoplasmosis usually are seen in fetuses exposed earlier in pregnancy, and there can be a 60% reduction in the rate of sequelae of infection if treated (Wilson and Remington, 1980). Long-term consequences of exposure are unpredictable. The incidence of contracting infection among seronegative women is 5%.

Although many groups have advocated routine prenatal screening and identification of seronegative women, universal screening has not been established because it has not been shown to be cost effective and laboratory measurements of antibody levels have been difficult to standardize and interpret. The advent of fetal blood sampling has improved the ability for diagnosing potentially affected fetuses.

At present, primary infection can be identified by any one of a number of antibody tests (Remington and Klein, 1995). To determine that the infection is primary, it is necessary to show a conversion of a titer from negative to positive or a rise in titer from low to high. The timing of the serologic test is important inasmuch as the peak of the titer may be missed if blood is drawn late after the clinical presentation. Because of the lack of sensitivity of many commonly used measurements of IgM, it also is important to use methods that are adequate in differentiating IgM toxoplasmosis from natural IgM, rheumatoid factor, and antinuclear antibody. Capture IgM, enzyme-linked immunosorbent assay (ELISA), and IgM-ISAGA are more sensitive measures. Remington and Klein (1995) indicated that any patient with a Sabin-Feldman dye test or an indirect fluorescent antibody (IFA) test titer of greater than 300 IU/ml or 1:1000 and an IgM IFA test titer of 1:80 or higher or a capture IgM ELISA of 2 or greater is presumed to have recently acquired infection. When primary infection is identified after 14 weeks' gestation, treatment should be instituted with pyrimethamine and sulfadiazine plus leucovorin. Safety of treatment with these drugs before 14 weeks has not been established. Prevention should be the goal, and advising pregnant women to avoid undercooked meat or contact with materials contaminated with cat feces is important.

Table 50-1 summarizes the current recommendations regarding evaluation and management of those infections already discussed that occur during pregnancy.

IMMUNIZATION

Immunization is important for all women of reproductive age, the objective should be to immunize women before pregnancy. In 1982 ACOG issued recommendations regarding immunization during pregnancy. The updated recommendations concluded that immunization during pregnancy should be reserved for the specific situations summarized in Table 50-2 and that if a pregnant woman requires an immunization, she should not receive vaccines containing live virus such as measles, mumps, or rubella. If a woman is in a endemic area and she is at high risk for exposure, then poliomyelitis and yellow fever vaccines may be adminis-

Table 50-1 Evaluation and management of common infectious diseases during pregnancy

Infectious disease	Clinical symptoms in pregnant woman	Clinical manifestations in fetus	Fetal infection rate	General guidelines for management
Cytomegalovirus	None	CMV infection, progressive deafness, learning disabilities, cerebral palsy, hydrocephalus, eye problems, increased risk of prematurity, LBW, IUGR	40%-50% in fetuses exposed to mother with primary infection	Hand washing/hygienic measures for high-risk groups (e.g., women working in day-care centers) No routine screening because no specific preventive treatment
Genital herpes simplex (HSV-2, HSV-1)	Painful vesicular lesions but can be asymptomatic carriers	First trimester: spontaneous abortion, severe congenital malformations Second and third trimesters: increase perinatal mortality	Possibly 8% in fetuses exposed to recurrent HSV	Inspection of female genital tract before delivery; if lesions present, delivery by cesaran section
Chlamydia and gonorrhea	Acute disease (see text) or asymptomatic carrier	? prematurity, PROM, IUGR, chorioamnionitis, disseminated infection		Screening with cervical cultures CDC advocates early in pregnancy; repeat during third trimester for high-risk women
Syphilis	Primary syphilis, secondary syphilis or asymptomatic	Congenital syphilis Increased risk for miscarriage and stillbirth		Screen all pregnant women with VRDL at first prenatal visit; repeat screening during second and third trimesters if high risk. Treat using standard protocols, and follow nontreponemal titers once a month for 3 mo. If there is not fourfold decrease, repeat treatment
Rubella (German measles)	Asymptomatic, slight fever, swollen lymph glands	Congenital rubella syndrome: cardiac defects, sensorineural and hearing loss, cataracts Risk for LBW, IUGR	Up to 50% during first 8 wk of pregnancy	Screening and immunization of all seronegative women of reproductive age; immunization contraindicated if pregnant or 3 mo. before conception because rubella vaccine is live attenuated virus
Varicella (chickenpox and zoster)	If contracted during pregnancy, high rate of varicella pneumonia and mortality	First trimester: ? association with limb hypoplasia, cutaneous scars, chorioretinitis, cataracts, cortical atrophy, microcephaly Within 5 days of onset of rash at delivery: neonatal varicella with associated high death rate	30% develop neonatal varicella if within 5 days of exposure at time of delivery	If exposed within 5 days of delivery, administer VZIG at delivery or within 24 hrs of delivery Screening for IgG antibody titers only if mother has negative history for chickenpox and has been exposed to infection. If seronegative, adminster VZIG after exposure
Parvovirus B19	Asymptomatic or constitutional symptoms and rash	Increased risk of nonimmune fetal hydrops before 20-wk gestation	Approximately 15% fetal death rate (United Kingdom study)	Offer IgM and IgG antibody testing. Counsel woman on risks to fetus. Monitor pregnancy with serial ultrasound and alpha-feto protein measurements
Toxoplasmosis	Asymptomatic	Seizures, hydrocephaly, microcephaly jaundice, chorioretinitis Increased risk of prematurity, LBW, IUGR		Treatment with pyrimethamine and sulfadiazine after 14 wk gestation. Routine prenatal screening impractical at this time. See text
Hepatitis B	Active disease; chronic carrier state	Acute fulminant hepatitis	10% during first trimester; 50%-60% during third trimester	Obtain serology in all pregnant women for HBsAg during first trimester; repeat if at high risk during third trimester and at delivery

continued

Table 50-1 Evaluation and management of common infectious diseases during pregnancy *(continued)*

Infectious disease	Clinical symptoms in pregnant woman	Clinical manifestations in fetus	Fetal infection rate	General guidelines for management
Hepatitis B *(continued)*				If positive, adminster 0.5 ml of hepatitis immune globulin during first 12 hr of life; then proceed with immunization with Heptavax during wk 1, 1 mo later, and at 6 mo.
Group B streptococcal infection	Asymptomatic carriers	Meningitis, neurologic complications, death	1 in 1000 live births develop neonatal sepsis	Pregnant women at high risk should be screened with vaginal and anorectal cultures and treated during labor with penicillin if positive, for GBS Screening all pregnant women during gestational wk 26-28 has been advocated by some but still remains controversial

Data from Remington JS, Klein JO, editors: *Infectious diseases of the fetus and newborn infant* ed 4, Philadelphia, 1995, WB Saunders.
LBW, low birth weight; IUGR, intrauterine growth retardation; PROM, premature rupture of membranes

Table 50-2 Immunization during pregnancy

Immunobiologic agent	Risk from disease to pregnant woman	Risk from disease to fetus or neonate	Type of immunizing agent	Risk from immunizing agent to fetus	Indications for immunization during pregnancy	Dose schedule	Comments
Live virus vaccines							
Measles	Significant morbidity, low mortality; not altered by pregnancy	Significant increase in abortion rate; may cause malformations	Live attenuated virus vaccine	None confirmed	Contraindicated (see immune globulins)	Single dose SC, preferably as measles-mumps-rubella*	Vaccination of susceptible women should be part of post-partum care
Mumps	Low morbidity and mortality; not altered by pregnancy	Probable increased rate of abortion in first trimester	Live attenuated virus vaccine	None confirmed	Contraindicated	Single dose SC, preferably as measles-, mumps-, rubella	Vaccination of susceptible women should be part of post-partum care
Poliomyelitis	No increased incidence in pregnancy, but may be more severe if it does occur	Anoxic fetal damage reported; 50% mortality in neonatal disease	Live attenuated virus (oral polio vaccine [OPV]) and enhanced, potency inactivated virus (e-IPV) vaccine†	None confirmed	Not routinely recomended for women in U.S., except persons at increased risk of exposure	Primary: 2 doses of e-IPV SC at 4-8 wk intervals and a 3rd dose 6-12 mos after the 2nd dose. Immediate protection: 1 dose OPV orally (in out-break setting)	Vaccine indicated for susceptible pregnant women traveling in endemic areas or in other high risk situations
Rubella	Low morbidity and mortality; not altered by pregnancy	High rate of abortion and congenital rubella syndrome	Live attenuated virus vaccine	None confirmed	Contraindicated	Single dose SC, preferably as measles—mumps-, rubella	Teratogenicity of vacine is theoretic, not confirmed to date; vaccination of susceptible women should be part of post-partum care

continued

Table 50-2 Immunization during pregnancy *(continued)*

Immunobiologic agent	Risk from disease to pregnant woman	Risk from disease to fetus or neonate	Type of immunizing agent	Risk from immunizing agent to fetus	Indications for immunization during pregnancy	Dose schedule	Comments
Live virus vaccines *(continued)*							
Yellow fever	Significant morbidity and mortality; not altered by pregnancy	Unknown	Live attenuated virus vaccine	Unknown	Contraindicated except if exposure is unavoidable	Single dose SC	Postponement of travel preferable to vaccination, if possible
Inactivated virus vaccines							
Influenza	Possible increase in morbidity and mortality during epidemic of new antigenic strain	Possible increased abortion rate; no malformations confirmed	Inactivated virus vaccine	None confirmed	Women with serious underlying diseases; public health authorities to be consulted for current recommendation	One dose IM every yr	
Rabies	Near 100% fatality; not altered by pregnancy	Determined by maternal disease	Killed virus vaccine	Unknown	Indications for prophylaxis not altered by pregnancy; each case considered individually	Public health authorities to be consulted for indications, dosage, and route of administration	
Hepatitis B	Possible increased severity during third trimester	Possible increase in abortion rate and prematurity; neonatal hepatitis can occur; high risk of newborn carrier state	Recombinant vaccine	None reported	Pre- and post-exposure for women at risk of infection	Three- or four-dose series IM	Used with hepatitis B immune globulin for some exposures; exposed newborn needs vaccination as soon as possible
Inactivated bacterial vaccines							
Cholera	Significant morbidity and mortality; more severe during third trimester	Increased risk of fetal death during third-trimester maternal illness	Killed bacterial vaccine	None confirmed	Indications not altered by pregnancy; vaccination recommended only in unusual outbreak situations	Single dose SC or IM, depending on manufacturer's recommendations when indicated	
Plague	Significant morbidity and mortality; not altered by pregnancy	Determined by maternal disease	Killed bacterial vaccine	None reported	Selective vaccination of exposed persons	Public health authorities to be consulted for indications, dosage, and route of administration	
Pneumococcus	No increased risk during pregnancy; no increase in severity of disease	Unknown	Polyvalent polysaccharide vaccine	No data available on use during pregnancy	Indications not altered by pregnancy; vaccine used only for high-risk individuals	In adults, 1 SC or IM dose only; consider repeat dose in 6 yrs for high-risk individuals	

continued

Table 50-2 Immunization during pregnancy *(continued)*

Immunobiologic agent	Risk from disease to pregnant woman	Risk from disease to fetus or neonate	Type of immunizing agent	Risk from immunizing agent to fetus	Indications for immunization during pregnancy	Dose schedule	Comments
Inactivated bacterial vaccines *(continued)*							
Typhoid	Significant morbidity and mortality; not altered by pregnancy	Unknown	Killed or live attenuated oral bacterial vaccine	None confirmed	Not recommended routinely except for close, continued exposure or travel to endemic areas	Killed: Primary: 2 injections SC at least 4 wks apart. Booster: Single dose SC or ID (depending on type of product used) every 3 yrs. Oral: Primary: 4 doses on alternate days. Booster: Schedule not yet determined	
Toxoids							
Tetanus, diphtheria	Severe morbidity; tetanus mortality 30%, diphtheria mortality 10%; unaltered by pregnancy	Neonatal tetanus mortality 60%	Combined tetanus-diphtheria toxoids preferred: adult tetanus-diphtheria formulation	None confirmed	Lack of primary series, or no booster within past 10 yrs	Primary: 2 doses IM at 1-2-mo interval with a 3rd dose 6-12 mos after the 2nd. Booster: Single dose IM every 10 yrs, after completio of primary series	Updating of immune status should be part of antepartum care
Specific immune globulins							
Hepatitis B	Possible increased severity during third trimester	Possible increase in abortion rate and prematurity; neonatal hepatitis can occur; high risk of carriage in newborn	Hepatitis B immune globulin	None reported	Postexposure prophylaxis	Depends on exposure; consult Immunization Practices Advisory Committee recommendations (IM)	Usually given with HBV vaccine; exposed newborn needs immediate postexposure prophylaxis
Rabies	Near 100% fatality; not altered by pregnancy	Determined by maternal disease	Rabies immune globulin	None reported	Postexposure prophylaxis	Half dose at injury site, half dose in deltoid	Used in conjunction with rabies killed virus vaccine
Tetanus	Severe morbidity; mortality 21%	Neonatal tetanus mortality 60%	Tetanus immune globulin	None reported	Postexposure prophylaxis	One dose IM	Used in conjunction with tetanus toxoid

continued

Table 50-2 Immunization during pregnancy *(continued)*

Immunobiologic agent	Risk from disease to pregnant woman	Risk from disease to fetus or neonate	Type of immunizing agent	Risk from immunizing agent to fetus	Indications for immunization during pregnancy	Dose schedule	Comments
Specific immune globulins *(continued)*							
Varicella	Possible increase in severe varicella pneumonia	Can cause congenital varicella with increased mortality in neonatal period; very rarely causes congenital defects	Varicella-zoster immune globulin (obtained from the American Red Cross)	None reported	Can be considered for healthy pregnant women exposed to varicella to protect against maternal, not congenital, infection	One dose IM within 96 hrs of exposure	Indicated also for newborns of mothers who developed varicella within 4 dys prior to delivery or 2 dys following delivery; approx. 90-95% of adults are immune to varicella; not indicated for prevention of congenital varicella
Standard immune globulins							
Hepatitis A	Possible increased severity during third trimester	Probable increse in abortion rate and prematurity; possible transmission to neonate at delivery if mother is incubating the virus or is acutely ill at that time	Standard immune globulin	None reported	Postexposure prophylaxis	0.02 ml/kg IM in one dose of immune globulin	Immune globulin should be given as soon as possible and within 2 wks of exposure; infants born to mothers who are incubating the virus or are acutely ill at delivery should receive one dose of 0.5 ml as soon as possible after birth
Measles	Significant morbidity, low mortality; not altered by pregnancy	Significant increase in abortion rate; may cause malformations	Standard immune globulin	None reported	Postexposure prophylaxis	0.25 ml/kg IM in one dose of immune globulin, up to 15 ml	Unclear if it prevents abortion; must be given within 6 dys of exposure

From ACOG technical bulletin, no. 160, Oct 1991.

SC, subcutaneously; PO, orally; IM, intramuscularly; ID, intradermally.

*Two doses necessary for adequate vaccination of students entering institutions of higher education, newly hired medical personnel, and international travelers.

†Inactivated polio vaccine recommended for nonimmunized adults at incrased risk.

tered. Routine vaccination with tetanus and diphtheria toxoids and influenza is safe during pregnancy. Because prolonged viral shedding after immunization can occur up to 3 months, women of reproductive age who receive live vaccines should be advised to use contraception to avoid pregnancy although fetuses with sequelae of infection from live virus vaccination have never been reported.

BIBLIOGRAPHY

General

Cefalo R, Moos M: *Preconceptional health care: a practical Guide,* ed 2, St Louis, 1995, Mosby.

Charles D: *Obstetrical and perinatal Infections,* St Louis, 1993, Mosby.

Hollingsworth DR, Resnik R: *Medical counseling before pregnancy,* New York, 1988, Churchill Livingstone.

Reilly K, Clemenson N: Infections complicating pregnancy, *Prim Care* 20:665, 1993.

Remington JS, Klein JO, editors: *Infectious diseases of the fetus and newborn infant,* 4 ed, Philadelphia, 1995, WB Saunders Co.

U.S. Preventive Health Task Force: *Guide to clinical preventive services: an assessment of the effectiveness of 169 interventions,* Baltimore, 1989, Williams & Wilkins.

Cytomegalovirus

Daffos F et al: Prenatal management of 746 pregnancies at risk for congenital toxoplasmosis, *N Engl J Med* 318:271, 1988.

Fowler KB et al: The outcome of congenital cytomegalovirus infection in relation to maternal antibody status, *N Engl J Med* 326:663, 1992.

Hunter K et al: Prenatal screening of pregnant women for infections due to cytomegalovirus, Epstein Barr, herpes, rubella and *Toxoplasma gondii, Am J Obstet Gyncol* 145:269, 1983.

Medearis D: CMV immunity: imperfect but protective, *N Engl J Med* 306:985, 1982.

Nankervis G et al: A prospective study of maternal cytomegalovirus infection and its effect on the fetus, *Am J Obstet Gynecol* 149:435, 1984.

Stagno S: Characteristics of CMV infection in pregnancy, *N Engl J Med* 313:1270, 1985.

Stagno S: Cytomegalovirus. In Remington JS, Klein JO, editors: *Infectious diseases of the Fetus and newborn infant,* ed 4, Philadelphia, 1995, WB Saunders.

Stagno S et al: Congenital cytomegalovirus infection: occurrence in an immune population, *N Engl J Med* 296:1254, 1977.

Stagno S et al: Congenital cytomegalovirus infection: the relative importance of primary and recurrent maternal infection, *N Engl J Med* 306:945, 1982.

Yow M, Demmler G: Congenital cytomegalovirus disease—20 years is long enough, *N Engl J Med* 326:702, 1992.

Group B streptococcal infection

American College of Obstetricians and Gynecologists: *Group B streptococcal infections in pregnancy* (Tech Bull No 170), Washington, DC, 1992, The College.

American College of Obstetricians and Gynecologists, Committee on Obstetric Practice: *Prevention of neonatal group B streptococcal infections,* (draft), Oct 7, 1994.

Baker CJ: From the National Institutes of Health: summary of the workshop in perinatal infections due to Group B streptococcus, *J Infect Dis* 136:137, 1977.

Boyer KM, Gotoff SP: Prevention of early onset neonatal group B streptococcal disease with selective intrapartum chemoprophylaxis, *N Engl J Med* 314:1665, 1986.

American Academy of Pediatrics, Committee on Infectious Diseases and Committee on Fetus and Newborn: Guidelines for prevention of group B streptococcal (GBS) infection by chemoprophylaxis, *Pediatrics* 90:775, 1992.

McKenzie H et al: Risk of preterm delivery in pregnant women with group B streptococcal urinary infections or urinary antibodies to group B streptococcal and *E. coli* antigens, *Br J Obstet Gynaecol* 101:107, 1994.

Minkoff HL, Mead P: An obstetric approach to the prevention of early onset group B beta-hemolytic streptococcal sepsis, *Am J Obstet Gyncol* 154:973, 1986.

Minkoff HL et al: Vaginal colonization with group B beta-hemolytic streptococcus as a risk factor for post-cesarean section febrile morbidity, *Am J Obstet Gynecol* 142:992, 1982.

Strickland D, Yeomans E, Hankins G: Cost effectiveness of intrapartum screening and treatment for maternal group B streptococci colonization, *Am J Obstet Gynecol* 163:4, 1990.

Yancey M et al: Peripartum infection associated with vaginal group B streptococcal colonization, *Obstet Gynecol* 84:816, 1994.

Hepatitis

American College of Obstetricians and Gynecologists: *Hepatitis in pregnancy* (Tech Bull No 174), Washington, DC, Nov 1992, The College.

Centers for Disease Control and Prevention: Maternal hepatitis B screening practices—California, Connecticut, Kansas, and United States, 1992-1993, *JAMA* 271:1819, 1994.

Immunization Practices Advisory Committee: Prevention of preinatal transmission of hepatitis B virus: prenatal screening of all pregnant women for hepatitis B surface antigen, *MMWR* 37:341, 1988.

Ohto H and the Vertical Transmission of Hepatitis C Virus Collaborative Study Group: Transmission of hepatitis C from mothers to infants, *N Engl J Med* 330:744, 1994.

Leikin E et al: Epidemiologic predictors of hepatitis C virus infection in pregnant women, *Obstet Gynecol* 84:529, 1994.

Silverman N et al: Hepatitis C virus in pregnancy: seroprevalence and risk factors in infection, *Am J Obstet Gynecol* 169:583, 1993.

Snydman D: Hepatitis in pregnancy, *N Engl J Med* 313:1398, 1985.

Zeldis J, Crumpacker C: Hepatitis. In Remington JS, Klein JO, editors: *Infectious disease of the fetus and newborn infant,* ed 4, Philadelphia, 1995, WB Saunders.

Herpes virus infections

Baker DA: Herpes and pregnancy: new management, *Clin Obstet Gynecol* 33:253, 1990.

Brown ZA et al: Genital herpes in pregnancy: risk factors associated with recurrences and asymptomatic viral shedding, *Am J Obstet Gynecol* 153:24, 1985.

Brown ZA et al: Effects on infants of a first episode of genital herpes during pregnancy, *N Engl J Med* 317:1246, 1987.

Brown ZA et al: Neonatal herpes simplex virus infection in relation to asymptomatic maternal infection at the time of labor, *N Engl J Med* 324:1247, 1991.

Cone RW et al: Frequent detection of genital herpes simplex virus DNA by polymerase chain reaction among pregnant women, *JAMA* 272:792, 1994.

Enders G et al: Consequences of varicella and herpes zoster in pregnancy: prospective study of 1739 cases, *Lancet* 343:1547, 1994.

Harger JA et al: Characteristics and management of pregnancy in women with genital herpes simplex virus infection, *Am J Obstet Gynecol* 145:784, 1983.

Kulhanjian JA et al: Identification of women at unsuspected risk of primary infection with herpes simplex virus type 2 during pregnancy, *N Engl J Med* 326:916, 1992.

Nahmias AJ et al: Perinatal risk associated with maternal genital herpes simplex virus infection, *Am J Obstet Gynecol* 110:285, 1971.

Paryani SG, Arvin AM: Intrauterine infection with varicella-zoster virus after maternal varicella, *N Engl J Med* 314:1542, 1986.

Prober CG: Herpetic vaginitis in 1933, *Clin Obstet Gynecol* 36:177, 1993.

Prober CG et al: Use of routine viral cultures at delivery to identify neonates exposed to herpes simplex virus, *N Engl J Med* 318:887, 1988.

Randolph AG, Washington AE, Prober CG: Cesarean delivery for women presenting with genital herpes lesions: efficacy, risks and costs, *JAMA* 270:77, 1993.

Spence M: Genital infections in pregnancy, *Med Clinic North Am* 61:139, 1977.

Stagno S, Whitley R: Herpesvirus infections of pregnancy. I. Cytomegalovirus and Epstein, Barr virus infections, *N Engl J Med* 313:1270, 1985.

Stagno S, Whitley R: Herpesvirus infections of pregnancy. II. Herpes simplex virus and varicella zoster virus infection, *N Engl J Med* 313:1327, 1985.

Parvovirus B19

Hall CJ: Parvovirus B19 infection in pregnancy, *Arch Dis Child* 71:F4, 1994.

Kirchner J: Erythema infectiosum and other parvovirus B19 infections, *Am Fam Phys* 50:335, 1994.

Public Health Laboratory Service Working Party on Fifth Disease: Prospective study of human parvovirus (B19) infection in pregnancy, 300:1166, 1990.

Torok T: Human parvovirus B19 infection in pregnancy, *Pediatr Infect Dis J* 9:772, 1990.

Torok T: Human parvovirus B19. In Remington JS, Klein JO, editors: *Infectious diseases of the fetus and newborn infant,* Philadelphia, 1995, WB Saunders.

Rubella

American College of Obstetricians and Gynecologists: *Rubella and pregnancy* (Tech Bull No 171), Washington, DC, 1992, The College.

Centers for Disease Control, Immunization Practices Advisory Committee: Increase in rubella and congenital rubella syndrome, United States 1988-1990, *MMWR* 40:93, 1991.

Cooper L, Preblud S, Alford C: Rubella. In Remington JS, Klein JO, editors: *Infectious disease of the fetus and newborn infant,* ed 4, Philadelphia, 1995, WB Saunders.

Miller E, Cradock-Watson JE, Pollack TM: Consequences of confirmed maternal rubella at successive stages of pregnancy, *Lancet* 2:781, 1982.

Syphilis

Centers for Disease Control: Guideline for the prevention and control of congenital syphilis, *MMWR* 37:51, 1988.

Centers for Disease Control: Sexually transmitted disease treatment guidelines, *MMWR* 38:5, 1989.

Dorfman DH, Glaser JH: Congenital syphilis presenting in infants after the newborn period, *N Engl J Med* 323:1299, 1990.

Ingall D, Sanchez P, Musher D: Syphilis. In Remington JS, Klein JO, editors: *Infectious Diseases of the fetus and newborn infant,* ed 4, Philadelphia: 1995, WB Saunders.

McFarlin B et al: Epidemic syphilis: maternal fators associated with congenital infection, *Am J Obstet Gynecol* 170:535, 1994.

Wendel GD Jr, et al: Penicillin allergy and desensitization in serious infections during pregnancy, *N Engl J Med* 312:1229, 1985.

Toxoplasmosis

American College of Obstetricians and Gynecologists: *Perinatal viral and perinatal infections* (Tech Bull No 177), Washington, DC, 1992, The College.

Guerina N, et al: Neonatal serologic screening and early treatment for congenital *Toxoplasma gondii* infection, *N Engl J Med* 330:1858, 1994.

McCabe R, Remington JS: Toxoplasmosis: the time has come, *N Engl J Med* 318:313, 1988 (editorial).

Wilson CB, Remington JS: What can be done to prevent congenital toxoplasmosis? *Am J Obstet Gynecol* 138:357, 1980.

Varicella

Enders G. et al: Consequences of varicella and herpes zoster in pregnancy: prospective study of 1739 cases, *Lancet* 343:1548, 1994.

Sison AV, Sever JL: Viral infections. In Charles D: *Obstetrical and perinatal infections,* St Louis: 1993, Mosby.

Immunization in pregnancy

American College of Obstetricians and Gynecologists: *Immunization during pregnancy* (Tech Bull No 64), Washington, DC, May 1982, The College.

American College of Physicians: Adult immunizations 1994, *Ann Intern Med* 121:540, 1994.

Fedson D: Adult vaccination: summary of the National Vaccine Advisory Committee Report, *JAMA* 272:1133, 1994.

51 Preeclampsia

Mari-Paule Thiet and Bruce B. Feinberg

Preeclampsia remains a major clinical problem and challenge in obstetrics. Complications from this disease result in a maternal mortality rate in the United States second only to that of pulmonary embolism. It is also a leading cause of fetal growth retardation, intrauterine fetal demise, and indicated preterm birth. Labeled the "disease of theories," preeclampsia continues to have an unknown cause. Worsening the dilemma, the only proven cure for the disease remains placental delivery. The inadequacy of effective therapeutic interventions largely stems from our limited understanding of the causative factor(s) and pathophysiologic features of the disease.

TERMINOLOGY

Since the disease is still poorly understood a variety of descriptive names have been used. These include pregnancy-induced hypertension, pregnancy-aggravated hypertension, preeclampsia, toxemia, preeclamptic toxemia, gestational hypertension, and edema-proteinuric-hypertensive gestosis. The Committee on Terminology of the American College of Obstetricians and Gynecologists groups patients as follows: (1) pregnancy-induced hypertension (hypertension without proteinuria), (2) preeclampsia (hypertension with proteinuria), and (3) eclampsia (preeclampsia with seizure activity).

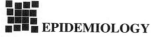

EPIDEMIOLOGY

Preeclampsia complicates 5% to 7% of pregnancies beyond 20 weeks' gestation. Eclampsia is much less frequent, occurring in 0.1% of pregnancies. The disorder is primarily a disease of primigravidas. Subsequent gestations of the same paternity are afforded some degree of adaptive protection from recurrence. If paternity changes, however, the risk of development of preeclampsia approaches that of the primigravida. Other risk factors for the development of preeclampsia include extremes of maternal age, gestations with large placental mass (e.g., twins, molar gestation), presence of underlying medical disorders (e.g., chronic hypertension, renal disease, autoimmune diseases, and diabetes mellitus) and a family history of preeclampsia (see box, below).

CAUSE

Although historically a variety of theories have been proposed the current areas of investigation focus on the following.

Abnormal eicosanoid metabolism

In vitro studies have demonstrated an increased thromboxane to prostacyclin ratio. The net effect of this imbalance leads to vasoconstriction. It is speculated that it may clinically lead to hypertension and end-organ changes associated with preeclampsia.

RISK FACTORS FOR PREECLAMPSIA

Primigravida
Extremes of maternal age
Gestations with large placental mass (e.g., twins)
Chronic hypertension
Diabetes
Renal disease
Autoimmune disease
Family history
Preclampsia in prior pregnancy

Circulating toxins

Recent reports demonstrate increased levels in circulating lipid peroxides in preeclamptic patients. This increase in lipid peroxides may inhibit endogenous nitric oxide, a potent vasodilator, eventually leading to vasoconstriction and clinical hypertension.

Endothelial cell injury

Vascular endothelial injury has been heralded recently as a consistent finding in preeclamptic pregnancies. The precise nature of the offending agent(s) resulting in endothelial cell damage has yet to be identified.

Immunologic factors

The clinical manifestations of preeclampsia could be attributed to an immune vasculitis caused by circulating immune complexes. A vasculitic cause unifies the preceding theories in the pathogenesis of preeclampsia. To date, however, the evidence supporting an immune complex vasculitis in preeclampsia is inconsistent.

DIAGNOSIS OF PREECLAMPSIA
Clinical presentation

Hypertension, proteinuria, and mild preeclampsia. Hypertension is defined as a blood pressure of 140/90 mm Hg, or a rise in systolic BP >30mm Hg, or a diastolic BP rise of 15 mm Hg over first trimester BP readings on two separate occasions at least 6 hours apart. The minimal proteinuric requirements are 300 mg in a 24-hour period or 100 mg/dl in at least two random urine samples 6 hours apart. Though many have traditionally included nondependent edema (e.g., facial, periorbital, hands) in their clinical criteria for preeclampsia, its presence is generally so common that it is not a clinically useful tool.

Preeclampsia has a wide clinical spectrum ranging from mild disease, such as minimal hypertension and proteinuria, to severe systemic disease. The overwhelming majority of patients with preeclampsia usually have mild disease, present in the late third trimester, and diagnosis is fairly straightforward.

Severe preeclampsia. Less frequent are patients with severe preeclampsia. Clinical indicators of severe preeclampsia may include diastolic hypertension >110 mm Hg, 5 g or more of urinary protein in a 24-hour period, visual disturbances, epigastric pain, headache, pulmonary edema, or oliguria (see box, below). Laboratory result abnormalities associated with severe preeclampsia may include elevated liver transaminases, thrombocytopenia, hyperbilirubinemia,

---

CRITERIA FOR SEVERE PREECLAMPSIA

Diastolic blood pressure >110 mm Hg
Proteinuria >5 g/24-hr collection
Visual disturbances, such as scotomata, blindness, diplopia
Headache
Epigastric pain
Pulmonary edema
Oliguria: <400 ml urine/24-hr collection
Laboratory abnormalities: elevated liver transaminases, serum creatinine, thrombocytopenia, hyperbilirubinemia
Fetal growth retardation

LABORATORY ASSESSMENT OF PREECLAMPSIA

Electrolytes
Serum creatinine level
Uric acid level
Liver transaminase levels
Complete blood count (including platelets)
Coagulation profile
24-hr Urine collection for total protein and creatinine clearance levels
Blood type and screen

---

and elevated serum uric acid levels and creatinine (see box, above). Fetal growth retardation may occasionally be the sole indicator of severe disease. **HELLP syndrome** is an acronym for hemolysis, elevated liver enzymes, and low platelets; it is usually an advanced stage of preeclampsia associated with disseminated intravascular coagulation. All of the findings listed reflect the systemic end-organ damage caused by preeclampsia.

Differential diagnosis

Since preeclampsia is a multiorgan system disease and is a clinical diagnosis its clinical and laboratory findings are often misdiagnosed as acute illnesses unrelated to pregnancy. As opposed to the typical mild and severe preeclamptics described previously, occasionally patients may have very atypical presentations. Liver or renal disease, cholecystitis, hemorrhage, immune thrombocytopenic purpura, epilepsy, and heart failure are not uncommon admitting diagnoses in patients with atypical severe preeclampsia. In evaluating a pregnant patient with any of the findings described the importance of considering preeclampsia as the primary diagnosis cannot be overemphasized (see box, below).

Complications of preeclampsia

Complications of preeclampsia result in a maternal mortality rate of 3/100,000 live births in the United States. Maternal morbidity may include central nervous system complications (e.g., strokes, seizures, intracerebral hemorrhage, and blindness), disseminated intravascular coagulation, hepatic failure

---

DIFFERENTIAL DIAGNOSIS FOR PREECLAMPSIA

Hepatobiliary disease: hepatitis, cholestasis, cholecystitis
Pancreatitis
Appendicitis
Renal disease: nephrotic syndrome, glomerulonephritis, renal failure, renal artery stenosis
Pheochromocytoma
Primary hyperaldosteronism
Systemic lupus erythematosus
Immune thrombocytopenic purpura
Thrombotic thrombocytopenic purpura
Hemolytic uremic syndrome
Epilepsy
CNS disease: cerebral tumor or hemorrhage, cerebritis, encephalitis
Hysteria

CNS, central nervous system.

or rupture, and abruptio placentae leading to maternal hemorrhage and acute renal failure. From a fetal perspective mortality rate markedly increases with rising maternal diastolic BP and proteinuria. For example, diastolic BP greater than 95 mm Hg are associated with a threefold rise in the fetal death rate. Fetal morbidity may include intrauterine growth retardation, fetal acidemia, and complications of iatrogenic preterm birth (e.g., respiratory distress syndrome, intraventricular hemorrhage, and necrotizing enterocolitis).

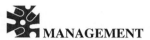

MANAGEMENT

Overview

The only definitive treatment for preeclampsia remains delivery. However, obstetric management is often influenced by the severity of the disease, gestational age at diagnosis, pulmonary maturation of the fetus, and "ripeness" of the maternal cervix. Depending on these factors, one considers conservative, expectant management versus a more aggressive interventional approach. If there is evidence of intrauterine fetal distress beyond viability, delivery is usually indicated regardless of the gestational age or fetal pulmonary maturity. Similarly if maternal findings suggest severe preeclampsia little is to be gained with conservative therapy. Serious maternal sequelae including acute renal failure, disseminated intravascular coagulation, HELLP syndrome, abruption, and eclampsia as well as intrauterine fetal death are markedly increased with conservative therapy of severe preeclampsia. Patients with preterm gestations and mild preeclampsia, however, can successfully continue their pregnancies for weeks with close maternal and fetal observation. Factors influencing early intervention in these patients include the subsequent development of severe preeclampsia, nonreassuring fetal surveillance findings, and evidence of fetal pulmonary maturation.

Antepartum conservative management of preeclampsia

Patients are generally hospitalized for bed rest and observation. BP, urine dipstick for protein, symptoms of severe preeclampsia, and fetal heart tones are monitored and recorded at least three times each day. The patient's weight is recorded daily. Twenty-four-hour urine protein collections are indicated for persistent urine dipstick results of 2+ or greater. Baseline liver and renal function tests, hematocrit, platelets, and coagulation studies are recommended. Repeat laboratory evaluation is based on clinical assessment of the patient's status. Weekly or semiweekly fetal surveillance, such as nonstress testing or fetal biophysical profile, is advised. Fetal ultrasound evaluation for interval growth and amniotic fluid volume is performed approximately every 2 to 3 weeks. The antepartum use of antihypertensive agents in preeclamptic patients being managed expectantly has not been shown to improve perinatal outcome and in fact may have deleterious effects. Controversy surrounds the use of glucocorticosteroids to enhance fetal lung maturity in these patients.

Decisions regarding delivery are as noted. In a patient with a poorly inducible cervix prostaglandin gel may be applied. Outright cesarean section is generally reserved for cases remote from immediate delivery with suspected fetal distress, when further fetal evaluation (e.g., fetal scalp sampling or fetal scalp electrode) is not possible or rapidly dete-

---

riorating maternal condition with an unfavorable cervical examination result or abnormal fetal presentation occurs.

Intrapartum management of preeclampsia

Use of magnesium sulfate. Despite recent controversy surrounding the use of phenytoin in preeclampsia, **magnesium sulfate** remains the obstetrician's drug of choice for the prevention of eclamptic seizures. It is administered when the decision to proceed with delivery is made. In the absence of renal disease an intravenous loading dose of 6 g is infused, followed by a 1 to 2 g/hr continuous maintenance dose (see box, above). Urine output should be monitored hourly as oliguria can lead to toxic serum levels. Signs of magnesium overdose include loss of deep tendon reflexes, visual blurring or diplopia, respiratory depression or paralysis, and, at levels greater than 25 mEq/L, cardiac arrest (Table 51-1). In the event of acute magnesium toxicity immediately discontinue magnesium infusion, maintain airway and oxygenation, and administer 1 g calcium gluconate slowly IV (over 3 minutes). Occasionally repeated doses of calcium gluconate may be required as well as mechanical ventilation.

Fluid balance. Careful monitoring of fluid balance is critical in these patients. Preeclampsia is associated with decreased intravascular volume, which can lead to oliguria. Unfortunately many patients also have capillary leak that predisposes them to pulmonary edema. A Foley catheter is helpful in monitoring urine output. Generally total hourly intravenous fluid rate is less than 100 ml/hr. If oliguria develops and is unresponsive to a 500-ml bolus of crystalloid, invasive hemodynamic monitoring with a Swan-Ganz catheter should be considered.

Treatment of hypertension. Intrapartum severe hypertension (persistent diastolic BP >110 mm Hg or systolic BP >180 mm Hg) may be controlled with **hydralazine** 5-10 mg IV push, then repeated every 20 minutes as needed to a total of 40 mg. It is important to recognize that the onset of action of hydralazine is not instantaneous and thus repeat doses should not be given more frequently than every 20

Table 51-1 Acute magnesium toxicity: signs and symptoms

Clinical findings	Serum level (mEq/L)
Seizure prophylaxis	4-7
Loss of deep tendon reflexes	10
Respiratory depression	12
Respiratory paralysis	15
Cardiac arrest	25

minutes to observe for hemodynamic effect. IV **labetalol** 20 mg initially then 40-80 mg every 10 minutes to a total of 300 mg may be administered as an alternative to hydralazine. A continuous IV infusion of 1-2 mg/min may be titrated to desired BP. Labetalol has the advantage of faster onset of action, causing less reflex tachycardia and hypotension than hydralazine. Care should be exercised not to reduce the BP either too abruptly or too far, as decreased intravascular volume and poor uteroplacental perfusion may lead to acute fetal distress. Continuous hemodynamic monitoring with an arterial line is recommended in patients requiring repeated parenteral doses of antihypertensive agents. Other agents useful in controlling acute hypertension include **nifedipine** 10-20 mg sublingual and IV **nitroglycerin** starting at 5 μg/min. Before delivery sodium nitroprusside is not recommended because of theoretic concerns regarding cyanide toxicity to the fetus.

Issues for labor and delivery. Anesthesia consultation in labor and delivery is strongly recommended. In general, epidural anesthesia may be used in preeclamptic patients, although again caution should be exercised to prevent significant sympathetic blockade and acute hypotension, which can result in acute fetal distress. If the patient manifests disseminated intravascular coagulation or thrombocytopenia then epidural anesthesia is to be avoided.

Continuous intrapartum fetal heart rate monitoring is advised as fetal acidemia secondary to poor uteroplacental perfusion is common in these patients. Patterns suggestive of fetal compromise include persistent tachycardia, decreased short- and long-term variability, and recurrent late decelerations not responsive to standard resuscitative measures. (See Table 51-2)

Postpartum management of preeclampsia

Most postpartum eclamptic seizures occur within the first 24 hours after delivery. Therefore magnesium sulfate seizure prophylaxis is continued during this period, whether the patient is delivered by cesarean section or vaginal delivery. Occasionally magnesium sulfate is continued for an additional 12 to 24 hours in patients considered at greatest risk for postpartum eclamptic seizures, such as those with signs of central nervous system (CNS) irritability. Intravenous fluid replacement (usually $\leq$100 ml/hr) should continue with close attention to intake and output data. Clinical and laboratory findings of preeclampsia may worsen immediately postpartum. However, usually signs and symptoms of preeclampsia begin to resolve within 24 to 48 hours postpartum and completely resolve within 1 to 2 weeks. In our experience the development of maternal diuresis often heralds the onset of resolution of this disease process. Patients with persistent hypertension (diastolic BP >110 mm Hg) may require short-term antihypertensive therapy. Diuretics and β-blockers are usually effective in postpartum BP management and have the added advantage of low cost. BP should be reassessed in 1 to 2 weeks after delivery, at which time the antihypertensive agent may be discontinued.

RECURRENCE OF PREECLAMPSIA IN SUBSEQUENT GESTATIONS

Patients diagnosed with preeclampsia in their first pregnancy are at increased risk for recurrent hypertensive disease in

Table 51-2 Summary table of intrapartum management of preeclampsia

Complication	Recommended intervention
Seizure prevention	Magnesium sulfate Loading dose: 6 g Maintenance dose: 1-2 g/hr continuous IV infusion
Fluid balance	Placement of Foley catheter Careful fluid monitoring with total IV fluid rate <100 ml/hr
Hypertension	Hydralazine 5-10 mg IV push, then repeated every 20 minutes as needed to total of 40 mg Labetalol 20 mg IV then 40-80 mg IV every 10 minutes to total of 300 mg, follow with IV infusion 1-2 mg/min if necessary titrated to desired BP Nifedipine 10-20 mg sublingual Nitroglycerin IV with starting dose 5 μg/min Consider arterial line
Labor and delivery	Anesthesia consultation Continuous intrapartum fetal heart rate monitoring

IV, intravenous; BP, blood pressure.

a subsequent pregnancy. Sibai et al. (1986) reported that, in women diagnosed with either severe preeclampsia or eclampsia in their first pregnancy, this recurrence risk can be as high as 45%. This risk is significantly higher in those patients having preeclampsia/eclampsia remote from term. There is some evidence that suggests a predisposition to the development of chronic hypertension in later life.

USE OF LOW-DOSE ASPIRIN IN THE PREVENTION OF PREECLAMPSIA

Since preeclampsia is associated with an increased thromboxane/prostacyclin ratio, selective blockade of platelet thromboxane production by low-dose aspirin (80 mg/day) has been evaluated. To date no studies verify therapeutic benefit to the use of low-dose aspirin in the management of existing preeclampsia. However, recent studies suggest a lower incidence of the development of preeclampsia when low-dose aspirin is given prophylactically to patients at risk for preeclampsia. These high-risk patients may include individuals with a prior history of preeclampsia (particularly remote from term), underlying vascular disorders, chronic hypertension, or chronic renal disease. In this patient population we recommended starting low-dose aspirin at 12 weeks' gestation and continuing its use through delivery.

IMPLICATIONS FOR DEVELOPMENT OF ADULT HYPERTENSION

The hypertensive effects of preeclampsia generally resolve within the first week postpartum. Occasionally patients require antihypertensive therapy up to 12 weeks postpartum. Controversy exists as to the correlation between the clinical diagnosis of preeclampsia and the subsequent development of chronic hypertension. It is recommended that women with a history of preeclampsia be advised of a slightly increased risk of chronic hypertension and have yearly BP evaluations.

BIBLIOGRAPHY

American College of Obstetricians and Gynecologists: *Management of Preeclampsia*, ACOG technical bulletin no. 91, Washington, DC, 1986.

Atrash HK et al: Maternal mortality in the United States: 1979-1986. *Obstet Gynecol* 76:1055, 1990.

Cunningham FG et al, editors: *Williams obstetrics,* ed 19, East Norwalk, Conn, 1993, Appleton & Lange.

Goodlin RC: Severe pre-eclampsia: another great imitator, *Am J Obstet Gynecol* 125:747, 1976.

Hubel CA et al: Lipid peroxidation in pregnancy: new perspectives on pre-eclampsia, *Am J Obstet Gynecol* 161:1025, 1989.

Martin JN et al: Pregnancy complicated by preeclampsia-eclampsia with the syndrome of hemolysis, elevated liver enzymes, and low platelet count: how rapid is postpartum recovery? *Obstet Gynecol* 76:737, 1990.

Roberts JM et al: Preeclampsia: an endothelial cell disorder, *Am J Obstet Gynecol* 161:1200, 1989.

Schiff E et al: The use of aspirin to prevent pregnancy-induced hypertension and lower the ratio of thromboxane A2 to prostacyclin in relatively high risk pregnancies, *N Engl J Med* 321:351, 1989.

Sibai BM, El-Nazer A, Gonzalez-Ruiz A: Severe preeclampsia-eclampsia in young primigravid women: subsequent pregnancy outcome and remote prognosis, *Am J Obstet Gynecol* 155:1011, 1986.

Sibai BM et al: Maternal and perinatal outcome of conservative management of severe preeclampsia in midtrimester, *Am J Obstet Gynecol* 152:32, 1985.

Walsh SW: Preeclampsia: an imbalance in placental prostacyclin and thromboxane production, *Am J Obstet Gynecol* 152:335, 1985.

52 Asthma in Pregnancy

Phyllis Jen

EFFECT OF ASTHMA IN PREGNANCY

The incidence of asthma during pregnancy is about 1%. The course of asthma in pregnant women is unpredictable: one third note no change, one third note improvement, and one third worsen. There is a tendency to repeat the same pattern with each pregnancy and a slight tendency for asthma to worsen in the third trimester. Asthma exacerbations during pregnancy can cause maternal hypoxia, hypocapnia, and alkalosis and resulting fetal hypoxia. Studies suggest that the severity of asthma during pregnancy (as indicated by steroid dependence) correlates with perinatal mortality, prematurity, and low birth weight. However, women who receive steroids and are able to avoid status asthmaticus have a better outcome than women who have status asthmaticus. Of note is that congenital abnormalities do not occur with increased frequency.

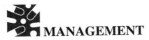 MANAGEMENT

Goals of management

The goals of managing the pregnant woman with asthma are similar to those for the nonpregnant woman. Most antiasthma medications are safe to use in pregnancy (see box, below). It should be emphasized that the possibility of an adverse outcome related to the asthma is minimized if status asthmaticus or uncontrolled bronchospasm can be prevented. An assessment of baseline pulmonary function should be made. Home monitoring of peak expiratory flow rates can often detect lung function changes before the onset of symptoms. If it has not already been done, an evaluation for allergy factors can be beneficial, although skin tests or immunotherapy should probably not be initiated during pregnancy. Ongoing allergic immunotherapy can be continued during pregnancy.

Choice of therapy

Chronic asthma. Women with chronic asthma maintained on medications should continue those medications that are safe to use during pregnancy. Medications should not be given unless necessary, especially during the first trimester. Medications considered to be reasonably safe with an acceptable track record and also those that are unsafe are listed in the box. The general treatment approach is to use beta-agonists, cromolyn, and steroids in various combinations depending upon the severity of the attack. Treatment approaches are summarized in Table 52-1.

Acute asthma. When a pregnant woman has an asthma exacerbation additional therapies are necessary. Rapid improvement of symptoms can often be achieved with inhaled beta-agonist therapy with minimal side effects. The addition of a spacer device can often improve delivery of the medication. Although definitive tests of safety during pregnancy are unavailable, beta-agonists such as terbutaline, albuterol, and metaproterenol are probably safe. However, because high-dose beta-agonists, even in the inhaled form, may inhibit uterine contractions, they should be avoided if possible in late pregnancy or at term. If symptoms cannot be controlled with inhaled beta-agonists, ephedrine and theophylline are safe to use in pregnancy, although transient neonatal tachycardia and irritability have been noted. The use of epinephrine is somewhat more controversial because of studies showing a slight reduction in placental blood flow, but is considered by many to be the treatment of choice for emergency use.

If an acute asthma exacerbation does not respond to bronchodilator therapy, oral corticosteroids should be used to speed remission and prevent status asthmaticus. A short course of steroids (<2 weeks) is not associated with any adverse outcomes. Patients with severe asthma requiring chronic steroids, however, have an increased incidence of premature delivery (<37 weeks) and low-birth-weight infants (<2500 g). Steroid-dependent asthmatics who experience status asthmaticus during pregnancy have an even greater incidence of low-birth-weight infants. This suggests that steroid therapy for pregnant women with severe asthma is appropriate and may improve fetal outcome by preventing status asthmaticus. Chronic inhaled steroid therapy for patients with less severe disease has been shown to reduce the frequency of acute exacerbations and to lower airway reactivity. There is no increased incidence of fetal mortality or congenital malformations when inhaled beclomethasone

---

SAFETY OF ASTHMA TREATMENTS DURING PREGNANCY

Drugs that are safe:
Theophylline, aminophylline
Ephedrine
Epinephrine
Cromolyn
Terbutaline, inhaled
Metaproterenol, inhaled
Beclomethasone, inhaled
Prednisone, hydrocortisone
Influenza vaccine
Antibiotics (penicillin analogs, cephalosporins, erythromycin)

Drugs that are unsafe:
Tetracycline
Quinolones
Iodide-containing expectorants
Barbiturate-containing asthma medications

Table 52-1 Management of asthma in pregnancy

Clinical presentation	Recommendations for treatment
Chronic	
Mild (symptoms 1-2 times/wk)	Inhaled beta$_2$-agonists 1-2 puffs q4h prn (terbutaline, metaproterenol, albuterol)
Moderate (symptoms more than 2 times/wk)	Inhaled beta$_2$-agonists 2 puffs qid
	Cromolyn 2 puffs qid
	Inhaled corticosteroid 2 puffs qid (beclomethasone)
Severe (daily symptoms)	Inhaled corticosteroid 2 puffs q2h
	Prednisone, at lowest effective dose
Acute exacerbation	Oxygen, fluids
	Albuterol nebulizer q30 min
	Terbutaline 0.25-0.5 mg SQ q30 min × 2 (preferable to epinephrine)
	Methyl prednisolone 80 mg IV q6h
Management during labor	Continue same medications
	For steroid-dependent patients, hydrocortisone 100 mg IV push
	If asthma symptoms increase during labor, treat as above for acute exacerbation

is used. A relationship between steroid use and cleft palate demonstrated in rabbits has not been found in humans. Cromolyn therapy can also reduce airway reactivity, especially in the atopic patient with seasonal disease. Adverse fetal effects have not been noted. Iodide-containing expectorants may cause fetal goiter and should be avoided. For a summary of management of acute asthma refer to Table 52-1.

Use of antibiotics and immunization. Antibiotics such as penicillins, cephalosporins, and erythromycin can be given to patients with infectious upper respiratory infections. Sulfa-containing antibiotics cross the placenta and when given near term can cause kernicterus. Tetracycline must be avoided because it causes staining of teeth and delayed fetal bone growth. Quinolones should also be avoided since this class of drugs has caused fetal arthropathy. Influenza immunization should be given, preferably in the second or third trimester.

Management during labor. Since minute ventilation can increase two times during labor, asthma symptoms should ideally be controlled before the onset of labor. Patients who are steroid-dependent or who have recently been on a prolonged course of steroids should receive stress-dose hydrocortisone coverage when labor begins.

BIBLIOGRAPHY

Fitzsimons R, Greenberger PA, Patterson R: Outcome of pregnancy in women requiring corticosteroids for severe asthma, *J Allergy Clin Immunol* 78(2):349, 1986.

Greenberger PA, Patterson R: Management of asthma during pregnancy, *N Engl J Med* 312(14):897, 1985.

Perlow JH et al: Severity of asthma and perinatal outcome, *Am J Obstet Gynecol* 167(4):963, 1992.

Schatz M et al: The course of asthma in pregnancy, postpartum and with successive pregnancies, *J Allergy Clin Immunol* 81(3):509, 1988.

53 Diabetes in Pregnancy

Michael F. Greene

Diabetes mellitus has always been recognized as a serious complication in pregnancy. Dr. Elliott Joslin's first published series of diabetes in pregnancy in 1915 (7 years before the discovery of insulin) detailed 10 pregnancies among 7 women. There were only three surviving children, and four of the women died. The prognosis for diabetic women and their offspring has improved steadily and dramatically since the introduction of insulin. The incidence of maternal mortality has become so small that it is difficult to measure. Significant morbidity such as hypoglycemia, diabetic ketoaci-

dosis, hypertension, and exacerbations of nephropathy and retinopathy still occur with greater frequency during pregnancy. Perinatal mortality is now less than one tenth of what it was shortly after insulin was introduced, but it is still twice that for the nondiabetic population. Although it is difficult to separate the elements of care for these patients to quantitate how each improvement has contributed to the improved prognosis for pregnancy, it is probably fair to say that no single intervention has been as important as improved metabolic control of the underlying disease.

PATHOPHYSIOLOGY
Metabolic changes associated with pregnancy

Compared with the nonpregnant state, normal pregnancy is associated with a fall in fasting blood glucose levels but a rise in postprandial glucose levels. The net result of these changes is a modest rise in mean daily blood glucose levels throughout pregnancy. These changes occur in the presence of insulin levels, which are elevated above nonpregnant levels and rise throughout pregnancy. The occurrence of relative postprandial hyperglycemia despite relatively high insulin levels is, by definition, insulin resistance and has led to the characterization of pregnancy as a "diabetogenic" state. The hormones chiefly responsible for the insulin resistance are cortisol, growth hormone, and chorionic somatomammotropin. Blood amino acid levels are lower during pregnancy than in the nonpregnant state. A relatively brief fast (overnight) during the later half of pregnancy will result in higher levels of the ketones acetoacetate and β-hydroxybutyrate than in the nonpregnant state. The rapid switch to fatty acids as an energy source after a brief fast, which is reflected by this ketone body formation, has been termed the *accelerated starvation* of pregnancy.

CLASSIFICATION OF DIABETES IN PREGNANCY

The problem of diabetes complicating pregnancy can be broadly classified into overt diabetes, which antedates pregnancy (either type I or type II), and gestational diabetes. A modification of the classification system originally proposed by White is presented in the box at right.

Gestational diabetes

Gestational diabetes mellitus (GDM) was redefined in 1984 as "carbohydrate intolerance of variable severity with onset or first recognition during the present pregnancy." The original definition of GDM by glucose tolerance testing in the 1960s was intended to identify women with relatively modest impairment of carbohydrate tolerance that developed later in pregnancy as a result of the physiologic changes of pregnancy. It was defined as glucose values two standard deviations above the mean for the population tested and validated by its association with an increased risk for the development of type II diabetes later in life. The new definition is so broad that it includes a wide variety of potentially very different patients. It includes patients with type II diabetes antedating pregnancy who possibly should have been receiving insulin or oral agents but who were not previously diagnosed. Harris (1988) found, for example, that at age 40 years, 8% of nonpregnant women had a degree of carbohydrate intolerance that would be classified as gestational diabetes. Occasionally type I diabetes develops coincidently during a young woman's pregnancy, and this too would be classified as gestational diabetes.

OVERT DIABETES
Maternal complications

Hypoglycemia. Early pregnancy frequently is associated with some degree of anorexia, nausea, and vomiting, as well as lower fasting glucose levels as previously mentioned. In diabetic women taking a fixed daily dose of insulin, these changes often result in an increased frequency of insulin reactions in early pregnancy. Intensively treated diabetic patients often have a diminished awareness of and response to hypo-

CLASSIFICATION OF DIABETES IN PREGNANCY	
GDM non–I Non–insulin-requiring gestational diabetes	Abnormal carbohydrate tolerance in pregnancy; no insulin required
GDM I Insulin-requiring gestational diabetes	Abnormal carbohydrate tolerance in pregnancy; insulin required
A	Abnormal carbohydrate tolerance before pregnancy; no insulin required before or during pregnancy
B	Insulin-requiring diabetes; onset after 20 years of age and duration less than 10 yr; no vascular complications
C	Insulin-requiring diabetes; onset 10-19 yr of age and duration less than 20 yr or duration 10-20 yr with onset after age 20
D	Insulin-requiring diabetes with either onset before 10 yr of age or duration greater than 20 yr regardless of age at onset or associated with background retinopathy or associated with chronic hypertension
F	Insulin-requiring diabetes with nephropathy (greater than 500-mg proteinuria per day)
R	Insulin-requiring diabetes with proliferative retinopathy
T	Insulin-requiring diabetes with renal transplant
H	Insulin-requiring diabetes with coronary artery disease

Modified from Hare JW and White P: *Diabetes Care* 3:394, 1980.

glycemia. Diamond et al. (1992) recently demonstrated this to be true for pregnant diabetic women too. They compared the response to hypoglycemia in nine intensively treated diabetic women and seven nonpregnant nondiabetic age-matched women using a hypoglycemic insulin clamp technique. They found that the counterregulatory hormonal responses of glucagon, epinephrine, and growth hormone did not begin to rise until lower levels of blood glucose were reached; they rose more slowly; and they did not reach the same maximum levels of response in the diabetic pregnant women as compared with the control subjects. Given the design of their study, it is impossible to determine the amount of difference caused as a result of pregnancy versus intensive insulin therapy.

The elevated progesterone levels of pregnancy are associated with delayed gastric emptying. In women with some degree of gastroparesis before pregnancy, this effect can be exacerbated. Delayed and unpredictable gastric emptying can make glycemic control, which depends on insulin injections timed to anticipate gastric emptying, difficult and result in wide swings in postprandial glucose values. At its worst in late pregnancy, it can lead to frequent vomiting, poor weight gain, and frequent hypoglycemia. Frequent vomiting of undigested meals 2 to 3 hours after eating is characteristic in these cases. Metoclopramide therapy has been quite helpful for these patients.

Severe hypoglycemia in the later half of pregnancy may be associated with a modest degree of fetal bradycardia—as low as 100 beats/min. This decrease reverses slowly as maternal blood glucose levels return to normal, with no obvious adverse consequences to the fetus. Recent data have suggested that overly zealous insulin therapy resulting in frequent symptomatic insulin reactions or chronic modest hypoglycemia may be associated with inadequate fetal growth.

Diabetic ketoacidosis. It is often said that women with type I diabetes are at increased risk for the development of diabetic ketoacidosis (DKA) during pregnancy, but the relationship is not clear. It is clear that during pregnancy DKA may develop at much lower blood glucose levels than would normally be a problem in nonpregnant women. Vomiting frequently is associated with DKA during pregnancy and may confuse the diagnosis if the observed ketonuria is attributed to starvation because of protracted vomiting. Although DKA always has the potential to become a life-threatening emergency, it is particularly threatening to the fetus in the later half of pregnancy. Fetal death rates as high as 50% have been observed. Treatment of DKA should be aggressive and no different in principle than for nonpregnant persons. DKA often induces premature labor and is associated with nonreassuring fetal heart rate patterns. Both problems are best treated by vigorously addressing the metabolic disorder.

Retinopathy. Virtually all patients with diabetes of sufficient duration eventually develop some degree of retinopathy. Duration of diabetes, degree of glycemic control, and diastolic blood pressure have all been shown to correlate with the risk for development and progression of retinopathy. There has been considerable controversy over the years regarding the role of pregnancy as a risk factor for diabetic retinopathy. The best prospective and controlled study of this issue was reported by Klein et al. (1990). Pregnant diabetic women were matched with nonpregnant control subjects and followed up in a similar fashion over comparable periods of time. Serial fundus photographs were obtained, and the degree of retinopathy was graded by ophthalmologists without knowledge of the pregnancy status of the patients. Serial tests of visual acuity also were performed. The ophthalmologists concluded that on the basis of the fundus photographs, progression of retinopathy was more likely to occur in pregnant women than in nonpregnant subjects. Furthermore, women with more advanced disease in early pregnancy were more likely to have more dramatic progression. Pregnant women were significantly more likely to suffer a deterioration in visual acuity than the nonpregnant control group. This difference was minimal, however, at long-term follow-up postpartum.

Several studies have shown, and the Diabetes Control and Complications Trial (DCCT) has recently confirmed, that intensification of metabolic control is associated with an exacerbation of diabetic retinopathy over the short term. To what degree the progression of retinopathy during pregnancy can be attributed to improved efforts at metabolic control versus pregnancy is speculative.

Nephropathy and hypertension. The microvascular diseases of diabetes have long been recognized to represent significant complications in pregnancy. As late as 1977,

Pederson, in the second edition of his book, recommended that women with nephropathy be counseled to avoid pregnancy because they and their offspring would do poorly. Nephropathy clearly has a negative impact on pregnancy, but considerable controversy exists regarding the effect of intercurrent pregnancy on the course of nephropathy. It has been easier to define the effect of nephropathy on pregnancy because the pregnancy outcome variables are discrete and reached in relatively short follow-up periods. It is considerably more difficult to assess the influence of pregnancy on the course of nephropathy because the necessary follow-up periods are much longer and because the natural history is for progressive deterioration with time.

The incidence of nephropathy among pregnant diabetic women has been increasing. This trend can be traced in three published series from the Joslin Clinic. In 1957 Oppe, Hsia, and Gellis reported a series of 31 women among 767 (4%) whose pregnancies were complicated by nephropathy. Kitzmiller et al. (1981) found 26 cases of nephropathy among 258 (10%) between 1975 and 1978. In the most recently published series of pregnancies progressing beyond 20 weeks in 1983 through 1987 there were 55 cases of nephropathy (and 4 renal transplantations) among 420 pregnancies, for an incidence of 14% (Greene et al., 1989).

Pregnancies among women with diabetic nephropathy are complicated by increased incidences of dense proteinuria, hypertension, hypoalbuminemia, anemia, prematurity, and perinatal mortality. The 40% increase in plasma volume and parallel increase in cardiac output that accompany pregnancy place increased demands on the kidneys. Nondiabetic women with normal kidneys and renal function increase their creatinine clearances by approximately 30% and lose increasing quantities of protein in their urine in the third trimester. Diabetic women without overt nephropathy whose urine dipstick results are negative for urine protein in the first trimester lose considerably more protein in their urine in the third trimester than do their nondiabetic counterparts. The increase in creatinine clearance can be dramatic and exaggerated (to 200 ml/min and more) for patients who enter pregnancy in the hyperfiltration phase of developing nephropathy. Diabetic women who begin pregnancy with established nephropathy (proteinuria greater than 500 mg/day) tend not to experience the characteristic rise in creatinine clearance and have even more dramatic progressive urinary protein loss. As many as 70% of these women will have proteinuria in excess of 3 g/day before delivery. This generally returns to prepregnancy values by 6 to 8 weeks after delivery in most of the patients. Not surprisingly, proteinuria of this magnitude frequently leads to significant hypoalbuminemia and dependent edema. Occasionally this results in anasarca and pulmonary edema, which is refractory to therapy and necessitates delivery.

Among all diabetic women with pregnancies progressing beyond 20 weeks reported from the Joslin Clinic, the incidence of chronic hypertension antedating pregnancy was 6%, but among women with nephropathy one third were hypertensive. In most series of diabetic women, approximately one quarter have clinically significant hypertension during pregnancy. Among women with nephropathy, however, two thirds have significant hypertensive complications. Preeclampsia is defined as hypertension with proteinuria and edema developing after 24 weeks of pregnancy. All of these patients have proteinuria, and clinically significant edema is virtually universal in the later half of pregnancy. The diagnosis of preeclampsia among the third of patients with chronic hypertension is thus rather arbitrary. Even in the other third of patients in whom hypertension develops during pregnancy, many follow a rather prolonged and relatively benign course. Clearly, patients with evidence of other organ system involvement such as hemolysis, thrombocytopenia, or hepatocellular necrosis have preeclampsia. In the absence of these other systemic signs, the definition is imprecise and of little clinical utility.

Anemia associated with nephropathy. Anemia is common and may be quite profound with hematocrit values in the low 20s. In the series of Reece et al. (1988), 42% of patients had hemoglobin concentrations of less than 10 g/dl. Kitzmiller et al. (1981) found a mean third-trimester hematocrit of 29%, and 58% of the patients had values below 30%. The anemia usually is normocytic and normochromic, and the standard evaluation usually is unrewarding. Recently, erythropoietin levels have been found to be inappropriately low in some of these patients, and they have responded dramatically to therapy with recombinant human erythropoietin. Care must be taken not to raise the hematocrit too high too quickly or significant hypertension may result.

Premature delivery. The incidence of delivery before 37 weeks in a general obstetric population is approximately 10%. Among diabetic women without nephropathy that risk is about 22%. In the series of Kitzmiller et al., 71% of the class F patients who did not spontaneously or electively abort delivered before 37 weeks. In the more recent Joslin Clinic series and that of Reece et al., that risk was 52% and 55%, respectively. In the Joslin series, almost one half of these premature deliveries (14/31) were the direct result of the development of apparent preeclampsia.

The outlook for survival for the fetuses of these patients has improved steadily, although it still does not equal that for infants of nondiabetic women or even that for other diabetic women. In the 1981 series of Kitzmiller et al. the perinatal mortality was 110/1000. Reece et al. reported a 60/1000 perinatal mortality rate for their 1975-1984 series. The perinatal mortality rate for the Joslin Clinic series of 1983-1987 was 70/1000 for the patients with nephropathy as compared with 27/1000 for the other patients in the series. These figures are comparable to a perinatal mortality rate in Massachusetts during this time of approximately 17/1000.

Treatment of hypertension in pregnancy. The antihypertensive agents traditionally used during pregnancy have been α-methyldopa and hydralazine. Although their use is safe during pregnancy, these agents are not particularly efficacious or well accepted by patients. Both must be given multiple times daily. In doses adequate to control significant hypertension, α-methyldopa often causes an unacceptable degree of somnolence. Hydralazine is ineffective as monotherapy in the outpatient setting but may be helpful when added to either α-methyldopa or a beta blocker. Neither drug is helpful in slowing the rate of progression of nephropathy or reducing proteinuria. **Beta blockers** have been used cautiously in diabetic patients because of concerns about damping the counterregulatory response to hypoglycemia. These agents, however, are quite effective in controlling hypertension; they are safe and efficacious during pregnancy, reduce proteinuria, seem to slow the progression of nephropathy, and are well

accepted by patients. **Metoprolol, atenolol,** and most recently **labetalol** are becoming the antihypertensive agents of choice during pregnancy. Metoprolol and atenolol have been used as the primary antihypertensive agents in prenatal patients at the Joslin Clinic for the past decade with minimal problems with hypoglycemia.

Angiotensin converting enzyme (ACE) inhibitors are now the drugs of first choice for treating nephropathy and its associated hypertension in diabetic patients. Unfortunately these drugs should not be used in pregnancy because they cause a constellation of severe fetal and neonatal problems. Fairly extensive evidence has accumulated that ACE inhibitors cause deficient calcification of the bones of the fetal skull (hypocalvaria) and renal tubular dysgenesis that can lead to oligohydramnios in utero and renal insufficiency, failure, and death in the neonatal period. Thus these agents should be avoided during pregnancy. The toxicity seems confined to late-pregnancy exposure, and there do not appear to be any adverse consequences to early first-trimester exposure. Patients receiving long-term ACE inhibitor therapy should discontinue its use as soon as pregnancy is diagnosed early in the first trimester and should be reassured that this brief exposure is not known to be harmful. Diuretics are not ordinarily used during pregnancy, but occasionally they may be necessary in nephropathic patients with significant volume overload or severe edema. They frequently are helpful in the puerperium to resolve edema. The use of calcium channel blockers during pregnancy has not been studied adequately to make any recommendations.

No antihypertensive therapy has ever been shown to reduce the incidence of preeclampsia superimposed on chronic hypertension. **Low-dose aspirin therapy (80 mg/day)** appears to reduce the incidence of preeclampsia in patients at high risk for its occurrence or recurrence. No studies to date have specifically addressed diabetes or diabetic nephropathy in pregnant women, but a study is currently in progress at several NIH-funded centers.

Obstetric and Perinatal Complications

Spontaneous abortion. The fertility of women with diabetes is unimpaired. There has been considerable debate, however, regarding the first-trimester spontaneous abortion rate among these women. It now seems clear that this rate is not increased for women in good metabolic control before and during very early pregnancy. The rate of first-trimester spontaneous abortions among clinically recognized pregnancies in the general population is 12% to 15%. The rate is the same for diabetic women with first-trimester glycosylated hemoglobin values up to 9 standard deviations above the nondiabetic mean. Several studies have now shown that first-trimester glycohemoglobin values greater than 9 standard deviations above the nondiabetic mean are associated with an increased incidence of spontaneous abortion. The poorest degrees of control are associated with a one-third risk of spontaneous abortion.

Major malformations. Most large series of births to women with diabetes mellitus report a 6% to 9% incidence of major congenital malformations, which is significantly higher than the 2% to 3% incidence in the general population. These malformations are now the single greatest source of perinatal mortality for infants of diabetic mothers (IDM), accounting for 50% of all perinatal deaths. The anomalies found among IDM span the range of the anomalies found in the nondiabetic population. The most common are cardiac abnormalities, neural tube defects (anencephaly and spina bifida), and urinary tract anomalies. Some of these have been reported to occur at rates that are 10 or more times higher than in the general population. Careful examination of a timetable for normal human development reveals that all of these anomalies arise within the first 6 weeks from fertilization, or 8 weeks from last menstrual period.

The first large series to demonstrate a relationship between first-trimester metabolic control and risk for anomalies was that of Miller et al. from the Joslin Clinic. The researchers found that when patients were ranked according to first-trimester glycohemoglobin values, those in the lower half had a risk for major malformation of just over 3% whereas those in the upper half had a risk of just over 20%. This was a highly statistically significant difference. Subsequently these findings have been confirmed in several other countries using a variety of glycosylated hemoglobin techniques, and these have been reviewed in detail elsewhere. Compilation of these data at the Joslin Clinic published in 1989 and ongoing studies, which include data from more than 700 diabetic gravidas, continues to support this relationship. The risk for major malformations does not rise with statistical significance from the 3% range until 12 standard deviations above the nondiabetic mean when the risk rises to 30% to 40%.

In summary, these data regarding the relationship between metabolic control and first-trimester events are both reassuring and worrisome for patients. They can be reassured that they do not need to be in perfect metabolic control to minimize their risks for spontaneous abortion and major malformations; good to fair control is adequate. Unfortunately, however, control is important. Women who conceive and spend the early first trimester in poor control face very high risks for spontaneous abortion and major malformation. In fact, at first trimester glycosylated hemoglobin values of 12 or more standard deviations above the mean, a spontaneous abortion, a major congenital malformation, and a nonmalformed live birth are approximately equally likely probabilities. Thus the single most important element of care for diabetic women to optimize perinatal outcome is to spend the first 6 postovulatory weeks of pregnancy in good metabolic control. For women whose diabetes is not always in good control, it can take several weeks of effort on the part of patients, dietitians, teaching nurses, and physicians in adjusting diet, insulin therapy, and exercise to achieve good control. If those efforts are not initiated until after women recognize their pregnancies, this critical period of early embryologic development frequently passes before good control can be achieved. It is critically important therefore that diabetic women plan their pregnancies, using appropriate contraception when necessary, to be certain that they enter pregnancy in as good metabolic control as possible.

Several studies have now been published that report the results of demonstration projects to enroll diabetic women into programs of preconception care to optimize metabolic control and reduce the malformation rate. All apparently have been successful in that attenders consistently demonstrate malformation rates of 1% to 2% whereas nonattenders have rates of 7% to 11%. These programs have been challenged on the basis that they may simply attract compliant women who would probably have entered pregnancy in good control regardless of the program, whereas noncompliant women do not voluntarily attend such programs. It has thus been argued that expensive health care resources are being thrown at women who need them least. It remains to be seen how successful these programs will be when applied to large populations.

Fetal death. Fifty years ago 25% of the fetuses of diabetic women died in utero near term. Most of these fetuses were macrosomic with no malformations and no obvious cause for death. These deaths were blamed on asphyxia, and their number declined in frequency over the decades as the general level of metabolic control improved even without understanding the physiology of these losses. The unexplained stillbirth rate on large academic services for diabetic women is now approximately 1/300 to 1/400. Although this is now a relatively rare event on large services, the pathophysiology of uteroplacental insufficiency remains important and may claim fetuses. Several factors may combine to render fetuses of diabetic women critically hypoxemic. Studies of placental perfusion using radiolabeled tracers have demonstrated a 35% to 45% decrease in uteroplacental blood flow index in diabetic women in general. This may be further exacerbated by microvascular disease. Glycosylated hemoglobin carries less oxygen molecule for molecule than does native hemoglobin. Furthermore, glycosylated hemoglobin binds that oxygen more tightly and releases it less well in the periphery at sites of lower oxygen tension, such as the placental bed. Hyperglycemic fetuses respond with hyperinsulinemia. Hyperinsulinemia in turn causes increased oxygen consumption in the fetus and results in an increased umbilical arteriovenous oxygen difference. These factors, which are associated with both acute and chronic hyperglycemia, may conspire to create a critical level of fetal hypoxemia.

Macrosomia

Excessive fetal growth (macrosomia) is characteristic of fetuses of diabetic women. In a general population, approximately 6% of delivered fetuses will weigh more than 4000 g whereas in most series of IDM 20% to 25% of fetuses will be that large. As many as 60% of IDM will be greater than the tenth percentile for their gestational ages. The standard explanation for this excessive growth is the *Pedersen hypothesis.* Maternal hyperglycemia readily becomes fetal hyperglycemia as glucose passes through the placenta by facilitated diffusion. The fetus responds with hyperinsulinemia. Insulin is the most important growth hormone of the fetus, causing accretion of fat, muscle, and bone. This has been further expanded to include consideration of transplacental passage of amino acids that can act as insulin secretagogues. Improved metabolic control can help to reduce but not eliminate macrosomia. Although it has been known for some time that insulin will not cross the placenta, recently it has been demonstrated that insulin–anti-insulin antigen-antibody complexes can cross the placenta into the fetal circulation. Furthermore, the level of these antigen-antibody complexes correlates with the degree of fetal macrosomia. This observation helps to explain the fact that a few diabetic women in excellent control nonetheless have very large fetuses.

Macrosomia is important because larger fetuses are more likely to require either operative pelvic or cesarean delivery. Operative deliveries expose the mothers to greater risks for morbidity. These large fetuses also are at increased risk for birth trauma.

GESTATIONAL DIABETES MELLITUS

The definition of GDM, as already discussed, encompasses a wide range of physiologic factors. Most of these patients, however, have a relatively mild degree of carbohydrate intolerance, which develops later in pregnancy as the result of the physiologic changes (insulin resistance) of late pregnancy. The issue of GDM is surrounded by considerable controversy. Questions have been raised regarding both the amount of morbidity and mortality that it causes, as well as the quantity and quality of the data, suggesting that these can be modified by screening and treatment. Perinatal mortality is so low that it has been, and likely will remain, impossible to demonstrate that GDM significantly increases the risk for perinatal mortality. As the result of a major meta-analysis of available studies published in 1989, Hunter and Keirse concluded that "except for research purposes, all forms of glucose tolerance testing should be stopped." It is becoming increasingly clear, however, that GDM is associated with macrosomia and its complications—operative delivery, birth trauma, and pregnancy-induced hypertension. The occurrence of GDM is so closely associated with both age and obesity on a population basis that it is almost impossible to separate them. The argument has been made that the obstetric complications associated with GDM are caused primarily by obesity, which also causes GDM.

Epidemiology

GDM originally was defined as glucose tolerance testing results two standard deviations above the mean; therefore the incidence of the abnormality was 2.5% by definition. Those original data were collected from a mixed population in Boston. Subsequently, it has become obvious that the specified degree of carbohydrate intolerance may be found at very different incidences in different populations. Native Americans from the Southwest and Mexican Americans, for example, have much higher incidences of GDM.

Screening

The major controversy surrounding GDM screening is identifying who should be screened biochemically with a glucose load. At present the American College of Obstetricians and Gynecologists recommends biochemical testing by means of a glucose load for patients with any of the following risk factors for GDM:

1. Maternal age 30 years or greater
2. Family history of diabetes
3. Previous macrosomic infant
4. Previous stillbirth
5. Previous malformed infant
6. Obesity
7. Hypertension
8. Glycosuria

The American Diabetes Association and the Centers for Disease Control and Prevention recommend universal screening of all pregnant women with a biochemical test regardless of risk factors.

A two-stage biochemical screening procedure is recommended. The response to a 50-g oral glucose load (glucose loading test [GLT]) is assessed by a venous plasma glucose determination 1 hour later. This glucose load can be administered in the fed or fasted state without prior dietary preparation. Values of 140 mg/dl or more should be followed by a full 3-hour 100-g oral glucose tolerance test (OGTT). This should be performed fasting after 3 days of dietary preparation with an unrestricted diet of at least 150 g of carbohydrate per day. The OGTT results are considered abnormal if two or more venous plasma glucose levels meet or exceed the following values: fasting 105 mg/dl, 1 hour 190 mg/dl, 2 hours 165 mg/dl, 3 hours 145 mg/dl. Attempts to use determinations of glycosylated serum proteins or hemoglobin as screening tests have been too insensitive. Islet cell antibodies are found only in a small number of women with GDM (2% to 38% depending on the assay used) and therefore are not useful in screening for the condition.

The insulin resistance of pregnancy increases with increasing gestational age; therefore the later in pregnancy that a population is tested, the greater the finding of abnormal carbohydrate tolerance. The later in pregnancy that a patient is diagnosed, however, the longer she may have had untreated carbohydrate intolerance and the less time there is left in pregnancy to attempt to improve outcome with proper therapy. Generally, patients should be screened once at 24 to 28 weeks of gestation.

The reproducibility of glucose tolerance testing is only fair. Only 40% of women with test results that are positive for GDM in one pregnancy will again have this finding in the next pregnancy. This fact has led many to criticize the validity of the testing procedure. As a practical matter, this means that women should be retested in subsequent pregnancies despite a prior pregnancy diagnosis of GDM. There are no data that address the question of whether this should be performed with use of GLT followed by OGTT or directly by OGTT.

MANAGEMENT

Pregnancy. A diet should be prescribed according to ideal body weight with 30 Kcal/kg in the first half of pregnancy and 35 Kcal/kg in the second half. Approximately 50% of the calories should be provided as carbohydrate, and 1.3 g of protein per kilogram of body weight are allowed. The remainder of the daily calorie requirement is allocated to fat.

Any serious effort at achieving euglycemia must include home capillary blood glucose self-monitoring. Patients who cannot maintain fasting blood glucose values below 105 mg/dl and 2-hour postprandial values below 120 mg/dl should be treated with insulin. The number of patients who require insulin is determined in part by the diligence with which patients comply with their diets and the frequency with which their blood glucoses are checked. Between 30% and 50% of patients require insulin.

Postpartum. The purpose of the original study of O'Sullivan and Mahan (1964) was to define the relationship between abnormal carbohydrate tolerance in pregnancy and the later development of diabetes. In their Boston population they found a 22% cumulative prevalence of diabetes 8 years after a pregnancy with OGTT results greater than two standard deviations above the mean. This compared with a 4%

prevalence for women with normal carbohydrate tolerance. Similar studies in various ethnic groups have been undertaken around the world confirming the relationship between GDM and later diabetes. Only the magnitude of the effect has varied. In Copenhagen, Damm et al. (1992) found a 17% prevalence of diabetes at follow-up (a mean of 6 years) in women who had non–insulin-requiring GDM. In Los Angeles, Kjos et al. (1991) found a 40% prevalence at 36 months' postpartum in an obese Mexican-American population. Among Zuni Indians in New Mexico, Benjamin et al. (1993) found a 30% prevalence at a mean of 4.8 years of follow-up.

Given the relatively high probability of developing diabetes within a short period after a pregnancy complicated by GDM, patients should be educated about the risk, its relationship to obesity, and the symptoms of diabetes mellitus. It has been suggested that all patients in whom the diagnosis of GDM has been made should be evaluated with a 75-g OGTT 6 to 12 weeks postpartum. The results should be interpreted according to the standard criteria of either the National Diabetes Data Group or the World Health Organization. If the results are abnormal, then the patient should be treated accordingly. If they are normal, then the patient should be reevaluated periodically, although there are no solid data on which to recommend a specific follow-up interval. Attempts have been made to identify specific factors in GDM that would be more highly predictive for the development of later diabetes. Although such factors as a particularly high fasting glucose or 2-hour value on an OGTT or the area under the glucose curve on an OGTT identify women at higher risk, they are not sufficiently discriminatory to be useful.

Contraception and future pregnancies also should be discussed with GDM women postpartum. Despite some concerns raised by an early report, intrauterine devices are both safe and effective in women with diabetes and with former GDM. Although data are limited, modern low-dose combination oral contraceptives also appear to be safe, inducing minimal changes in cardiovascular risk factor lipoprotein markers. As noted already, future pregnancies are at increased risk for GDM. The degree to which weight reduction can reduce the risk for GDM in subsequent pregnancies is speculative but should be considered for obese patients.

SUMMARY

Pregnancies complicated by diabetes mellitus require considerably more time and effort on the part of patients, primary care physicians, and obstetricians to ensure optimal outcomes. At present the perinatal mortality rate for diabetic women is still twice that for the general population. Further progress in reducing that rate will require planning pregnancies and improved preconception care to reduce the incidence of major congenital malformations. In this context it could be argued that the most important part of prenatal care for these patients is rendered by their primary care providers before conception.

BIBLIOGRAPHY

Barr M Jr, Cohen M Jr: ACE inhibitor fetopathy and hypocalvaria: the kidney-skull connection, *Teratology* 44:485, 1991.

Benjamin E et al: Diabetes in pregnancy in Zuni Indian women: prevalence and subsequent development of clinical diabetes after gestational diabetes, *Diabetes Care* 16:1231, 1993.

Catalano PM, Tyzbir ED, Sims EAH: Incidence and significance of islet cell antibodies in women with previous gestational diabetes, *Diabetes Care* 13:478, 1990.

Damm P et al: Predictive factors for the development of diabetes in women with previous gestational diabetes mellitus, *Am J Obstet Gynecol* 167:607, 1992.

Diamond MP et al: Impairment of counterregulatory hormone responses to hypoglycemia in pregnant women with insulin-dependent diabetes mellitus, *Am J Obstet Gynecol* 166:70, 1992.

Goldberg JD et al: Gestational diabetes: impact of home glucose monitoring on neonatal birth weight, *Am J Obstet Gynecol* 154:546, 1986.

Greene MF: Prevention and diagnosis of congenital anomalies in diabetic pregnancies. In Landon M, editor: *Clinics in perinatology,* Philadelphia, 1993, WB Saunders.

Greene MF et al: First-trimester hemoglobin A$_1$ and risk for major malformation and spontaneous abortion in diabetic pregnancy, *Teratology* 39:225, 1989.

Greene MF et al: Prematurity among insulin-requiring diabetic gravid women, *Am J Obstet Gynecol* 161:106, 1989.

Gregory R, Tattersall RB. Are diabetic pre-pregnancy clinics worthwhile? *Lancet* 340:656, 1992.

Hare JW and White P: Gestational diabetes and the white classification, *Diabetes Care* 3:394, 1980.

Harris MI: Gestational diabetes may represent discovery of preexisting glucose intolerance, *Diabetes Care* 11:402, 1988.

Hunter DJS, Keirse MJNC: Gestational diabetes. In Chalmers I, Enkin M, Keirse MJNC, editors: *Effective care in pregnancy and childbirth,* Oxford, 1989, Oxford University Press.

Imperiale TF, Petrulis AS: A meta-analysis of low-dose aspirin for the prevention of pregnancy-induced hypertension disease, *JAMA* 266:261, 1991.

Joslin EP: Pregnancy and diabetes mellitus, *Boston Med Surg J* 173:841, 1915.

Kitzmiller JL et al: Diabetic nephropathy and perinatal outcome, *Am J Obstet Gynecol* 141:741, 1981.

Kitzmiller JL et al: Preconception care of diabetes: glycemic control prevents congenital anomalies, *JAMA* 265:731, 1991.

Kjos SL et al: Serum lipids within 36 months of delivery in women with recent gestational diabetes, *Diabetes* 40:142, 1991.

Klein BEK et al: Effect of pregnancy on progression of diabetic retinopathy, *Diabetes Care* 13:34, 1990.

Madsen H, Ditzel J: Changes in red blood cell oxygen transport in diabetic pregnancy, *Am J Obstet Gynecol* 143:421, 1982.

Magee MS et al: Influence of diagnostic criteria on the incidence of gestational diabetes and perinatal morbidity, *JAMA* 269:609, 1993.

Metzger BE and the Organizing Committee: Summary and recommendations of the third international workshop-conference on gestational diabetes mellitus, *Diabetes* 40:197, 1991.

Miller E et al: Elevated maternal hemoglobin A$_{1C}$ in early pregnancy and major congenital anomalies in infants of diabetic mothers, *N Engl J Med* 304:1331, 1981.

Milley JR et al: The effect of insulin on ovine fetal oxygen extraction, *Am J Obstet Gynecol* 149:673, 1984.

Molsted-Pedersen L, Skouby SO, Damm P: Preconception counseling and contraception after gestational diabetes, *Diabetes* 40:147, 1991.

Oppe TE, Hsia DY-Y, Gellis SS: Pregnancy in the diabetic mother with nephritis, *Lancet* 1:353, 1957.

O'Sullivan JB, Mahan CM: Criteria for the oral glucose tolerance test in pregnancy, *Diabetes* 13:278, 1964.

Pedersen J: Problems and management. In *The pregnant diabetic and her newborn,* ed 2, Baltimore, 1977, Williams & Wilkins.

Petersen KR et al: Effects of contraceptive steroids on cardiovascular risk factors in women with insulin-dependent diabetes mellitus, *Am J Obstet Gynecol* 171:400, 1994.

Reece EA et al: Diabetic nephropathy: pregnancy performance and feto-maternal outcome, *Am J Obstet Gynecol* 159:56, 1988.

Rubinstein P et al: HLA antigens and islet cell antibodies in gestational diabetes, *Hum Immunol* 3:271, 1981.

Steel JM, Irvine WJ, Clarke BF: The significance of pancreatic islet cell antibody and abnormal glucose tolerance during pregnancy, *J Clin Lab Immunol* 4:83, 1980.

Ylinen K et al: Risk of minor and major fetal malformations in diabetics with high haemoglobin A$_{1C}$ values in early pregnancy, *Br Med J* 289:345, 1984.

54 Hypertension in Pregnancy

Michael F. Greene

The hypertensive disorders of pregnancy are responsible for a disproportionate amount of maternal and perinatal morbidity and mortality. Although routine prenatal care, recognition of hypertension, and intervention have made maternal mortality rare in the United States, it is the most common cause of maternal mortality in many developing nations. Proper diagnostic categorization of the various disorders can be difficult and confusing, while their management can be challenging. The fundamental reason for difficulties in diagnosis and management is incomplete understanding of the basic etiologic pathophysiology of preeclampsia. Despite incomplete knowledge, interventions are necessary to prevent serious complications.

PHYSIOLOGY
Cardiovascular changes with pregnancy

During normal pregnancy there is a 40% increase in intravascular volume and a 20% increase in cardiac output, but a fall in peripheral vascular resistance. This results in a net fall in blood pressure in the second trimester. In the third trimester these changes result in a rise in blood pressure to first-trimester levels. The fall in peripheral vascular resistance is associated with reduced vascular responsiveness to pressors, including catecholamines and angiotensin II. Although the data regarding serum levels of catecholamines are somewhat ambiguous, it is clear that serum levels of angiotensin II and aldosterone are elevated. The vascular refractoriness to pressors is likely mediated by the prostaglandin system, and some investigators have found the urinary excretion of prostaglandin E_2 (PGE_2) and its metabolites to be increased substantially in pregnant women compared with nonpregnant control subjects.

Classification of hypertensive disorders in pregnancy

Much of the confusion surrounding the treatment and prognosis for hypertension in pregnancy results from imprecision in its definition and diagnosis. Central to diagnosis is distinguishing hypertension that originates during pregnancy from hypertension that antedates pregnancy. If a patient is not seen for the first time until the midtrimester when blood pressure is normally somewhat lower, she may appear normotensive when she was really modestly hypertensive before pregnancy. The presence or absence of proteinuria is also a key diagnostic feature, and it cannot be assessed accurately without a 24-hour urine collection for quantitation. Semiquantitative urine protein diagnostic reagent dipsticks are not adequate (Kuo, Koumantakis, and Gallery, 1992).

During the 1980s the term *pregnancy-induced hypertension* (PIH) became popular, but it blurred some important distinctions and contributed more confusion than enlightenment. In 1990 the Working Group on High Blood Pressure in Pregnancy, convened by the National Heart, Lung and Blood Institute, reaffirmed the classification of hypertensive disorders in pregnancy proposed by the American College of Obstetricians and Gynecologists in 1972. That classification recognizes four diagnostic categories of hypertensive disorders in pregnancy:

1. Chronic hypertension
2. Preeclampsia-eclampsia
3. Preeclampsia superimposed on chronic hypertension
4. Transient hypertension

SPECIFIC HYPERTENSIVE DISORDERS
Chronic hypertension

Definition. Chronic hypertension is defined as hypertension (140/90 mm Hg or greater) that is observed before pregnancy or before 20 weeks' gestation. Retrospectively, patients whose hypertension persists beyond 42 days after delivery also are classified as having chronic hypertension. The vast majority of these patients have "essential" hypertension. A minority of these patients will have an assortment of relatively uncommon medical conditions complicated by hypertension, such as diabetic nephropathy, chronic glomerulonephritis, or systemic lupus erythematosus. A very small minority will have a variety of rare causes of hypertension, which are more or less surgically remediable, such as coarctation of the aorta, renal artery stenosis, Cushing's syndrome, or pheochromocytoma. The hallmark of chronic hypertension is that, although it may ameliorate postpartum, it persists beyond the puerperium.

Epidemiology. Estimates of the incidence of chronic hypertension among pregnant women are difficult to find. Most studies are not population based but rather cohort studies of the natural history of the disease in pregnancy or clinical trials. Both types of studies have accumulated cases from large population bases of unknown size with unknown percentages of ascertainment. From the difficulties encountered in obtaining significant numbers of patients for study, it can be inferred that the incidence is rather low. Even among women with diabetes mellitus antedating pregnancy, the incidence of chronic hypertension is only 6% (Greene et al., 1989). The demographic characteristics of the population influence the incidence as a result of the well-known associations with race and age.

Maternal and fetal complications. The most important complication of chronic hypertension in pregnancy is the increased risk for perinatal mortality. Much of this risk in turn is due to or associated with other complications such as superimposed preeclampsia, prematurity, abruptio placentae, and intrauterine growth retardation (IUGR). The increased risk for perinatal mortality has been recognized for decades and has generally been approximately three to four times the risk in the general population from which the hypertensive patients were drawn. In a recent study from Quebec, for example, the perinatal mortality was 45/1000 among 337 pregnancies in 298 hypertensive women whereas it was 12/1000 during the same period in the general pop-

Table 54-1 Incidence of intrauterine growth retardation ($<10^{th}$ percentile) among hypertensive patients

Reference	Type of hypertension	N	%
Lin et al., 1982	Virtually all had PE	34/157	21.6
Sibai, Abdella, and Anderson, 1983	Chronic HTN	10/190	5
Mabie, Pernoll, and Biswas, 1986	Chronic HTN and PE	7/21	32
	Chronic HTN	25/169	15
Ferrazzani et al., 1990	Chronic HTN	12/98	12
	Transient HTN	36/198	18
	PE	76/147	52
Rey and Couturier, 1994	Chronic HTN	52/337	15.5

HTN, hypertension; PE, preeclampsia.

Table 54-2 Chronic hypertension and risk of superimposed preeclampsia

Reference	%
Landesman et al., 1957	34
Kincaid-Smith, Bullen, and Mills, 1966	38
Leather et al., 1968	33
Sandstrom 1978	34
Curet and Olson, 1979	39
Welt et al., 1981	33
Sibai, Abdella, and Anderson, 1983	10
Rubin et al, 1983	26
Mabie, Pernoll, and Biswas, 1986	34
Sibai et al., 1990	16
Rey and Couturier, 1994	21

ulation (Rey and Couturier, 1994). Most of the increased risk for prematurity and cesarean section in these pregnancies is due to intervention to prevent stillbirth in the setting of IUGR, preeclampsia, abruptio placentae, or other perceived threat to fetal well-being. The incidence of IUGR, defined as birth weight less than the 10th centile for gestational age, has generally been reported to be 15% to 20% (Table 54-1). Estimates of the incidence of preeclampsia superimposed on chronic hypertension are often inaccurately high because patients recruited into studies relatively late in pregnancy are likely already to have some preeclampsia. Table 54-2 compiles the incidence of superimposed preeclampsia in patients with chronic hypertension in a number of studies. The incidence ranges from 10% to nearly 40%, with the best estimate being approximately 20%.

Patients with chronic hypertension frequently experience episodes of acutely elevated blood pressure, which some authors have termed "pregnancy aggravated" hypertensive episodes (Arias and Zamora, 1979). It is difficult to show that these episodes are the proximate cause of any maternal or fetal morbidity, but they are anxiety provoking for the physician and frequently result in hospitalization of the patient and additional antihypertensive therapy.

Management

Goals of therapy. Patients with severely elevated blood pressures should be treated to prevent the potential maternal consequences of severe hypertension such as cerebrovascular accidents. Similarly, patients with preexisting renal disease should be treated to protect their kidneys from further damage. Controversy arises regarding the advisability of treating mild chronic hypertension in patients without renal disease. The goals of antihypertensive therapy should be to reduce the risks of the aforementioned perinatal complications. In the past 25 years a large number of trials have been published with rather consistently disappointing results (Table 54-3).

Antihypertensive agents. Among the first agents used was *alpha-methyldopa (α-MD)* as epitomized in the studies of Leather et al. (1968) and Redman et al. (1976). Although these investigators were able to achieve adequate blood pressure control with α-MD and other agents, there was no significant impact on the incidence of superimposed preeclampsia, the mean birth weight, or the mean gestational age

at the time of delivery. It should be noted that the mean daily dose of α-MD necessary in the study of Redman, Beilin, and Bonnar (1977) was 1.9 g, with a maximum dose of 4 g/day. There were no adverse effects of the α-MD on either the mothers or their offspring followed through early childhood, thus firmly establishing its safety (Cockburn et al., 1982). Both studies found a reduced incidence of midtrimester loss associated with α-MD therapy. This was an unexpected finding with no obvious mechanism to explain it. Furthermore, no other studies have confirmed these initial studies.

The next group of drugs to be studied systematically comprised the *beta blockers*. Early reports suggested that they, particularly propranolol, were associated with a variety of fetal and neonatal complications, including IUGR and hypoglycemia. With the exception of one very small study of 15 patients treated with atenolol (Butters, Kennedy, and Rubin, 1990), hundreds of patients have been treated with metroprolol, atenolol, and oxprenolol without evidence for an increased incidence of these complications (see Table 54-3). Although the beta blockers were demonstrably efficacious in lowering blood pressure, they, like α-MD, produced no demonstrable improvement in perinatal outcome.

Most recently, labetalol, the combined alpha blocker and nonspecific beta blocker, has been studied in several large trials. The results of the trials indicate that labetalol is clearly both safe and effective for lowering blood pressure during pregnancy, but it does not improve perinatal outcome. It is clearly superior to α-MD in reducing pregnancy-aggravated hypertensive episodes and the frequency with which additional agents must be added to adequately control blood pressure.

The use of *calcium channel blockers* has been reported in some small series (Constantine et al., 1987). They appear to be safe and effective in reducing blood pressure, but there are not yet any trials to address their ability to change perinatal outcome. The use of *clonidine* has been reported in a small trial without convincing evidence that it improves perinatal outcome (Phippard et al., 1991).

Diuretic therapy during pregnancy should be discouraged. There is considerable literature to suggest that successful pregnancy is associated with adequate expansion of intravascular volume, whereas severe hypertension, IUGR, and perinatal mortality are associated with inadequate vol-

Table 54-3 Summary of major randomized controlled trials of antihypertensive therapy in pregnancy

Reference	Treatment (N)	Control (N)	Improved gestational age at delivery	Effect on IUGR incidence	Reduced PE
Leather et al., 1968	α-Methyldopa (52)	Routine care (48)	Yes	—	No
Redman et al., 1976	α-Methyldopa (117)	Routine care (125)	No	None	No
Sandstrom, 1978	Metoprolol (101)	Hydralazine (97)	No	None	No
Rubin et al., 1983	Atenolol (60)	Placebo (60)	No	None	Yes
Sibai et al., 1990	Labetalol (86)	No medication (90)	No	None	No
		α-Methyldopa (88)			
Pickles, Symonds, and Broughton Pipkin, 1989	Labetalol (70)	Placebo (74)	No	None	No
Plouin et al., 1988	Labetalol (91) Hydralazine prn	α-Methyldopa (85) Hydralazine prn	No	None	No
Hogstedt et al., 1985	Metoprolol plus hydralazine (82)	Routine care (79)	No	None	No
Fidler et al., 1983	Oxprenolol (50)	α-Methyldopa (50)	No	None	No
Plouin et al., 1990	Oxprenolol plus hydralazine (78)	Placebo (76)	Yes	None	No
Gallery, Ross, and Gyory, 1985	Oxprenolol (96) Hydralazine prn	α-Methyldopa (87) Hydralazine prn	No	Reduced	No
Butters, Kennedy, and Rubin, 1990	Atenolol (15)	Placebo (14)	No	Increased	—

IUGR, intrauterine growth retardation; PE, preeclampsia.

ume expansion. It is not clear whether adequate volume expansion is causal for optimal pregnancy outcome or whether both result from some more proximate physiologic cause. In a small series Sibai, Grossman, and Grossman (1984) have shown that patients who are maintained through pregnancy on their prepregnancy diuretic therapy fail to expand their blood volumes. The series was too small to recognize an adverse impact on perinatal outcome, nor was there evidence that if the diuretics had been discontinued, the blood volumes would have expanded. Nonetheless, diuretic therapy should be initiated during pregnancy only under unusual circumstances, such as pulmonary edema or anasarca associated with nephrotic syndrome, and not for blood pressure control. The issue of whether long-standing diuretic therapy, which is part of a balanced program of successful blood pressure control, should be discontinued with pregnancy is controversial. This author's practice is not to discontinue the therapy.

Angiotensin converting enzyme inhibitors deserve special mention because they are becoming very widely used in young diabetic women, and they should not be used during pregnancy. Although first-trimester exposure does not appear to be teratogenic, their use later in pregnancy can have devastating consequences, and the FDA has warned against their use in a *Medical Bulletin* issued in April 1992. Exposure in the second and third trimester has resulted in fetal renal tubular dysgenesis, oligohydramnios, severe IUGR, inadequate ossification of the calvarial plates, and transient or permanent neonatal renal insufficiency of severe or fatal degree (Barr and Cohen, 1991).

The use of *nitroprusside* should also be avoided during pregnancy. Animal studies have shown that the cyanide, which results from the metabolism of nitroprusside, can accumulate in the fetal compartment to toxic levels.

In summary, severe hypertension and hypertension associated with renal disease should be treated to prevent mater-

nal complications. Commonly used agents are summarized in Table 54-4. There is no convincing evidence, however, that treating hypertension during pregnancy reduces the incidence of IUGR, prematurity, superimposed preeclampsia, or perinatal mortality.

Prognosis. Women with chronic hypertension frequently experience exacerbation of their hypertension in late pregnancy. It usually requires several weeks after delivery for their blood pressure to return to prepregnancy levels. During that time they should be seen frequently because they may become hypotensive on the therapy that was increased in late pregnancy to control rising blood pressure.

A woman whose chronic hypertension complicates one pregnancy can expect subsequent pregnancies to be similarly affected. Complications of chronic hypertension, such as IUGR and superimposed preeclampsia, are more likely to recur in a patient (~20% for each) than to occur initially.

Preeclampsia-eclampsia

Definition. Preeclampsia is unique to pregnancy, requiring the presence of trophoblastic tissue, and seems unique to human beings without any naturally occurring animal models. It is classically defined as the triad of hypertension, proteinuria, and edema in pregnancy. Edema is so common during pregnancy however, affecting 50% to 80% of pregnancies, that it is considered normal. The clinical diagnosis of edema is subjective and impossible to standardize or quantitate. Attempts to distinguish between "normal edema" and "pathologic edema" on the basis of either the rate or timing of development or anatomic distribution have not been successful. Furthermore, the clinical assessment of edema has not been useful prognostically with respect to the risk for perinatal mortality. Edema, therefore, is not a very useful diagnostic sign.

Hypertension is diagnosed on both relative and absolute criteria. Compared with the average values before 20 weeks' gestation, a rise in systolic pressure of 30 mm Hg or more or

Table 54-4 Antihypertensive agents for use in pregnancy

Agent	Mechanism of action	Daily dose range (mg)	Dosing schedule	Comment
Methyldopa	Central sympatholytic	750-3000	tid-qid	Very safe. Slow onset of action. Often causes unacceptable degree of somnolence at therapeutic dose
Hydralazine	Direct relaxation of arterial smooth muscle	40-200	qid	Ineffective as chronic oral monotherapy. Useful when added to methyldopa or a beta blocker. Useful IV to acutely lower blood pressure (5 mg bolus at 15-min intervals or continuous infusion)
Metoprolol	Beta$_1$-blockade	100-400	bid	Effective, well tolerated, convenient dosing schedule
Atenolol	Beta$_1$-blockade	50-200	qd	Effective, well tolerated, convenient dosing schedule
Labetalol	Alpha blockade Beta$_1$- and beta$_2$-blockade	300-1200	tid-qid	Effective, well tolerated. Useful IV to acutely lower blood pressure (20-80 mg bolus at 20- to 30-min intervals or continuous infusion)
Nifedipine	Calcium channel blocker	30-120	tid	Seems safe and effective although least available data. Useful administered sublingually to acutely lower blood pressure

a rise in diastolic pressure of 15 mm Hg or more is considered hypertension. If blood pressure early in pregnancy is not known, then a value of 140/90 or greater beyond 20 weeks' gestation is considered hypertension.

Significant proteinuria is defined as greater than or equal to 300 mg protein in a 24-hour urine collection. The 95% upper confidence limit for protein loss in apparently normal women in the third trimester is 200 mg in 24 hours (Kuo, Koumantakis, and Gallery, 1992). This gives a small margin of separation between the normal range for the excretion rate and that which must be diagnosed as pathologic.

Attempts to grade preeclampsia as mild versus moderate have been arbitrary and not useful. There are generally accepted criteria for severe preeclampsia, with all other cases classified as mild. The presence of any of the following would be considered diagnostic of severe preeclampsia:

1. Blood pressure consistently in excess of 160 mm Hg systolic or 110 mm Hg diastolic
2. Dense proteinuria—various criteria ranging from 2 to 5 grams per day have been used
3. Oliguria or elevated serum creatinine levels (>1.2 mg/dl) in a patient previously known to have a normal serum creatinine
4. Thrombocytopenia (<100,000 per μl) and/or evidence of hemolysis
5. Epigastric pain and/or evidence of hepatocellular necrosis
6. Persistent headache and/or visual disturbance of apparently central origin
7. Retinal hemorrhages, exudates, or papilledema
8. Pulmonary edema
9. According to some authors, the presence of fetal growth retardation is a criterion

Eclampsia is diagnosed when a patient with preeclampsia develops seizures that cannot be attributed to another cause.

It is well recognized that eclamptic seizures may occur in mildly hypertensive patients with proteinuria and in hypertensive patients who have not yet developed proteinuria. The aforementioned criteria, therefore, should not be applied too rigidly in daily practice. A high index of suspicion should be maintained, and overdiagnosis is preferable to underdiagnosis if progression to eclampsia is to be avoided. It should be obvious from this discussion that preeclampsia is a clinical diagnosis based on a constellation of findings, none of which is specific. It could be difficult to distinguish the first occurrence of lupus nephritis in pregnancy from preeclampsia. In women with diabetic nephropathy with hypertension, proteinuria, and edema antedating pregnancy, the diagnosis of preeclampsia is entirely arbitrary in the absence of some complication indicating severe preeclampsia. Although not specific, a serum uric acid level, which rises disproportionately to the degree of renal dysfunction, may also be helpful in making the diagnosis of preeclampsia.

Incidence. Preeclampsia occurs in 4% to 10% of all pregnancies progressing beyond the first trimester. The actual incidence depends on the criteria used for diagnosis and the demographics of the population being studied. It is severalfold more common among primigravidas than it is in subsequent pregnancies (Eskenazi, Fenster, and Sidney, 1991). It is more common in young women because young women are more likely to be primigravidas, but when parity is controlled, youth does not seem to be a risk. Obesity and carbohydrate intolerance are also risk factors (Suhonen and Teramo, 1993). Advanced maternal age appears to be a risk factor, but this may be due to the association of chronic hypertension, obesity, and carbohydrate intolerance with advancing age and the risk for the superimposition of preeclampsia on chronic hypertension. Similarly, the higher incidence of preeclampsia among African-Americans may be due to their generally higher incidence of hypertension. The apparent relationship between low socioeconomic status and preeclampsia in the United States may be due to the relationship between race and socioeconomic status. In other countries, socioeconomic status does not appear to be a risk factor.

Eclampsia appears to be related to socioeconomic status. This probably is due to the fact that preeclampsia often can be prevented from developing into eclampsia by timely delivery in women receiving regular prenatal care. To the extent that women of lower socioeconomic status are more likely to receive less regular prenatal care, it is more likely that their preeclampsia will evolve into eclampsia.

A variety of medical and obstetric conditions cause a predisposition to preeclampsia. Women with insulin-requiring diabetes mellitus have a 20% to 40% risk of developing preeclampsia (Greene et al., 1989). Systemic lupus erythematosis and any preexisting renal disease increase the risk. Multiple gestations, hydatidiform moles, and hydropic fetuses of any cause also place women at high risk.

Maternal and fetal complications. Historically preeclampsia-eclampsia has been a major cause of maternal mortality. One of the most important benefits of routine prenatal care has been the early recognition of preeclampsia and intervention that now makes maternal mortality rare. Significant maternal morbidity, including intracranial hemorrhage, intrahepatic hemorrhage and rupture, abruptio placentae and hemorrhage, and renal cortical necrosis, can still result from severe preeclampsia.

A significant minority (10% to 15%) of patients with preeclampsia will develop a variant in which microangiopathic hemolysis, hepatocellular necrosis, or thrombocytopenia appear prior to or more prominently than hypertension and proteinuria. This variant, frequently referred to by the acronym HELLP (*H*emolysis, *E*levated *L*iver enzymes, and *L*ow *P*latelets syndrome), can be difficult to distinguish from a variety of other disease preocesses with which it overlaps. These include thrombotic thrombocytopenia purpura, hemolytic uremic syndrome, and systemic lupus erythematosis.

The cerebral circulation has the ability to autoregulate its own flow over a broad range of perfusion pressure. When the mean arterial pressure exceeds 140 mm Hg, however, that range is exceeded and hypertensive encephalopathy may result (Donaldson, 1978). Associated with this is severe arteriolar vasospasm that limits perfusion, which can result in ischemia, infarction, and petechial or gross hemorrhage. Petechial hemorrhages are frequently seen in the cerebral cortex of women dying of severe preeclampsia. They are particularly prone to occur in the occipital (visual) cortex and may be responsible for the visual phenomenon of scintillations, which are frequently described. It is generally difficult to interpret the significance of headache because it is such a common complaint, both in general and during pregnancy. In the setting of preeclampsia, however, headaches may be ominous signs, occurring in 85% of eclamptic women before their seizures.

Swelling of the liver causes stretching of Glisson's capsule and epigastric pain. In the setting of preeclampsia, epigastric pain usually is due to hepatic swelling, which may be associated with intrahepatic hemorrhage. If this progresses to hepatic rupture, it is associated with a very high fatality rate.

The healthy left ventricle, faced with increased afterload, is capable of responding with a substantial increase in work to maintain cardiac output. This ability is not infinite, however, and faced with sufficiently high afterload for a sufficiently long period of time, the left ventricle will fail and pulmonary edema will result. Most of the hemodynamic data obtained from preeclamptic women who have undergone invasive monitoring indicate that their left ventricles are healthy and respond normally to increased afterload. Thus pulmonary edema in the preeclamptic patient, which

occurs only rarely, is evidence of very severe disease. Much more commonly, pulmonary edema is seen in these patients as the result of overly zealous intravenous fluid therapy.

Perinatal mortality is significantly increased in preeclamptic women. Because of the generally low incidence of perinatal mortality, large numbers of patients must be studied to obtain reliable estimates of risk. The Collaborative Perinatal Project followed more than 50,000 mother-infant pairs from enrollment during pregnancy between 1959 and 1965 through the seventh year of the children. Analysis of that data showed the important influences of both hypertension and proteinuria on perinatal mortality. Although those data are now 30 years old, and the overall rate of perinatal mortality has fallen sharply during that time, the risk of perinatal mortality for normal women relative to hypertensive and proteinuric women probably has not changed. Those data show quite clearly that the risk for perinatal mortality increased progressively with increases in both diastolic blood pressure and proteinuria. The risk of IUGR also was increased in preeclampsia, and the risk for perinatal mortality dramatically increased among those IUGR fetuses.

Management. Preeclampsia is a progressive disorder for which the only cure is delivery of the fetus. Although it can be stated with confidence that preeclampsia will not resolve until after delivery, the rate of progression is entirely unpredictable. The period of mild preeclampsia from first diagnosis until the appearance of complications that warrant the diagnosis of "severe" or seizures indicating eclampsia can be quite prolonged. In patients with mild preeclampsia remote from term, expectant management is appropriate for the benefit of both the mother and the fetus. The mother benefits because the likelihood that she will have a successful pelvic delivery increases with increasing gestational age. The fetus benefits from increased maturity, which reduces the likelihood of complications in the nursery. Expectant management is not without risks however. The risk of stillbirth is everpresent for the fetus, and the mother could suffer an intracranial hemorrhage with permanent sequelae. The development of virtually any of the complications already listed as criteria for "severe" preeclampsia, with the exceptions of dense proteinura (Chua and Redman, 1992) and IUGR, is an indication for prompt delivery. All other patients should be managed expectantly when the neonatal risks of prematurity would be substantial. This risk-benefit analysis is dynamic and must be reevaluated frequently during the course of expectant management. Some of the most difficult decisions in obstetrics must be made in this setting.

A wide variety of therapies has been employed over the decades on the basis of an equally wide variety of theories regarding the pathophysiology of the disease to attempt to ameliorate the severity of preeclampsia and prevent eclampsia. These have included "lytic cocktails" of barbiturates and opiates, dietary therapy, antihypertensive therapy, volume expansion, dopamine, and others. Some have been harmful; none have been helpful. A detailed discussion of management is found in Chapter 51.

Preeclampsia superimposed on chronic hypertension

Current understanding is that the pathophysiology, potential complications, and management of preeclampsia superimposed on chronic hypertension are no different than those for preeclampsia. The prognosis for recurrence in subsequent pregnancies may be much higher however. Sibai, Mercer, and Sarinoglu (1991) have documented that in women with severe preeclampsia very early in pregnancy the recurrence risk in subsequent pregnancies may be as high as 65%. The use of low-dose aspirin for successful prophyphylaxis against the development of preeclampsia in patients at high risk has been reported and is discussed in the next section.

Transient hypertension

Definition. Transient hypertension is defined as hypertension of modest degree that first appears late in pregnancy or during the first 24 hours postpartum in a patient without evidence of preeclampsia or preexisting hypertension. There has been some difficulty in gaining recognition of this entity, which also has been termed *gestational hypertension* and *nonproteinuric pregnancy-induced hypertension*. The main argument against the utility of the diagnosis has been that a pregnancy can confidently be placed in this category only after it is over. Until then, the patient must be managed as though she were developing preeclampsia. Although there is certainly an element of truth to this argument, these patients often show characteristics that provide sufficient support for a prospective diagnosis. These patients tend to be older and more obese, with poorer carbohydrate tolerance and hyperinsulinemia (Solomon et al., 1994). The problem tends to recur in subsequent pregnancies. These patients tend to have family histories of hypertension and are more likely to develop chronic hypertension themselves. It is not associated with IUGR or other complications.

Management. Antihypertensive therapy is not indicated for patients with transient hypertension. Large randomized trials have failed to demonstrate any benefit to bed rest for these patients (Crowther, Bouwmeester, and Ashurst, 1992). An organized program of expectant outpatient management can provide excellent outcomes while minimizing drug therapy, inpatient admissions, and inductions of labor (Tuffnell et al., 1992). Generally these patients should be permitted to go to term and enter spontaneous labor with minimal intervention.

Aspirin therapy. There has been considerable interest in recent years in the potential for low-dose aspirin therapy to provide prophylaxis against preeclampsia, IUGR, and fetal demise. The theory behind the therapy has been that platelet activation, with thromboxane production and endothelial cell damage, is central both to the development of preeclampsia and to many cases of IUGR and fetal death as a result of "uteroplacental insufficiency." By disabling platelets with chronic low-dose aspirin therapy, it is hoped that this chain can be broken. Studies to date can be divided into two broad categories: those enrolling high-risk patients and those enrolling low-risk primigravidas. Differences among the studies in subject selection criteria, gestational age at initiation of therapy, and drugs used (some added dipyridamole to the aspirin) make grouping the data and direct comparisons difficult. In summary it is fair to say, however, that multiple studies of high-risk patients have rather uniformly shown a benefit to therapy in reducing the incidences of both preeclampsia and IUGR in the aspirin-treated groups. In contrast, the studies in low-risk women

have failed to demonstrate any benefit to aspirin therapy. One of the studies suggested that the aspirin may have caused an increased incidence of abruptio placentae (Sibai et al., 1993), but the other two do not confirm that risk. Taken together, the studies are reassuring that the aspirin is at worst not helpful but not harmful to mother or fetus.

Patients most likely to benefit from prophylactic aspirin therapy are those with a history of a prior episode of severe preeclampsia, especially early in pregnancy, and those with a history of IUGR caused by uteroplacental insufficiency, with or without fetal demise. A dose of 80 mg per day is adequate. The aspirin must be started before the development of any signs of preeclampsia or IUGR. The Collaborative Low-Dose Aspirin Study in Pregnancy showed that aspirin is ineffective if started after the development of signs of preeclampsia.

BIBLIOGRAPHY

Arias F, Zamora J: Antihypertensive treatment and pregnancy outcome in patients with mild chronic hypertension, *Obstet Gynecol* 53:489, 1979.

Barr M Jr, Cohen MM Jr: ACE inhibitor fetopathy and hypocalvaria: the kidney-skull connection, *Teratology* 44:485, 1991.

Beaufils M et al: Prevention of pre-eclampsia by early antiplatelet therapy, *Lancet* 1:840, 1985.

Benigni A et al: Effect of low-dose aspirin on fetal and maternal generation of thromboxane by platelets in women at risk for pregnancy-induced hypertension, *N Engl J Med* 321:357, 1989.

Butters L, Kennedy S, Rubin PC: Atenolol in essential hypertension during pregnancy, *Br Med J* 301:587, 1990.

Chua S, Redman CWG: Prognosis for pre-eclampsia complicated by 5 g or more of proteinuria in 24 hours, *Eur J Obstet Gynaecol Reprod Biol* 43:9, 1992.

Cockburn J et al: Final report of study on hypertension during pregnancy: the effects of specific treatment on the growth and development of the children, *Lancet* 1:647, 1982.

Collaborative Low-Dose Aspirin Study in Pregnancy Collaborative Group: CLASP: a randomised trial of low-dose aspirin for the prevention and treatment of pre-eclampsia among 9364 pregnant women, *Lancet* 343:619, 1994.

Constantine G et al: Nifedipine as a second line antihypertensive drug in pregnancy, *Br J Obstet Gynaecol* 94:1136, 1987.

Crowther CA, Bouwmeester AM, Ashurst HM: Does admission to hospital for bed rest prevent disease progression or improve fetal outcome in pregnancy complicated by non-proteinuric hypertension? *Br J Obstet Gynaecol* 99:13, 1992.

Curet LB, Olson RW: Evaluation of a program of bed rest in the treatment of chronic hypertension in pregnancy, *Obstet Gynecol* 53:336, 1979.

Donaldson JO: *Neurology of pregnancy*, Philadelphia, 1978, WB Saunders.

Eskenazi B, Fenster L, Sidney S: A multivariate analysis of risk factors for preeclampsia, *JAMA* 266:237, 1991.

Ferrazzani S et al: Proteinuria and outcome of 444 pregnancies complicated by hypertension, *Am J Obstet Gynecol* 162:366, 1990.

Fidler J et al: Randomised controlled comparative study of methyldopa and oxprenolol in treatment of hypertension in pregnancy, *Br Med J* 286:1927, 1983.

Friedman EA, Neff RK: *Pregnancy hypertension*, Littleton, Mass, 1977, PSG Publishing Co.

Gallery EDM, Ross MR, Gyory AZ: Antihypertensive treatment in pregnancy: analysis of different responses to oxprenolol and methyldopa, *Br Med J* 291:563, 1985.

Greene MF et al: Prematurity among insulin-requiring diabetic gravid women, *Am J Obstet Gynecol* 161:106, 1989.

Hauth JC et al: Low-dose aspirin therapy to prevent preeclampsia, *Am J Obstet Gynecol* 168:1083, 1993.

Hogstedt S et al: A prospective controlled trial of metoprolol-hydralazine treatment in hypertension during pregnancy, *Acta Obstet Gynecol Scand* 64:505, 1985.

Kincaid-Smith P, Bullen M, Mills J: Prolonged use of methyldopa in severe hypertension in pregnancy, *Br Med J* 1:274, 1966.

Kuo VS, Koumantakis G, Gallery EDM: Proteinuria and its assessment in normal and hypertensive pregnancy, *Am J Obstet Gynecol* 167:723, 1992.

Landesman R et al: Reserpine in toxemia of pregnancy, *Obstet Gynecol* 9:377, 1957.

Leather HM et al: A controlled trial of hypotensive agents in hypertension in pregnancy, *Lancet* 2:488, 1968.

Lin C-C et al: Fetal outcome in hypertensive disorders in pregnancy, *Am J Obstet Gynecol* 142:255, 1982.

Mabie WC, Pernoll ML, Biswas MK: Chronic hypertension in pregnancy, *Obstet Gynecol* 67:197, 1986.

Mathews DD: A randomized controlled trial of bed rest and sedation or normal activity and nonsedation in the management of non-albuminuric hypertension in late pregnancy, *Br J Obstet Gynaecol* 84:108, 1977.

McParland P, Pearce JM, Chamberlain GVP: Doppler ultrasound and aspirin in recognition and prevention of pregnancy-induced hypertension, *Lancet* 335:1552, 1990.

National High Blood Pressure Education Program: Working group report on high blood pressure in pregnancy, *Am J Obstet Gynecol* 163:1689, 1990.

Phippard A et al: Early blood pressure control improves pregnancy outcome in primigravid women with mild hypertension, *Med J Aust* 154:378, 1991.

Pickles CJ, Broughton Pipkin F, Symonds EM: A randomised placebo controlled trial of labetalol in the treatment of mild to moderate pregnancy induced hypertension, *Br J Obstet Gynaecol* 99:964, 1992.

Pickles CJ, Symonds EM, Broughton Pipkin F: The fetal outcome in a randomized double-blind controlled trial of labetalol versus placebo in pregnancy-induced hypertension, *Br J Obstet Gynaecol* 96:38, 1989.

Plouin P-F et al: Comparison of antihypertensive efficacy and perinatal safety of labetalol and methyldopa in the treatment of hypertension in pregnancy: a randomized controlled trial, *Br J Obstet Gynaecol* 95:868, 1988.

Plouin P-F et al: A randomized comparison of early with conservative use of antihypertensive drugs in the management of pregnancy-induced hypertension, *Br J Obstet Gynaecol* 97:134, 1990.

Redman CWG, Beilin LJ, Bonnar J: Treatment of hypertension in pregnancy with methyldopa: blood pressure control and side effects, *Br J Obstet Gynaecol* 84:419, 1977.

Redman CWG et al: Fetal outcome in trial of antihypertensive treatment in pregnancy, *Lancet* 2:753, 1976.

Rey E, Couturier A: The prognosis of pregnancy in women with chronic hypertension, *Am J Obstet Gynecol* 171:410, 1994.

Rubin PC et al: Placebo-controlled trial of atenolol in treatment of pregnancy-associated hypertension, *Lancet* 1:431, 1983.

Rubin PC et al: Obstetric aspects of the use in pregnancy-associated hypertension of the β-adrenoceptor antagonist atenolol, *Am J Obstet Gynecol* 150:389, 1984.

Sandstrom B: Antihypertensive treatment with the adrenergic beta-receptor blocker metoprolol during pregnancy, *Gynecol Obstet Invest* 9:195, 1978.

Schiff E et al: The use of aspirin to prevent pregnancy-induced hypertension and lower the ratio of thromboxane A_2 to prostacyclin in relatively high risk pregnancies, *N Engl J Med* 321:351, 1989.

Sibai BM, Abdella TN, Anderson GD: Pregnancy outcome in 211 patients with mild chronic hypertension, *Obstet Gynecol* 61:571, 1983.

Sibai BM, Grossman RA, Grossman HG: Effects of diuretics on plasma volume in pregnancies with long-term hypertension, *Am J Obstet Gynecol* 150:831, 1984.

Sibai BM, Mercer B, Sarinoglu C: Severe preeclampsia in the second trimester: recurrence risk and long-term prognosis, *Am J Obstet Gynecol* 165:1408, 1991.

Sibai BM et al: A comparison of no medication versus methyldopa or labetalol in chronic hypertension during pregnancy, *Am J Obstet Gynecol* 162:960, 1990.

Sibai BM et al: Prevention of preeclampsia with low-dose aspirin in healthy, nulliparous pregnant women, *N Engl J Med* 329:1213, 1993.

Solomon CG et al: Glucose intolerance as a predictor of hypertension in pregnancy, *Hypertension* 23:717, 1994.

Suhonen L, Teramo K: Hypertension and pre-eclampsia in women with gestational glucose intolerance, *Acta Obstet Gynecol Scand* 72:269, 1993.

Tuffnell DJ et al: Randomised controlled trial of day care for hypertension in pregnancy, *Lancet* 339:224, 1992.

Uzan S et al: Prevention of fetal growth retardation with low-dose aspirin: findings of the EPREDA trial, *Lancet* 337:1427, 1991.

Wallenburg HCS et al: Low-dose aspirin prevents pregnancy-induced hypertension and pre-eclampsia in angiotensin-sensitive primigravidae, *Lancet* 1:1, 1986.

Walsh SW: Preeclampsia: an imbalance in placental prostacyclin and thromboxane production, *Am J Obstet Gynecol* 152:335, 1985.

Welt SI et al: The effect of prophylactic management and therapeutics on hypertensive disease in pregnancy: preliminary studies, *Obstet Gynecol* 57:557, 1981.

---

55 Liver Disease in Pregnancy

Lori B. Olans and Jacqueline L. Wolf

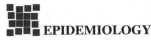

EPIDEMIOLOGY

Liver disease in pregnancy includes disorders present before pregnancy (which may be exacerbated during pregnancy) and those that may only occur during pregnancy. De novo liver function test abnormalities during pregnancy are uncommon, probably occurring in 5% or fewer of pregnant women in the United States. However, identification of their cause is important because of potential high maternal and fetal mortality rates if conditions such as acute fatty liver, preeclampsia, and hepatic rupture remain unrecognized and untreated. The focus of this chapter is a discussion of liver disorders unique to pregnancy.

CLASSIFICATION OF HEPATIC DISORDERS OF PREGNANCY

Hepatic disorders during pregnancy may be categorized as those occurring in the pregnant or nonpregnant state and those occurring only in the pregnant state. Those disorders that may occur independent of pregnancy, such as viral hepatitis and cholelithiasis, present special theraputic concerns for the mother and fetus during pregnancy. A discussion of these topics is beyond the scope of this chapter; see Chapters 14 and 50 for further information. Those disorders that occur only in the pregnant state include hyperemesis gravidarum, intrahepatic cholestasis of pregnancy, fatty liver of pregnancy, preeclampsia/eclampsia, HELLP syndrome

(*H*emolytic anemia, *E*levated *L*iver function test results, and *L*ow *P*latelet counts), and hepatic rupture.

LIVER FUNCTION TEST RESULTS DURING PREGNANCY

Many physiologic and systemic changes occur during pregnancy, and the liver is among the organs affected. Even in uncomplicated pregnancies liver function test results may differ from those in the nonpregnant state. For example, alkaline phosphatase level increases gradually during the first 7 months of pregnancy and then rises rapidly to peak at term. This elevation rarely exceeds two to four times the normal value and is principally of placental origin. In addition serum albumin concentration may be decreased to values 10% to 60% below normal, largely as a result of increased maternal blood volume during pregnancy. Levels of transaminases and bilirubin, however, are generally not altered by pregnancy (Table 55-1).

APPROACH TO THE PREGNANT PATIENT WITH ABNORMAL LIVER FUNCTION TEST RESULTS

History

The history obtained from a pregnant woman with abnormal liver function test findings should include several symptoms that may have different implications or less importance in the nonpregnant patient. The time of symptom onset in relation to the weeks of gestation provides an important clue to the cause of the test result abnormalities. Severe nausea and vomiting are the key features of hyperemesis gravidarium but when accompanied by headache and peripheral edema may indicate preeclampsia and, if accompanied by abdominal pain with or without hypotension in late pregnancy, may indicate hepatic rupture. Pruritis is the characteristic feature of intrahepatic cholestasis of pregnancy. It typically involves the palms of the hands and soles of the feet initially and then affects the rest of the body. Jaundice if present follows the pruritis. Abdominal pain is a significant symptom. One

should note the location of the pain; its duration; its character, that is, colicky, sharp or dull, insidious or sudden; factors that induce or relieve the pain; and other associated symptoms. Right upper quadrant and midabdominal pain has potential ominous implications, particularly in late pregnancy, when its occurrence may indicate acute fatty liver of pregnancy or hepatic rupture. Colicky pain with or without fever may indicate biliary colic or acute cholecystitis. Other symptoms important to elicit are headache, fever, peripheral edema, foamy urine, oliguria, insomnia, change in stools (i.e., acholia or diarrhea), malaise, weight loss or gain, dizziness, easy bruisability, or neurologic symptoms.

A history of the present and previous pregnancies may be helpful: multiple versus single fetus; multiparous versus primiparous; similar symptoms in previous pregnancies and time of onset of those symptoms; similar symptoms unassociated with pregnancies; and outcome of previous pregnancies (i.e., weight gain, maternal problems, weeks of gestation, health of newborn). Histories also should include symptoms with ingestion of oral contraceptive pills, drug ingestion or injection, previous blood transfusions, alcohol use, history of hepatitis or liver function test result abnormalities, diabetes mellitus, recent travel history, close contact with others with a similar illness, or pets at home. A family history of preeclampsia, oral contraceptive pill intolerance, pregnancy problems, or cholelithiasis is particularly pertinent.

Physical examination

Some of the common stigmata of liver disease on physical examination are found in the normal pregnant female. Because of physiologic and hormonal changes spider angioma and palmar erythema can be seen in a normal healthy pregnant female and do not in and of themselves indicate underlying liver abnormality. Jaundice, enlargement of the liver, tenderness of the liver, hepatic friction rub or bruit, splenomegaly, Murphy's sign, and excoriations are not normal in pregnancy. Other abnormal findings that may be associated with hepatic disorders of pregnancy are hypertension; orthostatic hypotension; peripheral edema; asterixes, hyperreflexia, or other neurologic findings; ecchymoses; and petechiae. The physical examination by itself is rarely diagnostic.

Diagnostic tests

Laboratory tests. The evaluation of abnormal liver function tests in pregnancy varies only slightly from that in nonpregnancy with the exception of limiting radiation exposure.

Blood tests should include a complete blood count (CBC) with hemoglobin, hematocrit, white blood cell count, and specific blood chemistries, including glucose, electrolytes, transaminases, lactic dehydrogenase, bilirubin, alkaline phosphastase, and uric acid levels. Also important are protime, partial thromboplastin time, and fibrinogen. Uric acid level elevation usually occurs in acute fatty liver of pregnancy and may occur in preeclampsia. Determination of serum bile acid levels, which may be elevated before the onset of or in conjunction with intrahepatic cholestasis of pregnancy (IHCP), is helpful if the diagnosis of IHCP is being considered. Measurement of amylase and lipase levels should be tested if abdominal pain or jaundice is present. If a viral cause is possible, one should obtain serologic results for hepatitis, including hepatitis A (immunoglobulin M [IgM]

Table 55-1 Liver function test results in normal pregnancy

Test	Effect	Trimester of maximum change
Albumin	↓10%-60%	2nd
γ–globulin	nl to sl↓	
Fibrinogen	↑50%	2nd
Transferrin	↑	3rd
Bilirubin	nl	
Alkaline phosphastase	2- to 4-fold ↑	3rd
SGOT/AST	nl	
SGPT/ALT	nl	
Cholesterol	2-fold ↑	3rd

Modified from Fallon HJ: Liver diseases. In Burrow and Ferris, editors: *Medical complications of pregnancy*, Philadelphia, 1988, WB Saunders. nl, normal; sl, slight; ↑ increase; ↓ decrease; SGOT/AST, serum glutamic-oxaloacetic transaminase/aspartate aminotransferase; SGPT/ALT, serum glutamic-pyruvic oxaloacetic transaminase/alanine aminotransferase.

and immunoglobin G [IgG]), hepatitis B (surface antigen, surface antibody, core antibody, and if surface antigen is present "e" antigen and "e" antibody), and hepatitis C. In certain circumstances delta-hepatitis antibody is indicated.

Other diagnostic tests. Abdominal ultrasound is safe in pregnancy and helpful in the evaluation of biliary tract disease, acute fatty liver of pregnancy, and hepatic rupture. However, if the finding is negative these diagnoses may not be ruled out. If there is a strong suspicion of biliary tract disease an endoscopic retrograde cannulation of the biliary ducts (ERCP) may be done safely with shielding by a skilled endoscopist. A computed tomographic (CT) scan may be more sensitive than ultrasound in detection of acute fatty liver and hepatic rupture but, if necessary for diagnosis, must be limited to one or two views because of the potential risk of radiation exposure to the fetus. The utility and safety in pregnancy of magnetic resonance imaging (MRI) scanning has yet to be determined conclusively. An angiogram is occasionally needed for the diagnosis of hepatic rupture.

Differential diagnosis

A complete discussion of the differential diagnosis is beyond the scope of this review. For a differential diagnosis by trimester of hepatic disorders most common in pregnancy and unique to pregnancy see Table 55-2.

LIVER DISORDERS SPECIFIC TO PREGNANCY
Hyperemesis gravidarum

Hyperemesis gravidarum occurs principally during the first trimester and has been rarely associated with abnormal liver function, particularly in women with extreme illness. The

Table 55-2 Differential diagnosis of common causes of transaminitis and/or jaundice in pregnancy

Trimester of pregnancy	Differential diagnosis
First	Hyperemesis gravidarum
	Gallstones
	Viral hepatitis
	Drug-induced hepatitis
	Intrahepatic cholestasis of pregnancy*
Second	Intrahepatic cholestasis of pregnancy
	Gallstones
	Viral hepatitis
	Drug-induced hepatitis
	Preeclampsia/eclampsia*
	HELLP syndrome*
Third	Intrahepatic cholestasis of pregnancy
	Preeclampsia/eclampsia
	HELLP syndrome
	Acute fatty liver of pregnancy
	Hepatic rupture
	Gallstones
	Viral hepatitis
	Drug-induced hepatitis

*Uncommon in this trimester.
HELLP, hemolytic anemia, elevated liver function test results, low platelet count.

clinical features of this disorder have been described elsewhere in this text (see Chapter 47) and include severe nausea and vomiting as well as dehydration, electrolyte disturbances, and ketosis. In affected women slight elevations in bilirubin, transaminase, or alkaline phosphatase levels may occur. In autopsy series liver histology is normal or show fatty infiltration, whereas in liver biopsy series the histologic findings are normal. Although the pathologic mechanism of liver injury is unknown the combined systemic effects of hypovolemia, malnutrition, and lactic acidosis are believed to play a role. Treatment is mainly supportive (Table 55-3).

Intrahepatic cholestasis of pregnancy

IHCP is a cholestatic disorder most common in the second and third trimesters of pregnancy. Pruritis, with or without jaundice, is a hallmark feature.

Epidemiology and risk factors. The incidence of IHCP has been difficult to estimate. It may be more common than previously suspected as a result of underreporting or failure to recognize mild cases. Incidence rates vary with geography and race. The highest incidence rate, 12% to 22%, has been reported in Chile among Araucanian Indians. Other reported incidence rates include 9% in Bolivia, 2% to 3% in Sweden, 0.2% to 0.8% in Australia, 0.2% in France, 0.13% in China, and 0.1% in Canada (Schorr-Lesnick and Dworkin, 1991; Van Dyke, 1990). Recent incidence rates in the United States and the United Kingdom are unknown. IHCP is extremely rare in black women: only one case has been reported in the literature (Vore, 1987).

Pathogenesis and cause. Family studies have suggested a dominant mode of mendelian transmission. Compared with those in control subjects, histocompatibility haplotypes human leukocyte antigen -B8 (HLA-B8) and HLA-BW-16 are more commonly found in affected women. IHCP has been more frequently observed in women with a family or previous medical history of IHCP or of cholestatic sensitivity to estrogens.

The cause of intrahepatic cholestasis of pregnancy has not been clearly delineated. A variety of theories and contributing factors have been postulated. Hormonal and genetic factors are suspected.

Women with intrahepatic cholestasis attributable to oral contraceptive use are more likely to develop IHCP. Furthermore rechallenging women with a history of IHCP by administering estrogens may precipitate pruritis and jaundice. This suggests a potential causative role for estrogens. The precise mechanism by which estrogens lead to cholestasis remains unclear. A variety of mechanisms have been proposed, including alteration of sodium-potassium–adenosine

Table 55-3 Hyperemesis gravidarum

Onset	Symptoms/signs	Laboratory tests
4-20 weeks	+Nausea +Vomiting	+Transaminase increase (1-2×) +Alkaline phosphatase increase (1-2×)
Usually 1st trimester		+Bilirubin increase (<5 mg/dl) +Urine ketone

triphosphatase (Na⁺/K⁺-ATPase) activity in hepatocyte plasma membranes, increase in cholesterol uptake by the liver leading to diminished membrane fluidity, and production of cholestatic metabolites.

Familial data have supported a heritable hepatic sensitivity to estrogens. The cause of IHCP is likely multifactorial with estrogens and genetics playing a major role. The contribution of opiate agonists, bile acids, and progesterones has been speculated and these theories remain to be proved.

Clinical presentation

History and physical examination. The spectrum of clinical illness varies from pruritis gravidarum, defined as diffuse itching, to severe cholestasis with accompanying jaundice. The onset of IHCP is most common in the third trimester although it has been reported as early as the second or, rarely, the first trimester (see Table 55-4).

PRURITIS. In almost all affected women the presenting symptom is pruritis, which can involve any part of the body, including the palms and soles. It tends to be particularly severe at night and may account for significant emotional distress resulting in insomnia, anorexia, and malaise. The pruritis generally resolves within 2 days of delivery and rarely extends beyond 2 weeks postpartum. Because of the intense itching another common physical finding is excoriations.

JAUNDICE AND OTHER SYMPTOMS. The frequency of jaundice associated with IHCP is approximately 25%. When jaundice occurs it generally follows the onset of pruritis by approximately 2 to 4 weeks and usually resolves by 1 to 2 weeks postpartum. Nausea, vomiting, and abdominal discomfort may rarely be associated with IHCP. Diarrhea caused by fat malabsorption may result from cholestasis.

Diagnostic tests. Laboratory tests reveal a variety of abnormalities. Serum bilirubin level, mostly direct, may be elevated but rarely exceeds 5 mg/dl. Alkaline phosphatase level may increase twofold, consistent with the normal rise in pregnancy. Transaminase levels can increase fourfold or, rarely, higher. Serum bile acid levels may increase 30 to 100-fold, and postprandial cholic acid 10- to 70-fold. Serum bile acid levels may represent the first or only sign of IHCP in women with pruritis but without other conventional liver function test abnormalities. Serum cholesterol, phospholipid, and triglyceride levels may also be elevated. Liver biopsy reveals cholestasis. Bile may be deposited within hepatocytes in a central-lobular pattern or may plug canaliculi. Minimal or no hepatocellular necrosis is present. It is not usually necessary to perform a liver biopsy since diagnosis can be made by history and physical examination.

Table 55-4 Intrahepatic cholestasis of pregnancy

Onset	Symptoms/signs	Laboratory tests
26 weeks to delivery	+Pruritis ± Jaundice	+Transaminase increase (1-4×) +Alkaline phosphatase level increase (1-2×) +Bilirubin level increase (<5 mg/dl)
Usually after 30 weeks		+Bile acid level increase (30-100×) ±Cholesterol level increase ± Triglyceride level increase

Maternal and fetal outcomes. Maternal outcome is benign when compared with that of infants. Pruritis, at times severe, resolves quickly after delivery. Although earlier series documented an increased risk of urinary tract infections and hemorrhage postpartum, these findings have not been reproduced in more recent studies. Steatorrhea-induced vitamin K deficiency was suggested but not proved as a contributing factor to postpartum hemorrhage. A long-term follow up study in Sweden has demonstrated an increased incidence of gallstones and gallbladder disease (Smith et al., 1991). There is no permanent liver damage to the mother postpartum.

Maternal intrahepatic cholestasis has been associated with an increased incidence of prematurity, perinatal deaths, fetal distress, and meconium staining of amniotic fluid. Elevated levels of bile acids, which are measurable in maternal blood, amniotic fluid, and umbilical cord blood, may contribute to the increased risk of poor fetal outcomes. Careful monitoring, particularly during the third trimester, for maternal and fetal well-being is recommended. Physicians should have a low threshold for early delivery if signs of fetal or maternal distress develop.

Management

Choice of therapy. Pruritis improves immediately after delivery. However, since IHCP does not significantly endanger maternal well-being, delivery before term is rarely first-line therapy. Instead management strategies have focused on symptomatic relief for the mother as well as careful monitoring for signs of fetal distress (see Table 55-5). General recommendations for alleviation of pruritis have included sleeping in a cool room and applying topical alcohol.

Antihistamines and phenobarbital have been ineffective in relieving pruritis. **Cholestyramine,** administered in maximum doses of 12 to 24 g/day, has met with variable success. Cholestyramine acts by binding bile acids in the intestinal lumen and thus decreasing systemic bile acid concentrations. It can produce relief within 1 to 2 weeks and usually works best in cases with moderately increased bile acid levels. Cholestyramine therapy may, however, aggravate malabsorption of fat-soluble nutrients.

S-Adenosyl-L-Methionine therapy showed promise in early studies for symptomatic and laboratory improvement in IHCP. This drug was thought to inactivate estrogen metabolites, increase membrane fluidity, and alter bile acid metabolism. However, in a subsequent double-blind, placebo-controlled trial no benefit could be demonstrated.

Table 55-5 Treatment regimens for IHCP

Drug	Dose/schedule	Precautions and side effects
Cholestyramine	4 gs 1-6 times/day	Constipation, flatulence, diarrhea, heartburn, abdominal discomfort; in large doses may interfere with absorption of fat-soluble vitamins; may interfere with absorption of other medications
Ursodeoxycholic acid (UDCA)	300 mg tid	Diarrhea

Ursodeoxycholic acid (UDCA) has been successfully to treat cholestatic liver disease and has shown promise in the treatment of IHCP. Its proposed mechanisms of action include modification of the bile acid pool by replacement of more hydrophobic and cytotoxic bile salts within hepatocyte membranes, inhibition of intestinal absorption of more hydrophobic bile acids, and modification of expression of major liver histocompatibility antigens. The largest published series using UDCA to treat IHCP includes eight patients with IHCP who received 10 days of open-label drug at a dose of 1 g/day in three divided doses. The drug was well tolerated with no adverse reactions. Patients' pruritis rapidly ameliorated and laboratory test results improved. Upon discontinuation of therapy in three patients symptoms recurred but responded well to resumption of treatment (Palma et al., 1992). In order to draw more definitive conclusions with regard to the efficacy of UDCA in IHCP and to delineate its longer-term effects on mother and infant, a randomized double-blind, placebo-controlled trial is needed. Although extensive studies have not been performed in humans, UDCA therapy has not contributed to fetal damage or postnatal growth alterations in pregnant mice or rabbits.

Dexamethasone has also shown promise as a potential therapy for IHCP. Through suppression of fetoplacental estrogen production, which may contribute to IHCP, dexamethasone therapy may lead to amelioration of symptoms. In one small series 10 women with IHCP received open-label oral dexamethasone at a dose of 12 mg/day for 7 days with subsequent gradual taper over 3 days (Hirvioja, Tuomala, and Vuori, 1992). After initiation of treatment pruritis was relieved, serum estrogen and total bile acid levels decreased, and liver function test results improved. No adverse reactions to the steroids were noted. In fact the authors noted a potential beneficial effect on fetal lung maturity in those infants who may be at risk for prematurity on the basis of maternal IHCP. Further clinical studies are needed before dexamethasone can be widely recommended for IHCP.

Acute fatty liver of pregnancy (AFLP)

Epidemiology and risk factors. Acute fatty liver of pregnancy is a rare and potentially fatal disease that generally occurs in the last trimester of pregnancy. Before 1980 the estimated incidence of AFLP was approximately one in a million pregnancies. More recent reports reveal an incidence of 1 in 13,328 deliveries. As with IHCP this increase in frequency is likely due to increased awareness as well as to recognition of mild cases.

AFLP is more commonly associated with primiparas, twin gestations, and male fetuses. Recently a genetic mode of inheritance in some patients has been suggested. AFLP does not generally recur in subsequent pregnancies although there is one case report of recurrence in the literature.

Pathogenesis and cause. Though its clinical manifestations are somewhat variable given the systemic nature of this disorder, histologically AFLP is characterized by a microvesicular fatty infiltrate of the liver.

The cause of AFLP in all patients is unknown. After the report of an infant homozygous for long-chain 3-hydroxyacyl-coenzyme dehydrogenase deficiency born to a heterozygous mother with acute fatty liver of pregnancy, a subsequent study has shown this association in some (7/10)

women with fatty liver of pregnancy. The same heterozygous trait was found in 4/4 fathers when the infant was homozygous and the mother heterozygous with AFLP (Tream et al., 1994). Some experts believe that AFLP and preeclampsia/eclampsia may be extremes of the same disorder. Nutritional factors, alterations in lipoprotein synthesis, and enzyme deficiencies in the urea cycle of mitochondria are among the many proposed mechanisms.

Clinical presentation

History and physical examination. AFLP generally occurs in the third trimester, usually between 32 and 38 weeks of gestation. It has been reported in the 26th week as well as in the postpartum period. Symptoms associated with AFLP may include headache, fatigue, malaise, nausea, vomiting, or abdominal discomfort. The abdominal discomfort may be localized to the midepigastrium or right upper quadrant or may be more diffuse. These prodromal manifestations may soon be followed by jaundice. Later or more severe stages include progressive liver failure with coagulopathy or encephalopathy and renal dysfunction with oliguria or uremia. In 20% to 40% of cases the onset of AFLP may be similar to the onset of preeclampsia with associated peripheral edema, hypertension, and proteinuria. The physical examination is rarely helpful diagnostically. (See Table 55-6.)

Diagnostic tests

LABORATORY TESTS. Laboratory test results are notable for cholestasis with mild to moderate elevations in transaminase levels. Bilirubin level may be normal early in the course and then rise if pregnancy is not terminated. Bilirubin level is rarely greater than 10 mg/dl. Alkaline phosphatase levels may be mildly elevated above those values found in normal pregnancies. Transaminase levels are almost always elevated but usually to values less than 500 U/L, thereby helping to distinguish AFLP from acute viral hepatitis. Hyperuricemia, principally resulting from impaired renal clearance, has been observed in approximately 80% of patients. Depending upon the severity and stage of AFLP other possible abnormal laboratory values include decreased platelet levels, elevated prothrombin time (PT) and partial thromboplastin time (PTT), microangiopathic changes on peripheral blood smear, leukocytosis, hypoglycemia, and elevated serum ammonia level.

RADIOGRAPHIC IMAGING. Radiographic imaging using ultrasound (US) or CT provides a noninvasive method for diag-

Table 55-6 Acute fatty liver of pregnancy

Onset	Symptoms/signs	Diagnostic tests
26 weeks to postpartum Usually after 32 weeks	+Nonspecific systemic symptoms +Right upper quadrant pain	+Transaminase level increase (1-5×) +Alkaline phospatase level increase (1-2×) +Bilirubin level increase (<10 mg/dl) +Uric acid level increase ± Platelet level decrease ± PT/PTT increase Increased echogenicity on ultrasound

PT, prothrombin time; PTT, partial thromboplastin time.

nosing AFLP especially if coagulopathy precludes liver biopsy. The US finding consistent with fatty infiltration of the liver is increased echogenicity, whereas CT demonstrates decreased attenuation. Although US is less expensive than CT, it is also less sensitive. CT, unlike US, however, carries a risk of radiation exposure to the unborn fetus. MRI has recently been used to image fatty infiltration of the liver, but its role in diagnosis remains undetermined.

LIVER BIOPSY. Liver biopsy may be key in making the diagnosis. If it is done, a frozen section is mandatory. The biopsy result is notable for microvesicular fatty infiltration detected only on frozen sections prepared with special fat stains such as oil-red-O. Fat is generally deposited in the cytoplasm of centrolobular hepatocytes. Inflammation and disarray of lobular hepatocytes as well as patchy cellular necrosis are commonly found. Although this pathology may make preeclampsia/eclampsia or viral hepatitis unlikely, these biopsy findings are not specific. They may be present in Reye's syndrome and in tetracycline or valproic acid toxicity. The transmission electron microscopic appearance of AFLP compared with that of Reye's syndrome is notable for subtle differences in hepatocyte mitochondria.

Maternal and fetal outcomes. Earlier studies demonstrated a poor prognosis in AFLP with maternal and fetal mortality rates approximating 85%. At present early diagnosis, rapid delivery after detection, and aggressive supportive care have decreased maternal and fetal mortality rates to 18% and 23%, respectively. Liver function test results improve soon after termination of pregnancy. If no aggressive action is taken, fulminant hepatic failure may develop and death may result.

Management. Early delivery is the mainstay of therapy and has improved maternal and fetal survival rates dramatically compared with those of continuation of pregnancy and medical management. Most women experience rapid improvement after delivery. There is one case reported of successful orthotopic liver transplant in a patient with AFLP that manifested fulminant hepatic failure despite delivery and intensive supportive care.

Preeclampsia/eclampsia

Epidemiology and risk factors. Preeclampsia is a systemic disorder in which the liver is one of the many target organs. It occurs in the second half of gestation and is characterized by hypertension, proteinuria, and edema.

Preeclampsia occurs in approximately 5% to 7% of pregnancies. It is generally a disease of primigravidas. Diabetes mellitus, hypertension, extremes of age (less than 20 years or greater than 45 years), and a family history of preeclampsia/eclampsia are all associated with an increased incidence of preeclampsia/eclampsia. Plural gestations, hydatiform mole, fetal hydrops, polyhydramnios, and inadequate prenatal care have also been shown to correlate with the occurrence of preeclampsia/eclampsia.

Chapter 51 discusses preeclampsia and eclampsia in detail. This discussion will focus on highlights, especially with respect to the liver abnormalities.

Pathogenesis and cause. The precise mechanism of preeclampsia/eclampsia is not understood. A variety of causes have been proposed to explain the occurrence of this multisystem disorder; they are outlined in Chapter 51. Hypotheses have included vasospasm, abnormal endothelial reactivity, and activation of coagulation.

Clinical presentation

History and physical examination. Characteristic clinical features associated with preeclampsia include the triad of hypertension, proteinuria, and edema. It traditionally occurs during the second half of gestation and usually during the third trimester. Symptoms, however, may occur in the postpartum period as well. Edema is not a rigid criterion since it is qualitative and complicates approximately 30% of normal pregnancies. Eclampsia includes the signs and symptoms of preeclampsia as well as convulsions or coma unrelated to other chronic cerebral conditions. The absence of pruritis and jaundice early in its course helps to distinguish preeclampsia from other liver disorders occurring during pregnancy. (See Table 55-7.)

Preeclamptics have been stratified into two categories, mild or severe, on the basis of the magnitude of blood pressure elevation and proteinuria. In the literature this distinction has been somewhat muddled by controversies regarding terminology and definitions. Preeclampsia/eclampsia is generally viewed as a multisystem disorder and may include renal, hematologic, hepatic, central nervous system (CNS), and fetal-placental involvement. In severe cases headaches, visual changes, abdominal pain, congestive heart failure, respiratory distress, or oliguria may occur. Although the liver may not be primarily involved in early preeclampsia it may become a target as the disease progresses.

Diagnostic tests. Abnormal liver function tests may be associated with preeclampsia. In early reports aspartate aminotransferase (AST) level was demonstrated to be abnormal in 84% of women with eclampsia, 50% with severe preeclampsia, and 24% with mild preeclampsia while alanine aminotransferase (ALT) level was demonstrated to be abnormal in 90% of women with eclampsia, 24% with severe preeclampsia, and 20% with mild preeclampsia (Chesley, 1978). The magnitude of transaminase level elevations may range from 5 to 100 times normal values. Bilirubin level is commonly normal; if it is elevated the value rarely exceeds 5 mg/dl. Abnormal hematologic parameters include thrombocytopenia, microangiopathic hemolytic anemia, and disseminated intravascular coagulation (DIC). Additionally uric acid levels are frequently elevated.

The diagnosis of preeclampsia with liver involvement is primarily clinical. Care must be taken to exclude other liver

Table 55-7 Preeclampsia

Onset	Symptoms/signs	Laboratory tests
20 weeks to delivery Usually late 2nd or 3rd trimester	+Nonspecific systemic symptoms +Hypertension +Edema	+Transaminase level increase (1-100×) ± Alkaline phosphatase level increase (1-2×) ± Bilirubin level increase (<5 mg/dl) +Uric acid level increase ± Platelet level decrease ± PT/PTT increase +Urine protein

PT, prothrombin time; PTT, partial thromboplastin time.

diseases associated with pregnancy, viral illness, and drug toxicity. Liver biopsy, although not required for diagnosis, may demonstrate periportal deposition of fibrin with associated hemorrhage. In severe cases hepatocellular injury may lead to necrosis.

Maternal and fetal outcomes. The major risks to the mother include cardiovascular, hepatic, respiratory, or renal failure, neurologic impairment, and hepatic rupture. The risks to the fetus include prematurity, fetal growth retardation, abruptio placentae, and low-birth-weight. Increased perinatal morbidity and mortality rates for the mother and fetus correlate with preterm delivery, severity of preeclampsia, multiple gestations, and preexisting maternal medical conditions such as hypertension. Perinatal morbidity and mortality rates in mild preeclampsia at term approximate those of normal pregnancies. The prognostic significance of liver function test abnormalities in mild preeclampsia is unclear. Some would argue that the finding of even mildly abnormal liver function tests demonstrates the presence of a systemic illness and should therefore change the classification of preeclampsia from mild to severe. This has prognostic importance since severe preeclampsia has higher associated morbidity and mortality rates than mild preeclampsia. However, there has never been a rigorous study demonstrating a correlation between abnormal liver function tests and maternal or fetal outcome.

Management. The primary goals in managing preeclampsia are maternal health followed by delivery of a healthy newborn. The unequivocal therapy for eclampsia and term preeclampsia is delivery. The management of mild and severe preeclamptics remote from term is more controversial with regard to hospitalization, antihypertensive therapy, and timing of delivery, as is outlined in Chapter 51. Hepatic dysfunction and associated liver function test result abnormalities generally improve rapidly after delivery.

HELLP syndrome

Epidemiology and risk factors. HELLP often occurs in the third trimester in association with preeclampsia/eclampsia but may occur independently.

HELLP occurs in approximately 0.2% to 0.6% of pregnancies. Although it is found in 4% to 12% of women with preeclampsia/eclampsia, it may occur in women with minimal or no signs of preeclampsia as well. In fact the absence of preeclampsia may lead to a delay in the clinical diagnosis of HELLP and in a subsequent therapeutic delivery. HELLP is more common in white multiparous women of older maternal age (mean age of 25 years) and generally occurs at approximately 32 weeks, although cases have been reported at or before 25 weeks. Onset occurs during the antepartum period in approximately two thirds of patients and in the postpartum period in approximately one third. In cases occurring after parturition, onset may extend from hours to days after delivery, although the majority appear within 48 hours. Signs and symptoms of preeclampsia may or may not be present before delivery. HELLP is unlikely to recur in subsequent pregnancies.

A detailed discussion of this syndrome appears in Chapter 51.

Pathogenesis and cause. The pathophysiologic characteristics of HELLP have not been clearly delineated. Like preeclampsia/eclampsia, HELLP is a multisystem disease involving the liver and may be due to abnormal vascular tone, vasospasm, or coagulation. A more complete description of potential causes is included in Chapter 51.

Clinical presentation

History and physical examination. Symptoms associated with HELLP include epigastric pain, nausea, vomiting, headache, weight gain, and edema. Hypertension may be absent in as many as 15% of patients. (See Table 55-8.)

Diagnostic tests. Laboratory test findings include moderate proteinuria, microangiopathic hemolytic anemia with associated depression in haptoglobin level and elevations in lactate dehydrogenase (LDH) and indirect bilirubin levels. Transaminase levels may be elevated to values as high as 4000 U/L although milder elevations are more often the norm. Platelet counts may be depressed to values of 6000 to 100,000 around the time of delivery. Platelet counts tend to normalize 5 days postpartum. PT, PTT, and fibrinogen level may be abnormal in a minority of cases. Hypertension and proteinuria, if present, may take up to 3 months to resolve. In one case report an abdominal ultrasound performed 24 hours before the onset of HELLP symptoms demonstrated echogenic lesions in the liver likely caused by hemorrhage or necrosis. Liver histologic features may demonstrate periportal or focal necrosis with hyaline deposits in sinusoids.

Maternal and fetal outcomes. Maternal and fetal outcomes do not correlate with the severity of liver involvement. Maternal mortality rates have ranged from 3% to 25%. Maternal morbidity has resulted from such problems as disseminated intravascular coagulation (DIC), abruptio placentae, and renal, cardiopulmonary, or hepatic failure. Depending upon the severity of the disease at the time of diagnosis the infant perinatal mortality rate has ranged from 10% to 60%. Infants are at increased risk for prematurity, intrauterine growth retardation, DIC, and thrombocytopenia.

Management. Prompt recognition and management are critical to the survival of mother and infant. In cases with early signs of maternal or fetal distress, delivery is clearly recommended. For other less clear-cut cases, the optimal time of delivery is somewhat controversial. Liver function test results may return to normal soon after delivery without long-term sequelae as long as the patient's course is relatively uncomplicated.

Hepatic rupture

Epidemiology and risk factors. Hepatic rupture is a relatively rare complication of pregnancy. It is reported in 1 to 77

Table 55-8 HELLP syndrome

Onset	Symptoms/signs	Laboratory tests
25 weeks to immediate postpartum Usually after 32 weeks	+Nonspecific systemic symptoms +Right upper quadrant pain	+Transaminase level increase (1-100×) ± Alkaline phosphatase level increase (1-2×) ± Bilirubin level (<5 mg/dl) +Uric acid level increase ± Platelet level decrease ± PT/PTT increase ± Urine protein

PT, prothrombin time; PTT, partial thromboplastin time.

of 100,000 deliveries. It may occur spontaneously or may be associated with an underlying hepatic abnormality. Preeclampsia/eclampsia is found in association with 80% of the cases of spontaneous rupture in pregnancy. Hepatic rupture in preeclamptic/eclamptic pregnancies occurs more commonly in older multigravidas. Hepatic rupture in pregnancy has more rarely been reported in association with hepatocellular carcinomas, adenomas, hemangiomas, hepatic abcesses, acute fatty liver of pregnancy, and HELLP. No recurrences of hepatic rupture in later pregnancies have been reported.

Pathogenesis and cause. The cause of spontaneous or secondary hepatic rupture in pregnancy is unknown. In cases with associated preeclampsia/eclampsia DIC has been thought to play a role. Yet rupture has been reported in pregnancies demonstrating only minimal or early signs of DIC.

Clinical presentation

History and physical examination. Hepatic rupture generally appears with acute abdominal pain and associated nausea and vomiting occurring during the last trimester or less commonly in the first 24 hours after delivery. Signs and symptoms of preeclampsia/eclampsia may be present if rupture is secondary. Soon afterward abdominal distention and hypovolemic shock ensue. Ruptures are generally limited to the right portion of the liver, although the left or both lobes may be involved. (See Table 55-9.)

Diagnostic tests. Liver function test results are often elevated with an associated anemia and consumptive thrombocytopenia with or without DIC. Useful diagnostic tests include abdominal US, CT, magnetic resonance imaging (MRI), and angiography. These imaging tests may be performed in preparation for surgery or intraoperatively.

Maternal and fetal outcomes. Maternal and fetal mortality rates are high. Maternal rates are estimated at 50% to 75%; fetal rates approximate 60%. Early recognition of hepatic rupture increases the chance of survival. The most frequent cause of maternal death after spontaneous rupture is hemorrhage. The mortality rate is lower in women with contained hematomas and in those who have prompt intervention. Fetal morbidity and mortality rates may be directly correlated with prematurity.

Management. Survival depends on early recognition and prompt surgical attention. In addition to delivery of the fetus surgical options have included direct pressure, evacuation, packing or hemostatic wrapping, application of topical hemostatic agents, oversewing lacerations, hepatic artery ligation, and partial hepatectomy. Angiographic embolization has been reported but works best when the rupture is limited to only one lobe.

Table 55-9 Hepatic rupture

Onset	Symptoms/signs	Laboratory tests
Late 2nd trimester to immediate postpartum Usually 3rd trimester	+Acute abdominal pain ±Nausea ±Vomiting	+Transaminase level increase (2-100×) +Alkaline phosphatase level increase ±Bilirubin level increase ±Platelet level decrease ±PT/PTT increase

PT, prothrombin time; PTT, partial thromboplastin time.

SUMMARY

The liver is among the many organs affected by the physiologic and hormonal changes that occur during pregnancy. Hepatic disorders diagnosed before pregnancy may be unaffected or exacerbated by the pregnant state. Liver disorders that are specific to pregnancy, including hyperemesis gravidarum, intrahepatic cholestasis of pregnancy, acute fatty liver of pregnancy, preeclampsia/eclampsia, HELLP, and hepatic rupture, may profoundly impact the morbidity and mortality rates of mother and fetus. Although an unequivocal diagnosis is often difficult to make, it should be attempted in a timely manner so that further treatment can be determined. After the diagnosis, maximizing the health of the mother and fetus will determine future management.

BIBLIOGRAPHY

Alexander J, Cuellar RE, Van Thiel DH: Toxemia of pregnancy and the liver, *Semin Liver Dis* 7(1):55, 1987.

Barron WM: The syndrome of preeclampsia, *Gastr Clin North Am* 21(4):851, 1992.

Barton JR, Sibai BM: Care of the pregnancy complicated by HELLP syndrome, *Gastr Clin North Am* 21(4):937, 1992.

Barton JR et al: Recurrent acute fatty liver of pregnancy. *Am J Obstet Gynecol* 163:534, 1990.

Chesley LC: *Hypertensive disorders in pregnancy,* New York, 1978, Appleton-Century-Crofts.

Fallon HJ: Liver disease. In Burrow G and Ferris T, editors: *Complications during pregnancy*, ed 3, Philadelphia, 1988, WB Saunders.

Farine D et al: Magnetic resonance imaging and computed tomography scan for the diagnosis of acute fatty liver of pregnancy, *Am J Perinatol* 7:316, 1990.

Fisk NM, Storey GN: Fetal outcome in obstetric cholestasis, *Br J Obstet Gynaecol* 95:1137, 1988.

Gitlin N: Liver disease in pregnancy. In Millward-Sadler GH, Wright R, Arthur MJP, editors: *Wright's liver and biliary disease: pathophysiology, diagnosis and management,* London, Philadelphia, 1992, WB Saunders.

Hirvioja ML, Tuimala R, Vuori J: The treatment of intrahepatic cholestasis of pregnancy by dexamethasone, *Br J Obstet Gynaecol* 99:109, 1992.

Johnson CD: Magnetic resonance imaging of the liver: current clinical applications, *Mayo Clin Proc* 68:147, 1993.

Jones EA, Bergasa NV: The pruritus of cholestasis and the opioid system, *JAMA* 268:3359, 1992.

Kaplan MM: Current concepts: acute fatty liver of pregnancy, *N Engl J Med* 313(6):367, 1985.

Loevinger EH et al: Hepatic rupture associated with pregnancy: treatment with transcatheter embolotherapy, *Obstet Gynecol* 65:281, 1985.

Lunzer M et al: Serum bile acid concentrations during pregnancy and their relationship to obstetric cholestasis, *Gastroenterology* 91:825, 1986.

Mabie WC et al: Computed tomography in acute fatty liver of pregnancy, *Am J Obstet Gynecol* 158:142, 1988.

Minuk GY, Lui RC, Kelly JK: Rupture of the liver associated with acute fatty liver of pregnancy, *Am J Gastroenterol* 82:457, 1987.

Ockner SA et al: Fulminant hepatic failure caused by acute fatty liver of pregnancy treated by orthotopic liver transplantation, *Hepatology* 11:59, 1990.

Palma J et al: Effects of ursodeoxycholic acid in patients with intrahepatic cholestasis of pregnancy, *Hepatology* 15:1043, 1992.

Palma J et al: Management of intrahepatic cholestasis in pregnancy, *Lancet* 339:1478, 1992.

Ribalta J et al: S-adenosyl-1-methionine in the treatment of patients with intrahepatic cholestasis of pregnancy: a randomized double-blind, placebo-controlled study with negative results, *Hepatology* 13:1084, 1991.

Riely CA et al: A reassessment based on observations in nine patients, *Ann Intern Med* 106:703, 1987.

Riely CA. Hepatic disease in pregnancy, *Am J Med* 96(suppl 1A):18,1994.

Rittenberry AB, Arnold CL, Taslimi MM: Hemostatic wrapping of ruptured liver in two postpartum patients, *Am J Obstet Gynecol* 165:705, 1991.

Schorr-Lesnick B, Dworkin B, Rosenthal WS: Hemolysis, elevated liver enzymes, and low platelets in pregnancy (HELLP syndrome): a case report and literature review, *Dig Dis Sci* 36:1649, 1991.

Schorr-Lesnick B et al. Liver diseases unique to pregnancy, *Am J Gastroenterol* 86:659, 1991.

Sibai BM: Pitfalls in diagnosis and management of preeclampsia, *Am J Obstet Gynecol* 159:1, 1988.

Sibai BM: Preeclampsia-eclampsia: maternal and perinatal outcomes, *Contemp Obstet Gynecol* 32:109, 1988.

Sibai BM:The HELLP syndrome (hemolysis, elevated liver enzymes, and low platelets): much ado about nothing? *Am J Obstet Gynecol* 162:311, 1990.

Sibai BM: Management of pre-eclampsia remote from term, *Eur Obstet* 42(S):S96, 1991.

Sibai BM et al: Pregnancy outcome in 303 cases with severe preeclampsia, *Obstet Gynecol* 64:319, 1984.

Smith LG et al: Spontaneous rupture of liver during pregnancy: current therapy, *Obstet Gynecol* 77:171, 1991.

Tream WR et al. Acute fatty liver of pregnancy and long chain 3-hydroxy-acyl-coenzyme A dehydrogenase deficiency. *Hepatology* 19:339, 1994.

Tream WR et al: Acute fatty liver of pregnancy (AFLP) and defects in fatty acid oxidation (FAO). *Gastroenterology* 106:1000, 1994.

Van Dyke RW: The liver in pregnancy. In Zakim D, Boyer TD, editors: *Hepatology: a textbook of liver disease*, Philadelphia, London, Toronto, Montreal, Sydney, Tokyo, 1990, WB Saunders.

Vore M: Estrogen cholestasis: membranes, metabolites, or receptors? *Gastroenterology* 93:643, 1987.

Wilson JA: Intrahepatic cholestasis of pregnancy with marked elevation of transaminases in a black American, *Dig Dis Sci* 32:665, 1987.

56 Nongynecologic Cancer in Pregnancy

Lawrence N. Shulman

Malignancy is not common in women of childbearing age, but it can occur, and when it does it presents serious problems for both the mother and the fetus. The pregnant woman generally receives her medical care from her obstetrician and her primary care physician. Fortunately in the vast majority of pregnant women, cancers will not develop, but making a diagnosis of cancer in the pregnant woman can be very difficult. Changes that normally occur in the breast during pregnancy may obscure a growing breast cancer. Fatigue and nonspecific constitutional complaints that may be signs of acute leukemia are frequently seen in the healthy pregnant woman. Hodgkin's disease in the mediastinum may manifest itself as cough and shortness of breath, symptoms that are nonspecific and commonly seen in the healthy pregnant patient. Therefore identifying the rare pregnant woman with cancer will be difficult and no specific guidelines can be offered other than to heed persistent complaints.

SPECIAL CONSIDERATIONS IN THE PREGNANT WOMAN WITH CANCER

When a pregnant woman is identified as having a cancer many special considerations need to be taken into account, including the following:

1. Difficulty in diagnosis and staging of the malignancy
2. Risk of the malignancy to the mother—specifically pace of the malignancy and its complications
3. Risk of therapeutic intervention to both the mother and the fetus
   a. Immediate effects
   b. Long-term implications

All of these factors must be carefully considered by a team composed of an obstetrician, a neonatologist, a hematologist-oncologist, and the primary care physician, as well as other supporting physicians, when indicated, including surgeons, radiation therapists, and radiologists. Close coop-

eration throughout the pregnancy and illness is essential for an optimal outcome for both mother and fetus. The box below lists some of the issues concerning the approach to the pregnant patient with cancer.

SPECIFIC MALIGNANCIES SEEN IN PREGNANCY

Though any malignancy can occur during pregnancy, those malignancies that affect young adults are most likely to coincide with pregnancy. Breast cancer, malignant lymphomas (Hodgkin's and non-Hodgkin's type), and acute leukemias are some of the more common malignancies seen in this age group. In this chapter we will deal specifically with these

---

APPROACH TO THE PREGNANT PATIENT WITH CANCER

Diagnosis—confirm with biopsy at earliest possible time

Stage disease—to determine implications for mother

Potential for organ compromise—Hodgkin's disease with compromise of the mediastinal structures, or acute leukemia with bone marrow effacement leading to neutropenia and fever

Interaction of pregnancy and cancer—breast cancer: difficulty in detecting breast mass and assessing extent of local involvement in the breast of the pregnant patient; concern about hormonal stimulation of tumor growth

Implications of treatment of the malignancy

Chemotherapy-induced neutropenia and risk of infection for mother and fetus

Risk of spontaneous abortion or stillbirth resulting from chemotherapy

Potential teratogenic effects of chemotherapy or radiation therapy on the fetus

Other potential toxicities of treatment on the fetus, such as the possibility of doxorubicin-induced cardiac damage

---

three diseases, not because others do not occur in pregnant women, but because these are among the more frequent cancers in pregnant women and because each raises important issues confronting the pregnant patient. Breast cancer is particularly difficult to detect during pregnancy, and the hormonal milieu of pregnancy may adversely affect its outcome. Hodgkin's disease is curable, even in an advanced stage, but can cause serious compromise of organ structures, particularly in the mediastinum. The acute leukemias have a major impact on immune defenses of the mother, which can lead to life-threatening infection for the mother and fetus.

Breast cancer

Epidemiology and risk factors. Though breast cancer increases in incidence with age, it does occur in women in their 20s, 30s, and 40s and, therefore, occasionally coincides with pregnancy. Even in young patients the majority of breast cancers occur in women with no family history and no identifiable risk factors. There are no data to suggest that pregnancy causes breast cancer. To the contrary, nulliparous women and women whose first pregnancy occurs late in life may be more likely to develop breast cancer. Breast cancer, though, poses special problems in detection, diagnosis, staging, and treatment when it occurs during pregnancy.

Problems with diagnosis. During pregnancy the breasts become engorged as a result of hormonal stimulation, and this is likely to make a growing breast cancer less obvious to a woman, even if she is accustomed to performing self–breast examination. Changes that occur as a result of a cancer may be ascribed to changes associated with pregnancy. The physician may also have difficulty detecting a mass in the breast of the pregnant patient and may be less likely to perform a biopsy of a suspicious lesion. He is unlikely to perform a mammogram as well, and mammography may not be very helpful in evaluating a mass in the dense breast of the pregnant patient. In a series reported from Memorial Sloan-Kettering Cancer Center, of those breast cancers diagnosed postpartum, in more than 50% of the patients a breast mass had been documented and followed but not diagnosed during pregnancy (Petrek, Dukoff, and Rogatko, 1991).

Staging and prognosis. It was suggested as early as 1880 that breast cancers occurring in pregnancy had a particularly dire prognosis, and in the 1940s Haagensen described 20 pregnant women with breast cancer and also commented on the advanced local and systemic manifestations of cancers in these patients as compared to nonpregnant patients. Others have not found breast cancers to have a particularly dire prognosis in pregnant women and have commented on the high percentage of estrogen-receptor-negative breast cancers (71%) in pregnant women in their series. It is possible, though, that the high estrogen levels in the pregnant patient cause false-negative estrogen-receptor assay results in the tumors of some of these women.

Prognosis is determined by the stage at the time of diagnosis. It is possible that cancers will grow to large size during pregnancy before detection and will have a higher risk of local and systemic dissemination before diagnosis and treatment. In the Memorial series patients who had the cancer diagnosed immediately postpartum had tumors that averaged 3.5 cm in size as compared to nonpregnant patients, whose tumors averaged 2.0 cm. Axillary lymph node involvement is the most predictive factor for the subsequent development of metastatic disease and ultimate death from breast cancer. Of women reported from the Memorial series who had breast cancer diagnosed postpartum, 64% had involvement of axillary lymph nodes, as compared to 38% for a group of nonpregnant women. Also of note was that an unexpectedly high number (7 of 63) of patients already had advanced breast cancer, with involvement of the skin, infraclavicular nodes, or supraclavicular nodes, or with distant metastases. A small number of the patients had definitive diagnosis and treatment before delivery and only 20% had axillary node involvement, suggesting that early detection and treatment are possible during pregnancy. Other series have confirmed the higher than expected incidence of axillary nodal involvement in patients who had breast cancer during pregnancy.

These findings probably mean breast cancers are difficult to detect when they are present in the breast of a pregnant women, as stated, and therefore are discovered at more advanced stages (larger size and more axillary node involvement). It is also possible that the hormonal milieu of the pregnant woman might lead to more rapid growth and dissemination of the cancer, since breast cancer cells sometimes have estrogen receptors present in them. This consideration becomes particularly troublesome when the diagnosis of breast cancer is made in a pregnant woman and there is the possibility that the continued pregnancy will cause rapid growth and spread of the cancer if left untreated. Whether the hormonal milieu of pregnancy truly stimulates breast cancers to grow and disseminate and worsens the prognosis of these patients remains controversial.

Techniques for diagnosis. If a cancer is suspected in a pregnant patient there now exist techniques to diagnosis the cancer without the need for general anesthesia. Percutaneous needle biopsy can be safely performed and, in experienced hands, will often succeed at making the diagnosis. If needle biopsy is unsuccessful then open biopsy under local anesthesia may be possible.

Management. Once the diagnosis is made the decisions about further diagnostic studies and treatment are difficult and need to be tailored to the individual, depending on the apparent extent of the cancer, the trimester of pregnancy, and the wishes of the mother and family. If the patient is near term, it may be possible to deliver the fetus if it is sufficiently mature, and then proceed with standard diagnostic studies and treatment. For the patient early in her pregnancy, therapeutic abortion is an option, and if it is rapidly performed the physician can subsequently evaluate and treat the patient in a manner similar to that for the nonpregnant breast cancer patient. If the patient does not desire an abortion or is too far advanced in her pregnancy for an abortion, then the decisions are particularly difficult. A patient diagnosed as 23 or 24 weeks of gestation is still 2 to 3 months from the time of preferred delivery, and during this period there may be substantial growth of the breast cancer if no treatment is instituted. If there are no apparent metastases and the cancer does not appear to be locally advanced (with involvement of the skin, infraclavicular nodes, or supraclavicular nodes), then modified radical mastectomy is an option, though it will necessitate general anesthesia. If the tumor appears small and there is no obvious axillary nodal involvement, simple excision with local anesthesia may be feasible, depending on the size of the tumor and the location within the breast. Breast or chest wall radiation therapy should be deferred until after delivery if possible. Though modest doses of radiation can be administered to the upper body with minimal "scatter" reaching the fetus, these doses are well below the usually acceptable antitumor doses used to control breast cancer.

If the cancer is locally advanced, preventing surgical management, or if there is distant metastatic disease, then ideal therapy consists of systemic chemotherapy. One would prefer not to administer chemotherapy to the pregnant woman, though it is feasible when necessary, as will be described. When possible the fetus should be delivered and chemotherapy begun postpartum.

Unfortunately it is often difficult to determine the size of a cancer and the extent of local tumor spread in the breast of a pregnant patient, and it may also be difficult to determine the significance of enlarged axillary nodes.

Hodgkin's disease

Hodgkin's disease most often occurs in patients in their 20s and 30s and therefore occasionally occurs in the pregnant patient. In this age group Hodgkin's disease is usually initially manifested by nodal enlargement in the cervical, supraclavicular, and mediastinal areas but can involve retroperitoneal nodes as well as visceral organs such as the liver and lung. Hodgkin's disease is a potentially curable illness even when disseminated, and management of the pregnant patient and her fetus should reflect this fact. In the nonpregnant patient treatment is governed by staging of the patient. Those with localized disease often receive radiation therapy only, and patients with more advanced and disseminated disease usually receive chemotherapy, with or without radiation therapy.

Diagnosis. When the pregnant patient is found to have lymphadenopathy in the cervical, supraclavicular, axillary, or inguinal nodal chains, then a biopsy under local anesthesia may yield the diagnosis. Once the diagnosis is made, an attempt can be made to "stage" the patient. Important areas to assess include the chest and retroperitoneum. Chest involvement occurs early in many young patients with Hodgkin's disease; if it is advanced it can cause embarrassment of the mediastinal structures, including tracheal or bronchial compression, obstruction of the superior vena cava, or other major veins of the chest or pericardial tamponade. Tracheal, vascular, and cardiac structures can usually be adequately and safely imaged with magnetic resonance imaging (MRI). The retroperitoneum can also be imaged with MRI or by ultrasound, with special attention to the kidneys and ureters, which can be obstructed by retroperitoneal adenopathy. Computed tomographic (CT) scans are often avoided in therapy of the pregnant patient because of the significant radiation dose administered during a scan.

Management. Approach to the pregnant patient with Hodgkin's disease is determined by the point in pregnancy that the patient has reached, the distribution and extent of the Hodgkin's disease in relation to vital organs, and the rate of growth of the lymphadenopathy. Hodgkin's disease can progress at extremely variable rates in both the pregnant and nonpregnant patient, and the rate of growth can often be assessed accurately after a week or two of observation.

In all patients it is critical to gather as much information about the extent of the disease as possible, as noted. If the patient is very early in her pregnancy, therapeutic abortion is an option. If the patient is near term, it is often possible merely to observe the patient until after delivery, when standard staging procedures and treatment can be carried out. If the patient is early in her pregnancy and does not desire a therapeutic abortion or is midway through the pregnancy, then treatment decisions depend on the extent of the Hodgkin's disease and its threat to important structures. Most frequent concerns are the mediastinal structures, particularly the central veins, trachea, and heart. If the extent of the disease is minimal and there is no impending compromise of vital structures the patient can be followed without specific treatment. If mediastinal adenopathy is beginning to obstruct major veins, the trachea, or major bronchi, or pericardial involvement is becoming critical, therapy is indicated. Often corticosteroids alone will sufficiently reduce the bulk of disease to remove the immediate danger and the response can be very rapid. Unfortunately the response to corticosteroids tends to be brief, though it can last weeks, and may be long enough to allow safe and successful delivery of the fetus. If further therapy is required low doses of radiation therapy can be administered to the mediastinal lymph nodes with little risk to the fetus.

Clinical outcome and prognosis. In a series of 15 pregnant patients with Hodgkin's disease reported by Stanford, three patients diagnosed early in pregnancy elected therapeutic abortion; 1 patient was followed without treatment until the seventh month, when she had induction and delivery, and the remaining 11 patients received some therapy during the pregnancy (Jacobs et al., 1981). Five of the patients became pregnant during treatment for Hodgkin's disease. Most patients received radiation therapy in doses of 1000 to 4000 cGy during the second and third trimesters, and all of these pregnancies resulted in normal babies. One patient received daily oral chlorambucil, an alkylating agent, throughout the 9 months of pregnancy, with no complications to mother or fetus. One patient who received high doses of radiation to the left breast (4435 cGy) had a spontaneous abortion. Thirteen of the 15 patients had no evidence of recurrent Hodgkin's disease at last follow-up observation. This small but important series of patients demonstrates that patients with Hodgkin's disease can be managed in a number of ways that will allow the mother to be cured of Hodgkin's disease and often have a successful pregnancy and healthy baby.

Acute leukemia

Both acute myelogenous leukemia and acute lymphoblastic leukemia can occur in young adults and sometimes in pregnant women. The chemotherapy usually administered for these diseases is not sterilizing; occasionally women being treated for acute leukemia become pregnant during therapy. Reynoso and colleagues reported 7 patients with concurrent pregnancy and acute leukemia and reviewed 51 other cases from the literature. Of the 58 cases, 35 were diagnosed as having acute myelogenous leukemia (AML), 16 as having acute lymphoblastic leukemia (ALL), 1 as having the blast phase of chronic myelogenous leukemia, and 6 acute leukemia, not otherwise specified. Both AML and ALL can be associated with elevated blast counts in the peripheral blood, which, if high enough, can result in leukostasis endangering the mother and fetus. In addition patients with AML or ALL often have severe suppression of normal hematopoiesis resulting in neutropenia, anemia, and thrombocytopenia that can pose a major immediate threat to both the mother and fetus. Therefore, patients with acute leukemia of either type often require urgent therapy and, in most circumstances, the pregnant patient cannot have therapy delayed for any significant period while awaiting fetal maturation to allow delivery. If infection occurs when the neutrophil count is very low as a result of leukemic infiltration of the bone marrow and resultant neutropenia, and antileukemic therapy is yet to be instituted, the mortality risk to mother and infant will be very high.

Management. Therapy of AML and ALL usually consists of intensive chemotherapy, which in itself will result in prolonged periods of neutropenia and thrombocytopenia before bone marrow recovery and, ideally, at a later date the attainment of remission with restoration of normal hematopoiesis. During the period of pancytopenia the patient is at significant risk for the development of life-threatening infection and hemorrhage. The risk of serious infection can be reduced by the administration of intravenous antibiotics when fever occurs, but in spite of broad-spectrum antibiotics infection can be lethal if the neutrophil count remains below $500/mm^3$. Hemorrhage from thrombocytopenia can usually be prevented with platelet transfusions but patients will occasionally become refractory to platelet product support and can suffer serious or fatal bleeding.

Clinical outcome and prognosis. Of the 58 patients reported by Reynoso and colleagues, two suffered spontaneous abortions, three elected therapeutic abortion, and four had stillbirths. Of the remaining patients about half delivered premature infants and the others carried to term. The major complications were related to neutropenia and infection, with severe maternal and fetal complications including sepsis, disseminated intravascular coagulation, and, in one case, fetal death.

As a general principle (though every patient and situation needs to be individualized) patients with AML or ALL diagnosed during pregnancy should be treated with standard chemotherapy regimens and the fetus should be delivered at the earliest possible time when blood counts are adequate. The choice of specific chemotherapy regimen and the timing of therapy and delivery will depend on the height of the circulating blast count, the compromise of normal hematopoiesis, and the stage of pregnancy.

EFFECTS OF THERAPY ON MOTHER AND FETUS
Chemotherapy

Many different chemotherapy agents are now available for use in the patient with malignancy and they have extremely varied properties, including pharmacokinetics, distribution, mechanisms of action, and toxicity. The most serious potential toxicity of chemotherapy administered to pregnant women is bone marrow suppression with resultant neutropenia and thrombocytopenia.

Bone marrow suppression
Neutropenia. When the neutrophil count is less than $500/mm^3$ the patient is at high risk for serious bacterial or fungal infection. If fever develops with a neutrophil count below this level, prompt institution of broad-spectrum intravenous antibiotics is indicated, even if there is no apparent infection or source of fever. The longer the neutrophil count remains below $500/mm^3$, the greater the risk of serious bacterial infection, and the longer the patient is treated with broad-spectrum antibiotics, the greater the risk of fungal infection. Even with prompt institution of intravenous antibiotics, infections can be lethal when the neutrophil count remains below $500/mm^3$; even if the condition is not lethal to the mother it can result in sepsis, hypotension, and loss of the fetus.

Thrombocytopenia. Thrombocytopenia can lead to serious spontaneous (nontraumatic) hemorrhage when the platelet count is below $20,000/mm^3$, but this can usually be prevented by platelet transfusions, which can usually raise the platelet count to safe levels. Occasionally alloimmunization to platelets will develop and the platelet count will persist at dangerous levels in spite of transfusions, and the patient will remain at risk for serious hemorrhage, including intracerebral and gastrointestinal bleeding.

Chemotherapy agents. In the following paragraphs some of the major classes of chemotherapeutic agents will be briefly mentioned. Extensive reviews of these agents are beyond the scope of this chapter and only major modes of action and potential toxicities of selected agents will be discussed.

Alkylating agents. Alkylating agents were among the first chemotherapeutic agents to be used against human malignancy, and in the 1960s these agents were first shown to be curative in Hodgkin's disease, even when it was discovered in advanced stages. These agents bind to deoxyribonucleic acid (DNA) bases, often at the N^7-guanine position, or the extracyclic oxygen, O^6-guanine. By binding at these and other sites on DNA the alkylating agents can prevent DNA replication, either by blocking DNA polymerase directly or by forming intrastrand or interstrand cross-links that prevent DNA polymerase from functioning normally. These agents can also cause configurational changes in DNA bases that can lead to DNA mispairing and mutagenesis. They are known to be mutagenic in humans and have been associated with the development of AML in patients receiving these agents for the treatment of other malignancies or nonmalignant conditions. It is presumed that these agents will cross the placenta and can cause bone marrow suppression in the fetus, as well as being potentially mutagenic to the fetus. Several patients reported in the literature support this concern.

Anthracyclines. The anthracyclines, including doxorubicin and daunorubicin, are used in the treatment of a wide variety of malignancies, including breast cancer, Hodgkin's disease, and the acute leukemias. These agents work by intercalating with DNA. They can cause significant, though transient, bone marrow suppression, particularly neutropenia.

When given in large, cumulative doses they may cause myocardial damage resulting in a cardiomyopathy that can be difficult to treat medically and has a very high mortality rate. Though the elderly are particularly prone to this complication, possibly because they often have underlying heart disease, there is now evidence that children receiving anthracyclines may be at risk of developing cardiomyopathies later in life. Lipshultz and colleagues reported that children treated with 228 mg/m^2 or more of doxorubicin had a 65% chance of developing either increased afterload or decreased contractility later in life, and that children below the age of 4 were at greater risk. This raises the question as to whether the fetus could be at significant risk of development of cardiac abnormalities if exposed to anthracyclines in utero.

There is debate whether the anthracyclines cross the placenta to the fetal circulation, and the theoretic risk exists that their use in the pregnant patient could lead to cardiomyopathy in the fetus that might not be manifested until later in life. Turchi and Villasis reported the results of 28 pregnancies in patients treated with anthracyclines during pregnancy. Twenty-four normal infants were born to these mothers, and bone marrow suppression was seen in an occasional infant, but cardiac disease was not reported.

Methotrexate. Methotrexate blocks the action of dihydrofolate reductase, an enzyme necessary to produce tetrahydrofolate, which is necessary, along with thymidylate synthetase, to produce thymidine nucleotides from uracil nucleotides. Without thymidine nucleotides DNA cannot replicate. Methotrexate, when administered in high dose, suppresses the bone marrow, leading to pancytopenia, and can also cause mucositis and diarrhea.

Methotrexate has been considered to be an abortifacient, possibly because of its effects on the placenta. In one study, when methotrexate was used in low doses in patients with rheumatic disease during the first trimester, of 10 pregnancies studied three resulted in spontaneous abortion, two in therapeutic abortion, and five in full-birth of term infants without obvious birth defects or impaired development.

Radiation therapy. The use of radiation therapy in a pregnant patient must take into account the anatomic location requiring radiation and its proximity to the fetus, the doses of radiation needed to control particular symptoms of the disease, and the trimester of pregnancy. As noted previously, in patients with Hodgkin's disease radiation therapy can apparently be safely administered to the mediastinum in doses between 1000 and 4000 cGy with beneficial effects to the mother and no apparent harmful effects to the fetus. Radiation should be administered in such a way as to minimize even small amounts of "scatter" radiation that might be absorbed by the fetal tissues and could be potentially mutagenic or sufficiently damaging to cause an abortion or stillbirth.

Most often, radiation therapy is likely to be used to shrink temporarily a tumor that is compromising a vital structure, as in mediastinal Hodgkin's disease causing tracheal compression and airway obstruction. In these circumstances well-planned radiation therapy can be lifesaving for the mother and for the fetus as well.

FETAL OUTCOME IN THE WOMAN WITH CANCER

Fetal outcome in the patient with cancer will depend on many factors, including the particular malignancy of the mother and the specific dangers posed by it to the mother and fetus, the stage of pregnancy when the malignancy is discovered, and the amount of time until the infant can be safely delivered, as well as the treatments required before the delivery of the infant.

Multiple reports suggest that the rate of spontaneous abortion increases in women treated for cancer during pregnan-

cy. Methotrexate and other agents appear to be implicated in this complication. In addition there is an increased incidence of low birth weight, a finding that may be influenced by attempts to deliver the fetus before term, though some infants have low birth weight adjusted for gestational age.

Myelosuppression of the fetus with neutropenia, thrombocytopenia, or both, is seen in approximately 30% of patients receiving chemotherapy in the 4 weeks before delivery, a time when the myelosuppressive effects of most chemotherapy are present. In some cases neonatal sepsis has resulted.

The rate of congenital abnormalities appears to increase in infants born to mothers who have received chemotherapy during pregnancy, particularly if administered in the first trimester. All chemotherapeutic agents are potentially mutagenic, but the alkylating agents are particularly so.

PREGNANCY IN THE WOMAN WITH A HISTORY OF TREATMENT FOR CANCER

For the woman who has been previously treated for a malignancy, has no evidence of active cancer, and has maintained her fertility, the decision to become pregnant is a complicated and difficult one. Many factors must be included in the discussion concerning a patient's desire to become pregnant, including the following:

1. Outcome of pregnancy—spontaneous abortion, prematurity and low birth weight, and birth defects
2. Prognosis of patient—likelihood of the cancer relapsing after pregnancy, leaving the child without a mother
3. Risk of relapse during pregnancy—implications for mother and fetus
4. Residual effects of disease and treatment on the mother—risk of infection and need for immunizations and cardiac and pulmonary complications

History of treatment

It appears that a pregnancy in a woman treated with chemotherapy and radiation therapy delivered more than a year before pregnancy is no more likely than a pregnancy in a normal woman to end in spontaneous abortion, result in premature birth, or result in birth defects. There may be an increased incidence of premature birth and low birth weight in women who conceive within a year of completing therapy, possibly because of the direct debilitating effects of treatment. Therefore for the fetus, previous treatment for cancer is not an adverse risk factor.

Prognosis of cancer

The prognosis for long-term remission and cure of the cancer is an important but difficult consideration. A woman with a very dire prognosis and a high likelihood of relapse in the near future may find herself dealing with recurrent cancer simultaneously with a pregnancy or during the early years of a child's life. If the relapse occurs after the pregnancy and the therapy for the relapsed cancer is unsuccessful, as is often the case with recurrent cancers of all types, then the child will be left without a mother. If the relapse occurs during pregnancy, all of the issues raised earlier in this chapter come into play, except that the prognosis for the cancer is likely to be worse and the woman may succumb to her cancer during pregnancy, before the fetus can be safely delivered. Prognosis varies and each woman must be made aware of her individual prognosis. Nonetheless, in a woman with an excellent prognosis cancer can recur, and in a woman with a poor prognosis it may not, so there is always a degree of uncertainty.

The issue of pregnancy after treatment for breast cancer is particularly complicated because of the concern that a pregnancy may cause a cancer to recur or may cause a breast cancer to grow more rapidly in the high-estrogen milieu of pregnancy. There is no evidence that pregnancy after treatment for breast cancer increases the chance of relapse from that cancer, or that the babies are more likely to have birth defects than the general population. It is possible that the cancer will grow more quickly in the high-estrogen state of pregnancy, but this is hard to quantitate or prove.

Other complications

Patients may also be left with other complications of their diseases or therapies. Patients with Hodgkin's disease, for instance, have an inherent defect in T-cell immunity even before therapy, and this defect persists throughout life, even if the patients are cured of their disease. They may lose their previous immunity to infectious agents such as rubella and may respond poorly to currently administered immunizations. Patients may also have lung disease from bleomycin or radiation therapy, cardiac disease from doxorubicin or radiation therapy, or many other complications of their previous treatments. All of these factors must be taken into account in counseling the woman who desires a pregnancy.

SUMMARY

Each patient who experiences a malignancy during pregnancy must be treated individually, and many concerns must be weighed before diagnostic and therapeutic decisions. The threat of the malignancy to the mother and, therefore, to the fetus must be ascertained. It is also essential to ascertain whether the malignancy is potentially curable since intensity of the therapy will vary, depending on treatment goals. Potentially curable patients generally are treated more intensively and more careful staging is required. Palliative therapy can often be less intensive and staging may not be as important.

The trimester of pregnancy in which the cancer is detected is obviously an essential part of the equation of any diagnostic and therapeutic decision.

Close cooperation among the obstetrician, the neonatologist, the hematologist-oncologist, and the primary care physician is essential in ensuring optimal outcome for both the mother and the fetus.

BIBLIOGRAPHY

Andrieu JM, Ochoa-Molina ME: Menstrual cycle, pregnancies and offspring before and after MOPP therapy for Hodgkin's disease, *Cancer* 52:435, 1983.

Blatt J et al: Pregnancy outcome following cancer chemotherapy, *Am J Med* 69:828, 1980.

DeVita VT et al: Curability of advanced Hodgkin's disease with chemotherapy: long-term follow-up of MOPP-treated patients at the National Cancer Institute, *Ann Intern Med* 92:587, 1980.

Feliu J et al: Acute leukemia and pregnancy, *Cancer* 61:580, 1988.

Gilliland J, Weinstein L: The effects of cancer chemotherapeutic agents on the developing fetus, *Obstet Gynecol Surv* 38:6, 1983.

Green DM, Hall B, Zevon MA: Pregnancy outcome after treatment for acute lymphoblastic leukemia during childhood or adolescence, *Cancer* 64:2335, 1989.

Haagensen CD, Stout AP: Carcinoma of the breast: criteria for operability, *Ann Surg* 118:859, 1943.

Jacobs C et al: Management of the pregnant patient with Hodgkin's disease, *Ann Intern Med* 95:669, 1981.

King RM et al: Carcinoma of the breast associated with pregnancy, *Surg Gynecol Obstet* 160:228, 1985.

Kozlowski RD et al: Outcome of first-trimester exposure to low-dose outcome methotrexate in eight patients with rheumatic disease, *Am J Med* 88:589, 1990.

Lacher MJ, Toner K: Pregnancies and menstrual function before and after combined radiation (RT) and chemotherapy (TVPP) for Hodgkin's disease, *Cancer Invest* 4:93, 1986.

Lipshultz SE et al: Late cardiac effects of doxorubicin therapy for acute lymphoblastic leukemia in childhood, *N Engl J Med* 324:808, 1991.

Mettlin C: Breast cancer risk factors: contributions to planning breast cancer control, *Cancer* 69:1904, 1992.

Mulvihill JJ et al: Pregnancy outcome in cancer patients: experience in a large cooperative group, *Cancer* 60:1143, 1987.

Nugent P, O'Connell TX: Breast cancer and pregnancy, *Arch Surg* 120:1221, 1985.

Petrek JA, Dukoff R, Rogatko A: Prognosis of pregnancy-associated breast cancer, *Cancer* 67:869, 1991.

Reynoso EE et al: Acute leukemia during pregnancy: the Toronto leukemia study group experience with long-term follow-up of children exposed in utero to chemotherapeutic agents, *J Clin Oncol* 5:1098, 1987.

Roboz J et al: Does doxorubicin cross the placenta? Lancet 2:1382, 1979.

Sutton R, Buzdar AU, Hortobagyi GN: Pregnancy and offspring after adjuvant chemotherapy in breast cancer patients, *Cancer* 65:847, 1990.

Trapido EJ: Age at first birth, parity and breast cancer risk, *Cancer* 51:946, 1983.

Treves H, Holleb AI: A report of 549 cases of breast cancer in women 35 years of age or younger, *Surg Gynecol Obstet* 107:271, 1958.

Tucker MA et al: Risk of second cancers after treatment for Hodgkin's disease, *N Engl J Med* 318:76 1988.

Turchi JJ, Villasis C: Anthracyclines in the treatment of malignancy in pregnancy, *Cancer* 61:435, 1988.

Zuazu J et al: Pregnancy outcome in hematologic malignancies, *Cancer* 67:703, 1991.

57 Seizures in Pregnancy

Phyllis Jen

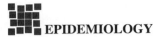

EPIDEMIOLOGY

Epilepsy is the most frequent neurologic problem encountered in pregnancy, occurring in 0.4% of all pregnancies. The majority (87%) of pregnant women with seizures during pregnancy have a history of seizure disorder, while 13% have a seizure for the first time during pregnancy. Pregnant women who have their first seizure during pregnancy should undergo immediate and thorough evaluation for underlying neurologic disease and should be treated with anticonvulsant medications.

In pregnant women with a history of epilepsy the frequency of seizures will remain approximately the same in 50%, will increase in 45%, and will decrease in 5%. Increased seizure frequency can occur for many reasons: metabolic and hormonal changes that alter drug levels, noncompliance with medications, sleep deprivation, and, possibly, hormonally mediated changes in seizure threshold.

RISK OF CONGENITAL MALFORMATIONS AND PERINATAL OUTCOME

Pregnant epileptic women may have twice the risk for an unfavorable outcome (perinatal death, low birth weight, microcephaly, mental retardation) compared with the general population. In all patients with epilepsy, both medicated and unmedicated, the risk of having a child with a congenital malformation is 1.25 times that of the general population. Factors that contribute to this risk include maternal epilepsy, the occurrence of seizures during pregnancy, and the teratogenicity of anticonvulsant therapy. The risk is lowest (1.8%) and approaches that of the general population in those women without seizures during pregnancy and taking no medications. Risk is 2.6% in those women with seizures but not taking medications, 11% in those without seizures but taking medications, and 12.7% in those who have seizures despite medications. It is important to realize that patients on medications are likely to have more severe epilepsy.

Congenital anomalies, either from the maternal epilepsy or from medications, can be major or minor anomalies. Major anomalies such as cardiac septal defects, skeletal abnormalities, mental retardation, and craniofacial clefts result from developmental derangements occurring in the first trimester. Minor anomalies include growth retardation or mild mental retardation. The **fetal hydantoin syndrome** has been characterized by craniofacial anomalies, mental retardation, low birth weight, and defective limbs. The exact relationship between hydantoin and the development of congenital anomalies, however, remains unclear since the syndrome has been noted in some children of epileptic women not taking any medications, as well as those taking carbamazepine, phenobarbital, and primidone.

Valproic acid and trimethadione are definitely teratogenic and should not be used during pregnancy. Congenital anomalies occur in 25% to 30% of pregnant women using trimethadione and neural tube defects occur frequently with valproic acid.

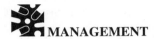

MANAGEMENT

Goals of management

The goal of management of epilepsy in pregnancy is to prevent seizures while judiciously administering anticonvulsant medications. No woman should receive medications unnecessarily. Medication withdrawal before pregnancy should be tried if a woman has been seizure-free for 2 years or has not had a grand mal seizure. A woman who has an active seizure disorder should understand that her risk of poor outcome or congenital anomalies is twice the normal rate and that seizures must be prevented. Patients on valproic acid or trimethadione must be taken off the medication unless all other agents have failed. The combination of ultrasound and α-fetoprotein testing can identify 90% of neural tube anomalies. If seizures are controlled there is no reason to try to switch to phenobarbital from among the other medications. The simplest regimen should be used, preferably with one drug.

Monitoring levels and treatment changes

Frequent monitoring of drug levels during pregnancy is essential, preferably at trough levels. Increased clearance of medications during pregnancy will require an increase in the dosage, especially in the third trimester. If dosages are being adjusted, levels should be checked weekly. If levels are in therapeutic range they should be rechecked monthly throughout pregnancy, then weekly after delivery. If seizures continue and compliance and sleep deprivation are not factors, then a second drug may need to be added.

Treatment of status epilepticus

Treatment of status epilepticus requires aggressive in-hospital treatment. Blood samples should be taken for analysis of glucose level, drug levels, toxic screen, electrolyte levels, and blood gas, and intravenous glucose should be given. Eclampsia should be ruled out. Adequate airway and oxygenation should be maintained, and precautions should be taken against aspiration. Valium 1-2 mg/min IV up to a maximum of 20 mg IV, or phenytoin up to 50 mg/min IV to a total of 18 mg/kg, can be used. If this fails to stop seizures, phenobarbital up to 100 mg/min IV can be given. Rarely, general anesthesia with halothane is required.

Bleeding problems in the newborn

Newborns of mothers on phenytoin or barbiturates may have decreased levels of vitamin K–dependent clotting factors and may experience bleeding problems soon after delivery. This can be prevented by giving oral vitamin K to the mother for 1 week before delivery and IV or IM vitamin K to the newborn after delivery. This may need to be continued if results of clotting studies are persistently abnormal in the neonate. Mothers can safely breastfeed while taking all anti-convulsants, except phenobarbital.

BIBLIOGRAPHY

Bjerkedal T, Egenaes J: Outcome of pregnancy in women with epilepsy, Norway 1967-78. In Janz D, Bossi L, Dam M, editors: *Epilepsy, pregnancy and the child,* New York, 1982, Raven Press.

Knight AH, Rhind EG: Epilepsy and pregnancy: a study of 153 pregnancies in 59 patients, *Epilepsia* 16:99, 1975.

Krumholz A: Epilepsy and pregnancy. In Goldstein PJ, editors: *Neurological disorders of pregnancy,* Mount Kisco, NY, 1986, Futura.

Nakane Y, Okuma T, Takahashi R: Multi-institutional study on teratogeincity and fetal toxicity of anti-epileptic drugs, *Epilepsia* 21:663, 1980.

Niswander KR, Gordon M: The women and their pregnancies, (DHEW publication no NIH 73-379, Washington DC, 1972, Government Printing Office.

58 Thromboembolic Disease in Pregnancy

Samuel Z. Goldhaber

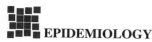

EPIDEMIOLOGY

Venous thromboembolic disease is an important preventable cause of maternal morbidity and mortality. In a Dutch cohort study venous thromboembolism appeared to be three times more common postpartum (23/10,000) than during pregnancy (7/10,000). In a British review the rate of venous thromboembolism during pregnancy was estimated to be 7/10,000 deliveries.

Kaunitz and colleagues noted that, until the 1970s, the classic triad for maternal death was hemorrhage, hypertensive disease of pregnancy, and obstetric infection. These investigators postulated that, in the United States, the increase in venous thromboembolism as the new leading cause of maternal mortality might be related either to overreporting on death certificates or to the difficulty of prevention, recognition, and treatment.

Although the overall U.S. maternal mortality rate is declining, pulmonary embolism (PE) continues to be the most common medical cause of maternal mortality associated with live births (Table 58-1). Risk factors for maternal mortality include increasing age, black race, unmarried status, low level of education, residence in the Northeast, and absence of prenatal care. It is likely that pregnancy alters the physiologic balance between coagulation and fibrinolysis, thus predisposing women to a hypercoagulable state, especially during the puerperium.

The overall maternal mortality ratio for the 8-year Center for Disease Control study from 1979 through 1986 was 9.1 deaths/100,000 live births. The ratio dropped steadily, from 10.9/100,000 in 1979 to 7.4/100,000 in 1986 (Fig. 58-1). For women whose pregnancy ended in a live birth, PE (mostly thrombotic) was the leading cause of death (Fig. 58-2). Other frequent causes were pregnancy-induced hypertension (PIH) (primarily central nervous system complications related to eclampsia and preeclampsia), hemorrhage (primarily postpartum uterine bleeding), and infection. Overall, the Center for Disease Control estimates that PE is the second most com-

Table 58-1 Cause of maternal death, by outcome of pregnancy, United States, 1978-1986

Cause of death	Outcome of pregnancy															
	Live birth		Stillbirth		Ectopic		Abortion*		Molar		Undelivered		Unknown		Total	
	No.	%	No.	%	No.	%	No.	%	No.	%	No.	%	No.	%	No.	%
Hemorrhage	249	18.3	89	33.9	305	88.9	43	34.8	2	14.3	30	20.5	81	20.7	799	30.2
PE	370	27.1	47	17.9	10	2.9	24	19.4	2	14.3	60	41.1	106	27.1	619	23.4
PIH	307	22.5	59	22.4	1	0.3	1	0.8	2	14.3	17	11.6	92	23.5	479	18.1
Infection	101	7.4	22	8.4	6	1.7	35	28.2	2	14.3	8	5.5	28	7.2	202	7.5
Cardiomyopathy	53	3.9	4	1.5	0	0.0	1	0.8	0	0.0	2	1.4	30	7.7	90	3.4
Anesthesia complications	65	4.8	3	1.1	4	1.2	11	8.9	0	0.0	0	0.0	3	0.8	86	3.3
Other	218	16.0	39	14.8	17	5.0	9	7.3	6	43.0	29	19.9	51	13.0	369	14.0
Total maternal deaths	1363	100.0	263	100.0	343	100.0	124	100.0	14	100.0	146	100.0	391	100.0	2644	100.0

From Centers for Disease Control, CDC Surveillance Summaries:*MMWR* 40 (no SS-2): 1991.
PE, pulmonary embolism; PIH, pregnancy-induced hypertension.
*Includes spontaneous and induced abortions.

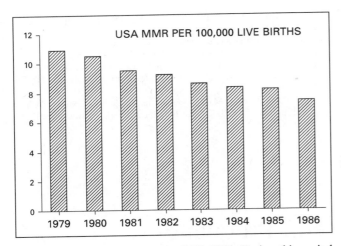

Fig. 58-1 USA maternal deaths 1979-1986. During this period there were 2644 maternal deaths/100,000 and 9.1 deaths/100,000 live births. MMR, maternal mortality rate. (From Morrison RB: Obstetrics. In Goldhaber SZ, editor: *Prevention of venous thromboembolism*, New York, 1993, Marcel Dekker.)

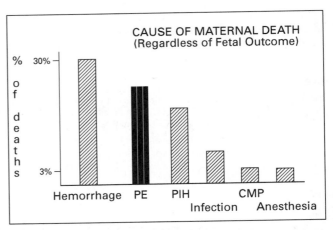

Fig. 58-3 Pulmonary embolism is the second most common medical cause of maternal death in the United States when all fetal outcomes are considered. PE, pulmonary embolism; PIH, pregnancy-induced hypertension; CMP, cardiomyopathy. (From Morrison RB: Obstetrics. In Goldhaber SZ, editor: *Prevention of venous thromboembolism*, New York, 1993, Marcel Dekker.)

mon medical cause of maternal death in the United States (Fig. 58-3).

CLINICAL PRESENTATION
History and physical examination

Deep venous thrombosis (DVT) often occurs without any symptoms or signs. When it is present, however, the major symptoms are leg pain, tenderness, and swelling, while the principal signs are leg edema, discomfort in the calf upon forced dorsiflexion of the foot (Homans' sign), venous distention of subcutaneous vessels, discoloration, or a palpable cord (i.e., thrombus). The symptoms and signs of DVT are often nonspecific and at times confusing in the pregnant patient. For example, leg swelling and leg cramps without clinical importance often occur in pregnancy and consequently can lead the clinician to overlook an evolving DVT.

Because these clinical features are not specific for DVT, a diagnosis based on physical findings is often incorrect. Therefore, clinical suspicion of DVT should prompt definitive evaluation with vascular imaging.

Diagnostic tests

Noninvasive imaging. During pregnancy, noninvasive imaging can be undertaken with high-resolution compression ultrasonography combined with color Doppler imaging as the initial diagnostic test. Contrast venography can usually be avoided. Compression ultrasonography of the legs has revolutionized screening for DVT, although its accuracy in asymptomatic pregnant women is uncertain. High-resolution B-mode ultrasonography is sensitive and specific for the detection of symptomatic proximal leg DVT, above the trifurcation of the calf veins. Color Doppler flow imaging combined with compression ultrasonography is available at most institutions and has been used to evaluate prospectively symptomatic patients who have suspected DVT during pregnancy. Gradient-echo magnetic resonance imaging (MRI) also appears to be a useful noninvasive modality to diagnose venous thrombosis. However, it is more expensive than leg ultrasonography and the resolution of MRI is inadequate for the assessment of suspected isolated calf vein thrombosis.

MANAGEMENT OF ACUTE VENOUS THROMBOSIS

Goals of management

For pregnant women with isolated calf vein thrombosis full-dose heparin anticoagulation should ordinarily be administered, just as for above-calf venous thrombosis. The underlying disease process is the same regardless of the anatomic location of the clot. If untreated, calf thrombi may propagate silently during pregnancy or the puerperium. For women contemplating pregnancy with prior isolated calf vein thrombosis the risk of recurrent venous thrombosis during

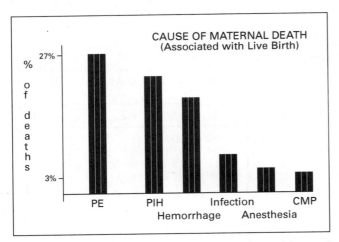

Fig. 58-2 Pulmonary embolism is the leading cause of maternal mortality associated with live births. PE, pulmonary embolism; PIH, pregnancy-induced hypertension; CMP, cardiomyopathy. (From Morrison RB: Obstetrics. In Goldhaber SZ, editor: *Prevention of venous thromboembolism*, New York, 1993, Marcel Dekker.)

pregnancy is probably similar to that for women with a prior above-calf venous thrombosis.

When a woman exhibits venous thrombosis or PE during pregnancy, an extensive evaluation for an underlying cause should be undertaken several months after delivery. Earlier diagnostic investigations may yield confusing results. For example, protein S levels ordinarily decline during pregnancy. However, one should obtain a molecular diagnostic test for a mutation in factor V, as well as lupus anticoagulant and anticardiolipin antibodies. If lupus anticoagulant is present or levels of anticardiolipin antibodies are elevated, a usual prescription is 81 mg of aspirin daily in addition to high-dose heparin.

Choice of therapy

Many physicians treat acute venous thrombosis with high-dose heparin, adjusted to maintain the activated partial thromboplastin time (PTT) between 1.5 and 2.5 times the upper limit of the control value. The heparin requirements to treat acute venous thrombosis appear to be greater during pregnancy than in the nonpregnant state. An initial intravenous bolus of 7500 to 10,000 units of heparin is administered during pregnancy, followed immediately by initiation of a continuous intravenous infusion of 1250 to 1500 U/hr of heparin. Four hours after starting the heparin infusion, a PTT is obtained to ensure that the heparin concentration is therapeutic. A subtherapeutic PTT is associated with recurrent thrombosis, whereas a supertherapeutic PTT is at most only weakly associated with an increased risk of bleeding. After 4 to 7 days of continuous intravenous heparin the patient usually begins self-injected, adjusted, high-dose subcutaneous heparin every 8 hours. The PTT is monitored, initially once daily, to ensure that the midpoint value obtained 4 hours after subcutaneous injection is between 1.5 and 2.5 times the upper limit of the control value. Alternatively, continuous infusion of heparin can be arranged for the patient on an ambulatory basis.

Heparin is continued throughout the pregnancy. After delivery overlap heparin with warfarin for about a week and adjust warfarin dosage to achieve a target International Normalized Ratio of 2.0 to 3.0. Then discontinue heparin treatment but maintain warfarin administration for at least 3 months postpartum. Before discontinuing warfarin repeat leg ultrasonography and perform impedance plethysmography. These tests may be useful in assessing the possibility of recurrent venous thrombosis after warfarin has been discontinued.

Graduated compression stockings are an important adjunctive therapy during pregnancy and postpartum to alleviate leg discomfort and help prevent postphlebitic syndrome. Generally, 30 to 40 mm Hg maternity-style pantyhose stockings are prescribed during pregnancy and patients are encouraged to wear these stockings when ambulatory. When recumbent at night, they can use a much less restrictive thigh-high stocking with 10 to 18 mm Hg of vascular compression.

We often invite pregnant patients with extensive venous thrombosis or pulmonary embolism and their "significant other" to participate in our physician–nurse-led Pulmonary Embolism Support Group. Our group meets for 75 minutes, once every 3 weeks, on a weeknight. We discuss medical questions about venous thrombosis if they arise. However, most of each session is devoted to exploring stresses and emotional and psychologic concerns shared by members of the group. Often, questions are raised that cannot be answered, such as "How do I know I won't suffer another blood clot if I stop taking anticoagulants?" or "How do I know that I won't have another blood clot if I get pregnant again?"

Overview

Physicians who treat women with an increased risk for DVT during pregnancy must consider several alternative pharmacologic and nonpharmacologic prophylactic strategies. Pharmacologic options include (1) subcutaneous heparin, (2) prednisone, and (3) low-dose aspirin. Nonpharmacologic options include mechanical measures such as use of graduated compression stockings and an intermittent pneumatic compression device. Another alternative is close follow-up observation without specific antenatal prophylaxis.

Currently, it is unclear which patients are most likely to benefit from intensive prophylactic measures. Likewise, the complications of these therapies, especially pharmacologic prophylaxis, have not been delineated precisely in this population. It appears that in about 10% of high-risk patients thromboembolic events will develop during pregnancy, even with the use of aggressive preventive strategies.

Choice of prophylaxis

No antenatal pharmacoprophylaxis. In a study of 24 women with one or more prior episodes of venous thromboembolism during pregnancy, routine antenatal prophylactic anticoagulation was withheld. After delivery, patients had anticoagulation for 6 weeks with heparin and/or warfarin. There were two spontaneous second trimester abortions and no perinatal losses. One patient may have had a PE antenatally. On the basis of this case series, Lao and colleagues advocated that antenatal prophylaxis not be given routinely to women who have suffered only one prior episode of venous thrombosis.

Heparin. Unfortunately when subcutaneous heparin is administered during pregnancy the rate of development of osteopenia is as high as 17%. Occasionally osteopenia can be debilitating and can manifest as multiple vertebral compression fractures. Bone demineralization appears to be related to the dose of heparin. Women who receive ≥20,000 U/day of heparin for more than 20 weeks are most susceptible, but even those treated 10 to 22 weeks may have osteopenia. Heparin-associated osteopenia can also develop even when low doses of 5000 units twice daily are administered for many weeks or months.

Some results of prolonged subcutaneous heparin administration are encouraging. In one study of 14 women with anticardiolipin antibodies (ACLAs) and prior abnormal pregnancy outcomes, heparin was started at an estimated gestational age of 10 weeks and was continued in an average daily total dose of 24,700 units per day for the duration of the pregnancy. Of 15 pregnancies 14 resulted in live births, on average at 36 weeks. Placental infarcts were fewer in treated cases than in previous deliveries. Heparin was well tolerated. None of the women experienced serious bleeding problems, thrombotic episodes, or osteoporotic fractures (Rosove, 1990).

Prednisone plus low-dose aspirin. In studies of women with lupus anticoagulant or ACLA and prior fetal loss, treatment with high-dose prednisone (at least 40 mg/day) and low-dose aspirin (75 to 81 mg/day) has been associated with improved fetal outcome. In a study comparing prednisone 40 mg/day versus low-dose heparin (both plus low-dose aspirin) among pregnant women with repeated fetal losses associated with antiphospholid antibodies, there was no difference between the two groups with respect to live birth rates. However, preterm delivery occurred more often among women randomly allocated to prednisone, and this was usually associated with premature rupture of the membranes or preeclampsia. It could not be determined whether the prednisone caused these adverse outcomes.

Low-dose aspirin. When aspirin is used during the first trimester of pregnancy, there does not appear to be an increased risk of fetal malformations. Moreover, newborns appear to have good clinical and biologic tolerance after mothers have ingested 60 to 80 mg/day of aspirin, beginning at 37 weeks of gestation. When aspirin (150 mg/day) was compared with placebo among pregnant mothers with a history of fetal growth retardation, mean birth weight was higher in the aspirin group and frequency of fetal growth retardation was halved. Of 156 women treated with low-dose aspirin eight had epistaxis or other minor bleeding compared with none on placebo. Other than minor bleeding aspirin had no side effects.

In a metaanalysis of women at high risk of PIH low-dose aspirin appeared to reduce the risk of PIH by two thirds. The risk of severe low birth weight was reduced by 44% in the aspirin group. The risk of cesarean section was reduced by 66%. There were no maternal or neonatal adverse effects associated with taking aspirin. However, low-dose aspirin has never been demonstrated to prevent venous thrombosis in pregnancy and the puerperium.

Warfarin. Only rarely is warfarin administered during pregnancy, because of the fear of teratogenicity. Warfarin-associated embryopathy is most likely to occur during weeks 6 to 12 of pregnancy. However, nursing mothers can safely take warfarin, although in the past they were advised against breastfeeding. The fear of transferring warfarin's anticoagulant effect to the baby has not been justified by careful studies.

Nonpharmacologic prophylaxis. The most commonly used nonpharmacologic measures are **graduated compression stockings** (GCS) and **intermittent pneumatic compression** (IPC) boots. Vascular compression with GCS or IPC boots is effective among surgical patients because it counters the otherwise unopposed *perioperative venodilatation* that appears to be causally related to postoperative venous thrombosis. Even among low-risk general surgery patients, GCS can reduce the frequency of venous thrombosis by more than 50% as compared to that among patients receiving no prophylaxis. As a result, GCS should be considered as first-line prophylaxis against PE in obstetric patients, except those with peripheral arterial occlusive disease, whose condition may be worsened by vascular compression.

IPC boots provide intermittent inflation of air-filled cuffs and prevent venous stasis in the legs; they also appear to stimulate the endogenous fibrinolytic system. Therefore, IPC should be considered among women at prolonged bed rest as a result of placenta previa and among those undergoing cesarean section.

It appears that GCS and IPC may work through somewhat different although complementary mechanisms. Thus these modalities can be used in combination in patients at moderate or high risk of venous thrombosis.

Variable prophylaxis. Our usual approach to venous thromboembolism prophylaxis is outlined in Table 58-2. Ordinarily, we withhold antenatal pharmacoprophylaxis among women with prior remote postpartum venous thrombosis or venous thrombosis unrelated to pregnancy. We also withhold antenatal pharmacoprophylaxis among women with a strong family history of venous thrombosis but no personal history of DVT or PE. These patients are encouraged to exercise 1 hour per day and to wear graduated compression stockings. However, our group *has* administered subcutaneous heparin to patients whom we considered clinically to be at high risk because of massive obesity, prolonged bed rest, quadriplegia, or prior first-trimester venous thrombosis. For patients with a severe bleeding tendency (e.g., placenta previa), we have prescribed mechanical prophylaxis (e.g., thigh-high sequential gradient ICP boots).

Postpartum, we often administer 4 to 6 weeks of warfarin to women whom we deem to be at high risk. We adjust the dose to a target international normalized ratio (INR) of 2.0 to 3.0.

APPROACH TO OBSTETRIC VENOUS THROMBOSIS PREVENTION

Each patient should be assessed individually for the risks of venous thromboembolism and should be managed with appropriate mechanical, pharmacologic, or combined prevention modalities. Our practice is to use mechanical prophylaxis with GCS, IPC devices, and exercise whenever feasible. For patients at high risk of venous thrombosis despite mechanical prophylaxis, or in whom expectation of compliance with vascular compression and exercise is not realistic, pharmacologic prophylaxis is used.

Prevention programs are designed to individualize each patient's risk factors throughout the pregnancy and postpartum. Often one finds that an initially excellent candidate for exercise and mechanical prophylaxis needs to be switched to pharmacologic prophylaxis with subcutaneous heparin during the last few months of pregnancy. The risk factors can change dramatically from one week to the next. Therefore, patients must return for frequent follow-up visits.

The patient's personal and family history is vital in determining the likelihood of an inherited hypercoagulable state. Familial history of thrombosis, repeated episodes of thromboembolism without a predisposing condition, and well-documented thromboembolism in adolescents and young adults are all clues in diagnosing the high-risk hypercoagulable patient. Prepregnancy counseling should include information about the potential risk of venous thrombosis and the possibility of transmitting the condition to offspring.

In rare circumstances, it might be recommended that a woman not become pregnant. Such conditions would include moderate or severe pulmonary hypertension caused by prior PE as well as a major allergic reaction (e.g., anaphylaxis) to heparin.

The decision to attempt or to forgo pregnancy should always be postponed until adequate counseling and consultation have been undertaken. Often there is no "right answer." Our Pulmonary Embolism Support Group is one venue in which patients grappling with such decisions can share their concerns and frustrations. Common questions

Table 58-2 Implementation of obstetric prophylaxis

Clinical history	Prevention approach
Noncompliant (e.g., poor understanding or inadequate family support)	Heparin
High-risk (e.g., massive obesity or prolonged bed rest)	Heparin
Quadriplegic	Heparin
Prior first-trimester DVT or PE	Heparin
Severe bleeding tendency (e.g., placenta previa)	Mechanical prophylaxis and exercise (e.g., thigh-high sequential gradient intermittent pneumatic compression boots)
Previous or remote postpartum PE	Exercise during pregnancy; heparin/warfarin in hospital followed by warfarin for 6 wks postpartum
Previous or remote VTE unrelated to pregnancy	Exercise/stockings/frequent follow-ups including leg ultrasound
Strong family history—no prior VTE	Exercise/stockings/frequent follow-ups including leg ultrasound
Cesarean section with a prior history of VTE	Mechanical prophylaxis during/after surgery (e.g., thigh-length sequential gradient intermittent pneumatic compression boots) during the hospital stay, heparin/warfarin in hospital followed by warfarin 6 wk postpartum

From Morrison RB: Obstetrics. In Goldhaber SZ, editor: *Prevention of venous thromboembolism,* New York, 1993, Marcel Dekker.
PE, pulmonary embolism; VTE, venous thromboembolism.

that patients ask are why they were stricken with venous thrombosis and whether they have an underlying coagulopathy or predisposing "bad genes."

Women with venous thromboembolism state repeatedly that they confront a paradox in their daily lives. Although they usually appear healthy, they have actually suffered a potentially life-threatening illness. Often a patient's youthful and healthy appearance may preclude the compassion and understanding they would receive if the illness were more outwardly apparent. In turn, the patients may feel hesitant to express their fears and feelings to close family and friends. We have found that by encouraging patients to express their underlying concerns, we can begin to address the psychosocial burden that usually accompanies the physical illness.

BIBLIOGRAPHY

Cowchock FS et al: Repeated fetal losses associated with antiphospholipid antibodies: a collaborative randomized trial comparing prednisone with low-dose heparin treatment, *Am J Obstet Gynecol* 166:1318, 1992.

Dahlman T, Lindvall N, Hellgren M: Osteopenia in pregnancy during long-term heparin treatment: a radiological study postpartum, *Br J Obstet Gynaecol* 97:221, 1990.

Dixon JE: Pregnancies complicated by previous thromboembolic disease, *Br J Hosp Med* 37:449, 1987.

Imperiale TF, Petrulis AS: A meta-analysis of low-dose aspirin for the prevention of pregnancy-induced hypertensive disease, *JAMA* 266:261, 1991.

Kaunitz AM et al: Causes of maternal mortality in the United States, *Obstet Gynecol* 65:605, 1985.

Koonin LM et al: Maternal mortality surveillance, United States, 1979-1986, *MMWR* 40(No.SS-2):1, 1991.

Lao TT et al: Prophylaxis of thromboembolism in pregnancy: an alternative, *Br J Obstet Gynaecol* 92:202, 1985.

McKenna R, Cole ER, Vasan U: Is warfarin sodium contraindicated in the lactating mother? *J Pediatr* 103:325, 1983.

Morrison RB: Obstetrics. In Goldhaber SZ, editor: *Prevention of venous thromboembolism,* New York, 1993, Marcel Dekker.

Orme M L'E et al: May mothers given warfarin breastfeed their infants? *Br Med J* 1:1564, 1977.

Polak JF: *Peripheral vascular sonography: a practical guide,* Baltimore, 1992, Williams & Wilkins.

Polak JF, Wilkinson DL: Ultrasonographic diagnosis of symptomatic deep venous thrombosis in pregnancy, *Am J Obstet Gynecol* 165:625, 1991.

Rosove MH: Heparin therapy for pregnant women with lupus anticoagulant or anticardiolipin antibodies, *Obstet Gynecol* 75:630, 1990.

Silveira LH et al: Prevention of anticardiolipin antibody-related pregnancy losses with prednisone and aspirin, *Am J Med* 93:403, 1992.

Spritzer CE et al: Deep venous thrombosis: experience with gradient-echo MR imaging in 66 patients, *Radiology* 177:235, 1990.

Treffers PE et al: Epidemiological observations of thrombo-embolic disease during pregnancy and in the puerperium, in 56,022 women, *Int J Gynaecol Obstet* 21:327, 1983.

Uzan S et al: Prevention of fetal growth retardation with low-dose aspirin: findings of the EPREDA trial, *Lancet* 337:1427, 1991.

Werler M, Mitchell AA, Shapiro S: The relation of aspirin use during the first trimester of pregnancy to congenital cardiac defects, *N Engl J Med* 321:1639, 1989.

59 Thyroid Disease in Pregnancy

Douglas S. Ross

ALTERATIONS IN MATERNAL THYROID FUNCTION DURING PREGNANCY

The most clinically significant change during pregnancy is a twofold to threefold increase in serum thyroxine binding globulin (TBG) levels. As a result total thyroxine (T_4) and triiodothyronine (T_3) concentrations in pregnant women are increased, while free thyroid hormone levels remain within the normal range (see Chapter 12). Serum thyroid-stimulating hormone (TSH) measurements are normal, although human chorionic gonadotropin (hCG) is a weak thyroid stimulator that may cause a slight rise in free thyroid hormone levels and a fall in serum TSH concentrations, usually within the normal range. The thyroid enlarges slightly during pregnancy; however, in areas of borderline iodine intake, a substantial goiter may develop.

THYROID FUNCTION IN THE FETUS

The fetal thyroid begins to concentrate iodine and produce iodinated thyronines by 10 to 12 weeks. TSH is also detectable as early as 10 weeks; however, negative feedback may not fully develop until the third trimester. Iodine, propylthiouracil (PTU), methimazole, thyrotropin-releasing hormone (TRH), and thyroid-stimulating and blocking immunoglobulins cross the placenta well, whereas there is minimal transfer of thyroid hormones and no transfer of maternal TSH. The neonate experiences a surge in serum TSH concentrations that lasts 48 hours; fetal and neonatal T_3 levels are lower than those of children and adults.

MATERNAL HYPOTHYROIDISM

Fertility is impaired in hypothyroidism. However, modern studies using TSH measurements suggest that 0.4% to 2.5% of pregnant women may have mild or subclinical hypothyroidism. Maternal hypothyroidism is associated with an increased risk of spontaneous abortion (twofold), stillbirths, placental abruption, preeclampsia, and motor and mental retardation in the neonate. Therefore, unless there are serious cardiovascular contraindications, pregnant hypothyroid patients should be started on full replacement doses of thyroid hormone with titration of dose to obtain a normal serum TSH level. Some studies have suggested that the risk of miscarriage is better correlated with thyroid autoantibody titers than thyroid hormone levels.

Hypothyroid women on replacement levothyroxine may require an increased dose during pregnancy, since hormone requirements are increased. TSH should be measured early during pregnancy, and levothyroxine dose retitrated to normalize serum TSH level. At least one more TSH measurement should be made later in pregnancy.

MATERNAL HYPERTHYROIDISM

Thyrotoxicosis complicates about 0.2% of all pregnancies. Most patients have Graves' disease; however, other causes of hyperthyroidism may be present (see Chapter 12), and trophoblastic disease must be considered as the cause of the hyperthyroidism. It is difficult to confirm the diagnosis of subacute lymphocytic thyroiditis in pregnancy since determination of the radioiodine uptake is contraindicated. One can assume that hyperthyroidism that spontaneously resolves is due to thyroiditis; however, pregnancy also has an ameliorating effect on Graves' hyperthyroidism, and flares are commonly seen postpartum.

Hyperthyroidism complicating pregnancy is best prevented by treating Graves' disease with radioiodine or surgery before pregnancy (see Chapter 12). Mild hyperthyroidism is generally well tolerated by mother and fetus, so the goal of therapy is to prevent overtreatment and accept mild hyperthyroidism. β-Blockers should be avoided except when essential because of possible intrauterine growth retardation. Radioiodine is absolutely contraindicated during pregnancy, and surgery is relatively contraindicated, so patients are managed with antithyroid drugs. Because of reports of a scalp defect, aplasia cutis, that occurs with methimazole therapy, PTU is the treatment of choice. PTU should be given in the smallest doses necessary to control significant hyperthyroid symptoms in order to prevent fetal goiter and hypothyroidism. Pregnant women on PTU should have monthly thyroid function tests. It is essential to appreciate the effects of TBG excess on total hormone values and to monitor free T_4 and T_3 concentrations, since TSH level may be subnormal throughout the pregnancy. Many patients can be weaned off PTU during the later stages of pregnancy as the hyperthyroidism becomes less severe. Levothyroxine should not be given with PTU, since it does not cross the placenta well and masks overtreatment.

FETAL AND NEONATAL HYPOTHYROIDISM

Excessive PTU therapy can lead to fetal hypothyroidism and goiter. Fetal goiter is rarely large enough to cause strangulation; however, this complication has been seen when pharmacologic iodine has been administered during pregnancy complicated by hyperthyroidism. Fetal thyroid size and fetal development should be monitored with ultrasound. Recently some have advocated percutaneous umbilical vein blood sampling for thyroid function tests. Intraamniotic or fetal intramuscular levothyroxine has been used to treat fetal hypothyroidism.

Congenital hypothyroidism complicates 1/4000 births and is now frequently assessed by neonatal screening. Children treated immediately after birth have normal development and usually have minimal neuropsychologic sequelae.

FETAL AND NEONATAL HYPERTHYROIDISM

Fetal and neonatal hyperthyroidism complicates about 2% of pregnancies in women with Graves' disease. The cause is transplacental transfer of thyroid-stimulating immunoglobulin (TSI). Mothers with a history of Graves' disease who have had their glands ablated (radioiodine or surgery) may still have significant TSI titers and give birth to children with thyrotoxicosis, even though they are euthyroid and having levothyroxine replacement therapy. TSI should be measured early in the second trimester of such women; most cases of neonatal Graves' disease have occurred in mothers who have TSI titers that exceed 500% of normal.

Fetal thyrotoxicosis can lead to craniosynostosis and retarded growth and intellect. Fetal ultrasound can detect goiter, advanced bone age, and poor development. Fetal heart rates greater than 160 may suggest fetal hyperthyroidism. PTU may be given to a euthyroid mother to treat fetal hyperthyroidism, aiming for a fetal heart rate of 140. Percutaneous umbilical vein sampling may be used to monitor thyroid function. Seven to 10 days after delivery, neonatal hyperthyroidism may result from persistent maternal TSI and falling PTU levels in the neonate.

THYROID NODULES DURING PREGNANCY

Thyroid scintigraphy is contraindicated during pregnancy. Fine needle aspiration can safely be done and will usually reassure patient and physician. Many small intrathyroidal papillary cancers can wait until after delivery for surgical excision with little risk to the patient. More aggressive neoplasms may require surgical intervention during pregnancy.

BIBLIOGRAPHY

Burrow GN: The management of thyrotoxicosis in pregnancy, *N Engl J Med* 313:562, 1985.

Mandel SJ et al: Increased need for thyroxine during pregnancy in women with primary hypothyroidism, *N Engl J Med* 323:91, 1990.

Perelman AH, Clemons RD: The fetus in maternal hyperthyroidism, *Thyroid* 2:225, 1992.

Zakarija M, McKenzie JM, Hoffman WH: Prediction and therapy of intrauterine and late-onset neonatal hyperthyroidism, *J Clin Endocrinol Metab* 62:368, 1986.

60 Urinary Tract Infections in Pregnancy

Stephanie A. Eisenstat

Urinary tract infections and acute pyelonephritis are common during pregnancy and pose a serious risk to the fetus. An association between urinary tract infections and increased risk of pyelonephritis development during pregnancy was reported in classic studies by Kass in 1960. Since that time multiple studies have confirmed that eradicating the urinary tract infection both decreases the risk of pyelonephritis and leads to improved fetal outcome. The relationship between bacteriuria and low birth weight was described by Kass in 1962. Data clearly demonstrate that screening for and then eradicating bacteriuria decrease the incidence of acute pyelonephritis and associated preterm birth.

This chapter summarizes the clinical recommendations regarding identification and treatment of bacteriuria, urinary tract infections, and pyelonephritis in pregnancy. A vast number of studies and books review this subject, with some key references listed at the end of this chapter. For more in-depth discussion on evaluation and management of acute dysuria in women, see Chapter 18.

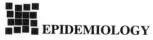 EPIDEMIOLOGY

Multiple studies estimate that the prevalence of bacteriuria is similar in pregnant and nonpregnant women: 2% to 11%. Risk factors for persistent bacteriuria include lower socioeconomic status, sickle cell trait, and documented bacteriuria at the first prenatal visit. Early studies by Kunin suggested that the incidence of bacteriuria increased with age. However, age does not appear to be a factor if the woman is pregnant; rather bacteriuria appears to be correlated with parity.

Women who have had more than three term pregnancies are at higher risk for bacteriuria.

Pyelonephritis occurs in 1% to 2% of all pregnancies and is one of the most serious infections in pregnancy. Preexisting bacteriuria is present in 60% of pregnant women.

DEFINITION

Bacteriuria, which can exist with or without symptoms of urinary tract infection, and is defined as the presence of more than 100,000 organisms/ml in a midstream clean-catch urine specimen (Kincaid-Smith, 1965). However, colony counts of less than 100,000/ml do not exclude infection; they may be low because of the timing of collection (Stamm et al., 1982). If the urinary bacterial colony count is greater than 10,000 organisms/ml but less than 100,000 organisms/ml, a repeat urine culture should be obtained. *Repeat* urine culture results of less than 100,000 organisms/ml should be considered bacteriuria in the pregnant woman. Acute cystitis is defined as a positive urine culture and is associated with symptoms of frequency, dysuria, and urgency. Symptoms of fever, chills, nausea, and flank pain usually indicate acute pyelonephritis. Among women with acute pyelonephritis, urine cultures are invariably positive, and in 10% blood cultures are positive for this condition (Cunningham, Morris, and Mickal,1973).

NORMAL PHYSIOLOGIC CHANGES DURING PREGNANCY

Various changes in the anatomy of the urinary tract during pregnancy predispose pregnant women to urinary tract infections and pyelonephritis. Dilation of the collecting system—renal calices, pelves, and ureters—begins during the first trimester and continues throughout pregnancy, probably a result of the dilating effect of progesterone on the smooth muscle of the tract. There is also an increase in renal length and compression of the bladder because of the enlarging of the uterus. These changes have been correlated with the increased risk of developing third-trimester pyelonephritis (Kreiger, 1986). Bacterial proliferation is promoted because of the urinary stasis, glycosuria, aminoaciduria, and incomplete emptying of the bladder.

PATHOGENS

The most common pathogens that cause bacteriuria and urinary tract infections in pregnancy are *Escherichia coli,* and *Klebsiella* and *Enterobacter* organisms (MacDonald et al., 1983). Other pathogens frequently isolated from women with bacteriuria include *Proteus mirabilis, Pseudomonas aeruginosa, Staphylococcus saphrophyticus,* enterococci, and group B beta-hemolytic streptococci (McNeeley, 1988). Group B beta-hemolytic streptococcal infection in the fetus can lead to severe morbidity and even death (see Chapter 50).

COMPLICATIONS OF BACTERIURIA

Acute pyelonephritis will develop during the pregnancy of 20% to 40% of pregnant women with bacteriuria. Bacteriuria is associated with acute pyelonephritis (usually occurring during the third trimester), anemia, toxemia, and chronic pyelonephritis in the mother. Acute pyelonephritis is more severe in pregnant women and has been associated with adult respiratory distress syndrome, hematologic abnormalities, renal insufficiency, and hypothalamic instability. For the infant there is an increased rate of prematurity and low birth weight, and some studies also suggest an increased rate of fetal infection, fetal wastage, and dorsal midline defects. Well-controlled studies have demonstrated that there is a marked reduction in the risk for pyelonephritis in women with bacteriuria who have been treated with antibiotics (Kincaid-Smith, 1965).

APPROACH TO THE PREGNANT PATIENT WITH URINARY TRACT INFECTION

Diagnostic tests

Because up to 11% of pregnant women have asymptomatic bacteriuria, the recommendation of the American College of Obstetricians and Gynecologists is to obtain a urine culture in all pregnant women during the first prenatal visit (preferably before 16 weeks' gestation). Because fewer than 1% of pregnant women acquire asymptomatic bacteriuria during pregnancy, it is unnecessary to repeat screening (Cox and Cunningham, 1993). However, if symptoms (frequency, dysuria) of urinary tract infection occur, a repeat urine culture is indicated. Unfortunately more cost-effective testing measures—such as urine dipstick, urine for nitrates, and urine for leukocytes—provide low sensitivity for identifying women with asymptomatic bacteriuria and therefore are not recommended as the initial screening measure. A Gram's stain of the urine yields high results but is expensive (Bachman et al., 1993).

The diagnosis of pyelonephritis is confirmed by positive urine culture and accompanying systemic symptoms (fever, rigors, chills, costovertebral angle–tenderness), or positive blood cultures or both.

Management

The goal of treatment is to eradicate the infection. The usual treatment is a complete course of antibiotics with follow-up cultures. Antibiotics cross the placenta; thus fetal safety needs to be considered. Standard therapies that are safe during pregnancy are noted in Table 60-1.

Choice of therapy

Asymptomatic bacteriuria or urinary tract infection. Asymptomatic bacteriuria and urinary tract infection must be treated. Options for therapy appear in Table 60-1. The pregnant woman with acute symptomatic infection should

Table 60-1 Choice of treatment for urinary tract infections during pregnancy

	First choice		Alternative	
	Drug	**Dosage**	**Drug**	**Dosage**
Asymptomatic Bacteriuria	Ampicillin	500 mg PO qid 7-10 days	Nitrofurantoin	100 mg PO 7-10 days
or				
Acute Cystourethritis	Cephalexin	250-500 mg PO qid 7-10 days	Sulfisoxazole	500 mg PO qid 7-10 days
Pyelonephritis				
*Acute**	Ampicillin	2 g IV q6h 7-14 days	Gentamicin	3-5 mg/kg/day q8h
	Cefazolin	1-2 g IV q6h 10-14 days	Tobramycin	3-5 mg/kg/day q8h
Chronic	Nitrofurantoin	50-100 mg PO hs for duration of pregnancy	Sulfisoxazole	500 mg PO bid for duration of pregnancy
Suppressive therapy*	Nitrofurantoin	100 mg hs		
	Sulfisoxazole	500 mg PO bid		
	Ampicillin	250 mg PO bid		

Modified from Kreiger J: *Urol Clin North Am* 13:685, 1986; McNeeley, *Clin Obstet Gynecol* 31:480, 1988.
*Intravenous until afebrile ≥48 hours, then consider oral therapy for total 10-14 day therapy. Follow-up urine culture; if positive, consider suppressive therapy.
**Complete 7-10 day course; if reinfected, then suppression for remainder of pregnancy.

be treated empirically until the results of urine culture are available. Traditionally 7- to 10-day courses have been used. Generally short course (1 or 3 day regimens) are not advised for pregnant women. Follow-up urine cultures 2 weeks after completion of treatment, are important to ensure that the infection is eradicated.

Pyelonephritis. Pregnant women with acute pyelonephritis should be treated with intravenous antibiotics. Because of the risk for severe complications with pyelonephritis during pregnancy, hospitalization is indicated. Fluid monitoring, rehydration, and fetal assessment are important. Because 30% of the women treated for pyelonephritis have persistent positive urine cultures, follow-up cultures and surveillance are important. If the urine culture remains positive for pyelonephritis and the patient's clinical condition is stable, suppressive therapy is indicated for the remainder of the pregnancy.

BIBLIOGRAPHY

Andriole VT, Patterson T: Epidemiology, natural history and management of urinary tract infections in pregnancy, *Med Clin North Am* 75:359, 1991.

Bachman J et al: A study of various tests to detect asymptomatic urinary tract infections in an obstetric population, *JAMA* 270:1971, 1993.

Cox S, Cunningham FG: Urinary tract infections. In Charles D, editor: *Obstetric and perinatal infections,* St Louis, 1993, Mosby.

Cunningham FG, Morris GB, Mickal A: Acute pyelonephritis in pregnancy: a clinical review, *Obstet Gynecol* 43:112, 1973.

Gilstrap et al: Renal infection and pregnancy outcome, *Am J Obstet Gynecol* 141:709, 1981.

Kass EH: Bacteriuria and pyelonephritis of pregnancy, *AMA Arch Intern Med* 105:194, 1960.

Kass EH: Pyelonephritis and bacteriuria: a major problem in preventive medicine, *Ann Intern Med* 56:46, 1962.

Kass EH: The role of unsuspected infection in the etiology of prematurity, *Clin Obstet Gynecol* 16:134, 1973.

Kincaid-Smith P: Bacteriuria and urinary tract infection in pregnancy, *Lancet* 1:395, 1965.

Kreiger J: Complications and treatment of urinary tract infections in pregnancy, *Urol Clin North Am* 13:685, 1986.

Kunin CM: An overview of urinary tract infections. In *Detection, prevention and management of urinary tract infections,* ed, 3 Philadelphia, 1979, Lea & Febiger.

Lindheineir MD, Katz AI: The kidney in pregnancy, *N Engl J Med* 283:1095, 1970.

MacDonald P et al: Summary of a workshop on maternal genitourinary infections and the outcome of pregnancy, *J Infect Dis* 147:596, 1983.

McNeeley SG: Treatment of urinary tract infections during pregnancy, *Clin Obstet Gynecol* 31:480, 1988.

Naeye R: Causes of the excessive rates of perinatal mortality and prematurity in pregnancies complicated by maternal urinary tract infections, *N Engl J Med* 300:819, 1979.

Pfau A, Sacks T: Effective prophylaxis for recurrent urinary tract infections during pregnancy, *Clin Infect Dis* 14:810, 1992.

Stamm WE et al: Diagnosis of coliform infection in acutely dysuric women, *N Engl J Med* 307:463, 1982.

Sweet RL: Bacteriuria and pyelonephritis during pregnancy, *Semin Perinatol* 1:25, 1977.

Waltzer W: The urinary tract in pregnancy, *Urol* 125:271, 19.. (review article).

Whalley P: Bacteriuria of pregnancy, *Am J Obstet Gynecol* 97:723, 1967.

Zinner H: Bacteriuria and babies revisited, *N Engl J Med* 300:853, 1979.

Zinner SH, Kass EH: Long term (10-14 years) follow-up of bacteriuria of pregnancy, *N Engl J Med* 285:820, 1971.

61 Use of Medications in Pregnancy and Lactation

Stephanie A. Eisenstat and Karen J. Carlson

Prescribing medications for a pregnant or lactating woman can be complicated by the risk of adverse effects on the fetus or in the infant if the mother is breastfeeding. The timing of medication use during pregnancy influences the potential risk. Often primary care clinicians avoid all medications during pregnancy because of fear of harm to the fetus and thus may undertreat certain medical conditions in the pregnant woman.

Difficult decisions—weighing the benefit to the pregnant or lactating woman against the potential risk to the fetus or infant—often must be made in the absence of adequate research data. Toxic effects of medications are most important during the first trimester, when the fetus is developing, and at the time of delivery, when medications may have an adverse effect on the course of labor or result in neonatal depression. Certain medications that are clearly detrimental during pregnancy are safe during the breastfeeding period (e.g., warfarin).

The purpose of this chapter is to summarize the major clinical issues in prescribing classes of medications not discussed elsewhere in this book. For a more detailed discussion of specific medications the reader is referred to standard references listed at the end of this chapter.

CLASSIFICATION OF MEDICATIONS

There are many problems in evaluating the effects of drugs in pregnancy and in implementing prospective studies. For many medications, research data are available only in animals. Many drugs have been released by the Food and Drug Administration (FDA) for which safety during pregnancy has not yet been established. To assist in the classification of medications the FDA developed a classification system based on known risk factors for the fetus (see box on the following page).

Category A drugs have been shown to be safe in the first trimester of pregnancy in controlled studies, and the potential

DRUG CLASSIFICATION SYSTEM OF THE FOOD AND DRUG ADMINISTRATION

A Controlled studies in women fail to demonstrate risk to fetus in first trimester and fetal harm remote

B Animal reproduction studies have not demonstrated risk to fetus, but no controlled studies in pregnant females; or animal studies have shown effect but no controlled studies in pregnant females

C Animal studies have revealed adverse effects in fetus; no controlled studies in women; *should be given only if potential benefit justifies risk*

D Evidence for fetal risk, but benefits may be acceptable in pregnant females despite risk (e.g., life-saving situation)

X Studies in animals and humans demonstrate fetal risk; contraindicated in pregnancy

Modified from Food and Drug Administration: *Federal Register* 44:37434, 1980

harm to the fetus is remote. The actual number of medications that fall into this category is small. **Category B** drugs are commonly used by physicians. For these medications, animal studies have revealed no detrimental effects in the fetus but no controlled studies in pregnant females exist, or detrimental effects found in animal studies have not been shown in controlled studies in pregnant women. **Category C** drugs are classified as such because animal studies demonstrate clear detrimental effects but there are no controlled studies in pregnant women. Because of the particular risk to the fetus, these drugs should be given only if potential benefit justifies the risk. **Category D** drugs have been shown to

have adverse effects for the fetus but in certain life-saving situations would be considered acceptable for use despite the risk to the fetus. **Category X** drugs are contraindicated in pregnancy because studies in animals and human beings have demonstrated severe fetal risk (see box, below).

TYPES OF MEDICATION
Analgesics

The appropriate medication for pain relief during pregnancy is a common clinical question for the primary care clinician. The pregnant woman may have a mild headache, backache, or other minor discomfort and may request advice on analgesic use. Generally, *acetominophen (Tylenol)* has been shown to be safe during pregnancy and lactation. Even though it crosses the placenta and is present in breast milk, controlled studies have shown that the levels attained in prescription doses are safe to the fetus. There is potential harm in very high doses such as those seen in overdose cases. When given close to the time of delivery, *salicylate (aspirin)* has the potential for increased bleeding abnormalities during labor and in the fetus because of the effect on platelets and the prolongation of the bleeding time (even with small doses). A few studies have suggested the occurrence of fetal malformations from first-trimester exposure, but this conclusion is controversial. The American Academy of Pediatrics recommends caution in prescribing aspirin. In some instances the use of aspirin may outweigh the potential risk, such as in the possible prevention of preeclampsia and the treatment of rheumatoid arthritis during pregnancy. *Ibuprofen* products (Motrin, Naprosyn) have been shown to be safe, but there is potential risk when used during the third trimester because of risk of bleeding (through prolongation of the bleeding time). Prolonged *narcotic* use can be a problem for the fetus because of the risk for respiratory depression or addiction, but in terms of risk for development of fetal malformations,

DRUGS CONTRAINDICATED IN PREGNANCY BECAUSE OF TOXICITY AND FETAL RISK (CATEGORY X)

Alcohol
Fetal alcohol syndrome

Diethylstilbestrol (DES)
Female offspring: anatomic anomalies of genital tract, adenosis, and clear cell carcinoma; increased risk of breast cancer
Male offspring: anatomic abnormalities, reproductive dysfunction, infertility, increased risk of testicular cancer

Disulfiram
Anomalies: *v*ertebral defects, imperforate *a*nus, *t*racheoesophageal fistula, and *r*adial and *r*enal dysplasia (VATER)

Folic acid agonists
Malformations

Isotretinoin
Severe malformations

Oral contraceptive pills
Increase cardiovascular defects, eye and ear anomalies

Quinine
CNS and limb defects

Trimethadione
Mental retardation, developmental delay, cleft palate/lip, intrauterine growth retardation; cardiac, urogenital, and skeletal abnormalities

Valproic acid
Neural tube defects, congenital heart disease, facial changes, developmental delay

Others
Measles, mumps, rubella vaccine (MMR)
Viral transmission to fetus
Radioactive iodine
Congenital hypothyroidism (cretinism)

Modified from Briggs G, Freeman RK, Yaffe SJ: *Drugs in pregnancy and lactation*, ed 3, Baltimore, 1990, Williams & Wilkins.

Table 61-1 Commonly used medications and their safety in pregnancy and lactation

Drug	Category	Pregnancy/fetal risk	Recommendation for use	
			Pregnancy	**Breastfeeding**
Acetaminophen	B	None in prescribed doses	Safe	Safe
Aspirin (during third trimester)	C	Possible fetal malformations	Caution	Caution
	D	Increased risk of neonatal hemorrhage		
Ibuprofen	B	None known	Safe	Safe
During third trimester	D			
Oxycodone	B	None	Safe	Caution
With prolonged use	D	Neonatal depression		
Codeine	C	Cardiac, circulatory malformations, pyloric stenosis inguinal hernia, cleft lip/palate	Caution	Caution
High dose at term	D	Neonatal depression		
Demerol	B	Neonatal depression	Safe	Safe

Modified from Briggs GC, Freeman RK, Yaffe SJ: *Drugs in pregnancy and lactation*, ed 3, Baltimore, 1990, Williams & Wilkins; Berkowitz R, Coustan D, Mochizuki T: *Handbook for prescribing medications during pregnancy*; ed 2, Boston, 1986, Little, Brown & Co.

all but codeine are considered safe. *Codeine* has been associated with fetal malformations, including circulatory and cardiac abnormalities, pyloric stenosis, inguinal hernia, and cleft lip and palate, and should be used with caution during pregnancy. *Demerol* is relatively safe and, except for the risk of neonatal depression in higher doses at the time of labor, is acceptable for use during pregnancy. All narcotic medications have abuse potential. Whether the potential for abuse is higher because of the effect of pregnancy on drug metabolism is unknown. Current recommendations for analgesic use are summarized in Table 61-1.

Asthma medications

For many medications commonly used in the treatment of asthma, the adverse effects on the fetus are unknown. There is no indication that the fetus suffers from serious effects except when exposed to corticosteroids. The potential detrimental effects from corticosteroids during the first trimester are not clearly delineated and may be greater for the oral preparations than for aerosolized forms. In addition, the risk of hypoxia to the fetus from an untreated episode of asthma is probably far greater than the risk from use of the medication during pregnancy. Beta adrenergic agonists and theophylline are safe for use during pregnancy. A summary of the commonly used medications and recommendations for use appears in Table 61-2. For a more detailed discussion on treatment of asthma in pregnancy see Chapter 52.

Antimicrobial agents

Most of the commonly used antimicrobial agents such as penicillin, dicloxacillin, and erythromyin (except for erythromycin estolate) are safe during pregnancy. Erythromycin estolate has been associated with cholestatic hepatitis in the pregnant woman and should be avoided. Ciprofloxacin has been shown to be embryotoxic, resulting in arthropathy in animals, and is contraindicated for use during pregnancy and lactation. Many clinicians avoid the use of ciprofloxacin in women of reproductive age because 50% of all pregnancies are unplanned and the detrimental effects of the drug are significant. Other contraindicated antibiotics are tetracycline (which causes dental dysplasia and inhibition of bone growth in the fetus) and trimethoprim-sulfamethoxazole (which is teratogenic in rats and increases the risk of kernicterus and hemolysis in the newborn). Antituberculous medications are all embryocidal in animals, but the benefit of treating active tuberculosis in the pregnant woman clearly outweighs the risk to the fetus. Recommendations for antibiotic use during pregnancy appear in Table 61-3.

Table 61-2 Commonly used antiasthmatic medications and their safety in pregnancy and lactation

Drug	Category	Pregnancy/fetal risk	Recommendation for use	
			Pregnancy	**Breastfeeding**
Beta adrenergic agonists	C	None	Safe	Safe
Steroid inhalers	C	Unknown	Use if medically indicated	Unknown
Oral steroids	C	Unknown	Use if medically indicated	Unknown
Cromolyn	B	None	Safe	Safe
Ipratropium (Atrovent)	B	None	Safe	Safe
Theophylline	C	None	Safe	Safe

Modified from Briggs GC, Freeman RK, Yaffe SJ: *Drugs in pregnancy and lactation*, ed 3, Baltimore, 1990, Williams & Wilkins; Berkowitz R, Coustan D, Mochizuki T: *Handbook for prescribing medications during pregnancy*, ed 2, Boston, 1986, Little, Brown & Co.

Table 61-3 Commonly used antimicrobial agents and their safety in pregnancy and lactation

Drug	Category	Pregnancy/fetal risk	Recommendation for use	
			Pregnancy	Breastfeeding
Antibacterial agents				
Penicillins	B	None	Safe	Safe
Dicloxacillin	B	None	Safe	Safe
Erythromycin				
Estolate	B	Cholestatic hepatitis in mother	Contraindicated	Safe
Others	B	None	Safe	Safe
Cephalosporins	B	None	Safe	Safe
Trimethoprim-sulfamethoxazole	C	Folate antagonism; teratogenic in rats; hemolysis in newborn; increased risk of kernicterus; teratogenic in animals	Use other options	Safe
Quinolones	C	Arthropathy in animals	Contraindicated	Contraindicated
Aminoglycosides	C	Eighth nerve toxicity	Use other options	Contraindicated
Tetracycline	D	Tooth discoloration and dysplasia; inhibition of bone growth in fetus	Contraindicated	Contraindicated
Vancomycin	C	Unknown—possible auditory and renal	Use other options	Contraindicated
Metronidazole	B	Unknown	Contraindicated in first trimester; safe in second and third trimesters	Safe
Antituberculous medications				
Isoniazid	C	Embryocidal	Caution	Caution
Rifampin	C	Teratogenic in animals	Caution	Caution
Ethambutol	B	None known—teratogenic in animals	Caution	Caution

Modified from Briggs GC, Freeman RK, Yaffe SJ: *Drugs in pregnancy and lactation*, ed 3, Baltimore, 1990, Williams & Wilkins; Berkowitz R, Coustan D, Mochizuki T: *Handbook for prescribing medications during pregnancy*, ed 2, Boston, 1986, Little, Brown & Co.

Anticoagulation therapy

Heparin does not cross the placenta and is therefore safe for use during pregnancy with respect to the fetus. *Warfarin (Coumadin)*, however, is not safe and is associated with the fetal warfarin embryopathy syndrome. The treatment of thromboembolic disorders of pregnancy is reviewed in Chapter 59. Unlike its use in pregnancy, Coumadin is the drug of choice during the breastfeeding period and does not pose undue threat to the fetus.

Anticonvulsant therapy

Treatment of seizure disorders is complicated in the pregnant woman because there are no safe anticonvulsant therapies. Physicians experienced in the management of these disorders should oversee anticonvulsant therapy during pregnancy. It is important to treat seizure disorders during pregnancy because of the risk of hypoxia to the fetus during a seizure. *Carba-*

mazepine (Tegretol) is considered the safest of the anticonvulsant therapies but is associated with multiple abnormalities, including craniofacial abnormalities, intrauterine growth retardation, microcephaly, and fingernail hypoplasia. *Phenytoin (Dilantin)* is associated with major birth defects as is *valproic acid (Depakene)*. The use of these medications in pregnancy is summarized in Table 61-4.

Nonprescription medications

Frequently pregnant women ask the primary care clinician about the safety of nonprescription medications. Most over-the-counter preparations are safe during pregnancy with the exception of certain antihistamines, aspirin, nonsteroidal antiinflammatory drugs (as previously described), certain antiacids, and cathartics. The safety of commonly used nonprescription medications is summarized in Table 61-5.

Table 61-4 Commonly used anticonvulsant medications and their safety in pregnancy and lactation

Drug	Category	Pregnancy/fetal risk	Recommendation for use	
			Pregnancy	Breastfeeding
Dilantin	D	Major birth defects; fetal hydantoin syndrome	Contraindicated	Caution
Phenobarbital	D	Risk of cleft palate and congenital heart disease; hemorrhagic disease in newborn	Contraindicated	Caution
Tegretol	C	Craniofacial abnormalities, IUGR, microcephaly, fingernail hypoplasia	Contraindicated	Caution
Valproic acid	X	Multiple malformations	Contraindicated	Safe

Modified from Briggs GC, Freeman RK, Yaffe SJ: *Drugs in pregnancy and lactation*, ed 3, Baltimore, 1990, Williams & Wilkins; Berkowitz R, Coustan D, Mochizuki T: *Handbook for prescribing medications during pregnancy*, ed 2, Boston, 1986, Little, Brown & Co.

Table 61-5 Commonly used nonprescription medications and their safety during pregnancy

Drug	Toxicity during pregnancy	
	First trimester	**Second and third trimesters**
Analgesics		
Acetaminophen (Tylenol)	Safe in recommended dose	Safe
Salicylates (aspirin)	Rare reports of malformations	Increased risk of neonatal hemorrhage
Ibuprofen (Motrin)	Safe	Risk of premature labor
Antihistamines*		
Dimenhydrinate (Dramamine)	Possibly teratogenic	Liver toxicity in fetus, premature labor
Diphenhydramine (Benadryl)	Oral clefts	
Clorpheniramine (Chlor-Trimeton)	Probably safe	Same as Dramamine
Pseudoephedrine (Sudafed)	Inguinal hernia, club foot	Safe
Bulk-forming agents		
Agar, bran, methycellulose, psyllium	Safe	Safe
Belladonna alkaloids	Safe	Safe
Cathartics		
Contact		
Anthracene	—	All but aloe safe; aloe stimulates fetal
Aloe, cascara, senna		intestines, resulting in increased meconium
Castor oil, bisacodyl	Safe	Safe
Saline		
Magnesium salts, Milk of magnesia, epsom salts	Safe	Safe
Mineral oil	Contraindicated	Contraindicated
Simethicone	Safe	Safe
Antacids		
Aluminum hydroxide	Risk of malformations	Safe
Calcium carbonate	Safe	Risk of fetal hypomagnesemia
Magnesium compounds	Unknown	Risk of fetal hypermagnesemia
Sodium bicarbonate	Contraindicated	Contraindicated because of increase in edema
Sympathomimetics		
Ephedrine, phenylephrine	Safe	Safe
Antitussive agent		
Dextromethorphan	Safe	Safe

Data from Berkowitz R, Coustan D, Mochizuki T: *Handbook for prescribing medications during pregnancy*, ed 2, Boston, 1986, Little, Brown & Co.
*Inhibit lactation.

BIBLIOGRAPHY

Berkowitz R, Coustan D, Mochizuki T: *Handbook for prescribing medications during pregnancy*, ed 2, Boston, 1986, Little, Brown & Co.

Briggs GC, Freeman RK, Yaffe SJ: *Drugs in pregnancy and lactation*, ed 3, Baltimore, 1990, Williams & Wilkins.

Cefalo R, Moos M: *Preconceptional health care: a practical guide*, St Louis, 1995, Mosby.

Cunningham FG et al: *Williams obstetrics*, ed 19, Norwalk, Conn, 1993, Appleton & Lange.

Hollingworth DR, Resnik R: *Medical counseling before pregnancy*, New York, 1988, Churchill Livingstone.

Lawrence RA: *Breastfeeding: a guide for the medical profession*, St Louis, 1989, Mosby.

Rayburn WF, Zuspan FP: *Drug therapy in obstetrics and gynecology*, ed 3, St Louis, 1992, Mosby.

62 Breastfeeding and Mastitis

Ruth A. Lawrence

Breastfeeding is recommended for all infants under ordinary circumstances throughout the world. Even if the mother's diet is not perfect it is still recommended, as the milk will be good. The health goals of the United States for the year 2000 include increasing the number of women who initiate breastfeeding to 75% and the number who are still breastfeeding 6 months postpartum to at least 50%. Early 1990 statistics indicate rates of 52.4% and 20.7%, respectively. Some of the difficulty in increasing the number of breastfeeding mothers in Western countries is related to a lack of understanding among medical professionals about lactation.

ANATOMY AND PHYSIOLOGY OF LACTATION

Understanding the anatomy and physiology of lactation is important for any practitioner who cares for women. By understanding the physiologic characteristics of successful lactation one can understand how to manage concurrent problems without interfering with the processing as well as facilitate the process when it is faltering.

The first rudimentary breast tissues appear in both male and female embryos at about 8 weeks gestation. The development of the breast in the fetus is used by neonatologists as one of the diagnostic landmarks to determine the gestational age of the infant at birth. After the development of a very rudimentary duct system and the presence of a small areolar and nipple at birth, the breast is essentially dormant throughout early childhood until puberty (Fig. 62-1). In the female breast development is one of the early signs of maturation. The nipple becomes more prominent and pigmented and is capable of becoming erect as the elastic tissue within it proliferates. The areola increases in circumference and pigmentation. The presence of a significant breast bud at puberty is an important sign of female development. With each menstrual cycle the ductal system responds to the hormone milieu, slowly increasing in size and complexity in the next few years. With each menstrual cycle there is a microscopic increase in the breast ductal system until the age of 28, unless pregnancy ensues. At the onset of pregnancy one of the early signs of conception that a woman perceives is the change in her breasts. The nipple and areola increase in pigmentation and prominence. Montgomery's tubercles become visible and begin to secrete sebaceous material to protect the nipple and areola. The ductal system begins to proliferate and continues to do so for the first 16 weeks of gestation until the areolar system is in place and the lacteal cells are capable of making milk.

The maternal body also builds up nutritional stores in the form of 8 to 10 pounds of tissue intended to provide nutritional support for the production of milk. Milk is not actively produced until the placenta is removed, thus eliminating the source of prolactin-inhibiting hormone.

After birth the normal infant is prepared to nurse at the breast. The infant is born with the correct reflexes: the rooting reflex to "find" the breast and latch on and the coordinated suck and swallow reflex. Breastfeeding for the mother is not a reflex and she needs to be taught how to position the infant on her breast and to trigger the infant's feeding reflexes.

Understanding the let-down reflex is basic to understanding human lactation (Fig. 62-2). When the infant suckles at the breast a signal is sent to the brain via the nervous system and the hypothalamus releases oxytocin and prolactin into the blood stream. The oxytocin stimulates the myoepithelium cells surrounding the ductal system in the breast to contract and that results in the ejection of milk through the nipple. During the first week or two postpartum until the uterus totally involutes the myoepithelial cells in the uterus also respond by contracting and tightening the uterine muscle (it may cause "after pains" for a day or so postpartum). As a result a lactating woman does not need methylergonovine maleate (Methergine) to control uterine bleeding postpartum. The release of oxytocin can also be triggered through other sensory pathways such as hearing the infant cry, see-

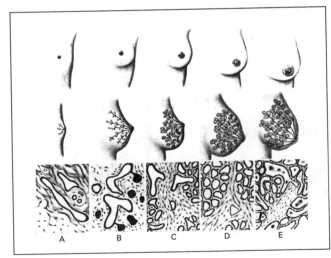

Fig. 62-1 Female breast from infancy to lactation with corresponding cross section and duct structure. **A, B,** and **C,** Gradual development of well-differentiated ductular and peripheral lobular-alveolar system. **D,** Ductular sprouting and intensified peripheral lobular-alveolar development in pregnancy. Glandular luminal cells begin actively synthesizing milk fat and proteins near term: only small amounts are released into lumen. **E,** With postpartum withdrawal of luteal and placental sex steroids and placental lactogen, prolactin is able to induce full secretory activity of alveolar cells and release of milk into alveoli and smaller ducts. (From Lawrence RA: *Breastfeeding: a guide for the medical profession,* ed 4, St Louis, 1994, Mosby-Year Book.)

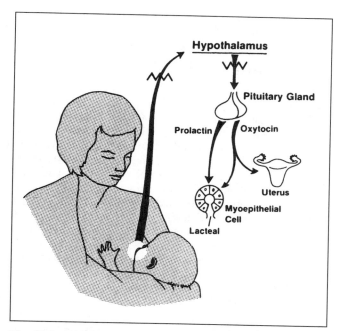

Fig. 62-2 Diagram of ejection reflex are. When the infant suckles the breast, mechanoreceptors in nipple and alveola are stimulated and a stimulus along nerve pathways to the hypothalamus, which stimulates the posterior pituitary to release oxytocin. Oxytocin is carried via the blood stream to breast and uterus. Oxytocin stimulates myoepithelial cells in the breast to contract and eject milk from the alveolus. Prolactin is responsible for milk production in the alveolus. Prolactin is secreted by the anterior pituitary gland in response to suckling. Stresses such as pain and anxiety can inhibit the let-down reflex. The sight or cry of an infant can stimulate the release of oxytocin but not of prolactin. (From Lawrence RA: *Breastfeeding: a guide for the medical profession,* ed 4, St Louis, 1994, Mosby-Year Book.)

ing the infant, or thinking about feeding time. The release of prolactin into the blood stream, on the other hand, stimulates the lacteal cells to make milk. It triggers the Golgi apparatus and reticuloendothelium to move nutrients into the lumen of the alveolus. Prolactin levels are high during pregnancy and lactation. It is the surge of prolactin doubling baseline levels that initiate milk production. Prolactin is released only when the breast is stimulated by suckling or manual or mechanical pumping but not by other sensory stimulus. Pain, stress, and anxiety interfere with let-down.

BENEFITS OF BREASTFEEDING
Nutrition and growth

The human infant, who is born the most immature of all mammals (except the marsupials), has a particularly immature brain and nervous system at birth. Thus in the early days, weeks, and months of life the brain will grow significantly. The brain doubles in size in the first year of life. This is reflected by the fact that the head circumference increases 4 inches in the first year and will only increase another 4 inches in the next 16 years. The constituents of human milk are specifically designed for optimal brain growth, as well as optimal physical growth. The nutritional benefits of human milk include the specific protein profile of ideal amino acids

that are easily digested and completely absorbed. Also easily digested, absorbed, and essential for brain growth are special fat components, including polyunsaturated fats, cholesterol, and docosahexaenoic acid (DHA). Human milk contains cholesterol, whereas infant formula has not contained cholesterol for several decades. Cholesterol is a vital, basic constituent of brain tissue, myelin, and many enzymes in the human body. The microminerals such as copper and zinc are in perfect proportion to infant needs. Human milk contains dozens of enzymes that interact during the digesting of the milk itself, as well as interacting with the mucosal layer of the gut to enhance its development and improve its use and absorption of nutrients.

Immunologic advantages

The infection protection provided by the immunoglobulins and other special constituents of human milk protects the newborn infant from gastrointestinal disease as well as respiratory disease, ear infections, and other general infections. In the third world this can be easily demonstrated by the fact that infants who are not breastfed have a 50% chance of dying from infection in the first year of life. The immunologic advantages of human milk are beginning to be recognized as science explores the intricacies of the immunologic protection provided. Epidemiologic studies have been published that reveal a protective effect of breastfeeding for at least 4 months against the childhood onset of diabetes, childhood cancers, Crohn's disease, and other gastrointestinal illnesses. An associated delayed onset of allergic symptoms, especially eczema and asthma, is also reported in infants who are exclusively breastfed.

ADVANTAGES TO THE MOTHER

The advantages to the mother who breastfeeds are related to the physiologic features of the postpartum period. Immediately breastfeeding decreases the potential for uterine hemorrhage and enhances the involution of the uterus. The uterus of the lactating woman returns to its prepregnant state much more quickly than that of the woman who does not breastfeed. The weight loss in the postpartum period associated with lactation in most cases exceeds the weight loss of women who do not breastfeed. Long-range studies of women who breastfeed suggest that there is a lessened potential for obesity associated with childbirth for those women who breastfeed. Other long-term advantages include a decreased incidence of breast cancer and a decreased incidence of long-term osteoporosis in women who breastfeed when compared to those who bear children and do not breastfeed. In psychologic studies women who breastfeed have higher self-esteem and mother their children differently. By understanding the tremendous benefits of breastfeeding to both the mother and infant, the clinician can better assess the risk/benefit ratio when confronted with a possible contraindication to breastfeeding, as the benefits usually far outweigh any risks.

DISADVANTAGES AND CONTRAINDICATIONS TO BREASTFEEDING

The only disadvantage to breastfeeding that has been documented is that only the mother can feed her infant. From the infant's standpoint, however, this means that the mother always gives the intimate attention the infant needs, and the important one-on-one relationship that was identified by Spitz many years ago in his studies of orphan children is protected by the mother's breastfeeding. A father who wishes to participate in his child's care has the very important task of providing nonnutrient cuddling. Infants may often need to be cuddled when they don't need to be fed. When a breastfeeding mother cuddles her baby the infant may root and nuzzle to be fed when feeding is not necessary. The infant smells the mother's milk. On the other hand when the father cuddles the infant the infant is not fed and settles down quickly.

The most common reason for a woman not to breastfeed is a lack of desire to do so. From a medical standpoint there are few clinical situations in which breastfeeding is not recommended. In industrialized countries today when there is an acceptable alternative, babies born to mothers who are human immunodeficiency virus (HIV)-positive should *not* be breastfed, according to the present understanding of the spread of the disease. Any infant born to a mother who is hepatitis B–positive should receive hepatitis immune globulin as well as the first of the series of three hepatitis vaccine immunizations. The infant can be breastfed after these two injections. When the mother has a medical disease that requires medications that might pass into the breast milk it is important to know whether the drug might be contraindicated for the infant (see box, below). When a physician is concerned about a medication in a lactating woman, specific information should be obtained from resources competent to provide information about lactation. Many resources that provide general information about medication do not give accurate information about the appearance of the compound in breast milk nor its risk to the infant.

The infant who has severe galactosemia at birth and is identified to have a deficiency of galactose-1-phosphate uridyl transferase does not tolerate lactose and thus cannot be breastfed. This infant must receive lactose-free formula.

MANAGEMENT IN THE IMMEDIATE POSTPARTUM PERIOD

Assuring good milk supply

The initiation of a good milk supply begins immediately after birth with the first feeding, which ideally takes place in the birthing area while the infant is alert and ready to suck-

le. After an hour or so of active, alert behavior the infant will drift off to sleep and be difficult to arouse to feed for 4 to 6 hours. Infants best latch on to the breast when they are alert and hungry, not when they are sleeping or exhausted from crying hard.

The postpartum hospital staff is responsible for assisting the nursing dyad, but the physician may be called upon to respond to maternal illness or concerns or to problems with the infant such as jaundice, excessive weight loss, or illness. An understanding of normal lactation is necessary to manage the problems without interfering with successful lactation. In general, the major cause of sore nipples and milk production problems can be solved by proper positioning at the breast and attention to suckling long enough to get the fat-laten hind milk. Introducing a bottle to the schedule in the first few weeks does not improve the milk production but diminishes it as the breast makes more milk in response to milk removal. The breast adapts to the infant's needs. As milk is made, more is produced.

Illness and breastfeeding

Minor illnesses in the mother such as bladder infection, endometritis, or mild toxemia are *not* a contraindication to breastfeeding. The milk in fact will provide the infant with mother's antibodies and protect against infection. Hypothyroidism and its treatment with thyroid hormone are *not* contraindications. Hyperthyroidism treated with propylthiouracil is *not* a contraindication, but the use of thiouracil and iodine should be avoided. Asthma that is controlled with inhalants or with low-dose corticosteroid is not a contraindication. When a mother has persistent toxemia, hypertension, or cardiovascular disease, diuretics, antihypertensives, and sedatives should be prescribed that have the least tendency to get into the milk (nadolol rather than captopril, furosemide rather than chlorothiazide, magnesium sulfate or phenobarbital rather than morphine).

Poor milk supply

The most common causes of poor milk supply are inadequate information on breastfeeding and the lack of support in the early initiation of lactation. Proper positioning at the breast with the infant facing the mother looking at the breast is fundamental to success: presenting the breast, supported by mother's hand, well back of the nipple so that the infant upon stimulus of the lower lip with the nipple opens wide and draws the breast into the mouth, elongating the areola into a teat that is compressed against the hard palate. The natural, undulating, or peristaltic motion of the tongue moves the milk from the ampulla of the duct to be ejected through the nipple. Initially it takes 2 to 3 minutes for the reflex to start the flow of milk. After the first week it occurs more quickly. It also takes a few minutes for the fat to get into the milk as the fat globules have to come together in the lacteal cells and pass into the lumen of the alveolus. The fat globule is enveloped by a membrane and suspended in the solution. The early milk at each feeding is low in fat, but the later or hind milk is rich in fat and thus in calories and fat-soluble vitamins. Infants who do not nurse long enough on one breast may not get this valuable nutrition and thus receive insufficient calories to gain weight. The physician's role is to rule out any true abnormality but also to instill con-

---

DRUGS THAT ARE CONTRAINDICATED DURING BREASTFEEDING	
Cyclophosphamide	Drugs of Abuse:
Cyclosporine	Amphetamine
Doxorubicin	Cocaine
Ergotamine	Heroin
Lithium	Marijuana
Methotrexate	Phencyclidine
Phencyclidine (PCP)	
Phenindione	

fidence in the mother and see that the mother is provided with the necessary support and encouragement through the trained office staff or nurse practitioner, who will attend to details and assure that the mother is psychologically supported. Fatigue is a common cause of a failing milk supply. Assessing the mother's opportunities for adequate rest is an initial step. Mothers may need to be taught how to nap when the infant naps and how to set priorities for other activities in the early postpartum period. The infant's needs come first until the milk supply is well established.

When poor milk supply, resulting in failure to thrive in the infant, is not solved by minor adjustments in positioning and timing, it requires a diagnostic evaluation to identify possible infant causes (see Fig. 62-3) and possible maternal causes. A complete history of the pregnancy, delivery, diet, and habits may identify a cause. The breasts should increase in size during pregnancy and the nipples and areolae become more pigmented. Lack of breast changes suggests a fundamental organ failure. If the breasts do not become mildly to moderately engorged postpartum and especially if there is excessive vaginal bleeding there may be retained placenta. A small amount of placental tissue may produce enough prolactin-inhibiting hormone to suppress full lactation. If the mother had a severe hemorrhage or crisis during delivery, the pituitary could have been shocked, producing transient or permanent hypopituitarism known as **Sheehan's syndrome.** The classic diagnostic finding in Sheehan's syndrome is failure of breasts to become engorged. Transient hypopituitarism may respond to the use of nasal spray oxytocin (Syntocin) to initiate lactation. A few drops are instilled onto the mother's nasal mucous membranes just before she puts the infant to the breast for a feeding. This will stimulate let-down and, when done with each feeding for 2 to 3 weeks, may lead to an increasing milk supply. Oxytocin (Syntocin) is available by prescription in 15-ml nasal spray containers or nasal drops.

Analysis of the blood levels of prolactin is available through most hospital laboratories by radioimmunoassay. The baseline level of prolactin gradually decreases over time postpartum from levels well above 100 ng/ml to just under 100 ng/ml; the normal range for nonpregnant nonlactators is usually 10 to 25 ng/ml. It is not the baseline that is diagnostic but the surge of prolactin produced by stimulus of the breast through infant suckling or mechanical breast pumping. The standard procedure is to insert an intravenous line with a heparin lock. Allow the mother to recover from the needle stick, which can elevate the prolactin level slightly; draw a baseline level; and then draw a second level after 10 minutes of full breast stimulus. The surge should double the baseline level. A failure to develop an adequate response to suckling suggests that prolactin insufficiency is responsible for the inadequate milk production.

Medical stimulus of prolactin has been demonstrated by maternal use of **meclopromide** (Reglan) 10 mg, three times a day. Published studies report use in women pumping to provide milk for their premature or ill infants who cannot nurse at the breast. It is also reported to be successful in women with faltering milk supply. Some medications, including bromocriptine and L-dopamine, suppress prolactin production, and their use could be the cause of the low prolactin levels. A complete history of all medications and ingestants may lead to the identification of a prolactin suppressant. This includes a review of natural foods, herbs, and teas, some of which may have potent pharmacologic action.

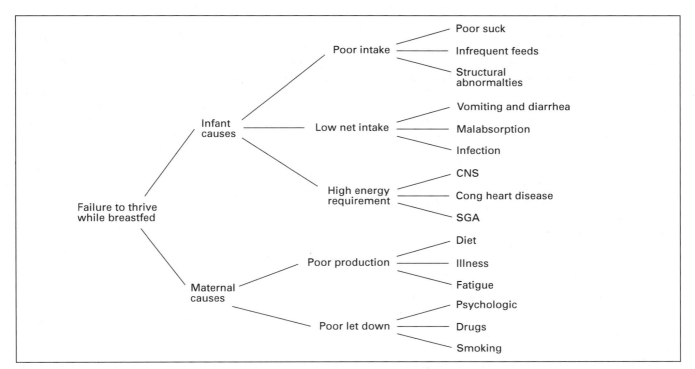

Fig. 62-3 Diagnostic flowchart for failure to thrive. (From Lawrence RA: *Breastfeeding: a guide for the medical profession*, ed 4, St Louis, 1994, Mosby-Year Book.)

Other diagnostic procedures to evaluate the mother's ability to produce milk include thyroid function studies, as hypothyroidism may be associated with inability to lactate. Conversely abnormal galactorrhea may also be associated with either hypothyroidism or hyperthyroidism.

Heavy smoking may interfere with let-down reflex. Excessive exercise may also result in diminished milk supply. Reports of increased lactic acid level in the milk after exercise have been associated with infant refusal of the breast. It has been noted, however, that if the first few milliliters of milk are expressed and discarded and the breast washed to remove any sweat there is no milk refusal.

MATERNAL DISEASE AND BREASTFEEDING
Diabetes mellitus

Diabetes mellitus is not a contraindication to breastfeeding. In fact a woman may experience some lowering of her insulin requirements during lactation. The diabetic makes good milk. Lactose production, which drives milk production, appears normal in the diabetic. The key to successful lactation in the diabetic is intake of adequate kilocalories. When insufficient calories are consumed (less than 2000 kcal for average weight women), milk production falters. Careful dietary guidance is essential to the diabetic, associated adjustment (usually lowering) of insulin level usually provides a feeling of well-being. Breastfeeding is an opportunity for the diabetic to do something special for her infant when she has been led to believe that her disease is a liability to the fetus in utero.

Seizure disorders

Women with seizure disorders may breastfeed their infants if their maintenance medications are those compatible with lactation. At birth the infant has some medication in the system, especially if a bolus was given during labor, and it may be necessary to supplement breastfeeding for a few days. Levels of phenytoin (Dilantin), phenobarbital, and valproic acid can be easily measured in the neonate. If not fully feeding the infant, the mother should pump and discard her milk to continue to develop her milk supply. The infant will require some substitute feeding of formula, preferably given by small medicine cup or dropper to prevent confusing the infant, because use of an artificial nipple may make it difficult for the infant to adjust to normal physiologic suckling at the breast. Usually after 2 to 3 days the infant can be fully breastfed. The small amount of medication that appears in the milk does not affect the infant. Valproic acid has milk/plasma ratios of 0.01 to 0.07 and is considered compatible with breastfeeding. If the infant is depressed and significant levels of phenobarbital or phenytoin are measurable

in the infant, breast and formula feedings can be alternated. This will allow the mother to provide some of the great benefits of her milk while maintaining her own self-esteem. The important goal of maternal medication is to keep her seizure-free.

Thromboembolic disease

A common postpartum complication is thromboembolic disease, which is discussed elsewhere in this text. When it occurs in the lactating women there are some important considerations. Heparin, because of its large molecular size, does not pass into the milk. Because it must be given parenterally it is impractical in most cases for home use. Coumarin or warfarin does not usually pass into milk and can be used. A monthly check of the infant's prothrombin time can confirm this. A dose of vitamin K will improve any lowered levels. Studies following infants whose mothers received coumarin and showing no anticoagulant effect in the infant are reported in the literature. On the other hand other anticoagulants, especially the synthetics, have been associated with problems in infants and are not recommended for the lactating woman.

POSTPARTUM MASTITIS
Acute mastitis

The acute onset of mastitis can occur anytime postpartum but is more common after 10 days and peaks in incidence at about 28 days. Rarely it occurs before delivery in association with nipple exercises and manipulations that some recommend to prepare the nipple for lactation. Table 62-1 illustrates the important features of mastitis compared to those of engorgement and plugged ducts.

Engorgement. Engorgement occurs early, is bilateral, and is not associated with systemic disease. Temperature is 101° or less. It can be treated with hot and cold compresses, warm showers that allow milk to drip freely, and, when all else fails, use of cabbage leaves. This historic remedy is carried out by placing cool fresh cabbage leaves on the breast until they fully wilt, replacing with fresh ones if necessary. The effect has no scientific explanation. Engorgement is a self-limited discomfort that peaks on the fifth to the seventh day postpartum and then resolves. It is worse in primiparas and in hospitalized or immobilized patients. It is important for the breasts to be gently massaged before a feeding to express a little milk to soften the areola. If this is not done, the infant cannot get a proper grasp and may clamp down on the nipple, causing considerable pain.

Plugged ducts. A plugged duct is a unilateral lump in the breast that is not hot, red, or very painful. It is usually treated with warm compresses and massage sufficient to remove the

Table 62-1 Comparison of findings of engorgement, plugged duct, and mastitis

Characteristics	Engorgement	Plugged duct	Mastitis
Onset	Gradual, immediately	Gradual, after feedings	Sudden, after 10 days postpartum
Site	Bilateral	Unilateral	Usually unilateral
Swelling and heat	Generalized	May shift/little or no heat	Localized, red, hot, and swollen
Pain	Generalized	Mild but localized	Intense but localized
Body temperature	<38.4° C	<38.4° C	>38.4° C
Systemic symptoms	Feels well	Feels well	Flulike symptoms

From Lawrence RA: *Breastfeeding: a guide for the medical profession,* ed 4, St Louis, 1994, Mosby-Year Book.

plug and allow the drainage of lobule involved. A patient with recurrent plugs should be evaluated for underlying disease.

Clinical presentation of acute mastitis

History and physical examination. Acute mastitis is usually unilateral, but if it is bilateral streptococcal infection should be considered and aggressive treatment for mother and infant undertaken. A wedge-shaped area of the breast is reddened, hot, swollen, and painful. The mother usually has a temperature $>101°$ F ($>38°$ C) and feels ill. The common causes are Staphylococcus and Escherichia coli organisms.

Management

CHOICE OF THERAPY. The treatment is first to continue breastfeeding on both breasts, taking care to "empty" the involved breast. Antibiotics such as dicloxacillin 500 mg q6 hr should be given for a minimum of 10 days, preferably 14 days. Strict instructions to continue the medication even though the patient feels better are important. A small amount of most antibiotics gets into the milk so a medication that can also be given directly to the infant is appropriate (avoid choloramphenicol and tetracycline).

Exhaustion is often the trigger point for mastitis so that complete care for mastitis is bed rest for the mother with feeding the infant her only responsibility until there is improvement. Local treatment includes hot or cold compresses, whichever gives the more relief of pain. Acetaminophen or ibuprofen safely provide relief of the local pain and generalized myalgia.

Recurrent and chronic mastitis

Inadequately treated mastitis can result in recurrent mastitis, which will continue to flare up every time antibiotics are discontinued. Early aggressive treatment of the initial bout of mastitis is the only way to prevent this. Recurrent mastitis quickly becomes chronic mastitis, which usually does not clear until the infant is weaned. In most cases, however, it is preferable to maintain the mother on low-dose antibiotics for the remainder of the lactation period. Erythromycin 250 mg twice daily is one treatment option.

Abscess

Abscess formation occurs when the initial mastitis is untreated or in some cases is inadequately treated. An abscess can be incised and drained without interfering with lactation. Milk may drain from the incision if a duct is cut in the procedure. It will heal while the infant continues to feed from the involved breast. The mother should press firmly over the incision with a sterile gauze square to minimize the flow of milk during a feeding.

Development of candidal vaginitis

Women who frequently harbor *Candida albicans* organisms vaginally are often subject to flare-ups of vaginal infection when taking antibiotics. Inflammation of the breast with *Candida albicans* organisms can occur, usually after a treated breast infection. The common description is burning pain when the infant suckles likened to being stabbed in the chest wall with a hot poker. A course of antifungal cream combined with cortisone rubbed into the nipples and areola after each feeding will usually clear the symptoms. Since the source may well have been the baby, the infant should also be treated with nystatin orally, whether or not the child has oral evidence of the disease or monilial diaper rash. This may require a call to the pediatrician.

LACTATION AFTER BREAST SURGERY

Augmentation mammoplasty as a surgical procedure is not a contraindication to breastfeeding. The procedure does not interrupt vital nerves or ducts. The presence of silicone implants has become a point of concern. The U.S. Food and Drug Administration (FDA) has not recommended removal of an implant unless it has ruptured or there are serious symptoms (pain or tissue contractions). The fact that silicone is in many other products besides implants has led to further investigations. The present position of the FDA does not limit breastfeeding. The underlying reason augmentation was necessary for a given woman may be inadequate glandular tissue; however, that can only be identified by initiating breastfeeding and measuring the ability to produce milk.

Reduction mammoplasty can be performed so that lactation can proceed without difficulty if the ducts are not cut and the nipple not removed and reimplanted. That information should be given to the woman before surgery while explaining the impact of the surgery, but if not then, at any time upon request of the patient. Women should be encouraged to ask questions before the procedure.

The removal of solitary lumps or cysts does not preclude breastfeeding. Fibrocystic disease is not a contraindication to breastfeeding. Breastfeeding after breast cancer is an individual matter that needs to be discussed with the woman's oncologist. The answer depends on the diagnosis and the pathologic characteristics of the tumor as well as of the lymph nodes and the need for additional treatment with irradiation or chemotherapy and length of time since surgery. Usually, pregnancy is not recommended for at least 5 years posttreatment. Breastfeeding on the remaining breast has been successful. It is possible to nourish an infant fully with one breast, as has been done for many other reasons including the preference of the infant. Whether lactation changes the probability of recurrence of the disease is not known, although 5-year survival rates in disease that was controlled before lactation are not reported to be different from those of women without pregnancy and lactation. As noted earlier breastfeeding appears to have a protective affect against cancer of the breast in large series.

BIBLIOGRAPHY

Brommage R, DeLuca HF: Regulation of bone mineral loss during lactation, *Am J Physiol* 248:E182, 1985.

Bryant CA: The impact of kin, friend and neighbor network on infant feeding practices, *Soc Sci Med* 16:1757, 1982.

Cumming RG, Klineberg RJ: Breastfeeding and other reproductive factors and the risk of hip fractures in elderly women, *Int J Epidemiol* 22:684, 1993.

Ferris AM et al: Lactation outcome in insulin-dependent diabetic women, *J Am Diet Assoc* 88:317, 1988.

Klaus M, Kennell J: Parent to infant bonding: setting the record straight, *J Pediatr* 102:575, 1983.

Lawrence RA: The pediatrician's role in infant feeding decision-making *Pediatr Rev* 14:265, 1993.

Lawrence RA: *Breastfeeding: a guide for the medical profession,* ed 4, St Louis, 1994, Mosby-Year Book.

Newton N: Psychologic differences between breast and bottle feeding, *Am J Clin Nutr* 24:993, 1971.

Report of the Surgeon General's workshop on breastfeeding and human lactation, Pub No HRS-D-MC 84-2, Washington, D.C., 1984, Department of Health and Human Services.

Ryan AS et al: Recent declines in breastfeeding in the United States, 1984 through 1989, *Pediatrics* 88:719, 1991.

Subcommittee on nutrition during lactation: *Nutrition during lactation* Washington, D.C., 1991, Institute of Medicine, National Academy of Sciences.

Wallace JP, Inbar G, Ernsthausen K: Infant acceptance of postexercise milk, *Pediatrics* 89:1245, 1992.

WHO/UNICEF: Protecting, promoting and supporting breastfeeding: the special role of maternity services: a joint WHO/UNICEF statement, Geneva, 1989, World Health Organization.

Woodward A, Hand K: Smoking and reduced duration of breastfeeding, *Med J Aust* 148:477, 1988.

Woodward A et al: Acute respiratory illness in Adelaide children: breastfeeding modifies the effect of passive smoking, *J Epidemiol Community Health* 44:224, 1990.

World Health Organization: *Contemporary patterns of breastfeeding, Report on the WHO Collaborative Study on Breastfeeding*, Geneva, 1981, World Health Organization.

Yoo K-Y et al: Independent protective effect of lactation against breast cancer: a case-control study in Japan, *Am J Epidemiol* 135:726, 1992.

63 Postpartum Psychiatric Disorders

Deborah A. Sichel

 EPIDEMIOLOGY

Postpartum psychiatric disorders comprise a number of different syndromes that involve the onset of either a mood or an anxiety disorder in the weeks or months after delivery. Each disorder is associated with a specific symptom constellation that suggests the clinical diagnosis. (For easy reference, see the tables within the text for each disorder.)

Although most studies have included disorders occurring up until 6 months postpartum, only the early onset disorders (i.e., onset within first 2 to 6 weeks postpartum) may actually reflect a neurochemical cause specific to the changing hormonal milieu of the postpartum period.

Kendall demonstrated the dramatic increase in hospital admissions for psychiatric disorders in the first 3 months after delivery, after which rates decline to those normally expected. This finding, together with the high recurrence rates for postpartum mood disorders, suggests a subgroup of women who may carry a genetic vulnerability to the rapidly changing hormonal milieu of the early puerpal period. Vulnerability to this particular hormonal state may be an important factor in distinguishing postpartum mood disorders from depressions that occur nonpuerperally or in men. In contrast, the later onset disorders (those occurring at 9 weeks postpartum or later) appear to be closely associated with psychosocial variables and may be less distinguishable from mood disorder occurring at other times. Increasing knowledge about neurohormonal kindling mechanisms may allow us to identify subgroups of women who may be especially vulnerable to the onset of disorders in the postpartum period. Prospective work is needed to clarify risk groups, possible neurohormonal causes, and other risk factors.

Early diagnosis and treatment may have significance for the well-being and development of the infant and other children dependent on the mother. Amply demonstrated are the emotional and cognitive disturbances in children of depressed mothers with potential for impaired family development.

Psychiatric mood disorders complicate 8% to 10% of all deliveries. More recent work has described the onset of anxiety disorder after delivery. Despite the large numbers of women affected, clinical recognition and diagnosis have been poor, partly because of misunderstanding of these disorders among psychiatric clinicians and further because pregnancy has been traditionally viewed as a period of well-being. Growing awareness among obstetricians and psychiatrists has sparked increasing interest in research, treatment, and prophylaxis of these disorders during pregnancy and the postpartum period. Psychiatric, obstetric, and pediatric training programs need to incorporate specific training for their staffs regarding the spectrum of psychiatric disorders linked to female reproductive function.

This chapter reviews the mood and anxiety disorders associated with childbirth.

PATHOPHYSIOLOGY

In women depression and anxiety disorders tend to appear and cluster predominantly in the childbearing years. There is a temporal relationship between psychiatric symptom emergence and periods of reproductive hormonal change including late luteal disorder and perimenopausal mood lability. Although newer hypotheses focus on the capacity of changing hormonal environments to impact at the neuroreceptor and neurotransmitter levels, producing symptoms characteristic of depression or anxiety disorder, no one comprehensive model has emerged to explain events fully.

Pregnancy is not always a period of emotional well-being. For some women with pregravid histories of affective or anxiety disorder, careful treatment planning is important before conception. For this population the postpartum period may in fact be one of substantial risk for worsening of symptoms. This finding is in contrast to epidemiologically derived studies that indicated that there was no difference in rates of depression in postpartum women and nonpregnant control subjects.

Biologic studies

Although numerous investigators have attempted to implicate estrogen, progesterone, cortisol, thyroid hormones, endorphins, neurotransmitters, neuroreceptors, enzymes, and vitamins as causes of these disorders, very few conclusive data have emerged. One of the problems of this research has been the "snapshot" approach, which merely takes a one-time picture of a rapidly changing physiologic milieu. Further, serum levels do not reflect neurochemical changes within the central nervous system. Studies have also been limited to the first 2 weeks postpartum and correlated with the "blues" phenomenon, so there is little information about women diagnosed with major depression or other disorders. One recent study in women with puerperal psychosis suggests evidence of altered dopaminergic activity, compared to that of normal women. More knowledge is needed about the multiple components of hormonal rates of change in the early postpartum period and impact on neuroreceptors.

Recent research indicates that changing estrogen and progesterone levels can impact negatively on monoaminergic pathways implicated in affective and anxiety disorders. It is very possible that the cause of some of these disorders lies in the *rates of change of hormones,* with little correlation with one specific serum level. Future investigation regarding neuroexcitatory or inhibitory effects may yield more significant evidence of causes.

RISK FACTORS FOR POSTPARTUM DEPRESSION

From a clinical standpoint evaluation of risk factors for emergence of anxiety and depression needs to begin with the first prenatal visit.

A brief set of questions at the first prenatal visit will detect genetic and personal clinical risk. The box below summarizes such questions.

An affirmative answer to any of these questions places a woman in a higher-risk group for a postpartum illness. Referral to psychiatry may be helpful to plan effective treatment interventions.

As the pregnancy progresses the obstetrician or nurse midwife should inquire about the onset of any mood changes or swings, anxiety, irritability, tearfulness, and the onset of sleep difficulties, such as inability to fall asleep, early waking, and inability to go back to sleep, that occur independently of physical discomfort or nocturia (see box, above right). Onset of these symptoms may indicate signs of early depression.

QUESTIONS TO DETECT WOMEN AT RISK FOR POSTPARTUM DEPRESSION

Is there a family history of depression, anxiety disorder, or alcohol abuse?

Is there a personal history of depression or anxiety disorder—even if this has been mild and has not come to the attention of a professional?*

Is there a past history of postpartum depression?

Has there been use of antianxiety or antidepressant medication in the past or present?

Is there a history of moderate to severe premenstrual mood changes?

---

*Many women may not know what depression is. Ask, "Have you ever noted a period of at least 2 weeks in your life when your mood was very sad and low and you lost interest in most of your usual activities? At that time did you note a change in your sleep pattern or appetite and concentration?

SIGNS OF EARLY DEPRESSION

Mood changes or swings
Anxiety
Irritability
Tearfulness
Onset of sleep difficulties
  Inability to fall asleep
  Early waking
  Inability to go back to sleep
Persistent sadness
Feelings of inflicting bodily harm
Suicidal thoughts

Irritability with mood lability frequently predominates over sadness in normal pregnancy. However, onset of these symptoms during the pregnancy correlates significantly with risk of postpartum depression.

Marital conflict, lack of an adequate social support network, work or other stressors, and obstetric complications are significant cofactors for some women, so that the cumulative effect of numerous stressors and a vulnerable biologic predisposition interact to produce disorder (see box, below). Loss of the woman's former life, roles, identity, and specific relationship with the husband may also constitute a particular stressor for a new mother.

The obstetrician or midwife can develop a profile of a woman "at risk" using these questions and noting these developing stressors that may contribute to the evolution of a postpartum illness. The following discussion will focus on the various syndromes, clinical symptoms, diagnosis, and preliminary treatments.

POSTPARTUM PSYCHIATRIC MOOD DISORDERS

The obstetric postpartum period is distinct from the psychiatric postpartum period. The obstetric period ends at 6 weeks with uterine involution. Emotional and maternal role development, however, continue for many months and may in fact take up to a year in a normal adjustment process. Superimposition of a major psychiatric illness on the family system may lead to significant family dysfunction that may be undiagnosed for years. Women at risk should be

---

COMMON STRESSORS FOR THE PREGNANT WOMAN

Issues with relationships
  Marital conflict
  Specific relationship with husband
  Conflicts at work
  Lack of adequate social support network

Issues with self-image
  Change of body habitus
  Loss of woman's former life and roles

Issues with pregnancy
  Obstetric complications
  Problems with fetal development

evaluated at 2 weeks postpartum and again at 6 weeks. All women should be given an opportunity to talk about how they are coping at their 6-week visit.

Maternity blues

Maternity blues is a self-limiting syndrome that affects 50% to 80% of women after delivery. Symptoms usually start on the second or third day after delivery, peak on the fifth to seventh day, and should start to remit by the second week. Symptoms include predominantly dysphoric mood with mood lability, crying, sleeping difficulty, anxiety, loss of appetite, and irritability. Treatment includes reassurance, support, and enlistment of the family in ensuring some periods of sleep for the new mother, even if she is breastfeeding. It is not detrimental to the breastfeeding relationship to introduce an occasional bottle of formula to allow the mother some badly needed sleep.

This syndrome differs from depression in that symptoms are mild, and it should remit by the third week postpartum. Suicidality is not a symptom of blues.

Complicated blues

Occasionally an extended period of the symptoms described continues into the fourth and fifth weeks postpartum. Strictly speaking this is no longer the "blues" and may fulfill criteria for major depression. However, for many women it resolves spontaneously at 4 to 8 weeks. Some clinicians have termed this particular phenomenon "complicated blues." Its clinical significance is that it may indicate a particularly vulnerable biologic diathesis to the hormonal changes that occur in the immediate puerperal period. After a subsequent pregnancy this may recur and not resolve spontaneously, thus constituting a major depression requiring active pharmacologic intervention.

Major nonpsychotic postpartum depression

Epidemiology. Major nonpsychotic depression denotes a nonpsychotic illness, meeting criteria for major depression, as delineated in the *Diagnostic and Statistical Manual of Mental Disorders (DSM-IV)*. Studies in North America and the United Kingdom indicate prevalence rates of between 6% and 16% at the 9-week postpartum point. In O'Hara's study this incidence was no different from that of the nonpregnant control group. Although these data challenged the belief that the postpartum period was a time of greater risk for depression than that of nonpregnant control subjects these figures were obtained from epidemiologically derived populations. The prediction and prevalence of disorder in clinically derived populations may, however, be considerably higher, suggesting that the postpartum period is one of increased risk for women with a previous history of anxiety or affective disorder or with a family history of affective or anxiety disorder. Prospective studies of pregnant women with pregravid histories of affective and anxiety disorders are under way to clarify prevalence, risk factors, and optimal treatment modalities for these groups of women.

History and symptom presentation. Though nonpsychotic postpartum depression was originally characterized as atypical depression, because of the predominant symptoms of agitation, anxiety, mood irritability, anger, and hostility, as opposed to a sad, slowed, and withdrawn presentation, current mood disorder criteria adequately cover this symptom constellation. The box below lists the characteristic symptoms of major nonpsychotic depression.

The onset of this depression may be in the acute puerperium (i.e., the first 1-2 weeks) or may follow a period of relative well-being and appear later, at 6 weeks, 8 weeks, or even later in the puerperium. Occasionally, even though the patient first appears at 6 to 8 weeks postpartum, an early onset can be found by history, documenting onset of symptoms from the first week postpartum. Timing of onset carries implications for pharmacologic prophylaxis in future pregnancies.

Diagnostic testing. Thyroid function levels should always be measured. Some prospective studies have revealed a 2% to 4% incidence of hypothyroidism in postpartum women.

Management

Goals of management. Treatment of the depression begins with an evaluation of severity of symptoms and suicide risk. It is a mistake to believe that the mother will not attempt to harm herself because of the presence of the baby. New mothers feel extremely fragile, and they frequently have the feeling that they have failed in this most fundamental of tasks, "the maternal role." Many women have fantasies of what a "good" mother they will be. Women from backgrounds of dysfunctional families are especially vulnerable. They desperately want to "redo" their difficult childhood and painfully feel the lack of a good parental role model. The interruption of the ongoing process of maternal role attainment by a depressive disorder fuels their sense of failure. If the mother is not safe at home or if a family member or friend is not available to provide supportive care through the fragile early pharmacologic stabilization period, then it may be better to hospitalize the mother. In England mother-baby units have been an important part of the treatment of the mother-baby dyad. Separation of mother and baby at these vital times may increase guilt and hinder recovery. The mother-baby unit treatment modality may soon become a reality in the United States with the development of a few pilot units at this time.

CHARACTERISTIC SYMPTOMS OF MAJOR POSTPARTUM NONPSYCHOTIC DEPRESSION

Mood lability
Tearfulness
Irritability, hostility, most often directed at spouse or partner
Poor concentration
Panic attacks
Agitation, fidgetiness, inability to sit still
Feelings of helplessness, hopelessness
Recurrent thoughts of guilt related to self-blame for the situation
No desire to hold or care for the baby
No desire to be left alone with the baby, fears about the baby's safety, frequent calls to the pediatrician, and inability to be reassured
Inability to fall asleep
Inability to stay asleep, waking even though baby may be asleep, and inability to fall asleep again
Poor appetite or excessive eating
Suicidal feelings or suicide plan

First steps in treatment depend on accurate diagnosis, pharmacologic stabilization, and safety considerations. Unipolar depression should be carefully distinguished from the depressive phase of a bipolar disorder since institution of an antidepressant in these situations often produces rapid cycling.

Choices of therapy

ANTIANXIETY MEDICATION. It is important to use antianxiety medication to settle the extreme agitation in the mother, such as **clonazepam** (Klonopin) in high doses: 1 mg three or four times a day. Clonazepam is preferable to the shorter-acting benzodiazepines (alprazolam, lorazepam, oxazepam) because of its greater potency and longer half-life. This dosage may cause some sedation and should be titrated to the woman's response.

ANTIDEPRESSANTS. Antidepressant medications should be started immediately. Tricyclics continue to be useful in the early phase. Frequently **nortryptiline** (Pamelor, Aventy) is used as a first line antidepressant since it will aid sleep in an agitated state, and blood levels within a specific therapeutic range may be measured. Newer antidepressants, such as **sertraline, fluoxetine, and paroxetine** (Zoloft, Prozac, Paxil) should be used with caution initially since they can occasionally produce added agitation.

Once some response to the tricyclic is seen, augmentation with the newer agents may be used. Frequently these disorders require use of two or more antidepressant agents concurrently. Occasionally electroconvulsive therapy may be needed for a treatment-resistant depression, followed by antidepressant therapy. Medication should be maintained for a least a year after remission of symptoms before a trial of taper is attempted to prevent relapse of illness.

Individual psychotherapy for the woman and her husband is highly recommended since the course through these times can be tumultuous and support is needed. Women frequently report that couple therapy becomes a necessity to facilitate communication after such an illness and to provide support and education for the husband.

Information about the potential for recurrence of this disorder through future pregnancies and in the postpartum period should be provided by psychiatrists knowledgeable in this area.

BREASTFEEDING AND TREATMENT FOR POSTPARTUM DEPRESSION. Breastfeeding can be continued if nortryptiline is used; new data suggest that it does not accumulate in the infant's serum. Breastfeeding is not advised with continued use of the benzodiazepines or lithium because of accumulation in the infant's serum. No breastfeeding data about the newer antidepressants and anxiolytics (bupropion, sertraline, fluoxetine, paroxetine) are available at this time so breastfeeding may have to be discontinued if these agents are used, until more data about safety are available.

Women should be more informed and prepared for premenstrual exacerbation of depression, which can sometimes be as severely symptomatic as the initial presenting symptoms. This usually diminishes in severity as the months progress.

Other treatment issues

CONTRACEPTION AND PROGESTERONE. Oral contraceptive agents may have to be avoided for the duration the woman uses antidepressant medication since they may exacerbate mood disorder. In bipolar depression patients, oral contraception may induce rapid cycling. Discussion of barrier methods and use of the intrauterine device for contraception while the woman is on antidepressant medication may be necessary. The use of progesterone in suppository form as a treatment for depression and premenstrual syndrome has gained popularity among women, gynecologists, and some psychiatrists. Unfortunately the data collection on progesterone use has been poor, and double-blind studies reveal no evidence of its efficacy. Other work suggests worsening of mood with progesterone. At this time progesterone use appears to be at best equal to use of placebo, and its use in the treatment of depression or premenstrual syndrome cannot be recommended.

Postpartum psychosis

Epidemiology. Postpartum psychosis is the most severe postpartum psychiatric disorder and generally occurs at a rate of 1 to 2/1000 births. Its onset is usually in the first 1 to 2 weeks after delivery.

History and symptom presentation. A careful history can often reveal onset within the first 48 hours. The most prominent symptoms at that time are restlessness and inability to sleep (see box, below). Postpartum staff often miss this early onset, believing that it is the excitement of the birth that has stimulated the restless behavior. The full-blown illness usually appears within the next 2 weeks.

Diagnostically this disorder shares features consistent with the acute onset of a manic phase of a bipolar illness. Many researchers believe that it a subtype of bipolar illness characteristically manifested with more puerperal episodes than nonpuerperal. Some investigators have described a waxing and waning course with some lucid periods, which probably represents a rapidly cycling diathesis, through a normal mood period.

Management. **Postpartum psychosis is a dangerous illness that carries a risk of infanticide and suicide and must be aggressively treated within a hospital setting.** Immediate institution of mood stabilizing agents (lithium, valproic acid, or carbamazepine) must be done in combination with use of antipsychotic drugs. Use of the more potent, less sedating agents (haloperidol, trifluperazine, fluphenazine, perphenazine) is preferable since the mother needs to be alert to the needs of the infant. Lorazepam or clonazepam is useful in the early phase to contain agitation.

Once a treatment response with these agents has been achieved, the emergence of a depressive phase may occur. Addition of antidepressants in low doses may be required for further stabilization. The same cautions about oral contraception apply in management of this disorder as in major depression.

Postpartum psychosis carries the highest risk of recurrence after future pregnancies, in some cases over 90%. Because of

---

CHARACTERISTIC SYMPTOMS OF POSTPARTUM PSYCHOSIS

Agitation	Delusions
Confusion	Paranoia
Hallucinations: auditory,	Inability to sleep
visual, tactile, olfactory	Poor appetite

the predictability of illness some researchers have advocated the prophylactic use of mood stabilizers instituted immediately after future deliveries, with encouraging results. The use of estrogen as a prophylactic agent is also being explored for this high-risk population, but remains experimental at this time.

Women who have a pregravid diagnosis of bipolar disorder are at high risk for an episode of decompensation postpartum but are also at more risk for psychotic episodes and worsening during pregnancy. A discussion of the management and treatment of this population is beyond the scope of this chapter, but comprehensive guidelines for pregnancy management have been recently reviewed (Cohen, 1992).

POSTPARTUM ANXIETY DISORDERS
Panic disorder

The course, impact, and prevalence of anxiety disorders related to pregnancy and the postpartum period have received little attention in the literature until now. Although some authors have noted improvement in panic symptoms during pregnancy, others have described severe worsening in the early postpartum period. A recent retrospective study of 49 women with histories of pregravid panic disorder revealed that although some women remained well during pregnancy, they did so while using antipanic pharmacotherapy (Cohen, 1992). Women with mild disorder demonstrated severe worsening in the early postpartum period, suggesting that it may represent a period of risk for women with pregravid disorder. Many of these women in fact demonstrated mild symptoms during their pregnancy but had not been undiagnosed.

History and symptom presentation. Worsening of panic characteristically occurred within the first 2 to 3 weeks after delivery, often escalating to several panic attacks a day, with significant intercurrent anxiety and functional impairment. Some women experienced a secondary depressive disorder. The classic symptoms of panic disorder are listed in the box below.

Management. The treatment of panic most commonly includes benzodiazepines. Clonazepam is the longest-acting and is preferred to the shorter-acting agents. Augmentation with antipanic tricyclics (imipramine, desipramine, nortryptiline) may be needed, as well as evaluation for the emergence of comorbid depression.

Behavioral and cognitive therapies are often necessary to augment pharmacotherapy and may help reduce dosages or allow tapering of pharmacotherapy at a later point.

Postpartum obsessive compulsive disorder

There is little information about the prevalence and course of obsessive compulsive disorder through pregnancy and the puerperium. In one recent retrospective report, 8 of 27 women were noted to have onset of obsessive compulsive symptoms after the birth of a child. Many of those women also reported fears of harm coming to their babies. A more detailed retrospective report describes the acute postpartum onset of obsessional symptoms in 15 women (Sichel et al., 1993). Features of this syndrome included a characteristic constellation of obsessive thoughts about harming their babies in various ways. Women reported thoughts of stabbing the babies, drowning them, throwing them from a window, and putting them into the microwave oven. None of these mothers was psychotic. Some exhibited avoidant behavior toward their infants. This presentation is unusual because none of these women demonstrated repetitive behavior such as checking or cleaning, along with the obsessional thoughts. One hypothesis about the emergence of this particular syndrome is the induction of a rapid, severe serotonin receptor dysfunction by the acute drop in levels of pregnancy hormones, particularly of estrogen.

The women responded to drug regimens of the serotonin reuptake inhibiting agents (fluoxetine, clomipramine) known for efficacy in treatment of obsessive compulsive disorder.

A summary of the postpartum psychiatric disorders appears in Table 63-1.

Women with pregravid obsessive compulsive disorder may be at risk for worsening during the pregnancy, and clinical experience reveals severe worsening in the postpartum period.

Currently prospective work is in progress to clarify risk groups, causes, treatment modalities, and potential prophylaxis.

The next decade promises to be an exciting period in the area of women's psychiatric health. New research is demonstrating more specifically the links between female reproductive function and emergence of and vulnerability to disorder. The unique neuroendocrine aspect of the menstrual cycle, pregnancy, and the postpartum period and the impact on mood and anxiety disorders necessitates a specific role for psychiatrists as integral caregivers on obstetric and gynecologic services. Leadership is needed from both psychiatric and obstetric staff to dispel ignorance and facilitate training for resident physicians so that early recognition and treatment of these disorders can occur, minimizing the extent of dysfunction for these families.

CHARACTERISTIC SYMPTOMS OF PANIC DISORDER	
Chest tightness/pain	Perioral numbness
Tremulousness	Feelings of unreality/sense of detachment
Sweating	
Palpitations	Dizziness
Hyperventilation	Fear of losing control
Tingling in the extremities	Fear of doom

BIBLIOGRAPHY

Buttolph ML, Holland A: Obsessive compulsive disorders in pregnancy and childbirth. In Jenike M, Baer L, Minichiello WE, editors: *Obsessive compulsive disorders, theory and practice,* Chicago, 1990, Yearbook Medical.

Cogill SR et al: Impact of maternal depression on cognitive development of young children, *Br J Psychol* 292:1165, 1986

Cohen LS: Use of psychotropic medications in pregnancy, *Currents,* p 5, Sept 1992.

Cohen LS et al: Impact of pregnancy and the puerperium on panic disorder, Proceedings of the Marce Society, Edinburgh, Sept 1992.

Cohen LS et al: Postpartum lithium prophylaxis in bipolar women, Presented at the Marce Society meeting, Eindhoven, Holland November, 1993.

Cox JL, Connor Y, Kendall RE: Prospective study of the psychiatric disorders of childbirth, *Br J Psychol* 140:111, 1982

Driscoll JW: Maternal parenthood and the grief process, *J Perinat Neonat Nurs* 4:1, 1990.

Driscoll JW: Transition to parenthood. In Fawcett CS, editor: *Family psychiatric nursing,* St. Louis, 1993, Mosby-Year Book.

Kendall RE, Chalmers JC, Platz: Epidemiology of puerperal psychoses, *Br J Psychol* 150:662, 1987.

Table 63-1 Summary of postpartum psychiatric disorders

	Symptoms	Onset	Resolution	Management
Postpartum mood disorders				
Maternity blues	Tearfulness Mood liability Anxiety Some difficulty with sleep	2-3 days post	2-3 wk delivery	Reassurance
Complicated blues	Same as above	Same as above	4-6 wk	Awareness for subsequent pregnancy
Major nonpsychotic depression	Agitation, anxiety Hopelessness Poor sleep Poor appetite Poor concentration Suicidal thoughts/plan	1-4 wk 8-12	After effective medications ? Hospitalization	Antidepressants Antianxiety drugs Counseling Contraception
Psychosis	Confusion/agitation Mania Hallucinations Delusions Paranoia	1-4 wk	Hospital	Mood stabilizers Antipsychotics Antianxiety drugs High recurrence rates Prophylaxis in future pregnancies
Postpartum anxiety disorders				
Panic disorder	Panic attacks Secondary mood disorder	1-6 wk	After effective medications	Antipanic medications Antidepressant
Obsessive compulsive disorder	Thoughts of harming infant Avoidant behavior Nonpsychotic secondary mood disorder	1-6 wk ? Later	After effective medications	SSRIs Clonazepam Counseling

Selective serotonin reuptake inhibitors.

Kumar R, Robson JM: A prospective study of emotional disorders in childbearing women, *Br J Psychol* 144:35, 1984.

O'Hara MW et al: A controlled prospective study postpartum mood disorders a comparison of childbearing and nonchildbearing women, *J Abnorm Psychol* 99:3, 1990.

Pitt B: Atypical depression following childbirth, *Br J Psychol* 114:1325, 1968.

Sichel DA et al: Postpartum obsessive compulsive disorder: a case series, *J Clin Psychol* 54:4, 1993.

Stewart D et al: Prophylactic lithium in puerperal psychosis: the experience of 3 centres, *Br J Psychol* 158:393, 1991.

Wieck et al: Incidence and clinical predictors of postnatal affective disorder in women with a history of bipolar or major depressive disorder, Proceedings of the Marce Society, Sept 1992

Wisner KL, Perel JM: Serum nortriptyline levels in nursing mothers and their infants *Am J Psychiatry* 148:9, 1991.

Zuckerman B et al: Maternal depressive symptoms during pregnancy and newborn irritability, *J Pelop Pediatr* 11(4):190, 1990.

64 Breast Cancer

Irene Kuter

Carcinoma of the breast is the most common cancer in women, accounting for 32% of female cancers (excluding nonmelanoma cancers of the skin). It is second only to lung cancer as a cause of cancer deaths in women, with an estimated 46,000 deaths in 1994. There has been a great deal of public concern about the high rate of breast cancer, which is heightened by the fact that its cause is unknown. In addition the lack of curative treatments for advanced disease (one in four women in whom breast cancer develops will die of it) has been alarming.

This chapter provides an overview of the epidemiology and management of breast cancer. Screening for breast cancer is discussed in Chapter 76, and evaluation of breast problems, including suspected cancer, in Chapter 30.

■ EPIDEMIOLOGY

Carcinoma of the breast, although predominantly a disease affecting women, can also occur in males. In 1994 there will be an estimated 182,000 new cases in women in the United States and 1000 new cases in men. After female gender, age is the most striking risk factor. One in nine women in the United States will develop breast cancer, assuming a life expectancy of 85.

A more useful statistic is the estimated risk of development of breast cancer at different ages (Fig. 64-1, Table 64-1). Despite the apparent "epidemic" of breast cancer it is reassuring that the risk of a diagnosis of breast cancer before age 50 remains relatively small. Nevertheless it has been estimated that 41% of woman-years lost to breast cancer are from women less than 50 years old.

It is well known that there has been a steady rise in breast cancer incidence in the United States since 1940; the incidence now is about two times greater (Fig. 64-2) than in 1940, although the mortality rate has remained unchanged. Although oncologists generally believe that they are seeing an increasing number of cases in young women, it has been shown that this is due to the absolute increase in the number of women less than 50 years old because of the "baby boom." There is, in fact, no significant increase in incidence in women under 50; the slow rise since 1940 is mostly in women above 50 years old.

There are several possible reasons for this increase, which approximates 1% per year. Over this period the mortality rate from many other causes has been declining. Because breast cancer is largely a disease of the older woman the number of women surviving to be at risk of development of the disease has therefore increased. It has been estimated that perhaps half of the increased incidence over the last five

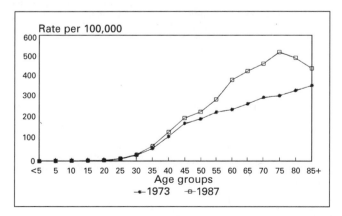

Fig. 64-1 Incidence of breast cancer as a function of age. (From Kessler LG: *Cancer* 69 (suppl 7):1896, 1992.)

Table 64-1 Estimated risk of development of breast cancer at different ages

| Current age | % Diagnosed with breast cancer by age*: | | |
	+10 yr	+20 yr	+30 yr
0	—	—	1/2500
10	—	1/2500	1/217
20	1/2500	1/217	1/51
30	1/238	1/52	1/24
40	1/66	1/26	1/15
50	1/43	1/18	1/12
60	1/29	1/15	1/11

Modified from Miller BA et al, editors: *SEER Cancer Statistics Review: 1973-1990,* National Cancer Institute, NIH Publication No 93-2789, 1993.
*Percentage of women diagnosed with breast cancer within 10, 20, or 30 years of their current age, if presently cancer-free.

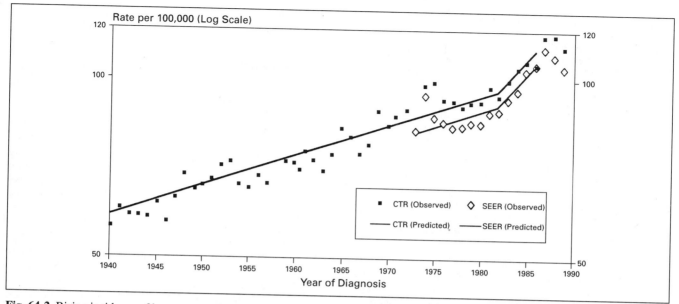

Fig. 64-2 Rising incidence of breast cancer in the United States since 1940. (From Miller BA, Feuer EJ, Hankey BF: *Ca—A Cancer Journal for Clinicians* 43:27, 1993.)

decades is secondary to increased longevity, but as much as half is due to a true increased incidence that is not fully understood. Over this period there have been many life-style changes in the U.S. population, such as improved nutrition, resulting in earlier menarche and increased commitment of women to careers with resulting delay in childbearing. Both of these are known risk factors for breast cancer and may account for some of the increased risk. Oral contraceptive pills do not seem to be responsible for the rise. To what extent environmental exposures can be implicated is not at all clear.

In addition to the gradual rise there has been a sharper increase in incidence since the early 1980s. This is thought to represent the impact of screening mammography with increased detection at an early stage of cancers that would have been discovered clinically at a later time. Consistent with the hypothesis that the accelerated increase in incidence over the last decade is due to increased screening is the observation that the increase has been in early-stage breast cancers, both ductal carcinoma in situ and small infiltrating carcinomas. There has in fact been a decrease in incidence of tumors greater than 2 cm and those associated with positive lymph nodes or metastases findings.

With the continued widespread use of screening mammography it is predicted that the incidence of new cases should drop as the prevalent cancers are detected and treated. Since 1987 there has been a slight decrease in incidence consistent with this hypothesis. Furthermore, mortality rates should decline after a lag of several years. Statisticians predict that a significant decrease in death rate should begin to be apparent in the middle to late 1990s as a result of widespread mammographic screening.

There is a striking variation in incidence of breast cancer throughout the world. Age-adjusted death rates vary from 1/100,000 to 29.3/100,000 with the highest rates seen in Europe, New Zealand, Canada, the United States, and Israel. The lowest rates are seen in Asian countries and Latin America. Studies of populations have demonstrated that this cannot be accounted for by genetic factors alone. Japanese who move to Hawaii or to the mainland United States experience an increasing risk with each generation, implicating life-style factors and environmental exposures as risk factors.

DETERMINING RISK

Although risk factors for breast cancer are much discussed, it should be remembered that 75% of women with breast cancer do not appear to have a high-risk profile. Some factors are clearly established, whereas others continue to be quite controversial. The worldwide variation in breast cancer rates suggests that there is hope that we may learn to modify risks by adjusting life-style and environment, but whether diet, hormonal profiles related to life-style factors, or environmental exposures are most important is still unknown.

When a possible risk factor is tested in a clinical trial the magnitude of the associated risk is often described in terms of relative risk. This is a numeric measure of the increased likelihood of acquiring breast cancer in the presence of a risk factor compared to the likelihood in the absence of that risk factor. A common misconception is that a relative risk of 2.0 translates into a twofold risk of acquiring breast cancer over that individual's lifetime. It should be noted, however, that the relative risk calculated is in reference to a matched individual at that age, followed over the duration of follow-up observation of that study. Thus, if a 40-year-old woman has a risk factor that is said to carry a relative risk of 1.3 and this was determined in a study that had a follow-up period of 10 years, this woman's risk of breast cancer is not (1 in 9) × 1.3 (equals 1 in 7) but rather (1 in 66) × 1.3 (equals 1 in 48) by age 50.

Risk factors

Genetic susceptibility. Although in a small number of families there is an inherited susceptibility to breast cancer,

Table 64-2 Relative risk of breast cancer according to family history

Mother or sister diagnosed with breast cancer	Increased risk (fold)
After menopause	
In one breast	1.2
In both breasts	4.0
Before menopause	
In one breast	1.8
In both breasts	8.8

making genetics the strongest risk factor for this disease, it is estimated that only about 5% of breast cancer is "familial." Familial breast cancer tends to occur in women at a younger age and to be bilateral. When assessing an individual's risk of breast cancer on the basis of family history it is important to focus on first-degree relatives and to determine whether breast cancer in the relatives was unilateral or bilateral, premenopausal or postmenopausal. Breast cancer occurring in a male in the family increases the chance that this family has a susceptibility gene. Table 64-2 gives a rough measure of relative risk to an individual based on characteristics of breast cancer in the family. Women who have a single relative with unilateral, postmenopausal breast cancer can be reassured that their risk is small, but a few women will be at very high risk and deserve special consideration in screening.

At least six familial syndromes associated with an increased risk of breast cancer have been described (Table 64-3). The best known of these are bilateral, premenopausal breast cancer and familial breast cancer associated with ovarian cancer, each of which is thought to be due to a mutation in a gene (BRCA1) on chromosome 17q. As more is understood about the genetics of these familial cancer syndromes, genetic screening will become an important part of management. It may soon be possible to screen individuals for inheritance of susceptibility genes. This will not only raise ethical questions but bring with it a need for emotional and psychologic support for those individuals found to inherit a mutated gene.

Predisposing benign breast condition. It has frequently been quoted that a previous history of biopsies of the breast for benign disease carries with it a risk of future breast cancer. This has caused inordinate anxiety among women. It is now clear that most benign breast disease is not a risk factor for breast cancer. In a classic study by Dupont and Page (Table 64-4) of 10,542 women who had biopsies showing benign breast disease, only the small group of women with atypical hyperplasia were found to be at high risk. If these women also had a positive family history in a first-degree relative, their risk doubled.

Thus most women who have had benign breast disease may be reassured that they are not at high risk of development of breast cancer. Women with atypical hyperplasia or with lobular carcinoma in situ (see later discussion) are counseled that they need careful follow-up observation because of their increased risk. It is reassuring, however, that their risk seems to attenuate with time. If a woman with proliferative disease without atypia has not had breast cancer in the first 10 years of follow-up observation, her risk falls to that of a woman without proliferative disease. For a woman who has atypical hyperplasia in whom breast cancer does not develop in the first 10 years of follow-up observation the risk also falls considerably thereafter.

Reproductive and hormonal factors. There is a small (approximately 1.3 times) increased risk of breast cancer associated with early menarche, late menopause, or nulliparity. It is believed that this risk is related to the increased number of ovulatory cycles experienced by these women with resulting stimulation of the breast epithelium by elevated estrogen levels. There is also a small increased risk associated with delay of first full-term pregnancy until after age 30. The longer the interval between menarche and the first full-term pregnancy, the higher the risk of future breast

Table 64-3 Familial syndromes associated with breast cancer

Name of syndrome	Defective gene	Other cancers	Other features
Li-Fraumeni (SBLA)	p53	Sarcoma, brain tumors, leukemia, adrenocortical carcinoma	—
Lynch type II	hMSH2 hMLH1	Colon, gastric, endometrial, genitourinary carcinomas	—
Bilateral premenopausal breast cancer	BRCA1		—
Breast/ovarian cancer	BRCA1	Ovarian	—
Cowden's disease	Unknown	Thyroid, colon carcinomas	Facial trichilemmomas, colonic polyps, papillomas of mouth and lips, acral keratoses, lipomas, uterine leiomyomata
Muir	Unknown	Basal cell and gastrointestinal carcinomas	Benign gastrointestinal tumors

Table 64-4 Risk of breast cancer in patients with benign breast disease

Diagnosis	No. of biopsies	% of benign lesions	% of evaluated biopsies
Benign specimens			
Nonproliferative disease	7,221	69.7	68.5
Proliferative disease without atypia	2768	26.7	26.2
Atypical hyperplasia	377	3.6	3.6
Total benign	10,366	100	98.3
Total carcinoma in situ	176		1.7
Total evaluated biopsies*	10,542		100

Type of benign breast disease	Relative risk of breast cancer
All patients	1.5
Nonproliferative disease	0.89
Proliferative disease	1.9
Proliferative disease without atypia	1.6
Proliferative disease with atypical hyperplasia	4.4
Proliferative disease with atypical hyperplasia, negative family history	3.5
Proliferative disease with atypical hyperplasia, positive family history	8.9

Data from Dupont WD, Page DL: *New Engl J Med* 312:146, 1985.

*The women who underwent 10,542 consecutive biopsies for a suspicion of breast cancer but who were found to have benign breast disease or carcinoma in situ were followed for a median of 17 years. Their relative risk of development of breast cancer as a function of histologic diagnosis of the original biopsy specimen was compared to that of a normal population of case-matched control women. Almost 70% of the women with benign breast disease were at no increased risk. The 4% who had atypical hyperplasia were at significantly increased risk and a positive family history increased that risk considerably.

cancer. Most striking, however, is the observation that an early full-term pregnancy is extraordinarily protective. A full-time pregnancy before age 15 results in a decreased relative risk of breast cancer to approximately 0.4 (Fig. 64-3). Lactation after pregnancy confers a small decrease in risk, but this benefit is lost after the menopause. Use of exogenous estrogens can increase a woman's risk of breast cancer, but the risk is small. It is estimated that only prolonged use carries a risk: 15 years of estrogen replacement therapy may elevate a woman's risk to 1.3 over the next 10 years. A small increased risk has also been noted to occur later in life for a woman who took diethylstilbestrol (DES) while pregnant.

Ionizing radiation exposure. From experience at Hiroshima, use of therapeutic irradiation of the chest, and use of fluoroscopy in patients with tuberculosis, it has become well established that ionizing radiation can increase the risk of breast cancer. The age of exposure is highly significant, with most of the risk occurring in women irradiated when under 25 years of age. It should be noted that the risk of therapeutic radiation used to treat primary breast cancer in conjunction with lumpectomy is associated with an acceptably small increased risk of contralateral breast cancer (relative risk 1.33 at 10 years). The risk of inducing a breast cancer by the use of screening mammography is negligibly small. It is estimated that perhaps less than one case per year per million women screened would be attributable to the radiation exposure.

Possible risk factors

There has been a very large number of other endogenous and exogenous risk factors proposed, consistent with the fact that we really have little idea of the cause of most breast cancer. There is an intriguing hypothesis that individual variations in **endogenous patterns of hormone metabolism,** which might be hereditary, could be associated with an increased risk. For example, elevated levels of the enzyme 16-α-hydroxylase,

which metabolizes estradiol to a more potent estrogen, has been suggested as a risk factor. Levels of **breast epithelial growth factors** other than estrogen may also play a role; for example, endogenous prolactin levels may be associated with an elevated risk but an association has never been proved.

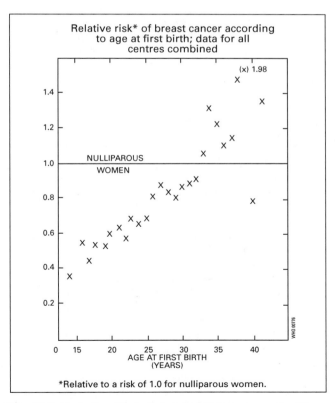

Fig. 64-3 Protective effect of an early full-term pregnancy. (From MacMahon B et al: *Bull WHO* 43:209, 1970.)

Multiple exogenous factors have been looked at critically. The **high-fat diet** theory emerged on the basis of epidemiologic studies showing a correlation between incidence of breast cancer in various countries and per capita fat consumption. However, it must be cautioned that correlation by no means implies causation, and many believe that fat intake per se is irrelevant but that another correlated factor is responsible.

Alcohol intake has been much in the press over the last few years. There is mounting evidence that daily intake of a moderate quantity of alcohol may be associated with an increased risk. Interestingly the increased risk mainly affects young women whose baseline risk is already low; thus it is unlikely to be a major risk factor. Recent clinical data have suggested that alcohol may cause increased risk through elevation of endogenous estrogen levels.

Oral contraceptive use does not, after decades of study, appear to lead to any significant increase in breast cancer incidence overall. However, recent reanalyses of old studies suggest that there may be an increased risk in certain subgroups. Women who have taken the oral contraceptive pill for prolonged periods (greater than 12 years) or women who took high-estrogen pills in their midteens may have an associated increased risk over the next two decades. Reassuringly, use for only a few years is extremely unlikely to affect risk significantly in the majority of women. It should be noted that the use of progestins as contraceptives must also be monitored for any increased risk of breast cancer because, in contrast to their action on the uterus, progestins act on breast tissue as a proliferative stimulus.

Many other putative agents have been examined such as smoking and use of hair dyes, and no definitive link has been proved. Although the risk factors discussed previously are important, we have not yet identified the major etiologic agent of breast cancer. Since genetic alterations in previously normal cells are a key component of carcinogenesis, exposure to chemical carcinogens is an obvious possible causal factor. There is much current interest in evaluating the relationship of environmental exposure to pesticides (which can be detected in body fat) to breast cancer risk, but at this time it is too early to conclude that these toxic agents can be implicated.

CLASSIFICATION OF BREAST CANCER

Figure 64-4 schematizes the subtypes of breast cancer and their frequency. The most common histologic type of breast cancer is "infiltrating ductal carcinoma, not otherwise specified," but there are several identifiable subtypes of infiltrating ductal carcinoma that may have a better or worse prognosis than the common type (e.g., mucinous infiltrating ductal carcinoma or tubular infiltrating ductal carcinoma, both of which have a more favorable prognosis).

Ductal carcinoma in situ (DCIS) is characterized by a proliferation of ductal cells, filling the ducts and spreading via the branching ductal network. Microcalcifications are often associated with DCIS within the ducts and can lead to early diagnosis on mammography before the disease spreads extensively through the ductal network or spawns an invasive cancer.

Infiltrating ductal cancer (IDC) is believed to arise by clonal evolution from DCIS and commonly appears as a mass or as a spiculated density on mammography. Small infiltrating ductal carcinomas can be found because of the microcalcifications in the ductal carcinoma in situ from which they arise. With increasing use of screening mammography there has been a gratifying rise in the detection of DCIS as a percentage of all ductal cancers as well as a shift to earlier stages of the invasive cancers that are found. This downstaging is the most important reason for the decrease in mortality rate seen with the use of screening mammography.

Infiltrating lobular carcinoma has distinctive histologic and clinical features. Unlike infiltrating ductal cancer, it does not show up easily on mammograms because it is not associated with microcalcifications and commonly infiltrates insidiously through the breast tissue without forming a discrete mass. It is common for infiltrating lobular carcinoma to appear as a diffusely thickened area of breast tissue.

Lobular carcinoma in situ (LCIS), whose name implies that it has malignant potential, is probably a form of hyperplasia and not a preinvasive neoplasm. Like atypical ductal hyperplasia, LCIS is a risk factor for the future development of DCIS or invasive carcinoma. It is frequently seen in both breasts, and the risk of future cancer is almost the same in the two breasts (approximately 20% to 25% lifetime risk).

MANAGEMENT OF PRIMARY BREAST CANCER

A patient newly diagnosed with breast cancer usually has various treatment options open to her. Because of the complexity of decision making and the need to integrate surgery, radiation therapy, and medical treatment, more and more breast cancer centers are being set up so that multidisciplinary consultations can be offered.

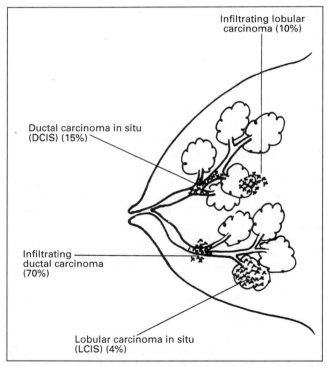

Fig. 64-4 Subtypes of breast cancer: Ductal carcinoma in situ is thought to be a precursor of invasive ductal carcinoma; lobular carcinoma is, in contrast, more akin to atypical hyperplasia and carries a risk of future ductal or invasive lobular carcinoma anywhere in the breast.

Surgical options

The rationale behind the Halsted radical mastectomy for primary breast cancer was that cancer was thought to grow like its namesake, the crab, sending out insidious infiltrating projections from the main mass into the surrounding normal tissue. Thus, Halsted reasoned, only a locally extensive surgical procedure had a chance of eradicating all traces of this insidious infiltration. Such was the power of Halsted's influence that, from the turn of the century until the mid-1970s, this mutilating surgery, in which the pectoralis major and minor muscles are sacrificed together with the breast and axillary lymph nodes, was standard treatment for breast cancer. Although it was hailed as a major advance in preventing local recurrences (which admittedly can be a major source of morbidity) the radical mastectomy failed to cure the majority of women, who succumbed to distant metastases.

Well-controlled clinical trials over the last several decades have supported a major change in how we use surgery to treat breast cancer. It is clear that the malignant cells in an invasive cancer can gain access to the bloodstream while the primary cancer is still small, and that the cells can also skip lymph nodes and embolize farther down the lymphatic chain. Thus axillary lymph nodes cannot be regarded as "filters" to trap all the cells that have escaped the breast. Axillary lymph node dissection is now regarded less as a therapeutic intervention and more as a staging operation to assess the extent of lymph node involvement by the cancer, which in turn gives an assessment of the likelihood that there has been systemic spread of the cancer cells. Recent studies using monoclonal antibodies have suggested that as many as 30% of women with early stage breast cancer have detectable micrometastases in the bone marrow at the time of initial surgery.

The goal of surgery is now merely to achieve local control of the primary tumor. "Cure" can only be achieved if the cancer is excised before distant metastases have been seeded or if adjuvant medical treatment is successful in eradicating these metastases. Clinical trials documented first that modified radical mastectomy (in which the pectoralis major muscle is spared) is equivalent to radical mastectomy in terms of long-term survival rate and local control, and then that "lumpectomy" with irradiation gives an identical survival rate with an acceptable local recurrence risk in the breast. When amputation of the breast is not performed, there will always be a chance of local recurrence within the breast, but if patients with increased risk of local failure are excluded (see later discussion) then this risk should be less than 5% and is acceptable to most women. Recurrence within the breast after lumpectomy and radiation therapy with the need for a "salvage" mastectomy has not influenced survival rate.

An NIH consensus report issued in 1990 upheld the position that lumpectomy with radiation was preferable to mastectomy because it has an equivalent long-term survival rate and spares the breast. Although the majority of women agree with this philosophy, some still choose mastectomy for a variety of reasons, which include an emotional wish to get rid of the cancerous breast, a fear of radiation, or simply a desire to have the treatment over and done with as quickly as possible. In other words most women can choose their surgical option on the basis of the side effects of the treatment with the knowledge that the chance of a cure will be the same, whichever they choose. For mastectomy the major side effect is obvious: physical loss of an appendage with its psychologic toll. Conservative surgery with radiation therapy will require several weeks (usually 5 or 6) of daily radiation treatments, some swelling and erythema of the breast during treatment (and this can sometimes last for months afterward), and the need for more intense follow-up surveillance to ensure that the cancer has not recurred in the breast. For some women the fear of finding recurrent disease in the breast is a major stress, but the majority of women are willing and able to deal with each of these side effects because of a strong motivation to avoid a mastectomy.

There are some women for whom breast conservation with radiation therapy is not a good choice. In some women, such as those who have more than one primary cancer in the breast or extensive lymphatic invasion, the risk of recurrence is unacceptably high. In others, such as those in whom the cancer is centrally located or is large in comparison to the size of the breast, the cosmetic outcome is likely to be poor. Studies are currently ongoing to see whether chemotherapy before surgery (neoadjuvant chemotherapy), which can render large or locally advanced breast cancers more easily operable, will in the long run give acceptable local control rates in the breast (when used with lumpectomy and irradiation). Initial reports are favorable.

Axillary dissection

Regardless of whether mastectomy or breast conservation is chosen, it is currently standard practice to dissect the ipsilateral axilla and remove levels I and II lymph nodes en bloc. Although clinical studies have documented that this axillary dissection can be delayed until such time as lymph nodes are palpable without adverse effect on survival rate, the extent of axillary lymph node involvement is the most important prognostic factor currently available, and decisions on adjuvant medical treatment (and eligibility for clinical research protocols) are made on the basis of what is found in the axilla. When the treatment will not be affected by the findings in the axilla (for example, an elderly patient with a large estrogen-receptor-positive cancer will receive tamoxifen whether or not the lymph nodes are positive) or when the morbidity risk of the general anesthesia required is likely to be considerable (for example, in an elderly woman with multiple medical problems) an argument can be made for *not* dissecting the axilla and treating the patient as if the nodes were involved.

Staging

The international TNM staging system is routinely used for staging breast cancer (Table 64-5). Figure 64-5 shows data from the SEER (*S*urveillance, *E*pidemiology, and *E*nd *R*esults) program of the National Cancer Institute relating survival to stage at diagnosis. It is important to note that the TNM system has been modified over the years, and certain clinical trial data may need to be reinterpreted with this in mind. For example, since 1988 the presence of an involved supraclavicular node has put a patient in stage IV because it has been found to connote a similar prognosis to that seen with distant metastases. Also in 1988, a $T_3N_0M_0$ cancer (tumor greater than 5 cm without lymph node involvement or distant metastases) was moved from stage IIIA to IIB because of SEER program data showing the 5-year survival rate of this group to be more in line with that of other stage II patients than others in stage IIIA.

Table 64-5 TNM staging system for breast cancer

Primary tumor (T)

T0	No evidence of primary tumor
Tis	Carcinoma in situ
T1	Tumor 2 cm or less in greatest dimension
T2	Tumor between 2 and 5 cm in greatest dimension
T3	Tumor more than 5 cm in greatest dimension
T4	Tumor of any size with any of the following:
	Extension to chest wall
	Edema or ulceration of skin of the breast
	Satellite skin nodules confined to the same breast
	Inflammatory carcinoma

Regional lymph nodes (N)

NX	Regional lymph nodes not assessed
N0	No regional lymph node metastasis
N1	Metastasis to movable ipsilateral axillary lymph node(s)
N2	Metastasis to ipsilateral axillary lymph node(s) fixed to one another or to other structures
N3	Metastasis to ipsilateral internal mammary lymph node(s)

Distant metastases

Mx	Presence of distant metastasis not assessed
M0	No distant metastasis
M1	Distant metastasis (includes metastasis to ipsilateral supraclavicular lymph node[s])

Stage grouping

Stage 0	Tis	N0	M0
Stage I	T1	N0	M0
Stage IIA	T0	N1	M0
	T1	N1	M0
	T2	N0	M0
Stage IIB	T2	N1	M0
	T3	N0	M0
Stage IIIA	T0	N2	M0
	T1	N2	M0
	T2	N2	M0
	T3	N1	M0
	T3	N2	M0
Stage IIIB	T4	Any N	M0
	Any T	N3	M0
Stage IV	Any T	Any N	M1

From Beahrs OH et al, editors: *Manual for staging of cancer*, ed 4, Philadelphia, 1992, Lippincott.

The role of radiologic evaluation in the staging of early breast cancer is controversial. One study showed that for clinical stage I disease, the yield of a bone scan was 0% and only 1.5% to 4% of clinical stage II disease had positive scan findings, whereas there was a 16% to 25% positive rate for clinical stage III disease. Another study looking at the role of liver scan results showed that only 5% were positive preoperatively but only 1% of patients had true positive study results; the others were false-positive results. Preoperative routine staging therefore should include bilateral mammograms (if not already done) to detect multicentric and bilateral lesions, chest radiographs, and liver function tests, including alkaline phosphatase. Most surgeons still

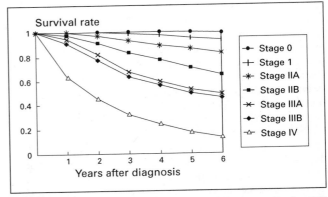

Fig. 64-5 Survival related to stage at diagnosis. (From Beahrs OH et al, editors: *Manual for staging of cancer*, ed 4, Philadelphia, 1992, Lippincott.

obtain a bone scan but there is a trend away from obtaining one for clinical stage I or II disease unless the alkaline phosphatase is elevated. Liver scans are no longer done routinely. If abnormal liver function test results are noted, an abdominal computed tomographic (CT) scan is done. A head CT scan is done only if signs or symptoms of central nervous system involvement are present.

Radiation therapy

If a mastectomy is performed as the primary surgery for an invasive breast cancer, radiation therapy is not routinely given unless the patient is deemed to be at high risk for local recurrence. Local radiation therapy, although effectively decreasing the local recurrence rate, has not convincingly been shown to improve survival rate. This is probably because mortality results from distant metastases and not from local recurrence. Patients at high risk for local recurrence include those who have close margins, extensive lymphatic invasion, more than four positive lymph nodes, or locally advanced disease (usually tumors greater than or equal to 5 cm).

If lumpectomy is the primary surgical treatment, radiation therapy is required for good local control. It is recommended that clear margins be obtained by lumpectomy, and radiation treatment be delivered in a dose of 4500 to 5000 cGy to the whole breast. If there is a close margin a boost may be necessary. If there is extracapsular invasion from involved axillary lymph nodes or if a large number of nodes are involved, axillary radiation therapy is also given. It is common for the patient to experience erythema and edema of the breast during and after irradiation. The swelling can last for a number of months and gradually diminishes. There may be a small risk of cancer in the contralateral breast from radiation scatter, but this increase in risk is currently judged to be acceptable (relative risk 1.19, rising to 1.33 at 10 years).

PROGNOSIS

The presence of positive axillary lymph nodes and their extent of involvement (number of nodes, level) are the single most important prognostic factors in patients with breast cancer. For example, a woman with a 1.5-cm invasive cancer may have a 10-year disease-free survival rate of 80% after local treatment alone if the lymph nodes are negative but only 50% if there are two or three axillary lymph nodes involved. Other factors that are in use to assess prognosis in early-stage breast cancer include tumor size, nuclear grade, histologic subtype, estrogen and progesterone receptor status, and presence of vascular invasion. However, there has been an explosion of information on prognostic factors in recent years. Some, such as ploidy analysis, initially appeared exciting but now do not seem to have independent prognostic value. Others, such as S-phase analysis (one of many assays that assess mitotic index as a measure of growth rate of the tumor), seem more likely to be useful clinically. The future roles of analyses of oncogene (e.g., Her-2/neu) expression, tumor suppressor gene (e.g., p53) expression, neovascularization, growth factor and growth factor receptor expression, and so on, hang in the balance at this time. It is unlikely that others, such as cathepsin-D, will have an important clinical role. Ideally an algorithm that will incorporate all the known prognostic factors and can be used to make decisions regarding adjuvant medical treatment will be constructed.

ADJUVANT SYSTEMIC THERAPY

Breast cancer is a chemotherapy-responsive disease. If the cancer has receptors for estrogen and progesterone, it is also responsive to hormone therapies. However, chemotherapy and hormonal therapy have not been curative for women who have established metastases. Clinical trials began nearly 50 years ago to try to improve the cure rate for breast cancer by giving chemotherapy early in the course of the disease, before distant disease is manifest, on the theory that the micrometastases inferred to be present at the time of the primary treatment might be eradicated and systemic relapse prevented.

The earliest trials included women with positive lymph nodes who were deemed to be at sufficiently high risk of relapse to justify experimental treatment. Perioperative or short postoperative courses, usually with single agents, were given at first. However, it was not until combination chemotherapy (cyclophosphamide, methotrexate, and 5-fluorouracil [5-FU] [CMF]) was given for a year or more postoperatively that impressive improvements in disease-free survival and overall survival rates were seen. In the first long-term follow-up evaluation of CMF, Bonadonna and colleagues reported that premenopausal women with positive axillary lymph nodes who were given CMF experienced a 17% improvement in relapse-free survival rate and a 14% improvement in overall survival rate at 10 years compared with untreated controls. With other groups reporting similar data, the NIH in 1985 issued a consensus conference report recommending that premenopausal women with positive axillary lymph nodes be given postoperative adjuvant chemotherapy as standard treatment. Postmenopausal women with positive axillary lymph nodes in the Bonadonna study gained only 6% improvement in relapse-free survival rate and 2% improvement in overall survival rate, and this small benefit was considered not significant enough for adjuvant chemotherapy to be offered routinely to this group. It was, however, not clear whether the less favorable results in the older women were due to underdosing with chemotherapy.

In contrast, for postmenopausal women with positive lymph nodes and cancers that were estrogen-receptor-positive (ER+), adjuvant hormonal therapy with tamoxifen was found to produce a remarkable improvement in disease-free survival and overall survival rates, comparable in fact to the effect of chemotherapy in the younger women. Interestingly tamoxifen was much less effective for premenopausal women with ER+ tumors, giving only a small benefit to this group. In 1985 therefore the NIH consensus conference committee recommended adjuvant tamoxifen for postmenopausal women who had ER+ tumors and positive lymph nodes but no adjuvant hormonal treatment for premenopausal women (who, as noted, were to have chemotherapy instead). Women with negative lymph nodes were thought to have a sufficiently favorable prognosis that adjuvant therapy was not advised because of the associated side effects.

Early Breast Cancer Trialists' Collaborative Group metaanalysis of adjuvant systemic therapies

Since the 1985 consensus conference report many new observations have been made on the role of adjuvant medical treatment. Many of these are summarized in a metaanalysis published in 1992 by the Early Breast Cancer Trialists' Collaborative Group (EBCTCG). This group assembled data from all known trials around the world of adjuvant treatment in breast cancer in which there were both a control and a treatment arm. One hundred and thirty-three trials involving 75,000 women were included. The main conclusions can be summarized as follows:

Adjuvant chemotherapy for women with positive lymph nodes. The significant benefit of adjuvant chemotherapy in premenopausal women was reaffirmed with a decrease in the annual recurrence rate of 36% and in the annual mortality rate of 25% compared with those of controls. Six months of polychemotherapy (CMF) were as good as 12 months (6 months of CMF can now be considered the "standard" against which all other adjuvant chemotherapy is judged). The survival benefit was greater at 10 years than at 5 years. In the postmenopausal group as a whole the benefits were indeed less, but still quite significant in the 50- to 59-year-old group. On the basis of this report chemotherapy has been offered more commonly to women in this age range, but hormonal therapy is still first choice in women above 60 years old.

Adjuvant hormonal therapy for women with positive lymph nodes. The substantial benefit of adjuvant tamoxifen in women more than 50 years old (30% decrease in annual recurrence rate, 20% decrease in annual mortality rate) and the relative lack of benefit in women less than 50 years old (12% decrease in annual recurrence rate, 6% decrease in annual mortality rate) were reaffirmed. Again the survival benefit was greater at 10 years than at 5 years. Comparison between studies showed that 2 years of tamoxifen were better than 1 year and treatment for more than 2 years was better still. Current studies are trying to assess the optimal duration of treatment. There was no added benefit from tamoxifen doses greater than 20 mg/day. Interestingly, although postmenopausal women with ER+ tumors derived the greatest benefit (23% decrease in annual mortality rate), there was still a substantial benefit in postmenopausal women with ER− tumors (16% decrease in annual mortality rate). The biologic significance of this is intriguing but as yet not fully understood. There was no benefit to premenopausal women with ER− tumors, however.

Adjuvant ovarian ablation. Most of the trials involving oophorectomy in the postoperative setting were conducted at a time when estrogen receptor analyses were not performed. As expected the metaanalysis showed no benefit derived from ovarian ablation in postmenopausal women, but a surprisingly significant benefit in premenopausal women. In this group the decreases in recurrence and mortality rates resulting from oophorectomy were comparable in magnitude to those seen with chemotherapy. These findings have stimulated a resurgence of interest in adjuvant oophorectomy and ovarian suppression in premenopausal patients.

Combination chemotherapy and hormonal therapy for women with positive lymph nodes. In women aged 50 to 69, for whom adjuvant tamoxifen therapy is more efficacious than adjuvant chemotherapy, it was shown that the combination of chemotherapy and tamoxifen was slightly more effective in decreasing recurrence rate than tamoxifen alone (although there was no effect on overall survival rate). For women aged less than 50 there are insufficient data to draw conclusions regarding combination therapy, but ongoing clinical trials are testing whether ovarian ablation or suppression in addition to chemotherapy is better than chemotherapy alone.

Adjuvant therapy for women with invasive cancer and negative lymph nodes. Since the recommendation in 1985 at the NIH Consensus Conference that women with negative lymph nodes not receive adjuvant systemic therapy, there have been many trials showing that these women do benefit from adjuvant therapy. The metaanalysis by the EBCTCG demonstrates that tamoxifen and chemotherapy will give the same percentage reduction in recurrence and mortality rates in node-negative as in node-positive women, but because the recurrence and mortality risks are significantly lower in the node-negative women the absolute benefits are also smaller. Thus a treatment that improves 10-year survival rate from 50% to 62% in a node-positive group (12% absolute benefit) might only improve survival from 90% to 92% (2% absolute benefit) in patients with small tumors and negative lymph nodes.

Logically, systemic therapy should be given to those "node-negative" women who are at sufficiently high risk to make the systemic chemotherapy worthwhile in terms of absolute benefit gained. The perfect algorithm that gives appropriate weighting to the various prognostic factors is not yet available. At present, most clinicians recommend adjuvant systemic therapy if the primary tumor is 2 cm or bigger and are more likely to recommend chemotherapy for an even smaller tumor if it is ER−, is high-grade, or has a high growth fraction. The relative importance of the various other prognostic factors is still controversial.

Side effects of chemotherapy

Six months of chemotherapy with "classic" CMF (cyclophosphamide, methotrexate, and 5-fluorouracil), a well-tolerated regimen with a good track record, is the standard against which other regimens are compared. This regimen usually causes only mild to moderate nausea in the majority of women, and usually only moderate alopecia and myelosuppression. Other troublesome side effects can include mucositis, conjunctivitis, tearing of the eyes, and unwelcome weight gain. Induction of menopause by chemotherapy is age-related, occurring in only 40% of women below 40 years old, but in over 90% of women above 40 years old. The risk of leukemia secondary to the chemotherapy is estimated to

be approximately 1%. The other regimen in common use is CAF, in which doxorubicin (Adriamycin) has been substituted for methotrexate. Although this regimen may be slightly more efficacious it is also more toxic. It causes more nausea and more complete alopecia and carries the risk of cardiac toxicity at high cumulative doses.

Side effects of tamoxifen

The only common side effects of tamoxifen are hot flashes and a mucoid vaginal discharge. With adjuvant therapy currently recommended for 5 years and the optimal duration unknown, long-term side effects must be considered. Luckily tamoxifen is not a pure antiestrogen. It is a mixed agonist/antagonist and has proestrogenic effects on several target organs. Its proestrogenic effect on the bones and the cardiovascular system gives some protection against osteoporotic bone loss, decreases cholesterol level, and decreases death of causes other than breast cancer (approximately 12% decrease, mostly attributable to a decrease in vascular events). Because it acts as an estrogen agonist on the endometrium, tamoxifen users experience an increased risk of endometrial cancer, but this small risk (roughly 1.1%, representing a 7.5-fold increase in their baseline risk) is more than counterbalanced in most women by the decreased risk of recurrence of breast cancer.

MANAGEMENT OF CARCINOMA IN SITU

Ductal carcinoma in situ

Ductal carcinoma in situ (DCIS) is a noninvasive type of breast cancer believed to be a precursor to infiltrating (invasive) ductal carcinoma. Once uncommon, it is being more frequently diagnosed now with the advent of screening mammography, because it is detectable on mammograms as microcalcifications even before a mass develops in the breast. Traditionally DCIS has been treated with mastectomy because this will guarantee that this noninvasive cancer will not recur, and historically an unacceptably high rate of recurrence in the breast (between 30% and 75%) has been noted with lumpectomy alone. As lumpectomy and radiation therapy became the accepted treatment for invasive cancer it was natural to ask whether a similar conservative approach might not be possible for small in situ ductal carcinomas. Recent clinical trials have been encouraging in this regard, and the current trend is to offer excision with radiation to selected women with small in situ tumors. It should be understood, however, that there will always be more risk associated with this approach because there will always be some risk of recurrence in the breast, and a proportion of these recurrences will be invasive. Each individual will therefore need to make a choice of treatment based, on the one hand, on the maximum peace of mind with a mastectomy and, on the other hand, the chance of avoiding a mastectomy but with a moderate risk of a recurrence in the breast that may be invasive and therefore associated with a small risk of life-threatening consequences.

Lobular carcinoma in situ

Lobular carcinoma in situ would better be described as lobular hyperplasia. Its presence signifies that the breast epithelium is abnormal and that the woman has an increased risk of development of invasive cancer in both breasts. The lifetime risk is approximately 20% to 25% in each breast. In the past some surgeons recommended bilateral mastectomy because of this bilateral risk. However, with good screening mammography it is now generally recommended that most women be followed carefully and surgical intervention offered only when indicated. For some women living with this fear will be unacceptable, whereas for others with mammographically dense breasts the sensitivity of radiography may not be acceptable. For these women bilateral simple mastectomy with or without reconstruction may be preferred.

FOLLOW-UP CARE OF THE WOMAN WITH EARLY-STAGE BREAST CANCER

If the primary treatment has been lumpectomy serial physical examinations and mammograms of the treated breast are essential to detect a recurrence. Usually the first follow-up mammogram will be obtained at 6 months after completion of irradiation. In the first year of follow-up observation physical examination is performed every 3 months, every 4 months in the second year, and then every 6 months thereafter. Although routine chest radiographs and bone scans used to be part of the routine follow-up care, clinical studies have shown no benefit in terms of outcome, and their routine use has been largely discontinued. Instead, attention is paid to symptoms, such as dry cough, exertional dyspnea, pleuritic chest pain, bony aches and pains, which may signify lung, pleural, or bony involvement. Blood tests to screen for bone (alkaline phosphatase) or liver dysfunction (liver function tests) are obtained every 6 months.

A currently controversial issue is that of estrogen replacement therapy in breast cancer survivors. It is widely believed that estrogens must be avoided at all costs in the woman with a history of breast cancer, but recently this has been challenged by a number of experts who point out that the evidence supporting an adverse effect of exogenous estrogens in women with a history of breast cancer is weak. In view of the tremendous benefits to the cardiovascular and skeletal systems that postmenopausal women receive from estrogen therapy, many are now calling for prospective randomized trials to assess the actual risk/benefit ratio of estrogen therapy in breast cancer survivors.

MANAGEMENT OF METASTATIC DISEASE

Although breast cancer can spread to any part of the body, the common sites for metastases are the bones, lung, liver, and pleura. It is also important to recognize the occasional involvement of the pericardium and intestine and (frequently late) involvement of brain or meninges. Unless recurrent disease is in the breast after a lumpectomy or is locoregional (i.e., in the chest wall or axilla on the side of the original mastectomy), there is no meaningful likelihood of a cure with standard therapy, and the goal of treatment is palliation.

Hormonal therapy

Unless the patient is in imminent danger of organ compromise from the metastases, hormone therapy is the treatment of choice in patients whose original cancer was positive for estrogen receptors, because in such cases the likelihood of a

response is 60% to 65%. Furthermore hormonal treatments have fewer side effects than chemotherapy. It was first noted by Beatson at the turn of the century that oophorectomy in premenopausal patients with breast cancer effected shrinkage of metastatic disease. Oophorectomy is still a valuable therapy for premenopausal women. Gonadotropin-releasing hormone (GnRH) agonists that lower estrogen levels by turning off ovarian function probably work equally well, but the once-a-month injections are expensive (approximately $200/month). In postmenopausal women tamoxifen, an antiestrogen, is the treatment of choice because it has fewer side effects, although similar response rates can be seen with megestrol acetate. Tamoxifen has been less well studied in premenopausal women, but some studies suggest that it is almost as efficacious as oophorectomy in this group. The mean time to response to hormonal therapy is approximately 2 months with the mean duration of response 1 to 2 years. Responses are more commonly seen in metastases in bone and soft tissue but less commonly in lung, liver, and brain. If a good response is obtained with the first endocrine treatment it is worth employing second-line hormonal therapy at the time of relapse with a likelihood of response of approximately 50%. Aminoglutethimide is a popular second-line (or third-line, after megestrol acetate) therapy in postmenopausal women. It inhibits adrenal synthesis of the hormones that are metabolized to estrogen in fat tissue. Because cortisol synthesis is suppressed, too, replacement glucocorticoid is usually given. Antiprogestins such as RU-486 are showing promise in preclinical and early clinical trials and may in the future add to our range of hormonal therapy options.

Chemotherapy

Chemotherapy is the systemic treatment of choice for patients with metastatic disease that is estrogen-receptor-negative (this group has less than 10% chance of a response to hormonal therapy) or for those whose disease is no longer responding to hormonal manipulation. Even for patients with metastatic disease that is estrogen-receptor-positive, chemotherapy is preferred if they have visceral involvement with imminent symptoms because hormonal therapy gives slow (1 to 2 months) responses compared with chemotherapy, which usually begins to shrink the tumors within a couple of weeks. Patients with hormone-refractory breast cancer can certainly have symptoms palliated by chemotherapy and can live longer with better quality of life. However, it is sobering to discover that, despite response rates greater than 75%, chemotherapy gives only temporary remissions in patients with metastatic breast cancer, and there is no meaningful long-term disease-free survival for these patients with standard therapy. The median duration of response to chemotherapy is 6 to 8 months, and the median survival after institution of chemotherapy is $1\frac{1}{2}$ to 2 years. There has not been any survival advantage to more aggressive regimens with high response rates, so it is common to use the gentlest, least toxic regimens first (e.g., CMF) and progress to more aggressive regimens (such as those containing anthracyclines such as doxorubicin) later. The latest of the drugs active against breast cancer is taxol, which is now being tested in combination with other drugs as first-line treatment of metastatic disease. It remains unlikely, however, that there will be any cures.

Autologous bone marrow transplantation

It is known that there is a dose-response relationship in the treatment of breast cancer with chemotherapy. It has been hypothesized that, whereas cure of metastatic disease does not seem possible with standard doses of chemotherapy, increasing the doses many times might be curative if the toxicity of the treatment could be lessened. When drugs such as the alkylating agents, whose dose-limiting toxicity is bone marrow suppression, are chosen a several-fold increase in delivered dose can be obtained if hematopoietic stem cells are harvested before administration of chemotherapy and returned to the patient after metabolism and excretion of the chemotherapy drugs. Autologous bone marrow transplantation (when the stem cells are harvested by marrow aspiration from the iliac bones) and autologous peripheral stem cell transplantation (when the stem cells are harvested from the peripheral blood after mobilization from the bone marrow by chemotherapy or growth factors) provide such a way of overcoming the devastating bone marrow suppression that would otherwise accompany such high-dose chemotherapy. In the early days of bone marrow transplantation for breast cancer, women who had widely metastatic disease and had been through several types of chemotherapy were recruited, but these women did poorly. Most had relapsed within 6 to 8 months and died within a year or so of transplantation. Currently the best candidates are considered to be young women with limited metastases who have had minimal previous chemotherapy and who show a good response to (induction) chemotherapy before transplantation conditioning. In some series, 20% of such highly selected women are disease-free several years after transplantation. Although these numbers are encouraging, the low percentage testifies to the fact that better drugs and new forms of treatment are needed.

CHEMOPREVENTION

One of the major areas of basic and clinical research in cancer currently is chemoprevention. There have been studies, for example, using retinoids in patients with head and neck cancer, in which the use of biologically active agents has decreased the risk of a new primary cancer. In breast cancer patients use of adjuvant tamoxifen has been shown to decrease the likelihood of a contralateral new primary breast cancer. A large multiinstitutional trial, NSABP-P1, is actively accruing 16,000 women at increased risk of breast cancer for randomization into placebo versus tamoxifen treatment arms to determine how protective tamoxifen might be. In Europe similar trials are ongoing and fenretinide, a retinoid derivative, is also being tested as a chemopreventive agent for breast cancer. Another study, at the University of Southern California, is treating women at high risk with GnRH analogues to suppress normal ovulation. These women receive supplementary low-dose estrogen and intermittent pulses of progesterone to minimize the adverse effects of estrogen deprivation and unopposed estrogen, respectively. If chemoprevention and modification of the environment could have a major impact on decreasing the rate of breast cancer, this would be a much more valuable contribution than the discovery of another new drug to treat metastatic disease.

BIBLIOGRAPHY

Adjuvant chemotherapy for breast cancer: NIH consensus development conference, September 9-11, 1985. *Cancer Treat Res* 60:375, 1992.

Beahrs OH et al, editors: *Manual for Staging of Cancer,* ed 4, Philadelphia, 1992, Lippincott.

Boring CC et al: Cancer statistics, 1994, *Ca—A Cancer Journal for Clinicians* 44:7, 1994.

Cobleigh MA et al: Estrogen replacement therapy in breast cancer survivors: a time for change, *JAMA* 272:540, 1994.

Dupont WD, Page DL: Risk factors for breast cancer in women with proliferative breast disease, *New Engl J Med* 312:146, 1985.

Early Breast Cancer Trialists' Collaborative Group: Systemic treatment of early breast cancer by hormonal, cytotoxic, or immune therapy. *Lancet* 339:1,71, 1992.

Fisher B et al: Endometrial cancer in tamoxifen-treated breast cancer patients: findings from the National Surgical Adjuvant Breast and Bowel Project (NSABP) B-14, *J Natl Cancer Inst* 86:527, 1994.

Kessler LG: The relationship between age and incidence of breast cancer, *Cancer* 69 (suppl 7):1896, 1992.

Lynch HT et al: Hereditary breast cancer and family cancer syndromes, *World J Surg* 18:21, 1994.

MacMahon B et al: Age at first birth and breast cancer risk, *Bull WHO* 43:209, 1970.

Miller BA, Feuer EJ, Hankey BF: Recent incidence trends for breast cancer in women and the relevance of early detection: an update, *Ca - A Cancer Journal for Clinicians* 43:27, 1993.

Miller et al, editors: *SEER Cancer Statistics Review: 1973-1990,* NIH Publication No 93-2789, Bethesda, Md, 1993, National Cancer Institute.

NIH consensus conference: Treatment of early-stage breast cancer, *JAMA* 265:391, 1991.

Pike MC, Spicer DV: The chemoprevention of breast cancer by reducing sex steroid exposure: perspectives from epidemiology, *J Cell Biochem* 17G (suppl):26, 1993.

Pike MC et al: Estrogens, progestogens, normal breast cell proliferation, and breast cancer risk, *Epidemiol Rev* 15:17, 1993.

Rosenberg L, Metzger LS, Palmer JR: Alcohol consumption and risk of breast cancer: a review of the epidemiologic evidence, *Epidemiol Rev* 15:133, 1993.

Thomas DB: Oral contraceptives and breast cancer, *J Natl Cancer Inst* 85:359, 1993 (commentary).

Vaughan WP: Autologous bone marrow transplantation in the treatment of breast cancer: clinical and technologic strategies, *Semin Oncol* 20(5 suppl 6):55, 1993.

Wong K, Henderson IC: Management of metastatic breast cancer, *World J Surg* 18:98, 1994.

Wynder EL et al: Dietary fat and breast cancer: where do we stand on the evidence? *J Clin Epidemiol* 47:217, 1994 (discussion 223).

65 Gynecologic Cancers

Iris Wertheim, Valena J. Soto-Wright, and Howard M. Goodman

CERVICAL CANCER

Cervical cancer is the third most common malignant disease of the female genital tract and is the only genital tract cancer for which an effective screening test has been established. Since the introduction of the Papanicolaou's test (Pap smear) in 1943 and the widespread institution of screening programs based on this test, there has been a decreasing incidence of and mortality from invasive cervical cancer. Although these improvements are not yet documented by results of randomized trials, they appear to be related to effective screening. (See Chapter 77 for further discussion.) In spite of the ease and efficacy of this test, it is expected that of 15,000 new cases to be diagnosed, 4600 women will die of cervical cancer.

Epidemiology and Etiology

Cervical neoplasia is believed to encompass a spectrum of disease ranging from preinvasive lesions (also known as dysplasia, cervical intraepithelial neoplasia, squamous intraepithelial lesion) to microinvasive cancer to frankly invasive disease. Preinvasive cervical cancer is believed to precede the development of invasive disease by about 10 years. The median age of diagnosis of invasive disease is 54 years, with a range extending from the teens to the ninth and tenth decades.

Risk factors

Multiple sex partners, early age of first intercourse, and prior history of sexually transmitted disease (STD) are all associated with an increased risk for cervical cancer, implicating a sexually transmitted factor in the pathogenesis. Human papillomavirus (HPV) is now thought to be causally related to the development of cervical neoplasia. Subtypes 16, 18, 31, 33, and 35 have been found in more than 90% of preinvasive cervical cancers. Cigarette smoking, independent of the other prognostic factors, is associated with an increased risk of cervical cancer. Of note is that cigarette smoke-related carcinogens are concentrated in the cervix and may account for this epidemiologic association. The use of oral contraceptives has been associated with an increased risk in some studies; however, many of these reports, which have been confounded by not correcting for the other sexually related prognostic factors, may not take into account the protective effects of barrier methods (see box, below right).

Natural history

Squamous cell carcinoma accounts for 80% to 90% of cervical cancer, and glandular tumors or adenocarcinomas account for the remainder. Of concern is that several reports have described these latter lesions in younger patients not usually considered to be at risk for cervical cancer. Tumor growth is described as **exophytic,** with a cauliflower-like appearance, or **endophytic,** with growth deep into the cervix and lower uterine segment that may result in a so-called barrel-shaped appearance of the cervix and uterus.

Early lesions may exhibit ulceration, induration, or granular areas of friable tissue, or they may be subclinical with no apparent abnormality visible with the naked eye. Colposcopic examination will reveal the changes of high-grade intraepithelial lesion and identify areas that suggest early invasion. Local spread to the vagina, as well as paracervical and parametrial tissue, may be followed by further tumor growth to the pelvic sidewall or to the mucosa of the bladder or rectum, or both. Lymphatic spread occurs in an orderly fashion to involve the external iliac, internal iliac, and obturator nodes and then to the secondary nodal regions of the common iliac and paraaortic regions. The scalene and inguinal nodes occasionally may be involved with more advanced disease. Hematogenous spread usually is associated with advanced or recurrent disease and, when present, may involve lung, liver, bone, or brain. Ovarian metastases are uncommon, thus allowing the option of preserving ovarian function in the young patient.

Clinical presentation

History and symptoms. The most common presenting symptom of cervical cancer is abnormal vaginal bleeding, which may manifest as menorrhagia or occur postcoitally, intermenstrually, or postmenopausally. Vaginal discharge, frequently pink-tinged or foul-smelling, or both, may be noted. On the basis of the population studied—specifically, the percentage of women in screening programs—a significant proportion of women may have abnormal findings on Pap smears and, it is hoped, early disease. Symptoms of advanced or recurrent disease include leg, back, or pelvic pain, usually related to nerve root or bony involvement. Persistent leg edema may develop secondary to extensive sidewall disease with compression of lymphatic or venous channels. Tumor growth also may be associated with hematuria, dysuria, rectal bleeding, or obstipation. The cause of death in most patients with advanced, recurrent, or untreated disease usually is hemorrhage from cervical and vaginal ulceration or renal failure from sidewall involvement and ureteral compromise.

Physical and pelvic examination. The size, mobility, and consistency of the cervix should be noted during bimanual examination. The cervix may look and feel entirely normal (occult disease) or may be replaced by a rock-hard or

---

RISK FACTORS FOR CERVICAL CANCER

Multiple sexual partners
Early age of first intercourse
Prior history of sexually transmitted disease
Infection with human papillomavirus
HIV infection
Cigarette smoking
Possibly oral contraceptives

friable tumor, appearing ulcerative or exophytic on visual examination. In general, the rectovaginal examination is considered a key element of the pelvic examination. It may be particularly helpful in assessing the cervix of postmenopausal women or in patients who have undergone multiple cervical procedures, in which the cervix has become flush with the vaginal apex as a result of atrophy.

Diagnostic tests

Pap smear

SCREENING. The American College of Obstetrics and Gynecology recommends that all patients have cytologic screening starting at age 18 years, or at the onset of sexual activity, in conjunction with annual bimanual pelvic examination. The optimal screening interval remains controversial, with some advocating a 2 to 3-year screening interval after two successive normal smear results in the absence of risk factors. For a more in-depth discussion of routine screening, see Chapter 77.

CLASSIFICATION OF PAP SMEAR FINDINGS. The Bethesda classification for cervical/vaginal cytologic findings recently has been adopted by most centers. This system reports Pap smear results in five categories: **normal, atypical cells of undetermined significance, low-grade squamous intraepithelial lesion, high-grade intraepithelial lesion,** or findings consistent with **invasive cancer.** Table 65-1 compares the Bethesda system to the prior Pap smear classifications.

MANAGEMENT OF ABNORMAL PAP SMEAR FINDINGS. The management of an abnormal Pap test result (see Table 65-2) requires a colposcopic examination of the cervix and vagina. The atypical smear may be referred for colposcopic evaluation although close follow-up with repeat smear in 3 to 4 months to confirm the abnormality is considered acceptable, with referral for colposcopic examination required for persistent atypia or for women with HIV sero-positivity. Patients whose Pap smears suggest the presence of squamous intraepithelial lesion or cells consistent with invasive cancer require colposcopic examination.

COLPOSCOPY. The colposcope is a binocular, stereoscopic operating microscope that provides strong illumination and 5- to 30-times magnification to permit identification of the epithelial and vascular changes associated with cervical neoplasia.

CHOICE OF THERAPY FOR PREINVASIVE DISEASE. Treatment is based on the colposcopic impression, histologic evidence of neoplasia, and anatomic location of disease. *The presence of a visible cervical lesion mandates obtaining a cervical biopsy specimen irrespective of cytologic results.*

Preinvasive disease, in general, is treated on an outpatient basis with preservation of fertility by use of such techniques as **cryocauterization, carbon dioxide laser,** or **electrosurgical loop excision** of the cervical transformation zone. The last involves that portion of the cervix that has undergone squamous metaplasia, which is the area evaluated by colposcopic examination and the site of origin of 80% to 90% of cervical neoplasia.

Management

Staging

Overview. Cervical cancer is staged clinically according to the tumor-staging system developed by the International Federation of Gynecology and Obstetrics (FIGO) (see box, on the following page). The initial evaluation as described earlier in this chapter should include a complete history and physical examination. For the purposes of staging, the clinician should order routine blood testing (CBC electrolytes, liver and kidney function tests), a chest radiograph, and an intravenous pyelogram. Skeletal radiographs and barium enema sometimes are clinically indicated, but they are not required for the staging of most tumors. A complete pelvic examination generally is performed with the patient under anesthesia at the time of cystoscopic and proctoscopic evaluation. Additional diagnostic tests such as a lymphangiogram, bone scan, computed tomography (CT) scan, and magnetic resonance imaging (MRI) may be useful for treatment planning. However, any additional information gained from these tests beyond that already acquired from the routine radiologic tests indicated earlier is not to be used in assignment of stage.

Staging system. In summary, *stage I* disease is confined to the cervix, *stage II* extends beyond the cervix but not to the pelvic sidewall or lower third of the vagina, *stage III* involves the pelvic sidewall or lower third of the vagina, and *stage IV* demonstrates spread beyond the pelvis or involvement of the mucosa of the bladder or rectum.

Choices of therapy. The treatment of cervical cancer depends on the stage of disease (Table 65-3).

Stage Ia (microinvasive disease). In the United States the Society of Gynecologic Oncologists has defined *microinvasive disease* as less than 3 mm of invasion into the cervical stroma and without evidence of lymphatic or vascular space invasion. This diagnosis corresponds to FIGO stage Ia, and patients can be treated with simple hysterectomy, performed

Table 65-1 Classification of Pap smear results

Original Pap system	Modern modification	Bethesda system
Class I: normal finding	Normal	No evidence of malignant cells
Class II: slightly suspicious for malignant lesion	Atypical cells present below the level of cervical neoplasia	Atypical cells of undetermined significance
Class III: moderately suspicious for (SIL), malignant lesion	Smear contains cells consistent with Intraepithelial neoplasia (CIN grade 1-3)	Squamous intraepithelial lesion (SIL), Low-grade: CIN 1 or changes of HPV
Class IV: highly suspicious for malignant lesion	Smear contains cells consistent with carcinoma in situ	Squamous intraepithelial lesion, high-grade, CIN 2 or 3
Class V: diagnosis consistent with malignant lesion	Smear contains cells consistent with invasive cancer	Smear consistent with invasion

CIN, cervical intraepithelial neoplasia; HPV, human papillomavirus; SIL, squamous intraepithelial lesion.

Table 65-2 Follow-up of abnormal Pap smear results

Pap smear result	Recommendation for follow-up
Negative for malignant cells	See guidelines for routine findings on Pap smear
No endocervical cells	If high risk, repeat within 1 mo If low risk, repeat at annual checkup Use cervical brush technique for improved sampling
Squamous metaplasia	Normal result
Atypia	Consider treatment for underlying infection Repeat in 3-4 mo unless positive for HIV If HIV-positive, refer directly for colposcopic examination If atypia still present, refer for colposcopic examination
Dysplasia	Refer for colposcopic examination

either abdominally or vaginally. These patients are believed to be at such minimal risk for parametrial or lymph node involvement that the additional morbidity of radical surgery and/or radiation therapy is not justified.

Stages Ib and IIa. These types of cancer may be treated either by radical hysterectomy with bilateral pelvic lymph node dissection or by radiation therapy.

RADICAL HYSTERECTOMY. Radical hysterectomy is a surgical technique that has little changed in the last 100 years. It involves resection of the uterus and cervix, their supporting elements (cardinal and uterosacral ligaments), the upper 2 to 3 cm of the vagina, and the regional lymph nodes in the pelvis and common iliac regions. The surgical approach has the advantage of preserving ovarian function in the younger patient, and it is associated with less postoperative sexual dysfunction than radiation therapy, which frequently is associated with vaginal fibrosis and stenosis. Vaginal dilators are prescribed by many centers, after radiation therapy to minimize these sequelae. A history of pelvic inflammatory disease or inflammatory bowel disease favors the surgical approach, thus avoiding the potential complications of radiation injury to the small bowel that may be fixed in the pelvis by adhesions.

RADIATION THERAPY. Radiation therapy is the conventional and highly efficacious treatment for patients with more advanced disease or in patients with early-stage disease who are not considered optimal candidates for the surgical approach because of excessive tumor size, coexisting medical illness, or obesity. Radiation therapy for cervical cancer involves a combination of external-beam therapy usually delivered to the entire pelvis by linear accelerators, followed by brachytherapy techniques with tandem and ovoids, or, on occasion, interstitial needles. The ability to cure a high percentage of patients with cervical cancer with radiation therapy is contingent on this latter aspect of therapy (brachytherapy), which permits safe administration of doses to the cervix and vagina in excess of 10,000 cGy while minimizing the amount of radiation to the more radiation-sensitive adjacent bladder and rectum.

Inoperable or metastatic disease

CHEMOTHERAPY. Chemotherapy usually has been reserved for patients with metastatic or recurrent disease. Active agents, commonly used in combination, include cisplatin,

FIGO STAGING SYSTEM FOR CANCER OF THE CERVIX

Stage I	Cancer confined to the cervix.
Stage Ia	Preclinical cancers that are diagnosed by use of microscopy.
Stage Ia1	Minimal microscopic evidence of stromal invasion.
Stage Ia2	Lesions detected microscopically that can be measured. Depth of invasion not more than 5 mm from the base of the epithelium from which it originates. Lateral spread not greater than 7 mm.
Stage Ib	Lesions of greater dimension than stage Ia2, whether seen clinically or not. Lymphatic or capillary space invasion does not alter stage but should be recorded for future reference.
Stage II	Cancer extension to the upper two thirds of the vagina or to the parametria, but not involving pelvic sidewall.
Stage IIa	No extension to the parametria.
Stage IIb	Extension to the parametria but not extending to the pelvic sidewall.
Stage III	Cancer extension to the lower third of the vagina or extension to the pelvic sidewall. Hydronephrosis or nonfunctioning kidney is automatic allotment to stage IIIb.
Stage IIIa	No extension to the pelvic sidewall.
Stage IIIb	Extension to pelvic sidewall, or hydronephrosis/nonfunctioning kidney.
Stage IV	Involvement of adjacent organs (bladder or rectum) or distant spread.
Stage IVa	Involvement of rectal or bladder mucosa.
Stage IVb	Distant metastases.

FIGO, International Federation of Gynecology and Obstetrics.

bleomycin, vincristine, 5-fluorouracil (5-FU), and ifosfamide. Although response rates ranging from 50% to 80% are routinely reported with combination therapy, durations of response are short, with survival benefits of 1 year or less for those patients who respond to treatment. Recently, combination therapy given initially or in a neoadjuvant fashion

Table 65-3 Treatment recommendations and survival for cervical cancer

Stage	Recommended treatment	Survival
Ia	Conservative hysterectomy*	99%
Ib-IIa	Radical hysterectomy and node dissection or radiation therapy	65-80%
IIb	Radiation therapy	50-60%
IIIa and b	Radiation therapy	30-35%
IVa	Radiation therapy or supraradical surgery	10-15%
IVb, inoperable metastatic	Chemotherapy or palliative radiation therapy	<10%

*May require more extensive treatment for some patients with Ia2 disease.

has been used in an attempt to obtain tumor shrinkage, thereby rendering some tumors surgically resectable or improving the ability of radiation therapy to achieve tumor control.

Prognosis, survival, and follow-up

Stage and tumor size are the most important clinical prognostic factors. Within each stage category, after correction for lesion volume, nodal status takes precedence as the most important prognostic factor. In stages IB and IIA disease, the survival of patients without involvement of the pelvic nodes is in excess of 85% at 5 years in contrast to 50% in patients with disease metastatic to these regional nodes. Worldwide survival rates for cervical carcinoma are as follows: stage I, 78%; stage II, 57%; stage III, 31%; and stage IV, 8%.

Patients usually are seen at 3-month intervals the first year after treatment, every 4 months the second year, at 6-month intervals to the 5-year mark, and thereafter at annual examinations. Sites at risk for recurrent disease include bone, lung, brain, upper portion of the abdomen, and the para-aortic lymph nodes, although in most recurrences the pelvis is the site affected. Risk of recurrence is directly related to stage of disease. Follow-up visits should include examinations of the supraclavicular and nodal regions of the groin, abdomen, and pelvis. A Pap smear is obtained at each visit. For all patients, radiologic studies should include a CT scan of the abdomen and pelvis and a chest radiograph at the 1-year mark. Further radiologic testing may be performed at the discretion of the treating clinician, usually involving annual CT scanning and chest radiographs for an additional 1 to 5 years. During the follow-up period for this and for other gynecologic malignancies, primary care issues and other cancer and noncancer-related screening procedures are recommended, such as mammography, blood pressure monitoring, and serum lipid screening. Patients usually are questioned regarding smoking habits and counseled accordingly (see Chapter 73).

ENDOMETRIAL CANCER
Epidemiology and risk factors

In the United States, endometrial cancer is the most common malignant disease of the female genital tract. It is estimated that 32,000 new cases of endometrial cancer were diagnosed in 1992, resulting in 5600 deaths. A woman's lifetime risk of developing endometrial cancer is 2% to 3%. This risk is modified by a history of early menarche, late menopause, nulliparity, obesity, anovulation, liver disease, or the use of unopposed exogenous estrogens (see box, above right). In contrast, high parity, smoking, and the use of oral contraceptives are associated with a decreased risk. This is a disease primarily of postmenopausal patients with the average age at diagnosis being 61 years. Hypertension and diabetes mellitus also are positively associated but may not be independent risk factors after correction for obesity. Women previously diagnosed with ovarian or breast cancer also are considered a high-risk group.

Pathophysiology

The pathophysiology of the epidemiologic factors is related to chronic unopposed estrogen stimulation of the endometrium that may result from increased production (estrogen-secreting tumors or obesity via increased peripheral conver-

RISK FACTOR FOR ENDOMETRIAL CANCER	
Early menarche	Liver disease
Late menopause	Use of unopposed estrogens
Nulliparity	Hypertension?
Obesity	Diabetes?
Anovulation	

sion of androstenedione to estrone by the aromatase reaction in adipose cells), decreased degradation (liver disease), or exogenous sources. The risk of developing endometrial cancer triples for those women who are 21 to 50 pounds overweight and is 10 times higher for those who are more than 50 pounds overweight. Conditions associated with anovulation also favor an estrogenic environment inasmuch as the ovarian theca cells are not stimulated to produce progesterone.

Clinical presentation

History and symptoms. The most common symptom of endometrial cancer is abnormal vaginal bleeding: postmenopausal bleeding, menorrhagia, intermenstrual, or postcoital bleeding (see box, below). In most patients, postmenopausal bleeding is the symptom most commonly associated with this disease. A watery vaginal discharge occasionally may be present. Pain is a somewhat uncommon presenting symptom, usually signifying either advanced disease or cervical stenosis, with resultant pyometra or hematometra. In rare cases, lower-extremity deep venous thrombosis is the only presenting symptom, in which initiation of heparin therapy uncovers an otherwise occult endometrial cancer.

Physical examination. Results of the physical examination may be normal in patients with endometrial cancer. The assessment should include documentation of height, weight, and blood pressure. The superficial lymph nodes (supraclavicular, axillary, and inguinal) must be palpated. Abdominal examination may reveal ascites, or it may show omental or hepatic metastases. The pelvic examination should include inspection and palpation of the vulva, vagina, and cervix to identify metastases and exclude other sources of bleeding. Bimanual and rectovaginal examination should assess uterine size, mobility, and the presence of adnexal or pelvic masses. A Pap smear should be obtained using a spatula on the ectocervix and a cytologic brush to sample the endocervical canal. A stool specimen should be tested for occult blood.

Diagnostic tests

Endometrial biopsy and dilation and curettage. The diagnosis of endometrial carcinoma must be established histologically with endometrial sampling obtained either by office endometrial biopsy or formal dilation and curettage

SYMPTOMS OF ENDOMETRIAL CANCER	
Abnormal vaginal bleeding	Vaginal discharge
Postmenopausal bleeding	Pelvic mass
Menorrhagia	Pain
Intermenstrual bleeding	
Postcoital bleeding	

(D&C) in patients with symptoms that suggest endometrial neoplasia: any abnormal vaginal bleeding, spotting, or staining. *It is the clinician's obligation to rule out endometrial cancer in all patients with these complaints.* D&C generally is reserved for patients in whom a biopsy cannot be obtained adequately in the office or in whom symptoms persist after negative biopsy results. Risks associated with either of these techniques include infection, uterine perforation, and patient discomfort; thus sampling is done for evaluation of symptoms and not as a screening technique.

Screening. There is currently no acceptable screening method to detect preclinical endometrial cancer. Pap smears are associated with an unacceptably high incidence of false-negative results in the presence of endometrial cancer—in excess of 80% in some reports. *Normal results of the Pap smear and pelvic examination cannot be relied on to rule out the presence of endometrial neoplasia.* The presence of either **atypical** or **normal endometrial cells** on a Pap smear in a menopausal patient is decidedly abnormal and warrants endometrial biopsy; Zucker, Kasdon, and Feldstein reported that about 20% of these patients will have endometrial pathology ranging from hyperplasia to polyp formation to carcinoma. Endometrial biopsy may be offered as a screening test to the patient at high risk (obese, diabetic, hypertensive) who understands the aforementioned risks. Preliminary reports in the literature advocate the use of vaginal probe ultrasound to facilitate selection of patients for endometrial biopsy on the basis of the appearance of the endometrial stripe. It must be emphasized that ultrasound evaluation adds to the cost and cannot be considered a substitute for a histologic diagnosis. The American College of Obstetricians and Gynecologists currently does not recommend routine screening of patients for this disease given the drawbacks of the screening techniques available and similarly does not support routine sampling of the endometrium before the initiation of hormone replacement therapy.

Management

Staging. In 1988 the International Federation of Gynecology and Obstetrics revised the staging of uterine cancer from clinical to surgical/pathologic (see box, above right), supporting the importance of early laparotomy in the management and evaluation of these patients.

Once the diagnosis of endometrial carcinoma is established by endometrial sampling, a preoperative assessment is performed, which should include a complete history and physical examination with special attention on the pelvic examination to possible sites of spread. In addition, a CBC is included in routine blood testing, and renal and liver chemistry and electrolyte levels are obtained, as well as a urinalysis, electrocardiogram (ECG), and a chest radiograph. This last test is helpful not only in assessing the patient's general medical state but in evaluating a common site of metastatic disease.

Preoperative radiotherapy. In the past after this pretreatment evaluation, most patients underwent radiation therapy, followed by exploration and hysterectomy. Although this sequence was widely employed, there were no data suggesting that the routine use of preoperative radiotherapy had a positive impact on survival. The Gynecologic Oncology Group developed protocols to study the natural history of this disease and the role of surgical/pathologic staging; the resul-

FIGO STAGING SYSTEM FOR CORPUS CANCER

Stage Ia Tumor limited to endometrium.
Stage Ib Invasion to less than one half the myometrium.
Stage Ic Invasion to greater than or equal to one half the myometrum.
Stage IIa Endocervical glandular involvement.
Stage IIb Cervical stromal invasion.
Stage IIIa Tumor involves serosa and/or adnexa, and/or positive peritoneal cytology.
Stage IIIb Vaginal metastases.
Stage IIIc Metastases to pelvic and/or paraaortic nodes.
Stage IVa Tumor invasion of bladder and/or bowel mucosa.
Stage IVb Distant metastases, including intraabdominal and/or inguinal nodes.

Notes to staging system
1. All cases are stratified by Grades 1, 2, and 3 on the basis of architectural pattern. Grade 1:5% or less of a nonsquamous or nonmorular solid growth pattern. Grade 2:6% to 50% of a nonsquamous or nonmorular growth pattern. Grade 3: more than 50% of a nonsquamous or nonmorular solid growth pattern.
2. Notable nuclear atypia, inappropriate for the architectural grade, raises the grade of a grade 1 or 2 tumor by 1.
3. Adenocarcinomas with squamous differentiation are graded according to the nuclear grade of the glandular component.
4. Patients treated primarily with radiation therapy should be staged by the FIGO clinical staging system of 1971.

tant data have greatly enhanced our understanding of this disease and the importance of surgical staging in tailoring treatment to the individual patient.

These studies have substantiated that tumor grade, depth of myometrial invasion, extrauterine disease, positive peritoneal cytologic findings and pelvic/paraaortic node metastasis—all of which cannot be reliably determined preoperatively—have prognostic significance that enables individualization of postoperative therapy.

Exploratory surgery and hysterectomy. Exploration, which is the initial step in the therapy of patients with endometrial cancer, usually is performed through a midline incision. Washings are obtained on entry, followed by a complete abdominal and pelvic exploration, with special attention to the liver, diaphragmatic surfaces, pelvic and paraaortic nodal areas, parametria, and adnexa. Total hysterectomy and bilateral salpingo-oophorectomy are performed. The uterus, which is opened intraoperatively, allows an assessment of myometrial invasion. Patients with high-grade tumors or deep myometrial invasion, or both, undergo nodal sampling. A small omental biopsy specimen may be obtained to complete operative staging. Stage assignment is made after pathologic evaluation of resected tissues.

Choice of therapy

Stage I. Most patients with endometrial cancer have stage I disease. The decision to administer postoperative radiation therapy is based on analysis of tumor grade and depth of myometrial invasion. Patients with low-grade disease or minimal myometrium invasion, or both, are at low risk for recurrence and require no adjuvant therapy. Patients with higher-grade disease or more extensive involvement of the myometrium receive whole-pelvis radiation therapy, which has been shown to decrease the risk of pelvic recurrence but has not demonstrated a clear survival advantage. Patients who fall into an intermediate risk category may receive postoperative vaginal radium or cesium therapy, which minimizes dose to the bladder and rectum, thus virtually eliminating side effects and, at the same time, minimizing the risk of vaginal apex recurrence. (See Table 65-4).

Stage II. Patients with stage II disease are considered to be at high risk (30% to 40%) for pelvic nodal involvement and pelvic recurrence. In general these patients are treated with postoperative pelvic radiation therapy.

Stage III. Patients with more extensive disease are generally treated with postoperative radiation therapy tailored to the sites of known disease and areas believed to be at high risk for recurrence. Patients with pelvic or paraaortic nodal spread are treated with pelvic or extended-field radiation therapy, respectively. Patients with evidence of peritoneal involvement may be considered candidates for whole abdominal radiation therapy.

Stage IV and recurrent disease. Patients with disease not amenable to surgical resection or radiotherapy require systemic therapy. Progestational agents, which reverse estrogen's trophic effects on the endometrium, have been used with response rates ranging from 10% to 30%. Higher response rates have been associated with increased differentiation and the presence of progesterone receptors. Poorly differentiated tumors in general do not respond to hormonal manipulation and require cytotoxic chemotherapy. Active agents include cisplatin, doxorubicin (Adriamycin), cyclophosphamide, and 5-fluorouracil (5-FU). Reported response rates for combined therapy range from 25% to 60%, with only modest impact on survival because of relatively short durations of response.

Prognosis, survival, and follow-up. The reported survival rates employing the FIGO clinical staging system of 1971 are 85% for stage I, 60% for stage II, 30% for stage III, and 10% for stage IV. Follow-up is as yet too short to report the incidence of 5-year survival based on the revised FIGO surgical pathologic staging system.

The posttreatment follow-up of patients very much depends on the extent of disease noted initially. In general,

all patients are seen at 3- to 4-month intervals the first year. Patients at low risk (stage I, well- or moderately well-differentiated tumors, minimal invasion) may then be seen at 3- to 6-month intervals until the 5-year mark is reached and annually thereafter. Patients at higher risk (deep invasion, poorly differentiated, advanced-stage disease) usually are seen at 3- to 4-month intervals for several years, then at 6-month intervals to the 5-year mark. In general, patients fitting into this last category are seen by the operating clinician or primary care provider and by a radiation or medical oncologist or both. These visits should include examinations of the supraclavicular and groin node regions, the abdomen, and pelvis. A Pap smear is performed at each visit. Major sites of recurrence include the pelvis, bone, brain, upper portion of the abdomen, and the lung, with the last representing the most common extrapelvic site. Again, radiologic testing should be based on risk. The patient at high risk as already defined, should undergo CT scanning and chest radiography annually to the 5-year mark. Patients at low risk for recurrence may have scans less frequently at the discretion of the treating physicians.

OVARIAN CANCER
Epidemiology

Cancer of the ovary is the second most common gynecologic malignant disease after cancer of the endometrium; however, it accounts for more deaths than the other gynecologic cancers combined. Overall, 1 in 70 women will develop ovarian cancer during her lifetime, with 24,000 new cases expected in 1994 in the United States. The incidence increases with age, from 1.4/100,000 in women younger than 40 years of age to 38/100,000 women older than 60 years of age, with a peak incidence at age 59 years. This disease is more commonly seen in the industrialized and developed countries, and it is more common in Caucasian than in African-American women.

Risk factors

Definite etiologic factors have not been identified; however, several risk factors have been proposed (see box, below). Women of low parity, decreased fertility, and late menopause are believed to be at higher risk. These factors apparently relate to incessant ovulation with its associated capsular rupture and inflammation of repair. Other factors increasing one's risk include a family history of ovarian, breast, or colon cancer, the use of talc on the perineum, and subclinical mumps before menarche. A study by Cramer and colleagues implicated a diet high in animal fat to be a risk factor as well.

Table 65-4 Treatment recommendations and survival in patients with uterine cancer

Stage	Recommended treatment	Survival (%)
I	Hysterectomy with or without radiation	85%
II	Hysterectomy and postoperative radiation	60%
III	Postoperative radiation Extended field radiation or ? whole abdominal radiation	30%
IV and metastatic disease	Progestational agents Chemotherapy: cisplatin, doxorubicin (Adriamycin), cyclophosphamide, 5-fluorouracil (5-FU)	10%

RISK FACTORS FOR OVARIAN CANCER

Low parity
Decreased fertility
Late menopause
Family history of ovarian, breast, or colon cancer
Use of talc on perineum
Subclinical mumps before menarche
Diet high in animal fat

Multiparity and the use of oral contraceptives appear to have a protective effect, believed to result from their association with decreased ovulatory events. A study from the Centers for Disease Control concluded that the use of the pill may decrease the lifetime risk of ovarian cancer by as much as 50%, and that this effect increases with duration of use and persists for several years after discontinuance. The use of oral contraceptives is the recommended birth control method for women at high risk for the development of ovarian cancer.

Tremendous attention recently has been given to the familial incidence of ovarian cancer, in part because of the recent death of the popular comedienne, Gilda Radner. Piver and colleagues reported that patients with one second-degree or one first-degree relative are believed to be at approximately two or four times the risk, respectively, of patients without a family history. Several studies have shown that women with multiple affected relatives are at substantially greater risk, perhaps as high as 50%, of developing ovarian cancer in their lifetime, with a tendency for the disease to occur at a much earlier age. As a result of these sorts of data, prophylactic oophorectomy has been advocated in patients with more than one first-degree relative affected. This usually is performed at completion of childbearing—optimally by age 35 years given the nature of familial ovarian cancer to occur at an early age.

Clinical presentation

History and symptoms. The high proportion of deaths that occur relative to the number of new cases is ascribed to a late presentation, early metastases, and ineffective screening. Typically the patient first consults a health care provider (frequently an internist or a family practitioner) complaining of vague abdominal pain or pressure, early satiety, anorexia, or dyspepsia, usually of about 4 to 6 weeks' duration. Nausea, vomiting, constipation, or increasing abdominal girth also may be described. With this constellation of findings the diagnosis of ovarian cancer must be considered, as well as primary gastrointestinal disease. It is not unusual for the patient to be totally asymptomatic at the time of consultation except for this latter complaint, or a mass may have been detected on routine pelvic examination or ultrasound study. At the time of diagnosis disease is confined to the ovaries in only 20% of cases.

Physical examination. Pertinent physical findings include a palpable abdominal or pelvic mass, often associated with nodularity in the cul de sac or a distended abdomen suggestive of bowel obstruction or ascites. Pleural effusion, supraclavicular or inguinal adenopathy, or an umbilical mass (**Sister Mary's** or **Sister Mary Joseph's nodule**) may be present. When the diagnosis of ovarian cancer is suspected, a careful physical examination with attention to these areas is mandatory. Although cervical cytologic findings obtained on speculum examination rarely contribute to the diagnosis of ovarian cancer per se, this assessment is essential to the complete gynecologic evaluation and of course may detect associated cervical, and on occasion, endometrial disease.

Diagnostic tests

Screening. There is currently no recommended or proved efficacious screening method for the detection of early ovarian cancer. Reports of the use of CA-125 serum testing,

transabdominal ultrasound, transvaginal ultrasound, and color Doppler flow analysis by means of vaginal sonography are appearing in the literature with increasing frequency. Although these tests have the ability to detect an early ovarian tumor, screening programs based on these studies are plagued by tremendous numbers of false-positive results, and thus low positive predictive values. The role of these sorts of testing regimens for the patient at high risk (patients with family history of ovarian cancer) is currently under study at a variety of centers worldwide.

Approach to the patient with a palpable adnexal mass. The approach varies according to the woman's age and reproductive status, as well as associated signs and symptoms (for a more in-depth discussion see Chapter 37). An ultrasound should be obtained to confirm the presence of and to help localize and characterize the mass. Within the reproductive age-group, most masses less than 7 to 8 cm in size are followed for one to two cycles with serial pelvic and ultrasound examinations to permit resolution of functional cysts that are so common in this age-group. Persistent masses, larger masses, other conditions that suggest malignancy, or associated symptoms requiring urgent surgery usually necessitate laparotomy. Because of the suppressive effects of oral contraceptives, patients on this regimen rarely have functional cysts, although occasional ovulatory events can occur with the lower-dose pills. This factor must be considered in evaluating patients who use this form of birth control. The clinician would have more cause to proceed to laparoscopy if a younger women taking oral contraceptive pills (OCPs) has a suspicious mass inasmuch as the likelihood of a functional cyst is extremely low. *In the prepubertal patient, and in women older than 40 years of age, an ovarian mass must be considered cancer until proved otherwise.* The exceptions to this rule include the small unilocular cyst, less than 5 cm in diameter, and unchanged in size over several examinations in the asymptomatic patient with an otherwise benign physical examination or the cysts found in the female neonate, which usually represent follicular stimulation from circulating placental human chorionic gonadotropin (hCG).

Exploratory laparotomy. Diagnosis of ovarian cancer requires histologic confirmation usually obtained at exploratory laparotomy. The inherent inability to diagnose this disease early and the impossibility of staging this condition clinically have lead to a surgical pathologic staging system as shown in the box, on the following page. Preoperative evaluation is undertaken in an attempt to support the presence of an ovarian primary that would require exploration, to rule out the presence of another primary that might obviate the need for surgery, to evaluate the general medical state of the patient who is likely to undergo exploration and cytoreductive surgery, and finally to help define surgical anatomy. This evaluation usually includes blood testing (CBC, SMAC-20, baseline CA-125, coagulation studies) urinalysis, ECG, chest radiograph, and CT scan of abdomen and pelvis. The CT scan helps define pelvic anatomy, the presence or absence of ureteral compromise, the status of lymph nodes and liver parenchyma, and the presence of ascites. Barium studies of the upper or lower gastrointestinal (GI) tracts, or both, may be performed for evaluation of severe symptoms arising from these areas. Generally they are not required inasmuch as formal bowel preparation is a

STAGING SYSTEM FOR CANCER OF THE OVARY

Stage I	Growth limited to the ovaries.
Stage Ia	Growth limited to one ovary, no ascites, washings negative, capsule intact, no tumor on the external surface.
Stage Ib	Growth limited to both ovaries, no ascites, washings negative, capsule intact, no tumor on the external surface.
Stage Ic	Tumor either stage Ia or Ib but with surface tumor, capsule rupture, or ascites or washings cytologically positive for cancer cells.
Stage II	Growth involving one or both ovaries with pelvic extension.
Stage IIa	Tumor extension to internal genitalia. No ascites, washings negative, ovarian capsules intact, no tumor on ovarian surfaces.
Stage IIb	Tumor extension to other pelvic structures. No ascites, washings negative, ovarian capsules intact, no tumor on ovarian surfaces.
Stage IIc	Tumor either Stage IIa or IIb but with surface tumor or capsule rupture, or ascites or washings cytologically positive for cancer cells.
Stage III	Tumor involving one or both ovaries with peritoneal implants outside the pelvis and/or positive retroperitoneal or inguinal nodes. Superficial liver metastases qualifies as stage III.
Stage IIIa	Tumor grossly limited to true pelvis, nodes negative, but with histologically confirmed microscopic seeding to abdominal peritoneal surfaces.
Stage IIIb	Tumor of one or both ovaries, nodes negative, with histologically confirmed implants of abdominal peritoneal surfaces, none exceeding 2 cm in diameter.
Stage IIIc	Abdominal implants greater than 2 cm and/or positive retroperitoneal or inguinal nodes.
Stage IV	Tumor extension beyond the peritoneal cavity. Cytologic evidence of a pleural effusion is required for assignment to stage IV. Intraparenchymal liver metastases.

procedural element in virtually all patients with a tentative diagnosis of ovarian cancer, thereby permitting resection of the GI tract if so required at exploration.

Pathology

Embryologic cell type of origin. It is useful to think of the classification of ovarian tumors in terms of embryologic cell type of origin (see box on the following page) **Epithelial ovarian tumors**, which account for 70% of all ovarian tumors and 90% of the cancers, arise from the ovarian capsular epithelium, itself derived from the coelomic epithelium. **Sex cord stromal tumors** arise from mesenchymal tissues and account for 5% of ovarian tumors and a similar percentage of the cancers. **Germ cell tumors** account for 25% of the tumors and perhaps 5% of the cancers. These percentages relate to patients in the adult population. In the pediatric population, epithelial ovarian tumors are less common, with germ cell tumors taking precedence.

Epithelial tumors are by far the most common. These can be divided into benign (**adenoma**), borderline malignant (**low malignant potential**), and frankly malignant (**adenocarcinoma**) lesions. Within these breakdowns are five histologic subtypes, each recapitulating a cell type found within the female genital tract, the lining of which is similarly derived from the embryonic coelom. **Serous lesions**, which resemble fallopian tube epithelium, account for the major portion of the total. **Mucinous tumors** resemble endocervical epithelium and account for 15% to 25% of the total. **Endometrioid tumors** of course are histologically similar to endometrium and constitute 15% to 20%. **Brenner tumors**, which consist of tissue that resembles transitional cell epithelium of the urinary tract, are relatively uncommon, accounting for perhaps 2% to 3% of the total. **Clear cell carcinoma** and undifferentiated carinomas make up the remaining 5% to 10%.

Natural history based on cell type. Benign epithelial ovarian tumors (cystadenomas or cystadenofibromas) tend to arise in any age-group and actually may grow to astounding size. Symptoms are related primarily to tumor size, not to specific histologic subtype, with resulting pressure on adjacent structures, or they may be caused by rupture, torsion, or hemorrhage, which may be associated with any ovarian mass. Treatment is surgical resection, with cure rates of 100% expected. These tumors require no adjuvant therapy. On rare occasions, mucinous cystadenomas may be associated with the later development of pseudomyxoma peritonei. Borderline ovarian cancers or ovarian cystadenomas of low malignant potential encompass an unusual type of ovarian neoplasm, histologically arising from any of the specified subtypes, which carries a prognosis significantly better than ovarian epithelial carcinomas but which still may recur and result in the patient's death. In general, these tumors are treated surgically with no evidence that adjuvant chemotherapy or radiation therapy is of any benefit. A discussion of these tumors is beyond the scope of this review, and the reader is referred to any gynecologic oncology text for more information. The remainder of this discussion focuses on epithelial ovarian carcinomas. In general, from a surgical and medical standpoint the management is the same regardless of histologic subtype.

Management

Surgical staging. After preoperative evaluation, patients undergo surgical exploration to establish the diagnosis, stage the disease, and permit surgical cytoreduction. This usually is performed through a midline incision that allows adequate exploration of the upper portion of the abdomen. If ascites is present, a sample is collected for cytologic evaluation. If there is no ascites, saline is instilled into the peritoneal cavity, then collected and sent for cytologic evaluation (washings). All peritoneal surfaces are visualized or palpated, with special attention to the omentum, appendix, liver, undersurfaces of the diaphragm, large and small bowel serosa and mesenteries, and the draining lymphatics in the pelvis and paraaortic areas. Appropriate biopsy specimens are obtained, with stage assigned per the FIGO staging system noted in the box above left.

Patients with disease apparently limited to the ovary usually undergo resection of the uterus, tubes, and ovaries, as well

PATHOLOGY OF TUMOR

Embryologic cell type of origin

Epithelial ovarian tumors: 70%

Types:

Adenoma
Low malignant potential
Adenocarcinoma

Further histologic classification:

Serous
Mucinous
Endometroid
Brenner
Clear cell and undifferentiated

Sex cord stromal tumors: 5%

Types of Granulosa cell

Thecoma
Fibroma
Sarcomas

Other types: Lymphoproliferative: 5%

Germ cell tumors: 20%

Types:

Teratoma
Dysgerminoma
Endodermal sinus tumor
Choriocarcinoma

---

as a staging procedure to identify occult spread. This includes washings, omental biopsy, random peritoneal biopsies, and lymph node sampling from the pelvic and paraaortic areas. Appendectomy has been recommended as part of the staging procedure inasmuch as this area may be involved occultly, and its resection carries virtually no additional morbidity. Patients who wish to maintain fertility may be treated in a conservative fashion with unilateral salpingo-oophorectomy and staging, thereby preserving the contralateral ovary, tube, and uterus for childbearing. Patients in whom more extensive disease is found after pathologic evaluation of the staging material may require reoperation to complete the resection. Thus a conservative approach is recommended only for the younger patient who understands the risks of this conservative approach. According to multiple studies, including one by Young and colleagues, patients proven to have disease confined to the ovaries, with grade 1 or 2 lesions, require no additional therapy, with survival in excess of 95% reported at 5 years. All other patients require adjuvant therapy.

Surgical cytoreduction. Patients with evidence of metastatic spread undergo surgical cytoreduction in an attempt to minimize residual disease. This procedure usually includes total hysterectomy, bilateral salpingo-oophorectomy, and omentectomy with gastrointestinal or urinary tract resection occasionally performed when resection of these areas will aid in achieving optimal cytoreduction, usually defined as the largest remaining nodule of disease not exceeding 2 cm in diameter. Multiple reports by Hacker and others suggest a higher response rate and improved survival in patients who have undergone optimal cytoreduction.

Chemotherapy and radiation. Except for the few patients with stage Ia or Ib—well- or moderately well-differentiated (grade 1 or 2) disease—virtually all patients are treated in an adjuvant fashion with chemotherapy or in certain circumstances with whole-abdomen radiotherapy. The latter technique is just as effective as chemotherapy in selected patients but is routinely employed only in a handful of centers. Treatment usually consists of combination chemotherapy employing either cisplatin or its analog carboplatin. The latter drug carries far less GI, renal, and neurologic toxicity, thereby permitting outpatient administration. The combination of carboplatin and cyclophosphamide administered for six cycles currently is the standard regimen in most centers, although Taxol has been moved up front in some centers.

Second-look surgery. It is extremely difficult to assess the status of disease in patients with ovarian cancer for the same reasons that patients tend to present to the physician with late-stage disease—lack of symptoms with minimal disease. CT scans, ultrasonographic and physical examination, and the use of serum markers, are not accurate enough to detect which patients have minimal disease at the completion of first-line chemotherapy. Thus second-look surgery was performed routinely for many years to evaluate the response to therapy, to stop treatment in those patients who had received a complete pathologic response, and to allow a change in therapy in unresponsive patients. Given the lack of efficacy of second-line regimens, there is no evidence that routine second-look surgery will affect overall survival. These procedures are, however, extremely helpful in assessing the efficacy of a new drug or combination, because they provide the first hard evidence of response data. With the advent of more effective second-line therapies, routine second-look surgery may again be practiced.

Salvage chemotherapy. Unfortunately, primary therapy is unsuccessful in most patients with epithelial ovarian cancer, thus salvage treatment is required. Current regimens include retreatment with platinum-containing regimens, with response rates in the 50% range attained; however, duration of response tends to be short. Other agents that can be effective in this disease in the salvage setting include hexamethylmelamine, ifosfamide, and Taxol. Taxol has recently gained tremendous press because of its apparent activity in patients resistant to cisplatin. Other techniques such as bone marrow transplantation or peripheral blood stem cell support are in developmental stages for treatment of patients with ovarian cancer.

Prognosis, survival, and follow-up

The overall prognosis for patients with ovarian cancer has little changed in the last 50 years in spite of the tremendous advances in the fields of gynecologic oncology, radiation therapy, chemotherapy and in other areas (Table 65-5). The major problem, as noted earlier, is stage distribution, with most patients diagnosed with advanced disease at initial presentation. Based on the conclusions of many studies, it is generally accepted that patients with disease confined to the ovary (stage Ia or Ib Grade 1 or 2) require no adjuvant chemotherapy, with survival in excess of 95% expected. Patients with high-risk stage I disease (Ic or Grade 3) usually are treated with adjuvant chemotherapy with survival in

Table 65-5 Treatment recommendations and survival in patients with ovarian cancer

Stage	Recommended treatment	Survival (5 yr)
Ia or Ib, grade 1 or 2	USO or TAH BSO Staging	95%
IC; Ia or Ib, grade 3	USO or TAH BSO Staging Chemotherapy	80%
II	TAH BSO Staging Cytoreduction Chemotherapy	50-70%
III	TAH BSO Staging Cytoreduction Chemotherapy Second look	20-30%
IV	Variable	3%

USO, unilateral salpingo-oophorectomy; TAH, total abdominal hysterectomy; BSO, bilateral salpingo-oophorectomy.

excess of 80% anticipated at 5 years. Survival falls off sharply with more advanced disease, in part based on the adequacy of surgical cytoreduction. Five-year survival rates of 50% to 60% and 20% to 30% may be anticipated for stages II and III disease, respectively.

Patients with ovarian cancer are considered at high risk for recurrence and generally are followed up very closely after completion of therapy. Office visits at 2- to 3-month intervals for 2 years is fairly standard, with CA-125 testing performed at least this frequently. Thereafter office visits may be scheduled less frequently at 3- to 6-month intervals to the 5-year mark. Less frequent visits may be recommended for the patient at low risk (stage I) at the discretion of the treating clinician. The abdominal cavity remains the site at greatest risk for the development of recurrent disease. CT scanning or ultrasonography at 6-month intervals for 2 to 3 years is commonly employed in the management of these women. Annual scans to the 5-year mark may be considered in the patient at high risk (advanced disease).

VULVAR CANCER
Epidemiology and risk factors
Vulvar cancer accounts for 5% of all gynecologic malignant disease and is the fourth most common cancer of the female genital tract after cancer of the endometrium, ovary, and cervix. The incidence of carcinoma in situ of the vulva is 0.7/100,000 and that of invasive cancer is 1.9/100,000. Preinvasive disease is seen predominantly in younger women whereas invasive carcinoma is predominantly a disease of the postmenopausal woman. Approximately 10% of patients with vulvar neoplasia, either invasive or in situ disease, have a synchronous primary neoplasm elsewhere, usually involving the lower genital tract, specifically the cervix. Patients with immunosuppression, diabetes, hypertension, and chronic vulvar dystrophies appear to be at increased risk for developing vulvar cancer.

Pathophysiology and preinvasive lesions
Suspected preinvasive lesions include a group of epithelial disorders of the vulva, previously termed **hyperplastic dystrophy** and currently referred to as **vulvar intraepithelial**

neoplasia (VIN). These lesions are graded I to III, depending on the proportion of the epithelial thickness involved by the neoplastic changes. In a manner similar to the grading of cervical dysplasia, minimal involvement is graded as VIN I, whereas essentially full-thickness involvement is graded as VIN III. Carcinoma in situ is synonymous with VIN III. The pathophysiologic basis for these disorders remains elusive. It is unclear to what degree chronic vulvovaginitis, metabolic disturbances, nutritional deficiencies, and autoimmune phenomena contribute to the development of dysplastic changes in the vulvar epithelium. Although invasive vulvar carcinoma is primarily a disease of the older patient, VIN is being diagnosed more frequently in younger age groups. This increased frequency appears to coincide with an increase in the frequency of such genital infections as human papillomavirus (HPV) and herpes simplex virus type 2. The younger patients with vulvar neoplasia frequently have lesions that exhibit the histologic changes associated with HPV and have a history of, or current infection with, condyloma whereas patients older than 50 years of age rarely demonstrate these associations.

There is conflicting evidence regarding the premalignant potential of these lesions. The spectrum of change from dysplasia through carcinoma in situ through invasive cancer has not been as well-defined for vulvar disease as for the corresponding lesions in the cervix. Actual rates of progression from VIN to invasive disease have not been established. Estimates range from 2% to 6%, with most reports indicating that progression is probably rare but is more likely to occur in older and immunocompromised patients. As with cervical neoplasia, there is an increased incidence of vulvar neoplasia and what appears to be increased progression from intraepithelial to invasive lesion in women exposed to HIV.

Clinical presentation
History and symptoms. Patients with vulvar neoplasia have pruritus, vulvar burning, pain, discharge, or bleeding. Pruritus is by far the most common complaint of patients with these diseases. Patients with more advanced invasive cancer also may have a mass involving either the vulva or groin, or they may have symptoms referable to involvement of adjacent structures—urethra, vagina, or anus.

Physical examination. Physical examination may reveal white, dark red, ulcerated, raised, warty, or nodular lesions. The labia majora is the most frequent site of a primary lesion, but the labia minora, clitoris, and perineum also must be carefully inspected. Sometimes the lesion is extensive or multifocal, and a site of primary origin is difficult to determine. *Visual examination alone is not adequate to diagnose virtually any vulvar lesion. In all cases definitive diagnosis requires a careful examination and biopsy.*

Diagnostic tests
Importance of biopsy. Long delays in diagnosis occur commonly in patients with persistent symptoms who are treated with a variety of creams and ointments for "vulvar inflammation" when a simple biopsy would confirm the presence of preinvasive or invasive vulvar neoplasia. Even in patients with a gross, ulcerative lesion visually "diagnostic" of cancer, biopsy is mandatory before treatment to rule out other ulcerative vulvar lesions such as Behcet's disease, lymphogranuloma venereum, chancroid, and herpes, any of which may become superinfected and be visually misdiag-

nosed as invasive cancer. Biopsy of all vulvar lesions is mandatory.

In most cases a biopsy specimen can be easily obtained in the office with local anesthesia and a routine dermal punch biopsy instrument. Before biopsy, a complete examination of the vulva is performed, with care taken to evaluate all surfaces and creases. Colposcopic examination may on occasion be helpful. Given the frequent association of other lower genital neoplasias, a Pap smear of the cervix should be taken and a complete pelvic examination completed. The suspicious area is infiltrated with lidocaine (Xylocaine), and the biopsy specimen is obtained with use of a small dermal punch (3 to 5 mm usually is adequate). Hemostasis can be achieved with the local application of silver nitrate or Monsel's solution (ferrous subsulfate), with suture rarely required.

Toluidine blue test. Some clinicians find the use of the toluidine blue test of benefit. Toluidine blue is a nuclear stain that lights up VIN lesions, which by definition contain nuclei in the superficial layers. A 1% aqueous solution of toluidine blue is applied, is allowed to dry, and is followed by application of a 1% solution of acetic acid, which washes away the excess stain. In practice, this test rarely is performed given the satisfactory results obtained by use of colposcopy.

Patients with extensive lesions, marked symptoms, or groin node enlargement should be referred for evaluation to a clinician with experience in dealing with vulvar disease.

Pathology

The most common type of vulvar cancer is squamous cell carcinoma, accounting for approximately 90% of all primary vulvar malignant disease. Basal cell carcinomas, adenocarcinomas (frequently involving Bartholin's gland), melanomas, verrucous carcinomas, sarcomas, and lymphoproliferative disorders account for the remainder. On occasion, an invasive adenocarcinoma arising from an area of Paget's disease of the vulva may be encountered.

Management

Vulvar intraepithelial neoplasia

Goals of management. The goal of treatment for intraepithelial disease (presumed preinvasive disease) is to eradicate the affected area. Clinical decision making in this area has been quite challenging inasmuch as the disease is often multifocal and occasionally quite extensive, and of course the probability of progression to invasive cancer is unknown.

Choice of therapy

5-FLUOROURACIL. Medical management with 5-fluorouracil (Efudex) may be helpful in reducing the size of the affected area; it also may be useful as a suppressive therapy if lesions are not eliminated after resection in patients with underlying immunosuppressive disorders. The clinician needs to counsel the patients extensively regarding the possible burning and ultimately ulceration that may occur with this treatment, but if therapy is regulated on the basis of side effects, a course of therapy usually is well tolerated.

SURGICAL EXCISION. Surgical excision by use of a wide local excision, extending to simple vulvectomy with or without skin graft, may be required for larger lesions. An alternative treatment is use of carbon dioxide laser vaporization. Although associated with more discomfort in the postoperative period, scar formation is minimal and healing usually is completed within 4 weeks. A disadvantage to the

laser approach is the absence of a surgical specimen. The clinician therefore must be comfortable that invasion has been ruled out before laser vaporization. Regardless of the therapy chosen, every effort should be made to obtain the least disfiguring, most cosmetically favorable result to minimize changes in body image and to ensure satisfactory sexual function.

Invasive vulvar carcinoma

Staging. Once a diagnosis of invasive vulvar cancer has been made, a staging evaluation provides data for assignment into the current FIGO staging system as noted in the box below. This system takes into consideration the natural history of vulvar cancer, which spreads primarily by local extension to neighboring structures and by lymphatic drainage to the inguinal and femoral nodes. Subsequently it spreads to the iliac and obturator nodes of the pelvis and then to the higher common iliac and paraaortic chains. Spread of labial lesions in particular tends to be to the ipsilateral lymph nodes. Central lesions—that is, periurethral, perineal, and clitoral lesions— have been seen to spread to contralateral lymphatics as well. Hematogenous spread and metastases to distant sites reflect late disease and are exceedingly rare without evidence of nodal metastases. The prior system was based on lesion size, involvement of adjacent structures, and clinical assessment of the inguinal lymph nodes. Because of the significant error associated with examination of this area, stage is now assigned based on histologic evidence of nodal involvement.

Choice of therapy

SURGICAL RESECTION. The standard procedure for the treatment of invasive disease has been surgical resection, specifically radical vulvectomy with bilateral groin node dissection as described by Taussig and Way in the 1940s. This procedure involves resection of the entirety of the vulva in continuity with the draining regional lymph nodes and bridging skin areas. Survival is excellent. However, the morbidity of the procedure, usually as a result of scarring and wound breakdown, is extensive, especially when one considers that many of these women are diagnosed in the seventh, eighth, or ninth decades of life. Delayed complications include lower-extremity edema secondary to chronic lymphatic obstruction, vaginal stricture or stenosis, and pelvic relaxation with the development of cystocele or rectocele.

FIGO STAGING SYSTEM FOR VULVAR CANCER

Stage I	Lesion less than or equal to 2 cm, confined to the vulva and/or perineum; no evidence of lymph node involvement.
Stage II	Lesion greater than 2 cm, confined to the vulva and/or perineum; no evidence of lymph node involvement.
Stage III	Lesion of any size, extending to the anus and/or lower urethra, and/or unilateral groin node involvement (confirmed histologically).
Stage IVa	Lesion of any size, extending to bladder, rectum, upper urethra, pelvic bones, and/or bilateral groin node involvement (confirmed histologically).
Stage IVb	Distant metastases or pelvic lymph node involvement.

RADICAL HEMIVULVECTOMY. In recent years individualization of treatment has been attempted in an effort to perform the most conservative operation feasible to minimize body image changes and functional morbidity, while at the same time achieving a similar cure rate as seen after formal radical vulvectomy. Radical local excision or radical hemivulvectomy with 2-cm margins about the lesion has a probability of cure as high as for radical vulvectomy, with dramatic decreases in wound breakdown and postoperative morbidity, and with excellent retention of function. In patients with localizing lesions, unilateral groin dissection may be performed, again minimizing surgical morbidity.

In a similar fashion, morbidity may be reduced by eliminating lymph node dissection in patients who do not appear to be at risk for nodal involvement. The disease in this group of women is termed *microinvasive vulvar cancer*, which is treatable by wide local excision alone. This classification has not as yet become part of the FIGO staging system. Patients with lesions less than 2 cm in diameter and with less than 1-mm stromal invasion appear to be at virtually no risk for nodal involvement, and they too may be treated in this more simple fashion. If there is ever a question regarding the need to evaluate the groin nodes, a limited superficial dissection may be combined with wide local excision, with minimal additional morbidity. Metastatic disease in these nodes suggests the need for more extensive resection, and its absence obviates the need for further surgery.

The status of the groin nodes is the major prognostic factor that guides the further management of these patients. In the absence of groin node involvement, the higher nodal chains are virtually never involved; thus treatment is completed and these patients generally do well. Involvement in this area is associated with a high recurrence rate, both in the groin and pelvis, and locally on the vulva as well, in addition to a significant decrement in overall survival. With histologic evidence of groin node involvement, postoperative radiation therapy usually is administered to the affected groin and whole pelvis.

Patients with more advanced disease (exceptionally large tumors or involvement of adjacent organs) not amenable to surgical excision—or in cases in which resection would require rectal or bladder resection with diversion—may undergo a combined modality approach with preoperative radiotherapy and/or chemotherapy to achieve tumor shrinkage and permit more conservative resection.

Prognosis, survival, and follow-up. The prognosis of patients with early diagnosis and tailored therapy is excellent, with survival rates in excess of 80% or 90% to be anticipated with stages I and II disease, respectively. Prognosis clearly is related to lesion size and the status of the regional lymph nodes. The cure rate in early-stage disease in which nodes are not affected exceeds 95% in some series. Survival in stage III disease may fall to 50% and to 10% with stage IV disease (see Table 65-6).

Most patients with vulvar cancer are diagnosed with early-stage disease, obviating the need for extensive radiologic testing in the follow-up period. Most recurrences are noted on the vulva and in the inguinal regions. Thus these areas are carefully examined at all visits, which are recommended at 3-month intervals the first year, then at 3- to 6-month intervals to 5 years, the frequency based on the extent

Table 65-6 Treatment recommendations and survival for patients with vulvar cancer

Stage	Recommended treatment	Survival(%)
I, II	Radical resection, radical local excision; radical hemivulvectomy; radical vulvectomy with groin node dissection	80-90
III	Radical vulvectomy and groin node dissection; radiation therapy	50
IV	Combined modality; radiation therapy; surgical resection; chemotherapy	10

of the initial lesion. Patients are carefully instructed to observe the vulva monthly, using palpation and hand mirrors, and to report any changes such as discolorations and lumps. They also are instructed to report any new or recurrent symptoms such as itching, burning, bleeding, or discharge. Radiologic screening, chest radiograph, and CT scan of the abdomen and pelvis usually are reserved for patients at high risk for recurrence (groin node involvement or extensive central disease).

Other malignant lesions of the vulva

Melanoma. Of all the nonsquamous cell cancers of the vulva, melanoma is the most frequent, comprising approximately 5% of primary vulvar cancers. The average age at presentation is 50 years, although melanoma may be seen in any age-group. These lesions may appear brown, black, or blue-black, raised or flat, with occasional satellite nodules surrounding the primary lesion. The most common sites are the clitoris and labia majora.

The FIGO staging system is not as useful for the management of melanoma because the natural history of this disease is significantly different from that of squamous cell carcinoma of the vulva. The most important prognostic factor for melanoma is depth of invasion. Various staging systems based on depth of invasion have been suggested over the years, with Clark's levels being the most common. It is generally believed that lesions corresponding to Clark level I or II—that is, less than 0.76 mm invasion—carry an excellent prognosis, with little likelihood of nodal metastases or local recurrence. Patients with deeper invasion or with evidence of groin node involvement usually succumb to disease.

The treatment of malignant melanoma of the vulva is primarily surgical, with most patients in the past treated with radical vulvectomy and bilateral groin node dissection. Recently it has become clear that patients are as well treated by more limited resection, with prognosis based on depth of invasion, not size of surgical margins. Similarly, nodal dissection appears to provide prognostic information only, with uniformly poor outcome achieved in patients with involved nodes.

Bartholin's gland carcinoma. Carcinoma arising in Bartholin's gland may be squamous cell, adenocarcinoma, or adenoid cystic carcinoma, the last a subtype specific to Bartholin's gland. These tumors account for approximately 2% of all vulvar cancers and are encountered primarily in the postmenopausal patient. The treatment, as with other vulvar cancers, is surgical, with prognosis based on the adequacy of the surgical margin and status of the regional lymph nodes.

Basal cell carcinoma. Basal cell carcinoma of the vulva is histologically and biologically similar to those found in other locations. It is a relatively rare lesion, accounting for 2% of all vulvar cancers. These tumors rarely metastasize to the regional nodes and are best treated with wide local excision, which provides an excellent prognosis.

Verrucous carcinoma. This rather rare cancer can arise in any site in the lower genital tract. It may grossly resemble genital warts and often is misdiagnosed as condyloma acuminata, in part as a result of inadequate depth of biopsy or sampling error in obtaining biopsy specimens in too few areas of an extensive lesion. It is a histologic variant of squamous cell carcinoma, and the treatment is again operative by wide local excision or vulvectomy. Five-year survival with early diagnosis and adequate excision approximates 95%, although there is a high tendency for local recurrence.

Paget's disease. Paget's disease of the vulva is an uncommon disease of postmenopausal women, with a median age at presentation of 65 years. Clinically, it appears raised, red, and velvety, with an occasional overlying pearly sheen. The lesion may be quite extensive, involving the mons pubis, thigh, or buttocks. Persistent weeping can be particularly troublesome. Paget's disease often extends beyond the lesion seen grossly. The usual treatment is surgical by wide excision or simple vulvectomy as required to attain surgical margins. Patients with Paget's disease are at risk for synchronous breast, cervix, or colon cancers and thus should undergo Pap testing, barium enema, or colonoscopy and mammography as part of their initial evaluation. Similarly, patients with Paget's disease are at risk for a carcinoma of the underlying skin appendages—thus the requirement for simple as opposed to skinning vulvectomy or laser vaporization as primary treatment. Local recurrences, which are common, are best treated with wide local excision.

SUMMARY

In spite of the dramatic—indeed explosive—advances in health care technology over the past several decades, our ability to cure advanced gynecologic cancers has little changed. The development of more effective screening tests and intelligent use of those currently available remain our best chance of conquering gynecologic cancer, placing the primary care provider in the key role of guiding the patient to early detection.

The cancer-related health checkup, as defined by the American Cancer Society, is recommended at 3-year intervals in women between the ages of 20 to 40 years and annually in all persons thereafter. The gynecologic aspects of this checkup are recommended by age 18 years in most women or at the onset of sexual activity. In women, this should include visualization of the vulva, vagina, and cervix, a Pap test, and bimanual pelvic examination, in addition to evaluations of the colon, thyroid, lymph nodes, oral cavity, skin, and breasts and counseling regarding smoking, diet, sun exposure, family history, and other personal factors. Many of these issues are addressed in other chapters in this book.

BIBLIOGRAPHY

American College of Obstetricians and Gynecologists: *Newsletter,* June 1984.

American College of Obstetricians and Gynecologists: *Report of task force on routine cancer screening: ACOG committee opinion 68,* Washington, DC, 1989, ACOG.

Amos CI et al: Age at onset for familial epithelial ovarian cancer, *JAMA* 268:1896, 1992.

Boring CC et al: Cancer statistics, 1994, *CA* 44:7, 1994.

Brand E et al: Controversies in the management of cervical adenocarcinoma, *Obstet Gynecol* 71:261, 1988.

Buxton EJ et al: Combination bleomycin, ifosfamide, and cisplain chemotherapy in cervical cancer, *JNCI* 81:359, 1989.

Centers for Disease Control and Steroid Hormone Study: Oral contraceptives and the risk of ovarian cancer, *JAMA* 249:1596, 1983.

Cramer DW et al: Dietary animal fat in relation to ovarian cancer risk, *Obstet Gynecol* 63:833, 1984.

Crum C: Vulvar intraepithelial neoplasia: histology and associated viral changes. In Wilkinson EJ, editor: *Pathology of the vulva and vagina,* New York, 1987, Churchill Livingstone.

Hacker NF et al: Primary cytoreductive surgery for epithelial ovarian cancer, *Obstet Gynecol* 61:413, 1983.

Lovecchio JL et al: Treatment of advanced or recurrent endometrial adenocarcinoma with cyclophosphamide, doxorubicin, *cis*-platinum, megestrol acetate, *Obstet Gynecol* 63:557, 1984.

Morley GW: Cancer of the vulva. In Knapp RC, Berkowitz RS, editors: *Gynecologic oncology,* New York, 1993, McGraw-Hill.

Morrow CP et al: Relationship between surgical-pathologic risk factors and outcome in clinical stages I-II carcinoma of the endometrium: a Gynecologic Group study, *Gynecol Oncol* 40:55, 1991.

1988 Bethesda system for reporting cervical/vaginal cytology, *JAMA* 262:931, 1989.

Piver MS et al: *The Gilda Radner familial ovarian cancer registry newsletter,* Buffalo, NY, 1990, Roswell Park Cancer Institute.

Taussig FJ: Cancer of the vulva: an analysis of 155 cases (1911-1940), *Am J Obstet Gynecol* 40:764, 1949.

Vousdon KH: Human papillomavirus and cervical carcinoma, *Cancer Cells* 1(2):43, 1989.

Way S: Carcinoma of the vulva, *Am J Obstet Gynecol* 79:692, 1960.

Young RC et al: Adjuvant therapy in stage I and stage II epithelial ovarian cancer, *N Engl J Med* 322:1021, 1990.

Zucker PK, Kasdon EJ, Feldstein ML: The validity of Pap smear parameters as predictors of endometrial pathology in menopausal women, *Cancer* 56:2256, 1985.

Part Three

Psychology and Behavioral Medicine

66 Alcohol and Drug Abuse

JudyAnn Bigby and Michele G. Cyr

Alcohol and other drug abuse has increasingly been recognized as a significant problem among patients seen by primary care physicians. Several aspects of this disorder, including the epidemiologic characteristics, the physiologic effects of alcohol and drugs, the social and medical consequences, and issues related to detection and management, distinguish it in women. This chapter will concentrate on these issues.

Substance abuse is used as a generic term in this chapter to describe abuse of and dependence on substances including alcohol, prescription and other licit drugs, and illicit drugs. Abuse of a substance is characterized as repetitive, chronic patterns of use associated with impairment of psychologic or social functioning and health. Dependence is characterized by loss of control of the use of a substance with evidence of tolerance (requiring increasing amounts of the substance to achieve the desired effects) or addiction (evidence of withdrawal when use of a substance decreases or ceases).

■ EPIDEMIOLOGY

Women comprise an estimated one third of all those having alcohol abuse or dependence (alcoholism) disorders in the United States, or approximately 4.6 million women, according to figures from 1991. Between 1967 and 1984 the percentage of women drinkers who reported problems related to alcohol increased from 1% to 3% and the percentage of heavy drinkers (four or more drinks on one occasion) from 26% to 34%. Approximately 5% of all women, compared to 8% of all men, reported using illicit drugs according to the National Institute on Drug Abuses's most recent national household survey. Over 8% of the women of childbearing age had used an illicit drug; marijuana was the most common. Women are prescibed psychotropic drugs at an earlier age and more frequently than men. They use and abuse prescription drugs at a higher rate than men. In addition, 30% to 70% of women alcoholics are codependent on other drugs, including sedatives and minor tranquilizers.

Use of substances varies according to race and ethnicity as well as socioeconomic status. Black women are more likely to abstain from alcohol than white women; Hispanic women report the highest rates of abstinence. Single, divorced, or separated women are more likely to drink heavily and experience alcohol-related problems than married or widowed women. Women who are college graduates are more likely to drink and to use cocaine than high school graduates. In some inner cities women's crack use is a major problem and exceeds men's.

The prevalence of substance abuse problems among women who consult medical care providers varies, depending on the setting. For example, 21% of women attending a clinic for the treatment of premenstrual disorders, 10% to 17% attending internal medicine or family medicine clinics, and 12% of those attending a private gynecology practice were substance abusers. The percentage of women with alcohol-related problems on inpatient services ranges from 8% to 12%, depending on the service. Recent surveys of women receiving prenatal and obstetric care provide some insight into the prevalence among women of problems related to drugs other than alcohol. In the study by Chasnoff and colleagues, 16% of pregnant women at public clinics and 13% at private offices had positive toxicologic screen findings for alcohol, opiates, cocaine, or marijuana.

Physicians frequently miss the diagnosis of substance abuse in patients and, even when they do recognize it, do not recommend treatment. Moore and colleagues found that only 30% to 60% of patients with substance abuse were identified through surgical, medical, and psychiatry services. The rate of recognition was 0% to 7% on the gynecology service. Physicians have been less likely to diagnose women than men with active drinking problems; in a study by Buchsbaum and others, 23.7% of women with drinking problems were recognized compared to 66.7% of men. Women may be more likely to seek or be referred for care in non–alcohol-specific settings such as mental health treatment centers.

CONSEQUENCES OF SUBSTANCE ABUSE
Social and psychologic consequences

Women suffer important social and psychologic consequences of substance abuse. Family and marital problems are more common among women, whereas job and legal problems are more commonly reported consequences in men. Women are more likely to have psychiatric diagnoses and to report a suicide attempt. They are more likely to be divorced after entering treatment (9 of 10 marriages in which the woman is alcoholic end in divorce compared to 1 of 10 in which the male is alcoholic) and report a fear of losing custody of their children as an important motivating factor for treatment.

Women who drink heavily or who are alcoholic are more likely to become victims of alcohol-related aggression such as rape. Younger women with substance abuse report particularly high rates of violence—48% report episodes of violence and 32% report rape or coerced sexual intercourse.

Women who abuse illicit substances are likely to depend on a male partner or significant other to supply the drug. Recent public concern about the effects of abused illicit substances on the fetus have prompted increased efforts to identify and legally address the use of illicit substances during pregnancy.

Medical consequences

Pathophysiology. There are significant differences in the way women and men metabolize alcohol. After a standard dose of alcohol adjusted according to body weight, women have higher blood alcohol levels than men. The higher proportion of body fat in women, changes in the absorption of alcohol with the menstrual cycle, and differences in the relative amounts of gastric alcohol dehydrogenase found in men and women account for this observation. These differences may explain the earlier appearance and increased severity of complications from drinking seen in women compared to men. For example, in spite of lower levels of consumption and later age for the onset of problem drinking, cirrhosis in women develops over a shorter period and women die at an earlier age. Both Native American and African-American women have particularly high rates of cirrhosis and death from cirrhosis.

Hypertension. The relationship between alcohol intake and hypertension has been well described. However, in women the relationship is best explained by a combination of factors—alcohol consumption, smoking, and age. Among women 45 to 69 years old, smokers demonstrate a steep correlation in diastolic and systolic blood pressure with alcohol consumption of 1.5 drinks or more each day.

Risk of breast cancer. Two major studies have reported an increased risk of breast cancer related to alcohol consumption among women already at risk for breast cancer. The relative risk was reported as 1.5 for women drinking 3 drinks each week. A metaanalysis of available data reported relative risk of 1.4 to 1.7 for women drinking 2 drinks each day, but another study did not confirm an association between alcohol consumption and breast cancer.

Gynecologic problems. Alcohol and other drug problems have been found at substantial rates among women consulting gynecologic practices. Higher rates of amenorrhea, dysfunctional uterine bleeding, dysmenorrhea, infertility, and premenstrual syndrome have been described among women who are heavy drinkers. Sexual dysfunction has also been reported at higher rates among women who abuse alcohol, opiates, cocaine, and other substances.

Fetal effects

Effect of alcohol. The fetal effects of alcohol and other drug use have been well described. The fetal alcohol syndrome represents the most severe complication and is one of the most important causes of mental retardation. Full-blown fetal alcohol syndrome results from heavy consumption of alcohol (more than 4 drinks a day) during pregnancy, but less severe effects, including learning disabilities and other subtle neurologic consequences, premature delivery, and low birth weight, result from more moderate consumption.

Effect of cocaine. Cocaine use during pregnancy is associated with abruptio placentae, placenta previa, intrauterine growth retardation, premature labor, and stillbirth. Birth defects such as neural tube defects and malformation of the genitourinary, gastrointestinal, and cardiovascular systems have been described. The effects of cocaine on the neuropsychologic development of children have been challenged because studies describing this problem have not controlled for nutritional, social, and other factors that may interfere with development. Marijuana use has been associated with impaired fetal growth.

Osteoporosis. Alcohol consumption is an important factor influencing osteoporosis and its complications. Women below the age of 65 who drank 2 to 6 ounces of alcohol each week were found to have an increased risk of hip fracture. This risk may be due to an increased incidence of falling and to the effects of alcohol on bone metabolism. The risk of hip fractures is also increased in those prescribed long-acting benzodiazepines.

Human immunodeficiency virus disease. More than 80% of cases of women with acquired immunodeficiency syndrome (AIDS) are associated with intravenous drug abuse. The minority involve injection drug use by the woman herself. Under the influence of alcohol or drugs women may engage in high-risk sexual encounters with people who are intravenous drug users and human immunodeficiency virus (HIV)-positive.

The prevalence of alcohol and drug problems among women who enter health care settings and the severe impact of social and medical consequences of alcohol and other drug use provide ample justification for screening, identification, and early intervention for alcohol and other drug problems among women in the primary care clinician's office.

SCREENING AND IDENTIFICATION
Screening

History and physical examination. Physicians who deliver primary care to women are in a unique position to educate women about the health effects of alcohol and other drugs, to identify women with problems, and to make appropriate referrals for treatment. In order to identify substance abuse, physicians should routinely screen patients and pursue possible problems among those women with risk factors for substance abuse.

Routine screening is often helpful in identifying patients with a diagnosis of substance abuse or those at risk for development of problems. Questions about the quantity and frequency of alcohol use are not sensitive or reliable in identifying alcoholism but provide a helpful entree to discuss the patient's use of alcohol. In addition, because of the high prevalence of polydrug use among women, it is important that physicians ask about use of prescription drugs as well as illicit drugs.

Specific questions to identify alcoholism. Questions that emphasize the adverse consequences of alcohol and drugs are helpful to identify patients with problems. The CAGE questions have been extensively studied in a variety of populations, and a finding of two affirmative responses has a sensitivity and specificity of 80% to 90% (see box, below). The questions are frequently modified to apply to other drugs. These questions emphasize the consequences of loss of control over alcohol or drug use, concern among family or friends, the feelings of the patient, and evidence for withdrawal from the substance. Any affirmative answer warrants a more detailed evaluation (e.g., "Why did you decide to cut down or stop? For how long were you able to stop drinking/using? Why did you start again? Who has expressed concern about your alcohol/drug use? What made you feel guilty? Have you ever experienced shakes, severe anxiety, tremulousness in the morning?").

CAGE QUESTIONS

Have you ever tried to *cut* down on your drinking?
Have you ever been *annoyed* by criticism of your drinking?
Have you ever felt *guilty* about your drinking?
Have you ever had an *eye opener*?

The CAGE questions and "Have you ever had a drinking problem?" were studied by Moulton and colleagues, and identified over 90% of women presenting an outpatient practice who had a positive screening result with more extensive questionnaires.

Clues to the diagnosis. In addition to routinely screening all patients, physicians should conduct a detailed substance use history and assess potential consequences in women with risk factors for substance abuse or potential signs or symptoms of substance abuse.

Risk factors for substance abuse include a family history, early onset of alcohol or drug use, a significant other with substance abuse, domestic violence, and a history of being prescribed a mood-altering drug.

Physical signs of dependence, end-stage organ damage, and abnormal laboratory test results are present in the *minority* of patients with alcohol or other drug problems and lack of them does not rule out a problem. Liver function tests and mean corpuscular volume are less sensitive and specific than the CAGE questionnaire.

The common early clues to the diagnosis of substance abuse are shown in the box at right. Other symptoms and signs of substance abuse such as stigmata of chronic liver disease, skin infections, recurrent pancreatitis, septal perforation, or endocarditis are late complications. Nicotine dependence, eating disorders, and a history of rape, incest, or molestation during childhood are conditions that have been associated with substance abuse in women.

After the physician has identified possible features of the history and physical examination consistent with substance abuse, it is important to share these concerns with the patient in a nonjudgmental, concerned fashion.

Making the diagnosis. The physician can confirm a diagnosis of substance abuse by gathering more information about the adverse consequences of substance use. It is important to ask specific questions about the relationship between substance use and family problems, problems with a spouse or significant other, job problems, legal and financial problems, and medical problems. For example, if a patient is having problems at home, expresses concern about a child's behavior, or mentions difficulty with a spouse, ask how drinking or drug use impacts on the problem. "Do you ever worry that you aren't taking good care of your son because of your drinking?" "Do you and your husband argue more when you've been drinking or using drugs?" Open-ended questions such as "Will you tell me more about your drinking/drug use?" are sometimes helpful, but often patients with substance abuse problems offer specific information only when asked directly.

Even after gathering more data about the patient's use of substances the physician may be unsure as to whether the patient has a problem. It is important to share that concern with the patient and develop a plan for follow-up and reevaluation. This might include a trial period of abstinence, controlled use within limits, or the patient's keeping a calendar of her use. The physician should make specific recommendations to the patient ("Limit your drinking to no more than 4 drinks per week and we will follow up in 4 weeks"). The physician should reassure the patient of his or her willingness to continue to have her as a patient regardless of whether she is able to follow the agreed upon plan. The

CLUES TO THE DIAGNOSIS OF SUBSTANCE ABUSE

Social

Family discord/problems
Requests for pain medications/tranquilizers
Requests for work excuses
Erratic behavior
Risky sexual encounters
Vague past medical history
Children with behavior problems

Findings

Unexplained/repeated trauma
Alcohol on breath
Unexplained tachycardia
Hypertension
Needle tracks
Weight loss

Symptoms

Anxiety/palpitations
Depression
Insomnia
Fatigue/lack of energy
Sexual dysfunction
Nonspecific abdominal complaints
Self-medication with alcohol
Complaints related to menstrual cycle, infertility, miscarriage

patient should be asked about her own concerns and they should be addressed as much as possible. When the patient returns, the information from the trial can provide further understanding of the patient's diagnosis. If the patient is able to follow through with the recommendations, she should continue to be followed and her use of alcohol and other drugs and the consequences of that use monitored. If the patient demonstrates an inability to cut down or stop as recommended, this may provide ample evidence of a problem. At this point the patient may agree to treatment.

MANAGEMENT

Developing a treatment plan

Patients who are at risk for substance abuse or who are engaging in hazardous or risky substance use benefit from education about the consequences of drinking and drug use. Women who are contemplating pregnancy and pregnant women should be informed about the effects of cigarettes, alcohol, and other drugs on the fetus.

Most experts suggest that for nonpregnant women 10 or fewer drinks each week represents nonrisky use (1 drink = 12 ounces of beer = 5 ounces of wine = 1.5 ounces of liquor). Recommendations about the safe use of illicit drugs are controversial. Although some individuals can use illicit drugs occasionally without adverse consequences, the risk of legal intervention and the consequences on family, school, and job make any illicit drug use risky. Pregnant women should be advised to follow their obstetrician's recommendations regarding alcohol use during pregnancy, as some obstetricians recommend total abstinence since it is unclear what the absolute safe use of alcohol is during pregnancy. Low birth weight and premature labor have been reported with drinking in the range of two or more drinks per day.

Potentially addictive medications should always be prescribed with caution, based on good medical judgment. All such prescriptions and the number of refills should be carefully documented in patients at high risk for or with a history of substance abuse. The diagnosis that warrants the prescription, the goals of treatment, and the expected duration of treatment should be documented and reviewed with the patient.

Once a substance abuse problem has been identified it is important that the physician express his concerns to the patient. It is important not to label the patient an alcoholic or drug addict but to link the negative consequences to her alcohol or drug use ("I am concerned that your problems at work, your difficulties with your husband, and your sleeping problem point to a problem with alcohol"). It is also important to inform the patient that there is help available for her problems. Tailor the treatment, taking into account the patient's individual situation. Men and women with comparable demographic characteristics at comparable stages of disease do equally well in treatment. However, it may be important to address issues of self-esteem, sexual abuse, sexism, and interpersonal relationships in treatment. It may be necessary to find treatment alternatives that address issues related to child care and other family responsibilities. In most states departments of public health keep track of all public and private substance abuse treatment programs.

Referral. Referral to a 12-step program such as Alcoholics Anonymous and follow-up treatment with the primary care physician may be appropriate first steps for the woman who has a stable social situation and no impending social disaster such as threat of lost custody, job loss, or divorce. Women respond better to self-help programs and to all-female groups. Physicians should make themselves familiar with the process of 12-step programs and refer patients to a meeting that is appropriate for them (an all-women's meeting, appropriate socioeconomic group, non-smoking, gay, etc.) During follow-up consultation the physician should encourage patients to learn new behavior to deal with stress, anxiety, anger, and so on, and to identify specific ways to maintain sobriety.

Individuals with significant medical problems, abusive home situations, legal problems, and a significant other with substance abuse should be referred for intense outpatient treatment or inpatient treatment. Family therapy is an important part of treatment in order to educate the family about the disease, to help them deal with the anger and anxiety directed at the patient, and to help them learn how to participate in the recovery process.

SUMMARY

Primary care providers are in a unique position to identify women with alcohol and other drug problems. Early identification can limit the adverse consequences of substance abuse. Physicians must pay attention to the differences in risk, alternative presentations, and treatment issues that are relevant to women.

BIBLIOGRAPHY

Ashley MJ et al: Morbidity in alcoholics: Evidence for accelerated development of physical disease in women, *Arch Intern Med* 137:883, 1977.

Baldwin DC et al: Substance use among senior medical students, *JAMA* 265:2074, 1991.

Bigby J: Negotiating treatment and monitoring recovery. In Barnes HN, Aronson MD, Delbanco TL, editors: *Alcoholism: a guide for the primary care physician,* New York, 1987, Springer-Verlag.

Buchsbaum DG et al: Physician detection of drinking problems in patients attending a general medicine practice, *J Gen Intern Med* 7:517, 1992.

Bush BT et al: Screening for alcohol abuse using the CAGE questionnaire, *Am J Med* 82:231, 1987.

Chasnoff I, Landress H, Barrett M: The prevalence of illicit drug or alcohol use during pregnancy and discrepancies in mandatory reporting in Pinellas County, Florida, *N Engl J Med* 322:1202, 1990.

Chavkin W: Mandatory treatment for drug use during pregnancy, *JAMA* 266:1556, 1991.

Moore RD et al: Prevalence, detection and treatment of alcoholism in hospitalized patients, *JAMA,* 261:403, 1989.

Moulton AW et al: Screening for alcoholism in women in an internal medicine practice, *Clin Res* 38:700A, 1990.

National Institute on Drug Abuse: Sample size and U.S. population size tables, In *National household survey on drug abuse: population estimates 1988,* Rockville, 1990, Department of Health and Human Services.

Piazza NJ, Urbka JL, Yeager RD: Telescoping of alcoholism in women alcoholics, *Int J Addict* 24(1):19, 1989.

Public Health Service: *Report of the Secretary's Task Force on Black and Minority Health.* Vol VII: *Chemical dependency and diabetes,* 1986, Rockville, Department of Health and Human Services.

Ray WA et al: Psychotropic drug use and the risk of hip fracture, *N Engl J Med* 316:363, 1987.

Svarstad BL et al: Gender differences in the acquisition of prescribed drugs, *Med Care* 25:1089, 1987.

Weisner C, Schmidt L: Gender disparities in treatment for alcohol problems, *JAMA* 268:1872, 1992.

Wilsnack RW, Wilsnack SC, Klassen AD: Women's drinking and drinking problems: patterns from 1981 national survey, *Am J Public Health* 74:1231, 1984.

Wilsnack SC et al: Predicting onset and chronicity of women's problem drinking: a five-year longitudinal analysis, *Am J Public Health* 81:305, 1991.

Zuckerman B et al: Effects of marijuana and cocaine use on fetal growth, *N Engl J Med* 320:262, 1989.

67 Depression

Carol Landau and Felise B. Milan

Depressive disorders are the most prevalent psychiatric diagnosis in women. It is often easy to underrecognize and sometimes inappropriately treat emotional disorders. Less than half of depressed patients seen in a primary care setting are properly diagnosed and treated. For these reasons primary care clinicians need to pay greater attention to detection and treatment of depression.

The psychiatric and, to a lesser extent, medical literature has recognized that women have particular issues in the area of depression. Unfortunately, historically the issues that received attention were *not* those relevant to most women. The orthodox psychoanalytic approach dominated psychiatric and psychologic training programs for many years and emphasized biologic factors to the neglect of such other issues as interpersonal or relationship issues. Most of the attention was given to women's menopausal symptoms and their relationship to depression. Therefore a great deal of attention was paid to the cessation of menstruation as the primary cause for depression. Numerous psychoanalytic writers, beginning with Deutsch in 1945, adopted this approach. Their significant error, however, was that there have never been any data to indicate that menopause was the peak time of depression in women from an epidemiologic standpoint. Focusing almost exclusively on menopause has caused more prevalent problems related to depression to be neglected. These include psychologic reactions to medical problems and procedures, substance abuse, and family issues, as well as other psychosocial factors.

There are at least two ways in which a primary care clinician can explore the issue of depression in women. The first is the basic diagnostic interview using criteria from *The Diagnostic and Statistical Manual of Mental Disorders (DSM-IV)* This chapter will address the issues of dysthymia and major depression, the most prevalent forms of depression in women. The *DSM-IV* includes at least five other categories of depressive disorders. The second approach is developmental; we will discuss it in a later section.

DEFINITIONS

Dysthymic disorder, once termed depressive neurosis, includes a lifelong tendency toward depressed mood. The following box details the criteria. The symptoms have existed in the patient most of the time for at least 2 years. Dysthymia also includes at least two of the signs or symptoms of a major depression. Thus by its definition, dysthymic disorder is a chronic problem. When it occurs during childhood it seems to occur equally often in both sexes. At the time of adolescence, however, the rate of depression in young women increases and reaches a 2:1 or 3:1 female to male ratio.

Major depressive disorder is an acute problem in which more frequent and severe symptoms present daily and interfere with functioning. The main symptom is depressed mood or loss of interest. The other diagnostic criteria are listed in the box on the following page. The average age of onset is in the late 20s and 30s, but it may occur at any time.

SYMPTOMS OF DYSTHYMIC DISORDER

1. Have you had a depressed mood for most of the day, more days than not, for at least 2 years?
2. Do you have, when you are depressed, at least *two* of the following?
   1. poor appetite or overeating
   2. insomnia or hypersomnia
   3. low energy or fatigue
   4. low self-esteem
   5. poor concentration or difficulty making decisions
   6. feelings of hopelessness
3. Have you ever had a manic episode—overly high amounts of energy, poor judgment? If so, you may have a bipolar disorder.
4. Are you taking medications that can cause depression? If so, check with your primary care doctor.

---

* If you have answered YES to questions 1 and 2, and NO to 3 and 4, you may have dysthymia.

Modified from *The diagnostic and statistical manual of mental disorders,* ed 4, Washington, DC, 1994, American Psychiatric Association.

DETERMINING RISK

Female gender is one of the primary risk factors for depression. The lifetime prevalence in women is anywhere from 9% to 26% and some researchers have suggested prevalence as high as 33%. In contrast, for males it is 7% to 12%. In terms of current point prevalence for females the rate of depression is anywhere between 5% and 10%, whereas for males it is between 2% and 3%. It is probable, then, that up to 1 of 10 women seen in a primary care practice may be suffering from a major depressive episode and thus depression merits the label "the common cold" of women's psychologic problems.

There has been much speculation as to why women have a tendency toward depression. Psychologic theories of depression such as the learned helplessness theory as well as the cognitive theory may well apply more to women than to men. With respect to sociodemographics we also know that women are more likely to experience poverty, physical and sexual abuse, lack of education, and job discrimination, and that these stressors have been found in some studies to precipitate depression.

In addition to possible biologic vulnerabilities psychosocial factors play a significant role. Weissman and her associates have documented the interpersonal nature of depression. The combination of women's investment in relationships and lack of power to effect change in those relationships may well account for higher rates of depression. These psychosocial factors in depression can be examined from a developmental perspective. This is the second approach to detecting major depression or dysthymic disorder in primary care to be discussed.

SYMPTOMS OF MAJOR DEPRESSIVE EPISODE

Have you had at least *five* of the following symptoms during the same 2-week period, and is this a *change* from your usual functioning?

1. depressed mood most of the day, nearly every day
-or-
2. markedly diminished interest or pleasure in all, or almost all, activities most of the day, nearly every day.
-and-
3. significant weight loss or weight gain when not dieting (e.g., more than 5% of body weight in a month), or decrease or increase in appetite nearly every day.
4. insomnia or hypersomnia nearly every day.
5. psychomotor agitation or retardation nearly every day.
6. fatigue or loss of energy nearly every day.
7. feelings of worthlessness or excessive or inappropriate guilt nearly every day.
8. diminished ability to think or concentrate, or indecisiveness, nearly every day.
9. recurrent thoughts of death (not just fear of dying), recurrent suicidal ideation without a specific plan, or a suicide attempt or a specific plan.

---

* If you answered YES to 1 or 2 and YES to four items from 3 to 9, you may be suffering from a major depressive episode.
Modified from *The diagnostic and statistical manual of mental disorders,* ed 4, Washington, DC, 1994, American Psychiatric Association.

Given the nature of medical problems and the long-term relationships that can develop between women patients and their health care providers, primary care clinicians have access to a tremendous amount of psychosocial information. By exploring relationship issues at the right time the clinician not only can provide better health care but may be able to detect depression, as well as other psychologic problems. The primary care clinician's ability to identify developmental issues as possible triggers for depression casts her in a unique role in the patient's life.

DEVELOPMENTAL ISSUES

Most people organize their lives around work issues and relationship issues. It is clear that even though women are now more likely to work outside the home they still psychologically organize their lives around family and relationship issues. Kaplan and her associates suggest that the best way to understand women's adult development is through a self-in-relationship model. Unlike models of male development, a female model of development postulates that women define themselves primarily through relationships with others—family members, friends, lovers, children. Thus any attempt to understand women's development, and especially depression, must place relationship issues at the center.

Young adulthood

During the early 20s most people form a significant relationship, often leading to marriage. Despite recent social and cultural changes, marriage or a committed relationship to a significant other is still the primary social bond for most women. The average age for first marriages for men and women is still in the early 20s.

The role of marital issues is critical in understanding depression in women. There has been a great deal of controversy with respect to the relationship between marriage and depression. Many studies suggest that the risk factors for depression include being married or divorced and having children below the age of 5 at home. The highest rates for major depression occur in women between the ages of 18 and 44. Other risk factors include having first-degree relatives who are depressed and living in an urban environment. Finally, many depressed patients are married to depressed spouses.

Weissman details the relationship issues in depression more clearly. She reported that, with respect to risk factors for depression, the rates are lowest for men and women who are married and getting along well with their spouses. Although women have higher rates of depression overall, the increased risk for major depression in unhappy marriage is nearly the same for men and women and is about 25-fold.

When looking at rates of depression it is interesting to note that the only category in which men outnumber women with respect to diagnosed depression is that of unemployment. Even given recent economic and social changes it is not surprising that a loss of or major problem in a job for a man might well have the same emotional impact as the loss of or a major problem in a marriage or significant relationship for a woman. Status issues are such that an unemployed man may feel devalued as does a woman who is divorced or in an unhappy marriage.

Although much literature has discussed the role of the traditional marriage in women's depression it is clear that divorced women also have high rates of depression. It should be noted that both of these categories of women, however, often bear the sole responsibility for the physical and emotional well-being of their children.

In screening for depression, if the primary care clinician were to ask a single question of a married woman, "Are you happily married?" might be the most useful. More subtle ways of getting to that issue could include "How are things going at home?" "Have there been any problems in the marriage?" "Tell me a little about your family life." It is usually more effective to use open-ended rather than closed questions. It is important for physicians to explore this issue with most patients, since it is often essential to the diagnosis of depression. Unfortunately this area is not explored often enough by physicians.

Developmental issues for women in their 20s and 30s include marriage, children, infertility, and divorce. It is not surprising that the average age of onset for a major depression is in the late 20s. Women tend to marry at the average age of about 24, and the peak stress of marital life occurs 7 years into the marriage. There is an association between marital discord and depression. Unhappily married women have been found to have higher levels of depressive symptoms than either happily married women or unmarried women.

With respect to lesbian relationships there are few large scale cross-sectional studies in this area. Clinical experience indicates some similarities. Unhappy relationships are correlated with depression. Social support appears to be a buffer to depression in lesbian women as well as other women but, because of discrimination, lesbians may have access to fewer social supports to provide this resource.

The thirties—family issues

Another issue facing women in their 20s and 30s is that of children. The shift in the family life goes from being a couple to being a family and, with recent changes in the work force, this often means a dual-career family. Many studies suggest that couples with young children feel more stress and pressure than any other group in the family life cycle. Ratings of life satisfaction tend to drop from high to average and remain there until the children leave home. Not surprisingly the couples who are most satisfied are those who have been married the longest, who want children a great deal, and who have outside resources including time, money, and social support.

It is clear that depression might strike women in this age group because of their dual roles as caretakers for children as well as full-time workers. One of the possible connections between depression and marriage may be feeling overwhelmed by and often conflicted over family responsibility. *The Second Shift*, by Hochschild and Machung, describes what the authors call a "stalled revolution." As the number of women in the work force grew, the necessary child care and help with responsibilities at home did not. Clinicians' experiences with depressed working mothers—married or single—document that most full-time working mothers spend an additional 20 hours each week on housework and child care. In contrast working fathers spend an additional 8 hours each week on these responsibilities. Women who work outside the home are no more likely to have help from their husbands than women who work at home full-time. Reviewing the daily schedule of many such women reveals a long history of sleep deprivation, excessive consumption of caffeine, and virtually no personal time. It should be noted, however, that despite these stresses there is a slightly greater risk of depression in women who are at home full-time than in those who work outside the home. This is probably true because of the access to social support at work and the wider range of sources of gratification.

Another growing problem for women in this age group is infertility. The most common psychologic issues associated with infertility include a feeling of loss of control, a feeling of helplessness, and problems in sexuality. It can also serve as a stress on the couple's relationship. In addition, the health care system itself may well have a negative impact on the couple. In fact much of the work with infertile couples is directed at helping them cope with numerous specialists. The primary care clinician can help couples understand all the information, laboratory tests, and procedures involved and can coordinate care. Women bear the brunt of the medical procedures and may feel the stigma of infertility more deeply than their male partners. The issue of potential loss can precipitate a depression at this time. Isolation is another problem associated with infertility. Attention should be paid to the couple's relationship and their access to social support. Psychotherapy and such self-help groups as RESOLVE can be extremely helpful. In addition to breaking the cycle of social isolation and feelings of secrecy RESOLVE can help couples explore the practical alternatives in coping with infertility.

A traumatic relationship issue of the late 20s and 30s is divorce. The growing population of separated and divorced individuals includes every age group but is most evident during young adulthood. Divorce is most likely to occur during the early years of marriage, in childless marriages, among those who marry young, and among people who have unhappy marriages in their family of origin. Divorce not only is a risk factor for depression but has implications for health care use. People going through divorce or separation are high users of health care services including office visits to primary care physicians. Thus it is important when dealing with a woman going through a marital separation or divorce to question her specifically about the areas of depression and anxiety. Other issues to be aware of include substance abuse and accidents, both of which may be more prevalent during separation and divorce.

Many women worry not only about their own future after divorce but about their children's futures as well. Wallerstein and Blakeslee documented that, even 10 years after a divorce, a full 30% of children are suffering from psychologic problems. In the end the responsibility for these children remains with their mothers over 90% of the time. On average, divorced mothers experience a 73% drop in their standard of living within the first year after divorce. It is particularly important, therefore, to ask female patients about the well-being of their children during and after a divorce. When the clinical setting permits, asking the children directly is recommended. One study revealed that less than 10% of the children going through a divorce had any adult other than their parents ask them about their feelings.

Midlife

With respect to the 40s and 50s, the primary issues are dealing with adolescent or adult children, divorce, menopause, medical problems, and the prospect of mortality. Previous discussions of women in midlife focused almost exclusively on menopause as if it were a single event and as if the biologic characteristics of menopause alone caused depression. Midlife is difficult to define. In addition to age midlife can be seen as a cognitive shift away from the time lived to the time left to be lived. Contrary to the myth, middle age is not the peak time for depression in women. Although there have been some studies that suggest that the midlife period is characterized by life crisis, others have not found this to be true.

McKinlay and McKinlay and their associates have conducted the definitive community-based study of menopausal women. Their study was cross-sectional, longitudinal, and involved a large sample of women. They found that depression, when it does occur, is correlated with the number of sources of worry in a woman's life. These stresses are often family-related. The time of midlife, when children may be adolescents, is correlated with a high level of marital distress. The adolescents' emotional outbursts and intensity of their relationships are often difficult to deal with. Midlife adults may find not only that they are in conflict with their children but that there may be disagreements between them as parents. An additional growing problem is the "refilled nest"—that of adult children returning to live at home because of economic or psychologic issues.

Within the life cycle, the second highest rate of divorce occurs during midlife. Divorce during midlife most frequently involves problems related to extramarital affairs. This may be particularly threatening to a midlife woman. In one study of those people divorcing at midlife 75% were found to have had long-term chronic unhappiness, but the divorce was delayed until the children left home.

Many middle-aged women do not experience a clinical depression but may become somewhat melancholy over impending health changes associated with midlife. Many women find that medical problems are beginning to occur for the first time. They may need to deal with high blood pressure and concerns about unwanted weight gain. Menopausal symptoms, which may be troubling in themselves, may be a reminder as well as a symbol of these changes. McKinlay's study of menopause found that depressed women were more likely to report menopausal symptoms. In a study by Neugarten and Kraines, 26% of menopausal women found not knowing what to expect during menopause the most troubling factor. This problem can be addressed by a primary care clinician's explaining the common problems of menopause.

A final issue of midlife is that women (as well as men) are beginning to focus on the finite nature of their lives. Women are also beginning to become concerned not only about their own mortality but about the possible death of their husband or partner. Their concern may be warranted as women are four times more likely than men to be widowed.

Older women

Elderly women are the fastest growing segment of our population. Estimates indicate that between 5% and 20% of the elderly are in need of mental health services. Factors that have been identified as causal in the development of psychiatric problems include stress, losses, maladaptive personality styles, and histories of psychiatric and physical illness. Depression is still the most common psychologic problem for older women. One difficulty in diagnosis is that many depressed women are preoccupied with physical symptoms or even somatic delusions when the depression itself may be the primary issue. Conversely, some evidence indicates that positive perceptions about health are protective and positively correlated with adjustment to the death of a spouse or divorce.

An interesting finding from one cross-sectional study was that men and women between the ages of 60 and 74 had the lowest prevalence of life crisis and self-reported psychic distress of any other generational group. Yet the elderly were more likely to be prescribed a psychotropic medication than any other age group: 44% of women had received a prescription in the past year. Of women in that age group 20% were taking psychotropic medications on a regular basis. Of men, 40% had received prescriptions in the past year and 17% were taking psychotropic medications on a regular basis. This finding may well be related to the fact that older people visit physicians more frequently. These prescribing patterns are problematic because there is a higher rate of adverse effects from psychotropic drugs in the elderly. It is not surprising, therefore, that one of the major clinical problems in the elderly is drug interactions.

EVALUATION

Careful consideration of the potential differential diagnoses is essential in the evaluation of the depressed patient. The following boxes list the possible medical conditions that include depression as a symptom and the major medications that cause depressive symptoms. When patients experience depression it is important to consider the possibility that one

---

MEDICAL CONDITIONS ASSOCIATED WITH DEPRESSION

Acquired immunodeficiency syndrome (AIDS)
Cancer
Coronary artery disease
Chronic fatigue
Chronic renal failure
Dementia
Diabetes
Fibromyalgia
Stroke
Thyroid disease

Modified from Depression Guideline Panel: *Depression in primary care: detection and diagnosis*, vol 1. Rockville, Md, 1993, US Department of Health and Human Services.

---

of these conditions could be involved. In general primary care clinicians are more likely to misdiagnose major depression than they are another diagnosis. In addition to using *DSM-IV* criteria the clinician can use one of the many self-report inventories for depression, the most common of which is the Beck Depression Inventory (BDI). This is a pen and pencil test and is easy to administer in the office as it takes the patient only 5 to 10 minutes to complete.

An additional consideration is alcohol and substance abuse. Many women use alcohol specifically to reduce stress. This has the unfortunate result of alleviating anxiety in the short run but potentially leading to an alcohol problem. In addition, clinical evidence suggests that use of alcohol in women has earlier and more severe medical complications. Therefore it is important to assess for the possibility of substance abuse carefully. There is a clear association between alcohol abuse and depression. In one study depression was found to be the strongest predictor of alcohol dependence. Multiple substance abuse is common. A study of Alcoholics Anonymous members found that 40% of the females were addicted to another drug as well, and for women below age 30 this figure was 60%. Alcohol and substance abuse are discussed in detail in Chapter 66.

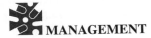 **MANAGEMENT**

Indications for referral

Every patient with depression should be evaluated for suicidality. Patients who have suicidal ideation with specific plans should immediately be referred for evaluation and treatment by a mental health professional to ascertain whether hospitalization is necessary. Other depressed patients who should be referred quickly for further evaluation and treatment include those with a psychotic depression, those with a history of treatment failures, and those who have severe vegetative symptoms.

Choice of therapy

The primary care physician can play a unique role in treating depression in women. With early identification and treatment depressive symptoms and morbidity can be reduced substantially. The first step is to determine whether the patient suffers from major depression or dysthymic disorder.

MEDICATIONS POSSIBLY ASSOCIATED WITH DEPRESSION*

Cardiovascular drugs
α-Methyldopa
Reserpine
Propranolol
Guanethidine
Clonidine
Thiazide diuretics
Digitalis

Hormones
Oral contraceptives
ACTH (corticotropin)
  and glucocorticoids
Anabolic steroids

Psychotropics
Benzodiazepines
Neuroleptics

Anticancer agents
Cycloserine

Antiinflammatory/antiinfective agents
Nonsteroidal antiinflammatory agents
Ethambutol
Disulfiram
Sulfonamides
Baclofen
Metoclopramide

Others
Cocaine (withdrawal)
Amphetamines (withdrawal)
L-dopa
Cimetidine
Ranitidine

Modified from Popkin MK: "Secondary" syndromes in DSM-IV: a review of the literature. In Frances AJ, Widiger T, editors: *DSM-IV sourcebook*, Washington, DC, American Psychiatric Press.
* These medications have been reported to induce depression in some cases. Not everyone receiving one of these will necessarily be depressed. The cause of depression in a depressed person receiving treatment is not necessarily the medication. This list indicates some medications that should be evaluated as possible causes of depression in particular patients.

If a major depressive episode is diagnosed then antidepressant medication is often indicated. Short-term psychotherapy is another alternative, and a combination of pharmacotherapy and psychotherapy is often ideal. Medication is indicated when the patient's symptoms are severe, when there is a family history of depression, if the patient has had three or more previous depressive episodes, and if the patient is experiencing symptoms of psychosis. Studies have shown that the antidepressants have equal effectiveness in treating depression. Therefore in choosing an antidepressant the primary care physician needs to consider the individual patient's concerns, the cost, and the side effect profile. The selective serotonin reuptake inhibitors (SSRIs), including fluoxetine (Prozac), sertraline (Zoloft), and paroxetine (Paxil), in general have a more favorable side-effect profile than the tricyclic antidepressants. The SSRIs tend to promote weight loss while the tricyclics may cause weight gain. This is important for patient education since many women are particularly concerned about weight gain and may have had problems tolerating tricyclics in the past.

The tricyclics also have significant anticholinergic side effects, and many have a sedative effect. Therefore if insomnia is a main target symptom one of the tricyclics taken at bedtime may have a more immediate benefit. Suicidality must be carefully considered when prescribing the tricyclics because ingestion of as little as a 10-day supply could be lethal. The SSRIs, on the other hand, have little to no potential for lethal overdose. Antidepressants have been clearly established as teratogens. Since many depressed women are in their childbearing years, this is a special risk.

The monoamine oxidase inhibitors (MAOIs) have been suggested for women whose depression has been refractory to treatment with other antidepressants. Given the interactions of the MAOIs with foods that are rich in the amino acid tyramine and with certain cold remedies, it is suggested that patients be referred to a psychiatrist for this treatment.

Compliance can be increased by a careful discussion of the potential side effects. Many of the side effects of the antidepressants are time-limited. It is important that the issue of addiction be discussed, since many women are concerned about it. It should be made clear that the antidepressants are not addictive and they should be contrasted with the anxiolytics.

One problem in management is that many patients have some component of anxiety as well as depression. Patients who have anxiety disorders can become depressed about their symptoms. Alternatively anxiety as a symptom can develop within a depressive disorder. One approach is to treat the primary disorder first and then reevaluate remaining symptoms. The physician should avoid the tendency to prescribe anxiolytics because of the lack of effectiveness in treating depression and because of the long-term additive potential.

Most women who are depressed have relationship and occupational issues as well. For these patients, and for patients suffering from dysthymic disorder, psychotherapy should be recommended. This will be most effective if the primary care clinician is familiar with psychotherapists who are sensitive to women's issues and who specialize in treating depression. This personalized approach will maximize the chance that a patient will follow through and benefit from the referral.

A large majority of depressed women report marital problems, and women who have more severe marital problems are more likely to experience relapse. If marital problems are detected by the clinician or identified by the patient marital psychotherapy should be the referral. It can be used independently or as an adjunct to use of antidepressant medication. Marital counseling has been shown to be effective in treating depressed women with marital discord.

Patients who are not severely depressed, who are dysthymic, or who refuse medication can benefit from psychotherapy. Short-term psychotherapy is indicated in many situations. This is also true for patients who have obvious social stressors. The psychotherapist should again be someone who is familiar with women's health and should specialize in one of the psychotherapies that have been shown to be effective with depression, including cognitive therapy, behavioral therapy, or an eclectic active form of psychotherapy. Psychodynamic therapy, since it usually does not focus on immediate symptom relief, has not been shown to be effective as a short-term treatment. Monthly or periodic visits to the primary care clinician should address the patient's involvement in psychotherapy. This will emphasize the importance of comprehensive treatment. Patient education materials such as McGrath's *When Feeling Bad Is Good* or the federal Depression Guideline Panel's *Depression is a Treatable Illness* are also helpful.

Monitoring

During the initial stage of pharmacologic treatment (approximately 1 month) patients should be seen every week in order to foster compliance, to adjust dosages, and to monitor side effects. One of the most common reasons for treatment failure is an inadequate dose, so it is important to try to reach a therapeutic dose before concluding that a medication trial failed. Close attention should be paid to dosage and side effects because of the effects of age, body weight, and body composition in women. After the acute phase periodic monthly or 6-week visits are adequate.

Perhaps the most important issue in monitoring is follow-up care. Since hopelessness and lethargy are part of depression, up to one third of patients may not follow through with a medication trial. The primary care clinician who is treating a depressed patient needs to take an active, educational approach.

Duration of treatment

The primary care physician is often confronted with the issue of when to discontinue antidepressant medication.

After one episode of major depression the traditional recommendation has been that antidepressant medication can be discontinued after 6 to 9 months. There is some evidence supporting use for 1 to 2 years.

Many experts feel that maintenance treatment will prevent a new episode of depression. Patients with three or more previous episodes of major depression should be considered for long-time antidepressant medication. Others suggest that this is also true for people who have had two episodes and one of the following: a positive family history of bipolar disorder, a history of recurrence within 1 year after previously effective medication was discontinued, onset of the first episode before age 20, or severe, sudden, or life-threatening episodes.

The decision about discontinuation of antidepressants should be made in collaboration with the patient. Tricyclic antidepressants should be tapered, whereas fluoxetine and other SSRIs can be discontinued without tapering. It is possible that patients will experience some mild sleep disturbances during the discontinuation. It is important to discuss with patients their own ability to monitor their depression so that they will be able to seek treatment again if they see that depression is recurring.

SUMMARY

Depressive disorders are among the most prevalent psychiatric disorders in women. The primary care clinician can use the *DSM-IV* criteria to provide early detection and treatment. In addition a developmental approach can help the clinician be sensitive to predictable changes and stressors in women's lives. Antidepressant medication can be extremely effective and many recommend combined pharmacotherapy with psychotherapy. Working closely with a mental health professional who specializes in treating depression is recommended.

BIBLIOGRAPHY

American Psychiatric Association: *Diagnostic and statistical manual of mental disorders*, ed 4, Washington DC, 1994, American Psychiatric Association.

Feldman HS, Lopez MA: *Developmental psychology for the health care professions:* Part 2. *Adulthood and aging*, Boulder, Colo, 1982, Westview Press.

Hochschild A, Machung A: The second shift: working parents and the revolution at home, New York, 1989, Viking Press.

Kaplan AG: The "self-in-relation": implications for depression in women, *Psychother Theory, Res Prac* 23:235, 1986.

McKinlay JB, McKinlay SM, Brambilla DJ: The relative contributions of endocrine changes and social circumstances to depression in mid-aged women, *J Health Soc Behav* 28:345, 1987.

Mellinger GD, et al: Psychic distress, life crisis and use of psychotherapeutic medication, *Arch Gen Psychol* 35:1045, 1978.

Neugarten BL, Kraines RJ: "Menopausal symptoms" in women of various ages, *Psychosom Med* 27:266, 1965.

Wallerstein JS, Blakeslee S: *Second chances: men, women and children a decade after divorce*, New York, 1989, Ticknor and Fields.

Weissman MM: Advances in psychiatric epidemiology: rates and risks for major depression, *Am J Public Health*, 77:445, 1987.

68 Domestic Violence

Stephanie A. Eisenstat

One in seven women who comes to the physician's office for general medical care has a history of domestic abuse; yet this history rarely is obtained during the office visit (Freund and Blackhall, 1990). Underdiagnosis of domestic abuse is a critical problem because the health consequences of domestic abuse are then undertreated. Significant morbidity, and sometimes mortality, ensues because of clinicians' failure to identify domestic abuse.

This chapter reviews the clinical presentation of domestic violence in the primary care setting, considers reasons for the difficulty in identification of clinical cases, and outlines strategies for evaluation and intervention for identified cases of domestic abuse.

A variety of guides has been developed by physician groups to help assist in the identification and evaluation of cases of domestic abuse. The available guides are listed at the end of this chapter.

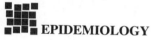

EPIDEMIOLOGY

Domestic abuse is a leading cause of morbidity and mortality in women. On the basis of national crime statistics an estimated 2 million women are battered each year in the United States. Because of underreporting the actual numbers probably are closer to 4 million. One in five women is the victim of a completed rape during her lifetime. According to a report issued by the Council on Scientific Affairs of the American Medical Association homicidal deaths resulting from one partner killing the other approached 40,000 from 1976 through 1986. More than half of these victims were women. In McLeer and Anwar's study of patients seeking emergency room treatment, one in three women was found to have a history of partner violence. One in six pregnant women was battered in a study by McFarlane and others of almost 700 pregnant women (see box, below).

DEFINITION AND CAUSE

Domestic violence has been defined by Flitcraft and associates as an ongoing, debilitating experience of *physical, psychologic,* and/or *sexual abuse* in the home, associated with increasing isolation from the outside world and limited personal freedom and accessibility to resources.

STATISTICS ON BATTERING

2-4 million women are battered per year
1 in 5 women is the victim of completed rape
1 in 4 women is physically abused
1 in 3 women seeking emergency room care has a history of partner violence
1 in 7 women coming to physicians' office for general medical care has a history of domestic abuse
1 in 6 pregnant women are battered every year

The aim of violence is to assert control and power. Figure 68-1, which illustrates the relationship between physical assaults, sexual assault, and other types of abusive and controlling behavior, was developed by the Duluth Domestic Abuse Intervention Project on the basis of discussions with more than 200 women. Often economic threats, emotional abuse, intimidation, isolation, and threats against the children occur along with the physical and sexual violence. Generally the severity, intensity, and frequency of the violent episodes increases as the abuser loses control and power over the victim. The physical abuse becomes recurrent and escalates in frequency and severity as illustrated in Fig. 68-2. The violence includes pushing, shoving, slapping, punching, kicking, choking, and assault with a weapon. The violent partner often refuses to help the victim when she is sick, and his behavior interferes with her obtaining proper medical treatment.

Psychologic abuse includes threats of harm, jealousy, possessiveness, and intimidation. Sexual abuse is any form of forced sex or sexual degradation.

RISK FACTORS

Although all women are at risk for domestic abuse, studies by Flitcraft have shown that some subgroups of women appear to be at higher risk (see box on the following page). Generally women who are single, young, and recently separated or divorced are at high risk. A history of alcohol or

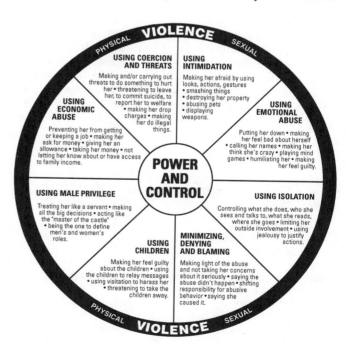

Fig. 68-1 Power and control wheel. (From Domestic Abuse Intervention Project, Duluth, Minn.)

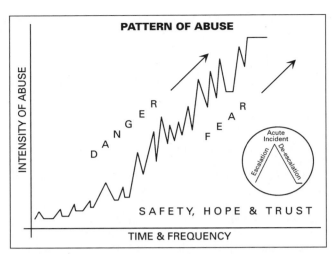

Fig. 68-2 Pattern of abuse. (From the New York State Office for the Prevention of Domestic Violence, 1990.)

substance abuse and mental illness in the patient or partner have been correlated with increased risk of domestic violence.

Pregnancy

A major risk factor is pregnancy. The incidence of domestic violence in pregnant patients was 8% in a study of a random sample at both private and public prenatal obstetric clinics by Helton, McFarlane, and Anderson and 7% to 11% in studies by Hilliard and Amaro of a nonrandom, university-based obstetric practices. According to Strauss and Gelles's review of the Second National Family Violence Survey, 15% of women in the first trimester of pregnancy and 17% of pregnant women during the second and third trimester pregnancy reported acts of domestic violence. For many women, the abuse starts during pregnancy, and according to McFarlane et al., for those with a prior history of partner abuse, the violence often escalates during pregnancy. The frequency, severity, and potential danger of homicide increase as well. A study of pregnant women by Bullock showed a higher rate of miscarriage and increased risk for low-birth-weight infants in pregnant women who were in abusive relationships. Other complications associated with battering during pregnancy are shown in the box, above right.

WOMEN AT RISK

Single women
Women who have been recently separated or divorced from their husband
Ages 17-28 years
History of alcohol or substance abuse; mental illness in patient or partner
Pregnant woman
History of childhood abuse

Modified from Alpert E et al: *Partner violence: how to recognize and treat victims of abuse—a guide for physicians,* Waltham, Mass, 1992, Massachusetts Medical Society.

ADVERSE PREGNANCY AND BIRTH OUTCOMES IN ABUSIVE RELATIONSHIPS

Miscarriage	Uterine rupture
Low birth weight	Premature rupture of membranes
Fetal fractures	Antepartum hemorrhage
Abruptio placentae	

History of childhood abuse

Studies by Flitcraft revealed that women with a history of childhood physical or sexual abuse were found to be at increased risk of experiencing domestic violence as adults. In addition, a correlation exists between child and wife abuse in the same family. In those families in which child abuse has been identified, outreach services should be offered to the wife as well.

BARRIERS TO IDENTIFICATION

For the clinician, dealing with cases of domestic abuse involves confronting difficult and ambiguous emotional circumstances. Sources of support and referral are not always readily available, and a number of barriers makes the accurate identification of domestic violence particularly difficult.

Patient barriers

Patients have misconceptions that interfere with their ability to tell the clinician about incidences of violence. The woman may think that the clinician is neither interested in her situation nor has the time to deal with it. Shame, guilt, and embarrassment can be overwhelming for the patient. Survivors of domestic violence report fear of the partner's reprisals, fear of threats to the children, and fear for their own safety. The battering of the woman's self-esteem results in the patient's perception that she deserves the abuse. Often there are financial threats as well as threats to the children.

Physician barriers

Physicians also face a number of barriers in dealing with cases of domestic abuse. Many clinicians hold deep-seated myths about abused patients (see box, below) that interfere with identification of these cases in the clinical setting. The reality for most of these women is that they are living in an environment of "terrorism" and because of the fear and manipulation on the part of the abuser, are unable to escape from the relationship. The patient does not provoke the violence. The abuser has a lack of impulse control and a need to

---

MYTHS ABOUT ABUSED PATIENTS

Violence is private
Patient can leave
Patient provokes violence
Problem of poor patients
Takes time to diagnose and intervene
Nothing can be done to prevent

Modified from Foley, Hoag, and Eliot: *Empowering battered women,* Boston, 1991, Massachusetts Coalition of Battered Women Services Groups.

control the partner. Cases of domestic abuse are seen in all socioeconomic and racial groups.

In addition to myths about these patients and intervention, the physician faces other barriers to identification. These include:

1. lack of education on strategies for identification and intervention
2. discomfort with dealing with the emotional aspects of the problem
3. lack of proper resources and referral networks.

In a small study of primary care physicians, Sugg and Inui explored the experience and attitudes of physicians with cases of domestic violence. The physicians identified lack of comfort with the problem, lack of time to deal with the problem, lack of resources and education, and a fear of offending the patient as barriers in diagnosis and treatment of the problem. Although clinicians are under time constraints, with proper training and access to resources, domestic violence cases can be identified and addressed in an efficient and effective manner.

HEALTH EFFECTS OF BATTERING

Although domestic violence happens in the home, the health and psychologic consequences of battering make it a priority for the primary care clinician. Battering has severe effects on the victim's health, well-being, and self-esteem. Obvious effects of domestic abuse are the physical trauma and potential risk of homicide. Abused women constitute 20% to 35% of all women who seek emergency room treatment for physical injuries. In addition to the physical trauma, continuous domestic abuse is associated with an increased risk for mental illness, alcoholism, substance abuse, and somatoform and eating disorders (see box, below).

There is evidence that domestic violence is associated with increased rates of physical and psychologic symptoms, hospitalizations, and substance abuse. Bergman and Brismar's controlled study of 117 women indicated higher rates of hospital utilization (Table 68-1), for trauma and for medical and gynecologic problems. The increased rates were particularly pronounced for inpatient hospitalizations for suicide attempts, gynecologic disorders, and observation (undefined disorders). The rates of mental illness, especially for depression, alcoholism, and substance abuse, were all increased in this study group as compared with the control group of women without a history of domestic violence (Table 68-2). The same correlation between prior sexual abuse and subsequent medical problems is suggested in a study by Springs and Friedrich as well.

In a study of 206 women seeking care at a gastroenterology practice for functional or organic disorders, 44% of

HEALTH EFFECTS OF ABUSE

Physical trauma
Mental illness
Increased risk for alcoholism and substance abuse
Somatoform disorder
Eating disorders

Table 68-1 Use of somatic hospital care during a period of 15 years (1973–1988) by battered women and age-matched control subjects

Reason for care	Battered Women (n =117)		Controls (n =117)	
	No. of women	No. of admissions	No. of women	No. of admissions
Surgical disorders (not trauma)	25	40*	19	22
Trauma	47†	70†	15	18
Gynecologic disorders	48†	91†	24	41
Induced abortion	20‡	22‡	7	8
Medical disorders	40†	71†	14	17
Suicide attempts	23†	55†	2	2
Observation	28†	71†	9	11
Total	90†	420†	58	119

From Bergman B, Brismar B: *Am J Public Health*, 81:1486, 1991.
*$p <0.05$.
†$p <0.01$.
‡$p <0.001$.

women reported sexual and physical abuse during childhood or adulthood (Drossman, 1990). Half of the abused women stated that some form of abuse was continuing into adulthood. Only about a third of these women told their physicians about the actual incidents of abuse. The group with a history of functional gastrointestinal complaints and physical abuse was four times more likely to have associated complaints such as diffuse pelvic pain, backaches, shortness of breath, and an increased rate of lifetime surgery. Despite multiple visits to the physician's office, fewer than 20% of the physicians were aware that the patients had experienced abuse. These findings are consistent with other clinical studies and reemphasize the need to suspect and identify cases of domestic violence especially if the woman manifests the particular spectrum of complaints in the following section.

Table 68-2 Diagnosis in psychiatric inpatient care of battered women and control subjects during 15 years (1973–1988)

Diagnoses	Battered women (n =117)		Control subjects (n =117)
	No.	%	
Depression	19	16*	0
Psychoses	10	9†	1
Alcoholism	27	23*	0
Drug addiction	10	9†	0
Suicide attempt	18	15*	0
Other and unspecified diagnosis	13	11†	0
Total number of psychiatric inpatients	69	59	1

From Bergman B, Brismar B: *Am J Public Health*, 81:1486, 1991.
*$p <0.01$.
†$p <0.001$.

CLINICAL PRESENTATION
History and symptoms

The interview. The first step in case identification is to ask the woman questions that will elicit a history of domestic violence. The box above lists common examples of such questions. It is important not to ask the question "Are you abused?" Studies have found that these women do not see themselves as "abused" and often will answer "no" to such a question but "yes" if the clinician asks "Has your partner ever hit you?"

It is important to make the patient feel comfortable, safe, and reassured. To promote this environment, it is important to interview the patient alone without the partner present and in a confidential manner. An explicit assurance of confidentiality by the clinician is important. The clinician should not break confidentiality by discussing the allegations with the patient's partner. Words such as "domestic violence," "abuse," or "battered" should not be used during interviews with patients. Because of their own perceptions of their situation, they will not necessary identify themselves as abused or in a relationship of domestic violence (see box, below). It also is important not to ask what the victim did to bring on the violence or why she has not left the relationship. Both statements are inappropriate and self-defeating.

The clinical presentation of the battered woman is *repeated physical injuries, medical complaints*, and *mental health problems.*

Physical trauma. The presenting complaints may clearly suggest battering with obvious physical trauma or they may be more obscure. Obvious clues to abuse include bilateral distribution of trauma in multiple areas, central distribution of injuries, bruises at different stages of healing, sexual assault, and trauma during pregnancy (see box, above right). Another clue to diagnosis is that the patient's *explanation* for the injury is often inconsistent with the *extent* of injury, and there may be a delay between the onset of the injury and presentation to the physician for treatment. The most common area of injury usually is the head and neck region as illustrated in Fig. 68-3, followed by the upper extremities, breast, back, and buttocks.

Somatic complaints and associated disorders. More subtle presentations include somatic complaints such as headaches, insomnia, fatigue, hyperventilation, and back or pelvic pain to list a few examples. A complaint of choking should prompt concern about the possibility of physical or sexual abuse. Eating disorders and other mental health problems are more common in women with a history of abuse.

A rare presentation is stroke in a young woman. Unexplained stroke in a young woman warrants further evaluation for suspected abuse. Lack of prenatal care and the physical or sexual abuse of the woman's children are other clues.

Common behaviors. Often women experiencing domestic violence are mistrustful of the primary care provider and fearful of reprisal from the abusive partner. This reaction is not totally unfounded inasmuch as studies have shown that violence by the partner may escalate after identification of the abuser. Dealing with this aspect of the problem is

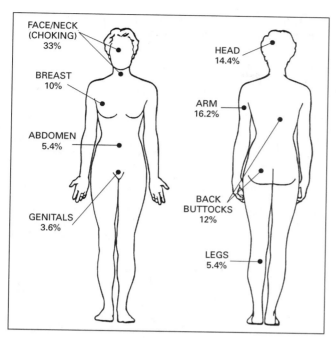

Fig. 68-3 Sites and percentages of abuse injuries. (From Helton A, Anderson E, McFarlane J: *Protocol of care for the battered woman,* White Plains, NY, 1986, March of Dimes Birth Defects Foundation.)

addressed in the next section. Because of fear and distrust, the profile of a woman who has a history of abuse may include evasive behavior, vague historic recollection, and anxious behavior during the interview. Frequent visits to the emergency room or outpatient office and an overly aggressive or attentive partner accompanying the woman should raise the clinician's suspicion for abuse. The box on the previous page lists these and other common behaviors seen in the battered woman.

Physical examination

A thorough documentation of the patient's account and complaints should be completed and a complete physical examination performed, with special attention to the areas of the patient's complaints. Any possible injuries should be photographed after informed consent. If domestic abuse is suspected, it is a good idea to contact a social worker, if one is available, as soon as possible to expedite the process of intervention.

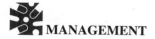 **MANAGEMENT**

Goals of management

The primary care clinician does not have to be an expert in the psychosocial aspects of domestic violence to effectively prevent future trauma and the development of associated medical disorders. The clinician's role is to diagnose and identify the problem, then to provide the appropriate referral network. It is important to investigate the various options available before facing a case of domestic violence and to have a general strategy and referral network in place. Resources are listed in Appendix X. If available, ideal intervention is interdisciplinary and involves social services and

---

nursing. The primary care physician's role is important in supporting the patient and validating the patient's experiences (see box, above).

Referral

Various options for action are available to the woman who has been subjected to domestic abuse (see box, below). In general, the process requires that the woman make a formal legal complaint against the abuser, which often is very difficult for her. As a competent adult she has the right to refuse intervention. It is important in these cases to keep the door open and to make sure that the woman knows her options and has available the appropriate telephone numbers to contact help when she is ready. Often after she has thought about the danger and the physical and psychologic trauma she has already endured, she is able to decide to take action. To maintain supportive contact it is helpful to arrange follow-up appointments with the primary care physician and any other social service advocates.

Restraining orders and shelters. The patient needs to be aware of the existence of shelters, the availability of law enforcement, and the method for obtaining legal restraining orders. Providing this information requires each physician to contact local agencies to determine local available resources. Many states now have strict laws and guidelines that protect all women in a familial or dating relationship, providing them the option to obtain an emergency, temporary, and/or permanent restraining order against the abuser. A permanent restraining order, which is valid up to 1 year, may be obtained through superior, probate, and family district or municipal court. In most states, if the batterer violates the restraining order or stalks the woman, the police must arrest him. The agencies associated with the "hotline" numbers listed in Appendix X should be able to provide this information. Many local groups for battered women have available information on shelters and state laws, as well as volunteers who serve as patient advocates.

Mandatory reporting. If violence is perpetrated against an elderly person, a child younger than 18 years of age, or a

MANDATORY REPORTING OF ABUSE

Children younger than 18 years of age
Elderly persons aged 60 years or older
Disabled persons
Sexual assault (without name identification)
Gunshot and stab wounds

disabled person, or if there is a sexual assault, the incident *must* be reported to state authorities (see box, above).

Assessment of safety. After the identification of domestic abuse, the episodes of abuse may escalate. Although it is not common for the abuser to be violent with clinical staff members, he may be more abusive to the patient. In discharge planning, it is important to assess the woman's safety. With the help of a social worker (if available), one should assess the *abuser's threats about homicide and suicide, depression, weapons possession, obsession with his partner, drug and alcohol consumption, access to the battered woman,* and the *degree of escalation of threats and violence.* The woman needs to understand her potential risk. Most women want to accept help, but the process of ending the relationship (however bad it is) is painful and difficult. If the woman is not ready to leave the abusive situation, even temporarily, every effort should be made to keep her options open and contact with the medical and social service system readily available.

For men who batter. There are in existence programs that provide counseling and intervention for the batterer. Unfortunately, the success of these programs is controversial, and more research data are needed to establish the efficacy of these programs. The initial intervention is to separate the patient from the violent situation and ensure that the woman (and her children) are in a safe environment. Available programs in each area can be obtained through the "hotline" numbers listed in Appendix X.

SUMMARY

Domestic violence is a common and often misdiagnosed problem in the primary care setting. It is important to screen women for violence first by asking the questions and then by intervening with support services. In addition to the psychosocial stresses caused by violence, these patients also have an increased risk of medical and psychiatric illness and require close medical follow-up. Alpert et al. developed the

RADAR

R Remember to ask routinely about partner violence.
A Ask directly about violence with questions such as "At any time has your partner hit you?"
   Interview in private.
D Document your findings.
A Assess your patient's safety.
R Review options with your patient.

From Alpert E et al: *Partner violence: how to recognize and treat victims of abuse—a guide for physicians,* Waltham, Mass, 1992, Massachusetts Medical Society.

acronym RADAR, which summarizes the important aspects in identification and intervention (see box, below left).

BIBLIOGRAPHY

Alpert E et al: *Partner violence: how to recognize and treat victims of abuse—a guide for physicians,* Waltham, Mass, 1992, Massachusetts Medical Society.

Amaro H et al: Violence during pregnancy and substance abuse, *Am J Public Health,* 80:575, 1990.

American College of Obstetricians and Gynecologists (ACOG): Washington, DC, *The battered woman* (Tech Bull 124), 1989, The College.

Atwood JD: Domestic violence: the role of alcohol, *JAMA* 265:460, 1991 (letter).

Benton DA: Battered women: why do they stay? *Health Care Women Int* 7:403, 1987.

Bergman B, Brismar B: A five year follow up study of 117 battered women, *Am J Public Health* 81:1486, 1991.

Bullock L, McFarlane J: The birth-weight/battering connection, *Am J Nurs,* p 1153, Sept 1989.

Bullock L et al: The prevalence and characteristics of battered women in a primary care setting, *Nurse Pract* 14:47, 1989.

Council on Scientific Affairs, American Medical Association: Violence against women: relevance for medical practitioners, *JAMA* 267:3184, 1992.

Drossman D et al: Sexual and physical abuse in women with functional or organic gastrointestinal disorders, *Ann Intern Med* 113:828, 1990.

Flitcraft AH: Violence, values and gender, *JAMA* 267:3194, 1992.

Flitcraft AH et al: *Diagnostic and treatment guidelines on domestic violence,* Chicago, 1992, American Medical Association.

Foley, Hoag, Eliot: *Empowering battered women: suggestions for health care providers,* Boston, 1991, Massachusetts Coalition of Battered Women Service Groups.

Freund KM, Blackhall LJ: Detection of domestic violence in a primary care setting, *Clin Res* 38:738A, 1990.

Gelles R: Violence and pregnancy: are pregnant women at greater risk of abuse? *J Marriage Fam* p 841, Aug 1988.

Gin N et al: Prevalence of domestic violence among patients in three ambulatory care internal medicine clinics, *J Gen Intern Med* 6:317, 1991.

Gottfried D: Medical aspects of domestic violence, *Conn Med* 267, May 1990.

Haber JD, Roos C: Effects of spousal abuse and/or sexual abuse in the development and maintenance of chronic pain in women, *Adv Pain Res Ther* 9:889, 1985.

Harrop-Griffiths J et al: The association between chronic pelvic pain, psychiatric diagnoses, and childhood sexual abuse, *Obstet Gynecol* 71:589, 1988.

Hasselt VN et al, editors: *Handbook of family violence,* New York, 1988, Plenum.

Helton A, McFarlane J, Anderson E: Battered and pregnant: a prevalence study, *Am J Public Health* 77:1337, 1987.

Helton A, Anderson E, McFarlane J: Protocol of care for the battered woman, White Plains, NY, 1986, March of Dimes Birth Defects Foundation.

Hillard PJ: Physical abuse in pregnancy, *Obstet Gynecol* 66:185, 1985.

King MC, Ryan J: Abused women: dispelling myths and encouraging intervention. In Foley, Hoag, Eliot, editors: *Empowering battered women: suggestions for the health care providers,* Boston, 1991, Massachusetts Coalition of Battered Women Service Groups.

Koss MP, Koss PG, Woodruff J: Deleterious effects of criminal victimization on women's health and medical utilization, *Arch Intern Med* 151:342, 1991.

Langan PA, Innes CA: *Preventing domestic violence against women.* Washington, DC, 1986, Department of Justice, Bureau of Justice Statistics.

McFarlane J et al: Assessing for abuse during pregnancy: severity and frequency of injuries and associated entry into prenatal care, *JAMA* 267:3176, 1992.

McLeer SV, Anwar R: A study of battered women presenting in an emergency department, *Am J Public Health* 79:65, 1989.

Newberger E et al: Pregnant women abuse and adverse birth outcome. In *Preterm birth: causes, prevention and treatment,* Elmsford, NY, 1990, Pergamon.

Newberger E et al: Abuse of pregnant women and adverse birth outcome: current knowledge and implications for practice, *JAMA* 267:2370, 1992.

Randall T: Hospital-wide program identifies battered women; offers assistance, *JAMA* 266:1177, 1991.

Randall T: Tools available for health care providers whose patients are at risk for domestic violence, *JAMA* 266:1179, 1991.

Randall T: Duluth takes firm stance against domestic violence; mandates abuser arrest, education, *JAMA* 266:1180, 1991.

Randall T: Domestic violence begets other problems of which physicians must be aware to be effective, *JAMA* 264:940, 1990.

Randall T: Domestic violence intervention calls for more than treating, *JAMA* 265:939, 1990.

Raymond C: Campaign alerts physicians to identify, assist victims of domestic violence, *JAMA* 261:963, 1989.

Schecter S: *Interviewing battered women: guidelines for the mental health practitioner in domestic violence cases,* Washington, DC, 1987, NCAV.

Springs F, Friedrich W: Health risk behaviors and medical sequelae of childhood sexual abuse, *Mayo Clin Proc* 67:527, 1992.

Reiter RC, Gambone JC: Demographic and historic variables in women with idiopathic chronic pelvic pain, *Obstet Gynecol* 75:428, 1990.

Reiter RC et al: Correlation between sexual abuse and somatization in women with somatic and nonsomatic chronic pelvic pain, *Am J Obstet Gynecol* 165:104, 1991.

Stark E et al: Wife abuse in the medical setting: an introduction for health personnel (monograph No 7), Washington DC, 1981, National Clearinghouse on Domestic Violence.

Straus MA, Gelles RJ: How violent are American families? Estimates from the national family violence resurvey and other studies. In Hotaling G et al, editors: *Family abuse and its consequences: new directions for research*, Newbury Park, Calif, 1988, Sage.

Straus MA, Gelles RJ, editors: *Physical violence in American families: risk factors and adaptions to violence in 8145 families*, New Brunswick, NJ, 1990, Transaction Books.

Straus MA, Gelles RJ, Steinmetz S: *Behind closed doors: violence in the American family*, New York, 1980, Doubleday.

Sugg N, Inui T: Primary care physicians' response to domestic violence: opening Pandora's box, *JAMA* 297:3157, 1992.

69 Eating Disorders

Nancy A. Rigotti

Anorexia nervosa and bulimia nervosa are psychiatric disorders of disturbed eating behavior that have serious medical consequences. Over 90% of cases occur in women. The task of the primary care physician is to recognize the syndromes, evaluate patients for medical complications, assist in ambulatory management, and determine when a patient requires hospitalization.

EPIDEMIOLOGY AND CLINICAL PRESENTATION

Anorexia nervosa is a syndrome of severe weight loss that results from inadequate food intake by individuals with no medical reason to lose weight. Instead an intense fear of becoming fat and a disturbance in body image lead to a refusal to maintain weight within a normal, healthy range for age and height. The American Psychiatric Association has developed criteria to guide diagnosis (see box on the following page). Weight loss can occur in two ways. About half of patients severely limit food intake (restricting subtype); a second group purges after eating, usually by vomiting or taking laxatives, and may also have eating binges (binge-eating/purging subtype). Both groups may exercise vigorously. Restricting anorexics are also likely to have obsessive-compulsive symptoms, whereas those who binge may have other impulse control problems, including substance abuse or sexual promiscuity. Patients with the purging subtype of anorexia nervosa have more medical problems and a worse prognosis than individuals with the restricting subtype.

Bulimia nervosa is an illness characterized by repeated episodes of binge eating, during which an individual rapidly consumes a large amount of high-calorie foods and feels unable to stop. To prevent weight gain after a binge, the bulimic patient either purges by inducing vomiting or taking laxatives or diuretics (purging subtype) or fasts or exercises for a prolonged period (nonpurging subtype). Bulimic patients fear losing control of their eating behavior and are ashamed when it happens. Binges must occur at least twice weekly for 3 months to meet diagnostic criteria for bulimia nervosa, but they may be repeated as often as several times daily. In severe cases there may be no regular eating pattern. The result of this behavior is frequent weight fluctuations but *not* severe weight loss.

There is considerable overlap between anorexia nervosa and bulimia nervosa. Preoccupation with food and body weight, a disturbed body image, poor self-esteem, and a fear of loss of control are hallmarks of both disorders. Symptoms of depression occur at a high rate in both conditions. Individuals may alternate between diagnoses during the course of the illness. Approximately half of anorexic patients have bulimic symptoms, and about half of patients with bulimia nervosa have a history of anorexia nervosa or have the symptoms during the illness. Nonetheless, the syndromes do differ in presentation. The emaciation of an anorexic patient often leads others to get her medical attention, even though she denies that she is ill. The physician then has the task of convincing the patient of the seriousness of her condition. In contrast, bulimics are aware that their behavior is abnormal, but shame leads them to conceal the problem. The bulimic's near-normal weight permits the illness to be hidden. Detection of surreptitious vomiting or laxative abuse is a challenge for the primary care physician.

Eating disorders start early in life. Anorexia nervosa usually begins during adolescence, with peaks occurring at ages 14 and 18, but it can appear before puberty or as late as midlife. The onset frequently coincides with a stressful life

DIAGNOSTIC CRITERIA FOR ANOREXIA NERVOSA AND BULIMIA NERVOSA

Anorexia nervosa

1. Refusal to maintain a minimal normal body weight for age and height, resulting in weight below 85% of that expected.

2. Intense fear of gaining weight or becoming fat, even though underweight.

3. Disturbance in the way in which body weight or shape is experienced, undue influence of body weight or shape in self-evaluation, or denial of the seriousness of current low weight.

4. Amenorrhea of ≥3 months.

Bulimia nervosa

1. Recurrent episodes of binge eating, characterized by:
   a. Eating a large amount of food within a discrete period of time, and
   b. Feeling a lack of control over eating during the episode.

2. Recurrent inappropriate compensatory behavior to avoid weight gain (e.g., self-induced vomiting, laxative or diuretic use, fasting, or excessive exercise).

3. Binge eating and compensatory behaviors occur an average of twice a week for 3 months.

4. Self-evaluation is unduly influenced by body shape and weight.

5. Symptoms occur when body weight is at least 85% of normal for age and height (e.g., patient does not have concurrent anorexia nervosa).

Modified from *Diagnostic and statistical manual of mental disorders,* ed 4, Washington, DC, 1994, American Psychiatric Association.

event such as separation from home or the loss of a loved one by illness, death, or divorce. Once considered a disorder of upper socioeconomic groups, it is now more evenly distributed across social strata. Bulimia nervosa begins in adolescence or young adulthood, with a peak incidence at age 18. Typically it begins during or after a diet.

Eating disorders appear to be increasing in prevalence. Approximately 0.5% to 1% of women between the ages of 15 and 30 have anorexia nervosa. Bulimia is more common, affecting 1% to 3% of adolescent and college age women. Many more women are preoccupied with food and weight, diet unnecessarily, and may even binge eat and purge occasionally without meeting the strict diagnostic criteria of anorexia nervosa or bulimia nervosa.

CAUSES AND PATHOGENESIS

The cause of anorexia nervosa and bulimia nervosa appears to be multifactorial, arising from an interplay of sociocultural, genetic, psychologic, and familial factors. Whatever the predisposing cause the immediate precipitant is usually a dissatisfaction with body shape that leads to dieting and then malnutrition. The physical and psychologic consequences of starvation help to perpetuate the illness. Even normal individuals who are experimentally starved develop food preoccupations, social withdrawal, loss of libido,

symptoms of depression, and temporary bingeing when they are refed.

The cultural pressure on women to be slender presumably explains the higher prevalence of eating disorders in Western societies and the female predominance of the disorders. Eating disorders rarely occur in societies that lack abundant food and do not value leanness in females. In the U.S. culture, eating disorders appear to be more prevalent in individuals for whom thinness is associated with professional success (e.g., dancers, gymnasts, figure skaters, long-distance runners, jockeys, models, and actors). However, cultural norms cannot explain why only some women have the illness.

Genetic, biologic, psychologic, or familial factors may contribute to an individual's vulnerability to development of an eating disorder. Twin studies suggest that anorexia nervosa may have an inherited component. Anorexic patients have well-documented neuroendocrine abnormalities, but the fact that these reverse with weight gain suggests that they are the consequence and not the cause of the starvation. The early age of onset of these disorders suggests that difficulties in emotional development or disturbed family dynamics are involved.

There is a strong association between eating disorders and mood disorders. Eating disorder patients have a high rate of comorbid depression, which may abate with weight gain. Affective disorders are more common in family members of individuals with eating disorders. Whether depression is a predisposing factor or a consequence of eating disorders is debated. Other psychiatric illnesses are also associated with eating disorders. Obsessive-compulsive disorder occurs in approximately 10% of anorexic patients. Bulimic patients have an increased rate of anxiety disorders, chemical dependency, and impulsive behavior such as overspending, shoplifting, sexual promiscuity, substance abuse, and self-mutilation. A history of sexual abuse has been reported in as many as one half of patients with anorexia and bulimia.

CLINICAL MANIFESTATIONS AND MEDICAL COMPLICATIONS
Anorexia nervosa

The presentation of the anorexic patient is remarkable for the lack of complaints despite emaciation. In contrast to patients who lose weight because of medical illness, the patient with anorexia nervosa is often unconcerned about, or even proud of, her weight loss. Unlike other starving individuals anorexics are usually not fatigued until malnutrition is advanced. Most are restless and physically active, and some exercise to excess. Patients may report difficulty sleeping, abdominal discomfort and bloating after eating, constipation, cold intolerance, and polyuria. Amenorrhea is uniformly present in females. Physical examination reveals an emaciated patient bundled in clothing. Skin is dry and may be pale (as a result of anemia) or yellow-tinged (as a result of carotenemia). Fine downy hair, termed *lanugo,* may cover face and arms. The female pattern of fat distribution disappears, but axillary and pubic hair are preserved. Bradycardia, hypotension, and hypothermia are common.

The physical consequences of anorexia nervosa are those of starvation. Inadequate nutrient intake results in a loss of fat stores and then atrophy of skeletal and cardiac muscle. Weight loss is accompanied by a compensatory slowing of metabolism mediated by thyroid hormone. This reduces energy expenditure and conserves body mass. In prepubertal patients skeletal growth, physical development, and sexual maturation stop. The signs and symptoms of anorexia nervosa reflect both the starvation and the homeostatic response. Anorexic patients who purge suffer additional physical consequences. Nearly all physical consequences are reversible with refeeding, but prepubertal patients may never grow to previously anticipated height.

The most serious medical consequences are cardiac arrhythmias, which may lead to sudden death. Prolonged QT intervals preceded death in one case series. A variety of other supraventricular and ventricular arrhythmias occur; sinus bradycardia is most common. Electrocardiographic changes include low voltage ST-segment depression and T-wave flattening. Cardiac muscle mass atrophies with starvation, but cardiac output is preserved and congestive heart failure does not occur. Echocardiography reveals mitral valve prolapse in up to one third of cases; it disappears with weight gain and is of no clinical significance.

Weight loss is also accompanied by widespread alterations in endocrine function. Thyroid hormone metabolism changes to slow metabolism and conserve body mass. Thyroxine is preferentially converted to the inactive reverse-triiodothyronine (reverse-T_3) rather than to the more potent triiodothyronine, as normally occurs. Thyroxine levels are in the low-normal range, but triiodothyronine levels are reduced, and anorexics have some clinical features suggesting hypothyroidism (such as bradycardia, hypothermia, dry skin, cold intolerance, and constipation). However, there is no compensatory rise in the level of thyroid-stimulating hormone (TSH). Patients are euthyroid and no treatment other than refeeding is necessary.

Starvation also leads to a reversible dysfunction of the hypothalamic-pituitary axis. A critical amount of body fat is necessary to initiate the cyclic gonadotropin release required for ovulation. Reduced gonadotropin secretion leads to anovulation, hypothalamic amenorrhea, and estrogen deficiency. Weight loss does not entirely explain the amenorrhea, because up to 25% of anorexics lose menses before losing much weight, and amenorrhea may persist after weight is regained. The hypothalamic-pituitary-adrenal axis is overactive, leading to elevated plasma cortisol levels that are not suppressed with administration of dexamethasone, but there are no clinical signs of Cushing's syndrome. Persistently elevated cortisol levels probably contribute to amenorrhea. Reduced vasopressin secretion from the posterior pituitary may occur and account for polyuria. The anorexic's hypothalamus defends core temperature poorly in the face of changes in environmental temperature, resulting in hypothermia.

Anorexics' diets are deficient in carbohydrates and total calories but, because protein and vitamin intake is relatively preserved, vitamin deficiencies and hypoalbuminemia are unusual. The metabolic slowing of anorexia nervosa is accompanied by characteristic changes. Gastrointestinal motility is slowed, explaining symptoms of abdominal bloating and constipation. A reversible bone marrow depression occurs, characterized by mild anemia (rarely caused by iron, folate, or vitamin B_{12} deficiency) and leukopenia (without immunosuppression). Cholesterol and carotene levels increase, reflecting an acquired defect in lipoprotein metabolism rather than excess dietary intake. Blood levels of glucose are normal or mildly reduced. However, when starvation is very advanced, severe hypoglycemia leading to coma and death has been reported. Mild elevations in liver enzyme levels and low serum zinc levels also occur in some patients. Electrolyte abnormalities are unusual in restricting anorexic patients; when present they generally indicate purging behavior.

Anorexic women have a reduced skeletal mass and an increased risk of fracture. The osteoporosis is multifactorial; estrogen deficiency, low dietary calcium intake, and excess cortisol probably all contribute. Bone density reductions have not been shown to reverse with refeeding, raising concerns that an episode of anorexia nervosa will predispose to osteoporosis later in life.

Bulimia nervosa

The medical consequences of bulimia nervosa are largely the consequence of the patient's purging, not her binge eating. Binge eating has few sequelae other than abdominal distention and discomfort. The complications of purging depend on the patient's specific behavior. Chronic vomiting can cause gastric and esophageal irritation and bleeding, and, rarely, Mallory-Weiss tears. Repeated regurgitation of stomach contents produces volume depletion and a hypochloremic metabolic alkalosis. Dizziness, syncope, thirst, orthostatic hypotension, and an elevated blood urea nitrogen (BUN) level occur in the volume-depleted patient. Renal compensation for the alkalosis and volume depletion leads to potassium depletion and hypokalemia, accompanied by low serum and urine chloride levels. Symptoms of hypokalemia are nonspecific: muscle cramps and weakness, paresthesias, polyuria, constipation. Arrhythmias, T-wave flattening, and U waves may be seen on the electrocardiogram. Reversible painless parotid gland swelling, often accompanied by hyperamylasemia, can occur with chronic vomiting. Repeated exposure of the teeth to stomach acid decalcifies enamel and leads to irreversible dental erosion. Abuse of emetine (ipecac) to induce vomiting causes a reversible myopathy of proximal skeletal muscle and a potentially fatal cardiomyopathy.

The abuse of laxatives may begin as a response to constipation and continue because of the temporary weight loss it causes. Weight loss is transient and secondary to fluid depletion rather than to reduced absorption of calories. Stimulant laxatives are often used. They increase colonic motility, producing abdominal cramps, watery diarrhea, and electrolyte loss. Volume depletion, hyponatremia, hypokalemia, and either metabolic acidosis or alkalosis may result. Hypocalcemia and hypomagnesemia have also been reported. Rapid fecal transit may irritate intestinal mucosa or hemorrhoids, causing rectal bleeding and even rectal prolapse. Rarely, chronic laxative abuse results in an immotile "cathartic colon" unable to produce bowel movements without stimulation. Usually, however, bowel function returns when laxative use stops.

Patients use diuretics more often to prevent fluid retention than to induce weight loss. Chronic use leads to a hypochloremic metabolic alkalosis, hypokalemia, volume depletion, and dilutional hyponatremia. In contrast to vomiters and laxative abusers, diuretic users do not have low urine sodium and chloride levels.

Even though bulimic women are not underweight, they may have menstrual irregularity or even a hypothalamic amenorrhea. The cause is not known, but elevations in serum cortisol level may be involved.

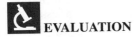

EVALUATION

Anorexia nervosa

Anorexia nervosa should be suspected when patients experience unexplained weight loss. A careful history usually suggests the diagnosis. The history should explore the patient's attitude toward her body shape, her weight loss, her desired weight, and her eating habits. A 24-hour dietary recall is more revealing than general questions about diet. Detailed weight and menstrual histories should be obtained, including the date and circumstances at the onset of weight loss, minimum and maximum weights, and recent weight changes. All patients should be asked about binge eating, vomiting, and use of laxatives, diuretics, diet pills, and emetics. The amount of daily exercise should be quantified. Patients should be asked about symptoms of malnutrition (fatigue, skin or hair changes), dehydration (lightheadedness, syncope, thirst), hypokalemia (cramps, weakness, paresthesias, polyuria, palpitations), and other symptoms common in purgers (heartburn, abdominal pain, rectal bleeding). Inquiry should also include questions about depressive symptoms, substance use, and physical or sexual abuse.

Physical examination, supplemented by laboratory studies, excludes other causes of weight loss and quantifies the severity of malnutrition and dehydration. A careful physical examination should include measurement of height, weight (without street clothing), temperature, and orthostatic vital signs. Laboratory investigation should include a complete blood count; BUN; levels of serum electrolytes, creatinine, and glucose; liver and thyroid function tests; and an electrocardiogram. If weight loss is severe, calcium, phosphorus, magnesium, and albumin levels should be measured. Mild abdominal discomfort and distension are common and do not need further evaluation; if symptoms are severe or accompanied by diarrhea, abdominal radiographs, barium studies, and stool examination may be indicated to exclude occult bowel disease. Bone densitometry should be considered for women who have been underweight and amenorrheic for 12 months.

Extensive evaluation of symptoms or laboratory or endocrinologic abnormalities common to anorexia is not necessary. However, if the clinical picture is atypical the physician must consider other causes of weight loss, including malignancy, chronic infection, intestinal disorders (malabsorption, inflammatory bowel disease, or hepatitis), and endocrinopathies (hyperthyroidism), panhypopituitarism, adrenal insufficiency, diabetes mellitus). Rarely, central nervous system tumors or seizure disorders mimic anorexia nervosa or bulimia; computed tomography or electroencephalography can exclude these diagnoses in patients wtih neurologic signs or symptoms. Psychiatric illnesses that can be confused with anorexia include depression, schizophrenia, and obsessive-compulsive disorder.

Bulimia nervosa

Making the diagnosis of bulimia requires maintaining a high index of suspicion, because binge eating and purging are easily concealed by a normal-weight woman. Clues include a preoccupation with weight and food, a history of frequent weight fluctuations, and complaints common to patients who purge and become dehydrated (dizziness, thirst, syncope) or hypokalemic (muscle cramps or weakness, paresthesias, polyuria). Vomiters may also have hematemesis or heartburn; laxative abusers may complain of constipation, rectal bleeding, and fluid retention. When the diagnosis is suspected the physician should ask directly and nonjudgmentally about bingeing and purging and assess serum electrolyte levels. A direct inquiry may elicit the history from a patient seeking help but ashamed to volunteer the information. Patients suspected of bulimia should also be asked about alcohol and substance use, depressive symptoms, and sexual or physical abuse.

Physical examination is often unrevealing, especially in patients with milder degrees of illness. The examination should include measurement of postural signs for evidence of volume depletion. Enlarged parotid glands, erosion of dental enamel, and scars on the dorsum of the hand used to induce vomiting (Russell's sign) are signs of chronic self-induced vomiting. Laboratory studies should include tests of serum and urine electrolytes; serum creatinine and BUN; and an electrocardiogram. Electrolyte levels are often normal early in the disease or in those who purge less often. The pattern of serum and urine electrolytes helps to determine the mode of purging. Calcium and magnesium levels should be measured in laxative abusers. Some patients who vomit deny that it is voluntary. Organic causes of chronic vomiting should be excluded in these cases with barium studies. The combination of unexplained hypochloremic alkalosis, concern about weight gain, and absence of other abnormality strongly suggests bulimia.

CHOICE OF THERAPY

The goals of treatment are (1) to restore weight in order to correct the physical and psychologic sequelae of malnutrition, (2) to control abnormal eating behavior, and (3) to prevent relapse by addressing the associated psychologic and family problems. Because the illness is multidimensional a multidisciplinary treatment approach, combining medical, nutritional, psychologic and pharmacologic therapies, is the standard of care for eating disorders.

Anorexia nervosa

Weight restoration is the first goal of treatment for patients with anorexia nervosa. Achieving this goal often requires hospitalization, ideally in a psychiatric unit experienced in treating eating disorders. Refeeding can usually be accomplished with a normal diet. Nasogastric tube feeding or parenteral nutrition is rarely necessary and best avoided because of the risk of complications. Inpatient treatment also includes medical monitoring, behavioral therapy that links desired activities to achievement of weight goals, supervised exercise, psychotherapy, and family therapy. This approach generally produces weight gain, but relapse is common. Outcome is best if the patient remains hospitalized until she has reached a normal weight. Some anorexic patients can gain weight as outpatients; they are less underweight, medically stable, highly motivated to change, and have a supportive environment. Close medical monitoring is necessary. If the patient does not gain weight within a few weeks, hospitalization is indicated.

A variety of medications, including antidepressants, antipsychotics, and appetite stimulants, have been tried for anorexia nervosa. Few have been subjected to placebo-controlled trials, and no drug has been demonstrated to be dramatically effective. Even though anorexic patients are often depressed, they respond poorly to antidepressants and are more prone to side effects. These drugs are best reserved for patients whose depression does not improve with weight gain.

Bulimia nervosa

Most bulimia nervosa patients can be treated as outpatients. Many types of psychologic treatments have been employed, but controlled studies are few. The best evidence supports cognitive-behavioral therapy, which helps patients monitor their behavior and alter their attitudes about weight and eating. Individual or group psychotherapy and family therapy are also commonly used. Treatment may be supplemented with support groups (e.g., Overeaters Anonymous). Substance abuse, if present, must be treated concurrently.

In contrast to their role in anorexia nervosa, antidepressants are effective in reducing the symptoms of bulimia nervosa, even in patients without coexistent depression. Placebo-controlled trials have demonstrated the efficacy of tricyclic agents (imipramine and desipramine), trazodone, fluoxetine, and monoamine oxidase inhibitors (phenelzine and isocarboxazid) in decreasing the frequency of binge eating and purging in bulimic patients. Drug treatment should supplement, not replace, psychologic treatment of bulimic patients.

NATURAL HISTORY AND PROGNOSIS

Anorexia nervosa has a variable course. Women may recover after a single episode, repeatedly gain and lose weight, or remain chronically underweight. More than half experience relapse after an initial hospitalization for weight gain. In studies following anorexic patients at least 4 years, 44% had a good outcome (weight returned to within 15% of recommended levels and menses resumed), 24% had a poor outcome (inadequate weight gain), and 28% had an intermediate outcome. Factors associated with poor outcome are lower weight, older age at presentation, longer duration of symptoms before treatment, and coexisting bulimia. Weight preoccupation, unusual eating behavior, and psychosocial problems often persist. Up to 40% of anorexic women develop bulimia and 15% to 25% of patients develop chronic anorexia nervosa. Because of the early age of onset of anorexia nervosa, physicians caring for adults are more likely to see women with a chronic syndrome.

Approximately 5% to 10% of patients with anorexia nervosa die, either of the consequences of starvation or by suicide. Most deaths are sudden, apparently caused by cardiac arrhythmias. Prolonged QT intervals may be a harbinger. Fatal hypoglycemic coma has also been reported. The risk of death increases with greater weight loss, especially when weight loss exceeds 30% of premorbid weight. Bulimic anorexics with metabolic abnormalities are probably also at higher risk.

Less is known about the natural history of bulimia nervosa, with or without treatment. The mortality rate appears to be lower than in anorexia nervosa, but the disorder can persist for years before and after it is discovered. Short-term prognosis is good: 70% of patients completing outpatient treatment programs achieve substantial symptom reduction, but 25% have a relapse within 6 months. The course is most often episodic with gradual improvement.

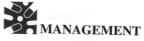

MANAGEMENT

Treating the patient with an eating disorder requires attention to both medical and psychosocial problems. For outpatient treatment the primary care physician usually works with a psychiatrist or psychologist to develop a coordinated treatment plan in which the primary care physician assumes responsibility for the patient's physical care while the psychiatrist coordinates psychosocial treatment. A dietitian is usually involved to monitor nutrition and provide counseling to help the patient learn to eat small, regular meals. The team approach eases the physician's burden when treating a patient who may deny the seriousness of the illness; can be deceptive, manipulative, and angry; and has difficulty trusting the physician. All caretakers must agree on overall goals and maintain contact with each other during the treatment.

The first challenge may be to convince an indifferent patient that treatment is necessary. The physician should inform the patient of the nature of the illness, its seriousness, and its potential complications. The patient should understand that anorexia is a life-threatening illness and that the first priority is to protect her life so that psychiatric treatment can proceed. For anorexics the necessity of weight gain to prevent long-term sequelae such as osteoporosis must be emphasized. Patients who purge should be educated about the consequences of their behavior, including the irreversible dental damage. The ineffectiveness of laxative or diuretic use for real weight loss should be explained. The connection between the eating disorder and any symptoms or laboratory abnormalities present should be pointed out.

The physician should set guidelines for outpatient management, (see box on the following page). It is helpful to make these explicit in a written contract signed by the physician and patient and shared with other caretakers. It should specify the conditions that must be met for outpatient medical treatment to continue; these usually include a minimum acceptable weight, maintenance of normal electrolyte levels, and regular psychologic and nutritional therapy. It should be understood that hospitalization will be required if these conditions are not met. The minimum weight is usually set at 30% below premorbid or ideal body weight. The weight goal is more difficult to determine and is often a point of disagreement between physician and patient. An estimate of desirable weight for height can be derived from standard tables. The weight goal should be at least 85% of this value and be a weight at which the patient has menstruated. It is usually close to the patient's premorbid weight. During treatment the patient's weight, vital signs, and serum electrolyte levels (if abnormal), should be monitored regularly— weekly if the patient is very underweight, less often as the condition stabilizes.

Refeeding the anorexic can lead to fluid retention and dependent edema, which complicate the interpretation of weight changes and alarm the patient. This is more common in patients who purge and are volume-depleted. Congestive heart failure has been reported with severe fluid retention,

GUIDELINES FOR MEDICAL MANAGEMENT

1. Assist in diagnosis by excluding other causes of weight loss or purging.
2. Assess the degree of malnutrition, dehydration, and electrolyte disturbance to determine whether hospitalization is necessary, (see box at right).
3. Coordinate management with psychologist or psychiatrist and dietitian.
4. Educate the patient about the medical complications of the illness.
5. Set guidelines for outpatient management:
   a. Minimum acceptable weight
   b. Weight goal (underweight patients)
   c. Rate of weight gain (1-2 lb/wk) for underweight patients
   d. Maintenance of normal electrolyte levels.
   e. Compliance with psychiatric and dietary therapy
6. Monitor weight, vital signs, and electrolyte levels regularly during treatment.
7. Treat hypokalemia with potassium chloride.
8. Prescribe a daily multivitamin.
9. Prescribe calcium supplements (1500 mg daily) for amenorrheic patients.
10. Consider bone densitometry and estrogen replacement therapy for patients underweight and amenorrheic for 12 months.
11. Consider a trial of antidepressants to control symptoms in bulimics.

INDICATIONS FOR HOSPITAL ADMISSION

Weight loss >30% of premorbid or ideal weight
Rapidly progressing weight loss
Cardiac arrhythmias
Persistent hypokalemia unresponsive to outpatient treatment
Severe depression or suicidal ideation
Behavior out of the patient's control (e.g, purging or exercise)

---

but it is rare. Refeeding too rapidly can lead to gastric dilatation and ileus. Transient elevation of liver function test results caused by fatty liver may also occur. To minimize these complications and prevent the development of binge eating, patients should regain weight slowly, at a rate of 1 to 2 pounds a week. A dietitian can formulate and monitor an eating plan. Nutritional supplements can be added if the patient is unable to gain weight at an acceptable rate. Although vitamin deficiencies are uncommon in anorexia nervosa, the marginal state of nutrition makes it prudent to recommend a daily multivitamin.

Complications of refeeding and rehydration should be anticipated and explained. Patients with pedal edema can be aided by support stockings, leg elevation, mild salt restriction, and reassurance that the condition is temporary. Diuretics should be avoided because of their potential for abuse. Congestive heart failure is treated in a conventional way. Patients with severe postprandial bloating caused by poor gastric emptying may benefit from metoclopramide.

Whether treatment with estrogen or calcium can prevent or reverse the bone loss associated with anorexia nervosa is not known, because randomized controlled trials have not yet been reported. However, it is reasonable to ensure that dietary calcium intake is adequate by prescribing supplements so that intake reaches 1500 mg per day. Women who have been amenorrheic for at least 12 months warrant consideration of bone densitometry and estrogen replacement

therapy. The doses used for postmenopausal patients may be better tolerated than oral contraceptives, which have higher estrogen doses and more side effects.

In bulimics or anorexics who purge, serum potassium levels and orthostatic vital signs must be monitored, and the patient instructed to eat potassium-rich foods. Maintaining normal electrolyte levels should be a condition of continued outpatient treatment. If the potassium level falls below normal despite dietary measures, supplemental potassium is indicated. This must be given as potassium chloride to correct the metabolic alkalosis that maintains the hypokalemia. Patients should be told to take the supplement at a time when purging does not occur; often this is at bedtime.

Patients who vomit should be referred for dental evaluation and informed about the irreversibility of enamel loss. Those using laxatives should be informed of the ineffectiveness of these agents for real weight loss and urged to stop, either abruptly or by gradual tapering. When laxative abuse stops, transient constipation, fluid retention, dependent edema, and weight gain are common. The reequilibration period may last several weeks. Fluid retention and edema also occur temporarily when diuretic use stops. To prevent constipation patients should increase dietary fiber intake and may benefit from fiber supplements or stool softeners. Physicians caring for bulimics should be alert to the possibility of drug and alcohol abuse, which is more common in these patients. A trial of tricyclic antidepressants should be considered for bulimic patients; this is usually coordinated with the psychiatrist.

INDICATIONS FOR HOSPITAL ADMISSION

The primary care physician should assess and then monitor the patient's physical state to determine whether hospitalization is necessary. Patients with severe degrees of weight loss, dehydration, metabolic derangement, and depression require hospital admission (see box, above).

BIBLIOGRAPHY

American Psychiatric Association: Practice guideline for eating disorder, *Am J Psychiatry* 150:212, 1993.
American Psychiatric Association: Eating disorders. In *Diagnostic and statistical manual of mental disorders,* ed 4, Washington DC, American Psychiatric Association.
Beumont PJV, Russell JD, Touyz SW: Treatment of anorexia nervosa. *Lancet* 341:1635, 1993.
Bo-Linn GW et al: Purging and calorie absorption in bulimic patients and normal women, *Ann Intern Med* 99:14, 1983.
Comerci GD: Medical complications of anorexia nervosa and bulimia nervosa, *Med Clin North Am* 74:1293, 1990.
Freund KM et al: Detection of bulimia in a primary care setting, *J Gen Intern Med* 8:236, 1993.
Garner DM: Pathogenesis of anorexia nervosa, *Lancet* 341:1631, 1993.

Gold PW et al: Abnormal hypothalamic-pituitary-adrenal function in anorexia nervosa, *N Engl J Med* 314:1335, 1986.

Herzog DB, Copeland PM: Eating disorders, *N Engl J Med* 313:295, 1985.

Humphries LL et al: Hyperamylasemia in patients with eating disorders, *Ann Intern Med* 106:50, 1987.

Isner JM et al: Anorexia nervosa and sudden death, *Ann Intern Med* 102:49, 1985.

Meyers DG et al: Mitral valve prolapse in anorexia nervosa, *Ann Intern Med* 105:384, 1986.

Mitchell JE et al: Medical complications and medical management of bulimia, *Ann Intern Med* 107:71, 1987.

Palmer EP, Guay AT: Reversible myopathy secondary to abuse of Ipecac in patients with major eating disorders, *N Engl J Med* 313:1457, 1985.

Rich LM et al: Hypoglycemic coma in anorexia nervosa: case report and review of the literature. *Arch Intern Med* 150:891, 1990.

Rigotti NA et al: The clinical course of osteoporosis in anorexia nervosa: a longitudinal study of cortical bone mass, *JAMA* 265:1133, 1991.

Salisbury JJ, Mitchell JE: Bone mineral density and anorexia nervosa in women, *Am J Psychiatry* 148:768, 1991.

Sharp CW, Freeman CPL: Medical complications of anorexia nervosa. *Br J Psychiatry* 162:452, 1993.

70 Fatigue and Chronic Fatigue Syndrome

Anthony L. Komaroff

CHRONIC FATIGUE

Nearly 15 million office visits per year in the United States are for the complaint of fatigue, and most of the patients seeking care are women. Indeed, many persons experience fatigue a lot of the time: in one British survey, 20% of adults said that they had "always felt tired" during the preceding month. The pace of life in the late twentieth century is fast. Far from evolving toward a "leisure society," we are working increasingly longer hours, with less time for relaxation. Moreover, some sleep physiologists believe that many citizens of the developed nations suffer from a chronic state of sleep deprivation.

Fatigue is one of those presenting complaints that physicians do not like to deal with. For one thing, the complaint of "fatigue" means different things to different patients: an unusual urge to sleep during the day, trouble finding the energy to start new tasks, difficulty concentrating, muscle weakness, or fatigability. Also, because many patients seen in a primary care practice are the anxious "worried well," a physician is likely to be skeptical that the patient's degree of fatigue is really beyond the normal life experience of every human being. In addition, attempts at treatment often are unsuccessful; thus, the physician is likely to feel a failure. Because patients seeking medical care for fatigue often have remarkable degrees of functional impairment, the physician is likely to feel even more discouraged at his or her inability to help the patient.

Sometimes patients seek medical care because of acute fatigue: a few weeks of fatigue that they believe is unusual for them and unexplained by physical, emotional, and intellectual stresses. Much more often, patients seek medical care for chronic fatigue, an unusual degree of fatigue that has lasted for many months or even longer. This chapter does not deal with acute fatigue but focuses only on chronic fatigue and one syndrome (the chronic fatigue syndrome) that involves a small fraction of all patients with chronic fatigue.

Causative factors

There are a variety of causes of fatigue, many of which are summarized in the box on the following page. Life-style factors (e.g., the pace of life, substance abuse) are at the top of the list, along with primary psychiatric disorders. Various well-characterized organic illnesses, as well as a few poorly understood illnesses, also can cause fatigue.

In the patient whose presenting complaint is chronic fatigue, the first question to consider is whether life-style factors are likely to explain the fatigue. The second question to consider is whether the patient is depressed: depression (often with associated anxiety or somatization disorder, or both) is a common cause of chronic fatigue. The depression may be "masked" and therefore difficult to diagnose. Because depression is a stigmatizing diagnosis in our society, patients may refrain from expressing feelings of sadness; rather, they may offer physical symptoms as the "ticket of entry" into the physician's office. If and when the physician makes the diagnosis of depression, the stigma attached to this illness may cause patients to have trouble accepting it. The diagnosis and treatment of depression, anxiety disorders, and somatization disorder in a primary care practice are covered in Chapters 67 and 74.

According to careful studies, well-characterized **organic diseases** of any type explain the complaint of fatigue in fewer than 10% of patients. Clinically, thyroid disease, various autoimmune disorders, and the chronic fatigue syndrome (CFS) are the most common organic causes of fatigue in women (CFS probably is an organic disease). They also can be difficult to diagnose. The physician thus is faced with a troublesome problem: although there is no organic disease present in most cases, a large number of diseases, each of which requires a number of different diagnostic tests to help establish the diagnosis, may be present. The question of when to order various diagnostic tests in the patient with fatigue is considered later in this chapter.

Unlike the autoimmune diseases and CFS, most of the other organic diseases listed in the following box usually are readily recognizable from findings of the history, physical examination, or laboratory testing. One is unlikely to miss fatigue caused by cardiac or respiratory insufficiency: the history indicates that the fatigue is worsened by physical challenge and becomes progressively more severe, and

SOME CAUSES OF FATIGUE

Physiologic
  Increased physical exertion
  Inadequate rest
  Sedentary life-style
  Environmental stress (noise, vibration, heat)
  New physical disability, recent illness, surgery, trauma

Habit patterns
  Caffeine habituation
  Alcoholism
  Other substance abuse

Psychosocial
  Depression
  Dysthymia and grief
  Anxiety-related disorders
  Stress reaction

Pregnancy

Autoimmune disorders
  Systemic lupus erythematosus
  Multiple sclerosis
  Thyroiditis (with or without thyroid dysfunction)
  Rheumatoid arthritis
  Myasthenia gravis

Sleep disorders
  Sleep apnea
  Narcolepsy

Infectious diseases
  Mononucleosis
  Human immunodeficiency virus infection
  Chronic hepatitis B or C virus infection
  Lyme disease
  Fungal disease
  Chronic parasitic infection
  Tuberculosis
  Subacute bacterial endocarditis

Endocrine disorders
  Hyperparathyroidism
  Hypothyroidism
  Apathetic "hyperthyroidism"

Endocrine disorders (cont'd)
  Adrenal insufficiency
  Cushing's syndrome
  Hypopituitarism
  Diabetes mellitus

Syndromes of uncertain etiology
  Chronic fatigue syndrome
  Fibromyalgia (fibrositis)
  Sarcoidosis
  Wegener's granulomatosis

Occult malignant disease

Hematologic problems
  Anemia
  Myeloproliferative syndromes

Hepatic disease
  Alcoholic hepatitis or cirrhosis

Cardiovascular disease
  Low output states
  "Silent" myocardial infarction
  Bradycardias
  Mitral valve dysfunction

Metabolic disorders
  Hyponatremia
  Hypokalemia
  Hypercalcemia

Renal disease
  Chronic renal failure

Respiratory disorders
  Chronic obstructive pulmonary disease

Miscellaneous
  Medications
  Autonomic overactivity
  Reactive hypoglycemia

Modified from Komaroff AL. In Branch WT Jr, editor, *Office practice of medicine,* ed 3, Philadelphia, 1994, WB Saunders.
* This list is not meant to be an exhaustive catalogue of every illness that can cause chronic fatigue; rather, it is intended to highlight some of the illnesses that most commonly do so.

physical signs usually are present. Weight loss, fever, pallor, and lymphadenopathy usually accompany the infectious, neoplastic, and hematologic diseases that produce fatigue. Chronic anemia usually is severe before it produces fatigue. Fortunately, many of these conditions can be suggested or diagnosed by inexpensive, routine blood tests.

A substantial fraction of patients do not have evidence of either organic or psychiatric causes of fatigue. Some organic illnesses that commonly produce fatigue may manifest initially in a less than full-blown form. **Multiple sclerosis (MS)** and **systemic lupus erythematosus (lupus)** are prime examples. Indeed, in many patients with mild MS or lupus, the predominant symptom for which they seek med-

ical care is fatigue rather than a focal neurologic deficit, a malar rash, or other characteristic manifestation of the illness. (See Chapter 26.)

Approach to the woman with chronic fatigue

History
Assessment of underlying psychiatric disorders. The assessment of underlying psychiatric disorders is detailed in Chapters 67 and 74 and is discussed only briefly here. When the patient with fatigue or other somatic symptoms is suffering from depression or anxiety, the interview serves as both a diagnostic and a therapeutic tool. The taking of the medical history, by exploring both organic and psychi-

Complete blood cell count
Manual differential white blood cell count (unless automated counts accurately determine atypical lymphocytes)
Erythrocyte sedimentation rate (Westergren method)
Chemistry panel, including assessment of renal and hepatic function and levels of glucose, electrolytes, calcium, phosphate, total cholesterol, albumin, and globulin
Thyroid function tests (highly sensitive TSH [thyroid-stimulating hormone] is sufficient)
Antinuclear antibodies and rheumatoid factor, if there are prominent arthralgias and myalgias
Urinalysis

Modified from Schluederberg et al: *Ann Intern Med* 117:325, 1992.

atric issues, can serve to make the patient aware of how his or her feelings relate to the symptoms, an essential first step in management. In attempting to elicit submerged information, it is important to remember that occult alcohol abuse (and other forms of substance abuse) often produces chronic fatigue, either directly as a result of chronic intoxication or indirectly through its disruptive effects on sleep or its production of inflammatory disease of the liver. Also, it appears that domestic violence, either in childhood or currently, can lead women to seek medical care for "unrelated" symptoms, such as fatigue. A simple interviewing technique can be based on the biopsychosocial approach developed by Engel.

Assessment of underlying organic disorders. Although underlying psychiatric disorders are common in patients with fatigue—and even though the interview may suggest that the patient has a current or lifetime psychiatric diagnosis—it is nevertheless important to assess the possible presence of concomitant organic illness. The depression itself can result from the patient's awareness of an impending or actual change in health status.

Diagnostic tests

Laboratory testing. In the patient with fatigue of modest severity and relatively short duration (e.g., 1 to 3 months) who probably is most typical of patients seeking medical care for fatigue, no laboratory testing may be warranted. This is particularly true when the patient clearly has enough life-style features to explain fatigue, when a psychologic disorder is deemed likely, and when no other symptoms suggest an organic abnormality.

When the fatigue has lasted 6 months or more or is significantly interfering with a patient's ability to work or maintain her primary responsibilities at work or at home, a modest screening evaluation is warranted to look for evidence of an underlying organic disorder. A panel of tests recently recommended by a National Institutes of Health conference is shown in the box above. Not all of these tests are highly sensitive for organic disease (e.g., erythrocyte sedimentation rate) nor highly specific for any particular disease. However, they serve as a useful screen for organic illness.

Management

There are no specific treatments for chronic fatigue. Instead, treatment follows from the differential diagnosis of fatigue. Thus treatment could include antidepressant therapy, immuno-

suppressive therapy of an underlying connective tissue disorder, a prescription to get more sleep, or other therapies.

CHRONIC FATIGUE SYNDROME
Definition

Chronic fatigue syndrome (CFS) is a syndrome, defined by a group of symptoms and signs, of uncertain etiology. Very few patients (perhaps fewer than 5%) of all patients who seek medical care for the complaint of chronic fatigue meet criteria for CFS.

CFS was first defined in 1988; the Centers for Disease Control (CDC) led the development of a working case definition that is summarized in Fig. 70-1. The CDC case definition relies entirely on a combination of symptoms and signs (not laboratory data) and on the exclusion of chronic active organic or psychiatric illnesses that can produce chronic fatigue.

Although CFS has been defined only recently, similar syndromes with different names have long been described in the medical literature. These include **neurasthenia** (or neurocirculatory asthenia), first described in the mid-nineteenth century; **myalgic encephalomyelitis** (ME) is a similar chronic fatiguing illness, typically occurring in epidemic form; **fibromyalgia,** originally called fibrositis, is an illness characterized by fatigue and chronic musculoskeletal pain, as well as tenderness at specific sites known as *tender points*; and **chronic mononucleosis,** a form of CFS that follows in the wake of classic acute infectious mononucleosis.

Causes

CFS probably is a heterogeneous collection of related disorders that all share certain pathogenic features and symptoms. It is unlikely to be, as is the acquired immunodeficiency syndrome (AIDS), a novel syndrome caused by a single new infectious agent. In recent years, research laboratories have reported a variety of abnormalities in patients with CFS, in contrast to healthy control subjects. In general, these studies indicate a state of chronic activation of the immune system, pathologic findings in the central nervous system, and an association with a variety of infectious agents. At the same time, it is fair to say that no clear model of the pathogenesis of the symptoms of CFS has yet emerged: it is not clear how specific is a variety of the abnormalities for CFS (as contrasted with other illnesses that produce chronic fatigue) nor whether the abnormalities actually account for the suffering experienced by patients.

A model for the pathogenesis of chronic fatigue syndrome

Many view CFS as primarily an immunologic disturbance, one that allows reactivation of latent and ineradicable infectious agents, particularly viruses. The reactivation of these viruses may only be an epiphenomenon. Alternatively, once secondarily reactivated, these viruses may contribute to the morbidity of CFS—directly, by damaging certain tissues (e.g., the pharyngeal mucosa) and indirectly, by eliciting an ongoing immunologic response in which a variety of cytokines are chronically elaborated, producing symptoms and signs such as fever, adenopathy, myalgias, arthralgias, mood and cognitive disorders, and sleep disorders, as already discussed.

What triggers the immune dysfunction in the first place? Many factors could do so: atopic disorders, new infection

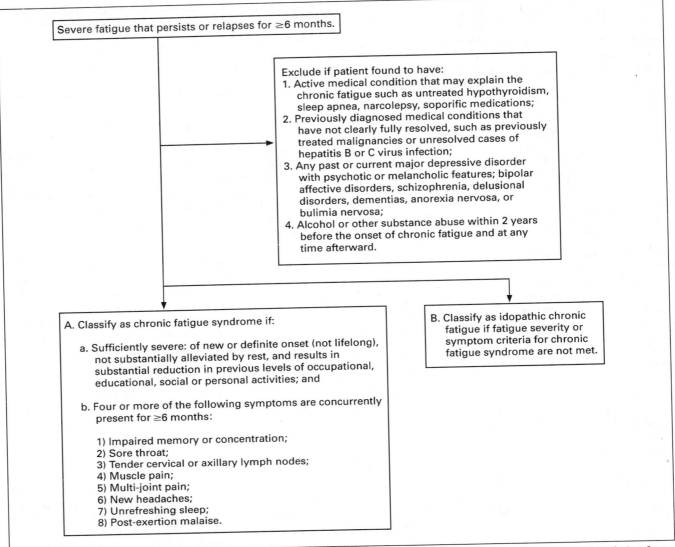

Severe fatigue that persists or relapses for ≥6 months.

Exclude if patient found to have:
1. Active medical condition that may explain the chronic fatigue such as untreated hypothyroidism, sleep apnea, narcolepsy, soporific medications;
2. Previously diagnosed medical conditions that have not clearly fully resolved, such as previously treated malignancies or unresolved cases of hepatitis B or C virus infection;
3. Any past or current major depressive disorder with psychotic or melancholic features; bipolar affective disorders, schizophrenia, delusional disorders, dementias, anorexia nervosa, or bulimia nervosa;
4. Alcohol or other substance abuse within 2 years before the onset of chronic fatigue and at any time afterward.

A. Classify as chronic fatigue syndrome if:

a. Sufficiently severe: of new or definite onset (not lifelong), not substantially alleviated by rest, and results in substantial reduction in previous levels of occupational, educational, social or personal activities; and

b. Four or more of the following symptoms are concurrently present for ≥6 months:

1) Impaired memory or concentration;
2) Sore throat;
3) Tender cervical or axillary lymph nodes;
4) Muscle pain;
5) Multi-joint pain;
6) New headaches;
7) Unrefreshing sleep;
8) Post-exertion malaise.

B. Classify as idopathic chronic fatigue if fatigue severity or symptom criteria for chronic fatigue syndrome are not met.

Fig. 70-1 Working case definition of chronic fatigue syndrome (Centers for Disease Control). (Modified from: Fukuda K et al: *Ann Intern Med* 121:953, 1994.)

with lymphotropic infectious agents, environmental toxins, stress, and even the biology of an underlying affective disorder. A recently described neuraxis abnormality that results in a basal hypocortisolism in CFS also could render the immune system "hyperresponsive" to antigenic stimulation, contributing to a state of chronic activation and partial exhaustion described in a later discussion. Clearly, like most illnesses, CFS seems likely to have multifactorial etiologic factors.

Why chronic fatigue syndrome especially affects women

In most studies of patients seeking medical care for chronic fatigue, and of that fraction who meet criteria for CFS, most patients are women. To put this observation in context, adult women more frequently seek medical care than do adult men for many medical conditions, although this is not true in childhood. There are many theories as to why women seek care more often for fatigue and for CFS, but none has been proved.

Proponents of the idea that fatigue and CFS are the somatic expression of psychic distress argue that the stresses of a woman's role in contemporary society are the explanation. They argue that women have an exhausting life-style that often requires major responsibilities both at work and at home. In addition, women remain subordinated and undervalued. Finally, women may be more likely than men to seek help for "nonemergent" conditions because in Western society, giving and receiving interpersonal support come more easily to women than to men.

Proponents of the idea that CFS represents primarily an organic illness—one that involves immune dysregulation—note that many immunologically mediated diseases occur predominantly in women. This is especially true of three diseases that can be confused with CFS: MS, lupus, and thyroiditis. Moreover, in animal models of autoimmune diseases it is typically the females of the species that become ill. Thus endocrinologic or other factors associated with female gender may predispose women to CFS.

Clinical presentation

History and symptoms. CFS is characterized by varying degrees of chronic fatigue and chronic or recurring fever, pharyngitis, myalgias, headache, arthralgias, paresthesias, depression, cognitive problems, and other symptoms. Table 70-1 presents a list of current experience with the presence of symptoms in more than 300 systematically studied patients.

Typically the chronic illness begins abruptly with an acute infectious-like syndrome that includes respiratory or gastrointestinal symptoms, or both, with associated fever, myalgias, and arthralgias. The chronic symptoms that are experienced regularly in the years *after* the acute onset of the illness clearly were not experienced regularly by these patients in the years *before* the onset of the illness. Virtually all patients perceive themselves to be impaired in some way. Some patients are completely disabled by the fatigue, muscular weakness, and pain.

Three features of CFS are particularly remarkable. The first is the sudden onset with a **flu-like illness.** The typical patient has been functioning very well, and then one day became acutely ill (patients often can remember the exact day and date). From that day forward, their lives change. The fact that the onset is so sudden, that it includes objective indicators of organic illness (e.g., fever, adenopathy), and that the change in a patient's functional status is so dramatic—all are in striking contrast to the much more common condition in which patients seek medical care for fatigue secondary to depression, describing symptoms that have occurred so gradually that it is difficult to pinpoint the time of onset.

A second remarkable feature of CFS is **postexertional malaise.** This is characterized not only by symptoms that could simply represent deconditioning—pain and weakness of the muscles involved in the exertion—but also by exacerbation of "systemic" symptoms, for example, fatigue, fevers, pharyngitis, adenopathy, and impaired cognition.

The third remarkable symptom is **night sweats.** These are recurring problems in nearly 50% of the patients studied. The night sweats are drenching, requiring changes of bedclothes and sheets. The night sweats are every bit as dramatic as can be seen with chronic infections (e.g., tuberculosis) or lymphoproliferative disorders. On those occasions when the patients take their temperatures, they are some-

Table 70-1 Frequency of symptoms and signs in chronic fatigue syndrome*

Symptom/sign	Frequency	Symptom/sign	Frequency
Fatigue	100%	Digits turn blue/white with cold, then red when warm	21%
Intermittently bedridden/shut-in	50%		
Regularly bedridden/shut-in	19%	**Neuropsychologic symptoms**	
		Awaken most mornings unrested	87%
Systemic symptoms		Difficulty concentrating, frequent and recurrent	83%
Night sweats, frequent and recurrent	50%	Headaches, new or different in character frequent and recurrent	76%
Unintentional weight loss (Median, 10 pounds)	49%	Unusually forgetful, frequent and recurrent	71%
Unintentional weight gain (Median, 15 pounds)	63%	Depression, by self-report	
Low-grade fever (by self-report), frequent and recurrent	36%	Following onset of CFS	68%
		Before onset of CFS	6%
Temperature >99.3° F, by examination†	30%	Anxiety, by self-report	
Temperature <97.0° F, by examination†	20%	Following onset of CFS	65%
		Before onset of CFS	12%
Respiratory tract symptoms		Alcohol regularly makes symptoms worse	59%
Sudden onset with "flu-like" illness	85%	Tingling/numbness in extremities, frequent and recurrent	57%
Swollen lymph glands in neck, frequent and recurrent	58%	Bright lights hurt eyes, frequent and recurrent	56%
Sore throat, frequent and recurrent	51%	Dizzy when move head suddenly frequent and recurrent	51%
Cough, frequent and recurrent	27%		
Palpable posterior cervical nodes†	54%	Visual blurring, frequent and recurrent	50%
		Impaired tandem gait, by examination†	23%
Musculoskeletal symptoms		Abnormal Romberg test, by examination†	22%
Muscles hurt, frequent and recurrent	89%	Impaired serial 7's test, by examination†	40%
Postexertional malaise, frequent and recurrent	88%		
Joints painful but not red/swollen, frequent and recurrent	75%	**Miscellaneous symptoms**	
		Premenstrual exacerbation of fatigue, frequent and recurrent	61%
Generalized muscle weakness, frequent and recurrent	70%	Nocturia, frequent and recurrent	46%
Morning stiffness, frequent and recurrent	58%	Nausea, frequent and recurrent	44%
Gelling, after sitting for hours, frequent and recurrent	56%	Sudden rapid heartbeat, frequent and recurrent	44%

*Summarized from formal studies of 320 patients as of April 1992. From Komaroff AL. In Straus SE, editor: *Chronic fatigue syndrome,* 1994, New York, Marcel Dekker.
†As detected on at least one physical examination.

times febrile but often have unusually low body temperatures (see following discussion).

A few patients with this disorder have had transient acute neurologic events, typically in the first 6 months of the illness: primary seizures, acute, profound ataxia, focal weakness, transient blindness, and unilateral paresthesias (not in a dermatomal distribution). Similar acute and transient neurologic events occasionally have been reported in outbreaks of myalgic encephalomyelitis as well.

The onset of the syndrome typically seems to be in young adulthood, although it also may begin in childhood or later in life. By definition (see Fig. 70-1), there is no evidence of rheumatologic, endocrinologic, infectious, malignant, or other chronic diseases. The diagnosis has been made about twice as often in women as in men.

Medical history. Most elements of the medical history are unremarkable in patients with CFS. However, there is a strikingly high frequency of atopic or allergic illness: 60% to 80% of patients with CFS have long-standing atopic disorders versus approximately 20% of the general population.

Physical examination. A few physical examination findings may be seen more often in CFS than in healthy persons, although this remains to be determined from controlled studies with blinded observers: fevers, unusually low basal body temperature (below 97° F), posterior cervical adenopathy, and abnormal findings on tests of balance (Romberg and tandem gait). Patients have detectable tender points with a frequency approaching that seen in fibromyalgia, and they occur much more often than in healthy control subjects. Therefore the finding of a significant number of tender points, along with the absence of tenderness at control sites, is evidence in favor of the diagnosis of CFS, although the absence of tender points does not rule out the diagnosis of CFS.

Diagnostic tests

Standard laboratory testing. Results of standard laboratory testing can be unremarkable. However, controlled studies have demonstrated that a few abnormalities may occur more frequently in CFS than in healthy control subjects of similar age and sex: atypical lymphocytosis, elevated alkaline phosphatase, lower levels of lactic dehydrogenase, and elevated total cholesterol values. None of these abnormalities is seen in more than 50% of patients with CFS; thus none constitutes a sufficiently sensitive diagnostic test. Moreover, each can be seen in other disorders; thus none is a sufficiently specific test.

Differential diagnosis. The differential diagnosis of CFS generally is the same as the differential diagnosis for chronic fatigue, as already discussed. Because patients with CFS typically have been more debilitated for a longer period of time than patients with chronic fatigue, the physician perceives a greater sense of urgency about making the proper diagnosis.

Immunologic testing. A large and growing literature reports immunologic abnormalities in patients with CFS. In general, the profile that is emerging indicates that in many patients with CFS all arms of the immune system can be chronically activated, with cytotoxic T lymphocytes and natural killer lymphocytes demonstrating an impaired function that could be interpreted as exhaustion secondary to a state of chronic activation. In sum, it appears that the immune system is chronically waging a battle against antigens that it perceives as foreign.

Although not all reports of immune function in CFS come to consistent conclusions, a few immunologic abnormalities have been found by multiple investigators, studying different groups of patients with CFS. First, the function of natural killer (NK) cells is impaired. NK cells play a central role in the immunologic containment of viral infections; thus their impairment of function in CFS is of particular interest. Second, about 30% to 45% of patients with CFS have circulating immune complexes, with a much higher frequency than is seen in healthy patients of the same age and sex. The immune complexes are present in low levels and without evidence of immune-complex–mediated disease. Third, there appears to be a higher number of B cells and T cells in an activated state in CFS, as manifested by the discovery of activation antigens on the cell surface. Fourth, several investigators also have reported T cell dysfunction, as reflected by anergy and reduced T cell lymphoproliferative responses after stimulation with various mitogens and antigens. Although these studies have all demonstrated objective differences in immunologic parameters between patients with CFS and healthy control subjects, more work needs to be done to determine whether these abnormalities also distinguish CFS from various organic and psychiatric diseases that also can produce chronic fatigue.

A widely held hypothesis is that the state of chronic immune activation leads to the most of the symptoms of CFS by causing a chronic "overproduction" of various immune system mediators—cytokines such as interferon-alpha, interleukin-6, tumor necrosis factor, interleukin-1, and interleukin-2. These cytokines can produce most of the symptoms characteristic of CFS: fatigue, fevers, adenopathy, myalgias, arthralgias, sleep disorders, cognitive impairment, and mood disorders. This hypothesis is actively being pursued by several research laboratories.

Neurologic studies. Several neuroimaging studies have compared findings in patients with CFS to those in healthy control subjects and to patients in various disease comparison groups, including acquired immunodeficiency syndrome (AIDS) encephalopathy, and major depression. Areas of abnormal signal in the subcortical white matter, and deeper structures, have been found by magnetic resonance imaging (MRI). The use of single photon emission computed tomography (SPECT) has shown diffuse impairment of perfusion and/or of central nervous system cellular function. Finally, preliminary reports have identified abnormalities on quantified electroencephalography more often in patients with CFS.

Neuroendocrine studies. An abnormality of the hypothalamic-pituitary-adrenocortical (HPA) axis has been demonstrated in CFS. The data indicate that in CFS there is diminished secretion by the hypothalamus of corticotropin-releasing hormone (CRH), leading to diminished secretion of adrenocorticotropic hormone (ACTH) by the pituitary, which results in diminished production of cortisol by the adrenal glands. This abnormality of the HPA axis is the opposite of what is seen in patients suffering from major depression.

Infectious disease studies. CFS typically begins suddenly with an infectious-like illness, although it apparently can begin after a variety of stressful noninfectious events (e.g., major surgery, accidents, and severe allergic reactions). CFS has been shown in some cases to follow in the wake of well-documented infection with Epstein-Barr virus infection, influenza virus infection, parvovirus infection, Lyme disease (in patients who have received adequate antibacterial treatment), and other infections. The aforementioned cases are important because they document that an acute infection can trigger CFS. They also demonstrate that CFS probably is not caused by a single infectious agent. However, these observations leave unexplained the pathogenetic mechanisms by which the *triggering* agent initiates the disease process, as well as the question of whether the infectious agent is necessary for the *perpetuation* of the process.

Several studies have incriminated the enteroviruses (coxsackieviruses, echoviruses, polioviruses) in some cases of CFS. Enteroviral nucleic acid has been found much more often in the muscle of patients with CFS than in healthy control subjects, and enteroviral antigen has been found more frequently in the stool and serum of patients with CFS. Enteroviruses can produce chronic, persistent infection and are both lymphotropic and neurotropic. They can be transmitted casually.

Human herpesvirus–6 (HHV-6) has been found to be actively replicating more often in patients with CFS than in matched healthy control subjects. The evidence indicates that reactivation of a long dormant infection with HHV-6, rather than new infection with HHV-6, is present in CFS. Thus the active HHV-6 infection most likely represents a secondary phenomenon in CFS. As such, it could be an epiphenomenon having nothing to do with the illness. Alternatively, even if the reactivation of HHV-6 is a secondary phenomenon, the reactivated virus could contribute to the symptoms of the illness: HHV-6 infects many target tissues that are affected in CFS: lymphocytes, pharyngeal cells, intestinal cells, glial cells, and probably neurons.

Several research teams are evaluating the possibility that novel **retroviruses** are involved in some cases of CFS. As of this writing, this research has not been informative and no direct evidence of a novel retrovirus has yet been found.

Psychologic studies. Most studies find that most patients with CFS *become* depressed and anxious after the onset (usually sudden) of their disorder. For many patients the depression and anxiety become the most debilitating parts of their illness. At the same time, these studies also indicate that a substantial fraction of patients with CFS (25% to 50%) have no evidence of any active psychiatric disorder since the onset of CFS.

By and large the studies find a higher frequency of psychiatric disorders in patients before they developed CFS than is found in the population at large: the average across-all-studies is around 30% (range, 20% to 50%) of CFS patients. On one hand, this past history of psychiatric disorders is greater than is found in the population at large (range, 5% to 10%); on the other hand, despite extensive psychiatric evaluation, no evidence of a preexisting psychiatric disorder can be found in most patients with CFS.

Although psychologic illness is not found in a substantial fraction of patients with CFS, it could well be playing a dominant role in the suffering of some patients with CFS. Even if CFS is triggered by an organic illness, such as an infection, the chronic illness that ensues could, in some

patients, reflect the reemergence of an underlying depression. Or it could indicate that the biologic underpinnings of depression somehow render one vulnerable to the "organic" abnormalities (e.g., the immunologic and virologic findings) seen in CFS. Or, in the individual patient, more than one of these factors may be operative.

Management

Choice of therapy

Low dose tricyclic agents. Randomized, controlled trials have shown that low-dose tricyclic drugs reduce the level of fatigue, musculoskeletal pain, and objectively demonstrable tender points in patients with fibromyalgia. Because CFS and fibromyalgia are similar, many physicians have tried the same therapy in CFS. No controlled trial of low-dose tricyclic agents has been mounted in CFS. However, it is the general anecdotal experience of most physicians that such treatment clearly improves the quality of sleep; as a consequence, perhaps, many patients state that their fatigue, myalgias, arthralgias, and cognitive problems also improve. The alpha-wave intrusion on delta wave–sleep disorder that has been found in both fibromyalgia and CFS improves with low-dose tricyclic therapy; thus there is objective confirmation of the experience reported by patients.

Amitriptyline or **doxepin** are the tricyclic drugs most often used for CFS; a typical regimen is 10 to 20 mg taken orally before bedtime. Of interest is that most patients with CFS cannot tolerate doses of tricyclic drugs usually used for depression (e.g., amitriptyline, 100 to 300 mg/day). Even with these very low doses, for about the first week of therapy, most patients with CFS report increased somnolence and fatigue in the morning. Patients should be warned of this transient adverse effect and urged to continue for at least 1 to 2 months before drawing any conclusions about the efficacy of the therapy.

In patients with concomitant depression and a sleep disorder, **sertraline,** 25 mg, or **fluoxetine,** 5 to 20 mg, each morning often is coupled with low-dose tricyclic drugs at bedtime. Low doses are achieved by cutting the capsules or tablets or suspending them in measured amounts of liquid, or both. As with tricyclic agents and all other central nervous system–active substances, patients with CFS often cannot tolerate usual doses of fluoxetine. Also, the sleep-disruptive potential of fluoxetine may be greater in CFS, leading to the recommendation that this medication be taken in the morning.

Treatment of a concomitant depression by psychotherapy or pharmacotherapy in patients with CFS often reduces the mood disorder; however, it rarely eliminates the fatigue, cognitive problems, myalgias, arthralgias, postexertional malaise, respiratory tract symptoms, fevers, and adenopathy. Cognitive behavior therapy has been helpful in some patients.

Other treatments. One antiviral agent, acyclovir, has been shown to be ineffective in CFS; however, it also has little in vitro effect on the viruses that have been associated with CFS. Controlled trials of gamma globulin have come to conflicting conclusions; at best, gamma globulin may offer a very brief and transient benefit, except in the unusual patients with CFS who also have a concomitant hypogammaglobulinemia and associated recurrent infections with encapsulated bacteria.

One randomized study reported a magnesium deficiency in CFS and a benefit from magnesium therapy; that study subsequently was subjected to much criticism. Although many patients take vitamins, there is no evidence that vitamins are helpful in CFS; one controlled trial found no evidence of benefit from vitamin B_{12} therapy. A large number of treatments, some of which have a reasonable conceptual basis, have been proposed but not studied. As with any illness for which no definitive therapy exists, a variety of unconventional therapies have been used. Also, frankly exploitative "quack" remedies are being promoted.

Nonpharmaceutical treatments. Patients should be encouraged to be as active as possible but to avoid activities that involve intensive physical or emotional stress. The role of exercise in CFS is controversial. Limbering exercises are recommended by nearly all physicians experienced in treating this disorder. Some physicians recommend a program of very gradually increasing aerobic exercises. In some patients, this seems to be well-tolerated, but in others it leads to relapses, including recurrence of fevers and adenopathy.

Pregnancy and chronic fatigue syndrome

As has been discussed, the most commonly prescribed treatment in CFS is low-dose tricyclic therapy. Although teratogenic effects from tricyclic agents (in doses that are equivalent to those used in human beings) have not been reported in animals, many tricyclic drugs cross the placenta, and occasional case reports of fetal abnormalities have led the FDA to recommend caution in the use of tricyclic drugs during pregnancy. These agents also can be excreted into breast milk, and the FDA cautions against tricyclic therapy in nursing mothers.

There is no evidence that CFS adversely affects either the pregnant woman or the fetus. No anecdotal or published data reveal any increase in the rate of fetal abnormalities or in the subsequent health, growth, and development of the children. Most women with CFS seem to feel somewhat better during the course of the pregnancy, although some clearly feel worse. In the first 6 to 9 months of the postpartum period, most women feel more fatigued but not more ill. That is, the energy required to deal with the needs of a new baby may be exhausting for the patient with CFS, just as it may be for a healthy person. However, the other symptoms of CFS—myalgias, arthralgias, sore throat, fevers—do not seem to regularly worsen. Indeed, many patients seem to receive a psychologic lift from childbearing because it demonstrates that they can be successful at one of life's most important challenges.

BIBLIOGRAPHY

Ahmed SA, Talal N: Sex hormones and autoimmune rheumatic disorders, *Scand J Rheumatol* 18:69, 1989.
Bates DW et al: Clinical laboratory test findings in patients with the chronic fatigue syndrome, *Arch Intern Med* 155:97, 1995.
Buchwald D, Komaroff AL: Review of laboratory findings for patients with chronic fatigue syndrome, *Rev Infect Dis* 13:S12, 1991.
Buchwald D et al: A chronic illness characterized by fatigue, neurologic and immunologic disorders, and active human herpesvirus type 6 infection, *Ann Intern Med* 116:103, 1992.
Butler S et al: Cognitive behaviour therapy in chronic fatigue syndrome, *J Neurol Neurosurg Psychiatry* 54:153, 1991.
Cox B et al: *The health and lifestyle survey,* London, 1987, Health Promotion Research Trust.
Dement W: *The sleepwatchers,* Stanford, Calif, 1992, Stanford University Press.
Demitrack MA et al: Evidence for impaired activation of the hypothalamic-pituitary-adrenal axis in patients with chronic fatigue syndrome, *J Clin Endocrinol Metab* 73:1224, 1991.
Engel GL: The need for a new medical model: a challenge for biomedicine, *Science* 196:129, 1977.
Fukuda K et al: The chronic fatigue syndrome: a comprehensive approach to its definition and study, *Ann Intern Med* 121:953, 1994.
Goldenberg DL: Fibromyalgia syndrome: an emerging but controversial condition, *JAMA* 257:2782, 1987.
Goldenberg DL, Felson DT, Dinerman H: A randomized, controlled trial of amitriptyline and naproxen in the treatment of patients with fibromyalgia, *Arthritis, Rheum* 29:1371, 1986.
Gow JW et al: Enteroviral RNA sequences detected by polymerase chain reaction in muscle of patients with postviral fatigue syndrome, *Br Med J* 302:692, 1991.
Hickie I et al: The psychiatric status of patients with the chronic fatigue syndrome, *Br J Psychiatry* 156:534, 1990.
Holmes GP et al: Chronic fatigue syndrome: a working case definition, *Ann Intern Med* 108:387, 1988.
Klimas NG et al: Immunologic abnormalities in chronic fatigue syndrome, *J Clin Microbiol* 28:1403, 1990.
Komaroff AL, Buchwald D: Symptoms and signs of chronic fatigue syndrome, *Rev Infect Dis* 13:S8, 1991.
Kroenke K, Arrington ME, Mangelsdorff AD: The prevalence of symptoms in medical outpatients and the adequacy of therapy, *Arch Intern Med* 150:1685, 1990.
Kroenke K et al: Chronic fatigue in primary care: prevalence, patient characteristics, and outcome, *JAMA* 260:929, 1988.
Landay AL et al: Chronic fatigue syndrome: clinical condition associated with immune activation, *Lancet* 338:707, 1991.
Lloyd AR et al: Immunological abnormalities in the chronic fatigue syndrome, *Med J Aust* 151:122, 1989.
Schluederberg A et al: Chronic fatigue syndrome research: definition and medical outcome assessment, *Ann Intern Med* 117:325, 1992.
Schor JB: The *overworked American: the unexpected decline of leisure,* New York, 1992, Basic Books.
Schwartz RB et al: SPECT imaging of the brain: comparison of findings in patients with chronic fatigue syndrome, AIDS dementia complex, and major unipolar depression, *Am J Roentgen* 162:943, 1994.
Straus SE et al: Persisting illness and fatigue in adults with evidence of Epstein-Barr virus infection, *Ann Intern Med* 102:7-16, 1985.
Verbrugge LM, Wingard DL: Sex differentials in health and mortality, *Women Health* 12:103, 1987.
Wessely S, Powell R: Fatigue syndromes: a comparison of chronic "postviral" fatigue with neuromuscular and affective disorders, *J Neurol Neurosurg Psychiatry* 52:940, 1989.
Whiteside TL, Herberman RB: The role of natural killer cells in human disease, *Clin Immunol Immunopathol* 53:1, 1989.

71 Obesity

Susan Cummings

While the image of the ideal woman in the United States has become thinner, women have on average become heavier in the past 20 years. Using the standard weight/height charts, approximately 35% of white females and 60% of African-American females are overweight or obese by middle age. With heavy cultural pressures toward thinness, there is a preoccupation with body size that makes many woman vulnerable to claims for weight loss programs and willing to try new weight loss techniques very readily.

It is important that the primary care physician have expertise in the management of obesity because women patients frequently have concerns about overweight. In addition, obesity is associated with increased health risks such as increased mortality rate and development or exacerbation of several chronic degenerative diseases. There is also a body of evidence suggesting that weight cyclers ("yo-yo dieters") are at risk of development of coronary artery disease because of repeated diet cycles.

This chapter outlines an approach to overweight and obesity in primary care practice. The practitioner needs to understand the health impairments related to obesity in order to target patients who need intervention, to be able to assess the degree of overweight and define reasonable treatment goals, and to be familiar with the range of available treatments and their effectiveness.

EPIDEMIOLOGY

An increase in body weight of 20% or more above desirable body weight constitutes an established health hazard. On the basis of this definition of obesity, an estimated 34 million persons in the United States are overweight. Among adults 20 to 74 years of age 24% of men and 27% of women are overweight. In 1993 the NIH Technology Assessment Conference Panel reported that as many as 40% of women and 24% of men are trying to lose weight at any given time.

The prevalence of overweight increases with age in both men and women. However, in men the peak prevalence occurs between 45 and 54 years of age, whereas in women prevalence continues to increase throughout the entire age range, reaching a peak in 65- to 74-year-old women. More women than men are in the upper range of body weight distribution associated with obesity. Among women African-Americans and Hispanics have a higher prevalence of overweight. This difference may be related to genetic as well as cultural factors.

Health problems of obesity

The health hazards of obesity are listed in Table 71-1. Obesity is associated with an increased risk of a cluster of disorders referred to as Syndrome X, which includes insulin resistance, glucose intolerance, hyperinsulinemia, hypertension, increased very-low-density lipoprotein (VLDL) level, and decreased high-density lipoprotein (HDL) level. Obesity also increases the risk of pulmonary disorders, gallstones, cholecystitis, osteoarthritis, gout, and certain forms of cancer.

Scientific evidence for benefits associated with weight reduction is more limited than might be expected. Some patients will be motivated by the knowledge that weight loss can prevent the onset of hypertension and that the same may be true for diabetes mellitus. Weight loss has clearly been shown to improve diabetic control and blood pressure control in diabetic and hypertensive women. Better functional status, less pain, and greater social role function occur after weight loss in very obese individuals.

The evidence linking weight loss with decreased mortality rate is meager. Weight loss attempts may themselves carry some risk. Although the data on the physical effects of

Table 71-1 Health hazards of obesity*

Disorder	Magnitude of risk	Comments
Hypertension	8-fold increase	Risk increase greatest in women below 40
Stroke	3- to 4-fold increase	Risk increase greatest in women below 40
Hyperlipidemia	Every 10% increase in weight associated with 12 mg/dl increase in cholesterol level	Effect less marked in women than men
Coronary artery disease	2- to 3-fold increase	Epidemiologic studies in women document increased risk even with mild to moderate overweight
Diabetes	3- to 10-fold increase	Risk increases with severity of obesity
Gallstones	3- to 4-fold increase	Yearly incidence >1% in women ≥40% overweight
Respiratory disorders	Not well quantified	Decreased vital capacity and compliance Higher rates of sleep apnea with increasing obesity
Cancer	Mortality ratio 1.55	Higher rates of endometrial, gall bladder, cervical, ovarian, and breast cancers in obese women
Gout	Not well quantified	Increased risk in women seen only when ≥40% overweight
Arthritis	3-fold increase	Prevalence of osteoarthritis increases from 0.4% to 1.45% in obese women

*Obesity indicates 20% or more above ideal body weight determined by actuarial tables, unless otherwise specified.

weight cycling are inconclusive, there may be an effect on energy metabolism resulting in faster weight regain. More data are needed on the negative psychologic and physical health effects of weight cycling

PATHOPHYSIOLOGY

An understanding of the cause of obesity will assist the practitioner in setting appropriate treatment goals for individual patients. Obesity occurs when there is an imbalance in the energy balance equation: intake is too high and/or expenditure is too low. Why this imbalance occurs is unclear. Research to date suggests that it is a complex problem reflecting genetic factors, physiologic and psychologic conditions, and environmental, cultural, and socioeconomic factors.

Biologic factors

There is clear evidence that there are many biologic factors that can cause weight gain (or regain) that are not under the individual's control.

Family membership is a significant determinant of energy expenditure independent of body composition, age, or gender. Epidemiologic studies of identical and fraternal twins show that body fatness is under strong genetic control. If one parent is obese the offspring have a 40% chance of becoming obese; if both parents are obese, the risk to the child is 80%.

The role of size and number of fat cells (adipocytes) has also been studied. Hypertrophic obesity is caused by enlargement of fat cells; hyperplastic obesity is caused by an increased number of fat cells. Fat cell proliferation occurs in children (ages 12 to 18 months), in adolescents (ages 12 to 16 years), and in adults when usual body weight is exceeded by 40% to 60%. Once formed, adipocytes become permanent, allowing one to store more fat. Adolescent-onset obesity is generally associated with hyperplastic obesity and greater body weight as an adult. Those persons with hyperplastic obesity are less likely to reach or maintain an ideal body weight. Hypertrophic obesity associated with adult onset or mild obesity (20% to 40% overweight) is more often reversible.

Other biologic factors that have been investigated are metabolic factors, including metabolic rate, thermic effect of food, and exercise-induced thermogenesis. Impairment in physiologic mechanisms that signal satiety may explain why some patients have difficulty internally regulating their food intake.

On the basis of what is known of the biologic factors associated with obesity, factors that are predictive of a poor response to weight reduction down to an "ideal body weight" are positive family history and adolescent onset. For these patients it is especially important to set realistic weight goals.

Psychosocial and environmental factors

The intense societal focus on thinness encouraged by the commercial weight loss industry and the advertising media creates unrealistic expectations about desirable body weight and produces an environment conducive to dangerous eating disorders. A 1986 *Psychology Today* survey on appearance and weight reported that more than 50% of women surveyed were unhappy with their weight. Women's self-image of body size and specific body parts such as the waist and hips is consistently exaggerated. For many women the intense social pressures to achieve thinness cause much psychologic dissatisfaction and distorted body image.

Some overweight women appear to increase eating in response to stress, anxiety, depression, or low self-esteem and body image. Other external regulatory factors, such as the local environment and the sight, smell, and taste of food, also influence eating behavior. On the basis of a study of the responses to these cues it has been proposed that whereas internal mechanisms primarily govern the lean individual's appetite, external variables are more important for some obese persons.

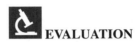 EVALUATION

History

The interview is the first step in gathering baseline data. The interview should be conducted with sensitivity to the patient's possible embarrassment and lifetime struggle with her weight. The interview is a good time to build rapport that will enhance the patient's long-term success. If the physician is going to recommend treatment, it is especially important to establish a patient-physician partnership based on shared responsibility.

Questions are directed toward the possible causes of the patient's obesity, the presence or risk of medical complications, and any behavioral, psychologic, nutritional, and environmental considerations that have influenced the patient's obesity. The patient's history of dieting and physical activity should also be addressed. Women should be asked about gestational diabetes and episodes of toxemia. (See box on the following page)

To date there is no diet assessment tool available for the primary care clinician to incorporate into an office visit. The USDA Food Guide Pyramid is a useful tool for both assessing intake and educating the patient about food choices (Fig. 71-1). It can be used for all age groups. Reviewing each food group with the patient and asking how much and how often she eats foods from each food group will assist in identifying gross dietary deficiencies or excesses.

Screening for underlying causes of obesity involves taking a medication history and screening for certain endocrinopathies. Medications commonly associated with increased food intake and weight gain included tricyclic antidepressants, antipsychotics (including chlorpromazine and haloperidol), certain antihistamines (notably cyproheptadine [Periactin]), and corticosteroids. Hypothyroidism (see Chapter 12) and polycystic ovary syndrome (see Chapter 9) are endocrine disorders frequently associated with obesity in women.

A subgroup of obese women exhibit binge eating. Screening to identify these patients will assist in making appropriate treatment recommendations. Although data are limited, various studies suggest that obese binge eaters report more restrictive dieting and feel less capable of maintaining their diet; experience more hunger and a higher tendency toward disinhibition of eating; show more obsessive-compulsive thinking, anxiety, self-doubt, and guilt; report

EVALUATION OF THE OVERWEIGHT OR OBESE WOMAN

Interview

Age of onset
Family history
Environmental influences
Previous diets and results
Stress levels
Eating behaviors
  Binging
  Skipping meals
Eating disorders
  Bulimia
  Diuretic/laxative abuse
Physical activity
  Duration/intensity of exercise
  Activities of daily living
Symptoms or medical diagnosis influenced by obesity
Gestational diabetes; toxemia
Stage of change
  Precontemplation, contemplation, motivation/preparation, action, maintenance/relapse

Anthropometric indices

Growth chart (adolescents)
% Desirable weight
Body mass index
Waist-to-hip ratio

Physical examination and diagnostic tests

Blood pressure
Cancer screening
  breast, endometrial, cervical, and ovarian
Osteoarthritis
Lipids
ECG
TSH

Modified from Blackburn, GL: Medical treatment of obesity, Harvard Medical School Continuing Education Conference: Multidisciplinary Approach to Obesity, Boston, Mass, 1991.
ECG, electrocardiogram; TSH, thyroid-stimulating hormone.

more depression; and have an increased prevalence of psychiatric disorders, especially affective disorders.

Measurement

To assess weight status in the adolescent growth charts are used to compare weight for height, and changes in usual growth pattern are noted (taking into account the normal adolescent growth spurt).

Anthropometric indices used in adults that are practical for use in the office are (1) weight compared to standard tables, (2) body mass index, and (3) waist-to-hip ratio. Weight compared to standard tables is expressed as percentage overweight. The National Institute of Health has defined obesity as above 120% of desirable weight. A major limitation of weight tables is that they do not take into account ethnic differences nor account for body composition. The weights identified as ideal body weights for men and women may not be appropriate for the patient who has hyperplastic obesity or who has been a chronic dieter, as even if the ideal weight can be achieved, long-term maintenance of the lower weight is unlikely.

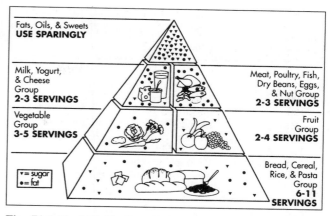

Fig. 71-1 Food Guide Pyramid: guide to daily food choices. (From Nelson, JK: *Diet manual: a handbook of nutrition practices*, US Dept of Agriculture, US Dept of Health and Human Services.)

Body mass index (BMI) (weight [kg]/height [m²]) (Fig. 71-2, Table 71-2), an index of body mass that is normalized for height, correlates highly with body fat percentage and is the most widely used measure. BMI is relatively higher than percentage overweight for shorter persons and lower for taller persons. The National Institute of Health Consensus Conference found that the risk to health begins when the BMI exceeds 27. Intervention becomes more strongly indicated with a BMI greater than 30, which corresponds with

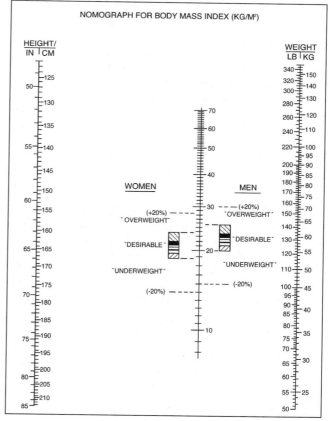

Fig. 71-2 Nomogram for body mass index. (From Bray GA: *Obesity in America*, NIH Publication No 79-359, November 1979.)

Table 71-2 Medical classification of obesity using body mass index

Desirable weight (%)	Definition	Grade of obesity	Excess fat (lbs/kgs)	BMI (kg/m2)
Men				
225	Super morbid obesity	6	173/79	≥50
200	Morbid obesity	5	139/63	45
180	Super obesity	4	111/50	40
160	Medically significant obesity	3	83/38	35
135	Obesity	2	48/22	30
110	Overweight	1	14/6	25
100	Desirable weight	0	0	22
70	Medically significant starvation	−3	−5/−7[†]	15
Women				
245	Super morbid obesity	6	158/72	≥50
220	Morbid obesity	5	131/59	45
195	Super obesity	4	103/47	40
170	Medically significant obesity	3	76/34	35
145	Obesity	2	49/22	30
120	Overweight	1	22/10	25
100	Desirable weight	0	0	21
75	Medically significant starvation	−3	−20/−9[†]	15

Developed by the Nutrition/Metabolism Laboratory, Cancer Research Institute, Boston, Mass.
* Medical risk of obesity is further modified by concurrent illness(es), complicating organ dysfunction, body fat distribution, velocity of weight change, and age. Relative risk varies from 2- to 15-fold. % desirable weight = % desirable body weight −154 pounds for (70 inch) reference man; 120 pounds for (64 inch) reference woman (1980 Recommended Dietary Allowance Table). Excess fat (pounds), assuming 90% of excess body weight is fat. BMI, body mass index (weight/height^2).
† Assuming 75% of weight loss in simple semistarvation is body fat.

an increased mortality ratio. For average women severe obesity is present if BMI = 40 kg/m^2 (corresponding roughly to 100 lb overweight) and defines a level of obesity where active intervention may be indicated.

Waist-to-hip ratio can be measured by measuring the smallest area around the waist (with the patient's stomach relaxed), measuring the widest area around the hips, and dividing the measurement of the hips into the waist measurement. A ratio greater than 0.8 in women age 40 to 59 has been associated with increased health risks of diabetes mellitus, hypertension, and gallbladder disease. Age and obesity level have been shown to be two important determinants of body fat distribution. For a given level of obesity a younger woman will have relatively more weight in the hip area, whereas older women will have relatively more weight in the stomach area. Above-the-waist fat distribution (termed "android") is more highly correlated with increased health risks, below-the-waist fat distribution (termed "gynoid") is not (Fig. 71-3). Women with upper body obesity may be more likely to improve their waist-to-hip ratio with weight loss; waist-to-hip ratio in lower body obesity tends to remain constant with weight loss.

Physical examination and diagnostic tests

The primary purpose of the physical examination and laboratory testing is to detect consequences of obesity: hypertension, osteoarthritis, disorders of carbohydrate metabolism, and hyperlipidemia. If there is a clinical suspicion of hypothyroidism, a thyroid-stimulating hormone (TSH) level is the most sensitive screening test. Other laboratory testing (for example, for polycystic ovary syndrome or gout) is dictated by the clinical history and physical examination.

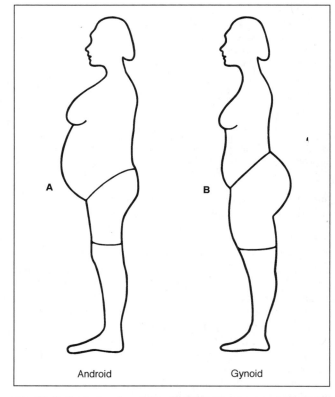

Fig. 71-3 Central and peripheral obesity in women. *A*, Android, abdominal, or upper-body pattern of body fat distribution. *B*, Gynoid, femoral, or lower body pattern of body fat distribution. (Modified from Davidson J and DiGirolamo M: Non-insulin dependent diabetes mellitus. In *Clinical diabetes mellitus*, New York, 1991, Thieme Medical Publishers.)

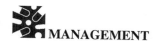

MANAGEMENT

Goals of management

Should all women who consult the primary care physician wanting to lose weight be encouraged to do so? The advisability of dieting should be questioned for women who are adolescents, have little weight to lose, or have a history of weight cycling.

Adolescence is a critical time for growth and development, both physically and psychosocially. Emphasis on thinness and dieting can lead to eating disorders or a lifetime of poor self-image and diet cycling. Because adolescence is a time of rapid growth and development it is important for the mildly overweight adolescent to be educated about the expected weight changes during this time. Emphasis should be placed on healthy food choices and increased activity rather than dieting. For the severely overweight adolescent family therapy should be considered.

The adult woman who has too little weight to lose (<10% above ideal body weight) is at larger risk of losing excessive lean body mass and should not be encouraged to pursue weight loss.

Some women have been weight cycling for so many years that dieting has become a way of life, marked by little success at maintaining a lower weight and a rebound to a higher weight after each diet effort. These women are often extremely sensitive about their weight and have a low sense of self-efficacy. If there are no medical problems, education about healthy eating and increased activity is appropriate regardless of the individual's weight. However, if the patient is at increased risk of development of a chronic disease associated with her obesity or already has a chronic disease, treatment may be indicated.

Extreme care should be taken in the initiation of a weight loss regimen. It is most important that women have an empathetic clinician who listens to their concerns and is able to establish a long-term relationship that provides support, education, and motivation. The most important factor is that the woman accept responsibility for her weight and be empowered to make decisions based on knowledge and self-control rather than guilt, willpower, and fear.

There is evidence that the health benefits of weight loss occur during the first 10% to 20% of excess body fat lost. Sharing this information with the woman may relieve her of the often overwhelming feeling of having to achieve an ideal body weight and may provide a motivation for weight loss.

Attention should be given to whether or not the patient desires weight loss and is ready, motivated, and willing to make the necessary commitments. The stage paradigm is a proactive and interactive model for behavior change that can be used to assess a patient's readiness for making changes and provide guidelines for professional intervention (see box, above right).

For the patient who is ready to take action, identifying short- and long-term goals is important. Goals should be positive, feasible, and specific. Often the patient may need the physician's guidance in setting these goals. Current recommendations are that treatment of obesity should set an initial goal of no more than 10% weight loss. Once this weight has been maintained for 1 year a goal of losing an additional

---

THE PROCESS OF HOW PEOPLE CHANGE

Stages of change

1. **Precontemplation**—unaware of, denies, or minimizes the problem

   Needs: confrontation and information

2. **Contemplation**—aware of problem, but weighing costs and benefits of change

   Needs: gentle confrontation, information and rationale to change, clarification of notions (often has misinformation)

3. **Motivation/preparation**—has decided to make change, plans to do so within next month, or has limited action to data collection or information gathering

   Needs: strategies for making change, goal setting

4. **Action**—plan is in progress; attitudinal and behavioral changes have begun

   Needs: tools and techniques to implement goals, positive reinforcement

5. **Maintenance/relapse**—action maintained over 6 months (maintenance) or return to old habits (relapse)

   Maintenance is most difficult stage; if maintained for 6 months, prognosis good: "A lapse does not a relapse make."

   Needs: tools for successful maintenance, feedback and encouragement

   Self-monitoring: checklist for each day (food intake, exercise)

   Coping skills and stress management

   Support systems

   Cognitive restructuring

Modified from Prochaska J, DiClemente C, Norcross J: *Am Psychol* 47(9):1102, 1992.

10%, if necessary, can be set. A 20% reduction in body weight will reduce fat cell hypertrophy and achieve normal energy metabolism. It will also reduce risk for chronic diseases such as hypertension, coronary artery disease, diabetes, and degenerative arthritis. Reasonable goals can include stopping weight gains (increases may be due to medications, physical impairment causing decreased activity, or stresses that may be triggering binge eating, for example) and stabilizing weight, particularly for the weight cycler.

It is useful to summarize the highlights of the interview by addressing biologic and environmental factors, social support and psychologic status, and timing of changes (see box on the following page). In this way the clinician has the opportunity to let the patient know she or he has been listening and sets the stage for appropriate goal setting and treatment interventions.

Choice of therapy

It has been reported that most persons who lose weight regain all of the lost weight by the end of 5 years. However, the discouraging long-term outcome should not suggest that treatment for obesity is neither cost-effective nor warranted. There are no data available on those persons who lose weight on their own and manage to keep the weight off; few data from hospital-based programs; and no data from commercial weight loss programs. Most of the data available come from university-based research settings that may inherently attract more refractory cases of obesity.

FORMULATING A PLAN

B—Biologic factors: "You have been overweight since adolescence and both of your parents are obese; it will be a little more difficult for you to lose weight and we certainly should not expect you to be at an ideal body weight."

E—Environmental factors: "You told me that you have been sedentary on your new job and that you do not have the time to cook so you depend on fast foods for many of your meals. These factors do have an effect on your weight and cholesterol, and fortunately, unlike your biologic factors, these are under your control. Today there are many low-fat food choices even for the busy person who doesn't have time to cook."

S—Social support and psychologic status: "Since your children are also concerned for your health, you can talk to them about your need to control your weight and that it would be helpful if they did not bring the chips, pizzas, etc., into the house."

T—Timing: "You stated that this is a good time for you to focus on losing weight and that your high cholesterol and the way you have been feeling are motivating you to take some action. Are you able to commit to a weekly program at this time? If so, I can make some recommendations. In the meantime, how do you feel about keeping a diet diary and finding acceptable low-fat alternatives? I recommend that you purchase a low-fat cookbook."

Self-guided weight loss

For the patient who has adult onset obesity, is on no medications, has no risk factors for chronic disease, and attributes weight gain to environmental factors, an appropriate first step would be to outline realistic exercise and nutritional goals. An emphasis on adequate calories (no fewer than 1000 kcal/day) should be coupled with an exercise program that may include both aerobic activity for fat burning and strength training to increase lean body mass. Using the visual aid of the Food Guide Pyramid the clinician can teach the patient how to build a healthy diet using starches, fruits, and vegetables as the base of the diet, meeting calcium needs by incorporating low-fat or nonfat milk and/or yogurt (300 mg calcium/8 oz), and complementing these foods with protein (10% to 15% of total calories: about 4 to 6 oz/day for women). Simple sugars and fats are at the top of the pyramid and are included less frequently in a healthy low-calorie meal plan. For weight management no more than 20% of total calories from fat is recommended. For a 1200- to 1500-calorie plan this would be 27 to 33 g of fat/day; on an 1800-calorie meal plan this would be 44 g of fat/day. The clinician may suggest the patient keep a food diary and record total fat intake by using a fat gram counter book and reading food labels.

For women who are following a self-guided weight loss program periodic visits to the primary care clinician can be important for monitoring progress and providing external reinforcement for weight loss and maintenance.

Individual and group programs

Many researchers believe that matching patients to an appropriate program may increase their chances for success and decrease any risks that may be associated with the weight loss process. Women should be encouraged to choose a program that focuses on nutritious food choices, exercise, activities of daily living, reversing of cognitive distortions around eating behavior, and ongoing support.

For the woman who has weight-cycled all her adult life, treatment should focus on halting the weight cycling and stabilizing her weight. If there are obesity-related health problems, deemphasizing weight and focusing on healthy eating and activity may be most beneficial.

Counseling about exercise and providing an exercise prescription are important. Exercise has a beneficial effect on body fat composition by reducing the waist-to-hip ratio and increasing lean body mass, thereby increasing basal metabolic rate. There is substantial evidence that overweight women who are active have lower rates of morbidity and mortality than those who are sedentary.

Patients with a long history of dieting often carry guilt about not being able to stick to a diet or about regaining the weight back after each attempt. Decreased self-esteem, self-confidence, and self-efficacy have been associated with chronic dieting. Empowering these patients to take control and make choices based on accurate information and self-control is important. An interdisciplinary team consisting of the physician, a dietitian, and a behavioral psychologist is very helpful for such patients.

For women identified as having a binge-eating disorder, cognitive/behavioral therapy has been among the most successful of the behavioral/psychologic approaches. This model postulates that irrational beliefs and fears lead to negative emotional states that produce "out of control" behavior, reinforcing initial beliefs. Referral to a group or individual program that incorporates cognitive/behavioral therapy may be particularly helpful for this subgroup of women.

For women referred to any individual or group program, monitoring in a primary care setting may be of benefit for adjustment of medications, assessment of the clinical effects of weight loss, and screening for symptoms related to gallbladder disease, the risk of which is increased by certain diets. To reduce the risk of gallbladder disease the diet should provide adequate amounts of protein and fat (14 g of protein and 10 of fat at one meal at least once daily to ensure adequate gallbladder contraction); weight loss should be limited to 2% or less per week; and the diet limited to 12 weeks or less in duration.

Balanced deficit diets

Balanced deficit diets are designed to cause a calorie deficit that will induce weight loss. Balanced deficit diets are incorporated into self-diets, self-help programs, worksite programs, commercial programs, hospital-based programs, and private counseling sessions.

Balanced deficit diets are considered to be generally safe for individuals who are 10% to 40% overweight. The calorie content is usually between 900 and 1500 calories to produce a weight loss of approximately 1 to 2 lb/wk. Low-fat diets consisting of 10% to 20% of total calories from fat focus on fat-gram counting rather than calorie counting. Adult-onset obesity may respond to a balanced-deficit diet consisting of fewer than 20% calories from fat, with emphasis on distribution of calories throughout the day, adequate protein, and increased exercise.

Providing a balanced deficit diet alone does not address the issues of external regulation of food intake and may, in fact, contribute to weight cycling. A nondiet approach with emphasis on internal versus external regulation of food intake, mindful eating, and cognitive restructuring may be a more effective approach for some patients (combined with psychologic therapy when indicated.

Very-low-calorie diets

Very-low-calorie diets (VLCDs) were developed to provide larger and more rapid short-term weight loss than the standard low-calorie diets, while avoiding the dangers and adverse effects of total fasting. A VLCD can be defined as a hypocaloric diet containing 800 calories or less per day and 0.8 to 1.5 g of protein/kg of ideal body weight/day. VLCDs are given in a form that completely replaces usual food intake (liquid formulations or food-based protein-sparing modified fasts using lean meat, fish, and fowl). The liquid formulations contain all the necessary nutrients while the food-based fast must incorporate vitamin and mineral supplements. Usually these diets are given for 12 to 16 weeks.

VLCDs should be restricted to women ages 18 to 65 years who are more than 30% above ideal weight and who have failed to maintain weight loss on more conservative diet programs. Contraindications to VLCDs are recent myocardial infarction; history of cerebrovascular, renal, or hepatic disease; cancer; type I diabetes; and pregnancy. Patients should also be screened for bulimia, depression, acute psychiatric disturbance, and substance abuse disorder.

Persons undergoing a VLCD program should be medically monitored weekly. Multidisciplinary care including nutrition education and life-style modification may increase successful long-term maintenance. A recent NIH Consensus Conference on Voluntary Weight Loss and Control concluded that "VLCDs are helpful in obtaining and maintaining weight loss for 2 to 3 years in some persons when used in conjunction with behavioral modification and an exercise program."

Medical therapy

The role of medical therapy in the management of obesity is evolving. In the past the potential for abuse has limited clinical use of appetite-suppressant drugs for weight control. Newer serotonergic agents appear to be equally effective for appetite suppression with little or no potential for abuse. Randomized trials of fenfluramine (Pondimin) and fluoxetine (Prozac) have shown that these agents are more effective than placebo in producing weight loss. However, weight regain occurs after withdrawal of medication. Weintraub's widely publicized randomized trial of fenfluramine combined with phentermine showed a significant weight reduction compared to that of a program combining behavior modification, exercise, and diet; the effect persisted for over 3 years.

Although there is a growing body of evidence that serotonergic appetite-suppressant drugs are effective and safe, weight loss benefits are relatively small, weight regain follows treatment withdrawal, and drugs may too easily become a substitute for patient education, exercise, and good nutrition. Long-term drug therapy may be appropriate for consideration in patients with a long history of weight loss and regain, particularly those who already have complications of obesity.

There are some practical considerations in the use of medical therapy for obesity. Most current licensing regulations limit the pharmacologic treatment of obesity to short periods, most commonly 12 to 16 weeks. Fluoxetine is not currently approved in the United States for the treatment of obesity. Early studies have shown weight loss during the first 8 weeks of fluoxetine treatment, followed by weight regain after 16 to 20 weeks in some patients. Fenfluramine is available in two forms. Dex-fenfluramine, the more widely studied, is not available in the United States; the prescribing of D,L-fenfluramine, a Schedule IV substance, is subject to regulation. References providing detailed information on the effectiveness and clinical use of serotonergic agents are listed in the bibliography.

Surgery

Surgery may be considered in selected women with severe obesity that has proved refractory to more conservative treatment. Although the long-term effects of current surgical treatment have not been well-defined, the substantial physical and psychosocial hazards of obesity may justify their use in some cases. Candidates for surgery include women with severe obesity (BMI greater than 40 kg/m^2 or approximately 100 lb overweight) and some individuals with less severe obesity (BMI between 35 and 40 kg/m^2) associated with serious cardiopulmonary disease. Evaluation of surgical candidacy should be made by a multidisciplinary team and should consider the patient's motivation, risk of surgical complications, and willingness to participate in lifetime medical surveillance.

Two surgical procedures that reduce gastric size, vertical banded gastroplasty and gastric bypass procedures, currently account for the majority of operations for obesity. The gastric bypass procedure produces a greater weight loss on average but carries a higher risk for complication.

Both procedures produce substantial weight reduction. Approximately 50% of excess weight is lost during the first year after surgery, with a nadir occurring at 18 to 24 months. Some weight regain after 2 years is often seen. Comorbid conditions and psychosocial functioning often improve, though the duration of improvement has not been established. Long-term complications include micronutrient deficiencies (especially vitamin B$_{12}$, folate, and iron) and the dumping syndrome.

Eighty percent of patients who undergo surgery for obesity are women of reproductive age. Pregnancy should be avoided until weight has stabilized a year or two after surgery. Women who become pregnant after gastric reduction procedures should be closely monitored during pregnancy to ensure adequate weight gain and nutritional support for the fetus.

Prognosis

Factors associated with successful weight loss are self-monitoring, goal setting, social support, and length of treatment. Factors associated with successful maintenance are physical activity, self-monitoring, and continued contact with the program. The psychologic effects of physical activity have the greatest impact: enhanced self-concept, general self-efficacy, and reduced anxiety, stress, and depression. Successful maintainers typically achieve a weight that is about halfway between presenting weight and ideal body weight.

SUMMARY

Obesity has come to be recognized as a complex phenomenon that entails more than excess body fat. Obesity is caused by genetic, biologic, and environmental factors. A thorough assessment including an interview, anthropometric indices, and a physical examination will provide information that will allow the physician to individualize treatment and set appropriate goals. A desirable intervention plan considers the patient's physical and psychosocial status as well as her weight and dieting history.

Treatment for obesity is evolving. Balanced deficit diets, coupled with exercise and behavior modification, have been the standard approach. For severely overweight patients for whom traditional diets have been unsuccessful (particularly those with complications of obesity), very-low-calorie diets, medical treatment, and surgery are treatment options.

It is important that the patient have the confidence and desire to adopt a new life-style. The patient can be empowered through the recognition of the complexity of her personal needs. Often an interdisciplinary team or an integrated program is the best approach. Success is measured not just by absolute weight loss but also by stabilization of a weight cycler's weight or halting of weight gains, and by decreasing of risk for chronic disease.

BIBLIOGRAPHY

Bray GA: Use and abuse of appetite-suppressant drugs in the treatment of obesity, *Ann Intern Med* 119:707, 1993.

Brownell KD, Stunkard AJ, Albaum JM: Evaluation and modification of exercise patterns in the natural environment, *Am J Psychiatry* 137:1540, 1980.

Brownell KD, Wadden TA: The heterogeneity of obesity: fitting treatments to individuals, *Behav Ther* 22:153, 1991.

Consensus Development Conference Panel: Gastrointestinal surgery for severe obesity: Consensus Development Conference statement, *Ann Intern Med* 115:956, 1991.

Elliot DL, Goldberg L, Girard DE: Clinical reviews obesity: pathophysiology and practical management, *J Gen Intern Med* 2:188, 1987.

Gormally J, et al: The assessment of binge eating severity among obese persons, *Addict Behav* 7:47, 1982.

Grilo CM, Brownell KD, Stunkard AJ: The metabolic and psychological importance of exercise in weight control. In Stunkard AJ, Wadden TA, editors: *Obesity: theory and therapy,* ed 2, New York, 1993. Raven.

Hirsch J, Leibel RL: A biological basis for human obesity, *J Clin Endocrinol Metab* 73:1153, 1991.

Kanders BS, Blackburn GL: Reducing primary risk factors by therapeutic weight loss. In Wadden TA, Van Itallie, editors: *Treatment of the seriously obese patient,* New York, 1992, Guilford Press.

Marcus MD, Wing RR, Hopkins J: Obese binge eaters: affect, cognitions, and response to behavioral weight control, *J Consult Clin Psychol* 55:433, 1988.

Marcus MD et al: A double-blind, placebo-controlled trial of fluoxetine plus behavior modification in the treatment of obese binge-eaters and non-binge-eaters, *Am J Psychiatry* 147:876, 1990.

Peeke PM: Health risks of obesity for women, Health Watch 2000 Conference, February 1992.

Prochaska J, DiClemente C, Norcross J: In search of how people change: applications to addictive behaviors, *Am Psycholog* 47(9):1102, 1992.

Slochower JA: *Excessive eating: the role of emotions and environment.* New York, 1982, Human Sciences Press.

Technology Assessment Conference, Methods of Voluntary Weight Loss and Control, *Ann Intern Med* 116(11):942, 1992.

VanItallie TB: Health implications of overweight and obesity in the United States, *Ann Intern Med* 103:983, 1985.

Wadden TA, Foster GD: Behavioral assessment and treatment of markedly obese patients, In Wadden TA, Van Itallie TB, editors: *Treatment of the seriously obese patient.* New York, 1992, Guilford Press.

Weintraub M et al: Long-term weight control study: I-VII, *Clin Parmacol Ther* 39:501, 1985.

Williamson DF: Descriptive epidemiology of body weight and weight change in U.S. adults, *Ann Intern Med* 119(7 pt 2):646, 1993.

---

72 Sexual Assault

Stephanie A. Eisenstat

Sexual assault against women is common, with one in six women reporting a history of sexual assault. It carries both short-term and long-term physical and psychologic effects. The term *rape* is a legal term, not a medical one. The trauma inflicted brings the patient in contact with the health care system, and for the clinician it is important to know how to evaluate victims of a rape and to develop strategies for dealing with both the short- and long-term consequences of sexual assault. This chapter addresses the physician's role and responsibility in dealing with a woman who has experienced sexual assault and outlines protocol for evaluation and management. A few reviews have been published on management of the victim of sexual assault, and they are listed in the bibliography at the end of this chapter. The following discussion highlights the important principles in evaluation and management and draws on the information in these reviews.

DEFINITION

Rape is a legal term, the definition of which has changed over the years and varies from state to state. Rape is now defined as the "nonconsensual sexual penetration of an adolescent or adult obtained by physical force, by threat of bodily harm, or when the victim is incapable of giving consent by virtue of mental illness, mental retardation or intoxication" (Searles and Berger, 1987).

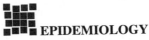 **EPIDEMIOLOGY**

Sexual assault is one of the most common crimes against women. One in five adult women, one in six college women, and one in eight adolescent girls have been sexually assaulted over their lifetime, as reported from national crime statistics from the U.S. Department of Justice. These numbers are likely underestimated because of the hesitancy of rape victims to report the sexual assault; 39% of rape victims report having sustained physical injury, and only 54% of these women receive medical care for the injuries (Harlow, 1989).

HEALTH CONSEQUENCES
Rape trauma syndrome

Rape trauma syndrome is the psychologic reaction of the rape trauma victim which is characterized by two major phases after sexual assault (see box, below). The first phase of shock and disbelief can last from 6 weeks to a few months, with the woman displaying either intense fear and anxiety and crying episodes or the opposite, with little display of emotion. Frightening recollections of the assault may be associated with generalized hypersensitivity to environmental stimuli. The second phase is delayed and involves a psychologic reorganization, a long-term process that can last a few months or indefinitely. The woman develops various coping strategies to deal with activities of daily living and to integrate the experience and thus achieve psychologic recovery. Flashbacks, phobias, and depression still may occur, in addition to gynecologic and somatic complaints. Sexual dysfunction is common. There appears to be a time inbetween these two phases when the woman enters a phase of denial and gives the outward appearance of coping. During this period, medical symptoms may develop or intensify, causing the woman to seek medical attention, but she may not inform the clinician of the sexual assault because of intense shame and guilt. It is important for clinicians to ask patients directly during the interview about a history of sexual assault.

Medical disorders

Any sexual assault or trauma can lead to the development of chronic physical complaints and an increased risk for serious mental illness such as depression or suicidal impulses (see box, above right). Somatic complaints include extreme fatigue, abdominal pain, nausea, headaches, and gynecologic and menstrual complaints. A constant concern is the

---

MEDICAL DISORDERS ASSOCIATED WITH SEXUAL ASSAULT

Depression
Substance abuse
Gastrointestinal complaints
Headaches
Insomnia
Gynecologic and menstrual complaints

---

development of sexually transmitted diseases, pregnancy, and HIV infection. Frequent utilization of primary medical care for up to 2 years after the assault is common.

Sexual assault during pregnancy

Sexual assault often occurs during pregnancy although the exact incidence is difficult to estimate because of underreporting. Overall pregnancy outcome has been found to be normal in small retrospective studies of pregnant women who have been sexually assaulted; however, there is an increased risk for low-birth-weight infants and premature delivery. In these studies pregnant women had the same incidence of vulvar, oral, and anal penetration as matched nonpregnant sexual assault victims, but they experienced less truncal injuries if the assault occurred after 20 weeks' gestation. There was a higher incidence of sexually transmitted diseases, urinary tract infections, and vaginitis. It is important in the evaluation of sexual assault during pregnancy to remember that pregnancy and its effect on the vaginal flora do not preclude the collection or interpretation of clinical or forensic evidence, and every effort should be made to collect the appropriate specimens. Prophylaxis against sexually transmitted disease also is important (see management section).

 EVALUATION

Goals

The physician's responsibility in evaluating a woman who has been sexually assaulted is to stabilize her medical condition and then to document the history and physical evidence clearly in the medical record, to assess the patient's psychologic state, and to provide prophylactic therapy to prevent sexually transmitted disease and pregnancy (see box on the following page). It is important to avoid judgmental statements to the patient. It is not the role of the physician to determine whether or not the rape has occurred.

History and symptoms

The interview. Ensuring confidentiality and privacy is important when the clinician interviews the victim of sexual assault. One needs to obtain informed consent before proceeding with the history, physical examination, and collection of specimens for physical evidence. A clear explanation for the process and protocol for evaluation is reassuring and helpful. An overt statement that the patient is safe is often necessary. It is helpful if a rape counselor is present during the history and physical examination (see box on the following page).

RAPE TRAUMA SYNDROME

Acute phase (may last hours to days)
Paralysis of patient's coping mechanisms
Shock, denial, disbelief
Classic triad:
  Haunting, intrusive recollections
  Numbing of feelings
  Generalized hypersensitivity to environmental stimuli
Body pain, insomnia
Vaginal discharge, pain or itching, and rectal pain
Depression, anxiety, and mood swings

Delayed (organizational) phase (may occur months to years after assault)
Flashbacks, nightmares
Phobias and depression
Gynecologic and menstrual complaints
Somatic complaints: extreme fatigue, abdominal pain, nausea, headaches
Sexual dysfunction
Serious psychosocial dysfunction with increased risk of suicide and substance abuse

From Burgess AW, Holmstrom LL. In Burgess AW, Holmstrom LL, editors: *Rape: victims of crisis,* Bowie, Md, 1974, Robert J Brady.

**PHYSICIANS' RESPONSIBILITIES IN DEALING WITH
A WOMAN WHO IS A VICTIM OF SEXUAL ASSAULT**

Medical

Obtain accurate gynecologic history.
Assess and treat physical injuries.
Obtain appropriate cultures and treat any existing infections.
Provide therapy to prevent unwanted conception.
Provide counseling.
Arrange for follow-up medical care and counseling.

Legal

Provide accurate recording of events.
Document injuries.
Collect samples.
Report to authorities as required.

From American College of Obstetricians and Gynecologists: *Int J Gynecol Obstet* 42:67, 1993.

History. The key events in the history are summarized in the box, above right. Reassuring the patient and explaining the reasoning behind the questions can be helpful. Often the woman feels shame and humiliation because she may think she caused the assault. Assurance and support help the victim. It is important to document the age of the patient, date and time of assault, circumstance of the assault, and details of the contact. The activities of the victim after the assault and a general medical and gynecologic history should be ascertained. It also is important to assess the patient's psychologic status, coping strategies, and support systems. The history should be clearly documented, and judgmental statements should be avoided (see box, below right). Many emergency room settings have rape evaluation kits to help in the appropriate documentation, or these can be obtained from the local crime forensics laboratories.

Physical examination

A complete physical examination should be performed with particular focus on the area of injury. The woman is asked to disrobe over paper sheets on which any debris or fibers can be collected. Her clothes are then placed in labeled paper bags to avoid contamination. Careful collection of specimens for evidence should be performed as listed in the box on the following page. After collection the specimens should be locked in a safe place until the police can remove them. Photographs should be taken if necessary and with informed consent. Because as many as 67% of victims have external extragenital trauma, a careful examination for lacerations, abrasions, and bruising should then be completed. Common sites for external trauma include the mouth, throat, wrist, arms, breast, and thighs. Bite marks also are common and should be examined for.

INITIAL INTERVIEW

Ensure confidentiality.   Ensure safety.
Obtain informed consent.   Obtain rape counselor.
Explain protocol and procedures.

KEY FACTORS IN THE HISTORY

Accurate account of events
Objective description for documentation
Thorough sexual and gynecologic history:
  Pregnancy history
  Use of contraception
  Date of last menstrual period
Assessment of emotional status, coping strategies, and
  support

Gynecologic examination. A complete gynecologic examination, including a rectal examination, should be performed, and the use of lubricants, which can be spermicidal, should be avoided. Genital trauma should be asertained by visual examination. Staining with toluidine can help in the detection of subtle tears. Because determining subtle genital trauma can be difficult, some clinicians have advocated the use of colposcopy to determine genital trauma in rape victims. Given the potential psychologic trauma of a colposcopic examination, more controlled studies on its use should to be undertaken. Aspiration of the posterior vaginal fornices after normal saline wash should be performed if no obvious secretions can be identified and collected. After collection, the aspirate should be suspended in warm normal saline and examined for the presence of sperm, documenting both the number and motility per high-power field. The rest of the aspirate is then sent to a forensics laboratory to be tested for acid phosphatase. High concentrations of the enzyme is associated with recent coitus. The sample also should be assayed for the glycoprotein p30, which is present in seminal fluid, and for genetic testing. A few studies have used prostate specific antigen (PSA) as a marker, but further studies are needed before its use can be recommended.

If there is a delay in transport of the specimens, they should be kept refrigerated. In addition to the complete gynecologic examination, a particular emphasis should be placed on the examination of the perineal and inner thigh area. This is accomplished with a Wood's lamp to detect semen stains. Areas of fluorescence should then be swabbed with saline-moistened cotton swabs and smeared on a slide to examine for the presence of sperm. Culture specimens for *Neisseria gonorrhoeae* and *Chlamydia trachomatis* should be obtained from all sites of entry. Pap smear and pubic hair sampling should be completed. Combing of the pubic hair increases the yield of the assailant's hair samples. Samples of the patient's hair should be clipped and stored.

MEDICAL DOCUMENTATION

Do not use "rape" or "sexual assault" because these are legal
  terms.
Use terms such as "consistent with the use of force."
Collect physical evidence as soon as possible.
Document physical and emotional condition.
Document thorough history and physical examination.

KEY FACTORS IN PHYSICAL EXAMINATION

Collect clothing

Complete physical examination
To include photographs and drawings of injured areas

Skin examination
Cuts, bruises, bite marks

Head and neck examination
Oral secretions for acid phosphatase
Injuries as a result of oral penetration
Culture for gonorrhea

Genitourinary examination
Pubic hair combing and sampling
Vaginal secretions and cervical mucus:
Motile sperm
Acid phosphatase
Glycoprotein p30
DNA fingerprinting by wet or dry swab
Pap smear
Cultures for gonorrhea and chlamydia
Complete pelvic examination for gynecologic injury, trauma, and foreign objects

Rectal examination
Examination for trauma
Culture for gonorrhea
Collect secretion for motile sperm and acid phosphastase if indicated

KEY DIAGNOSTIC TESTS

Cultures

Pharyngeal
Gonorrhea
Chlamydia

Vaginal/cervical
Gonorrhea
Chlamydia
Trichomonas
Herpes simplex

Rectal
Gonorrhea
Chlamydia
Herpes simplex
Fingernail scrapings

Other tests
Pregnancy test
Baseline VDRL for syphilis
Serologic tests:
Herpes simplex virus
Hepatitis B
HIV
Cytomegalovirus
Saliva for major blood group antigen

Diagnostic tests

In addition to cultures (pharyngeal swabs for gonorrhea and chlamydia, vaginal/cervical swabs for gonorrhea, chlamydia, *Trichomonas vaginalis*, and herpes simplex virus and rectal swabs for gonorrhea, chlamydia, and herpes simplex), certain blood tests should be obtained (see the box, above right). These include pregnancy test (serum human chorionic gonadotropin) and a baseline VDRL (or rapid plasma reagin [RPR]) for syphilis. Many clinicians also obtain serologic data for herpes simplex virus, hepatitis B, cytomegalovirus, and, with consent, baseline HIV testing. Seroconversion for HIV infection can occur up to 1 year after exposure and therefore is repeated at 3-month intervals for 1 year. It also is necessary to collect (1) saliva for the major blood group antigen and (2) scrapings from the woman's fingernails.

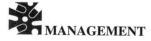

MANAGEMENT
Choice of therapy

Prophylaxis for sexually transmitted diseases and HIV. According to the Centers for Disease Control, up to 6% to 12% of victims contract gonorrhea and chlamydial infection, and 3% of victims contract syphilis. Trichomonal infection and bacterial vaginosis also are frequently contracted. Therefore prophylaxis for gonorrhea and chlamydia and testing for syphilis are indicated for all victims of sexual assault. Treatment for trichomonal infection and bacteri-

al vaginosis has been recommended by the Centers for Disease Control as well. The standard treatment protocols are listed in Table 72-1. Recommendations for the pregnant woman are included.

If the assailant is thought to be in a high-risk category for hepatitis B or if the victim has experienced vaginal or anal assault with bleeding, hepatitis B immune globulin (HBIG 0.06 ml/kg IM) should be given and repeated in 1 month if the patient shows seronegativity (Dunn and Gilchrist, 1993). An alternative approach is to give a single dose of HBIG and then initiate hepatitis B vaccination for both short-term and long-term protection (CDC, 1993).

No data are available on the risk of contracting HIV after a sexual assault, and there are no present recommendations regarding prophylaxis with zidovudine (AZT). Women should be counseled regarding HIV transmission and safe sex practices. If the woman desires testing for HIV, it should be done at the time of the assault, then every 3 to 4 months up to 1 year before assurance can be given regarding seroconversion. Generally, seroconversion occurs within 6 months after exposure to HIV. For more details regarding HIV, see Chapter 16.

Prevention of pregnancy. Pregnancy occurs in 5% of all fertile female victims. The patient should be offered the "morning-after pill" for prevention of pregnancy, unless by history the woman is menstruating or is known to be pregnant. It should be offered regardless of the woman's cycle phase at the time of the assault. Standard regimen is two orally administered combination contraceptive pills, usually 50 μg estrogen each (such as Ovral) immediately and again 12 hours later. The "morning-after pill" is effective within 72 hours of the assault. This and other options for pregnancy prevention appear in the box on the following page. For a more detailed discussion on the morning-after pill, see Chapter 27.

Counseling and follow-up. Rape counseling is very important for the victim and should be arranged at the time of evaluation (see box on the following page). Follow-up medical evaluation should be arranged within 72 hours of the initial assault to assess bruising and the woman's psychologic state, followed by another evaluation within 2 weeks. Often the victim of sexual assault develops symptoms such

Table 72-1 Management of sexual assault: treatment guidelines for sexually transmitted diseases

Disease	Prophylactic antibiotics Recommended treatment	Alternatives
Gonorrhea Pharyngeal, rectal Urogenital	Ceftriaxone 250 mg IM once	Cefixime 400 mg PO once Spectinomycin 2 g IM once*
Pregnancy	Same	Same
Chlamydia Urethral, cervical, rectal	Doxycycline 100 mg PO bid × 7 days	Azithromycin 1 g PO once[†] Erythromycin 500 mg PO qid × 7 days
Pregnancy	Erythromycin 500 mg PO qid × 7 days	Erythromycin ethylsuccinate 800 mg PO qid × 7 days[‡] Amoxicillin 500 mg PO tid × 7 days
Trichomonas	Metronidazole (Flagyl) 2 g PO once	Flagyl 500 mg PO bid × 7 days
Pregnancy First trimester Second and third trimesters	Wait until after first trimester, then treat Oral Flagyl	
Bacterial vaginosis	Flagyl 500 mg PO bid × 7 days	Clindamycin cream 2%, 1 vaginal application qhs × 7 days Clindamycin 300 mg PO bid × 7 days Flagyl 2 g PO once
Pregnancy First trimester Second and third trimesters	Clindamycin cream Oral or vaginal Flagyl	
Hepatitis B immune globulin[§]	0.06 ml/kg single IM dose within 14 days of exposure	
Vaccination[§]	Three doses, each 1 ml IM in the deltoid muscle at 0, 1, 6 mo	

Modified from Centers for Disease Control and Prevention: *MMWR* 42 (No RR-14):3184, 1993.
*Not effective against pharyngeal gonorrhea nor against incubating syphilis.
[†]Safety during pregnancy not been established.
[‡]Can switch to 250 mg PO qid for 14 days if not tolerated; erythromycin estolate is contraindicated during pregnancy.
[§]Both safe in pregnancy.

as gastrointestinal complaints, headaches, insomnia, nightmares, eating disorders, and irritability, which are not directly related to the physical injuries but are a result of the severe psychologic trauma. Characteristics of posttraumatic stress syndrome may develop, such as flashbacks, sensitivity to certain stimuli, hypersensitivity, and difficulty with concentration.

A VDRL for syphilis and other serologic tests (see box, below) should be repeated after 3 to 4 weeks. HIV testing should be completed with informed consent every 3 months for the first year after the assault. Pregnancy counseling and safe sex practices should be completed at the time of the assault and readdressed at each follow-up visit.

OPTIONS FOR PREGNANCY PROPHYLAXIS

No immediate therapy; wait until next menses before performing repeat pregnancy test
No immediate therapy; repeat serum pregnancy test in 1 week
Prescribe:
"Morning-after" pill
   Ethinyl estradiol–norgestrel (Ovral) (50 μg estrogen) 2 tablets at time victim is seen, then 2 tablets in 12 hr
   or
Ethinyl estradiol 5 mg PO × 5 days
   or
Conjugated equine estrogen 20-30 mg PO qd × 5 days
   or
Diethylstilbestrol 25 mg PO bid × 5 days

Modified from American College of Obstetricians and Gynecologists: *Int J Gynecol Obstet* 42:67, 1993; Beebe D: *Am Fam Physician* 43:2041, 1991.

SUMMARY

Sexual assault is common and requires both short-term intervention and long-term support. It is important to evaluate the victim thoroughly and document both the history and

---

SEXUAL ASSAULT FOLLOW-UP

Provide rape counseling.
See patient within 72 hours to assess delayed bruising and coping.
See patient again in 1-2 weeks for counseling and follow-up.
Provide pregnancy counseling.
Repeat serologic tests in 3-4 weeks.
Repeat HIV testing in 3-6 months.

physical findings clearly in the medical record. Collection of specimens is important for legal reasons, and procedures and protocols should be explained to the patient. Most hospitals have standard rape protocol kits for this purpose. Prophylaxis for sexually transmitted diseases and pregnancy should be completed. Finally, because of the psychologic trauma and development of associated medical disorders, these women should have close medical follow-up from their primary medical care team and the support of rape counselors.

BIBLIOGRAPHY

American College of Obstetricians and Gynecologists: Sexual assault (ACOG Tech Bull No 172), *Int J Gynecol Obstet* 42:67, 1993.

Beckman CR, Groetzinger LL: Treating sexual assault victims: a protocol for health professionals, *Female Patient* 14 (5):78, 1989.

Beebe D: Emergency management of the adult female rape victim, *Am Fam Physician* 43:2041, 1991.

Beebe D: Initial assessment of rape victim, *J Miss State Med Assoc* 32(11):403, 1991.

Burgess AW, Holmstrom LL: Rape trauma syndrome. In Burgess AW, Holmstrom LL, editors: *Rape: victims of crisis,* Bowie, 1974, Robert J. Brady.

Centers for Disease Control and Prevention: 1993 sexually transmitted diseases treatment guidelines, *MMWR* 42 (No RR-14):1, 1993.

Council on Scientific Affairs: Violence against women: relevance for medical practitioners, *JAMA* 267:3184, 1992.

Dunn S, Gilchrist V: Sexual assault, *Prim Care* 20:359, 1993.

Dupre: Sexual assault, *Obstet Gynecol Surv* 48:640, 1993.

Elam AL, Ray VG: Sexually related trauma: a review, *Ann Emerg Med* 15:576, 1986.

Enos WF, Beyer JC: Management of the rape victim, *Am Fam Physician* 18:97, 1978.

Forman B: Psychotherapy with rape victims. *Psychotherapy: Theory, Research, and Practice,* 17:304, 1980.

Forster G: Rape and sexually transmitted diseases, *Br J Hosp Med* 47:94, 1992.

Geist R: Sexually related trauma, *Emerg Med Clin North Am* 6:439, 1988.

Gostin: HIV testing, counseling and prophylaxis after sexual assault, *JAMA* 271:1436, 1994.

Harlow CW: *Injuries from crime,* Washington, DC, 1989, Department of Justice, Bureau of Justice Statistics.

Hendricks-Matthews: Survivors of abuse: health care issues, *Prim Care* 20:391, 1993.

Hendricks-Matthews: Recognition of sexual abuse, *J Am Board Fam Pract* 6:511, 1993.

Hicks DJ: Sexual battery: management of the rape victim. In Sciarra JJ, editor: *Gynecology and obstetrics,* vol 6, Philadelphia, 1990, Harper & Row.

Hicks DJ, Minkin MJ, Solola A: Examining the rape victim, *Patient Care* 20(8):98, 1986.

Hochbaum SR: The evaluation and treatment of the sexually assaulted patient, *Emerg Med Clin North Am* 5:601, 1987.

Jenny C et al: Sexually transmitted diseases in victims of rape, *N Engl J Med* 322:713, 1990.

Kobernick ME, Seifert S, Sanders AB: Emergency department management of the sexual assault victim, *J Emerg Med* 2:205, 1985.

Koss MP: Hidden rape: sexual aggression and victimization in a national sample of students in higher education. In Burgess AW, editor: *Rape and sexual assault,* New York, 1988, Garland Publishing.

Koss MP: The women's mental health research agaenda: violence against women, *Am Psychol* 45:374, 1990.

Koss MP, Harvey M: The rape victim: clinical and community approaches to treatment, Beverly Hills, Calif, 1991, Sage Publications.

Koss MP, Koss, PG, Woodruff WJ: Relation of criminal victimization to health perceptions among women medical patients, *J Consult Clin Psychol* 58:147, 1990.

Koss MP, Woodruff WJ, Koss PG: Deleterious effects of criminal victimization on women's health and medical utilization, *Arch Intern Med* 151:342, 1991.

Mishell DR Jr: Contraception, sterilization and pregnancy termination. In Herbst AL et al, editors: *Comprehensive gynecology,* ed 2, St Louis, 1992, Mosby.

Patel HC: Colposcopy and rape, *Am J Obstet Gynecol* 168:1334, 1993.

Rambow B et al: Female sexual assault: medical and legal implications, *Ann Emerg Med* 21:727, 1992.

Resick P et al: Adjustment in victims of sexual assault, *J Consult Clin Psychol* 49:705, 1981.

Roach BA, Vladutru AO: Prostatic specific antigen and prostatic acid phosphatase measured by radioimmunoassay in vaginal washings from cases of suspected sexual assault, *Clin Chim Acta* 216:199, 1993 (letter).

Ruckman L: Victims of rape: the physician's role in treatment, *Curr Opinion Obstet Gynecol* 5:721, 1993.

Satin A et al: Sexual assault in pregnancy, *Obstet Gynecol* 77:710, 1991.

Satin A et al: The prevalence of sexual assault: a survey of 2404 puerperal women, *Am J Obstet Gynecol* 167:973, 1992.

Schwarcz SK, Whittington WL: Sexual assault and sexually transmitted diseases: detection and management in adults and children, *Rev Infect Dis* 12 (suppl 6):S682, 1990.

Searles P, Berger RJ: The current status of rape reform legislation: an examination of state statues, *Wom Rights Law Reporter* 9:25, 1987.

Slaughter L, Brown C: Colposcopy to establish physical findings in rape victims, *Am J Obstet Gyncol* 166:83, 1992.

US Senate Committee on the Judiciary: *Violence against women: the increase of rape in America 1990—majority report,* Washington, DC, 1991, Library of Congress.

Department of Justice, Federal Bureau of Investigation: *Uniform crime reports for the United States,* Washington, DC, 1988, US Government Printing Office.

Young W et al and the New Hampshire Sexual Assault Medical Examination Protocol Project Committee: Sexual assault: review of a national model protocol for forensic and medical evaluation, *Obstet Gynecol* 80:878, 1992.

73 Smoking Cessation

Nancy A. Rigotti and Lela Polivogianis

Cigarette smoking is a major health hazard for women. It is the leading preventable cause of death for both women and men in the United States, responsible for an estimated 419,000 deaths each year, or one in every five deaths. Primary care physicians take care of the health consequences of their patients' tobacco use. It is equally important for them to prevent smoking-related disease by addressing the smoking habits of their patients.

EPIDEMIOLOGY
Patterns of tobacco use

Cigarette smoking in the United States and its health consequences are largely twentieth-century phenomena. Smoking was uncommon before 1900, rose rapidly in the first half of the century, and peaked in 1965, when 40% of adult Americans smoked cigarettes. Since then smoking rates have declined, reflecting growing public awareness of the health risks of tobacco use. By 1992 adult smoking prevalence had fallen to 26%. This decline is primarily attributable to smoking cessation. Smoking initiation rates have not decreased since 1980, despite a concurrent fall in smoking prevalence. In both sexes smoking starts during childhood and adolescence; 90% of smokers begin to smoke before the age of 20.

These aggregate data conceal dramatic differences in the smoking patterns of men and women that have led to substantial gender differences in smoking-related disease mortality. American women did not take up smoking in large numbers until World War II, three decades later than men. When smoking prevalence peaked in 1965, only 32% of adult women smoked, compared to 50% of men. After 1965 smoking rates fell four times faster in men than in women. The result has been a convergence in the smoking rates of men and women. By 1992, 24% of adult women and 28% of men smoked cigarettes. A marked gender difference persists in the use of other tobacco products. Few women smoke cigars or pipes or use smokeless tobacco.

The narrowing of the gender gap in smoking is primarily attributable to sex differences in smoking initiation rates, which have fallen less rapidly in young women than in young men. Currently adolescent girls and boys are smoking at the same rates, but during the 1980s more females than males began to smoke. In contrast, women smokers have quit at approximately the same rate as male smokers since 1965. By 1989, 43% of women who had ever smoked had quit smoking, as compared to 49% of men.

In the United States smoking is more closely linked to education than it is to age, race, occupation, or any other sociodemographic factor. Smoking is inversely related to educational attainment in both women and men. In 1992 smoking prevalence in women ranged from 13% among college graduates to 27% among high school dropouts. Because less educated women are more likely to start smoking and less likely to stop than their better educated peers,

this disparity is likely to increase. Educational attainment is a marker for socioeconomic status, and these data indicate that smoking is a problem becoming concentrated in lower socioeconomic groups.

Young people, aged 25 to 44, have the highest smoking rates; 30% of them smoked in 1992. Smoking varies by occupational status in men, with higher rates in blue-collar than white-collar workers, but this relationship is weaker in women. Racial differences in smoking are also smaller in women than men; in 1992 the prevalence of smoking was 19% in Hispanic women, 23% in black women, and 25% in white women.

HEALTH CONSEQUENCES OF TOBACCO USE

Epidemiologic studies of the health consequences of tobacco use were first conducted in men because of their higher smoking rates. Subsequent studies in women have confirmed that the relationships identified for male smokers hold for female smokers. In short, women who smoke like men get sick and die like men. In addition, smoking poses health risks for women that are not shared with men.

Cigarette smoking increases the overall mortality and morbidity rates of both women and men. Approximately 106,000 deaths in women in 1985 were attributable to smoking, representing 25% of all female deaths. In both sexes smoking is a cause of cardiovascular disease (including myocardial infarction and sudden death), cerebrovascular disease, peripheral vascular disease, chronic obstructive pulmonary disease, and cancers of the lung, larynx, oral cavity, and esophagus. Middle-aged women who smoke are three times more likely to die of coronary artery disease and five times more likely to die of a stroke than are nonsmoking women. Women who smoke are over 10 times more likely to die of lung cancer, laryngeal cancer, esophageal cancer, and chronic obstructive pulmonary disease than are nonsmoking women.

Lung cancer, once a rare disease in women, has increased dramatically since 1950. Between 1960 and 1986 the lung cancer mortality rate increased more than fourfold among women smokers, while it did not change in nonsmoking women. By 1986 lung cancer surpassed breast cancer to become the leading cause of cancer death in women. Smoking accounted for 21% of cancer deaths in women in 1991, and 79% of female lung cancer deaths. Cigarette smokers also have higher rates of cancers of the bladder, pancreas, kidney, and stomach. Smoking interacts with alcohol to increase the risk of laryngeal, oral cavity, and esophageal cancers in both sexes. Tobacco interacts with asbestos and other occupational exposures to increase cancer risk greatly.

Smokers have higher rates of peptic ulcer disease, poorer ulcer healing, and higher recurrence rates than nonsmokers. They are more susceptible to upper respiratory infections and have more cataracts than nonsmokers. The majority of residential fire deaths are caused by smoking. There is no safe level of tobacco use. Smoking as few as 1 to 4 cigarettes per day increases the risk of myocardial infarction and cardiovascular mortality in women. Smoking cigarettes with reduced tar and nicotine content does not protect against the health hazards of smoking.

The health hazards of smoking are not limited to those suffered by smokers. Nonsmokers are harmed by chronic exposure to environmental tobacco smoke (ETS). The children of parents who smoke have more serious respiratory infections during infancy and childhood, more respiratory symptoms, and a higher rate of chronic otitis media and asthma than the children of nonsmokers. Nonsmoking women whose husbands smoke have a higher lung cancer risk than nonsmoking women whose husbands do not smoke. A 1993 Environmental Protection Agency report summarized the evidence regarding the health effects of passive smoking and identified ETS as a carcinogen, responsible for approximately 3000 lung cancer deaths each year in U.S. nonsmokers. Passive smoke exposure may also increase nonsmokers' risk of coronary heart disease.

SPECIAL HEALTH CONCERNS FOR WOMEN

American women enjoy a longer life expectancy than men. It has been suggested that women's greater longevity is a consequence of their lower smoking rates during the first half of this century. As women's and men's smoking patterns converge, the female advantage in life expectancy can be expected to diminish. Additionally, women who smoke have health risks not shared with male smokers; these relate to pregnancy, oral contraceptives, cervical cancer, and osteoporosis.

Smoking is associated with many **pregnancy complications.** It is a cause of low-birth-weight (<2500 g) infants. Babies born to smokers weigh, on average, 200 g (7 oz) less than babies of nonsmoking mothers. This is primarily attributable to intrauterine growth retardation (IUGR), although smoking in pregnancy also increases the risk of preterm delivery. Smoking is the major known cause of IUGR in the developed world, responsible for an estimated 30% of cases. Other adverse pregnancy outcomes linked to smoking are miscarriage (spontaneous abortion), stillbirth, and neonatal death. Placenta previa, abruptio placentae, and bleeding occur more often in smokers than nonsmokers, suggesting that smoking impairs placental function.

Smoking during pregnancy affects children even after birth. Sudden infant death syndrome is two to four times more common in infants born to mothers who smoked during pregnancy. Cognitive deficits and developmental problems in childhood have also been linked to maternal smoking during pregnancy, but these studies have potential confounding factors and the relationships are not clearly causal. The adverse health effects of smoking extend to reproductive function before pregnancy. Smoking has been associated with reduced fertility in both men and women, though a causal link remains to be established.

Oral contraceptive use compounds a woman smoker's risk of serious cardiovascular disease. Women smokers who use the pill have a substantially increased risk of subarachnoid hemorrhage and stroke, and their risk of myocardial infarction rises 10-fold.

Cervical cancer rates are higher in smokers than in nonsmokers. The excess risk conferred by smoking is independent of other factors known to increase cervical cancer risk. Adding biologic plausibility to this association is the discovery that components of tobacco smoke can be isolated from the cervical mucus of smokers. Cervical cancer rates are lower in ex-smokers than in current smokers, suggesting that risk is reversible after smoking cessation.

Menopause occurs 1 to 2 years earlier in women who smoke than in nonsmoking women. Former smokers have menopause at the same age as those who have never smoked. The mechanism is uncertain; suggestions include alteration in estrogen metabolism or a direct toxic effect of tobacco on the ovary.

Some, but not all, studies link smoking with reduced bone mass and **osteoporosis.** There is also conflicting evidence about whether smokers have a higher risk of osteoporotic fracture than nonsmokers. Women who smoke are thinner and have an earlier menopause than nonsmokers; both are risk factors for osteoporosis. Smoking may also have an antiestrogen effect. A large cohort study of women in Framingham, Massachusetts, reported that estrogen replacement protected nonsmokers but did not protect smokers from osteoporotic hip fractures.

Smokers have more prominent **skin wrinkling** than nonsmokers, an association independent of sun exposure. Although this effect is not limited to women, it may be of greater concern to women, reflecting the stronger cultural emphasis for women to have a youthful appearance.

HEALTH BENEFITS OF SMOKING CESSATION

Epidemiologic data demonstrate that smoking cessation has health benefits for women and men of all ages. Even those who stop smoking after the age of 65 or who quit after the development of a smoking-related disease derive benefit. Smoking cessation decreases the risk of lung cancer and other cancers, heart attack, stroke, chronic lung disease, and peptic ulcer disease. After 10 to 15 years of abstinence, smokers' overall mortality rate approaches that of persons who never smoked. The cardiovascular risk reduction occurs more rapidly than the risk reduction for lung cancer or overall mortality. Half of the excess risk of cardiovascular mortality is eliminated in the first year of quitting, whereas for lung cancer 30% to 50% of the excess risk is still evident 10 years after quitting and some excess risk remains after 15 years.

The benefits of stopping smoking translate into a longer life expectancy for former smokers, as compared with continuing smokers. The degree to which former smokers benefit from cessation depends on their previous lifetime dose of tobacco, their health status at the time of quitting, and the elapsed time since quitting. Smokers who benefit the most are those who quit when they are younger, have fewer pack-years of tobacco exposure, and are free of smoking-related disease. The health benefits of smoking cessation far exceed any risks from the small weight gain that occurs with cessation.

The benefits of smoking cessation for both sexes were summarized in the 1990 Surgeon General's Report on Smoking. A subsequent report from the Nurses' Health Study, which followed a cohort study of over 100,000 female nurses, confirmed that women benefit as much as men from quitting smoking. In that study former smokers had a 24% reduction in cardiovascular death rates within 2 years of quitting. The risks of total mortality, cardiovascular mortality, and total cancer mortality among former smokers approached the level of that for persons who had never smoked after 10 to 14 years of abstinence. Benefits of cessation were present regardless of daily cigarette consumption or the age at which smoking started.

Smoking cessation reverses the hazards of smoking to the fetus. Women who stop smoking before pregnancy or during the first 3 to 4 months of gestation have infants who weigh the same as those born to women who never smoked. Pregnant smokers who stop smoking at any time up to the 30th week of gestation have infants with higher birth weights than women who smoke throughout pregnancy. Reducing daily cigarette consumption without quitting smoking is of less benefit in preventing low birth weight.

SMOKING CESSATION

Approximately half of living Americans who ever smoked have quit smoking. According to surveys a majority of the remaining smokers would like to stop smoking and have made at least one serious attempt to do so. Older studies suggested that female smokers have more difficulty quitting smoking than male smokers do. Recent data indicate that men and women are equally likely to try to quit and to succeed in quitting. However, the process of quitting differs in men and women. Issues of particular importance for women include weight concerns, social support, and mood disorders.

Surveys of former smokers reveal how and why smokers stop smoking. The reason most often cited by former smokers for stopping smoking is fear of illness. However, awareness of health risks is not sufficient to motivate smoking cessation. Over 90% of current smokers know that smoking is harmful to health yet they continue to smoke. Many smokers rationalize that they are immune to the health risks of smoking until these risks become personally salient. Current symptoms (e.g., cough, breathlessness, chest pain), even if they represent minor illness rather than the onset of a smoking-related disease, stimulate change in smoking behavior more powerfully than does fear of future disease. Illness in a family member may also motivate smoking cessation. Another frequently cited reason for quitting is growing social pressure from work, family, and friends not to smoke.

In surveys 90% of former smokers say that they quit on their own. Most quit abruptly ("cold turkey"), although smokers can progressively reduce daily cigarette intake in preparation for quitting. A variety of programs are available to smokers who seek help. The best evidence for efficacy supports behavior modification programs; hypnosis is poorly evaluated, and acupuncture is not effective for smoking cessation.

The majority of former smokers did not succeed in stopping on their first try. About 30% of smokers who attend formal programs are not smoking 1 year later; most resume smoking within 3 months. Behavioral scientists liken smoking cessation to a learning process rather than to a discrete episode of willpower. Smokers learn from mistakes made during a prior attempt to quit and thereby increase the likelihood that the next attempt will succeed. Psychologists have identified a series of cognitive stages through which smokers pass as they move toward nonsmoking: (1) initial lack of interest in quitting, (2) thinking about health risks and contemplating quitting, (3) actively preparing to quit within the next month, (4) currently taking action to stop smoking, and (5) maintained nonsmoking.

MANAGEMENT OF BARRIERS TO SMOKING CESSATION

Nicotine withdrawal syndrome

Cigarettes and other tobacco products are addicting. Evidence summarized in the 1988 Surgeon General's Report on Smoking identified nicotine as the addictive drug in tobacco that is capable of creating tolerance, physical dependence, and a withdrawal syndrome in habitual users. Nicotine withdrawal symptoms include (1) cravings for a cigarette; (2) irritability, anxiety, impatience, and anger; (3) difficulty concentrating; (4) excessive hunger; and (5) sleep disturbance. These symptoms begin within a few hours of the last cigarette, peak 48 to 72 hours later, diminish rapidly during the first week of abstinence, and wane further in subsequent weeks. The severity of nicotine withdrawal is variable and related to the level of prior nicotine intake. Other than craving for a cigarette, the symptoms are nonspecific, and many smokers fail to recognize them as nicotine withdrawal. Gender differences in nicotine withdrawal have not been identified. Some evidence indicates that nicotine withdrawal symptoms are more severe during the luteal phase of a woman's menstrual cycle, but there is no evidence that quitting smoking is more likely to succeed at any particular point in the menstrual cycle.

The discomfort of nicotine withdrawal is one reason why smokers fail in their efforts to stop. Nicotine replacement therapy relieves the symptoms, but pharmacologic treatment is not mandatory, because mild symptoms can be managed with behavioral methods.

Behavioral factors

The attractiveness of smoking is attributable to more than nicotine dependence. Smoking is also a habit, a behavior that has become an integral part of a daily routine. Smokers come to associate cigarettes with enjoyable activities, such as finishing a meal or having a cup of coffee. These actions trigger the desire for a cigarette in smokers who are trying to quit. Smokers also use cigarettes to cope with stress and negative emotions such as anger, anxiety, loneliness, or frustration. Quitting smoking represents the loss of a valuable coping tool, one that may be especially important for women, for whom the direct expression of anger is less socially sanctioned.

Behavior modification strategies address these barriers to quitting smoking and are effective in aiding smoking cessation. Smokers monitor their cigarette intake to identify cues to smoking, change their habits to break the link between the trigger and smoking, and learn to anticipate and handle urges to smoke that occur. The skills can be taught in formal group programs or packaged into booklets or videotapes for at-home use.

Weight and smoking cessation

Smokers weigh 5 to 10 lb less than nonsmokers of comparable age and height. When smokers quit 80% of them gain weight. The average weight gain of 5 lb (2.3 kg) poses a minimal health risk, especially when compared with the benefits of smoking cessation. Women gain more weight than men; their average weight gain in one national sample was 8 lb (3.8 kg). Though many women fear large weight gains, only about 10% gain more than 25 lb after cessation. Heavier smokers (>25 cigarettes/day) gain more than lighter smokers. The mechanism is incompletely understood, but a nicotine-related decrease in metabolic rate and possibly increases in food intake appear to be largely responsible. The weight gain occurs in both sexes, but survey data reveal that it concerns female smokers more than male smokers, presumably because women experience greater cultural pressure to be slender. Although weight gain has been considered a trigger to relapse, some studies show that successful abstainers gain more weight than relapsers. Smokers who quit using nicotine gum gain less weight than those who quit with a placebo, though weight gain may just be delayed until after gum use stops. The effect of the nicotine patch on weight gain is contradictory across studies. Behavior modification approaches to avoiding weight gain have neither achieved this goal nor increased smoking cessation rates.

The best approach to the problem may be a change in attitude. Smokers may realize that, although some weight gain is likely, the amount is less than they fear. Accepting a small increase in weight until smoking cessation is secure is a better strategy than attempting to stop smoking and lose weight simultaneously. The chance of a large weight gain may be reduced by avoiding high-calorie snacks and increasing physical activity during smoking cessation. Nicotine gum may provide a way to avoid or at least delay weight gain.

Social support

Women with nonsmoking spouses are more likely to quit than women whose partners smoke. Smokers whose efforts to stop are supported by partners, family, and friends are more likely to succeed than smokers without this support. This is especially true for women smokers. Those who live with smokers can ask them to restrict smoking to outdoor areas or to limited areas of the home, in order to provide a smoke-free area in the home. Formal cessation programs provide an additional source of social support.

Mood disorders

Stopping smoking represents a loss for many smokers. Cigarettes have been reliable "companions" as well as coping tools. Transient sadness is common and requires no special treatment. Acknowledgment that this is normal can be helpful.

There is, however, growing evidence of an association between smoking and mood disorders. Smokers have more depressive symptoms than nonsmokers and are more likely to have a history of major depression. Smokers with depression are less likely to stop smoking than nondepressed smokers. There are case reports that smoking cessation precipitated depression in smokers with a history of major depression and that resumption of smoking restored mood. These observations suggest that some smokers use nicotine to regulate mood. Clinicians should be alert to the possibility of depression in smokers. If present it should be treated before cessation is attempted. Smokers with a history of depression should be watched for the reemergence of symptoms during smoking cessation. Close attention to the possibility of mood disorders may be particularly important for women smokers, because depression is a more common diagnosis in women than in men.

Substance abuse

Smokers of both sexes use more drugs—including coffee and alcohol—than nonsmokers. Because alcohol is frequently an ingredient in relapse situations, smokers attempting to quit are commonly advised to avoid alcohol temporarily after quitting. Smoking increases caffeine excretion. Smokers who stop should be advised to reduce caffeine intake to avoid increased blood levels and jitteriness. There is a high rate of smoking among abusers of alcohol, cocaine, and heroin. Depression and substance abuse should be considered as potential comorbid disorders in smokers who repeatedly try and fail to quit.

PHYSICIAN'S ROLE

The optimal way for women to avoid the health hazards of tobacco is not to smoke. Because smoking behavior begins so early, preventing smoking is a task for physicians who care for children and adolescents. The challenge for physicians taking care of adult women is smoking cessation. Physicians have the opportunity to intervene with smokers, because each year they see an estimated 70% of the 23 million American women who smoke. Primary care physicians have the advantage of repeated contact with smokers. Physicians have the additional opportunity of seeing smokers at times when symptoms have made them concerned about their health, and therefore, more likely to change their smoking behavior. For example, the diagnosis of coronary artery disease motivates behavior change in both sexes. Approximately one third of smokers stop smoking after a myocardial infarction, and this proportion can be increased with brief counseling delivered by a physician or nurse. For women, pregnancy encourages smoking cessation. Approximately 30% of female smokers stop smoking while pregnant, though many resume smoking after delivery. Other smoking-related conditions may also provide "teachable moments" when smokers are more receptive to advice to stop smoking.

Although physicians report advising most patients to stop smoking, fewer than half of smokers recall having ever received this advice. Providing brief advice to stop smoking to all patients seen in the office increases patients' smoking cessation rates, as demonstrated in a randomized controlled trial of British general practitioners. Although advice to quit is effective, several randomized controlled trials in general internal medicine and family practices have demonstrated that supplementing advice with brief counseling is more effective. Programs shown to be effective consist of brief structured counseling during which the physician asks the patient to set a quit date, provides written materials, offers nicotine replacement, and schedules a follow-up visit. Randomized trials have also demonstrated that counseling smokers during routine prenatal visits increases smoking cessation rates during pregnancy. Cost-effectiveness analyses demonstrate that counseling smokers in office practice is at least as cost-effective as other accepted medical practices and that counseling smokers as part of prenatal care is cost-saving.

SMOKING CESSATION COUNSELING FOR OFFICE PRACTICE

The primary care of adult women should include a routine assessment of smoking status in all patients, strong advice to all smokers to quit, and assistance for those smokers who are ready to stop. The National Cancer Institute has organized the common elements of effective smoking cessation counseling programs into a four-step protocol intended to require approximately 3 minutes of an office visit.

Ask

Physicians should routinely ask all patients at every visit whether they smoke cigarettes (see box, below). Those who smoke should be asked whether they are interested in quitting smoking. This permits the physician to determine the smoker's readiness to change. Categorizing smokers in this way is a clinically useful approach that helps the physician

---

SMOKING CESSATION COUNSELING PROTOCOL FOR PHYSICIANS

Ask about smoking at every visit.
  "Do you smoke?"
  "Are you interested in stopping smoking?"

Advise every smoker to stop.
  Make advice clear: "Stopping smoking now is the most important action you can take to stay healthy."
  Tailor advice to the patient's clinical situation (symptoms or family history).

Assist the smoker in stopping smoking.
  For smokers ready to quit:
  Ask smoker to set a "quit date."
  Provide self-help material to take home.
  Consider nicotine replacement therapy.
  Consider referral to a formal cessation program.
  For smokers not ready to quit:
  Discuss advantages and barriers to cessation, from smoker's viewpoint.
  Provide motivational booklet to take home.
  Advise smoker to avoid exposing family members to passive smoke.
  Indicate willingness to help when the smoker is ready.
  Ask again about smoking at the next visit.

Arrange follow-up visits.
  Make follow-up appointment 1 week after quit date.
  At follow-up, ask about smoking status.
  For smokers who have quit:
  Congratulate!
  Ask smoker to identify future high-risk situations.
  Rehearse coping strategies for future high-risk situations.
  For smokers who have not quit:
  Ask, "What were you were doing when you had that first cigarette?"
  Ask, "What did you learn from the experience?"
  Ask smoker to set a new "quit date."

Modified from Glynn TJ, Manley MW: How to help your patients stop smoking, National Cancer Institute, NIH Publication No 89-3064, 1989.

---

to determine what counseling strategy is appropriate and to set achievable goals for that encounter. Although the clinician's overall goal is to assist the smoker to stop permanently, a realistic goal for a single office visit is to move the smoker to the next stage of readiness to stop smoking.

Advise

Regardless of a smoker's degree of interest in quitting it is the physician's responsibility to deliver clear advice to each smoker about the importance of stopping smoking. The message should be strong and unequivocal, such as "Quitting smoking now is the most important action you can take to live a long and healthy life." If appropriate, advice should be tailored to the clinical situation, either current symptoms or family history. For example, the smoker can be informed that she will have fewer colds, less asthma, or a healthier baby if she stops smoking. Advice is more effective when phrased in a positive way (e.g., emphasizing the benefits to be gained from quitting rather than the harms of continuing to smoke).

Assist

The third step is to assist the smoker in quitting smoking. The physician's approach should vary according to the smoker's readiness to stop smoking.

If the smoker is interested in quitting smoking, the physician should ask her whether she is ready to set a "quit date," a date within the next 4 weeks when she will stop smoking. If so the date should be recorded in the chart and on material given to the patient to take home. The physician should discuss with the patient what approach is most likely to be successful. A stepped-care model of smoking treatment can guide the physician in making this recommendation. For smokers making a first attempt to quit the physician should assist the patient in quitting on her own; this can be done most simply by providing a take-home booklet containing standard behavioral modification strategies (see box on the following page). Alternatively, this information could be provided by office staff or, a videotape. The physician should be prepared to discuss management of barriers to cessation, if the smoker asks.

More intensive treatment is indicated for smokers who have been unsuccessful in previous attempts to quit. Options at this second level are referral to a formal smoking cessation program and prescription of nicotine replacement therapy. Smoking cessation programs provide intensive training in behavioral smoking cessation skills combined with social support from the counselor and other group members. Social support may be particularly valuable for women smokers. Nicotine replacement therapy is appropriate for smokers likely to have severe nicotine withdrawl symptoms. These are the smokers who suffered nicotine withdrawal symptoms on previous attempts to quit or who are likely to have them because they smoke >25 cigarettes daily, have their first cigarette within 30 minutes of awakening, or are uncomfortable when forced to refrain from smoking for more than a few hours. Combinations of nicotine replacement and a behavioral counseling program are more effective than either one alone.

For the smoker not interested in quitting or not ready to set a quit date, the physician should ask what the smoker considers the benefits and harms of smoking are for her.

From an understanding of the patients' perspective the physician can provide missing information about health risks and correct misconceptions about the process of smoking cessation. The discussion should focus on short-term benefits rather than distant risks, and the physician should be prepared to discuss common barriers to smoking cessation. The clinician should advise the smoker not to expose family members to passive smoke (e.g., not smoke inside her home if nonsmokers are present), provide a take-home booklet about smoking cessation, and indicate his or her future availability to help the smoker when she is ready to quit.

Follow-up

Randomized trials have demonstrated that offering follow-up visits to discuss smoking increases the success of physician counseling. The smoker should be asked to return shortly after her quit date to monitor progress; this is especially important for smokers using nicotine replacement.

If the smoker has stopped smoking at the follow-up visit she should be congratulated heartily but warned that continued vigilance is necessary to maintain abstinence. The level of nicotine withdrawal symptoms should be assessed and, if indicated, treated. To prevent relapse to smoking the patient should be asked to identify future situations in which she anticipates difficulty remaining abstinent. The physician can help her to plan and rehearse coping strategies for these times. Further follow-up visits or telephone calls should be offered.

If the smoker has not been able to remain abstinent since the quit date, the physician's role is to redefine an experience that the smoker feels has been a failure into a partial success. The smokers can be told that even one day without cigarettes is the first step toward quitting and reminded that it takes time to learn to quit just as it took time to learn to smoke. In order to help the smoker learn from the experience, the physician should ask in detail about the circum-

stances surrounding the first cigarette smoked after the quit date. The smoker should be asked what she learned from the experience that can be used for her next attempt to quit. Finally, she should be asked whether she is ready to set a new quit date.

Office environment

Smoking counseling in an office need not and should not be limited to the physician's actions. A systemwide approach is as effective as a physician-focused model, and it reduces the burden on a busy physician. In this model the physician's primary role is to provide advice to stop smoking and discuss the setting of a quit date. The patient's smoking status is assessed before the physician sees the patient. The same staff member who checks weight or blood pressure can ask about smoking and label the chart to remind the physician to discuss smoking. Studies demonstrate that simple reminder systems such as this increase the amount of time physicians spend counseling smokers. Office personnel build on physician advice to provide counseling, medication instruction, or referrals to outside programs.

PHARMACOLOGIC TREATMENT
Nicotine replacement therapy

The rationale of nicotine replacement is to supply nicotine in a form other than tobacco in order to block the symptoms of nicotine withdrawal in smokers attempting to quit (Table 73-1). Nicotine replacement permits the smoker to break the smoking habit first and taper off nicotine later. Two forms of nicotine replacement are currently approved for use in the United States, nicotine polacrilex (i.e., a gum) and a transdermal skin patch. Both produce relatively constant blood levels of nicotine, a substantially different pattern of exposure from fluctuating nicotine levels produced by cigarette smoking. The nicotine supplied by the gum or patch is sufficient to block nicotine withdrawal symptoms but not to reproduce the pleasures of smoking.

Randomized placebo-controlled trials demonstrate that nicotine gum and patch each reduce nicotine withdrawal symptoms and increase smoking cessation rates. A meta-analysis of nicotine patch trials found that the patch more than doubled smoking cessation rates, compared to placebo, though the cessation rates in individual trials varied widely. A metaanalysis of nicotine gum demonstrated its effectiveness in special clinics treating smokers, but not when used in medical settings. The effectiveness of both products depends on the instruction and counseling that accompany it. This is particularly true for the gum, which requires careful instruction for proper use. Compliance is less of a problem with the nicotine patch. However, effective use of either product requires that the physician provide the smoker with concurrent behavioral counseling of some type to teach her how to break the cigarette habit.

Both products have been used safely, even in smokers with stable coronary artery disease. Contraindications to nicotine replacement include acute or recent cardiovascular events (myocardial infarction, unstable angina, or serious arrhythmias). Anecdotal reports of myocardial infarction in patients who were smoking while using the patch were not borne out by more careful study, but smoking is contraindicated in patch users; it increases blood nicotine levels and, more important, is not a pattern of behavior that leads to

Table 73-1 Nicotine replacement products

Brand name (manufacturer)	Nicotine content (mg)	Dosage per day	Recommendation duration of use
Transdermal nicotine patch			
Habitrol (*Ciba-Geigy*)			
21 mg	52.5	21 mg/24 hr	4-8 weeks
14 mg	35.0	14 mg/24 hr	2-4 weeks
7 mg	17.5	7 mg/24 hr	2-4 weeks
Nicoderm (*Marion Merrell Dow*)			
21 mg	114.0	21 mg/24 hr	4-8 weeks
14 mg	78.0	14 mg/24 hr	2-4 weeks
7 mg	36.0	7 mg/24 hr	2-4 weeks
Nicotrol (*Parke-Davis*)			
15 mg	24.9	15 mg/16 hr	4-12 weeks
10 mg	16.6	10 mg/16 hr	2-4 weeks
5 mg	8.3	5 mg/16 hr	2-4 weeks
Prostep (*Lederle*)			
22 mg	30.0	22 mg/24 hr	4-8 weeks
11 mg	15.0	11 mg/24 hr	2-4 weeks
Nicotine gum			
Nicorette 2 mg (*Marion Merrell Dow*)	2.0	9-12 pieces/day* (maximum 30)	2-3 months (maximum 6)
Nicorette DS (*Marion Merrell Dow*)	4.0	9-12 pieces/day* (maximum 20)	2-3 months (maximum 6)

Modified from Nicotine Patches, *Med Lett* 34:37, 1992.
*Chew as needed or 1 piece every 1-2 hours while awake.

smoking cessation. The gum is contraindicated in patients with temporomandibular disease; the patch is contraindicated in patients with widespread skin eruptions. The safety of either product in pregnancy is not established. Nicotine replacement is almost certainly safer than smoking cigarettes, but medicolegal concerns have limited its use. Clinicians have generally reserved nicotine replacement therapy for use in pregnant patients who have failed a behavioral stop-smoking program, and have prescribed it only after documenting a risk-benefit discussion with the patient.

Transdermal nicotine patch

The nicotine patch continuously releases a fixed dose, which is absorbed through the skin. Each of the four products available is more effective than placebo in relieving withdrawal symptoms and promoting smoking cessation. No studies have directly compared different patches; therefore there are insufficient data to recommend any one patch as most effective or most safe. The most common side effect is local skin irritation, which rarely requires discontinuation of treatment and can be treated with topical steroids. Vivid dreams, insomnia, and nervousness have also been reported; they can be managed by removing the patch at bedtime or using a lower-dose patch.

The smoker applies the first patch on the morning of her quit day and applies a new patch to rotating skin sites each morning afterward. Three products are intended for 24-hour use; the fourth is removed after 16 hours (e.g., at bedtime). Smokers started on the patch should be monitored after 1 week to assess level of withdrawal symptoms and to screen for smoking during patch use. Most patches are available in three sizes to permit tapering, and most manufacturers recommend that patch use continue for 2 to 3 months. Lower starting doses are recommended for patients who weigh less than 100 lb or smoke fewer than 10 cigarettes each day. Long-term dependence on the nicotine patch appears to be uncommon.

Nicotine gum

Nicotine gum is available in 2 mg and 4 mg strengths. Careful instruction in proper chewing technique is essential to allow it to be effective and to prevent side effects; for this reason, compliance is more problematic than with the nicotine patch. The gum should not be chewed like regular gum. A piece is chewed only long enough to release nicotine, producing a peppery taste, then placed between the gums and buccal mucosa to allow nicotine absorption. After 30 minutes it is discarded. No liquid should be drunk while the gum is in the mouth, and acidic beverages (e.g., coffee) avoided for 1 to 2 hours before gum use. Side effects are common but minor; they include those related to nicotine (nausea, dyspepsia, hiccups, dizziness) and to chewing (sore jaw, mouth ulcers).

The product is approved for use as needed to handle urges to smoke; however, its effect is slower than that of smoking. Most patients chew fewer than the recommended 9 to 12 pieces daily. Consequently some clinicians use fixed-dose schedules (e.g., chewing one piece for the first 30 minutes of every hour) to achieve adequate blood nicotine levels to prevent withdrawal. Approximately 5% to 10% of gum users develop long-term dependence on the gum.

Other pharmacologic agents

Clonidine, a centrally acting α-adrenergic agonist, is used to treat craving for psychoactive drugs other than nicotine. In randomized, placebo-controlled trials both oral and transdermal clonidine reduced withdrawal symptoms, but there is inconsistent evidence that either product increases smoking cessation rates long-term. Clonidine is not approved for use as an aid for smoking cessation.

There is no evidence to support the use of tranquilizers or benzodiazepines for smoking cessation. The growing awareness of the link between smoking and mood disorders has stimulated interest in use of antidepressants, especially fluoxetine and other selective serotonin reuptake inhibitors, to treat smoking in individuals with a history of depression. Until more is known, it is appropriate to use these agents to treat depression in a smoker and to continue their use when the patient attempts to stop smoking. Whether they have any role in smokers who are not currently depressed is not known.

BIBLIOGRAPHY

Bartecchi CE, MacKenzie TK, Schrier RW: The human cost of tobacco use, *N Engl J Med* 330:907, 975, 1994.
Benowitz NL: Nicotine replacement therapy during pregnancy, *JAMA* 266:3174, 3177, 1991.
Cohen SJ et al: Encouraging primary care physicians to help smokers quit: a randomized controlled trial, *Ann Intern Med* 110:648, 1989.
Cummings SR et al: Training physicians in counseling about smoking cessation: a randomized trial of the "Quit for Life" program, *Ann Intern Med* 110:641, 1989.
Fiore MC et al: The effectiveness of the nicotine patch for smoking cessation: a meta-analysis, *JAMA* 271:1940, 1994.
Fiore MC et al: Tobacco dependence and the nicotine patch: guidelines for effective use, *JAMA* 268:2687, 1992.
Fontham ETH et al: Environmental tobacco smoke and lung cancer in nonsmoking women: a multicenter study, *JAMA* 271:1752, 1994.
Glassman A: Cigarette smoking: implications for psychiatric illness, *Am J Psychiatry* 150:546, 1993.
Glynn TJ, Manley MW: *How to help your patients stop smoking: a National Cancer Institute manual for physicians,* US Department of Health and Human Services, Public Health Service, National Institutes of Health, National Cancer Institute, Division of Cancer Prevention and Control. NIH Publication No. 89-3064, 1989.
Hollis JF et al: Nurse-assisted counseling for smokers in primary care, *Ann Intern Med* 118:521, 1993.
Kawachi I et al: Smoking cessation in relation to total mortality rates in women: a prospective cohort study, *Ann Intern Med* 119:992, 1993.
Kiel DP et al: Smoking eliminates the protective effect of oral estrogens on the risk for hip fracture among women, *Ann Intern Med* 116:716, 1992.
Lam W et al: Meta-analysis of randomized controlled trials of nicotine chewing gum, *Lancet* 2:27, 1987.
Manley MW, Epps RP, Glynn IJ: The clinician's role in promoting smoking cessation among clinic patients, *Med Clin North Am* 76:477, 1992.
Nicotine Patches, *Med Lett* 34:37, 1992.
Russell MAH et al: Effect of a general practitioner's advice against smoking, *Br Med J* 2:231, 1979.
Sexton M, Hebel JR: A clinical trial of change in maternal smoking and its effect on birth weight, *JAMA* 251:911, 1984.
U.S. Department of Health and Human Services: *Reducing the health consequences of smoking: 25 years of progress: a report of the Surgeon General,* US DHHS, Public Health Service, Centers for Disease Control, Office on Smoking and Health. DHHS Publication No (CDC) 89-8411, 1989.
U.S. Department of Health and Human Services: *The health benefits of smoking cessation: a report of the Surgeon General,* US DHHS, Public Health Service, Centers for Disease Control, Office on Smoking and Health, DHHS Publication No (CDC) 90-8416, 1990.
Williamson DF et al: Smoking cessation and severity of weight gain in a national cohort, *N Engl J Med* 324:739, 1991.
Wilson DM et al: A randomized trial of a family physician intervention for smoking cessation, *JAMA* 260:1570, 1988.

74 Somatoform Disorders

Felise B. Milan and Carol Landau

Depression is perhaps the most prevalent psychologic problem encountered in the primary care of women. Closely related and often more difficult for the primary care provider to manage is the overlap between depression and the somatoform disorders, which are also diagnosed more often in women than in men. In primary care settings depression is one of the most common disorders underlying somatization and somatization is one of the most common disorders underlying depression.

It is estimated that from 30% to 50% of people who are diagnosed with somatoform disorders either are dysthymic or are suffering from a major depression. The reported frequency varies depending on the studies' clinical setting (primary care versus psychiatric clinic) and the diagnostic criteria used. For example, in defining the criteria for somatization, some studies have included as somatic complaints insomnia, anorexia, and loss of libido, all of which are classic major depressive symptoms.

One striking study found that of 60 women who met the *Diagnostic and Statistical Manual of Mental Disorders (DSM-IV)* criteria for somatization disorder, 90% also met criteria for a major affective disorder. A number of studies have attempted to identify which characteristics make patients with depression more likely to somatize. When gender and sex were examined depressed older women appear to have an increased tendency to somatize.

In an attempt to understand the atypical presentation of these patients some have referred to somatic symptoms as "depressive equivalents" and have used such terms as "masked depression" and "atypical depression" to describe this clinical picture. Masked depression is defined as a depressive illness in which somatic symptoms mask the mood and cognitive components of the disorder. The low rate of recognition of depression in primary care settings may be at least partially explained by the fact that some of the patients do not exhibit the expected mood disturbance.

There are many other explanations for why depressed patients may have somatic symptoms. Patients who are aware of their depressed moods may choose to focus on somatic symptoms to avoid a discussion of their underlying problems, which may be felt to be stigmatizing. Other patients are convinced that their somatic symptoms represent a primary physical illness to which their depression is secondary. There are also patients who may lack the ability to identify and express emotions (*alexithymia*) and therefore rely on physical symptoms to express feelings.

An association between depression and somatization has also been found in those patients with somatization disorder. Several studies have shown high rates of comorbid depression in patients in primary care (55%), psychiatric outpatient (85%), psychiatric inpatient (95%), and community (65%) settings.

Furthermore, patients with somatization disorder have been found to have high rates of comorbid generalized anxiety disorder (35%) and panic disorder (25%). The overlap between somatization and anxiety is complicated. As with depressed patients, anxious patients may experience any number of somatic symptoms. These symptoms are usually secondary to autonomic hyperactivity such as palpitations, diarrhea, flushing, and diaphoresis. In addition anxiety and emotional arousal seem to increase patients' sensitivity to bodily sensations. Several studies have found anxious patients to have a decreased tolerance for pain. Patients with panic disorder may focus on their somatic complaints and deny feelings of anxiety. One study of patients with panic disorder referred from a primary care service found their presenting complaints to be epigastric pain (28%), tachycardia (25%), chest pain (22%), dizziness or vertigo (18%), shortness of breath (13%), headache (11%), and syncope (9%) (Katon, 1984).

DEFINITIONS

The concept of somatization has been defined by Lipowski as "a tendency to experience and communicate somatic distress and somatic symptoms unaccounted for by relevant pathological findings and to attribute them to physical illness and to seek medical help for them." Kaplan defines it as "the patient's experience of sensory bodily complaints when psychological or social problems are present and when there is no presently measurable pathophysiologic disturbance sufficient to explain the symptoms." The terms *somatization* and *hypochondriasis* are often used interchangeably and, although the two processes may often occur together, the concepts are somewhat different. Both disorders involve patients who may amplify physical signs or sensations, who may seek medical care for these concerns, and who are without any clinical evidence of disease. Hypochondriacs, however, are preoccupied with the belief or fear that they have a serious illness. This belief persists despite medical reassurance. Another distinguishing feature of hypochondriasis is a relatively equal distribution over both genders, whereas somatization is seen almost exclusively in women.

Many authors who have written about somatization in primary care have expressed the view that somatization should not be conceptualized as a distinct diagnostic entity. They suggest that it is an illness-focused behavior style with multiple causes that may be associated with a number of different disorders. It can occur in a wide spectrum of patients, from those with severe psychiatric comorbidity to those who only somatize in response to extreme emotional distress.

Transient somatization and hypochondriasis are often seen in medical students who have gained a limited understanding of pathophysiology during a period of emotional and physical stress. In such students symptoms that previously had been dismissed are then attributed to some dreaded disease discussed in class. Individuals undergoing an acute grief reaction may also experience transient somatization or hypochondriasis.

Somatization can also occur in the presence of disease or be precipitated by the diagnosis of a serious or chronic illness, which then produces a heightened concern about bodily processes and physical sensations. Whereas for some, somatization is transient behavior present only in times of distress, for others it is a deeply ingrained way of dealing with the world.

In an attempt to standardize the identification of these patients within psychiatric research settings, *DSM-IV* has divided the somatoform disorders into categories with distinct diagnostic criteria. The somatoform disorders outlined by *DSM-IV* include body dysmorphic disorder, conversion disorder, hypochondriasis, somatization disorder (formerly Briquet's syndrome), somatoform pain disorder, and undifferentiated somatoform disorder.

Body dysmorphic disorder and conversion disorder are rarely seen in the primary care setting and will not be discussed here. The box below presents the *DSM-IV* criteria for hypochondriasis. There is a considerable amount of overlap among the other somatoform disorders (somatization disorder, somatoform pain, and undifferentiated somatoform disorder) (see boxes on the following page). This chapter focuses on somatization disorder and somatoform pain disorder because of their prevalence in the primary care setting and their overwhelming predominance among women.

Somatization disorder

The essential features of somatization disorder are the chronicity of the illness and the multiplicity of the somatic

---

DIAGNOSTIC CRITERIA FOR HYPOCHONDRIASIS

A. Preoccupation with fears of having, or the idea that one has, a serious disease, based on the person's misinterpretation of bodily symptoms.

B. The preoccupation persists despite appropriate medical evaluation and reassurance.

C. The belief in Criterion *A* is not of delusional intensity (as in Delusional Disorder, Somatic Type) and is not restricted to a circumscribed concern about appearance (as in Body Dysmorphic Disorder).

D. The preoccupation causes clinically significant distress or impairment in social, occupational, or other important areas of functioning.

E. The duration of the disturbance is at least 6 months.

F. The preoccupation is not better accounted for by Generalized Anxiety Disorder, Obsessive-Compulsive Disorder, Panic Disorder, a Major Depressive Episode, Separation Anxiety, or another Somatoform Disorder

From the *Diagnostic and statistical manual of mental disorders*, ed 4, Washington DC, 1994, American Psychiatric Association.

DIAGNOSTIC CRITERIA FOR PAIN DISORDER

A. Pain in one or more anatomic sites is the predominant focus of the clinical presentation and is of sufficient severity to warrant clinical attention.

B. The pain causes clinically significant distress or impairment in social, occupational, or other important areas of functioning.

C. Psychologic factors are judged to have an important role in the onset, severity, exacerbation, or maintenance of the pain.

D. The symptom or deficit is not intentionally produced or feigned (as in Factitious Disorder or Malingering).

E. The pain is not better accounted for by a Mood, Anxiety, or Psychotic Disorder and does not meet criteria for Dyspareunia.

From the *Diagnostic and statistical manual of mental disorders*, ed 4, Washington DC, 1994, American Psychiatric Association.

complaints. The disorder begins before the age of 30, often in the teen years. The lifetime prevalence rates have been reported to range from 0.2% to 2.0% among women; the disorder is rarely diagnosed in men. Female first-degree biologic relatives of women with somatization disorder have a higher than expected incidence of the disorder (10% to 20%). Male relatives of these women show an increased risk of substance abuse and antisocial personality disorders. Results from adoption studies have indicated that both genetic and environmental factors contribute to the development of this disorder. Frequently patients with this disorder have taken or are taking multiple psychoactive prescription medications and are at risk for psychoactive substance abuse disorders. The course of somatization disorder tends to be chronic, with some fluctuation in severity; spontaneous remission is rare.

DIAGNOSTIC CRITERIA FOR UNDIFFERENTIATED SOMATOFORM DISORDER

A. One or more physical complaints (e.g., fatigue, loss of appetite, gastrointestinal or urinary complaints).

B. Either **(1)** or **(2)**:
(1) after appropriate investigation, the symptoms cannot be fully explained by a known general medical condition or the direct effects of a substance (e.g., a drug of abuse, a medication)
(2) when there is a related general medical condition, the physical complaints or resulting social or occupational impairment is in excess of what would be expected from the history, physical examination, or laboratory findings

C. The symptoms cause clinically significant distress or impairment in social, occupational, or other important areas of functioning.

D. The duration of the disturbance is at least 6 months.

E. The disturbance is not better accounted for by another mental disorder (e.g., another Somatoform Disorder, Sexual Dysfunction, Mood Disorder, Anxiety Disorder, Sleep Disorder, or Psychotic Disorder).

F. The symptom is not intentionally produced or feigned (as in Factitious Disorder or Malingering).

From the *Diagnostic and statistical manual of mental disorders*, ed 4, Washington DC, 1994, American Psychiatric Association.

Pain disorder

Formerly known as psychogenic or somatoform pain disorder, this disorder has as its essential feature chronic preoccupation (greater than 6 months) with pain that is inconsistent with or out of proportion to physical findings. There is sometimes evidence of a temporal relationship between ini-

DIAGNOSTIC CRITERIA FOR SOMATIZATION DISORDER

A. A history of many physical complaints beginning before age 30 years that occur over a period of several years and result in treatment being sought or significant impairment in social, occupational, or other important areas of functioning.

B. Each of the following criteria must have been met, with individual symptoms occurring at any time during the course of the disturbance:
(1) *four pain symptoms:* a history of pain related to at least four different sites or functions (e.g., head, abdomen, back, joints, extremities, chest, rectum, during menstruation, during sexual intercourse, or during urination)
(2) *two gastrointestinal symptoms:* a history of at least two gastrointestinal symptoms other than pain (e.g., nausea, bloating, vomiting other than during pregnancy, diarrhea, or intolerance of several different foods)
(3) *one sexual symptom:* a history of at least one sexual or reproductive symptom other than pain (e.g., sexual indifference, erectile or ejaculatory dysfunction, irregular menses, excessive menstrual bleeding, vomiting throughout pregnancy)
(4) *one pseudoneurologic symptom:* a history of at least one symptom or deficit suggesting a neurologic condition not limited to pain (conversion symptoms such as impaired coordination or balance, paralysis or localized weakness, difficulty swallowing or lump in throat, aphonia, urinary retention, hallucinations, loss of touch or pain sensation, double vision, blindness, deafness seizures; dissociative symptoms such as amnesia; or loss of consciousness other than fainting)

C. Either **(1)** or **(2)**:
(1) after appropriate investigation, each of the symptoms in *B* cannot be fully explained by a known general medical condition or the direct effects of a substance (e.g., a drug of abuse, a medication)
(2) when there is a related general medical condition, the physical complaints or resulting social or occupational impairment are in excess of what would be expected from the history, physical examination, or laboratory findings

D. The symptoms are not intentionally produced or feigned (as in Factitious Disorder or Malingering).

From the *Diagnostic and statistical manual of mental disorders*, ed 4, Washington DC, 1994, American Psychiatric Association.

tiation or exacerbation of symptoms and psychosocial stressors. For some patients the pain has symbolic significance or may serve as unconscious punishment. For example, a patient with unresolved guilt over placing her mother in a nursing home may begin to experience chest pain after her mother dies of a myocardial infarction.

Onset can occur at any age but most frequently is in midlife. In almost half of the cases the pain develops immediately after a physical trauma. The pain then may increase in severity over weeks or months, often resulting in a decreasing level of functioning. Patients will often stop working, seek disability compensation, and increasingly take on the sick role. These patients are also at risk for dependence on narcotic analgesics and often undergo numerous invasive surgical procedures.

Comorbid depression is so frequent that some have suggested that somatoform pain disorder is a variant of depressive disorder and that it can be successfully treated with antidepressant medication. Although the overall prevalence of the disorder is unclear, the ratio of females to males is 2:1.

CAUSES OF SOMATOFORM DISORDERS

Many different theoretic explanations for somatization have been proposed. We will consider four theories of cause: psychodynamic, personality-based, neurobiologic, and behavioral.

Psychodynamic theories of somatization have been eloquently described by Engel (1959). The basic premise of these theories is that patients' symptoms are symbolic, expressing an underlying conflict. As an example, a common clinical scenario is a patient whose symptom represents punishment that serves to ease unconscious feelings of guilt.

As evidence for the role of personality in somatization Smith (1986) found that somatizers had frequent concurrent personality disorders. Barsky (1979) has described "the somatizing personality" and discussed three different personality themes and the role that somatizing may play within these different personality styles. There are the masochistic patients whose symptoms fulfill their need for suffering and self-sacrifice. The passive-aggressive personality style is often indirectly hostile and their illness is consistent with their feelings of having been deprived and wronged by the world. Finally, the patients with dependent personality style often use illness behavior to maneuver themselves into the position of needing care and their health care provider into the role of caregiver.

Patients with borderline personality disorders sometimes appear in the primary care setting with severe somatization disorder. They frequently have seen multiple practitioners and have often been dismissed by some. The patient with borderline personality disorder and somatization disorder is probably one of the most difficult for the primary care physician to treat.

Neurobiologic theories of somatization basically posit that some individuals may have a constitutional predisposition to misinterpret and amplify bodily sensations. The proposed mechanism for this is an underlying abnormality of the central nervous system within the sensory pathways that alters patients' perceptions and cognitions of bodily symptoms.

Behavioral theories maintain that all behaviors evolve and are perpetuated by environmental factors. Somatization can be conceptualized as abnormal illness behavior that is learned during childhood and reinforced throughout life. In fact, in some dysfunctional families somatization is the only behavior that receives positive reinforcement. Women with one of the somatoform disorders often report a positive family history for somatization. They describe families in which a family member's illness behavior was a significant ingredient in the family system or a family that used expression of somatic complaints as a means of communicating.

This family dynamic is frequently a function of cultural beliefs and attitudes. Many cultures discourage the direct expression of emotion or attach stigma to particular psychiatric disorders such as depression and anxiety. The tendency to generalize and dramatize somatic complaints has been shown to be related to one's cultural background. Many cultures attribute different meanings to symptoms that may be a cause of concern for the patient.

Both familial and cultural factors may play a role in situations in which symptoms are being reinforced and perpetuated by the patient's secondary gain. These secondary gains may include increased support and caring from one or more family members, relief from certain responsibilities including work inside or outside the home, and monetary gain such as disability compensation or anticipated compensation from litigation. In a fairly common scenario a woman experiences an acute low back injury that requires that she stay home at rest for several weeks. During this period her husband spends more time at home and less time with his friends. He becomes more involved in the care of their children, helps with the household chores, and communicates more actively with his spouse. For the woman staying at home with her children may be more consistent with her cultural traditions and her pain elicits greater attention and sympathy from family members. The more chronic the disability becomes the more maladaptive behaviors the patient and her family have acquired and the greater the investment in continuing the symptom.

A history of childhood physical or sexual abuse is one environmental factor that may be particularly important in women with somatization disorders. Among some populations of patients seen for the treatment of chronic pain the frequency of past abuse has been as high as 50%. Several studies have documented associations of chronic pelvic pain and functional gastrointestinal disorders in women with a history of abuse. Chapter 13 and Chapter 38 consider these subjects in greater detail.

 EVALUATION

The diagnosis of somatization involves more than just ruling out physical disorders that would explain patients' symptoms. By obtaining a thorough history and listening carefully for the signs of somatization the diagnosis of somatization can be made concurrently with the appropriate medical evaluation. Recognizing the diagnosis early may also prevent many unnecessary diagnostic tests and procedures.

The central issues in somatization are the complaint of multiple unexplained symptoms or unexplained pain coupled with overwhelming concern about the underlying cause of the symptom(s). One clue to somatization is the expression of a great deal of concern regarding the authenticity of symptoms. Women with somatization disorders have usually undergone many medical evaluations in the past by physicians who they felt did not take their symptoms seriously. Many will vehemently insist on finding a physical cause for their symptoms and deny the influence of any psychosocial factors despite what seem to be related life events and situational stressors.

Their medical history is often characterized by accounts of multiple inconclusive tests and unsuccessful therapies or "much doctoring and little curing." Women with somatization have often undergone one or more of the following surgical procedures: laparoscopy, hysterectomy, laminectomy, or cholecystectomy.

The quantity and nature of the symptoms reported may offer a clue to the diagnosis of somatization. Women who somatize will list many symptoms involving multiple organ systems. The symptoms may also be vaguely described ("I feel weak all over"), bizarre in nature ("the pain starts in my hair"), or inconsistent ("I've had this headache 24 hours a day, every day for the last 10 years"). Despite a rather dramatic style of presentation these women may deny any emotional disturbance ("If not for this pain my life would be absolutely perfect!").

Another clue to the diagnosis has been described in patients with somatization as "disease syndrome–illness behavior discrepancy." These patients' reactions to being told that they are healthy is not one of relief but of displeasure. They seem happiest when informed of a "real" or medical diagnosis regardless of the consequences.

It is helpful for clinicians to recognize the emotional reactions they may have to somatizing patients. Groves noted that somatizing patients can stimulate feelings of aversion, fear, guilt, inadequacy, and malice in their physicians. It is common to feel overwhelmed early in a patient encounter by the number of the complaints and the extensive medical history, frustrated by the vague descriptions, and angry at the patients themselves. Anger may be felt in response to the patient's anger and to the constant demands for a diagnosis before an adequate assessment can be completed. There is often a struggle for control of the interview with feelings of dissatisfaction in both patient and clinician.

There are several strategies that are usually helpful when the diagnosis of somatization is suspected:

1. Explore the patient's beliefs about the illness—beliefs about both cause and treatment.
2. Start at the beginning. Find out what was going on in the patient's life when the symptoms first started and when she last felt well.
3. Assess how the symptom or symptoms have interfered with the patient's life.
4. Elicit what the patient hopes you will do for her, making sure to distinguish the goals of symptom management from cure or diagnosis.

Although asking these questions is always important in the evaluation of any patient's complaints, they can be especially useful in uncovering the psychogenic origin of symptoms in patients with somatization.

DIFFERENTIAL DIAGNOSIS

Once somatization has been recognized it is always important to evaluate the patient for associated affective disorders.

Other disorders that need to be considered in the differential diagnosis of the somatoform disorders are malingering, factitious illness, and Munchausen's syndrome (Table 74-1). Malingerers are knowingly "faking" their symptoms for some clear benefit such as avoidance of imprisonment. In factitious illness the patient creates physical evidence of illness (such as a false reading on a thermometer) in order to take on the sick role. These patients are often women in the health care field. Munchausen's syndrome is quite rare and occurs primarily in men. These patients typically go from hospital to hospital feigning serious illness that often requires invasive procedures or surgical intervention. Their stories are well rehearsed and often quite believable. Patients with Munchausen's syndrome and those with factitious illness often have severe psychopathologic conditions and require psychiatric evaluation.

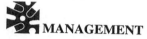

MANAGEMENT

The major determinant of management and prognosis is the time course of the patient's disorder.

Women who have recently experienced a somatoform disorder in response to a major life stressor have a very good prognosis and often respond to reassurance and education about the somatization process. The most important objective of treatment is to prevent the acute disorder from becoming a more chronic problem. The physician should help the patient identify how these symptoms are affecting her life, the stressors that precipitated the symptoms, and ways to handle the emotions associated with those stressors.

Women who have a history of a lifelong pattern of somatization have a much worse prognosis and are much more difficult to treat. The key principle of treatment involves setting realistic goals for both the patient and the provider (see box on the following page).

Goals of management

The most important goal for the physician and the patient to discuss and agree upon is that of symptom management rather than symptom cure. These patients and often their physicians are frequently frustrated and disappointed by unrealistic expectations of complete symptom resolution. With improved management of their symptoms, improved coping and socialization skills, and increased insight into their problems, these patients may achieve improved domestic and occupational functioning. In addition the physician may be able to help the patient avoid unnecessary surgical procedures, avoid dependence on addicting medications, and use the medical system more appropriately. Patients who have regularly scheduled visits with their primary care provider will not need to use the emergency room or call their provider as frequently.

While helping the patient to achieve these goals it is important that the physician set firm limits and negotiate an arrangement with the patient with which he or she is comfortable. The physician should also increase awareness of and ability to manage many of the negative emotions that may be elicited by the patient.

Initial management. The initial tasks are explaining the diagnosis to the patient and reassuring her that she does not have a serious or life-threatening disease. Empathic com-

Table 74-1 Differential diagnosis

Syndrome	Malingering	Factitious Disorder	Munchausen's syndrome
Clinical description	Feigns illness for clear primary benefit (avoid army, jail, etc.)	Creates false evidence of disease (i.e., heating thermometer)	Creates detailed story consistent with serious illness—history of many surgeries, many MDs in many locations
Risk factors	Male >females	Females >>> males; health care workers	Male >>female
Underlying psychopathology	Possible sociopathy	Major psychopathology	Major pathology
Treatment	Nonjudgmental confrontation, open discussion of issues	Psychiatric referral	Psychiatric referral

munication of this information is essential with all patients. Approaches that may be especially useful with somatizing patients include legitimizing the seriousness of the symptom to the patient ("It is clear how incapacitating this pain has been for you"), expressing respect for whatever adaptive behavior the patient has exhibited ("I'm impressed that you've been able to continue working considering how uncomfortable you are"), reflecting the emotions the patient expresses about their situation ("You are clearly very upset about how these headaches are affecting your marriage"), and expressing support and partnership in helping the patient address her concerns ("I want you to know that I will work with you and do what I can to help make things better for you").

When attempting to reassure these patients, it is important not to dispute the presence or severity of their symptoms. Rather than saying "Your symptoms are not serious and there's nothing wrong with you," it may be more effective to say, "I understand how serious these symptoms are to you but the good news is that I don't think they represent a progressive or life-threatening illness."

GOALS OF MANAGEMENT

For the patient

Achieve better management of symptom(s) (not cure)
Improve occupational and domestic functioning
Avoid unnecessary surgery and procedures
Avoid dependence on potentially addicting medications, i.e., narcotics and benzodiazepines
Improve overall health status through improvement of healthy behaviors
Improve coping and socialization skills
Decrease medical overutilization
Gain insight into the connection between emotions and symptoms

For the physician

Help patient to achieve goals above
Use limit setting to achieve an arrangement that is comfortable (office visits, phone calls, etc.)
Improve awareness and handling of emotional reactions to patient such as anger, frustration, and feelings of inadequacy

For reassurance to be effective it is also important that it comes after the patient feels that the physician has all the necessary information. It is better to postpone giving reassurance until after a full history and physical examination have been completed even when patients ask for it early in an evaluation.

When discussing the formulation, the message to give should depend on how ready the patient is to accept a psychologic diagnosis. For the patients who seem ready to accept this idea it is useful to explain the connection between emotions and physical symptoms sensitively, using examples from everyday life, such as the sweaty palms and dry mouth that may accompany stage fright, the role of stress in the development of gastric ulcers, and the commonness of tension as a cause of headaches.

To those who are more resistant to these ideas it is useful to explain their problems in more scientific terms, emphasizing the physiologic nature of the mind-body connection. One approach that has been successful involves explaining how the "chemicals in the brain" (referring to neurotransmitters) are altered by our emotions and in turn affect the functioning of the entire body. This oversimplified but not untrue concept can provide a framework acceptable to both the physician and the patient.

There are somatizing patients who will resist all attempts at making any connection between emotions and somatic complaints. These patients may benefit from receiving a descriptive diagnosis—one that describes their symptoms but does not carry with it unwarranted implications. It is possible to satisfy some patients needs for a diagnostic label with descriptions such as abnormal gastrointestinal motility, muscle contraction headaches, and hyperventilation syndrome.

Long-term management. Once a relationship with the somatizing patient has been established it is important for the physician to recognize that it is tremendously therapeutic for the patient to have an objective, caring individual listen empathically to her problems. In the context of this relationship it is important to reinforce the discussion of emotions and psychosocial stressors positively with active listening and questioning, while negatively reinforcing the expression of somatic complaints.

Frequent but time-limited visits that are regularly scheduled independent of changes in symptoms can serve to change the patient's orientation toward physician utilization. Ideally patients will feel that they do not need to have new complaints in order to see their physicians. Strictly limiting the time available for each visit is important. If there are long lists of symptoms and concerns it is useful to begin each visit by negotiating which one or two symptoms the patient wishes to discuss in the time available.

Although each symptom should be taken seriously and possible organic diseases ruled out when indicated, limits should be set with regard to referrals to specialists. Physicians need to decide what arrangement is acceptable to them and communicate that to the patient. Many physicians will make it clear to their patients that frequent self-referral could lead to termination from their practice.

The patient may gradually come to accept the association between her emotional reactions and physical complaints. At that time the primary care provider may consider referring the patient for psychotherapy. Headaches, chronic back pain, and other forms of chronic pain can be effectively treated with behavioral methods (such as relaxation techniques and biofeedback) and cognitive psychotherapy.

Pharmacologic therapy

In general somatoform disorders are not effectively treated with medication. It may be beneficial, however, to treat specific target symptoms or clearly defined affective disorders such as major depression, generalized anxiety disorder, and panic disorder. Although many patients with somatization disorder may complain of nonspecific feelings of anxiety, treatment with benzodiazepines should be avoided as these symptoms of anxiety are almost always chronic and may provide the patient with some stimulus to deal with the emotional component of their problem.

There are two exceptions to this general principle. The first exception is chronic somatoform pain disorder. Chronic pain, as mentioned previously, has been approached by some as an indication of depression and has been successfully treated with tricyclic antidepressants. Narcotic analgesics should be avoided.

The other exception is monosymptomatic hypochondriasis, which some consider a variant of obsessive-compulsive disorder. Therefore the selective serotonergic receptor uptake inhibitors (SSRIs) (fluoxetine, sertraline, and paroxetine) and clomipramine (the tricyclic with the greatest amount of serotonergic activity) have been used to treat this disorder.

SUMMARY

Somatization disorder, somatoform pain disorder, and the more general illness behavior of somatization are very frequently seen in women in the primary care setting. The overlap of these disorders with the affective disorders and several of the personality disorders makes their recognition and management very difficult. There are definite signs of somatization in these patients' histories. The most important clue is a history of multiple complaints with multiple evaluations and few explanations. Obtaining a family history of somatization and a history of physical or sexual abuse can also be very helpful in making the diagnosis. Once the diagnosis is made and empathically communicated to the patient the physician-patient relationship may be tremendously therapeutic. With frequent, time-limited, regularly scheduled visits the physician can often redirect the patient's focus from her somatic symptoms to her emotional distress. It is important to avoid pharmacologic therapy in these patients unless there is a clearly defined disorder or target symptom to be treated. Physicians can reduce much of the frustration felt by both the patients and themselves by setting realistic goals, aiming for management of symptoms and not cure.

BIBLIOGRAPHY

American Psychiatric Association: *Diagnostic and statistical manual of mental disorders*, ed 4, Washington DC, 1994, American Psychiatric Association.

Barsky AJ III: Patients who amplify bodily sensations, *Ann Intern Med* 91:63, 1979.

Berry J, Storandt M, Coyne A: Age and sex differences in somatic complaints associated with depression, *J Gerontol* 39:465, 1984.

Engel GL: Psychogenic pain and the pain prone patient, *Am J Med* 26:899, 1959.

Groves JE: Taking care of the hateful patient, *N Engl J Med* 298:883, 1978.

Kaplan C, Lipkin M, Jr, Gordon G: Somatization in primary care: patients with unexplained and vexing medical complaints, *J Gen Intern Med* 3:177, 1988.

Katon W: Panic disorder and somatization, *Am J Med* 77:101, 1984.

Lipowski Z: Somatization and depression, *Psychosomatics* 31(1):13, 1990.

Morrison J, Herbstein J: Secondary affective disorders in women with somatization disorder, *Compr Psychol* 29:433, 1988.

Smith RG, Monson R, Ray D: Patients with multiple unexplained symptoms: their characteristics, functional health, and health care utilization, *Arch Intern Med* 146:69, 1986.

75 Stress Management

Kathleen Hubbs Ulman

In recent years the role of stress in the development and course of illness has been increasingly recognized and integrated into the overall understanding of health in our culture. Experts define stress in several ways: (1) as a stimulus, acute or chronic, that requires adaptation or (2) as the altered state that is the result of inadequate adaptation to a life event.

Recent studies of the relationship between stress and health suggest that the increase in risk of illness for an individual is mediated by several psychosocial factors. The key factors are the meaning of an individual's life situation, adaptation to stress as determined by an individual's personality and coping style, and the influence of an individual's characteristic psychologic reactions on general physiologic functioning and, in particular, the immune system.

As with much medical and psychologic research men were the subjects of the majority of the initial studies of stress. Only in the past few decades have women been included as subjects in studies concerning the effects of work, personal life, personality, coping style, and emotional functioning on health. This research has shown that the circumstances under which women experience psychologic and physical distress are sometimes different from those that influence men. In addition, psycholinguistic theory and research have shown gender differences in the ways in which men and women present and discuss physical and emotional symptoms with their physicians.

The primary care physician can increase the recognition of the role of stress in the symptoms of women patients by learning about the role of stress in illness in general and understanding the risk factors associated with increased illness in women, in particular. In addition, the primary care physician can increase the likelihood of diagnosing a stress-related illness in female patients by listening carefully to a woman's description of symptoms and asking for information regarding the context of her life, general mood, and sense of satisfaction with her life. During the information-gathering portion of the examination it is important for the physician to convey to the patient a sense of understanding and acceptance of her situation. Women in particular respond more positively to a physician's recommendations if they feel understood and listened to rather than labeled.

Once the stress in a woman's life is diagnosed and acknowledged by both patient and physician the primary care physician can provide basic counseling in methods to reduce stress. All suggested changes should be carefully outlined in detail. The physician's prescription for stress-reducing life-style changes such as exercise, recreation, or increased social contact has great power for women who have been socialized to put others' needs first. Some women will only be able to initiate stress-reducing changes and set limits on demands of family and work by invoking the authority of their physician. For patients with more complicated situations, the primary care physician can supplement the basic counseling with an appropriate psychiatric referral (see box, below).

EPIDEMIOLOGY AND RISK FACTORS FOR STRESS

Prevalence

It is well established in the medical literature that at a given age men have increased rates of mortality and life-threatening illness, while women have increased rates of morbidity and nonfatal chronic conditions. Thus men die at a younger age, and women have more chronic illness that interferes with everyday functioning and impairs their quality of life. Women are twice as likely as men to suffer from depression, another risk factor for increased morbidity rate. Women also have increased rates of symptom reporting and increased use of medication and medical services.

Epidemiologic studies suggest that biologic factors play a primary role in the sex differences in mortality rate, whereas social factors play a major role in the sex differences in morbidity rate. In U.S. society women are more vulnerable to the social factors associated with increased risk of nonfatal chronic conditions. These risk factors will be enumerated in the following section.

Risk factors for stress

Men and women. Psychosocial factors that compromise health can be divided into acute and chronic categories (see the box on the following page). The acute stressors may be external events such as loss of employment, sudden illness, death of a loved one, rape, or a natural disaster. Chronic stressors may be any ongoing aversive situation that requires adaptation such as marital problems, divorce, conflict at work, economic pressure, a history of childhood trauma, chronic medical problem in a family member or oneself, or emotional problem such as anxiety or depression.

Research on the impact of acute stressors such as natural disasters and unexpected events shows that most people recover and do well after such events. Recovery depends in

---

ORDER OF PSYCHOSOCIAL INTERVENTIONS

Diagnose stress.
Suggest appropriate environmental and behavior change.
Schedule follow-up visit to evaluate change.
With appropriate change:
  Reinforce change.
  Consider referral to counseling for further exploration and change.
  Refer cases of incest and rape for counseling.
No appropriate change:
  Refer for counseling with follow-up evaluation.

RISK FACTORS FOR HEALTH IMPAIRMENT: MEN AND WOMEN

Acute

Loss of employment
Assault
Natural disaster

Chronic

Personal:
  Marital conflict
  Recent separation
  Bereavement
  Loneliness
  Dissatisfaction with one's life
  Type A personality
  History of incest
  History of physical abuse
Work-related:
  Job with little control
  Dissatisfaction with one's job
Work and personal:
  Roles with irregular schedules
  Roles with little time pressure
  Roles with great time pressure
  Roles with decreased responsibility
  Roles with decreased activity

part on how the acute stressor fits into the worldview of the individual and how it meshes with her history. If the individual feels that the event can be understood within her expectations for her life, the event is less likely to cause prolonged distress. However, if the event drastically challenges the individual's view of the world and interferes with the individual's sense of control, the experience can be traumatic and have psychologic and physical consequences. For example, if a woman believes that death is part of a greater scheme and that she will see her loved one after her death, she may move from a state of shock and distress caused by the unexpected death of her husband to a state of acceptance and adaptation more quickly and completely than someone who feels that death is random. If a woman is raped in her own home, her general sense of where she is safe in the world has been violated. For a while she may feel in constant danger and will remain in a continual state of arousal and distress. The longer she stays in this state of arousal and distress the more likely it is that her health may suffer. The length of time in which she remains in a state of physical arousal will depend in part on her history, her style of coping, and the psychosocial context of her life.

There are some areas of similarity in the effects of chronic stress on health risk for both sexes. For men and women alike dissatisfaction with one's life and roles is associated with ill health. It is the individual's subjective reactions to his or her roles that have impact on health rather than the exact job or life position. Roles associated with less responsibility and less activity are associated with ill health. In addition roles that include either great or little time pressure are associated with increased health risk. In contrast, increased role involvements or responsibilities for men and women are not associated with increased health risks.

Rather, involvement in an activity that has value and meaning for the individual at a level of responsibility that matches his or her temperament and physical and emotional capacity is associated with decreased health risk.

Personality and coping style are thought to play a role in the impact of stressful events or roles on health. For many years a type A personality style has been associated with increased risk for heart disease in men. This personality style includes a chronic sense of time urgency. Kobasa (1987) found that individuals who shared three characteristics she called stress-hardiness had a decreased risk of ill health when subjected to stress. These characteristics are (1) a strong sense of commitment to life and work, (2) a sense of control over one's life, and (3) a perception of life changes as a challenge.

Women

Roles. The type and variety of roles a woman enjoys have an influence on her health. Married employed parents have the best health profiles. Employment contributes the most health protection to married women. In contrast, marriage contributes the most protection to men. Unemployed married women above age 40 have the poorest health.

As stated previously, women's increased risk of morbidity has been attributed to social factors related in part to women's roles. Many women tend to be dissatisfied with their primary roles, which they often see as having low status. They also tend to have fewer roles and thus decreased opportunities to derive gratification and enjoyment from a number of sources. Women's traditional roles include characteristics associated with increased morbidity rate such as low income, irregular time schedules, and low or high time pressure. Women who pursue advanced career opportunities of their choice may enjoy some protection from these health risks. However, career women with children often have irregular time schedules and high time pressure.

Social context. The generality of the increased health protection afforded by roles is influenced by the context of a woman's life at home and at work. The amount of physical help a married woman receives at home and the amount of emotional support and validation she receives in her marriage influence her health. In addition, the degree to which others depend on her for care and nurturance influences a woman's vulnerability to ill health. Too few or too many demands from others increase a woman's health risk. Depression in mothers increases as the number of children increases and the age of the youngest child decreases.

The quality of a woman's relationships at home and at work is an important factor related to her health and her satisfaction with her roles. For a woman, a supportive relationship must be one in which she can confide her feelings as well as provide caring. Depression in women is often associated with unequal relationships in which women provide much care and nurturance and receive little affirmation and support in return. Thus involvement in large social networks where many individuals depend on a woman for help and give little in return increases her health risk.

The impact of employment on a woman's health depends on the conditions of her work and her feelings about her work. A woman who works out of economic necessity in a clerical job with little control or satisfaction enjoys much less health protection than a woman who has chosen to work, who finds work relationships supportive, or who is in a career of her choice.

Women are also vulnerable to particular stressors in our culture such as violence, rape, incest, sexual objectification, and economic problems that increase risk of morbidity. Hamilton (1994) reported that young women who have been sexually objectified and treated as adornments demonstrate symptoms of stress and have an increased vulnerability to depression. Often stressors such as rape and incest are accompanied by shame, which promotes isolation, impedes the use of social and medical resources, and thus increases health risk. Pennybaker (1993) found that women who had experienced childhood trauma and had not confided in anyone saw physicians more often than those who had discussed the trauma with someone.

Sex role socialization and psychologic development of women. Women's psychologic development is profoundly impacted by our culture's definition of a desirable woman as being attractive, nurturing, selfless, and peace-making. The development of self-esteem is impaired in young females as they become aware of the devaluation and categorization of women as second-class citizens by virtue of their biologic characteristics. Socialization encourages women to be compliant with social expectations and to neglect their own sensations and perceptions of events in favor of responding to others' needs. As a consequence many adult women today derive self-esteem from and organize their identity around pleasing and caring for others. They are encouraged to locate the control of their lives in others' needs and are thus disconnected from their own perceptions and needs. This difficulty in separating herself from the needs and distress of those around her makes it difficult for a woman to set limits on others to attend to her own emotional or physical needs and puts her at risk for ill health.

Difficulty in setting limits occurs for many women both at home with their families and at work. Women in professional careers are not immune from this difficulty of setting limits. Yet according to Lawler and Schmidt (1992), the ability to see oneself, rather than external events, as the source of decisions and control of one's life is the very aspect of "stress-hardiness" that appears to be most protective of women's health. Thus women's tendency in our culture to see themselves and their lives as determined by external forces contributes to an increased health risk.

Personality style and identity. The degree to which a woman's roles fit with her views of herself as a woman influences her health. As stated previously the personality traits associated with stress-hardiness are incompatible with the ways women are socialized in our society. In addition the direct and strong expression of anger is discouraged in women. Yet repressed anger increases heart rate and blood pressure in women as well as men. Thomas and Williams (1991) report that the more a woman can discuss anger directly at work or at home rather than suppress it or use it to blame others, the better her health. Women with less traditional sex role norms are better able to negotiate for themselves and to express anger than women who identify with a traditional female sex role.

Roles, social context, and sex role norms can come together to provide increased health risk for women. According to Haynes and Feinleib (1980) working women do not as a whole have an increased incidence of heart disease. However, clerical workers have almost twice the rate of coronary heart disease (CHD) of women who work in the home. The factors associated with CHD for clerical workers are suppressed hostility, a nonsupportive boss, and decreased job mobility. The highest rate of CHD is in clerical workers with children who are married to blue-collar workers. Women with traditional sex role norms whose spouses offer only minimal task sharing and who do not have a supportive confidante are at the greatest risk for health problems.

A list of risk factors for health impairment in women is shown in the box, below.

PATHOPHYSIOLOGY

Life situations that include loss or conflict are often associated with decreased immune system functioning and with increased symptoms of ill health or with a more severe course of an illness. According to Kiecolt-Glaser (1987), individuals in a distressed marital relationship or those recently separated have decreased immune function as measured by percentage of natural killer cells. The degree of decreased immune function is related to the amount of attachment to the spouse and to the length of separation. The longer the individual has been separated the more likely the immune function will return to normal. Other studies have indicated that loneliness and bereavement are related to poor immune functioning. Finding a new partner is associated with increased immune function for separated and divorced people.

It appears that having a supportive social network in which a woman can express her feelings and experience a sense of understanding and respect promotes good immune functioning and may interact with other physiologic factors to influence the course of an illness. The act of putting feelings into symbolic expression, particularly words, relieves

---

RISK FACTORS FOR HEALTH IMPAIRMENT: WOMEN

Acute
  Rape

Chronic
  Personal:
    Intimate relationship with unsupportive mate
    Friendships that are not supportive
    Family relationships that are not supportive
    Family relationships that require extra help and support
    Sick spouse, child, or parent
    Personality that suppresses anger
    Several young children
    Lack of sharing of domestic chores
  Work:
    Unsupportive boss
    Work in clerical job out of economic necessity
    Decreased job mobility
  Overall:
    Unemployed, married, and more than 40 years old
    Clerical worker with children and married to blue-collar
      worker

distress and diminishes risk of ill health. Pennybaker (1993) has found that writing about feelings associated with current stressful situations or past traumas improves immune function, decreases physician visits, and decreases subjective distress. Individuals who have not discussed their feelings about unpleasant situations or traumas demonstrate the largest increases in immune functioning as a result of writing about feelings. Holding back feelings may heighten autonomic system activity, which, over time, leads to changes in immune functioning. Individuals with a medical illness who participate in individual or group psychotherapy demonstrate decreased use of medication, decreased number of office visits, and increased immune functioning.

DIFFERENTIAL DIAGNOSIS

The diagnosis of either acute or ongoing stress in a medical patient is complex and often not definitive. Yet a timely diagnosis and appropriate interventions are important parts of a patient's overall care and may increase the rate of recovery from an acute illness, prevent the development of an ongoing chronic condition, or stabilize a chronic disease, thereby significantly improving the quality of life and decreasing physician office visits and medication use. The primary care clinician may be the only person in contact with the patient who is in a position to make the diagnosis and initiate the appropriate intervention. When evaluating a patient for stress-related problems the possibility of a depression or anxiety disorder should always be considered. Often these can be diagnosed and treated concurrently with the evaluation and treatment of stress.

Stress can influence any system and aggravate any chronic disease. Thus the diagnosis cannot be made on the basis of a specific constellation of symptoms. The process of diagnosing stress-related problems is further complicated by the fact that patients often do not recognize that they are stressed. The presence of symptoms that may be related to stress can be suspected when the total picture does not make sense: when for example an infection persists or reappears repeatedly despite recommended treatment, or a chronic disease has an unexpected flare-up. The diagnosis is often made by using a combination of knowledge of known risk factors and knowledge of the particular patient's medical history and life situation.

In addition to evaluating the presence of known risk factors, the clinician can look for the presence of behaviors associated with emotional distress such as sleep disturbance, changes in eating, increased alcohol consumption, changes in balance of time spent in work or recreation, and changes in amount of time spent with others. When such changes are present the possibility of a depression or anxiety disorder should be considered. The clinician should also inquire about factors known to be protective of health such as the ability to devote some time to work or hobbies that are meaningful, time spent relaxing, and availability of a supportive network of friends. Such questions as "How many people depend on you?" "Whom do you talk to?" "Do you have someone to confide in?" "Whom can you ask to take over when you need help?" often provide important information.

Clinical presentation

Women whose lives involve the level of distress that might compromise their health will present themselves in the physician's office in several ways. The presentation will depend, in part, on the woman's personality, her understanding of her symptoms, and her situation.

The insightful patient. A woman who recognizes the connection between symptoms and stress will often start her visit with the statement that some physical symptoms are bothering her and she is also going through a difficult time in her life. She often wants reassurance that the symptoms are connected to stress and not a more serious illness. She may also want assistance in the form of listening or a referral for counseling. The difficulty with such patients is that in spite of the stress there also may be more serious physical problems that need to be evaluated and treated. Thus the physician should not be too easily swayed by the patient's self-diagnosis of stress.

The naive patient. Another common presentation is that of a woman who has a list of physical complaints such as tiredness, stiff neck, and stomach pains that have developed in the past year. In response to questioning, she states that a relative is dying and her husband recently lost his job. She has not connected her symptoms with her life situation but does acknowledge she is experiencing psychologic distress. Her ability to experience and acknowledge psychologic distress will make it easier for the physician to make the diagnosis and for the patient to assume some responsibility to initiate new behaviors to take care of herself.

The stoical patient. One of the more difficult presentations is that of a woman who describes a variety of symptoms that are causing her significant physical distress. All physical and laboratory findings are normal. Upon questioning she maintains that emotionally she is fine in spite of the fact that she has had significant losses or changes in her life in the past year. It is in relation to this type of patient that knowledge of the known risk factors associated with ill health in women is important. This woman is not able to perceive or acknowledge that the circumstances of her life are putting her at risk. Often some of these women are opposed to acknowledging the influence of the overall context of their lives on their health because they need to see themselves as being invulnerable to stress and as having the capacity to weather any life circumstance with no emotional or physical sequelae. Chapter 74 provides a more detailed discussion of somatization.

The denying patient. Another type of presentation is given by a woman who does not expect much out of her life. This woman's identity is derived from taking care of others. She has little or no appreciation of her own needs. Her personality and view of herself do not allow for active assessment of the situation or interventions to ameliorate the condition for herself. Often this type of patient just wants her symptoms treated and does not want to embark on any exploration of her life situation because she fears any disruption of her sense of self or of close relationships.

A complicated situation in which the contribution of stress is often not recognized is that of a woman who has an acute life-threatening illness such as a myocardial infarction or a serious exacerbation of a chronic illness such as diabetes or asthma. The patient's medical condition is so serious that the initial focus must be on stabilization and treatment of symptoms. However, even when medical treatment is instituted her condition may remain unstable or she may not return to her previous level of health. This lack of expected progress or relapse should be a red flag to the physician to explore the role of stress in the patient's recuperation and adjustment to her illness. For such a patient the diagnosis of the contribution of stress to her serious medical condition is essential to the outcome of her disease. The woman's life situation may include several risk factors associated with diminished health, such as an abusive marriage, single parenthood, inability to enlist the help of her husband in order to decrease her responsibilities at home, absence of a confidante, and presence of a history of childhood sexual trauma.

For such patients two types of psychosocial interventions may be useful. The first is an overall evaluation of her day-to-day life with consideration of whether there is anyone to help her and whether she continues to care for others such as her husband, children, and other relatives in spite of her serious medical difficulties. This is often particularly characteristic of older couples with traditional life-styles. Women with serious medical conditions may continue to take total responsibility for their own and their husband's care and may not mention this to their physician unless directly asked. In such cases some form of counseling that includes the spouse and other family members may be useful.

The second type of intervention is to provide the opportunity for the woman to talk about previously unexpressed feelings with a confidante, a therapist, or a support group. Such a process can bring about increased self-esteem, an increase in an internal sense of control, and an increase in options that provide a woman with a sense that she can exert control over her day-to-day life by asking others for help and initiating activities that are gratifying and rewarding for her. As stated previously, having a supportive network and talking to a confidante increase immune function and thus may contribute to the stabilization of a serious chronic medical condition.

THERAPY AND MANAGEMENT

Once the physician has determined that a woman's symptoms are in part stress-related, several types of intervention are available. The particular intervention or combination of interventions chosen will depend on the symptom pattern, the patient's life circumstances, and the patient's personality (see box, above right).

One of the most useful treatment strategies is to change the individual's environment when possible. Areas that can be changed include increasing the amount of help with physical responsibilities, decreasing the burden of responsibilities involved in caring for others, rearranging the daily schedule to make it less stressful, increasing opportunities for care for the patient, and arranging changes in the physical environment if appropriate.

The second type of useful treatment strategy is to change the patient's behavior and psychologic functioning. One major mode of behavior change is to stop behavior that perpetuates the stressful experience. This might include improved nutrition, changes in sleep routine, improved time management, decrease in alcohol use, and decreased exposure to stressful relationships or tasks. Another behavioral intervention is to introduce behavior that produces a state of

---

| STRESS-REDUCING INTERVENTIONS |

Change environment
Reducing external stress such as noise, pollution
Reducing stimulation at home
When possible reducing stimulation at work
Reducing threats to physical safety
Ensuring fulfillment of basic physical needs

Change behavior
Nutrition
Exercise
Alcohol consumption
Sleep
Relaxation, meditation, or hypnosis
Reduced exposure to conflicted situations
Time management

Change psychologic functioning
Increasing awareness of options
Increasing awareness of possibility of internal change
Increasing sense of validity of limit setting
Increasing awareness of feelings
Increasing verbal expression of feelings
Increasing confidence in one's perceptions

---

relaxation such as training in relaxation, meditation, self-hypnosis or introduction of exercise in the appropriate amount.

The introduction of opportunities to change psychologic functioning and self-esteem is the third form of intervention to reduce stress. Examples include encouragement of increased time spent in validating and supportive relationships, increase in meaningful responsibilities, and expression of emotion in writing or in person to the appropriate people.

One result of a discussion of possible behavioral and psychologic changes is to increase the patient's awareness of the possibility of change and the existence of alternatives. Such a discussion also conveys to the patient that her physician sees her as worthy of having her needs taken seriously and as being able to take active control over some aspects of her life.

The degree to which the clinician will be able to discuss these possible changes with a patient will depend on available time and severity of illness. However, it is important for the clinician to remember that direct advice from the physician or from other clinicians in authoritative roles can be very effective in empowering a woman to make changes that have a positive influence on her health. Many women who experience stress-related health problems have low self-esteem, have been socialized to derive their self-esteem from caring from others, and may be in a personal or work relationship that continues to encourage them to neglect themselves. Often they have become disconnected from their own perceptions and lack the belief that they can take their needs into account and still be valued.

Straightforward prescriptions for life-style changes are very important. The physician's authority gives the patient permission and validation to set limits on the demands of others and to engage in stress-reducing behaviors. Although statements such as "You must find time to exercise each week" may seem simple, the physician may be the first person or at least the only person in her current life who conveys to her a sense of worthiness and entitlement to self-care.

The final option for behavior and psychologic change is to refer for counseling. Counseling will provide an opportunity for the patient to receive validation, to organize her thoughts and feelings into words, to discuss feelings and memories of events that may never before have been shared, and to become aware of options for change—all factors that have been demonstrated to reduce health risks and improve immune function.

Indications for referral

The primary care clinician can help the woman initiate changes to reduce her level of stress. Initially the clinician can suggest behavior changes (e.g., exercise, recreation, alcohol intake, or family care responsibilities) with a return visit in a month. The return visit will give the clinician an opportunity to assess the ability of the patient to initiate changes in her life. If the appropriate behavior changes have been made, the clinician and patient can assess the degree of symptom relief that the patient has obtained from these changes. If the degree of relief is satisfactory, the patient can be encouraged to continue the new behavior and return for follow-up evaluation in several months.

If the degree of relief is not satisfactory, in spite of the behavior changes the patient may be referred for further help such as relaxation training, hypnosis, or a stress management group. If the patient is interested in exploring the role of her psychologic functioning and feelings in the development of the stress-related symptoms a referral for psychotherapy can be considered. The possibility of an unrecognized depression or anxiety disorder should also be evaluated. The diagnosis of depression or anxiety does not exclude further recommendations for stress reduction.

If at the follow-up visit it is determined that behavior changes have not been initiated, the clinician should gently explore the reasons why. Often underlying issues that may prevent the implementation of such changes will become evident. For example, a woman may be so out of touch with signals from her body that the word *relaxation* has no meaning to her; a patient may have used excessive activity as a means of distracting herself from intolerable feelings and may not be able to relax until she begins to address the intolerable feelings; or a woman may be so dependent on her husband or others for approval that she may be unable to set limits in order to care for herself. Again the possibility of an underlying depression must be considered. When a patient is unable to initiate behavior changes a referral for psychotherapy is appropriate for the exploration and treatment of obstacles to change. A referral for behavior therapy or relaxation training may fail until the underlying obstacles to change are identified and changed. If the patient feels she might be able to initiate behavior changes in the context of increased support a referral to a support group or stress management group could be made. However, with a patient who has demonstrated difficulty with initiation a follow-up to the referral is recommended.

SUMMARY

Women are vulnerable to diminished health and are at risk for illness in our society because of their vulnerability to violence and because of their focus on providing nurturance for others as a source of self-esteem in a society that does not value that role. Visiting a physician for ill health is acceptable to women in their roles as nurturers. Thus physicians need to understand the importance to women patients of their suggestions and prescriptions for change and use them to help women care for themselves and set limits on others. It is vital that physicians who treat women appreciate the value of indicating to women patients in a variety of ways that the balance of rewards and demands in their lives has an impact on their physical and psychologic well-being.

BIBLIOGRAPHY

Belle D: Gender differences in the social moderators of stress. In Barnett RC, Biener L, Baruch GK, editors: *Gender and stress,* New York, 1987, The Free Press.

Frankenhauser M, Lundberg U, Chesney M, editors: *Women, work, and health: stress and opportunities,* New York, 1991, Plenum Press.

Hamilton JA: Objectification experiences in relational orientation predict depression in women. Unpublished paper presented at American Psychological Association meeting Psychosocial Factors in Women's Health: Creating an Agenda for the 21st Century, Washington, D.C., May 1994.

Haynes SG, Feinlieb M: Women, work, and coronary heart disease: findings from the Framingham heart study, *Am J Public Health* 70:133, 1980.

Kiecolt-Glaser JK et al: Marital quality, marital disruption, and immune function, *Psychosom Med* 49:13, 1987.

Kobasa SCO: Stress responses and personality. In Barnett RC, Biener L., Baruch GK, editors: *Gender and stress,* New York, 1987, The Free Press.

Lawler KA, Schmidt LA: A prospective study of women's health: the effects of stress, hardiness, locus of control, type A behavior, and physiological reactivity, *Women Health* 19:27, 1992.

Pennybaker JW: Putting stress into words: health, linguistic, and therapeutic implications, *Behav Res Ther* 31:539, 1993.

Thomas SP, Williams R: Relationships among perceived stress, trait anger, modes of anger expression, and health status of college men and women, *Nurs Research* 40:303, 1991.

Ulman KH: Group psychotherapy with the medically ill. In Kaplan HI, Sadock BJ, editors: *Comprehensive group psychotherapy,* Baltimore, 1993, Williams & Wilkins.

Vanfossen BE: Sex differences in the mental health effects of spouse support and equity, *J Health Soc Behav* 22:130, 1981.

Verbrugge LM: Role burdens and physical health of women and men, *Women Health* 11:47, 1986.

Woods NF: Women's lives: pressure and pleasure, conflict and support. *Health Care Women Int* 8:109, 1987.

Wortman CB et al: Stress, coping, and health: conceptual issues and directions for future research. In Friedman HS, editor: *Hostility, coping and health,* Washington, D.C., 1992, American Psychological Association.

Part Four

Preventive Medicine

76 Breast Cancer Screening

Susan E. Bennett

Women and their physicians are more worried about breast cancer than at any time in the past. With great frequency women read and hear about the breast cancer "epidemic," which conjures visions of certain doom, particularly for those at highest risk, and gives rise to the false perception that enormous forces are being amassed to combat this disease. Thus women hope and expect screening tests to be powerful tools with perfect sensitivity and specificity. They expect to have breast cancer detected at an early stage with certain survival if they follow screening recommendations. Their health providers, however, know that screening is limited, although many are unsure about the efficacy of various screening tests. Many clinicians harbor doubts about their ability to palpate breast abnormalities and this can result in overreliance on mammography. Finally, physicians know that many women hold unrealistic hopes for breast cancer screening and fear that patients will be angry and possibly litigious if screening fails to detect cancer in the earliest stages. Much will be accomplished if physicians better understand the goals and limitations of screening for breast cancer and convey these facts to women.

EPIDEMIOLOGY

Breast cancer is the most common malignancy for women in North America and Europe. The incidence of breast cancer is increasing in South America, Australia, and Asia; second-generation immigrants to high-incidence countries are acquiring breast cancer at higher rates than women in their parents' countries of origin. Although increased detection of breast cancer accounts for some of the rising incidence, it dies not account for all of the increase. In North America (and most populations studied worldwide) the incidence of breast cancer is increasing by 1% to 2% each year. As a result the estimated lifetime risk of development of breast cancer has increased from 1:11 to 1:8; this estimate, however, is based on the presumption that women will live to age 110 and roughly one third of the predicted cancers will occur after age 75.

Table 76-1 shows that absolute risk is age-dependent and is perhaps a less threatening way to predict risk. According to this model the risk of acquiring breast cancer in the forties is 1:1000, whereas the risk for a woman in her fifties is 1:500. The risk of dying of breast cancer before age 75 is only 2.5%. Breast cancer risk is race-dependent as well as age-dependent: the cumulative probability of a white woman's

having breast cancer by age 75 is 8.2%, whereas that for African-American women is 7.0% and that for Hispanic-American women is 4.8%. The cumulative risk among Japanese-American women of development of breast cancer is 5.4%. It is important for women and their physicians to understand that all women are at risk for breast cancer. Three quarters of women with breast cancer have no identifiable risk factors. Understanding this concept and some basic facts about the pathophysiologic characteristics of breast cancer helps the clinician to make decisions about screening frequency and tests.

PATHOPHYSIOLOGY

It has been well established that survival of breast cancer is inversely proportional to the size of the primary tumor and to the number of axillary lymph nodes involved with metastases. The mastectomy originated on the basis of this evidence and the belief that breast cancer did not undergo hematogenous dissemination until local lymph nodes were invaded. However, studies documented that breast cancer sometimes recurred in women with localized breast cancer after mastectomy and that survival was independent of the number of lymph nodes removed at mastectomy.

Table 76-1 Probability of eventually developing and dying of breast cancer*

Age interval	Risk of developing breast cancer (%)	Risk of developing invasive breast cancer (%)	Risk of dying of breast cancer (%)
Birth-110	10.2	9.8	3.6
20-30	0.04	0.04	0.00
20-40	0.49	0.42	0.09
20-110	10.34	9.94	3.05
35-45	0.88	0.83	0.14
35-55	2.53	2.37	0.56
35-110	10.27	9.82	3.56
50-60	1.95	1.86	0.33
50-70	4.67	4.48	1.04
50-110	8.96	8.66	2.75
65-75	3.17	3.08	0.43
65-85	5.48	5.29	1.01
65-110	6.53	6.29	1.53

*White females.
Seidman H et al: *Ca-A Journal for Clinicians*, 35:36, 1985.

An aggressive subset of tumors were identified in a study of the natural history of breast cancer. Approximately 40% of breast cancers appear to be *aggressive*, with a relative mortality rate of 25% each year. *Lead time bias* based on the existence of an aggressive subset of breast cancers confounds the results of screening studies, in that early detection lengthens the time between diagnosis and death without altering the outcome.

Approximately 60% of breast cancers appear to be *indolent*, with a relative mortality rate of 2.5% each year. These malignancies either grow very slowly, undergoing late hematogenous dissemination, or appear histologically malignant while behaving clinically benignly. *Length bias* based on the existence of an indolent subset also confounds studies of screening by detecting preclinical tumors that would have remained undetected and, perhaps, harmless. A recent study reported evidence that, after adjusting for tumor size, cancers detected by screening had lower malignant potential than control cases. Controlled, prospective studies of screening for breast cancer have been carried out over the past three decades with long follow-up periods; lead time and length bias become less important as study groups are followed over many years.

EARLY DETECTION BY MAMMOGRAPHY

Table 76-2 lists the large-scale, prospective, controlled completed studies of screening mammography only or mammography plus clinical breast examination (CBE). The screening intervals, length of follow-up observation, and ages included in the studies vary. Screening mammography reduces the breast cancer mortality rate for women above 50 years of age but not for women who are younger. The average reduction in mortality rate attributed to screening primarily by mammography is 30% for women above 50 years of age. This is a significant reduction but smaller than most believe; a 30% reduction in mortality rate does *not* mean that one in three women screened will be spared a breast cancer death. On making a case against screening Strabanek claimed that a 30% reduc-

tion in mortality rate means that there will be one less death each year for every 15,000 women screened.

For women less than 50 years old screening mammography with or without clinical breast examination (CBE) has *not* been demonstrated to reduce breast cancer mortality rate. The only exception to this is at 18 years of follow-up observation in the Health Insurance Plan of Greater New York (HIP) study, where a trend of survival appears for women who entered screening in their forties. Two completed studies and preliminary results from the National Breast Screening Study of Canada actually reported a *higher* mortality rate of breast cancer among younger women screened with mammography. Some hypothesize that false-negative mammogram results falsely reassure patients and their physicians in the face of a palpable breast abnormality. Others wonder whether breast malignancies detected by mammography are less likely to be treated with adjuvant chemotherapy than cases presenting outside screening because they are smaller and appear less life-threatening. Thus there is no consensus about when to commence screening average-risk women with mammography; evidence for screening before age 50 is lacking in all but one study at almost two decades after screening. For now it can be concluded that screening mammography has a modest but significant impact on breast cancer mortality rate for women between the ages of 50 and 70. There has not been a study of screening after age 70. Because the risk of acquiring breast cancer increases with advancing age the decision about screening cessation should be determined on an individual basis.

EARLY DETECTION BY CLINICAL BREAST EXAMINATION

Does CBE make an independent contribution to screening? The sensitivity of mammography has been calculated to be as high as 70%, compared to 50% for CBE. In the HIP study a large proportion of cancers found at screening were detected by CBE alone. In the Breast Cancer Detection Demonstration project however, with improved mammographic technique, less than 10% of cancers were palpable but invisible on mammography. This was the finding that lead European investigators to design studies of screening with mammography only. It was an appealing concept that clinicians could defer to mammography rather than depend on an often inconclusive breast examination, especially in premenopausal women whose breasts are dense with fibronodular changes. In the Nijmegen study, investigators carried out a retrospective study of cancers that appeared in the intervals between screening mammograms. In this study one-view mammography was performed every 2 years without CBE. Using estimates of doubling time and tumor size at diagnosis they showed that one third of these interval cancers would have been palpable at the time of screening mammography.

Although CBE is reported to have a lower sensitivity than mammography, sensitivity improves with experience and search time. In the Canadian National Breast Screening Study (NBSS) where CBE sensitivity approached that of mammography, clinicians estimated that each breast examination averaged 10 minutes. In a recent controlled study, clinicians trained to detect small lumps in silicone breast models improved their sensitivities from a mean of 57% to

Table 76-2 Controlled trials of screening for breast cancer by mammography (MAM) and clinical breast examination (CBE)

Study	Test/frequency	Follow-up observation	Reduced mortality rate Age <50	Reduced mortality rate Age >50
HIP	CBE + MAM/1 year	10 years	None	40%
HIP	CBE + MAM/1 year	18 years	25%*	23%
Sweden	MAM/2-3 years	9 years	None	31%
Malmo	MAM/1.5-2 years	9 years	None	20%*
Nijmegen	MAM/2 years	6 years	None	52%
Florence	MAM/2.5 years	12 years	None	70%
DOM	MAM + CBE	6 years	NA†	70%
UK	MAM + CBE	7 years	None	17%

HIP, Health Insurance Plan of Greater New York; Sweden, Swedish Two-county Study; Malmo, Malmo Study, Sweden; Nimegen, case-control study, Nimegen, the Netherlands; Florence, case-control study, Florence, Italy; DOM, case-control study, Ultrecht, the Netherlands; UK, United Kingdom Study, Edinburgh component.
*Findings do not achieve statistical significance.
†Not applicable as study was limited to women over 50 years old.

63%. Thus screening is best accomplished with a combination of mammography and a *proficient* CBE. Furthermore, for premenopausal women with dense breast tissue that reduces the sensitivity of mammography, CBE is probably a better test to detect breast cancer.

EARLY DETECTION BY BREAST SELF-EXAMINATION

Is there a role for breast self-examination (BSE) in screening for breast cancer? To date there has not been a controlled, prospective study documenting that BSE reduces breast cancer mortality rate. Two such studies are in progress in Russia and Great Britain. Although both studies reported smaller tumors with less axillary lymph node involvement at diagnosis among women trained in BSE compared to control cases, mortality rate has not yet been affected. Retrospective studies reported lower breast cancer mortality rates among women who practice BSE than women who denied BSE practice, and a much higher self-detection rate among women reporting some BSE. A controlled, prospective study demonstrated that BSE instruction improved the detection of small lumps in silicone breast models from a baseline sensitivity of 45% to 67%, and that improved proficiency persisted for 1 year of follow-up study. In the NBSS compliance in practicing BSE at least 12 times a year improved from 20% to 64% as a result of brief episodes of repeated BSE instruction.

Thus, although BSE has not been shown to reduce breast cancer mortality rate, the potential for it to do so exists. It seems prudent to instruct women briefly in some form of BSE at the time of periodic screening. Encouraging women to become accustomed to their breast texture by simply palpating their breasts while bathing is a strategy many clinicians adopt, as it is much less threatening than asking women to search for lumps. Without formal proficiency training women do not know the difference between a discrete breast lump and fibroglandular lumpiness; an attempt to practice formal BSE under these circumstances simply results in anxiety and lack of confidence.

RISKS AND DRAWBACKS OF SCREENING

What are the drawbacks to screening? Although there were initial concerns about inducing radiogenic carcinomas with mammography, the potential hazard attributable to radiation exposure from a modern mammogram is considered to be negligible for women older than 40. Radiation hazard is greatest among women in the second and third decades of life and should be avoided whenever possible.

The primary drawback of screening mammography is its low positive predictive value, estimated to be 8.6% in the Canadian National Breast Screening Study; this means that screening incurs a large number of benign biopsies. Biopsies are expensive, use health resources, and inevitably cause emotional trauma for women and their families.

False-negative mammogram results may falsely reassure women and their doctors, so that they ignore breast lumps that become palpable in the months after screening. A false-negative mammography result in the case of a palpable breast lump (especially in younger women) was among the primary causes of delayed diagnosis of breast cancer in a study by the Physician Insurers Association of America.

Table 76-3 Costs and benefits from screening 100,000 women age 50-59

Item	Program		
	Single-view mammography alone biennially	Double-view mammography plus physical examination biennially	Physical examination alone annually
Mortality reduction years 3-7 (%)	40	60	42
Cost of screens ($)	5,075,400	9,047,500	7,768,650
Cost of extra biopsies ($)	2,886,900	2,886,900	942,540
Total costs ($)	7,962,300	11,934,400	8,711,190
Savings from averted deaths ($)	3,724,600	5,586,900	3,910,800
Net cost ($)	4,237,700	6,347,500	4,800,390
PYLS*	1705	2558	1790
Cost per PYLS ($)	2,485	2,481	2,682

From Miller AB: Early detection of breast cancer. In Harris JR et al, editors: *Breast diseases*, ed 2, Philadelphia, 1991, JB Lippincott.
PYLS, potential years of life saved to age 70.

The primary drawback to screening CBE and BSE is the low sensitivity associated with lack of experience or training. Although there is a limit to tactile abilities clinicians and patients have learned to detect lumps smaller than 1 centimeter. Educational programs to improve proficiency are, however, costly and hard to come by. The lack of demonstrated efficacy in BSE does not yet justify the cost of such program.

Does the benefit of screening outweigh the drawbacks? Table 76-3 illustrates an analysis of the costs and benefits of mass screening for women in their fifties. The estimated cost for each potential year of life saved to age 70 is $2500. As a society we have decided that the benefit is worth the cost. Table 76-4 compares screening recommendations of the American Cancer Society (ACS), United States Preventive Services Task Force, Sweden, and the United Kingdom. It is apparent that the United States has a more ambitious screening program than other countries, although the benefits of other screening programs may be equivalent to those of the U.S. Future studies must focus on the question of screening fre-

Table 76-4 Recommendations for screening mammography

Age Group (years)	ACS	USPSTF	Sweden	UK	Evidence from controlled trials*
	Frequency of mammography (years)				
<40	once	0	0	0	No evidence of benefit
40-49	1-2	0	1.5	0	No early but possible late benefit
50-64	1	1	2	3	Benefit established
>64	1	1	2	0	Benefit established to age 70

ACS, American Cancer Society; USPSTF, United States Preventive Services Task Force; Sweden, Swedish Board of Welfare; UK, United Kingdom.
*See Table 76-2.

quency, ages for commencing and terminating screening, and lower-cost screening. It is also apparent that a better screening test for early detection of breast cancer needs to be developed, or primary prevention of breast cancer needs to be improved.

SUMMARY

In summary, on the basis of the results of clinical trials and weighing of the benefits against the drawbacks of screening, recommendations for screening for breast cancer are as follows:

1. All women between the ages of 50 and 70 should have annual CBE and mammography at least every two years.
2. Average-risk women between 40 and 50 years of age and over 70 years of age should have annual CBE. For women who desire mammography despite the lack of established efficacy mammography should be done annually for women in their forties and every 2 years for women over 70 years of age.
3. High-risk women should have annual mammography and CBE commencing at age 35, or 5 years earlier than the age at which their first-degree relative acquired breast cancer.
4. All women should be briefly instructed in BSE at the periodic health examination and should be encouraged to practice some form of BSE at least once a month.

BIBLIOGRAPHY

Baines CJ, Miller AB, Bassett AA: Physical examination. Its role as a single screening modality in the Canadian National Breast Screening Study, *Cancer* 63:1816, 1989.

Baines CJ, To T: Changes in breast self-examination behavior achieved by 89,835 participants in the Canadian National Breast Screening Study, *Cancer* 66:570, 1990.

Baines CJ et al: Sensitivity and specificity of first screen mammography in the Canadian National Breast Screening Study: a preliminary report from five centers, *Radiology* 160:295, 1986.

Baker LH. Breast cancer detection demonstration project: five year summary report, *Cancer* 32:194, 1982.

Bennett SE et al: Effectiveness of methods used to teach breast self-examination, *Am J Prev Med* 6:208, 1990.

Campbell HS et al: Improving physicians' and nurses' clinical breast examination: a randomized controled trial, *Am J Prev Med* 7:1, 1991.

Cole PH et al: So-called interval cancers of the breast: pathologic and radiologic analysis of sixty-four cases, *Cancer* 49:2527, 1982.

Council on Scientific Affairs: Mammographic screening in asymptomatic women aged 40 years and older, *JAMA* 261:2535, 1989.

Eddy DM: Screening for breast cancer, *Ann Intern Med* 111:389, 1989.

Fisher B, Slack NH: Number of lymph nodes examined and the prognosis of breast carcinoma, *Surg Gynecol Obstet* 131:79, 1970.

Foster RS, Costanza MC: Breast self-examination and breast cancer survival, *Cancer* 53:999, 1984.

Fox M: On the diagnosis and treatment of breast cancer, *JAMA* 24:489, 1979.

Haagensen DC. *Diseases of the breast,* Philadelphia, 1971, WB Saunders.

Harris JR et al, editor: *Breast diseases,* ed 2, Philadelphia, 1991, JB Lippincott.

Klemi PJ et al: Aggressiveness of breast cancers found with and without screening, *Br Med J* 304:467, 1992.

Liff JM et al: Does increased detection account for the rising incidence of breast cancer? *Am J Public Health* 81:462, 1991.

Seidman H et al: Probabilities of eventually developing or dying of cancer— United States, *Ca-A Cancer Journal for Clinicians* 35:36, 1985.

Shapiro S: Evidence on screening for breast cancer from a randomized trial, *Cancer* 39:2772, 1977.

Strabanek P: The case against, *Br Med J* 297:971, 1988.

Trombly ST: The breast cancer "epidemic," *Forum* 13(3):2, 1992.

77 Cervical Cancer and Human Papillomavirus

Ellen E. Sheets

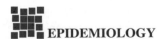

EPIDEMIOLOGY

Because of the natural history of invasive cervical cancer, which includes a lengthy preinvasive stage and an easy to perform, readily available screening test, it has long been thought that this disease is preventable. In the United States approximately 13,000 new cases and 7000 deaths occur yearly as a result of this disease. However, the numbers worldwide are still very high, approximately 400,000 new cases yearly, making it second only to breast cancer as the documented cause of cancer death among women. Every study that evaluates the role of cervical cytologic screening shows a significant decrease in the occurrence and mortality rates of cervical cancer.

The incidence of cervical cancer varies according to race. In the United States the incidence rate for blacks, Hispanics, and Native Americans is approximately twice that of whites. The risk of Asians is similar to that of whites. Interestingly results from the 1987 U.S. National Health Interview Survey indicate that blacks are screened at rates comparable to or higher than those for whites through age 69. Hispanics have a lower screening rate than whites. Why blacks have a higher incidence rate is unknown.

Age appears to alter the incidence of invasive cervical cancer worldwide. Studies show that the age-related pattern is for women to decrease their use of cervical cytologic screening as their age increases. This coincides with an age-related increase in the incidence of invasive cervical cancer. Most studies grouped patients by age, before 65 and after 65, but the greatest difference occurred between those women 44 years of age or younger and those 65 years of age or older.

Geography also appears to play a role in incidence of this disease. High rates of cervical cancer are found in the Caribbean and Latin America. Annual incidence rates are greater than 20/100,000 women in Latin America compared to 2 to 5/100,000 in the United States. Other regions with high incidences are Hong Kong, parts of India, Denmark, Romania, and the Northwest Territories of Canada. Whether these differences represent deficiencies of screening or general health care, artifact, or areas with higher rates of causal factors are not clear. Further, it is possible that the causative factors involved in cervical cancer affect the population in these areas differently.

RISK FACTORS FOR CERVICAL CANCER
Sexual factors

It is not a recent idea that cervical cancer is sexually transmitted. One of the first reports supporting this idea was the 1842 report of Rigoni-Stern, who noted that married (i.e., sexually active) women had a greater risk of development of cervical cancer than cloistered women. Since then there have been numerous accounts of sexually related risk factors. These factors have been pared down to early sexual activity (before age 17) and numerous sexual partners (greater than five). Other factors, such as associated sexually transmitted diseases, poor sexual hygiene, and contact with a high-risk male, have variably been related to cervical cancer development. Not all studies support these other factors, and their importance is most probably a reflection of the primary risk factors. The role of the high-risk male was suggested by studies of men whose consorts had cervical cancer, whose subsequent consorts were at higher risk of development of cervical cancer.

Smoking

When trying to assess the risk of nonsexual factors, studies must be controlled for the major sexual risk factors. Recent U.S. studies looking at the role of smoking have indicated a 50% higher risk of development of cervical cancer among smokers than among comparably matched control subjects. In addition the risk appears to increase the longer one smokes, the more one smokes, and with use of unfiltered cigarettes.

Diet

Although dietary factors have not been as extensively studies as other risk factors, there appears to be a general trend. When confounding factors are controlled for it appears that those women whose diet is deficient in vitamin A or C are at greater risk for cervical cancer. Less solid are data implicating folic acid deficiency as a risk factor. These factors may explain the regional variation in cervical cancer incidence.

Oral contraceptives

As a result of confounding factors the role of contraceptive method in cervical carcinogensis is difficult to evaluate. Traditional risk factors require controls as well as the contraceptive method. Women who use barrier contraceptives may have more protection than those who do not. Studies that control for all of these factors indicate that the longer a woman uses the pill, the greater her risk of cervical cancer becomes. Overall relative adjusted risk from the World Health Organization (WHO) Collaborative Study of Neoplasia and Steroid Contraceptives for pill users was 1.2. The same group found a 1.5 relative adjusted risk when the pill was used for 5 years or more.

PATHOPHYSIOLOGY
Role of sexual function

Since the 1840s when intercourse was identified as a risk factor for development of cervical cancer virtually every substance that could be transmitted sexually had its moment as hypothesized causative agent. The traditional sexually transmitted diseases gonorrhea and syphilis, sperm deoxyribonucleic acid (DNA), trichomoniasis, herpes simplex virus-2 (HSV-2), Epstein-Barr virus, and now human papillomavirus (HPV) have been implicated at some time. None is still considered a possible cause except the sexually transmitted viruses.

Although herpes was the first considered, its role has never been consistently supported either by culture finding or by sophisticated DNA hybridization methods. In the early 1970s several case-controlled studies compared the prevalence of serum antibodies to HSV-2. The control subjects had a lower rate of positivity than high-risk patients. Unfortunately these studies were complicated by cross-reactivity to HSV-1. Also one point value could not determine whether HSV-2 infection preceded the development of cervical cancer. Therefore the best assessment of HSV-2 data thus far is to assume that its presence indicates that sexual activity most likely has occurred.

Role of human papillomavirus

An association between human papillomavirus (HPV)-induced lesions and preinvasive disease of the female lower reproductive tract was first noted in 1976. Then exophytic and flat condylomata were seen in conjunction with cervical intraepithelial neoplasia (CIN) and some cases of invasive cervical cancer. Immunochemical studies using antibodies that reacted to exophytic condylomata antigens revealed proteins associated with HPV in preinvasive cervical lesions. This finding has only been strengthened with the isolation first of HPV 6 DNA and subsequent DNA types. Using DNA hybridization techniques a strong association has been found between the presence of HPV DNA and preinvasive and invasive cervical disease. Late in the 1980s it became apparent that HPV DNA can integrate into host cell DNA. Integration seems to correlate strongly with increasing grades of CIN and with invasive cervical cancer. No final step between HPV infection and development of invasive cervical cancer has been determined.

Transition from precancerous to cancerous lesions

Initially the Papanicolaou's (Pap) smear was developed to identify those patients with early, asymptomatic cervical cancer in the hope that they would be more amenable to intervention. It was not until the 1960s that Pap smear screening for preinvasive cervical disease was established. Then preinvasive cervical disease was broken down into different degrees of abnormality, such that mild dysplasia (abnormal growth), moderate dysplasia and severe dysplasia were separate, defined categories. Later in the 1960s the hypothesis that preinvasive disease of the cervix represented a continuity of change was proposed and the term *cervical intraepithelial neoplasia* was coined. This idea that preinvasive cervical disease could move forward to invasive cancer or back to normal epithelium is taken for granted today. However, it formed the basis of our limited understanding of how invasive cervical cancer develops. What causes the initial change from normal epithelium to abnormal is the basis of intense research. In general HPV is felt to be intimately involved in the process. Other environmental or genetic factors probably play a role but currently remain undefined.

HUMAN PAPILLOMAVIRUS EPIDEMIOLOGY
Historical aspects

Descriptions of clinical lesions that we now know were caused by HPV have been in the literature since antiquity. These lesions even then were thought to be transmitted sexually. Since the isolation of HPV 6 DNA in 1980 an explosion of knowledge about HPV has occurred. The vast majority of these data were accumulated by using molecular biologic techniques. The reason such sophisticated science is needed is that HPV will not grow in cell culture. Although advances in DNA techniques have helped the lack of a culture system for HPV has certainly constrained the limits of our knowledge.

Definition of human papillomavirus type

Human papillomaviruses will only grow within human epithelium. However, different viral types appear to have preferences for certain regions of epithelium. A type is defined by the extent of its DNA homology with other, previously isolated HPV DNA types. To be a new type it must have less than 50% DNA homology with other known types. This homology is measured in a standard liquid hybridization assay. Classification is then based on DNA analysis and predilection for certain epithelium. There are now 60 known HPV types. In general the important ones in the human reproductive tract are HPV 6, 11, 16, 18, 31, 33, and 35, 39, 42, 43, 44, 45, 50, and 51 to 60. If HPV-related lesions are separated into two groups, low-risk (condylomata, low-grade CIN) versus high-risk (high-grade CIN, invasive cancer), certain HPV types are associated with each group. Types 6, 11, and 42 are found in low-risk lesions, and 16, 18, 33, 35, and 39 in high-risk lesions.

Natural history of human papillomavirus infection

Although other methods of transmission cannot be fully excluded, studies as early as the 1950s have supported a sexual route of HPV infection. Servicemen returning home who had condylomata gave the infection to their consorts within 6 weeks to 3 months. This type of lesion is overwhelmingly associated with HPV 6. The incubation period for other HPV viruses is not as well defined.

To define the natural history of a disease it must be followed without treatment for a period. Studies usually confirm the cytologic or colposcopic impression of HPV-related infection by biopsy. Then patients are followed by colposcopy and Pap smears unless progression of the lesion is suspected. What these studies have uncovered is the fluctuating course of infection. In the low-grade preinvasive disease group between 20% and 60% of the lesions spontaneously regress. As the degree of CIN increases the chance of spontaneous lesion regression starts to decrease.

Prospective studies have revealed that HPV-infected women can fluctuate between clinically evident infections and subclinical or latent infections. Clinically evident infections are defined as those that can be demonstrated by clinical diagnostic methods. Either Pap smear, colposcopy, or tissue biopsy will reveal evidence of the infection. Subclinical or latent infections are defined as those cases in which no evidence of HPV infection can be documented except by HPV DNA analysis. As a result of the complexity involved in defining subclinical infections no well-documented data

exist as to their clinical significance or long-term prognosis. Even the rate of progression to clinically evident infection is not known. These problems with latent infections become important clinically when large-scale screening for the presence of HPV is considered. If HPV DNA is detected in clinically asymptomatic women the prognosis of this finding remains unknown.

Methods of human papillomavirus detection

Methods that detect the presence of HPV can be divided into two groups: those that will detect only clinically evident infection and those that will detect both clinical and subclinical diseases. For the clinically evident infection Pap smears and histologic examination detect the presence of HPV-related lesions. Any other proof that HPV is indeed present thus far relies on DNA analysis. Until HPV can be grown in a culture system some type of DNA analysis will be necessary to detect subclinical disease and to confirm documentation of its presence in clinically evident infection.

Thus far, the methods of clinical detection rely on characteristic findings on cytologic or histologic review. These methods, although documented as highly reliable for the presence of HPV DNA, will not reveal the HPV type that is associated with the lesion. Cytologic evidence is defined as the presence of koliocytic changes through tissue associated with preinvasive or invasive disease. Histologic counterparts exist for koliocytic changes and preinvasive disease. Some progress has been made in defining morphologic changes that can be associated with HPV 16, which is commonly thought to be strongly associated with high-grade CIN.

Categories of DNA studies can be made by using the sensitivity of the assay as the basis for distinction. In order of increasing sensitivity there is in situ hybridization (detects 10 to 50 HPV gene copies per cell), southern blot hybridization (detects less than one HPV gene copy per cell), and polymerase chain reaction (detects one HPV gene per 100,000 cells). Even such sophisticated techniques cannot be viewed as 100% accurate. This is due to variations in any given laboratory's ability to perform and interpret these techniques, and detection is subject to sampling error. HPV DNA is not equally distributed within the lower reproductive tract epithelium, and it is possible to obtain different results from different epithelial areas within the same patient. Most investigators try to use at least two different DNA techniques for any study.

Factors involved in prevalence of human papillomavirus

Determining the prevalence of HPV is fraught with many problems. These problems range from the characteristics of the group being screened to the method of detection and the age of the patient group. Every study looking at the issue of prevalence has to define these parameters.

It would be helpful to determine the background rate of HPV infection in humans. This has been approached by evaluating low-risk women, that is, those who do not have risk factors for cervical cancer. The problem with this approach is that it is not entirely clear that the risks for HPV infection mirror those for cervical cancer. Studies have focused on women who do not have any clinical evidence of HPV infection. Unfortunately these studies were not always controlled for cervical cancer risk factors. Also it is difficult to screen large asymptomatic groups through methods that require tissue or even cytologic specimens. Some progress has been made with serologic techniques, but these methods are extremely time consuming and labor intensive.

Once the characteristics of the study group have been defined, then the method of detection becomes a factor. The lack of standardization of these methods has hampered the ability to compare studies and subsequent rates of infection. Generally the overall rate of asymptomatic infection detected by clinical methods ranges from 2% to 5%. If polymerase chain reaction (PCR) is used then up to 80% of the asymptomatic population harbors this virus.

Most studies have indicated that the peak infection rate occurs at about 20 years of age. There appears to be a stabilization of the rate at about 10% after the age of 40. This infection rate most likely will vary if risk factors for cervical cancer are applied to each group. However, large prospective studies have not addressed both issues thus far. Also, as the population ages these values may change.

Role of human papillomavirus types in cervical cancer development

There is no doubt that world-wide data support a strong causal role between HPV infection and the development of preinvasive and invasive cervical disease. Common factors associated with HPV infections and cervical cancer can be summarized as follows:

1. HPV is a sexually transmitted disease and has the same associated risk factors as those known to predispose women to cervical cancer.
2. HPV is involved in all facets of benign, preinvasive, and invasive disease.
3. HPV infection shares the same natural history as that of CIN (potential to progress to invasive disease if left untreated).
4. Data support a long latency period for HPV infection in both sexes.
5. HPV type and physical state of the virus (i.e., integration versus episomal state) appears to be related to the malignant potential of the virus.
6. HPV probably does not act alone in cervical carcinogenesis but requires some form of cofactor.
7. HPV infections appear to vary in their clinical course if the immunologic status of the host is altered.

Of all the HPV types, type 16 has had the strongest association. Its presence in high-grade CIN and invasive squamous cervical cancer is generally reported as 80% to 95%. Further, it has been found that HPV 16 becomes integrated into the host cell DNA. It is believed that integration represents a significant step in the subsequent development of high-grade preinvasive and invasive disease. Obviously the viral DNA's ability to affect host cell function will be markedly changed with this development. Although it affects the incidence of invasive disease there are no geographic differences in the incidence of HPV 16 in cervical cancer. Age, however, does seem to affect the incidence of HPV 16. Recent data suggest that if all factors related to HPV infection and cervical carcinogenesis are controlled, HPV 16 is not independent of increasing patient age. The

effect of age is interesting and requires further study. Increasing age also parallels the natural history of CIN and invasive disease.

SCREENING
History of Papanicolaou's smear

Papanicolaou's smear was developed by Dr. George Papanicolaou in the 1930s. Widespread usage for screening started in the 1940s and, as previously discussed, it was initially used as a tool to identify those patients who had asymptomatic cervical cancer. Since the 1960s when preinvasive disease became defined, there have been an explosion of preinvasive disease and a significant decrease in incidence of invasive cancer and mortality rate of this disease.

The Pap smear process depends on collecting exfoliated cervical cells by scraping the cervical epithelium. Falsely negative Pap smear results can be caused by improper scraping technique and lack of exfoliation of the cervical cells. Marked improvement occurs when the clinician uses an endocervical brush in addition to an Ayer's wooden or plastic spatula. Air-drying artifact is reduced if the endocervical specimen is plated before the cervical scrape. Other reasons for false-negative Pap smear results are improper fixation or staining of the cells and incorrect interpretation. False-negative rates of 20% to 57% have been reported.

Significance of screening

It is estimated that screening women 20 to 65 years old every 3 years will decrease the incidence and mortality rates of invasive cervical cancer by approximately 90%. Factors that affect the mortality rate of cervical cancer include the population's natural incidence of the disease, the preclinical stage duration, the sensitivity and specificity of the screening process, and the quality of treatment available for preinvasive and invasive diagnoses. Studies have evaluated the age at which screening should start, the frequency with which it should be done, the age when screening should cease, and the appropriate personnel to perform the screening examination.

There seems to be little debate when a woman should start to undergo periodic screening. Most would agree that once regular intercourse has started the risk for development of preinvasive disease is present. How often a Pap smear should be done after initiation of periodic screening is not clear (Table 77-1). The American College of Obstetricians and Gynecologists in conjunction with several other major cancer organizations have recently recommended that every woman should have a yearly Pap smear and pelvic examination starting at age 18 or at the onset of sexual activity. Screening should occur yearly for 3 years. If the results are normal the physician can recommend that the screening interval be extended. There has been much debate as to the cost-effectiveness of this approach. Eddy's data indicate that screening once every 1 to 2 years as compared to every 3 years increases the effectiveness by less than 5%. His data clearly show that as screening becomes more frequent, the cost and inconvenience that result from unnecessary diagnostic procedures grow. One concern clinically is that if women do not have annual Pap smears they also will not have annual bimanual examinations. Therefore, screening for other gynecologic problems as well as ovarian cancer (for which there is no other adequate screening protocol) will not

Table 77-1 Recommendations for routine Papanicolaou's smear screening for cervical cancer

Group	Age to start	Interval to repeat	Age to stop	Other comments
National Institute's Health Consensus Conference on Cervical Cancer Screening, 1980	18 or onset sexual activity	1-3 years after 2 normal, consecutive annual results	60 if previous screening adequate and Pap smears negative findings	
Canadian Task Force on Cervical Cancer, 1991	18 or onset sexual activity	1-3 years after 2 normal, consecutive annual results	69 and stop if all previous screen results were normal	
American College of Obstetricians and Gynecologists, 1989	18 or onset of sexual activity	Annually for 3 consecutive years then at physician recommend interval	No recommendation	Annual bimanual pelvic examination
United States Preventive Health Task Force, 1989	Onset of sexual activity	1-3 years on physician recommendation based on risk factors	65 if physician can document consistently normal previous pap smear results	
National Cancer Institute, 1990	18 or onset sexual activity	After 3 normal consecutive annual results, repeat less frequently	No recommendation	

American College of Obstetrics and Gynecology Committee Opinion: *Report of the task force on routine cancer screening,* Washington, DC, 1989, American College of Obstetrics and Gynecology;
Report of a national workshop on screening for cancer of the cervix, *Can Med Assoc J* 145 (10):1301, 1991.
Fink DJ: Change in American Cancer Society checkup guidelines for detection of cervical cancer, *Cancer* 38:127, 1988.
Guide to clinical preventive services: an assessment of the effectiveness of 169 interventions: report of the U.S. Preventive Services Task Force, Baltimore, 1989, William and Wilkins.
McPhee SJ, Bird JA: Implementation of cancer prevention guidelines in clinical practice, *J Gen Int Med (Suppl):* 116, 1990.
HIV, human immunodeficiency virus.

be completed. There are no consistant recommendations for how often to perform the bimanual examination or whether the bimanual examination is a sensitive screening procedure.

Studies have retrospectively looked at the interval between diagnosis of cervical cancer and the previous pap smear. Uncontrolled data from New York State assessed the interval from the last Pap smear and the onset of cervical cancer in 261 women diagnosed from 1983 to 1985. These data indicated that 54% had an interval of greater than 3 years between last Pap smear and diagnosis of disease. When case-controlled study situations were evaluated it was found that the overall number of Pap smears was inversely related to the risk of disease. Although the exact number varied most patients received significant protection from cervical cancer when the interval of screening was 4 or fewer years. When compared to those patients who were never screened those who had at least three Pap smears had the risk of development of cervical cancer decreased by 90%. Interestingly those patients whose Pap smears were done by an obstetrician-gynecologist had significantly less chance of development of invasive cancer over any specific interval evaluated. This finding may be related to the introduction of the cervical brush.

Unfortunately large retrospective studies show that screening decreases as age increases. Estimates of never-screened women age 65 years or older are as high as 63%. Even more unfortunate are the retrospective data that indicate that close to 80% of these unscreened women had seen a medical practitioner within the past 2 years, with greater than 90% indicating visits within the past 5 years. These data, along with data indicating that only 11% of women realize that Pap smears are done to prevent cervical cancer, indicates how important it is to educate women and primary care providers. When using a mathematical model to pre-

dict reductions in mortality rate by instituting triennial screening in women over 65 years old approximately a 74% reduction would occur. Still there is no consensus when a patient should stop having routine Pap smear screening. Although there is a documented increased risk of development of cervical cancer as age increases, a patient who has had frequent, negative Pap smear results before the age of 65 benefits less from routine screening after age 65. Since a large percentage of patients in this age group have not been either screened or screened regularly, it seems prudent to extend periodic testing beyond age 65. Again a physician should make such a decision.

Cost-effectiveness of screening

It is essentially a given that mass screening programs for the prevention of cervical cancer will use the Pap smear as the screening tool. However, the question of whether a Pap smear is the appropriate tool has to be asked. Cervical cytologic testing generally yields an abnormal result around 5% of the time. When cervical colposcopy is used as a primary screening tool, an additional 6% of preinvasive lesions is found. This leads to an overall rate of 11%. It appears that those lesions that were not detected by cytologic examination alone repesented small lesions occupying less than two quadrants of the cervix. Larger lesions were uniformly identified by Pap smear. Because Pap smear is less than half the cost of colposcopy, further data on the clinical potential of these smaller lesions will be necessary before routine colposcopy should be advocated as a screening tool.

When using the Pap smear as the screening tool essentially all the studies indicate that the more frequent the screening, the most common it will be that unnecessary diagnostic and treatment procedures will be done. In comparing the cost of screening to the cost of treating and supporting invasive disease, screening programs that decrease the incidence of invasive disease will be cost-effective. It is estimated that the relative risk of development of cervical cancer when comparing those never screened with those screened at least once, is 0.32.

It becomes more difficult to choose more frequent screening and to determine where the cut-offs will be in terms of disease avoided versus cost. It is clear from the literature that an interval of 2 to 3 years provides excellent protection against development of invasive disease although it is more costly for each life year saved. The problem that clinicians face is that Pap smear results, and even subsequent evaluation by colposcopy and histologic testing, have no ability to predict which woman is really at risk for development of cervical cancer.

Recommendations for routine Pap smear screening

The current recommendations for when to perform screening Pap smears appear in Table 77-1. The standard of care generally adheres to the recommendations by the American College of Obstetricians and Gynecologists and the United States Preventive Health Task Force.

APPROACH TO WOMAN WITH AN ABNORMAL PAP SMEAR RESULT

Follow-up of abnormal Pap smear results

The results of the screening Pap smear will determine the recommendations and advice the clinician gives to the woman. Table 77-2 summarizes the current recommendations for follow-up of an abnormal Pap smear result.

If the Pap smear result is **negative for malignant cells** and is an adequate sample (judged by the presence of endocervical cells) then the clinican should follow the guidelines for routine Pap smear screening outlined in Table 77-1. It is important to know what endocervical cells are present to assure an adequate sampling. If the **endocervical cells are not present** then the clinician should schedule the repeat Pap smear on the basis of the risk of development of disease for the particular woman. For instance if the woman has multiple risk factors and therefore is at increased risk for the development of cervical dysplasia and cancer, one generally repeats the Pap smear not less than 6 weeks or more than 3 months after the inadequate sample. If the patient is at low risk, then it is appropriate to recommend that the Pap smear be repeated at the annual visit.

There are some results on Pap smears, such as **squamous metaplasia,** that are considered normal and require no intervention other than following the guidelines for routine Pap smear screening.

The finding of **atypia** is abnormal. However, except for women who are HIV-positive, the Pap smear is generally repeated in 3 to 4 months and any underlying infection, such as trichomonas or gardnerella is treated. If the woman is HIV-positive referral to a gynecologist for colposcopy is indicated.

Finally, a finding of **dysplasia** or **squamous intraepithelial lesion** requires referral for colposcopy. (See Plate 12 of the front feature section.) Because of the cross-over of the risk factors (i.e., sexual activity) between HPV and HIV exposure, women with dysplasia should be screened for all HIV risk factors. Testing should be considered when appropriate or on the request of the patient.

SUMMARY

Women should be screened for cervical cancer and its precursors. Routine Pap smear screening will decrease the indicence and mortality rates of cervical cancer. Data clearly support a Pap smear every 3 years for women age 20 to 65. Whether it is cost-effective to decrease the screening interval or extend screening beyond age 65 is not entirely apparent.

Another factor that can reduce the incidence and mortality rates of cervical cancer is education of the medical practitioner and patient about cervical cancer risk factors, and the benefits of screening. Decrease of the number of women who smoke will lead to a decrease in cervical cancer development. Other, less well-defined factors, such as the role of diet and oral contraceptives, would benefit from further study. Increasing the number of women who are routinely screened will also lead to a reduction in the incidence of cervical cancer.

The evidence that suggests a causal role for HPV in the development of preinvasive and invasive cervical disease is strong. Most of these data stem from molecular biologic data identifying the presence and physical state of HPV DNA. However, molecular data indicate a high prevalence rate for HPV infection and thus the idea that HPV requires some type of cofactor. The epidemiologic data for smoking, use of oral contraceptives, and geographic differences in disease incidence support the role of a possible cofactor. What the cofactor(s) may be will be an area of research in the 1990s.

Table 77-2 Follow-up of abnormal Pap smear results

Pap smear result	Recommendation for follow-up
Negative for malignant cells	See guidelines for routine Pap smear
No endocervical cells	If high risk, repeat within 1 month
	If low risk, repeat at annual check-up
	Use cervical brush technique for improved sampling
Squamous metaplasia	Normal result
Atypia	Consider treatment for underlying infection
	Repeat in 3-4 months unless HIV-positive
	If HIV-positive, refer directly for colposcopy
	If atypia still present on repeat smear in normal host, refer for colposcopy
Dysplasia	Refer for colposcopy

Modified from the Algorithm for follow-up of abnormal Pap Smear results, 1988, Harvard Community Health Plan.

BIBLIOGRAPHY

American College of Obstetrics and Gynecology Committee Opinion: *Report of the task force on routine cancer screening,* Washington DC, 1989, American College of Obstetrics and Gynecology.
Bosch FX et al: Second international workshop on the epidemiology of cervical cancer and human papillomavirus, *Int J Cancer* 52:171, 1992.
Eddy DM: Screening for cervical cancer, *Ann Intern Med* 113:214, 1990.
Fahs MC et al: Cost effectiveness of cervical cancer screening for the elderly, *Ann Intern Med* 117:520, 1992.

Fletcher A: Screening for cancer of the cervix in elderly women, Lancet 335:97, 1990.

Fink DJ: Change in American Cancer Society checkup guidelines for detection of cervical cancer, *Cancer* 38:127, 1988.

Giles JA et al: Colposcopic assessment of the accuracy of cervical cytology screening, *Br Med J* 296:1099, 1988.

Guide to clinical preventive services: an assessment of the effectiveness of 169 interventions: report of the U.S. Preventive Services Task Force, Baltimore, 1989, William & Wilkins.

Harlan LC, Bernstein AM, Kessler LG: Cervical cancer screening: who is not screened and why? *Am J Public Health* 81:885, 1991.

Klassen AC, Celentano DD, Brookmeyer R: Variation in the duration of protection given by screening using the pap test for cervical cancer, *J Clin Epidemiol* 42:1003, 1989.

Koopmanschap MA, van Ineveld BM, Miltenburg TE: Costs of home care for advanced breast and cervical cancer in relation to cost-effectiveness of screening, *Soc Sci Med* 35:979, 1992.

McPhee SJ, Bird JA: Implementation of cancer prevention guidelines in clinical practice, *J Gen Int Med* (Suppl): 116, 1990.

Meanwell CA: The epidemiology of human papillomavirus infection in relation to cervical cancer, *Cancer Surv* 7:481, 1988.

Nasca PC et al: An epidemiologic study of pap screening histories in women with invasive carcinomas of the uterine cervix, *NY State J Med* 91:152, 1991.

Parazzini F et al: Screening practices and invasive cervical cancer risk in different age strata, *Gynecol Oncol* 38:76, 1990.

Reeves WC, Rawls WE, Brinton LA: Epidemiology of genital papillomaviruses and cervical cancer, *Rev Infect Dis* 11:426, 1989.

Report of a national workshop on screening for cancer of the cervix, *Can Med Assoc J* 145(10):1301, 1991.

Schiffman MH: Recent progress in defining the epidemiology of human papillomavirus infection and cervical neoplasia. *J Nat Cancer Inst* 84:394, 1992.

Schwartz M et al: Woman's knowledge and experience of cervical screening: a failure of health education and medical organization, *Community Med* 11:279, 1989.

Syrjanen KJ: Epidemiology of human papillomavirus (HPV) infections and their associations with genital squamous cell cancer, APMIS 97:957, 1989.

Syrjanen K, Syrjanen S: Epidemiology of human papilloma virus infections and genital neoplasia. *Scan J Infect Dis [Suppl]* 69:7, 1990.

van Ballegooijen M et al: Diagnostic and treatment procedures induced by cervical cancer screening, *Eur J Cancer* 26:941, 1990.

van der Graaf Y, et al: The effectiveness of cervical screening: a population-based case-control study, *J Clin Epidemiol* 41:21, 1988.

---

78 Endometrial, Ovarian, and Vulvar Cancer

Karen J. Carlson

In the course of providing routine care, the primary care clinician has the opportunity to screen asymptomatic women for common gynecologic malignancies. The value of the Papanicolaou's (Pap) smear for early detection of cervical neoplasia is well supported by a body of indirect evidence (Chapter 77). There is less scientific information to document the benefit of screening for other malignancies of the female genital tract, including endometrial, ovarian, and vulvar cancers. This chapter provides an overview of the epidemiology and risk factors for these diseases, reviews screening procedures suitable for the primary care setting, and provides recommendations for screening based on the available evidence for its effectiveness. The focus of this chapter is screening of the asymptomatic woman. The approach to women with symptoms warranting evaluation of endometrial cancer (Chapter 28), ovarian cancer (Chapter 37), or vulvar cancer (Chapter 31) is discussed elsewhere.

ENDOMETRIAL CANCER
Epidemiology

Endometrial cancer is the most common gynecologic malignancy (Table 78-1). Its incidence has increased in the past two decades, probably as a result of the growth in use of estrogen replacement therapy as well as the aging of the population. The incidence of endometrial cancer increases with age (Fig. 78-1), with an average age at diagnosis of 63 years. The mortality rate from endometrial cancer has fallen slightly over the past 20 years, and it is a less important cause of cancer deaths than other gynecologic malignancies (Fig. 78-2). Five-year survival rate for all stages combined is approximately 80% for white women and 55% for African-American women.

The risk factors for endometrial cancer (see the box on the following page) reflect a strong role for an excess of estrogen relative to progesterone in the biologic mechanism of the disease. These factors include obesity, chronic anovulation, nulliparity, late menopause, and unopposed estrogen therapy. Obesity is associated with a threefold increase in risk from excess weight of 25 to 50 pounds. The evidence for a familial association of endometrial cancer is relatively weak, except in rare kindreds with a hereditary syndrome of colon, endometrial, and ovarian cancer. Other risk factors reflect underlying immune compromise. The use of tamoxifen has been shown to increase endometrial cancer risk approximately twofold after 2 years of use. The risk of endometrial cancer is reduced by use of the oral contraceptive pill and by pregnancy.

Table 78-1 Estimated incidence and deaths from gynecologic cancers in the United States, 1994

Site	New Cancer Cases	Deaths
Endometrium	31,000	5900
Cervix	15,000	4600
Ovary	24,000	13,600
Other genital sites	5300	1100

Estimates based on rates from Surveillance, Epidemiology, and End Results (SEER) Program, National Cancer Institute.

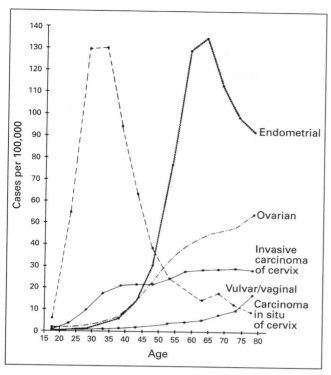

Fig. 78-1 Age-specific incidence of gynecologic cancers in women in the United States. (From Knapp RC, Berkowitz RS: *Gynecologic oncology,* New York, 1986, Macmillan.)

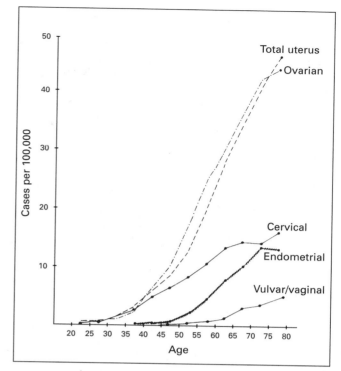

Fig. 78-2 Age-specific mortality rate of gynecologic cancers in women in the United States. (From Knapp RC, Berkowitz RS: *Gynecologic oncology,* New York, 1986, Macmillan.)

Screening techniques

The Pap smear is a relatively insensitive technique for early detection of endometrial cancer. However, if benign endometrial cells are observed on a Pap smear in a postmenopausal woman further evaluation with endometrial sampling is necessary.

Endometrial sampling has a high correlation with the results of formal dilation and curettage for detection of endometrial cancer. A variety of sampling methods are available for use in the outpatient setting. Methods that provide tissue specimens are more accurate than those that yield cytologic specimens; however, the cytologic techniques produce less discomfort and are easier to use in the ambulatory setting. The sensitivity of cytologic sampling methods (measured in women with vaginal bleeding) ranges

from 80% to 100% for detection of endometrial carcinoma and 35% to 45% for detection of endometrial hyperplasia. A single large cohort study of cytologic screening in asymptomatic women demonstrated an apparent sensitivity of 80% for detection of cancer (Koss et al., 1984).

The utility of transvaginal ultrasound in early detection of endometrial cancer has not been established. Preliminary studies indicate that the thickness of the endometrial stripe correlates well with the presence of endometrial hyperplasia and carcinoma. An endometrial thickness of less than 4 mm reliably indicates an atrophic endometrium in postmenopausal women; however, a thickness of 5 to 8 mm cannot distinguish proliferative from hyperplastic endometrium or endometrial carcinoma. In a postmenopausal woman not receiving hormone replacement therapy an endometrial thickness greater than 8 mm requires evaluation with endometrial biopsy.

Effectiveness of screening

There are sparse data to support routine screening of asymptomatic average-risk women for endometrial cancer. In the largest study of cytologic screening for endometrial cancer, in which the prevalence of cancer was 7/1000, the positive predictive value of screening was 17% to 20% (Koss et al., 1984). Thus 80% of women with a positive screening test result would be free of cancer but would be required to undergo further evaluation (such as dilation and curettage). There have been no randomized trials of screening using endometrial sampling, and no formal cost-effectiveness analyses of cytologic screening or transvaginal sonography have been published.

RISK FACTORS FOR ENDOMETRIAL CANCER	
Increased risk	**Decreased risk**
Obesity	Oral contraceptive pill
Nulliparity	Pregnancy
Late menopause	
Unopposed estrogen	
Chronic anovulation	
Family history of endometrial cancer	
History of breast, colon, or ovarian cancer	
History of diabetes	
History of radiation	
Tamoxifen	

In women with one or more risk factors for endometrial cancer the appropriate role of screening has not been defined. The exception is for women receiving unopposed estrogen replacement therapy, for whom consensus supports performance of annual endometrial biopsy. There has been a single study of cytologic screening in women at increased risk, which demonstrated a prevalence of preinvasive endometrial abnormality in 6% of diabetic women ages 45 to 69 years compared to 1% of women with hypertension (Gronroos et al., 1993).

Recommendations

Routine screening for endometrial cancer in asymptomatic women is not recommended. Women receiving unopposed estrogen replacement therapy should undergo periodic endometrial biopsy (see Chapter 36). In asymptomatic postmenopausal women with risk factors for endometrial cancer such as obesity or diabetes, routine screening with endometrial sampling is not recommended.

OVARIAN CANCER
Epidemiology

Ovarian cancer is the most common cause of death from a gynecologic malignancy (see Table 78-1). Mortality rate from the disease has increased only slightly over the past two decades. The incidence of ovarian cancer increases with age; the average age at clinical presentation is 59 years.

Aside from age the strongest risk factor for ovarian cancer identified to date is familial evidence of ovarian cancer (Table 78-2), which is present in about 7% of women with the disease. The two types of familial patterns of ovarian cancer are associated with different magnitudes of risk. The rare hereditary ovarian cancer syndromes, which may have an autosomal dominant mode of inheritance, can be associated with a lifetime risk of ovarian cancer as high as 50%. Clues to a hereditary ovarian cancer syndrome include the occurrence of ovarian, breast, endometrial, or colorectal cancers in several members of two or more generations of the family and presentation of ovarian cancer at an earlier age than the average of 59 years.

Much more common is a family history of ovarian cancer in a single first-degree or second-degree relative. Such a history is associated with a modest increase in absolute risk of the disease.

Table 78-2 Risk factors for ovarian cancer

Risk factor	Relative risk	Lifetime risk for ovarian cancer,%*
No risk factors	1.0	1.2
Hereditary ovarian cancer syndrome	Unknown	Up to 50
One relative with ovarian cancer	3.1	3.7
Two or three relatives with ovarian cancer	4.6	5.5
Oral contraceptive pill use	0.65	0.8
Pregnancy	0.5	0.6

Modified from Carlson KJ et al: *Ann Intern Med* 121:124, 1994.
*Risk for cancer in a 50-year-old woman.

Two factors have been strongly associated with a substantially decreased risk of ovarian cancer in epidemiologic studies: oral contraceptive pill use and parity (Table 78-2).

Screening techniques

The pelvic examination has been the traditional method of screening for ovarian cancer in the primary care setting. However, its value for the early detection of ovarian cancer has never been established. Some of the published studies of the pelvic examination for screening asymptomatic women suggest that an examination by a highly skilled examiner may identify early-stage ovarian cancer.

Pelvic ultrasonography by the transabdominal or transvaginal route has been investigated as a screening technique for ovarian cancer. The sensitivity of ultrasound for the detection of ovarian cancer (all stages combined) is 80% to 90%, and its specificity is 93% to 94%. Color-flow Doppler imaging is under study as a method for improving the specificity of ultrasonography.

The CA125 radioimmunoassay measures a tumor marker detectable in the serum of approximately 80% of women with ovarian cancer and in some with endometrial and pancreatic malignancies. Serum CA125 level may also be elevated in benign gynecologic conditions, including endometriosis, leiomyomas, benign ovarian cysts, and pelvic inflammatory disease. Most studies of CA125 for ovarian cancer screening have focused on postmenopausal women. The specificity of CA125 (defining an abnormal level as 35 U/ml or greater) in these studies ranges from 98% to 99%.

Effectiveness of screening

The feasibility of either ultrasonography or CA125 for screening has been limited by the relatively high false-positive rate of both tests. In an average-risk population of women 50 years and older, the positive predictive value of annual pelvic ultrasonography is less than 1%; thus only 1 woman in 100 with an ultrasound result suggestive of malignancy would actually have ovarian cancer. The predictive value of CA125 in a similar population is also unacceptably low (3%). The adverse consequences of false-positive test results are considerable because of the need for invasive diagnostic tests (laparotomy or laparoscopy) to evaluate suspected ovarian cancer.

In women with a family history of ovarian cancer in one relative, the prevalence of ovarian cancer is higher, and the predictive value of screening with CA125 is increased to approximately 10%. The predictive value of CA125 or ultrasonography in women with the rare hereditary ovarian cancer syndromes is unknown. In clinical practice a policy of screening female members of such families with CA125 and ultrasound is often followed because of the very high lifetime risk of malignancy. However, there are no randomized trials to determine whether mortality rate of ovarian cancer is decreased by screening in this or any other population of women.

Ongoing research on the combination of CA125 and ultrasound, the use of serial CA125 tests, or a combination of tumor markers may identify effective strategies for use of these techniques in screening asymptomatic women. A screening protocol for postmenopausal women evaluated by Jacobs et al. (1993), using CA125 as the primary screening test followed by ultrasound for those with abnormal CA125 levels, achieved a positive predictive value of 27%.

Recommendations

The available scientific evidence does not support screening for ovarian cancer with ultrasound or CA125 in premenopausal and postmenopausal women without a family history of ovarian cancer. For women with a family history of ovarian cancer in one or more relatives without evidence of a hereditary cancer syndrome, routine screening is not recommended. Individualized decisions about screening can be made after such women are counseled about their individual risk (considering age, parity, and history of oral contraceptive pill use) and advised of the potential adverse effects of screening. Because of the high risk of ovarian cancer in women from families with the rare hereditary ovarian cancer syndromes, referral to a gynecologic oncologist for follow-up evaluation is appropriate.

VULVAR CANCER
Epidemiology

Vulvar cancer is a relatively rare cause of cancer death in women (see Fig. 78-2). Invasive vulvar cancer largely occurs in older women; the average age at diagnosis is 70 years. Five-year survival rate for all stages combined is approximately 55%.

There is growing evidence that vulvar carcinoma may comprise two distinct clinical subsets. The first, occurring primarily in younger women, is related to sexually transmitted factors, principally human papillomavirus (HPV). Twenty to thirty percent of vulvar cancers subjected to histopathologic analysis contain HPV. The pathogenesis for the majority of vulvar carcinomas, which occur in older women, is less clear. A strong link between vulvar cancer and chronic vulvar inflammatory disease (also known as vulvar dystrophies) has been established. However, the risk of future vulvar carcinoma in women with hyperplastic or atrophic vulvar diseases has been reported at less than 5%, suggesting that in the great majority of women with these diseases cancer will not develop. Epidemiologic evidence for an association with other diseases (such as diabetes) is inconclusive.

Screening techniques

The most important screening technique for the primary care clinician is careful inspection of the vulva. Any white, reddened, ulcerated, nodular, fissured, or abnormal raised pigmented area should undergo biopsy.

Effectiveness of screening

There are no studies to determine whether early detection of vulvar cancer by screening is associated with reduced mortality rate from the disease.

Recommendations

Careful inspection of the vulva should be part of a pelvic examination performed for other reasons, such as cervical cancer screening. The epidemiologic associations of vulvar cancer suggest that the vulvar examination is particularly important in women with HPV and those with chronic vulvar inflammatory diseases. The value of periodic vulvar examination in women without risk factors who are not undergoing pelvic examination for other reasons has not been established.

BIBLIOGRAPHY

Canadian Task Force on the Periodic Health Examination: The periodic health examination. 1. Introduction. 2. 1987 Update, *Can Med Assoc J* 138:617, 1988.

Carlson KJ, Skates SJ, Singer DE: Screening for ovarian cancer, *Ann Intern Med* 121:124, 1994.

Crum CP: Carcinoma of the vulva: epidemiology and pathogenesis, *Obstet Gynecol* 79:448, 1992.

Gronroos M et al. Mass screening for endometrial cancer directed in risk groups of patients with diabetes and patients with hypertension, *Cancer* 71:1279, 1993.

Jacobs I et al: Prevalence screening for ovarian cancer in postmenopausal women by CA125 measurement and ultrasonography, *Br Med J* 306:1030, 1993.

Knapp RC, Berkowitz RS: *Gynecologic Oncology,* New York, 1986, Macmillan.

Koss LG et al: Detection of endometrial carcinoma and hyperplasia in asymptomatic women, *Obstet Gynecol* 64:1, 1984.

Pritchard KI: Screening for endometrial cancer: is it effective? *Ann Intern Med* 110:177, 1989.

U.S. Preventive Services Task Force: *Guide to clinical preventive services: An assessment of the effectiveness of 169 interventions,* Baltimore, 1989, Williams & Wilkins.

Varner RE et al: Transvaginal sonography of the endometrium in postmenopausal women, *Obstet Gynecol* 78:195, 1991.

Vuopala S: Diagnostic accuracy and clinical application of cytological and histological methods for investigating endometrial carcinoma, *Acta Scand Obstet Gynecol* 70 (suppl):1, 1977.

Section II

Other Preventive Issues

79 Occupational Hazards

L. Christine Oliver, Jennifer Helmick, and Carolyn S. Langer

On September 6, 1991, 25 workers were killed and 55 injured in an attempt to escape a fire that broke out in a chicken processing plant in Hamlet, North Carolina. Contributing to the high death toll were the lack of automatic heat-detection sprinkler systems and a fire evacuation plan, as well as blocked fire doors that failed to meet national safety standards. The plant had not undergone a safety inspection in the 11 years of its existence. Many of those killed were women. This unnecessary tragedy was reminiscent of the fire at the Triangle Shirtwaist Company in New York City on March 25, 1911. The fire killed 145 employees trapped in the burning building. Most of them were women.

In 1970 the Occupational Safety and Health Act (OSHA) was signed in to law. The purpose of the act was to ensure, insofar as possible, a safe and healthful workplace for every working American and to preserve human resources. Increasingly, working Americans are women. In 1975 female participation in the civilian labor force was 46.3%; it is estimated that the rate in 1995 will be 60.3%. Women will make up over half of the country's civilian work force.

Historically, women have been employed primarily in the service industries, in clerical jobs, and in semiskilled work in manufacturing industries. Female workers predominate in the retail trades; males predominate in the wholesale trades. Women also have occupied a larger proportion of nonconstruction low-paying unskilled jobs, such as those in the poultry processing industry. U.S. Department of Labor Bureau of Labor statistics for 1989 identified the poultry processing industry as second only to ship building and repair in the number of serious illnesses and injuries for each 100 workers. In the same year nine industries with ≥100,000 injury cases each were identified. These industries included eating and drinking establishments, retail grocery stores, hospitals, nursing and personal care facilities, department stores, and hotels and motels. These are industries in which female employees are likely to predominate.

Occupational disease is preventable. As a leading federal agency for prevention the Center for Disease Control (CDC) has categorized its approaches to injury and disease prevention on the basis of (1) delivery of prevention technologies and (2) timing of intervention by stage of disease or injury. Both approaches rely heavily on the primary care physician (1) to detect and reduce causal risk factors, such as lead exposure or poorly designed computer work stations; (2) to detect and appropriately treat disease at an early stage; and (3) to organize and deliver relevant tertiary health care. In the case of occupational injury or disease the latter includes rehabilitative services that minimize morbidity and allow for return to work at the same job in a different capacity or at a different job altogether. In many cases the accomplishment of these tasks will require a joint effort of the primary care physician and public health professionals, government and labor union officials, and employers.

This chapter discusses diagnosis of occupational disease, using a system-oriented approach to highlight occupational diseases for which women are at special risk. Legal and ethical issues are discussed in the context of the female worker and the attendant responsibilities of her primary care physician.

DIAGNOSIS OF OCCUPATIONAL DISEASE

Symptoms and physical findings in cases of occupational illness, disease, and injury are not unlike those seen in cases of disease and injury unrelated to work. Laboratory test results are rarely specific. For the clinician then the key to diagnosis is the *occupational history*. In addition to allowing correct diagnosis the occupational history promotes proper treatment, prevents worsening of disease or unnecessary development of iatrogenic disease, prevents the occurrence of disease in similarly exposed co-workers, and contributes to a database that allows a better understanding of the epidemiologic characteristics of occupational disease and injury.

Individuals may present clinical evidence of illness or disease or a history of work at a job that is potentially hazardous, on the basis of either an airborne or surface exposure or an ergonomic or physical hazard, such as heavy lifting or noise. In both cases the occupational history is the same. A chronologic lifetime work history is ideal and may be necessary in cases of known or suspected disease with long latency, such as asbestosis or asbestos-related lung cancer. In general a shorter and more focused history is sufficient for the primary care physician. If occupational disease is diagnosed or strongly suspected on the basis of the history or laboratory findings the physician may wish to refer the patient to an occupational physician in situations such as the following: (1) diagnosis depends on a more detailed evaluation of the workplace; (2) elimination of the causal exposure is possible only if the patient leaves her place of employment and a higher level of certainty regarding diagnosis is desired; or (3) the patient desires to file a workers compensation claim or suit against a third party and a medical opinion or legal testimony from the diagnosing physician will be required.

What is your present job?
What was your previous job?
What was the job you worked at the longest?

For risk assessment

Job title and job description
Tasks performed
Exposures (e.g., chemical, dust, gas, fumes): type and level
Adequacy of work area ventilation
Availability of personal protective equipment (e.g., gloves, respirators)

For evaluation of symptoms

Correlation between symptoms and known health effects of exposures
Temporal association of symptoms with work
Occurrence of symptoms or disease in coworkers

Critical components of the occupational history for the primary care clinician are shown in the box above. For each job years of hire and termination, as well as total duration of employment, are needed. Both job *title* and job *description* should be obtained. General estimates of level (e.g., mild, moderate, heavy) by the patient are useful in overall exposure assessment.

Of critical importance, particularly with regard to short-latency disease or illness such as asthma or angina, is an understanding of the temporal association of symptoms with work. Questions about severity of symptoms during the workday and workweek, at night and over the weekend, and on vacation will help elicit this information. Also important is information about occurrence of illness, disease, or injury among co-workers—particularly co-workers with the same job. Turnover rate may provide indirect information about the health and safety of the workplace.

Under the OSHA Hazards Communication Standard (29 Code of Federal Regulations 1910.1200), both employees and their physicians have a "right to know" what chemicals are in their workplace. This information exists in the form of Material Safety Data Sheets (MSDS). These give both generic and brand names, chemical composition, reported acute and chronic health effects, and steps to be taken in the event of overexposure. Because MSDSs are required only for chemicals and because employers may resist providing MSDSs it is useful to obtain additional information from other sources (see the section, Resources). Information about exposures may be obtained on the basis of reported job and nature of work; and information about health effects, on the basis of exposures. Examples are shown in Table 79-1. When assessing the potential for exposure to hazards all routes of exposure should be considered, including transdermal, inhalation, and ingestion.

OCCUPATIONAL HEALTH HAZARDS FOR WOMEN BY SYSTEM
Respiratory

Occupational lung disease is one of the nation's 10 leading causes of work-related illness and disease. Although it does not preferentially affect women it is a major cause of morbidity among female workers. Causes include inhaled organic and inorganic dusts, irritants, vapors, gases, and

Table 79-1 Occupational respiratory hazards

Site of effect	Causal agents	Disease process	Typical exposures in women
Lung parenchyma	Irritant gases (e.g., chlorine, nitrogen dioxide, ammonia)	Pulmonary edema Pneumonitis	Cleaning, laboratory work, welding
	Organic dusts (e.g., thermophilic actinomycetes)	Hypersensitivity pneumonitis (acute phase) Fibrosis, granulomatosis (chronic phase)	Farming, clerical work
	Inorganic dusts (e.g., asbestos, silica)	Pulmonary restriction	Textile manufacture, construction, household contact
	Metals (e.g., beryllium, cobalt)	Pulmonary restriction or obstruction; granuloma formation	Electronics, tool and die manufacture, ceramics manufacture
Airways	Irritants, gases, fumes, dust	Bronchitis	Laboratory work, construction, cleaning
	High-molecular-weight particles (e.g., wheat, rye flour, enzymes)	Asthma	Detergent manufacture, baking, shellfish processing
	Low-molecular-weight compounds (e.g., toluene diisocyanate)	Asthma	Paint, polyurethane, and plastics manufacture
	Irritants, gases, fumes (e.g., nitrogen oxides)	Asthma	Welding
	Metals (e.g., cobalt, platinum, nickel)	Asthma	Welding, tool and die manufacture
	Inadequate ventilation ("sick building syndrome")	Rhinitis, laryngitis, cough, bronchospasm	Clerical, service jobs

fumes, as well as work in inadequately ventilated buildings. Both upper and lower respiratory tracts may be affected. Latency may be short (e.g., asthma, rhinitis, acute pulmonary beryllium disease) or long (e.g., asbestosis, exposure-related lung cancer). In the past interstitial fibrosis of the lung has been the major type of occupational lung disease seen in the clinical setting; it is likely to be supplanted by occupational asthma in the coming decades as exposure to such agents as asbestos and coal dust diminishes and new chemicals with the potential to induce bronchospasm are introduced in the workplace.

Categorization by effect. The workplace exposures described may affect the lung interstitium, the airways, the pleura, and the nasal mucosa and sinuses. Effects on the lung parenchyma include inflammation, fibrosis, and granuloma formation. Causal agents and respiratory effects are summarized in Table 79-1. In the case of irritant gases such as phosgene and NO_2, exposure may antedate the onset of pulmonary edema by 12 to 24 hours. The degree of penetration into the lung is inversely related to water solubility, so that gases with less solubility, such as NO_2, penetrate deeply into the lung, whereas those with greater solubility, such as ammonia, are deposited higher in the respiratory tract.

Hypersensitivity pneumonitis may be acute, including shortness of breath, cough, chest pain, and fever. If the illness is not diagnosed and exposure continues a chronic form of the disease may develop, with granuloma formation and irreversible fibrosis. **Asbestosis, silicosis,** and **coal workers' pneumoconiosis** have characteristic radiographic and pathologic pictures. Latency is generally 10 years or more and may vary by level of exposure.

Work-related airways disease includes industrial bronchitis and reversible and irreversible airways obstruction. Industrial bronchitis is characterized by cough and sputum, worse at work. It is a nonspecific manifestation of airway irritation and inflammation and may occur in association with exposure to irritants, gases, fumes, and dust. **Occupational asthma** is reversible airway obstruction related to exposure to a wide variety of substances found in the workplace. **Reactive airways dysfunction syndrome** (RADS) is an example of reversible airway obstruction that may occur after a single or limited number of exposures to relatively high levels of irritant gases and fumes. Symptoms often persist for years after exposure. Because of the variable nature of airway obstruction and the possibility of normal lung function when the patient is on optimal medication, clinical assessment of disability from work is particularly difficult with asthma. It may be that there is disability without demonstrable physiologic impairment at given points in time.

Among the first case reports of **pulmonary beryllium disease** were those from a group of women exposed to beryllium during the course of work in fluorescent light bulb manufacture. In addition to the lung parenchyma, beryllium may affect the airways, producing an obstructive physiologic defect. Clinically and pathologically, pulmonary beryllium disease resembles sarcoidosis. Distinguishing features are history of exposure and blast transformation of lymphocytes in the lung lavage on exposure to beryllium salts in vitro. Similarly, cobalt may affect either the airways or the lung parenchyma, causing asthma or so-called hard metals

disease. The latter is characterized by the presence of multinucleated giant cells in the lung and lung lavage.

A constellation of respiratory health effects has been reported among workers in buildings with inadequate ventilation—so-called sick building syndrome. Symptoms include rhinitis, laryngitis, cough, and wheeze. Identified causal factors include formaldehyde and other volatile organic hydrocarbon vapors from carpeting, draperies, and upholstered furniture; fiberglass dust from ceiling tiles and insulation material; low relative humidity; diesel fumes from outside traffic; and environmental tobacco smoke. To the extent that many jobs held by women are clerical and service, women are at particular risk for the development of this problem.

Musculoskeletal

Musculoskeletal disorders rank as the leading cause of disability in the United States for work-age individuals. At least 50% of the work force will be affected by musculoskeletal injuries at some point in their careers. These include "acute and chronic injuries to muscles, tendons, ligaments, nerves, joints, bones, and supporting vasculature." Injuries most commonly involve the back, cervical spine, and upper extremities and are usually characterized by the structure affected (e.g., tendonitis, synovitis, bursitis).

Musculoskeletal injuries result from biomechanical stresses that exceed the worker's physical capabilities and limitations (see box, below). Primary risk factors include heavy lifting, repetitive motion, vibration, poor posture, and excessive bending, twisting, reaching, pushing, and pulling. Secondary factors include age, gender, strength, physical fitness, fatigue, trauma, emotional stress, and preexisting conditions such as degenerative changes. Women may be particularly prone to musculoskeletal injuries because many work stations, tools, and types of protective gear are designed for the average male body stature and physical capacity.

Despite indications that the *average* female tolerates lower maximum weights and forces than the *average* male, physical capacities vary widely among *individual* males and

---

RISK FACTORS FOR OCCUPATIONAL MUSCULOSKELETAL DISORDERS

Primary risk factors

Heavy lifting
Repetitive motion
Vibration
Poor posture
Excessive bending, twisting, reaching, pushing, pulling

Secondary risk factors

Age
Gender
Strength and physical fitness
Fatigue
Trauma
Emotional stress
Preexisting conditions (e.g., degenerative arthritis)

---

females. Therefore employers should use sound ergonomic principles that seek to fit specific jobs to individual workers, whether male or female. Mechanical aides and work station and tool redesign represent the most effective ways to reduce the risk of musculoskeletal injuries in the workplace. Examples include use of conveyor belts, hoists, lift tables, proper work-surface heights, and contoured hand grips on tools.

Employee selection by type of job is a less suitable method for prevention of musculoskeletal injuries in the workplace. Selection criteria may be discriminatory, unrelated to actual job demands, or poorly predictive of potential for injury. For example, radiographs of the lumbosacral region, once widely used as a screening tool, have been invalidated as a predictor for back injuries in workers.

Physicians who treat workers for musculoskeletal injuries should inquire beyond job titles into specific job tasks with particular emphasis on frequency, intensity, duration, and direction of biomechanical forces to which patients are exposed. Careful exploration of work station conditions and job demands not only will assist in identifying the cause of many work-related musculoskeletal disorders but may lead to useful insights into prevention and job modification through ergonomic interventions. Carpal tunnel syndrome, an occupational musculoskeletal disorder common in women, is discussed in detail in Chapter 24.

Reproductive

The National Institute for Occupational Safety and Health (NIOSH) has ranked disorders of the reproductive system among the nation's 10 leading categories of work-related injuries and illnesses. Reproductive hazards include any chemical, physical, or biologic agent that can harm the reproductive system or a developing fetus or child. For women the effects of reproductive hazards can include one or more of the following: altered menstrual function; decreased libido; reduced fertility; adverse pregnancy outcomes (e.g., spontaneous abortion, preterm birth, low birth weight, structural abnormality, or functional deficiency); breast milk contamination; and childhood cancer in offspring.

Chemical hazards. Table 79-2 lists some of the known or suspected reproductive hazards in the workplace, typical jobs in which these chemicals are used, and their potential reproductive effects. Although the table lists potential effects on the female reproductive system only, most reproductive hazards affect both the male and female reproductive systems.

The physician should use caution when comparing results of workplace monitoring to legal standards for occupational exposure. Most of the 60,000 chemicals in commercial use have not been thoroughly evaluated for reproductive or developmental toxicity. Only four agents have been regulated in part to prevent reproductive damage (lead, radiation, dibromochloropropane, ethylene oxide), and these regulations may not be sufficiently protective. NIOSH has issued Recommended Exposure Limits that, although not legally enforceable, provide guidelines for estimating safe exposure limits.

Physical hazards. Exposure to several physical agents can result in adverse reproductive and developmental effects. Ionizing radiation is in widespread use in occupations in medicine, industry, government, and nuclear fuel operations. Depending on dose, exposure to ionizing radiation during pregnancy can result in birth defects, mental retardation, childhood leukemia, and other childhood cancers in offspring. Radiation exposure before implantation of the fetus is not likely to result in birth defects, however, because either the death of the conceptus or total effective repair will occur.

With the widespread use of computers in the past decade, there has been growing concern about the reproductive effects of video display terminals (VDTs). To date the majority of epidemiologic data, including those from a well-designed study by NIOSH, do not support a significant association between VDT use and spontaneous abortion. Although VDTs produce a minimal amount of ionizing radiation, they also emit very low-frequency (VLF) and extremely low-frequency (ELF) radiation, which have been shown in some experimental studies to cause biologic damage. Other characteristics of jobs involving prolonged use of VDTs include stress and ergonomic factors that may contribute to potential adverse reproductive outcome. Because little is known about the effects of low-frequency electromagnetic fields on humans, users of VDTs should minimize their exposure by taking the following precautions: (1) maintaining a minimum distance of 18 inches from the screen, (2) ensuring proper ergonomic design of the work station, and (3) taking periodic breaks to prevent eye and musculoskeletal strain.

Little information is available on human reproductive effects of occupational exposure to noise. In animal studies, pregnancy-rate reduction has been a consistently reported effect of noise, and noise exposure is associated with increased embryolethality and fetolethality.

Physically strenuous work may be safe until late in pregnancy for a healthy woman who receives adequate nutrition and prenatal care. There is growing evidence, however, that repetitive heavy lifting in the last trimester can cause uterine contractions. The American Medical Association has issued guidelines for continuation of various job tasks during pregnancy.

Biologic hazards. Several infectious agents that may be acquired in the workplace can cause intrauterine infections, produce teratogenic effects in an embryo or fetus, infect offspring through contamination of breast milk, or act as abortifacients. These agents include the rubella virus, cytomegalovirus, hepatitis B, human immunodeficiency virus, human parvovirus B19 (fifth disease), and chickenpox. Workers exposed to infectious disease include health care workers, housekeepers, laundry workers, laboratory workers, day care workers, teachers, workers in contact with animals and animal products, and sanitation workers.

Counseling women regarding pregnancy. Many reproductive hazards can exert teratogenic effects before a woman is aware of pregnancy (Fig. 79-1). For this reason it is desirable to identify and eliminate or reduce exposure to workplace reproductive hazards before conception. Because of increasing evidence of male-mediated effects on the fetus a woman planning a pregnancy should be informed that her partner's exposure to chemicals in the workplace may result in adverse reproductive outcome.

The frequency, timing, duration, and intensity of exposure must all be taken into account in assessing potential

Table 79-2 Potential reproductive hazards in the workplace

Occupational hazard	Types of jobs	Potential effects on female reproductive system and pregnancy
Arsenic and arsine	Jobs involving use of pesticides, herbicides, metal alloys, special glasses and enamels, antifouling paints, semiconductor devices, and printed circuits	Birth defects and low birth weight in offspring, breast milk contamination
Anesthetic gases	Dental workers, health care workers, chemical workers	Spontaneous abortion, stillbirths, birth defects
Benzene	Chemical manufacture, paint and varnish removal, laboratory workers	Mutagenesis. In animal studies: teratogenesis in offspring of exposed animals
Cadmium	Paint pigment making, artists, electrical workers, welding, metal machining	Menstrual irregularities, spontaneous abortion, stillbirth, breast milk contamination
Carbon disulfide	Electrical, hospital and health care, laboratory, refinery, pesticide, textile, and rubber workers	Menstrual irregularities, fetotoxicity, spontaneous abortion. In animal studies: birth defects, behavioral changes in offspring
Carbon monoxide	Tunnel workers, traffic police, auto repair, fork lift operators, truck drivers, firefighters, workers exposed to environmental tobacco smoke	Low birth weight and birth defects in offspring, increased fetal or infant death, decreased fertility
Chlordane, heptachlor	Manufacture and use of pesticides	Possible blood disorders and childhood cancer in offspring; in animal studies: mutagenesis, decreased fertility
Chlorpyrifox	Manufacture and use of pesticides	Decreased fertility
Cytotoxics, antineoplastics	Health care workers	Spontaneous abortion, birth defects in offspring of women treated with these drugs, mutagenesis, breast milk contamination
2,4 Dichlorophenoxy-acetic acid (2,4,D)	Manufacture and use of pesticides	In animal studies; birth defects
Ethylene oxide (ETO)	Hospital and health care workers, food workers, chemical workers, manufacture and use of pesticides	Mutagenesis; in animal studies: decreased fertility, birth defects, fetolethality
Formaldehyde	Pathology laboratory workers, cosmetic/plastic resin manufacture, textile workers, work involving use of particle board or adhesive	Menstrual irregularities, mutagenesis
Glycol ethers (e.g., 2-Methoxy-ethanol)	Electronic and semiconductor workers, auto workers, general manufacturing	Spontaneous abortion, decreased fertility; in animal studies: birth defects
Lindane	Manufacture and use of pesticides	Possible brain damage in offspring; in animal studies: possible death of offspring
Lead	Bridge painters, house painters and deleaders, people who work with stained glass or ceramics, auto radiator repair workers, welders	Menstrual irregularities, decreased fertility, birth defects, stillbirth, brain defects in offspring (e.g., hyperactivity, learning disabilities)
Mercury	Dental and health care workers, electrical workers, pharmaceutical and chemical workers, manufacture and use of pesticides, thermometer manufacture	Menstrual irregularities, spontaneous abortion, breast milk contamination; in animal studies: decreased fertility, birth defects, damage to developing fetus, stillbirth
Methyethyl ketone (MEK, 2-butanone)	Many manufacturing jobs, including plastics, textiles, paints	Damage to developing fetus
Methylene chloride	Furniture stripping, chemical manufacturing	Breast milk contamination; in animal studies: birth defects, mutagenesis
Perchloroethylene (tetrachloroethylene)	Dry cleaners, degreasers	Breast milk contamination; in animal studies: fetotoxicity
Styrene	Plastics workers, paper workers	Menstrual irregularities, decreased fertility
Toluene	Chemical and general manufacturing, laboratory workers	Spontaneous abortion; in animal studies: fetotoxicity, fetolethality
1,1,1 trichloroethane (methyl chloroform)	Manufacturing	In animal studies: fetotoxicity, birth defects, mutagenesis
Trichloroethylene	Electronics	In animal studies: birth defects, impaired growth in offspring
Xylene	Laboratory workers, plastics manufacture, synthetic textiles, paints, lacquers, varnishes, adhesives, cements, pharmaceuticals	Menstrual irregularities; in animal studies: fetotoxicity

Modified from Massachusetts Coalition for Occupational Safety and Health: *Confronting reproductive health hazards on the job,* 1992.

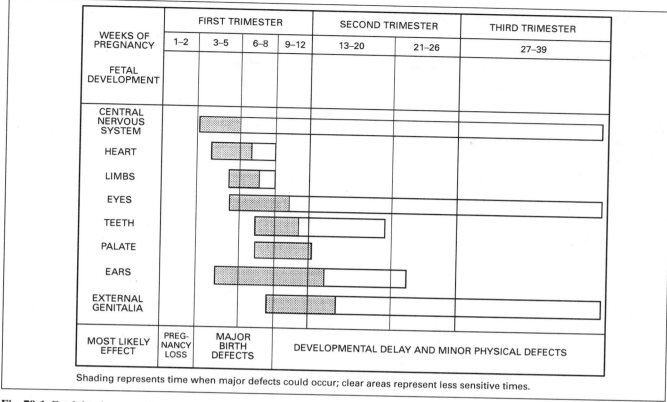

WEEKS OF PREGNANCY	FIRST TRIMESTER				SECOND TRIMESTER		THIRD TRIMESTER
	1–2	3–5	6–8	9–12	13–20	21–26	27–39
FETAL DEVELOPMENT							
CENTRAL NERVOUS SYSTEM							
HEART							
LIMBS							
EYES							
TEETH							
PALATE							
EARS							
EXTERNAL GENITALIA							
MOST LIKELY EFFECT	PREG-NANCY LOSS	MAJOR BIRTH DEFECTS	DEVELOPMENTAL DELAY AND MINOR PHYSICAL DEFECTS				

Shading represents time when major defects could occur; clear areas represent less sensitive times.

Fig. 79-1 Fetal development: times when a fetus can be most susceptible to defects (From *Confronting reproductive health hazards on the job*, 1992, MassCosh.)

reproductive outcome. For example, exposures that occur within the first 8 weeks of pregnancy are more likely to cause major morphologic abnormalities and result in loss of the conceptus; those that occur later are more likely to cause physiologic and minor morphologic abnormalities that allow carrying the fetus to term but result in birth defects (Fig. 79-1). It is important that the primary care physician counsel women who are considering pregnancy about the potentially devastating effects of some exposures during the early stages of pregnancy and about the importance of an occupational and environmental exposure assessment before conception.

The physician may be asked to make suggestions for improvements in the work environment to protect worker health. The "hierarchy of controls" is applicable to reproductive hazards, like all workplace hazards. Eliminating the hazard (e.g., substituting a safer chemical) is the most effective control strategy. Engineering controls (e.g., well-maintained local exhaust ventilation or enclosure of the work process) are less effective but can significantly reduce exposure. Use of personal protective equipment (e.g., respirators, protective clothing) is the least effective control strategy but may be necessary on a short-term basis.

If exposure cannot be controlled satisfactorily the physician may need to assist the patient in obtaining a temporary job transfer or leave. It is essential to be aware of the economic consequences of these options for the patient: how a leave or transfer will affect income, seniority, health insurance, disability payments; and whether she is guaranteed a

job upon return from leave. By law the employer may not treat requests by pregnant women for job transfers and leaves differently from requests by other workers.

LEGAL ISSUES IN WOMEN'S OCCUPATIONAL HEALTH

As women continue to enter the work force in unprecedented numbers and to assume broader roles in traditionally male occupations it is important that primary care practitioners understand the statutory, regulatory, and judicial mechanisms that protect female workers from occupational exposures and gender-based employment discrimination. Such knowledge will allow appropriate counseling of patients and employers and appropriate referral of patients to outside resources for assistance when necessary.

OSHA and regulatory protection

OSHA was established in 1970 to "ensure so far as possible every working man and woman in the Nation safe and healthful working conditions." Under the general duty clause (Section 5(a)(1)) of the OSHA Act, employers must provide places of employment "which are free from recognized hazards that are causing or are likely to cause death or serious harm" to employees. The standard setting provision of Section 6(b) authorizes the secretary of labor to promulgate any occupational safety and health standard "dealing with toxic materials or harmful physical agents" and to "set the standard which most adequately assures . . . that no employee will suffer material impairment of health or functional capacity." OSHA is empowered with the authority and responsibility for enforcement of the act.

The Hazards Communication Standard

OSHA promulgated the Hazards Communication Standard (HCS) in 1987 to provide for the transmission of information about the hazards of chemicals in the workplace to employers and employees. Under the HCS employers must (1) ensure that each container of hazardous chemicals is labeled with the identity and toxicity of the contained chemical, (2) "provide employees with information and training on hazardous chemicals in their work area" at the time of initial assignment and whenever a new chemical is introduced, and (3) maintain and ensure employee access to this information.

Antidiscrimination legislation

Despite differences in male and female body stature, muscle strength, and childbearing capacity there are few situations that justify different treatment of women in the workplace. The Civil Rights Act of 1964 (Title VII) explicitly prohibits sex-based discrimination with respect to hiring, discharge, compensation, terms, privileges, and other conditions of employment. This act was further amended by the Pregnancy Discrimination Act of 1978 to prohibit sex-based discrimination on the basis of pregnancy, childbirth, or related medical conditions, except in those circumstances in which sex is a bona fide occupational qualification reasonably necessary to the normal operation of that particular business or enterprise. Such a job qualification must relate to the essence or the central mission of the employer's business. Thus an employer may legitimately refuse to hire females for jobs in which "male" attributes lie at the core of the job (e.g., as models for men's clothing). Otherwise, when individual women or the class of women possess the necessary job-related skills and aptitudes they must receive equal treatment in employment decisions.

Fetal protection policies

Despite the provisions of the Civil Rights Act of 1964 and the Pregnancy Discrimination Act of 1978, employers persisted throughout the 1980s in discriminating against female workers through the institution of fetal protection policies. These policies were in fact practices implemented by employers—typically through workplace exclusion policies—to minimize occupational exposures that potentially could result in adverse pregnancy outcomes. For example, in 1982 Johnson Controls, a lead battery manufacturer, instituted a fetal protection policy that excluded women of all ages from jobs that involved potential lead exposure—creating an exception only for those women who presented medical documentation of sterility.

In 1991 the U.S. Supreme Court invalidated fetal protection policies in a landmark decision called *International Union, UAW v. Johnson Controls, Inc.* The court declared these policies to be a form of discrimination based on gender because they did not apply equally to the reproductive capacity of male and female employees. The court further held that sex was not a bona fide occupational qualification because sex and childbearing capacity did not relate to the central mission of the employer's business. Thus, despite employers' concerns about fetal safety (and potential tort liability), the court concluded that "decisions about the welfare of future children must be left to the parents who conceive, bear, support, and raise them rather than to the employers who hire those parents."

The Americans with Disabilities Act

Title I of the Americans with Disabilities Act (ADA) prohibits all employment practices that discriminate against the disabled. The act creates an exception when reasonable accomodation of disabled workers is not feasible and their disability poses a direct threat to them or to others. The ADA applies to all employers with 15 or more employees.

The ADA defines *disability* as (1) a physical or mental impairment that limits one or more major life activities, (2) a history of such impairment, or (3) *being regarded as* having such an impairment. The ADA has little impact on gender discrimination because of the act's interpretation of a physical impairment ("any physiological disorder, or condition, cosmetic disfigurement, or anatomical loss affecting one or more . . . body systems") and its emphasis on the nature, severity, and duration of impairment. For example, a pregnant woman is not protected under the ADA because pregnancy is not the result of a physiologic disorder and is only a temporary condition.

The primary care physician should be aware that the ADA prohibits (1) preoffer medical examinations and (2) divulgence of specific diagnoses or disabilities to the employer. Thus, although employers may administer preoffer nonmedical tests (such as agility testing) that are job-related, they may not require a medical examination until the applicant has been given a job offer that is contingent only on passing the medical examination. During the postoffer medical examination the physician must determine whether the applicant meets the employer's health and safety requirements but may only disclose to the employer directly relevant information about functional ability and limitations (e.g., permissible disclosure: "Applicant should not work at heights"; prohibited disclosure: "Poorly controlled epilepsy"). The employer is then responsible for making determinations about feasibility of reasonable accommodation.

Legal remedies available to workers

Government regulations proactively address health and safety issues by establishing safe standards for the workplace. In contrast, legal remedies provide compensation after an injury has occurred. In theory such compensation provides incentives for a safe and healthful workplace. Legal remedies available to workers include **workers' compensation** (WC) and remedy under the **tort system.** WC is a no-fault system instituted in the United States in the 1920s and is based on systems operative in Great Britain and the Republic of Germany. It represents a compromise between labor and industry whereby the employee (the "first" party) gives up her right to sue the employer (the "second" party), and the employer automatically accepts the employee's claim of a work-related injury or disease. Thus the employee is automatically entitled to certain benefits after incurring an occupational injury or disease, irrespective of fault. The employer on the other hand is protected from unpredictable jury awards that may be not only compensatory but also punitive.

Although WC may provide reasonable compensation in cases of work-related injury the system fails to provide adequate restitution for occupational diseases—particularly those with long latencies and those without pathognomonic features, such as asthma and infertility. The bases for litigation are usually causality and the existence or extent of disability from work. The worker must prove that the injury or illness "arose out of or in the course of employment." To be compensable, however, a disorder must not only be causally related to work but also produce disability and, as a corollary, a reduction in earning capacity. For example, infertility, impotence, or miscarriage arising out of a workplace injury or exposure does not necessarily produce disability or diminish employment opportunities. Therefore some states may not adequately compensate workers for these conditions unless the WC laws make specific provisions for such effects as "loss of reproductive function/organs."

Tort remedies. In cases in which employees are injured or disease results from action of a "third" party, remedy is available under the toxic torts system. Employees may sue the third party under negligence or strict liability doctrines. An example is the case of asbestos. Because asbestos manufacturers negligently failed to place warning labels on asbestos-containing products put into workplaces or used in the manufacture of end products, workers exposed to asbestos in workplaces have successfully sued these manufacturers, even though they were barred by the exclusive remedy provisions of WC law from suing their employers. Tort law, unlike WC, provides compensation for injury in the absence of demonstrable impairment and disability. Tort cases are adjudicated in a court of law, where a jury determines the award.

Role of the health care provider. Primary care physicians who recognize the statutory, regulatory, and judicial avenues available to workers can significantly improve the occupational health of their patients. Because of the legal remedies available to workers the physician caring for a patient with work-related disease or injury has responsibilities that extend beyond simple diagnosis and treatment. These include (1) determination of nature and extent of impairment/disability, (2) determination of causality, (3) provision of written opinion regarding diagnosis and causality, (4) provision of examining physician testimony at a deposition or in a court of law, and (5) facilitation of workplace evaluation in some cases. By definition *causality* in medical-legal terms means "more likely than not," or with greater than 50% certainty. For example, in order to diagnose occupational asthma in a patient with reversible airway obstruction the primary care physician must believe that, more likely than not, exposure to a chemical or fume at work was causally related to the development or worsening of asthma.

Providing a written opinion is important because statutes of limitation begin to run under both WC and tort law at the time a diagnosis of occupational disease is made. Notice in writing to the patient prevents subsequent ambiguity regarding time of diagnosis. Such ambiguity may bar a worker from a remedy to which she is entitled.

RESOURCES		
Regulatory agencies	
Occupational Safety and Health Administration	Standard setting and enforcement, etc.
NIOSH	Research and recommendations re: standards
State Department of Labor	Worksite inspections by request
Hotlines	
Pregnancy Environmental Hotline	
State Poison Control Networks	
Computer data bases	
Toxline	Contains >400,000 references
Reprotox	Contains information on effects of >600 substances on reproductive health

Health care professionals must appreciate the limitations of regulation and legal remedies in the prevention of workplace injuries and illnesses. A careful understanding of women's occupational health issues and early consultation with patients and their employers may avert the development of occupational disease or injury, thus obviating the need for regulatory enforcement action and legal remedies.

RESOURCES

Resources available to the primary care physician caring for a patient with known or suspected occupational illness, injury, or disease are summarized in the box, above. The state committees on occupational safety and health, or COSH groups, are organizations that have been formed in many states to educate workers and others, including health care providers, about occupational safety and health. These COSH groups are a valuable source of written material about the potential adverse health effects of specific jobs and exposures. Additionally they often provide safety and health training for workers. In Massachusetts the Reproductive Hazards Center and Occupational Health Program at the University of Massachusetts Medical Center in Worcester provides (1) patient care related to the reproductive effects of potentially hazardous exposures for women and men, (2) telephone consultation, and (3) educational services for health care providers and employees or workers.

BIBLIOGRAPHY

American Medical Association Council on Scientific Affairs: Effects of pregnancy on work performance, *JAMA* 251:1995, 1984.

BLS survey of occupational injuries and illnesses for 1989 shows no significant improvement; OSHA disappointed no reduction. In Dreger M, editor: *ACOM report: monthly newsletter* January 1991.

Massachusetts Coalition for Occupational Safety and Health: *Confronting reproductive health hazards on the job: a guide for workers.* Boston, 1992, Mass Cosh.

Messite J, Bond MB: Occupational health considerations for women at work. In Zenz C, editor: *Occupational medicine: principles and practical applications,* Chicago, 1988, Year Book Medical.

Office of Technology Assessment: *Reproductive hazards in the workplace,* OTA-BA-266, Washington, DC, 1985, Government Printing Office.

Oleinich A et al: Current methods of estimating severity for occupational injuries and illnesses: data from the 1986 Michigan comprehensive conpensable injury and illness database, *Am J Industr Med* 23:231, 1993.

Oliver LC, Stoeckle JD: Prevention and evaluation of occupational respiratory disease. In: Goroll AH, May LA, Mulley AC, editors: *Primary*

care medicine: office evaluation and management of the adult patient, Philadelphia, 1987, JB Lippincott.

Paul M, editor: *Occupational and environmental reproductive hazards,* Baltimore, 1993, Williams & Wilkins.

Paul M, Himmelstein J: Reproductive hazards in the workplace: what the practitioner needs to know about chemical exposures, *Obstet Gynecol* 71:921, 1988.

Proposed national strategy for the prevention of leading work-related diseases and injuries, DHHS (NIOSH) Publication No 89, 1986.

Teutsch SM: A framework for assessing the effectiveness of disease and injury prevention, *MMWR* 41:1, 1992.

80 Screening and Immunization Guidelines

Barbara J. Woo

This chapter presents the current guidelines for screening interventions and immunizations in adult women. Principles of screening are reviewed to provide a foundation for clinicians to devise their own recommendations for individual patients when discordance between authorities exists or when available data to support a preventive measure effectively are limited. Screening for cervical, ovarian, and breast cancer is considered in greater detail in Chapters 76-78. Chapters 11 and 50 include material on screening for osteoporosis and immunizations during pregnancy.

The concept of the periodic comprehensive physical examination was developed at the turn of the century and has remained one of the most common reasons for a visit to the doctor today. Many women still expect an annual checkup, complete with a comprehensive physical examination, Papanicolaou's smear, and battery of blood tests. In the last 15 years, however, the rationale for this long-standing practice has been challenged. Physicians have gradually been convinced that many screening interventions are not beneficial as these maneuvers have been subjected to more scientific scrutiny. Furthermore, third-party payers are forcing both doctors and patients to be more wary of indiscriminate use of screening maneuvers when they refuse to pay for certain screening procedures and annual check-ups.

SCREENING GUIDELINES
Principles of screening

The objective of a screening maneuver is to reduce morbidity and mortality rates of a given disease in a defined population at a reasonable cost. In order for this to occur, the target disease and screening tool must meet the following criteria:

1. The disease must have a significant burden of suffering in terms of prevalence, morbidity, and mortality.
2. The disease must have an asymptomatic period during which detection and treatment can yield a therapeutic result superior to that obtained by delaying treatment until symptoms appear.
3. The screening test must be sufficiently sensitive, specific, safe, and acceptable to the patient and must be available at a reasonable cost.

Clinicians should be critical when evaluating a screening program as screening tests are not without risks, discomfort to patients, and costs. A false-positive test result can lead to further expensive and risky diagnostic procedures and cause unnecessary anxiety. If the test provides a false-negative result, it can promote false reassurance and a possible delay in subsequent diagnosis of the disease. In order to minimize false-negative and false-positive findings the test must have reasonable sensitivity and specificity. The **sensitivity** of the test indicates the proportion of persons with the condition who correctly test positive for the disease. If the test lacks sensitivity, cases will be missed and false-negative findings will occur. The **specificity** of the test indicates the proportion of persons without the disease who correctly test negative. If the test lacks specificity it will cause an unacceptable number of healthy persons to have false-positive test results.

Besides ensuring adequate sensitivity and specificity, another way to improve the effectiveness of a test and reduce the number of false-positive findings is to screen a population with a higher prevalence of disease. For this reason many screening tests are recommended only for certain individuals who fall within a certain age or risk factor profile for a particular condition.

When evaluating the effectiveness of a screening program one must be wary of the pitfalls of bias that may exaggerate the benefits of screening. **Lead time bias** occurs when survival appears to be prolonged because screening simply advances the time of diagnosis. The time of death is not actually postponed. **Length time bias** may also create the illusion of improved survival. A screening test tends to detect a disproportionate number of indolent forms of the disease that have a longer window of detection. These cases detected by screening, therefore, may falsely appear to have an improved survival rate.

Development of screening guidelines

In the last 20 years a concerted effort has taken place to develop screening guidelines based on more scientific data. The Canadian Task Force (CTF) was one of the first authorities to rigorously outline and apply the screening principles discussed above to evaluate the usefulness of individual preventive maneuvers. For each preventive intervention the existing literature was reviewed and evaluated. The studies that were subject to less bias and misinterpretation were given more weight. For instance, randomized controlled trials were relied upon more strongly than cohort studies or expert opinions. On the basis of their review of the available literature, the authorities then devised a quality-of-evidence profile for each intervention (see the box, below). Using this assessment of the literature the CTF created a 5-point strength of recommendation scale in an attempt to translate the science into a clinical recommendation (see the box, at right). The A, B, D, and E recommendations reflect good evidence for the inclusion or exclusion of a screening tool in a physician's practice. Unfortunately many screening tests are given C rankings, indicating that there is poor evidence for inclusion or exclusion of the procedure, but that recommendations can be made on other grounds. In some instances a maneuver may be described as clinically prudent despite the lack of convincing evidence of effectiveness if it is not associated with significant harm or cost. In other areas a recommendation against the procedure is made even if the quality of evidence to exclude the procedure is poor, because of high cost, risk of the procedure, or a high false-positive rate. Finally, when the reviewers judge that there is inadequate evidence to make a recommendation for or against a procedure they leave the decision to the individual judgment of the clinician.

In the last decade many revisions by the CTF and guidelines by other groups have come about. In 1989, using the same criteria and process as the CTF, the United States Preventive Services Task Force (USPSTF) published the most comprehensive set of guidelines assessing the effectiveness of 169 screening interventions. The following text compares and contrasts the recommendations of the CTF, USPSTF, American College of Physicians (ACP), American Cancer Society (ACS), and other authorities. Given the high cost of screening and the high cost of treating potentially preventable diseases, it is clear that much research needs to be done to evaluate screening procedures and guide clinicians more effectively.

Screening guidelines

History and physical examination. The annual comprehensive physical examination is no longer recommended by

---

QUALITY OF EVIDENCE

I: Evidence obtained from at least one properly-designed randomized controlled trial.

II: Evidence obtained from well designed cohort or case-control analytic studies, preferably from more than one center or research group.

II-2: Evidence obtained from comparisons between times or places with or without the intervention. Dramatic results in uncontrolled experiments (such as the results of the introduction of penicillin in the 1940s) could also be regarded as this type of evidence.

III: Opinions of respected authorities, based on clinical experience, descriptive studies or reports of expert committees.

From Canadian Task Force on the Periodic Health Examination: *Can Med Assoc J* 121:1195, 1979.

STRENGTH OF RECOMMENDATIONS

A. There is good evidence to support the recommendation that the condition be specifically considered in a periodic health examination.

B. There is fair evidence to support the recommendation that the condition be specifically considered in a periodic health examination.

C. There is poor evidence regarding the inclusion of the condition in a periodic health examination, and recommendations may be made on other grounds.

D. There is fair evidence to support the recommendation that the condition be excluded from consideration in a periodic health examination.

E. There is good evidence to support the recommendation that the condition be excluded from consideration in a periodic health examination.

From Canadian Task Force on the Periodic Health Examination: *Can Med Assoc J* 121:1195, 1979.

---

most authorities. Advocates of these examinations emphasize the benefits of establishment of the physician-patient relationship and opportunities for immunizations and counseling. Opponents argue that the annual health check-up is not cost-effective, has not been shown to reduce morbidity and mortality rates, and may convey a sense of false reassurance to patients. Most physicians, however, would not argue the utility of a *baseline* history and physical examination. Although there are no data to support this as a cost-effective screening procedure, knowledge of a patient's medications, allergies, current and past medical history, health habits, and social and family history is essential to the provision of preventive medical care.

Counseling. Poor health habits contribute to almost half of the deaths attributable to the leading causes of mortality in adults. Although further research is necessary, good evidence already exists demonstrating the benefit of counseling on diet, smoking cessation, and exercise for the primary prevention of disease. Counseling is likely to be the most effective clinician-mediated interventon of all preventive maneuvers. Even if counseling has limited success at changing behavior, it is likely to have a significant impact on overall morbidity and mortality rates given the prevalence of diseases with which poor health habits are associated. As clinicians, we should spend more time counseling about diet, exercise, seat belt use, safe sexual practices, smoking, and alcohol abuse.

Self breast examination, clinical breast examination, and mammography. It is clear that breast cancer meets the criteria as a target disease for screening. It has a high prevalence, it has high morbidity and mortality rates, and there is convincing evidence that screening can reduce mortality from breast cancer. The extent to which the three screening tools can help, how often screening needs to be done, and at what age screening should start and end are somewhat controversial. The quality of evidence and strength of recommendation for clinical breast examination and mammography in women age 50 to 59 are very strong. For patients 60 and over the data and recommendation for screening are fair. The controversy primarily exists for women ages 40 to 49. Unfortunately, the studies have not been consistent in their results and even the individual interpretation of a single study can vary, depending on which method of analysis is used. For these reasons the recommendations for patients in their forties differ among authorities. Authorities such as the CTF, ACP, and USPSTF do not believe that the evidence shows a beneficial reduction in mortality rate, and that the cost, radiation exposure, and risks of false-positive results incurred by mammography are not justified for women ages 40 to 49. Other groups, such as the ACS, are of the opinion that the data are persuasive enough to recommend mammography to these women. (See Chapter 76 for a more detailed discussion of breast cancer screening.)

The **self breast examination (SBE)** is the least efficacious of the screening maneuvers; however, the procedure itself is inexpensive and not associated with any risks. The ACS and National Cancer Institute recommend monthly SBE despite the poor sensitivity and specificity of the test. The USPSTF and the CTF, however, do not make a recommendation for or against SBE. Because of the potential for false-positive results to cause unnecessary doctors visits, testing, and anxiety, their recommendation is less aggressive than that of the ACS. The ACS recommends a **clinician breast examination** every 3 years for ages 20 to 40 and then yearly thereafter. For women who have a family history of breast cancer they recommend more frequent examinations starting at age 20. The ACP, CTF, and USPSTF recommend yearly clinical breast examinations beginning at age 40. For women with a family history of premenopausal breast cancer in a first-degree relative, screening with clinical breast examination should begin at age 35.

The ACP and CTF recommend yearly **mammograms** starting at age 50. The USPSTF recommends them every 1 to 2 years for ages 50 to 75. The ACS recommends mammography every 1 to 2 years for ages 40 to 50 and then yearly thereafter. (Their previous recommendation of a baseline study between ages 35 and 39 was deleted in 1992.) For patients with a family history of premenopausal breast cancer or at "high risk," the ACP recommends yearly mammograms beginning at age 40 and the USPSTF and CTF at age 35.

Pelvic examination. The pelvic examination as a separate screening tool apart from the Papanicolaou's (Pap) smear is not considered by many of the authorities. The USPSTF does *not* recommend the pelvic examination as a screening tool for ovarian cancer. The poor sensitivity and specificity of the examination and the lack of evidence that detection of an ovarian cancer by palpation is likely to improve overall survival rate are responsible for their recommendation. They do state, however, that it is clinically prudent to examine the uterine adnexa when performing gynecologic examinations for other reasons. The ACS, as well as the NCI, American College of Obstetricians and Gynecologists (ACOG), and American Medical Association (AMA), recommend a pelvic examination or bimanual examination every 1 to 3 years with the Pap smear for ages 18 to 40 and every year after age 40. The ACS recommends the pelvic examination because "bimanual palpation of the ovaries is the only examination that currently meets the American Cancer Society's criteria of feasibility, practicality, reasonable cost, and low risk." The ACP and CTF do not consider the pelvic examination in their recommendations for ovarian cancer screening. (See Chapter 78 for further details on screening for ovarian cancer.)

Papanicolaou's smear. A large body of evidence has accumulated supporting the efficacy of the Pap smear in decreasing morbidity and mortality rates from cervical cancer. Screening should reduce the incidence and mortality rate of this disease by 60% to 90%. All authorities, therefore, agree on regular Pap smears; however, the frequency of the test and the age at which Pap smears can be discontinued are undetermined.

The ACS recommends that all women who are or who have been sexually active or who have reached age 18 should have an annual Pap smear and pelvic examination. After a woman has had three or more consecutive satisfactory normal test results the Pap smear may be performed every 1 to 3 years at the discretion of her physician. The ACS did not recommend an age to discontinue testing. The CTF recommends Pap smears every 3 years after two normal test results for women when they become sexually active or at age 18, then every 5 years from age 36 to 74. The USPSTF recommends Pap smears every 1 to 3 years beginning at age 18 or when the woman becomes sexually active. At age 65, Pap smears may be discontinued if the physician can document consistently normal Pap smear results in the previous 10 years. All groups recommend more frequent testing if high risk conditions exist such as early onset of sexual activity or multiple sexual partners. (See Chapter 77 for further details on screening for cervical cancer.)

Rectal examination, stool for occult blood, and sigmoidoscopy. Colorectal cancer is common, with serious associated morbidity and mortality rates, and therefore is a disease targeted for screening. Unfortunately, the available screening tools are suboptimal. The **rectal examination** has limited usefulness given that less than 10% of colorectal cancers are within reach of a digital examination. The efficacy of screening for colorectal cancer with **fecal occult blood testing** had been inconclusive until the Minnesota Colon Cancer Control Study published its results in 1993. This prospective randomized trial of over 46,000 subjects demonstrated a 33% reduction in mortality rate from colorectal cancer in patients screened with annual fecal occult blood tests compared to that of a control group. The study did use a protocol of rehydration of slides, which increases the sensitivity of the test from 80.8% to 92.2%, although at the cost of reducing the specificity from 97.7% to 90.4%. Hence, although more false-positive results were caused by this practice of rehydration, it was also partially responsible for the significant decrease in mortality rate and therefore should be done to maximize the efficacy of the test.

As for **sigmoidoscopy,** no convincing randomized controlled trials support improved survival rate from screening; therefore many authorities believe that the expense, risk, and inconvenience to the patient do not support a global recommendation for the procedure until more conclusive data are available. On the other hand, given the high burden of suffering from colorectal cancer and the indirect evidence that screening should be efficacious, authorities such as the ACS and ACP believe that enough evidence exists to warrant screening with sigmoidoscopy, until proof exists otherwise. In fact a recent case-control study at the Kaiser Permanente Program has demonstrated a significant decrease in mortality rate with screening by rigid sigmoidoscopy. The benefit was only seen for patients with cancers that were within reach of the sigmoidoscope. No benefit was found for colon cancers beyond the reach of the device and therefore confounding variables were thought to be unlikely.

Currently the ACS recommends rectal examinations annually beginning at age 50, testing of stool for occult blood annually beginning at age 40, and sigmoidoscopy every 3 to 5 years at age 50 after two initial normal annual examination findings. The ACP supports the recommendations of the ACS in regard to stool for occult blood and sigmoidoscopy. They do not comment on the rectal examination for colorectal screening. The USPSTF does not recommend the rectal examination given its limited efficacy at detecting colorectal cancers. Both the USPSTF and CTF currently state that there is insufficient evidence to recommend for or against fecal occult blood testing or sigmoidoscopy in asymptomatic persons. They also state that there is insufficient evidence to warrant stopping this practice where it already exists. The USPSTF and CTF recommendations in effect leave the decision to screen for colorectal cancer up to the individual practitioner and patient. Given the recent data published by the Minnesota group regarding fecal occult blood testing and the Kaiser group regarding sigmoidoscopy it is likely that they will rethink their recommendations and endorse these screening measures more strongly. Most authorities do consider the data adequate to recommend screening with sigmoidoscopy to patients aged 40 and older with a first-degree relative with colorectal cancer; a personal history of endometrial, ovarian, or breast cancer; or a previous diagnosis of inflammatory bowel disease, adenomatous polyps, or colorectal cancer. Periodic colonoscopy is recommended for all persons with a family history of familial polyposis.

IMMUNIZATION RECOMMENDATIONS

Unlike the uncertainty of efficacy for many of the screening tools outlined, the effectiveness of immunizations has clearly been demonstrated for the control of many infectious diseases. Unfortunately immunizations are often a low priority for primary care physicians, with the result that only a minority of patients are properly immunized. Patients may also be unaware of the need for immunizations or be concerned about side effects. It is therefore imperative that all clinicians be aware of the recommendations and make certain that a thorough immunization history is completed. Information regarding risk factors secondary to life-style and occupational exposures and travel history should also be detailed.

Adverse reactions to immunizations are very rare. Contraindications to the routinely used adult vaccines include the following:

- Anaphylactic reactions to eggs: measles, mumps, and influenza vaccines are prepared from viruses grown in embryonated eggs and therefore have small quantities of egg proteins
- Anaphylactic reactions to neomycin (MMR-containing vaccines)
- Known hypersensitivity to preservatives or stabilizers in the vaccines
- Live vaccines (especially rubella) during pregnancy; inactive vaccines are considered safe

- Live vaccines in immunocompromised hosts (i.e., lymphoma, leukemia, chemotherapy, symptomatic human immunodeficiency virus [HIV] infection); low-dose steroids in any form are usually not immunosuppressive

Misconceptions about contraindications deserve special mention as they prevent clinicians from appropriately vaccinating their patients. As outlined by the Centers for Disease Control the following are *not* contraindications:

- Reaction to a previous vaccination that involved only localized soreness, redness, or swelling or temperature less than 40.5° C.
- Mild acute upper respiratory or gastrointestinal illness with fever less than 38° C
- Current antibiotic therapy or convalescent phase of illness
- Pregnancy of a household contact
- Recent exposure to an infectious disease
- Breastfeeding
  History of nonspecific allergies or relatives with allergies
- Allergies to penicillin
- Family history of an adverse event after vaccination

General recommendations on Immunization in the United States are primarily those of the Immunization Practices Advisory Committee of the Center for Disease Control. Six vaccines are recommended for routine use in adults living in the United States (see Table 80-1).

Specific guidelines

Tetanus-diphtheria. Approximately 40% of patients above age 60 lack protection to tetanus and diphtheria. Correspondingly, most cases occur in elderly patients. One should ensure that all elderly patients have received a primary series of three shots.

If the primary vaccination schedule has been interrupted or delayed, there is no need to restart a series. An adequate level of immunity will still be reached on completion of the primary series.

For clean, minor wound management, patients should receive a tetanus booster if they have not had one in 10 years or have not completed a primary series. For more serious wounds patients should receive a booster if more than 5 years has passed since their last booster or primary series was completed. If they have not completed a primary series or their immunization status is unknown, they should also receive tetanus immune globulin.

Measles. All persons born before 1957 are considered immune. Because of recent outbreaks of measles a second dose of live vaccine should be considered for young adults entering college, travelers to foreign countries, or health care workers. It is recommended that women vaccinated for measles receive the combined or mumps, measles, and rubella (MMR) vaccine if there is any uncertainty about immunity to any one of these diseases. Even if immunity exists already there is little risk to the combined vaccine.

Rubella. Approximately 10% to 15% of young adults are susceptible to rubella. Outbreaks have occurred in schools and hospitals. If infection occurs early in pregnancy, the sequelae may include fetal abnormalities, miscarriages, and

Table 80-1 Routine vaccines for adults

Vaccine	Indicated for	Dosage	Contraindications	Adverse
Tetanus-diphtheria (toxoid)	All adults Never immunized	Booster every 10 yrs of 0.5 m IM Primary series 3 doses 0.5 ml IM at 0, 1-2 mo, then 6-12 mo	Neurologic reaction or hypersensitivity to previous dose	Local pain and swelling can be more severe if boosters given <5 years apart
Measles (live vaccine)	Unimmunized born after 1956 Previously immunized with one dose, for college entry, health care workers, and foreign travel	2 doses 0.5 ml SC at least 1 mo apart 1 dose 0.5 ml SC	Egg allergy; hypersensitivity to neomycin; pregnancy; immunocompromised patients	Low-grade fever; rash, local pain, and swelling in patients previously immunized
Rubella (attenuated live virus grown in human diploid cells)	Unimmunized young women and health care workers	1 dose 0.5 ml SC	Pregnancy; immunocompromised patients; hypersensitivity to neomycin	Arthralgias in 40% of non-immune adults
Hepatitis B (noninfectious recombinant hepatitis B surface antigen)	High-risk patients and health care workers	3 doses 1 ml IM in the deltoid, second dose after 1 month, third dose 6 months after first dose; higher dose for immunocompromised and dialysis patients	None	Local soreness
Influenza (inactivated whole or virus subunits, grown in chick embryo cells)	High-risk patients, health care workers, and all more than 65 years old	1 dose 0.5 ml IM annually	Egg allergy	Infrequent fevers, chills, myalgia lasting 1-2 days
Pneumococcal (Capsular polysaccharide from 23 types)	High-risk patients and more than 65 years old	1 dose 0.5 ml IM		Local soreness in approx. 50% of patients

Modified from *Med Lett* 32(19), 1990.

stillbirths. All women of childbearing age and health care workers should be either empirically vaccinated if no documentation exists regarding previous immunization or tested serologically for rubella antibodies. Those who receive the vaccine should be counseled not to become pregnant for 3 months. Although studies have not shown fetal problems in women inadvertently vaccinated during pregnancy, the vaccine should be avoided in pregnant women. It is recommended that patients requiring rubella vaccination receive the combined MMR vaccine if any uncertainty exists about their immunity to measles or mumps as there is little risk to the combined vaccine.

Hepatitis B. High-risk women include intravenous drug abusers, heterosexual women with multiple sexual partners, recipients of certain blood products, and health care workers with frequent exposure to bodily fluids. The three-dose vaccination series confers immunity to 90% to 95% of healthy young adults. Protection exists for at least 7 years despite the fact that antibody levels can fall or even become undetectable. Therefore routine serologic testing for antibody levels and booster shots are not currently recommended.

More studies will be necessary to determine the duration of protection and when and whether boosters will be necessary.

Influenza. Annual vaccination each fall is indicated for all women over 65 years of age; those with chronic cardiac or pulmonary disease, diabetes, renal disease, or immuno-supression; and inhabitants of chronic-care facilities or nursing homes. All health care workers who are capable of transmitting infection to high-risk patients should also be immunized. Since fear of side effects is a common barrier to patients' receiving the flu vaccine, one can reassure these patients that a randomized trial comparing a saline injection to a flu vaccination had no difference in rates of systemic side effects. Amantadine prophylaxis against influenza A virus should also be considered as an adjunct to the vaccine when community outbreaks exist. It should be given for 2 weeks until antibodies from the vaccine appear. A dose of 100 mg/day is considered adequate. A dosage higher than this should not be used in elderly patients.

Pneumococcus. Pneumococcal vaccination should be given to all candidates for the influenza vaccine. In addition, women with asplenia, chronic liver disease, or alcoholism should be vaccinated. Pregnant women at high risk may be vaccinated, although it is preferable to wait until after the first trimester.

The issue of revaccination has not been fully resolved. High-risk patients vaccinated before 1983, when only the 14-valent vaccine was available, should be considered for revaccination with the 23-valent vaccine for increased coverage of pneumococcal serotypes. Antibody titers may begin to fall after several years; hence, for patients at greatest risk (i.e., asplenic patients) revaccination is recommended every 6 years. Revaccination should be considered for patients with serious cardiopulmonary or liver disease as well. Finally, for patients with nephrotic syndrome and renal failure, revaccination after 3 to 5 years is recommended because of rapidly declining antibody levels. (See Chapter 50 for further details on immunizations during pregnancy.)

BIBLIOGRAPHY

American College of Physicians Task Force on Adult Immunization: Guide for Adult Immunization, ed 2, Philadelphia, 1990, American College of Physicians.

Canadian Task Force on the Periodic Health Examination: The periodic health examination, *Can Med Assoc J*, 121:1193, 1979.

Dodd GD: American Cancer Society guidelines on screening for breast cancer: an overview, *Ca-A Cancer J Clin* 42(3):177, 1992.

Eddy DM: Screening for breast cancer, *Ann Intern Med* 111:389, 1989.

Eddy DM: Screening for cervical cancer, *Ann Intern Med* 113:214, 1990.

Eddy DM: Screening for colorectal cancer, *Ann Intern Med* 113:373, 1990.

Hayward RS et al: Preventive care guidelines, *Ann Intern Med* 114:758, 1991.

Immunization Practices Advisory Committee: General recommendations on immunization, *MMWR* 38:205, 1989.

Levin B, Murphy GP: Revision in American Cancer Society recommendations for the early detection of colorectal cancer, *Ca-A Cancer J Clin* 42(5):296, 1992.

Mandel JS et al: Reducing mortality from colorectal cancer by screening for fecal occult blood, *N Engl J Med* 328:1365, 1993.

Margolis KL et al: Frequency of adverse reactions to influenza vaccine in the elderly: a randomized, placebo-controlled trial, *JAMA* 264(9):1139, 1990.

Med Lett Routine immunization for adults, 32:54, 1990.

Mettlin C, Dodd GD: The American Cancer Society guidelines for the cancer related check-up: an update, *Ca-A Cancer J Clin* 41(5):179, 1991.

Ransohoff DF, Lang CA: Screening for colorectal cancer, *N Engl J Med* 325(1):37, 1991.

Selby JV et al: A case-control study of screening sigmoidoscopy and mortality from colorectal cancer, *N Engl J Med* 326:653, 1992.

Selby JV et al: Effect of fecal occult blood testing on mortality from colorectal cancer, *Ann Intern Med* 118:1, 1993.

U.S. Preventive Services Task Force: Guide to clinical preventive services: an assessment of the effectiveness of 169 interventions. Baltimore, 1989, Williams & Wilkins.

I Laboratory Reference Values

ENDOCRINOLOGIC NORMAL VALUES

Hormone and metabolite normal values

Adrenocorticotropin (ACTH), serum	15-100 pg/ml	
Aldosterone (mean ± standard deviation)		
Serum		
210 mEq/day sodium diet		
Supine	48 ± 29 pg/ml	
Upright (2 hr)	65 ± 23 pg/ml	
110 mEq/day sodium diet		
Supine	107 ± 45 pg/ml	
Upright (2 hr)	532 ± 228 pg/ml	
Urine	5-19 μg/24 hr	
Calcitonin, serum		
Basal	0.15-0.35 ng/ml	
Stimulated	<0.6 ng/ml	
Catecholamines, free urinary	<110 μg/24 hr	
Chorionic gonadotropin, serum		
Pregnancy		
First month	10-10,000 mIU/ml	
Second and third months	10,000-100,000 mIU/ml	
Second trimester	10,000-30,000 mIU/ml	
Third trimester	5000-15,000 mIU/ml	
Nonpregnant	<3 mIU/ml	
Cortisol		
Serum		
8 AM	5-25 μg/dl	
8 PM	<10 μg/dl	
Cosyntropin stimulation (30-90 min after 0.25 mg cosyntropin intramuscularly or intravenously)	>10 μg/dl rise over baseline	
Overnight suppression (8 AM serum cortisol after 1 mg dexamethasone orally at 11 PM)	≤5 μg/dl	
Urine	20-70 μg/24 hr	
C peptide, serum	0.28-0.63 pmol/ml	
11-Deoxycortisol, serum		
Basal	0-1.4 μg/dl	
Metyrapone stimulation (30 mg/kg orally 8 hr prior to level)	>7.5 μg/dl	
Epinephrine, plasma	<35 pg/ml	
Estradiol, serum		
Male	20-50 pg/ml	
Female	25-200 pg/ml	

Estrogens, urine (increased during pregnancy; decreased after menopause)	*Male*	*Female*
Total	4-25 μg/24 hr	5-100 μg/24 hr
Estriol	1-11 μg/24 hr	0-65 μg/24 hr
Estradiol	0-6 μg/24 hr	0-14 μg/24 hr
Estrone	3-8 μg/24 hr	4-31 μg/24 hr
Etiocholanolone, serum	<1.2 μg/dl	
Follicle-stimulating hormone, serum		
Male	2-18 mIU/ml	

continued

Hormone and metabolite normal values—cont'd

Female
    Follicular phase   5-20 mIU/ml
    Peak midcycle   30-50 mIU/ml
    Luteal phase   5-15 mIU/ml
    Postmenopausal   >50 mIU/ml
Free thyroxine index, serum   1-4 ng/dl
Gastrin, serum (fasting)   30-200 pg/ml
Growth hormone, serum
  Adult, fasting   <5 ng/ml
  Glucose load (100 g orally)   <5 ng/ml
  Levodopa stimulation (500 mg orally   >5 ng/ml rise over baseline within 2 hr
    in a fasting state)
17-Hydroxycorticosteroids, urine
  Male   2-12 mg/24 hr
  Female   2-8 mg/24 hr
5'-Hydroxyindoleacetic acid   2-9 mg/24 hr
  (5'-HIAA), urine
Insulin, plasma
  Fasting   6-20 μU/ml
  Hypoglycemia (serum glucose <50 mg/dl)   <5 μU/ml
17-Ketosteroids, urine
  Under 8 years old   0-2 mg/24 hr
  Adolescent   0-18 mg/24 hr
  Adult
    Male   8-18 mg/24 hr
    Female   5-15 mg/24 hr
Luteinizing hormone, serum
  Male adult   2-18 mIU/ml
  Female adult
    Basal   5-22 mIU/ml
    Ovulation   30-250 mIU/ml
    Postmenopausal   >30 mIU/ml
Metanephrines, urine   <1.3 mg/24 hr
Norepinephrine
  Plasma   150-450 pg/ml
  Urine   <100 μg/24 hr
Parathyroid hormone, serum
  C-terminal   150-350 pg/ml
  N-terminal   230-630 pg/ml
Pregnanediol, urine
  Female
    Follicular phase   <1.5 mg/24 hr
    Luteal phase   2.0-4.2 mg/24 hr
    Postmenopausal   0.2-1.0 mg/24 hr
  Male   <1.5 mg/24 hr
Progesterone, serum
  Female
    Follicular phase   0.02-0.9 ng/ml
    Luteal phase   6-30 ng/ml
  Male   <2 ng/ml
Prolactin, serum
  Nonpregnant
    Day   5-25-ng/ml
    Night   20-40 ng/ml
  Pregnant   150-200 ng/ml
Radioactive iodine (^{131}I) uptake (RAIU)   5%-25% at 24 hr (varies with iodine intake)
Renin activity, plasma (mean ± standard deviation)
  Normal diet
    Supine   1.1 ± 0.8 ng/ml/hr
    Upright   1.9 ± 1.7 ng/ml/hr
  Low-sodium diet
    Supine   2.7 ± 1.8 ng/ml/hr
    Upright   6.6 ± 2.5 ng/ml/hr
  Diuretics and low-sodium diet   10.0 ± 3.7 ng/ml/hr
Testosterone, total plasma
  Bound

continued

Hormone and metabolite normal values—cont'd

Adolescent male	<100 ng/dl
Adult male	300-1100 ng/dl
Female	25-90 ng/dl
Unbound	
Adult male	3-24 ng/dl
Female	0.09-1.30 ng/dl
Thyroid-stimulating hormone, serum	<10 μU/ml
Thyroxine (T_4), serum	
Total	4-11 μg/dl
Free	0.8-2.4 ng/dl
Thyroxine-binding globulin capacity, serum	15-25 μg T_4/dl
Thyroxine index, free	1-4 ng/dl
Triiodothyronine (T_3), serum	70-190 ng/dl
T_3 resin uptake	25%-45%
Vanillylmandelic acid (VMA), urine	1-8 mg/24 hr

From Stein: *Internal medicine,* ed 4, St Louis, 1994, Mosby.

Endocrine function tests

Adrenal gland

Glucocorticoid suppression: overnight dexamethasone suppression test (8 AM serum cortisol after 1 mg dexamethasone orally at 11 PM) — ≤5 μg/dl

Glucocorticoid stimulation: cosyntropin stimulation test (serum cortisol 30-90 min after 0.25 mg cosyntropin intramuscularly or intravenously) — >10 μg/ml more than baseline serum cortisol

Metyrapone test, single dose (8 AM serum deoxycortisol after 30 mg/kg metyrapone orally at midnight) — >7.5 μg/dl

Aldosterone suppression: sodium depletion test (urine aldosterone collected on day 3 of 200 mEq day/sodium diet) — <20 μg/24 hr

Pancreas

Glucose tolerance test* serum glucose after 100 g glucose orally)

60 min after ingestion	<180 mg/dl
90 min after ingestion	<160 mg/dl
120 min after ingestion	<125 mg/dl

Pituitary gland

Adrenocorticotropic hormone (ACTH) stimulation. See Adrenal gland, Metyrapone test

Growth hormone stimulation: insulin tolerance test (serum growth hormone after 0.1 U/kg regular insulin intravenously after an overnight fast to induce a 50% fall in serum glucose concentration or symptomatic hypoglycemia) — >5 ng/ml rise over baseline

Levodopa test (serum growth hormone after 0.5 g levodopa orally while fasting) — >5 ng/ml rise over baseline within 2 hr

Growth hormone suppression: glucose tolerance test (serum growth hormone after 100 g glucose orally after 8 hr fast) — <5 ng/ml within 2 hr

Luteinizing hormone (LH) stimulation: gonadotropin-releasing hormone (GnRH) test (serum LH after 100 μg GnRH intravenously or intramuscularly) — 4- to 6-fold rise over baseline

Thyroid-stimulating hormone (TSH) stimulation: thyrotropin-releasing hormone (TRH) stimulation test (serum TSH after 400 μg TRH intraveneously) — >2-fold rise over baseline within 2 hr

Thyroid gland

Radioactive iodine uptake (RAIU) suppression test (RAIU on day 7 after 25 μg triiodothyronine orally 4 times daily) — <10% to <50% baseline

Thyrotropin-releasing hormone (TRH) stimulation test. See Pituitary gland, Thyroid-stimulating hormone (TSH) stimulation

From Stein: *Internal medicine,* ed 4, St Louis, 1994, Mosby.
*Add 10 mg/dl for each decade over 50 years of age.

HEMATOLOGIC NORMAL VALUES

Differential cell count of bone marrow

Myeloid cells		
Neutrophilic series		
Myeloblasts	0.3%-5.0%	
Promyelocytes	1%-8%	
Myelocytes	5%-19%	
Metamyelocytes	9%-24%	
Bands	9%-15%	
Segmented cells	7%-30%	
Eosinophil precursors	0.5%-3.0%	
Eosinophils	0.5%-4.0%	
Basophilic series	0.2%-0.7%	
Erythroid cells		
Pronormoblasts	1%-8%	
Basophilic normoblasts		
Polychromatophilic normoblasts	7%-32%	
Orthochromatic normoblasts		
Megakaryocytes	0.1%	
Lymphoreticular cells		
Lymphocytes	3%-17%	
Plasma cells	0%-2%	
Reticulum cells	0.1%-2.0%	
Monocytes	0.5%-5.0%	
Myeloid/erythroid ratio	0.6-2.7	
Acid hemolysis test (Ham)	No hemolysis	
Carboxyhemoglobin		
Nonsmoker	<1%	
Smoker	2.1%-4.2%	
Cold hemolysis test (Donath-Landsteiner)	No hemolysis	
Complete blood count		
Erythrocyte life span		
Normal	120 days	
^{51}Cr-labeled half-life	28 days	
Erythropoietin by radioimmunoassay	9-33 mU/dl	
Ferritin, serum		
Male	15-200 μg/L	
Female	12-150 μg/L	
Folate, RBC	120-670 ng/ml	
Fragility, osmotic		
Hemolysis begins 0.45%-0.38% NaCl		
Hemolysis completed 0.33%-0.30% NaCl		
Haptoglobin, serum	100-300 mg/dl	
Hemoglobin		
Hemoglobin A_{1c}	0%-5% of total	
Hemoglobin A_2 by column	2%-3% of total	
Hemoglobin, fetal	<1% of total	
Hemoglobin, plasma	0%-5% of total	
Hemoglobin, serum	2-3 mg/ml	
Iron, serum		
Male	75-175 μg/dl	
Female	65-165 μg/dl	
Iron-binding capacity, total serum (TIBC)	250-450 μg/dl	
Iron turnover rate (plasma)	20-42 mg/24 hr	
Leukocyte alkaline phosphatase (LAP) score	30-150	
Methemoglobin	<1.8%	
Reticulocytes		
Schilling test (urinary excretion of radiolabeled vitamin B_{12} after "flushing" intramuscular injection of B_{12})	6%-30% of oral dose within 24 hr	
Sedimentation rate	*Male*	*Female*
Wintrobe	0-5 mm/hr	0-15 mm/hr
Westergren	0-15 mm/hr	0-20 mm/hr
Transferrin saturation, serum	20%-50%	

continued

Differential cell count of bone marrow—cont'd

Volume	*Male*	*Female*
Blood	52-83 ml/kg	50-75 ml/kg
Plasma	25-43 ml/kg	28-45 ml/kg
Red cell	20-36 ml/kg	19-31 ml/kg

Complete blood count

Parameter	Male	Female
Plasma	25-43 ml/kg	28-45 ml/kg
Hematocrit (%)	40-52	38-48
Hemoglobin (g/dl)	13.5-18.0	12-16
Erythrocyte count ($\times 10^{12}$ cells/L)	4.6-6.2	4.2-5.4
Reticulocyte count (%)	0.6-2.6	0.4-2.4
MCV (fL)	82-98	82-98
MCH (pg)	27-32	27-32
MCHC (g/dl)	32-36	32-36
WBC ($\times 10^9$ cells/L)	4.5-11.0	4.5-11.0
Segmented neutrophils	1.8-7.7	1.8-7.7
Average (%)	40-60	40-60
Bands (cells)	0-0.3	0-0.3
Average (%)	0-3	0-3
Eosinophils (cells $\times 10^9$/L)	0-0.5	0-0.5
Average (%)	0-5	0-5
Basophils (cells $\times 10^9$/L)	0-0.2	0-0.2
Average (%)	0-1	0-1
Lymphocytes (cells $\times 10^9$/L)	1.0-4.8	1.0-4.8
Average (%)	20-45	20-45
Monocytes (cells $\times 10^9$/L)	0-0.8	0-0.8
Average (%)	2-6	2-6
Platelet count (cells $\times 10^9$/L)	150-350	150-350

From Stein: *Internal medicine*, ed 4, St Louis, 1994, Mosby.

Coagulation normal values

Template bleeding time	3.5-7.5 min
Clot retraction, qualitative	Apparent in 30-60 min; complete in 24 hr, usually in 6 hr
Coagulation time (Lee-White)	
Glass tubes	5-15 min
Siliconized tubes	20-60 min
Euglobulin lysis time	120-240 min
Factors II, V, VII, VIII, IX, X, XI, or XII	100% or 1.0 unit/ml
Fibrin degradation products	<10 μg/ml or titer $\leq$1.4
Fibrinogen	200-400 mg/ml
Partial thromboplastin time, activated	20-40 sec
Prothrombin time (PT)	11-14 sec
Thrombin time	10-15 sec
Whole blood clot lysis time	>24 hr

From Stein: *Internal medicine*, ed 4, St Louis, 1994, Mosby.

SERUM NORMAL VALUES

Acetoacetate	0.3-2.0 mg/dl
Acid phosphatase	0-0.8 U/ml
Acid phosphatase, prostatic	2.5-12.0 IU/L
Albumin	3.0-5.5 g/dl
Aldolase	1-6 IU/L
Alkaline phosphatase	
15-20 years	40-200 IU/L
20-101 years	35-125 IU/L
Alpha$_1$-antitrypsin	200-500 mg/dl
ALT	0-40 IU/L
Ammonia	11-35 μmol/L
Amylase, serum	2-20 U/L
Anion gap	8-12 mEq/L (mmol/L)
Ascorbic acid	0.4-1.5 mg/dl
AST	5-40 IU/L
Bilirubin	
Total	0.2-1.2 mg/dl
Direct	0-0.4 mg/dl
Calcium, serum	8.7-10.6 mg/dl
Carbon dioxide, total	18-30 mEq/L (mmol/L)
Carcinoembryonic antigen, serum	<2.5 μg/L
Carotene (carotenoids)	50-300 μg/dl
C3 complement	55-120 mg/dl
C4 complement	14-51 mg/dl
Ceruloplasmin	15-60 mg/dl
Chloride, serum	95-105 mEq/L (mmol/L)
Cholesterol, total	
12-19 years	120-230 mg/dl
20-29 years	120-240 mg/dl
30-39 years	140-270 mg/dl
40-49 years	150-310 mg/dl
50-59 years	160-330 mg/dl
Copper	100-200 μg/dl
Creatine kinase, total	20-200 IU/L
Creatine kinase, isoenzymes	
MM fraction	94%-95%
MB fraction	0%-5%
BB fraction	0%-2%
Normal values in	
Heart	80% MM, 20% MB
Brain	100% BB
Skeletal, muscle	95% MM, 2% MB
Creatinine, serum	
Female adult	0.5-1.3 mg/dl
Male adult	0.7-1.5 mg/dl
Delta-aminolevulinic acid (ALA)	<200 μg/dl
α-Fetoprotein, serum	<40 μg/L
Folate, serum	1.9-14.0 ng/ml
Gamma-glutamyl transpeptidase	
Male	12-38 IU/L
Female	9-31 IU/L
Gastrin	150 pg/ml
Glucose, serum (fasting)	70-115 mg/dl
Glucose-6-phosphate dehydrogenase	5-10 IU/g Hb
G6PD screen, qualitative	Negative
Haptoglobin	100-300 mg/dl
Hemoglobin A$_2$	0%-4% of total Hb
Hemoglobin F	0%-2% of total Hb
Immunoglobulin, quantitation	
IgG	700-1500 mg/dl
IaA	70-400 mg/dl

continued

SERUM NORMAL VALUES—cont'd

IgM	
Male	30-250 mg/dl
Female	30-300 mg/dl
IgD	0-40 mg/dl
Insulin, fasting	6-20 μU/ml
Iron-binding capacity	250-400 μg/dl
Iron, total, serum	40-150 μg/dl
Lactic acid	0.6-1.8 mEq/L
LDH, serum	20-220 IU/L
LDH isoenzymes	
LDH_1	20%-34%
LDH_2	28%-41%
LDH_3	15%-25%
LDH_4	3%-12%
LDH_5	6%-15%
Leucine aminopeptidase (LAP)	30-55 IU/L
Lipase	4-24 IU/dl
Magnesium, serum	1.5-2.5 mEq/L
5'-Nucleotidase	0.3-3.2 Bodansky units
Osmolality, serum	278-305 mOsm/kg serum water
Phenylalanine	3 mg/dl
Phosphorus, inorganic, serum	2.0-4.3 mg/dl
Potassium, plasma	3.1-4.3 mEq/L
Potassium, serum	3.5-5.2 mEq/L
Protein, total, serum	
2-55 years	5.0-8.0 g/dl
55-101 years	6.0-8.3 g/dl
Protein electrophoresis, serum	
Albumin	3.2-5.2 g/dl
Alpha$_1$	0.6-1.0 g/dl
Alpha$_2$	0.6-1.0 g/dl
Beta	0.6-1.2 g/dl
Gamma	0.7-1.5 g/dl
Sodium, serum	135-145 mEq/L
Sulfate	0.5-1.5 mg/dl
T_3 uptake	25%-45%
T_4	4-11 μg/dl
Triglycerides	
2-29 years	10-140 mg/dl
30-39 years	20-150 mg/dl
40-49 years	20-160 mg/dl
50-59 years	20-190 mg/dl
60-101 years	20-200 mg/dl
Urea nitrogen, serum	
2-65 years	5-22 mg/dl
Male	10-38 mg/dl
Female	8-26 mg/dl
Uric acid	
10-59 years	
Male	2.5-9.0 mg/dl
Female	2.0-8.0 mg/dl
60-101 years	
Male	2.5-9.0 mg/dl
Female	2.5-9.0 mg/dl
Viscosity	1.4-1.8 (serum compared to H_2O)
Vitamin A	0.15-0.60 μg/ml
Vitamin B_{12}	200-850 pg/ml

From Stein: *Internal medicine*, ed 4, St Louis, 1994, Mosby.

URINE NORMAL VALUES

Acidity, titratable	20-40 mEq/24 hr
Ammonia	30-50 mEq/24 hr
Amylase	35-260 Somogyi units/hr
Bence Jones protein	None detected
Bilirubin	None detected
Calcium	
Unrestricted diet	<300 mg/24 hr (men)
	<250 mg/24 hr (women)
Low-calcium diet (200 mg/day for 3 days)	<150 mg/24 hr
Chloride	120-240 mEq/24 hr (varies with dietary intake)
Copper	0-32 μg/24 hr
Creatine	
Male	0-40 mg/24 hr
Female	0-100 mg/24 hr
Creatinine	1.0-1.6 g/24 hr or 15-25 mg/kg body weight/24 hr
Cysteine, qualitative	Negative
Delta-aminolevulinic acid	1.3-7.0 mg/24 hr
Glucose	
Qualitative	None detected
Quantitative	16-300 mg/24 hr
Hemoglobin	None detected
Hemogentisic acid	None detected
Iron	40-140 μg/24 hr
Lead	0-120 μg/24 hr
Myoglobin	None detected
Osmolality	50-1200 mOsm/L
pH	4.6-8.0
Phenylpyruvic acid, qualitative	None detected
Phosphorus	0.8-2.0 g/24 hr
Porphobilinogen	
Qualitative	None detected
Quantitative	0-2.4 mg/24 hr
Porphyrins	
Coproporphyrin	50-250 μg/24 hr
Uroporphyrin	10-30 μg/24 hr
Potassium	25-100 mEq/24 hr
Protein	
Qualitative	None detected
Quantitative	10-150 mg/24 hr
Sodium	130-260 mEq/24 hr (varies with dietary sodium intake)
Specific gravity	1.003-1.030
Uric acid	80-976 mg/24 hr
Urobilinogen	0.05-3.5 mg/24 hr <1.0 Ehrlich units/2 hr

From Stein: *Internal medicine*, ed 4, St Louis, 1994, Mosby.

II Adult Weight for Height Tables

METROPOLITAN WEIGHT* AND HEIGHT† TABLES (1983)

Weight					Height	
Pounds			**Kilograms**			
Average	**Range**		**Average**	**Range**	**Feet**	**Centimeters**
117	102–131		53.2	46.4–59.5	4'9"	145
119	103–134		54.1	46.8–60.9	4'10"	147
121	104–137		55.0	47.3–62.3	4'11"	150
123	106–140		56.0	48.2–63.6	5'0"	152
126	108–143		57.3	49.1–65.0	5'1"	155
129	111–147		58.6	50.5–66.8	5'2"	158
133	114–151		60.5	51.8–68.6	5'3"	160
136	117–155		61.8	53.2–70.4	5'4"	163
140	120–159		63.6	54.5–72.3	5'5"	165
143	123–163		65.0	55.9–74.1	5'6"	168
147	126–167		66.8	57.3–75.9	5'7"	170
150	129–170		68.2	58.6–77.3	5'8"	173
153	132–173		69.5	60.0–78.6	5'9"	175
156	135–176		70.9	61.4–80.0	5'10"	178
159	138–179		72.3	62.7–81.4	5'11"	180
—	—		—	—	6'0"	183
—	—		—	—	6'1"	185
—	—		—	—	6'2"	188
—	—		—	—	6'3"	191

Modified from 1979 Build Study Society of Actuaries and Association of Life Insurance Medical Directors of America, 1980, Metropolitan Life Insurance Company.

*Weights are at ages 25 to 59 yr based on lowest mortality. Weight is in pounds (indoor clothing weighing 3 lb).

†The table is adjusted to reflect subject *without shoes* for height measurement.

U.S. DEPARTMENT OF AGRICULTURE, U.S. DEPARTMENT OF HEALTH AND HUMAN SERVICES ACCEPTABLE WEIGHTS FOR ADULTS

Height*	Weight in Pounds[†‡]	
	19-34 yr	35 yr and older
5'0"	97–128	108–138
5'1"	101–132	111–143
5'2"	104–137	115–148
5'3"	107–141	119–152
5'4"	111–146	122–157
5'5"	114–150	126–162
5'6"	118–155	130–167
5'7"	121–160	134–172
5'8"	125–164	138–178
5'9"	129–169	142–183
5'10"	132–174	146–188
5'11"	136–179	151–194
6'0"	140–184	155–199
6'1"	144–189	159–205
6'2"	148–195	164–210
6'3"	152–200	168–216
6'4"	156–205	173–222
6'5"	160–211	177–228
6'6"	164–216	182–234

From Human Nutrition Information Service, US Department of Agriculture: *Report of the Dietary Guidelines Advisory Committee on the dietary guidelines for Americans*—1990, Hyattsville, Md, June 1990, US Government Printing Office.
*Without shoes.
[†]Without clothes.
[‡]The higher weights in the ranges generally apply to men, who tend to have more muscle and bone; the lower weights more often apply to women, who have less muscle and bone.

III Recommended Dietary Allowances

FOOD AND NUTRITION BOARD, NATIONAL ACADEMY OF SCIENCES—NATIONAL RESEARCH COUNCIL RECOMMENDED DIETARY ALLOWANCES,* REVISED 1989 (DESIGNED FOR THE MAINTENANCE OF GOOD NUTRITION OF PRACTICALLY ALL HEALTHY PEOPLE IN THE UNITED STATES)

| Category | | | | | | | | Fat-soluble vitamins | | | |
	Age (yr) Condition	Weight† (kg)	Weight† (lb)	Height† (cm)	Height† (in)	Protein (g)	Vitamin A (μg RE)‡	Vitamin D (μg)§	Vitamin E (mg α-TE)"	Vitamin K (μg)
Women	11–14	46	101	157	62	46	800	10	8	45
	15–18	55	120	163	64	44	800	10	8	55
	19–24	58	128	164	65	46	800	10	8	60
	25–50	63	138	163	64	50	800	5	8	65
	51+	65	143	160	63	50	800	5	8	65
Pregnant						60	800	10	10	65
Lactating	First 6 mo					65	1300	10	12	65
	Second 6 mo					62	1200	10	11	65

Modified from National Academy of Sciences: *Recommended Dietary Allowances*, ed 10. Copyright 1989 by the National Academy of Sciences. Courtesy of the National Academy Press, Washington, DC.

*The allowances, expressed as average daily intakes over time, are intended to provide for individual variations among most normal persons as they live in the United States under usual environmental stresses. Diets should be based on a variety of common foods to provide other nutrients for which human requirements have been less well defined.

†Weights and heights of Reference Adults are actual medians for the U.S. population of the designated age, as reported by NHANES II. The median weights and heights of those under 19 years of age were taken from Hamill et al. (1979). The use of these figures does not imply that the height-to-weight ratios are ideal.

‡Retinol equivalents. 1 retinol equivalent = 1 μg retinol or 6 μg β-carotene.

§As cholecalciferol. 10 μg cholecalciferol = 400 IU of vitamin D.

"α-Tocopherol equivalents. 1 mg d-α tocopherol = 1 α-TE.

Water-soluble vitamins							Minerals						
Vitamin C (mg)	Thiamin (mg)	Ribo-flavin (mg)	Niacin (mg NE)[¶]	Vitamin B$_6$ (mg)	Folate (μg)	Vitamin B$_{12}$ (μg)	Calcium (mg)	Phos-phorus (mg)	Mag-nesium (mg)	Iron (mg)	Zinc (mg)	Iodine (μg)	Sele-nium (μg)
50	1.1	1.3	15	1.4	150	2.0	1200	1200	280	15	12	150	45
60	1.1	1.3	15	1.5	180	2.0	1200	1200	300	15	12	150	50
60	1.1	1.3	15	1.6	180	2.0	1200	1200	280	15	12	150	55
60	1.1	1.3	15	1.6	180	2.0	800	800	280	15	12	150	55
60	1.0	1.2	13	1.6	180	2.0	800	800	280	10	12	150	55
70	1.5	1.6	17	2.2	400	2.2	1200	1200	320	30	15	175	65
95	1.6	1.8	20	2.1	280	2.6	1200	1200	355	15	19	200	75
90	1.6	1.7	20	2.1	260	2.6	1200	1200	340	15	16	200	75

[¶]1 NE (niacin equivalent) is equal to 1 mg of niacin or 60 mg of dietary tryptophan.

IV Calcium

FOOD SOURCES OF CALCIUM

	Serving size	(mg)
Sardines	3 oz	372
Milk, skim	1 cup	300
Milk, whole	1 cup	290
Milk, buttermilk	1 cup	296
Cheese, cheddar	1 oz	210
Cheese, American	1 slice	195
Cheese, mozzarella	1 oz	163
Turnip greens, cooked	$2/_3$ cup	184
Salmon	3 oz	167
Custard	$1/_2$ cup	161
Tofu	3 oz	128
Ice cream	$1/_2$ cup	99
Shrimp	3 oz	98
Spinach, cooked	$1/_2$ cup	88
Broccoli, cooked	$1/_2$ cup	68
Peanuts, roasted, with husks	$2/_3$ cup	68
Green beans, cooked	$1/_2$ cup	62
Egg, poached	1 large	51
Beans, cooked	$1/_2$ cup	50
Cottage cheese	$1/_4$ cup	38
Almonds	12 nuts	38
Perrier water	1 cup	32
Cream cheese	1 oz	23
Fish, broiled	$4^1/_2$ oz	20
Bread, enriched white	1 slice	20
Wheat cereal, flakes	1 cup	12

From Cefalo RC, Moos M-K: *Preconceptional health care: a practical guide*, ed 2, St Louis, 1995, Mosby.

ELEMENTAL CALCIUM AVAILABLE IN SOME OVER-THE-COUNTER SUPPLEMENTS

Brand	Amount of calcium carbonate (mg)	Amount of elemental calcium (mg)
Os-Cal 500	1250	500
Tums (low sodium)	500	200
Tums (extra strength)	750	300

From Cefalo RC, Moos M-K: *Preconceptional health care: a practical guide*, ed 2, St Louis, 1995, Mosby.

V Iron

FOOD SOURCES OF IRON

	Serving size	Iron (mg)
Calf liver, cooked	$3^{1}/_{2}$ oz	14.2
Liverwurst	3 oz	8.7
Chicken livers, cooked	$3^{1}/_{2}$ oz	8.5
Prune juice	$^{1}/_{2}$ cup	5.2
Ground beef, lean, cooked	$3^{1}/_{2}$ oz	3.8
Chickpeas	$^{1}/_{2}$ cup	3.0
Steak, cooked	3 oz	2.7
Raisins	$^{1}/_{2}$ cup	2.5
Molasses	1 tablespoon	2.3
Prunes, large	4	2.2
Kidney beans	$^{1}/_{2}$ cup	2.2
Spinach, cooked	$^{1}/_{2}$ cup	2.0
Chicken	$^{1}/_{4}$	1.8
Turkey	3 oz	1.5
Apricots, dried	4 halves	1.3
Avocado	$^{1}/_{2}$	1.3
Egg	1	1.1
Blueberries	$^{5}/_{8}$ cup	1.0
Bread, whole wheat	1 slice	0.8
Bread, enriched white	1 slice	0.6
Dry cereal	Read label; varies widely	

From Cefalo RC, Moos M-K: *Preconceptional health care: a practical guide*, ed 2, St Louis, 1995, Mosby.

IRON SUPPLEMENTS

	Amount of elemental iron (%)	Dose containing 60 mg of elemental iron (mg)
Ferrous sulfate	20	300
Ferrous fumarate	32.5	185
Ferrous gluconate	11	545

From Cefalo RC, Moos M-K: *Preconceptional health care: a practical guide,* ed 2, St Louis, 1995, Mosby.

VI Summary of Drug Interactions with Oral Contraceptives

Drugs that interfere with oral contraceptive efficacy
    Drugs that reduce efficacy
        Anticonvulsants
            Phenytoin, phenobarbital, methylphenobarbital, primidone, carbamazepine, ethosuximide
        Antibiotics
            Rifampin (proven)
            Ampicillin, tetracycline, other broad-spectrum antibiotics (possibly)
            Griseofulvin (possibly)
    Drugs that increase plasma levels of contraceptive steroids
        Ascorbic acid
Oral contraceptives that interfere with the metabolism of other drugs
    Increase plasma levels of the following drugs:
        Benzodiazepines
        Theophylline and caffeine
        Cyclosporine
        Metaprolol
        Phenazone
        Prednisolone
        Ethanol (possibly)
    Decrease plasma levels of the following drugs:
        Aspirin
        Clofibric acid
        Morphine
        Paracetamol
        Temazepam

From Rayburn WF, Zuspan FP: *Drug therapy in obstetrics and gynecology*, ed 3, St Louis, 1993, Mosby. Data from Back O, Orme ML'E: *Clin Pharmacokinet* 18:472, 1990.

VII   Possible Effects of Oral Contraceptives on Laboratory Tests*

Laboratory test	Effects	Probable mechanism
Serum, plasma, blood		
Albumin	Slightly decreased	Decreased hepatic synthesis
Aldosterone	Increased	Activates renin-angiotensin system
Amylase	Slightly increased (common)	Not established
	Markedly increased (rare)	Pancreatitis
Antinuclear antibodies	Become detectable	Not established
Bilirubin	Increased (rare)	Reduced secretion into bile
Ceruloplasmin	Increased	Increased hepatic synthesis
Cholinesterase	Decreased	Decreased hepatic synthesis
Coagulation factors	Increased II, VII, IX, X	Increased synthesis
Cortisol	Increased	Increased cortisol-binding globulin
Fibrinogen	Increased	Increased hepatic synthesis
Folate	Decreased or no change	Decreased folate absorption
Glucose tolerance tests	Small decrease in tolerance	Several mechanisms proposed
γ-Glutamyl transpeptidase	Increased	Altered secretion in bile
Haptoglobin	Decreased	Decreased hepatic synthesis
HDL cholesterol	Increased with estrogens and decreased with progestins	Not established
Iron-binding capacity	Increased	Increased transferrin levels
Magnesium	Decreased or no change	Decreased bone resorption
Phosphatase, alkaline	Increased (rare)	Altered secretion in bile
Plasminogen	Increased	Increased hepatic synthesis
Platelets	Slightly increased	Not established
Prolactin	Increased	Not established
Renin activity	Increased	Increased synthesis of renin substrate
Thyroxine (total)	Increased	Increased thyroxine-binding globulin
Transaminases	Slightly increased	Not established
Transferrin	Increased	Increased hepatic synthesis
Triglycerides	Increased	Increased synthesis
Triiodothyronine resin uptake	Decreased	Increased thyroxine-binding globulin
Vitamin A	Increased	Increased retinol-binding protein
Vitamin B_{12}	Decreased	Not established
Zinc	Decreased	Shift of zinc into erythrocyte
Urine		
δ-Aminolevulinic acid	Increased	Increased hepatic synthesis
Ascorbic acid	Decreased or no change	Not established
Bacteria	Increased incidence of bacteriuria	Not established
Calcium	Decreased	Decreased bone resorption
Cortisol (free)	Unchanged	
Porphyrins	Increased (may precipitate porphyria in susceptible patients)	Increased δ-aminolevulinic acid synthetase
17-Hydroxycorticosteroid	Slightly decreased or no change	Increased binding proteins
17-Ketosteroid	Slightly decreased or no change	Increased binding proteins

From Rayburn WF, Zuspan FP: *Drug therapy in obstetrics and gynecology*, ed 3, St Louis, 1993, Mosby.
*These effects are thought to be dose dependent and uncommon with the use of low-dose preparations.

VIII Human Chorionic Gonadotropin

METHODS FOR MEASUREMENT OF HUMAN CHORIONIC GONADOTROPIN

Method	Type of analysis	Principle
QUALITATIVE ASSAYS		
Slide tests	Agglutination inhibition	Colored latex or other visible particles (red blood cells) coated with hCG, antibodies to hCG, and urine are mixed with particles.
		Negative urine results in visible agglutination; presence of hCG in urine inhibits agglutination (or protein flocculation).
Tube tests	Same as preceding method	Same as preceding method 1; reaction occurs in tube.
Immunoenzymatic concentration tests	Sandwich immunometric assay	Solid-phase, double-antibody sandwich ELISA in which hCG binds to antibody. Enzyme-labeled antibody added, and residual activity directly related to hCG concentration.
QUANTITATIVE ASSAYS—SERUM AND URINE		
Radioimmunoassay (RIA)	Competitive inhibition	Radiolabeled (radioactive iodine, ^{125}I) hCG competes with sample analyte for binding to anti-hCG.
		Increased hCG in sample, decreased bound radioactivity.
Enzyme-linked immunosorbent assay (ELISA)	Sandwich immunometric assay	Enzyme-labeled anti-hCG reacts with sample hCG bound to solid-phase anti-hCG. Amount of bound enzyme activity directly proportional to amount of hCG in sample.

From Kaplan LA, Pesce AJ: *Clinical chemistry: theory, analysis, and correlation*, ed 2, St Louis, 1989, Mosby.

Use	Comments
QUALITATIVE ASSAYS	
Was frequently used as stat urinary pregnancy test; urine	Least sensitive of all hCG methods; most rapid (2-3 min)
Was sometimes used for stat urine pregnancy tests; urine	More sensitive than slide; some approach upper limit of sensitivity of RIA methods; 45-120 min per assay
Has become assay of choice, has speed of "slide" and sensitivity of "tube" with a colored end point; urine and serum	Reported sensitivity 20-50 mU/ml, 5- to 15-min assay; many forms: membrane, bead, paddle, dipstick, coated tube.
QUANTITATIVE ASSAYS—SERUM AND URINE	
Infrequently used as stat procedure; serum or urine	Most sensitive hCG assay available; 40-60 min per assay
Most frequently used assay; serum and urine	Reported sensitivity of 2-10 U/ml; assay time 1-3 hr

From Kaplan LA, Pesce AJ: *Clinical chemistry: theory, analysis, and correlation*, ed 2, St Louis, 1989, Mosby.

VALUES OF SERUM HUMAN CHORIONIC GONADOTROPIN WITH GESTATIONAL AGE

Gestational age	hCG (mU/ml)
0.2-1 wk	5-50
1-2 wk	50-500
2-3 wk	100-5000
3-4 wk	500-10,000
4-5 wk	1000-50,000
5-6 wk	10,000-100,000
6-8 wk	15,000-200,000
2-3 mo	10,000-100,000

From Kaplan LA, Pesce AJ: *Clinical Chemistry: theory analysis, and correlation*, ed 2, St Louis, 1989, Mosby.

IX Contraception

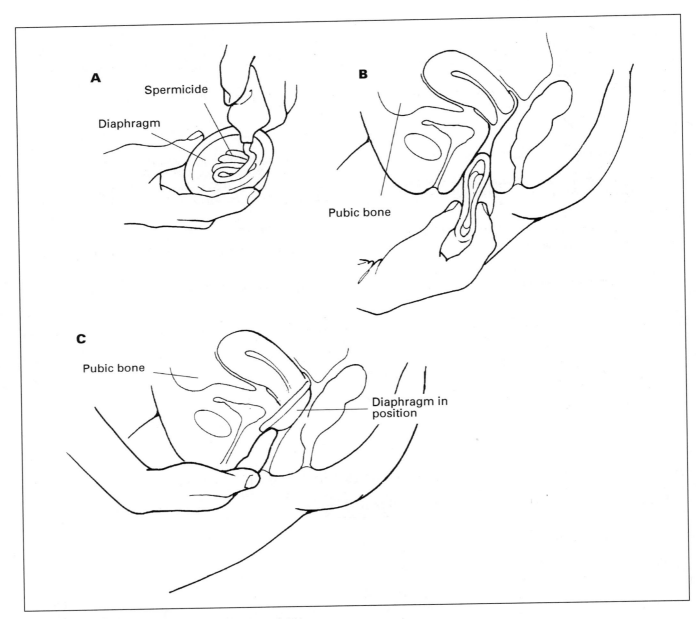

How to insert a diaphragm. (Courtesy Harriet Greenfield.)

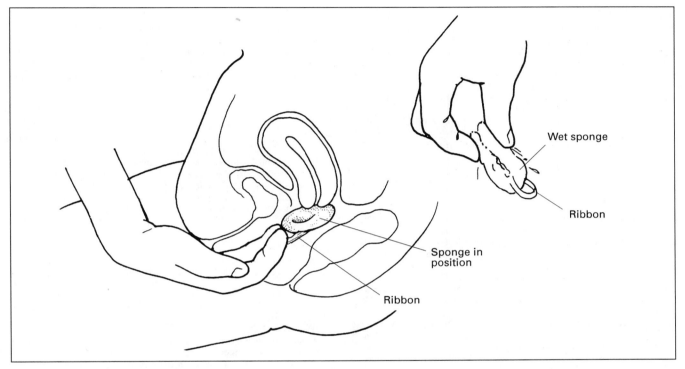

How to insert the contraceptive sponge. (Courtesy Harriet Greenfield.)

X Resources

ALCOHOLISM

National Clearinghouse for Alcohol and Drug Information (NCADI), PO Box 2345, Rockville, MD 20852, 1-800-729-6686.

National Council on Alcoholism and Drug Dependence, Inc., 12 West 21st Street, 8th Floor, New York, NY, 10010, 1-800-NCA-CALL.

Materials on alcoholism, fetal alcohol syndrome.

Relapse Prevention Hotline, 1-800-RELAPSE.

Self-Help Groups: AA, Al-Anon, Adult Children of Alcoholics, Narcotics Anonymous, Women for Sobriety.

Listings of meetings can be obtained from headquarter offices with telephone numbers in local directories.

The National Institute on Drug Abuse, Treatment referral hotline 1-800-662-4357.

For drug treatment facilities in local communities.

DEPRESSION

American Association of Suicidology, 2459 South Ave. Denver, CO 80222.

For those who have experienced the suicide of someone close.

Depression after delivery, PO Box 1281, Morrisville, PA 19067, (215)295-3994. A resource, not a counselling service. Information request line: 1-800-944-4773.

For women experiencing postpartum depression.

Depression/Awareness, Recognition and Treatment (D/ART), National Institute of Mental Health, Room 15C-05, 5600 Fishers Lane, Rockville, MD 20857.

A federal government/private sector effort to inform primary health care providers, mental health specialists, and the general public about the most up-to-date treatments for depressive illness.

National Depressive and Manic Depression Association, Merchandise Mart, PO Box 3395, Chicago, IL 60654.

For depressed persons and their families.

National Foundation for Depressive Illness, Inc., PO Box 2257, New York, NY 10611, 1-800-248-4344.

Provides referrals to support groups.

PMS Access, PO Box 9326, Madison, WI 53715, 1-800-222-4PMS.

For information on PMS, PMS clinics, support groups.

The National Alliance for the Mentally Ill, 2101 Wilson Blvd., Suite 302, Arlington, VA 22201, (703)524-7600, 1-800-950-6264.

Provides information, emotional support, and advocacy through local and state affiliates for families.

PREGNANCY

American College of Obstetricians and Gynecologists (ACOG), 409 12th Street SW, Washington DC 20024-2188, 1-800-673-8444.

For educational pamphlets on subjects related to women's health.

Healthy Mother, Healthy Babies Coalition (or state chapters) 409 12th Street SW, Room 309, Washington DC 20024, (202)638-5577.

Information and education to improve maternal/infant health.

Local Planned Parenthood Clinic 1-800-230-PLAN(7526).

VIOLENCE

Child Help–Child Abuse Hotline, 1-800-422-4453.

Clearinghouse on Child Abuse and Neglect Information, PO Box 1182, Washington DC 20013, (703)821-2086.

Legal Aid Societies. Numbers are listed in local phone directories.

Local Rape Crisis Center, 1-800-656-HOPE(4673).

National Coalition Against Domestic Violence (NCADV), PO Box 15127, Washington DC 20003-0127, 1-800-333-SAFE.

A national organization of shelters and support service for battered women and their children.

National Organization for Women (NOW), 1000 16th Street NW, Suite 700, Washington DC 20036, (202)331-0066.

Parents United, 232 East Gish Rd., 1st floor, San Jose, CA 95112, (408)453-7616.

For abused children and for adults who were abused as children.

Index

Page numbers in italics indicate illustrations; *t* indicates tables.

Neurologic studies in chronic fatigue syndrome diagnosis, 454
Neurologic syndromes in systemic lupus erythematosus, 192
 management of, 195
Neurology, 148-156
Neuropathic diseases, venous disease differentiated from, 37
Neutropenia
 from chemotherapy, 371-372
 immune, 104
Nicotine gum, 476
Nicotine patch, transdermal, 476
Nicotine replacement therapy, 475-476
Nicotine withdrawal syndrome, 472
Nicotinic acid in hypercholesterolemia management, 20
Nifedipine
 for incontinence, 243t
 for intrapartum hypertension, 344
 in pregnancy, 357t
Night pain in rheumatologic disorders, 159
Night sweats in chronic fatigue syndrome, 453-454
Nimodipine in stroke management, 31
Nipple
 dermatitis of, 224
 discharge from, 223-224
Nitrofurantoin for urinary tract infections in pregnancy, 383t
Nitroglycerin for intrapartum hypertension, 344
Nitroprusside for chronic hypertension in pregnancy, 356
Nodules, thyroid, 77-78
Nonatherosclerotic vascular disease, 34-35
 atherosclerosis differentiated from, 36
Nonsteroidal antiinflammatory drugs (NSAIDs)
 in abortive treatment of headache, 151, 152t
 for dysmenorrhea, 265
 for osteoarthritis, 170
 for rheumatoid arthritis, 186-187
Nortriptiline for postpartum depression, 397
Nuck's canal, cyst of, epidermal inclusion cyst differentiated from, 226
Nutrition
 bone loss and, 65
 during preconception, 307-314
Nutritional factors in osteoporosis prevention and treatment, 68-69

O

Obesity, 457-464
 epidemiology of, 457-458
 evaluation of, 458-460
 health problems of, 457-458
 management of, 461-463
 medical classification of, 450t
 pathophysiology of, 458
 as risk factor for coronary artery disease, 9
Obsessive compulsive disorder, postpartum, 398
Occlusive arterial disease, venous disease differentiated from, 37
Occupational asthma, 508
Occupational disease, diagnosis of, 506-507
Occupational hazards, 506-513
 legal issues in, 511-513
 musculoskeletal, 508-509
 reproductive, 509-511
 respiratory, 507-508
Ocular infection, gonococcal, 117
Oligomenorrhea, 210, 215
Oncology, 400-423; *see also* Cancer
Oophorectomy
 for breast cancer, 407-408
 hysterectomy and, 301

Oral contraceptives, 202-204
 amenorrhea and, 204
 breakthrough bleeding and, 203-204
 breast cancer and, 203
 breast cancer risk and, 404
 cardiovascular disease and, 202-203
 cervical cancer and, 497
 cervical dysplasia and, 203
 combination, 202
  for dysfunctional uterine bleeding in adolescence, 230
  for idiopathic anovulation, 232
  for menorrhagia, 231
 contraindications to, 203
 diabetes and, 46-47
 for diabetic women, 203
 drug interactions with, 204, 534
 for dysfunctional uterine bleeding from premature ovarian failure, 232
 for dysmenorrhea, 265
 effects of, on laboratory tests, 535
 gallbladder disease and, 203
 glucose intolerance and, 203
 hepatic adenomas and, 203
 for hyperandrogenism, 56-57
 hyperlipidemia and, 21-22
 hypertension and, 203
 for hypertensive women, 203
 lipid abnormalities and, 203
 low-dose, for idiopathic anovulation in perimenopausal women, 232
 management issues for, 203-204
 mechanism of action of, 202
 for migraine headache patients, 203
 morning-after, 204
 nausea and, 204
 for postpartum women, 203
 in premenstrual syndrome management, 269
 progestin-only, 202
 as risk factor
  for coronary artery disease, 9
  for stroke, 29
 risks of, 202-203
 side effects of, 204
 smoking and, 471
 for women over 40, 203
Orgasmic dysfunction, 271
 prognosis for, 273
 treatment techniques for, 273
Ornade for incontinence, 243t
Orthopedic interventions for osteoarthritis, 171-172
OSHA, regulatory protection and, 511-512
Osteoarthritis, 167-172
 carpal metacarpal
  clinical presentation of, 174
  epidemiology of, 172
  management of, 174
  pathophysiology of, 173
 cervical, 6
 clinical presentation of, 169-170
  management of, 170-172
 definition of, 167
 differential diagnosis of, 168-169
 epidemiology of, 167
 of knee
  clinical presentation of, 177
  management of, 178
 management of, 170-172
 osteophytes and, 168
 pathophysiology of, 167-168
 physiology of, 167
 rheumatoid arthritis differentiated from, 183

 risk factors for, 167
 thoracic, 6
Osteoarthrosis, 167
Osteomalacia, 64
 classification of, 66
Osteopenia, 64
 in hyperprolactinemia, 60
Osteophytes, osteoarthritis and, 168
Osteoporosis, 64-71
 classification of, 65, 66
 epidemiology of, 64
 estrogen replacement therapy and, 253
 evaluation of, 65-68
 fall prevention in, 71
 menopause and, 251
 pathophysiology of, 64-65
 prevention of, 68-71
 smoking and, 471
 substance abuse and, 428
 treatment of, 68-71
Osteotomy, tibial, for osteoarthritis, 171
Outflow tract disorders, amenorrhea from, 215
 management of, 220
Ovarian hyperstimulation syndrome, acute renal failure in pregnancy from, 142-143
Ovary(ies)
 ablation of, for breast cancer, 407-408
 agenesis of, amenorrhea from, 216-217
 cancer of, 257, 416-420, 504-505
  clinical presentation of, 417-418
  epidemiology of, 416, 504
  follow-up in, 420
  management of, 418-419
  pathology of, 418
  prognosis for, 419-420
  risk factors for, 416-417
  screening for, 504-505
  staging system for, 418
  survival with, 419-420
 cyst of, functional, 257
 cystadenomas of, 257
 enlarged, postmenopausal, 258
 failure of
  amenorrhea from, 215-217
  management of, 220
  dysfunctional uterine bleeding from, management of, 232
Overflow incontinence, 241
 management of, 243
Ovulation kit, 212
Ovulatory cycle
 abnormal vaginal bleeding in, 210
 disorders of, amenorrhea from, 215-218
  management of, 220-221
 dysfunctional uterine bleeding in, 230-231
 evidence of, 208
 status of, determination of, in evaluation of abnormal vaginal bleeding, 211-212
Oxybutynin chloride for incontinence, 243t
Oxycodone in pregnancy and lactation, 385t
Oxytocin to induce abortion, 290

P

Paget's disease
 of breast, 42, 224
 of vulva, 423
Pain
 abdominal, abuse and, 84
 breast, cyclic, 222-223
 joint, in rheumatoid arthritis, 180
 knee, 176-178
 lower back, 174-176
 neurogenic, in rheumatologic disorders, 159
 night, in rheumatoid disorders, 159